the calorie carb and fat bible

The UK's Most Comprehensive Calorie Counter

Juliette Kellow BSc RD, Lyndel Costain BSc RD & Rebecca Walton

The Calorie, Carb & Fat Bible

© Weight Loss Resources 2019
Lyndel Costain's contributions © Lyndel Costain

Published by:
Weight Loss Resources Ltd
2C Flag Business Exchange
Vicarage Farm Road
Peterborough
PE1 5TX.

Tel: 01733 345592
www.weightlossresources.co.uk

Companies and other organisations wishing to make bulk purchases of the Calorie, Carb and Fat Bible should contact their local bookstore or Weight Loss Resources direct.

ISBN 978-1-1904512-24-0

Authors: Lyndel Costain BSc RD
          Juliette Kellow BSc RD
          Rebecca Walton, Weight Loss Resources

Database Editor: Sam Holt
Design and Layout: Joanne Putney

Printed and bound in the UK by Bonacia Ltd
www.bookprintinguk.com

Contents

Losing weight – the easy way

Juliette Kellow BSc RD

PIZZA, curries, chocolate, chips and the odd glass of wine! Imagine being told the best diet to help you lose weight can include all these foods and more. It sounds too good to be true, doesn't it? But the truth is, these are exactly the types of foods you can still enjoy if you opt to lose weight by counting calories.

But you'd be forgiven for not knowing you can still eat all your favourite foods *and* lose weight. In recent years, endless trendy diets have helped to make dieting a complicated business. Added to this, an increasing number of celebrities and so-called nutrition experts have helped mislead us into thinking that dieting is all about restriction and denial. Is it any wonder then that most of us have been left feeling downright confused and miserable about what we should and shouldn't be eating to shift those pounds?

Dieting doesn't have to be a complicated or unhappy experience. In fact, there's really only one word you need to remember if you want to shift those pounds healthily and still eat all your favourite foods. And that's CALORIE!

It's calories that count

When it comes to losing weight, there's no getting away from the fact that it's calories that count. Ask any qualified nutrition expert or dietitian for advice on dropping pounds and you'll receive the same reply: quite simply you need to create a calorie deficit or shortfall. In other words, you need to take in fewer calories than you use up so that your body has to draw on its fat stores to provide it with the energy it needs to function properly. The result: you start losing fat and the pounds start to drop off!

Fortunately, it couldn't be easier to create this calorie deficit. Regardless of your age, weight, sex, genetic make up, lifestyle or eating habits, losing weight is as simple as reducing your daily calorie intake slightly by modifying your diet and using up a few more calories by being slightly more active each day.

Better still, it's a complete myth that you need to change your eating and exercise habits dramatically. You'll notice I've said you need to reduce your calorie intake 'slightly' and be 'slightly' more active. It really is just LITTLE differences between the amount of calories we take in and the amount we use up that make BIG differences to our waistline over time. For example, you only need to consume one can of cola more than you need each day to gain a stone in a year. It's no wonder then that people say excess weight tends to 'creep up on them'.

10 simple food swaps you can make every day (and won't even notice!)

Make these simple swaps every day and in just 4 weeks you'll lose 7lb!

SWAP THIS...	FOR THIS...	SAVE...
300ml full-fat milk (195 calories)	300ml skimmed milk (100 calories)	95 calories
1tsp butter (35 calories)	1tsp low-fat spread (20 calories)	15 calories
1tbsp vegetable oil (100 calories)	10 sprays of a spray oil (10 calories)	90 calories
1tsp sugar (16 calories)	Artificial sweetener (2 calories)	14 calories
1tbsp mayonnaise (105 calories)	1tbsp fat-free dressing (10 calories)	95 calories
Regular sandwich (600 calories)	Low-fat sandwich (350 calories)	250 calories
Can of cola (135 calories)	Can of diet cola (1 calorie)	134 calories
Large (50g) packet of crisps (250 calories)	Small (25g) packet of crisps (125 calories)	125 calories
1 chocolate digestive (85 calories)	1 small chocolate chip cookie (55 calories)	30 calories
1 slice thick-cut wholemeal bread (95 calories)	1 slice medium-cut wholemeal bread (75 calories)	20 calories
	TOTAL CALORIE SAVING:	868 calories

The good news is the reverse is also true. You only need to swap that daily can of cola for the diet version or a glass of sparking water and you'll lose a stone in a year – it really is as easy as that!

Of course, most people don't want to wait a year to shift a stone. But there's more good news. To lose 1lb of fat each week you need to create a calorie deficit of just 500 calories a day. That might sound like a lot, but you can achieve this by simply swapping a croissant for a wholemeal fruit scone, a regular sandwich for a low-fat variety, a glass of dry white wine for a gin and slimline tonic and using low-fat spread on two slices of toast instead of butter. It is also important to become more active and increase your level of exercise; simply walking a little more will help. Losing 1lb a week, amounts to a stone in 14 weeks, or just under 4 stone in a year!

Taking control of calories

By now you've seen it really is calories that count when it comes to shifting those pounds.

A calorie-controlled diet is one of the few that allows you to include anything, whether it's pizza, wine or chocolate. A healthy diet means including a wide range of foods *(see 'Healthy Eating Made Easy' page 32).*

And that's where this book can really help. Gone are the days when it was virtually impossible to obtain information about the calorie contents of foods. This book provides calorie information for more than 22,000 different branded and unbranded UK foods so that counting calories has never been easier.

The benefits of counting calories

- *It's guaranteed to help you lose weight providing you stick to your daily calorie allowance*

- *You can include favourite foods*

- *No foods are banned*

- *It's a great way to lose weight slowly and steadily*

- *Nutrition experts agree that it's a proven way to lose weight*

Calorie counting made easy

Forget weird and wacky science, complicated diet rules and endless lists of foods to fill up on or avoid every day! Counting calories to lose weight couldn't be easier. Quite simply, you set yourself a daily calorie allowance to help you lose between ½-2lb (¼-1kg) a week and then add up the calories of everything you eat and drink each day, making sure you don't go over your limit.

To prevent hunger from kicking in, it's best to spread your daily calorie allowance evenly throughout the day, allowing a certain amount of calories for breakfast, lunch, dinner and one or two snacks. For example, if you are allowed 1,500 calories a day, you could have 300 calories for breakfast, 400 calories for lunch, 500 calories for dinner and two snacks or treats of 150 calories each. You'll find more detailed information on p26-31 (Your step-by-step guide to using this book and shifting those pounds).

QUESTION
What affects the calorie content of a food?

ANSWER:
Fat, protein, carbohydrate and alcohol all provide the body with calories, but in varying amounts:

- *1g fat provides 9 calories*

- *1g alcohol provides 7 calories*

- *1g protein provides 4 calories*

- *1g carbohydrate provides 3.75 calories*

The calorie content of a food depends on the amount of fat, protein and carbohydrate it contains. Because fat provides more than twice as many calories as an equal quantity of protein or carbohydrate, in general, foods that are high in fat tend to contain more calories. This explains why 100g of chips (189 calories) contains more than twice as many calories as 100g of boiled potato (72 calories).

DIET MYTH:
Food eaten late at night stops you losing weight

DIET FACT:
It's not eating in the evening that stops you losing weight. It's consuming too many calories throughout the day that will be your dieting downfall! Providing you stick to your daily calorie allowance you'll lose weight, regardless of when you consume those calories. Nevertheless, it's a good idea to spread your calorie allowance throughout the day to prevent hunger from kicking in, which leaves you reaching for high-calorie snack foods.

Eat for good health

While calories might be the buzz word when it comes to shifting those pounds, it's nevertheless important to make sure your diet is healthy, balanced and contains all the nutrients you need for good health. Yes, you can still lose weight by eating nothing but chocolate, crisps and biscuits providing you stick to your calorie allowance, but you'll never find a nutrition expert or dietitian recommending this. And there are plenty of good reasons why.

To start with, an unbalanced diet is likely to be lacking in essential nutrients such as protein, vitamins, minerals and fibre, in the long term putting you at risk of nutritional deficiencies. Secondly, research proves that filling up on foods that are high in saturated fat and/or salt and sugar can lead to many different health problems. But most importantly, when it comes to losing weight, it's almost impossible to stick to a daily calorie allowance if you're only eating high-calorie foods.

Filling up on lower-calorie foods also means you'll be able to eat far more with the result that you're not constantly left feeling unsatisfied. For example, six chocolates from a selection box contain around 300 calories, a lot of saturated fat and sugar, few nutrients – and are eaten in just six mouthfuls! For 300 calories, you could have a grilled skinless chicken breast (packed with protein and zinc), a large salad with fat-free dressing (a great source of fibre, vitamins and minerals), a slice of wholemeal bread with low-fat spread (rich in fibre and B vitamins) and a satsuma (an excellent source of vitamin C). That's a lot more food that will take you a lot more time to eat! Not convinced? Then put six chocolates on one plate, and the chicken, salad, bread and fruit on another!

Bottom line: while slightly reducing your calorie intake is the key to losing weight, you'll be healthier and far more likely to keep those pounds off if you do it by eating a healthy diet *(see 'Healthy Eating Made Easy' page 32)*.

Eight steps to a healthy diet

1 *Base your meals on starchy foods.*

2 *Eat lots of fruit and vegetables.*

3 *Eat more fish.*

4 *Cut down on saturated fat and sugar.*

5 *Try to eat less salt - no more than 6g a day.*

6 *Get active and try to be a healthy weight.*

7 *Drink plenty of water.*

8 *Don't skip breakfast.*

SOURCE: www.nhs.uk/live-well/eat-well/eight-tips-for-healthy-eating/

Fat facts

Generally speaking, opting for foods that are low in fat can help slash your calorie intake considerably, for example, swapping full-fat milk for skimmed, switching from butter to a low-fat spread, not frying food in oil and chopping the fat off meat and poultry. But don't be fooled into believing that all foods described as 'low-fat' or 'fat-free' are automatically low in calories or calorie-free. In fact, some low-fat products may actually be higher in calories than standard products, thanks to them containing extra sugars and thickeners to boost the flavour and texture. The solution: always check the calorie content of low-fat foods, especially for things like cakes, biscuits, crisps, ice creams and ready meals. You might be surprised to find there's little difference in the calorie content when compared to the standard product.

Uncovering fat claims on food labels

Many products may lure you into believing they're a great choice if you're trying to cut fat, but you need to read between the lines on the labels if you want to be sure you're making the best choice. Here's the lowdown on what to look for:

LOW FAT	by law the food must contain less than 3g of fat per 100g for solids. These foods are generally a good choice if you're trying to lose weight.
REDUCED FAT	by law the food must contain 30 percent less fat than a similar standard product. This doesn't mean the product is low-fat (or low-calorie) though! For example, reduced-fat cheese may still contain 14g fat per 100g.
FAT FREE	the food must contain no more than 0.5g of fat per 100g or 100ml. Foods labelled as Virtually Fat Free must contain less than 0.3g fat per 100g. These foods are generally a good choice if you're trying to lose weight.
LESS THAN 8% FAT	this means the product contains less than 8g fat per 100g. It's only foods labelled 'less than 3% fat' that are a true low-fat choice.
X% FAT FREE	claims expressed as X% Fat Free shall be prohibited.
LIGHT OR LITE	claims stating a product is 'light' or 'lite' follows the same conditions as those set for the term 'reduced'.

10 easy ways to slash fat (and calories)

1 Eat fewer fried foods – grill, boil, bake, poach, steam, roast without added fat or microwave instead.

2 Don't add butter, lard, margarine or oil to food during preparation or cooking.

3 Use spreads sparingly. Butter and margarine contain the same amount of calories and fat – only low fat spreads contain less.

4 Choose boiled or jacket potatoes instead of chips or roast potatoes.

5 Cut off all visible fat from meat and remove the skin from chicken before cooking.

6 Don't eat too many fatty meat products such as sausages, burgers, pies and pastry products.

7 Use semi-skimmed or skimmed milk instead of full-fat milk.

8 Try low-fat or reduced-fat varieties of cheese such as reduced-fat Cheddar, low-fat soft cheese or cottage cheese.

9 Eat fewer high-fat foods such as crisps, chocolates, cakes, pastries and biscuits.

10 Don't add cream to puddings, sauces or coffee.

Getting Ready for Weight Loss Success

Lyndel Costain BSc RD

THIS BOOK not only provides tools to help you understand more about what you eat and how active you are, but guidance on how to use this information to develop a weight loss plan to suit your needs. Getting in the right frame of mind will also be a key part of your weight control journey, especially if you've lost weight before, only to watch the pounds pile back on.

The fact is that most people who want to lose weight know what to do. But often there is something that keeps stopping them from keeping up healthier habits. The same may be true for you. So what's going on? For many it's a lack of readiness. When the next diet comes along with its tempting promises it's so easy to just jump on board. But if you have struggled with your weight for a while, will that diet actually help you to recognise and change the thoughts and actions that have stopped you shifting the pounds for good?

Check out your attitude to weight loss programmes

Before starting any new weight loss programme, including the Weight Loss Resources approach, ask yourself:

Am I starting out thinking that I like myself as a person right now?	(YES or NO)
OR I feel I can only like myself once I lose weight?	(YES or NO)
Do I want to stop overeating, but at the same time find myself justifying it – in other words I want to be able to eat what I want, but with no consequences?	(YES or NO)
Do I believe that I need to take long-term responsibility for my weight?	(YES or NO)
OR Am I relying on 'it' (the diet) to do it for me?	(YES or NO)

Keep these questions, and your replies, in mind as you read through this chapter.

Next Steps

You may have already assessed the healthiness of your weight using the BMI guide on page 37. If not, why not do it now, remembering that the tools are a guide only. The important thing is to consider a weight at which you are healthy and comfortable – and which is realistic for the life you lead *(see opposite - What is a healthy weight?)*.

The next step is to have a long hard think about why you want to lose weight. Consider all the possible benefits, not just those related to how you look. Psychologists have found that if we focus only on appearance we are less likely to succeed in the long-term. This is because it so often reflects low self-esteem or self-worth – which can sabotage success – as it saps confidence and keeps us stuck in destructive thought patterns. Identifying key motivations other than simply how you look - such as health and other aspects of physical and emotional well being - is like saying that you're an OK person right now, and worth making changes for. Making healthy lifestyle choices also has the knock on effect of boosting self-esteem further.

Write down your reasons for wanting to lose weight in your Personal Plan *(see page 42)* – so you can refer back to them. This can be especially helpful when the going gets tough. It may help to think of it in terms of what your weight is stopping you from doing now. Here's some examples: to feel more confident; so I can play more comfortably with my kids; my healthier diet will give me more energy; to improve my fertility.

What is a Healthy Weight?

With all the mixed messages in the media it can be easy to get a distorted view about whether your weight is healthy or not. However, as the BMI charts suggest, there is no single 'ideal' weight for anybody. Research also shows that modest amounts of weight loss can be very beneficial to health and are easier to keep off. Therefore, health professionals now encourage us to aim for a weight loss of 5-10%. The ideal rate of weight loss is no more than 1-2 pounds (0.5-1kg) per week – so averaging a pound a week is great, and realistic progress.

The health benefits of modest weight loss include:

- *Reduced risk of developing heart disease, stroke and certain cancers*

- *Reduced risk of developing diabetes and helping to manage diabetes*

- *Improvements in blood pressure*

- *Improvements in mobility, back pain and joint pain*

- *Improvements with fertility problems and polycystic ovarian syndrome*

- *Less breathlessness and sleep/snoring problems*

- *Increased self esteem and control over eating*

- *Feeling fitter and have more energy*

Are You Really Ready to Lose Weight?

When you think of losing weight, it's easy just to think of what weight you'd like to get to. But weight loss only happens as a result of making changes to your usual eating and activity patterns – which allow you to consume fewer calories than you burn *(see 'It's calories that count' page 5)*.

So here comes the next big question. Are you really ready to do it? Have you thought about the implications of your decision? If you have lost weight in the past, and put it all back on - have you thought about why that was? And how confident do you feel about being successful this time?

To help you answer these questions, try these short exercises.

Where would you place yourself on the following scales?

Importance

How important is it to you, to make the changes that will allow you to lose weight?

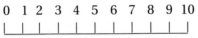

Not at all important   Extremely important

If you ranked yourself over half way along the scale then move on to the next question. If you were half way or less along the scale, you may not be mentally ready to make the required changes to lose weight. To further explore this, go to *'The Pros and Cons of Weight Loss' (page 17)*.

Confidence

How confident are you in your ability to make the changes that will allow you to lose weight?

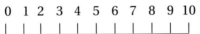

Not at all confident   Extremely confident

Now ask yourself (regarding your confidence ratings):

1. Why did I place myself here?

2. What is stopping me moving further up the scale (if anything)?

3. What things, information, support would help me move further up the scale? (if not near 10)

If you aren't sure about answers to question 3, then keep reading for some pointers.

The Pros and Cons of Weight Loss

Making lifestyle changes to lose weight is simpler if there are lots of clear benefits or pros, for example, clothes fit again, more energy, helps back pain - but there will also be associated downsides or cons. For example, some may feel it interferes with their social life, or don't have the time to plan meals or check food labels. Or overeating can help, if only temporarily, as a way of coping with unwanted feelings. Being overweight allows some people to feel strong and assertive, or to control their partner's jealousy. So in these cases there are downsides to losing weight, even if the person says they are desperate to do it.

If you are aware of the possible downsides, as well as the pros, you will be better prepared to deal with potential conflicts. Understanding what could be (or were with past weight loss efforts) barriers to success gives you the chance to address them. This boosts confidence in your ability to succeed this time, which in turn maintains your motivation.

Have a go at weighing up the pros and cons using the charts below and on page 18. Some examples are included. If you decide that the pros outweigh the cons, then great. You can also use the cons as potential barriers to plan strategies for *(see page 42)*. If you find it's the other way around, this may not be the best time to actively lose weight. Try the exercise again in a month or so.

Making Lifestyle Changes to Lose Weight Now

CONS *e.g. Must limit eating out, take aways*	PROS *e.g. Feel more energetic, slimmer*

Not Making Changes Now – how would I feel in 6 months time?

PROS *e.g. Haven't had to worry about failing;* *Still able to eat take aways a lot*	CONS *e.g. Perhaps gained more weight;* *Still don't like how I look and feel*

To change your weight, first change your mind

To lose weight you may already have a list of things to change, such as eating more fruit and veg, calculating your daily calorie intake, going for a walk each morning or buying low fat options. Others could also give you tips to try. But knowing what to do isn't the same as feeling motivated or able to do it. To be effective, you have to believe the changes are relevant, do-able and worth it.

What you think, affects how you feel, and in turn the actions you take.

Self-efficacy

In fact, research is telling us that one of the most important factors that influences weight loss success are your feelings of 'self-efficacy'. Self-efficacy is a term used in psychology to describe a person's belief that any action they take will have an effect on the outcome. It reflects our inner expectation that what we do will lead to the results we want. Not surprisingly, high levels of self-efficacy can enhance motivation, and allow us to deal better with uncertainty and conflict, and recovery from setbacks. But low levels, can reduce our motivation. We fear that whatever we do will not bring about our desired goal. This can lead self-defeating thoughts or 'self-talk', which make it hard to deal with set-backs, meaning we are more likely to give up. Here's some examples.

Examples: Low self-efficacy

'No matter how carefully I diet, I don't lose weight ...'

'I have eaten that chocolate and as usual blown my diet, so I may as well give up now.'

'I had a rich dessert – I have no willpower to say no. I can't stand not being able to eat what I want.'

If you have a strong sense of self-efficacy, your mindset and 'self-talk' will be more like:

Examples: High self-efficacy

'I know from previous weight loss attempts, that if I stay focussed on what I am doing I do lose weight. I have always expected to lose too much too quickly which frustrates me. I know that I will lose weight if I keep making the right changes, and this time it is important to me.'

'The chocolate bar won't ruin my diet, but if I think it has and keep on eating, then my negative self-talk will. So I will get back on track.'

*'Losing weight is very important to me, so I **can** make better food choices. After all, the world won't stop if I say no to dessert, and I will feel great afterwards. If I think about it, I am not hungry so would just feel bloated and guilty if I ate it.'*

Willpower is a Skill

Many people feel that they just need plenty of willpower or a good telling off to lose weight. But willpower isn't something you have or you don't have. Willpower is a skill. Like the dessert example on page 19, it's a sign that you've made a conscious choice to do something, because you believe the benefits outweigh any downsides. In reality everything we do is preceded by a thought. This includes everything we eat. It just may not seem like it because our actions often feel automatic *(see 'Look out for trigger eating' page 21).*

When it comes to weight loss, developing a range of skills – including choosing lower calorie options, coping with negative self-talk and managing things that don't go to plan - will boost your sense of self-efficacy to make the changes you want. This is especially important because we live in such a weight-promoting environment.

Our weight-promoting environment

We are constantly surrounded by tempting food, stresses that can trigger comfort eating and labour-saving devices that make it easy not to be physically active. In other words, the environment we live in makes it easy to gain weight, unless we stop and think about the food choices we make and how much exercise we do. In fact, to stay a healthy weight/maintain our weight, just about all of us need to make conscious lifestyle choices everyday. This isn't 'dieting' but just part of taking care of ourselves in the environment we live in.

It is also true that some people find it more of a challenge than others to manage their weight, thanks to genetic differences in factors such as appetite control, spontaneous activity level and emotional responses to food – rather than metabolic rate, as is often believed. The good news is that with a healthy diet and active lifestyle a healthier weight can still be achieved. But do talk to your doctor if you feel you need additional support.

Coping with Common Slimming Saboteurs

Lyndel Costain BSc RD

Look out for 'trigger' eating

Much of the overeating we do or cravings we have are actually down to unconscious, habitual, responses to a variety of triggers. These triggers can be external, such as the sight or smell of food, or internal and emotion-led, such as a response to stress, anger, boredom or emptiness. Your food diary (see page 43) helps you to recognise 'trigger' or 'non-hungry' eating which gives you the chance to think twice before you eat (see below).

Get some support

A big part of your success will be having someone to support you. It could be a friend, partner, health professional, health club or website. Let them know how they can help you most.

Make lapses your ally

Don't let a lapse throw you off course. You can't be, nor need to be perfect all the time. Doing well 80-90% of the time is great progress. Lapses are a normal part of change. Rather than feel you have failed and give up, look at what you can learn from a difficult day or week and use it to find helpful solutions for the future.

Understand why you eat

When I ask people what prompts them to eat, hunger usually comes down near the bottom of their list of reasons. Some people struggle to remember or appreciate what true hunger feels like. We are lucky that we have plenty of food to eat in our society. But its constant presence makes it harder to control what we eat, especially if it brings us comfort or joy.

If you ever find yourself in the fridge even though you've recently eaten, then you know hunger isn't the reason but some other trigger. The urge to eat can be so automatic that you feel you lack willpower or are out of control. But it is in fact a learned or conditioned response. A bit like Pavlov's dogs. He rang a bell every time he fed them, and from then on, whenever they heard the bell ring they were 'conditioned' to salivate in anticipation of food.

Because this 'non-hungry' eating is learned, you can reprogramme your response to the situations or feelings that trigger it. The first step is to identify when these urges strike. When you find yourself eating when you aren't hungry ask yourself 'why do I want to eat, what am I feeling?' If you aren't sure think back to what was happening before you ate. Then ask yourself if there is another way you can feel better without food. Or you could chat to your urge to eat in a friendly way, telling it that you don't want to give into it, you have a planned meal coming soon, and it's merely a learned response. Whatever strategy you choose, the more often you break into your urges to eat, the weaker their hold becomes.

Practise positive self-talk

Self-talk may be positive and constructive (like your guardian angel) or negative and irrational (like having a destructive devil on your shoulder).

If you've had on-off battles with your weight over the years, it's highly likely that the 'devil' is there more often. 'All or nothing' self-talk for example, 'I ate a "bad food" so have broken my diet', can make you feel like a failure which, can then trigger you into the action of overeating and/or totally giving up (see 'Diet-binge cycle' page 23). One of the most powerful things about it is that the last thoughts we have are what stays in our mind. So if we think 'I still look fat' or 'I will never be slim', these feelings stay with us.

To change your self-talk for the better, the trick is to first recognise it's happening (keeping a diary really helps, see Keep a Food Diary, page 29). Then turn it around into a positive version of the same events (see Self-efficacy, page 18) where the resulting action was to feel good and stay on track. Reshaping negative self-talk helps you to boost your self-esteem and feelings of self-efficacy, and with it change your self-definition - from someone who can't 'lose weight' or 'do this or that', to someone 'who can'. And when you believe you can…

The Diet – Binge Cycle

If this cycle looks familiar, use positive self-talk, and a more flexible dietary approach, to help you break free.

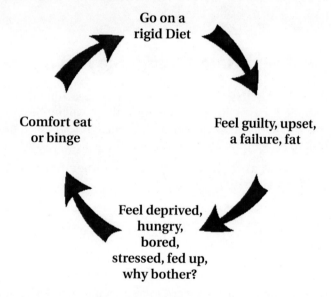

Go on a rigid Diet

Feel guilty, upset, a failure, fat

Feel deprived, hungry, bored, stressed, fed up, why bother?

Comfort eat or binge

Really choose what you want to eat

This skill is like your personal brake. It also helps you to manage 'trigger/ non-hungry' eating and weaken its hold. It legalises food and stops you feeling deprived. It helps you to regularly remind yourself why you are making changes to your eating habits, which keeps motivation high. But it doesn't just happen. Like all skills it requires practise. Sometimes it will work well for you, other times it won't – but overall it will help. Basically, ask yourself if you really want to eat that food in front of you. This becomes the prompt for you to make a conscious choice, weighing up the pros and cons or consequences of making that choice, and feeling free to have it, reject it or just eat some. Remembering all the while that you can eat this food another time if you want to.

Action Planning

Successful people don't just wait for things to happen. They believe in themselves, plan ahead, take action and then refine their plan until it gets, and keeps on getting the results they want. Successful slimmers use a very similar approach. They don't rely on quick-fixes or magic formulas, but glean information from reliable sources to develop a plan or approach that suits their needs, tastes and lifestyle. Thinking of weight management as a lifelong project, which has a weight loss phase and a weight maintenance phase, is also a route to success.

When the Going Gets Tough - Staying on Track

If things start to go off track, don't panic. Learning new habits takes time. And life is never straightforward so there will be times when it all seems too much, or negative 'self- talk' creeps in to try and drag you back into old ways. So if the going gets tough:

- Value what you've achieved so far, rather than only focus on what you plan to do.

- Look back at your reasons to lose weight and refer to the list often.

- Don't expect to change too much, too quickly. Take things a step at a time.

- Accept difficulties as part of the learning and skill building process.

- Enjoy a non-food reward for achieving your goals (including maintaining your weight).

- Use recipes and meal ideas to keep things interesting.

- Talk to your supporters and get plenty of encouragement. This is really vital!

Strategies of Successful Slimmers

Thanks to research conducted by large studies such as the US National Weight Control Registry and the German Lean Habits Study, we now know more about what works best for people who have lost weight and successfully kept it off. So be inspired!

The key elements of success are to:

- Believe that you can control your weight and the changes involved are really worth it.
- Stay realistic and value what you have achieved rather than dwell on a weight you 'dream' of being.
- Be more active – plan ways to fit activity into your daily life – aim for 1 hour of walking daily.
- Plan ahead for regular meals and snacks, starting with breakfast.
- Choose a balanced, low-fat diet with plenty of fruit and vegetables *(see Healthy Eating Made Easy, page 32).*
- Watch portion size and limit fast food.
- Sit down to eat and take time over meals, paying attention to what you are eating.
- Have a flexible approach – plan in and enjoy some favourite foods without guilt.
- Recognise and address 'all or nothing' thinking and other negative 'self-talk'.
- Keep making conscious choices.
- Learn to confront problems rather than eat, drink, sleep or wish they would go away.
- Enlist ongoing help and support from family, friends, professionals or websites.
- Regularly (at least once a week but not more than once daily) check your weight.
- Take action before your weight increases by more than 4-5lb (2kg).
- Accept that your weight management skills need to be kept up long-term.
- Take heart from successful slimmers, who say that it gets easier over time.

Your step-by-step guide to using this book and shifting those pounds

Juliette Kellow BSc RD and Rebecca Walton

1. Find your healthy weight

Use the weight charts, body mass index table and information on pages 36-43 to determine the right weight for you. Then set yourself a weight to aim for. Research shows it really helps if you make losing 10% of your weight your first overall target. It also brings important health benefits too *(see 'What is a Healthy Weight?' page 15)*. You can break this down into smaller manageable steps, for example, 3kg/6.5lbs at a time. If 10% is too much, then go for a 5% loss – this has important health benefits too. In fact, just keeping your weight stable is a great achievement these days, because of our weight-promoting environment *(see page 20)*.

Waist Management

In addition to BMI, another important way to assess your weight is by measuring your waist just above belly button level. It is especially useful for men as they tend to carry more excess weight around their bellies, but women should test it out too. Having excess weight around your middle (known as being 'apple-shaped') increases your risk of heart disease and type 2 diabetes. A simple way to stay aware of your waist is according to how well, or otherwise, skirts and trousers fit. Talk to your doctor about any weight and health concerns.

WAIST MEASUREMENT

	Increased Health Risk	High Risk to Health
Women	32-35in (81-88cm)	more than 35in (88cm)
Men	37-40in (94-102cm)	more than 40in (102cm)

---

2. Set a realistic time scale

With today's hectic lifestyles, everything tends to happen at breakneck speed, so it's no wonder that when it comes to losing weight, most of us want to shift those pounds in an instant. But it's probably taken years to accumulate that extra weight, with the result that it's unrealistic to expect to lose the excess in just a few weeks! Instead, prepare yourself to lose weight slowly and steadily. It's far healthier to lose weight like this. But better still, research shows you'll be far more likely to maintain your new, lower weight.

If you only have a small amount of weight to lose, aim for a weight loss of around 1lb (½kg) a week. But if you have more than 2 stone (28kg) to lose, you may prefer to aim for 2lb (1kg) each week. Remember though, it's better to keep going at 1lb (½kg) a week than to give up because trying to lose 2lb (1kg) a week is making you miserable! The following words may help you to keep your goal in perspective:

'Never give up on a goal because of the time it will take to achieve it – the time will pass anyway.'

Weight Fluctuations

Weight typically fluctuates on a day to day basis. You know that shock/horror feeling when you weigh yourself in the morning then later in the day, or after a meal out, and it looks like youve gained pounds in hours! But this is due to fluid not fat changes. Real changes in body fat can only happen more gradually (remember, to gain 1lb you need to eat 3500 calories more than you usually do). Don't be confused either by seemingly very rapid weight loss in the first week or so.

When calorie intake is initially cut back, the body's carbohydrate stores in the liver and muscles (known as glycogen) are used up. Glycogen is stored with three times its weight in water, meaning that rapid losses of 4.5- 6.6lb (2 -3 kg) are possible. These stores can be just as rapidly refilled if normal eating is resumed. True weight loss happens more gradually and this book helps you to lose weight at the steady and healthy rate of no more than 1-2 lbs per week.

3. Calculate your calorie allowance

Use the calorie tables on pages 39-40 to find out how many calories you need each day to maintain your current weight. Then use the table below to discover the amount of calories you need to subtract from this amount every day to lose weight at your chosen rate. For example, a 35 year-old woman who is moderately active and weighs 12 stone (76kg) needs 2,188 calories a day to keep her weight steady. If she wants to lose ½lb (¼kg) a week, she needs 250 calories less each day, giving her a daily calorie allowance of 1,938 calories. If she wants to lose 1lb (½kg) a week, she needs 500 calories less each day, giving her a daily calorie allowance of 1,688 calories, and so on.

TO LOSE...	Cut your daily calorie intake by	In three months you could lose...	In six months you could lose...	In one year you could lose...
½lb a week	250	6.5lb	13lb	1st 12lb
1lb a week	500	13lb	1st 12lb	3st 10lb
1½lb a week	750	1st 5.5lb	2st 11lb	5st 8lb
2lb a week	1,000	1st 12lb	3st 10lb	7st 6lb

TO LOSE...	Cut your daily calorie intake by	In three months you could lose...	In six months you could lose...	In one year you could lose...
¼kg a week	250	3.25kg	6.5kg	13kg
½kg a week	500	6.5kg	13kg	26kg
¾kg a week	750	9.75kg	19.5kg	39kg
1kg a week	1,000	13kg	26kg	52kg

4. Keep a food diary

Writing down what you eat and drink and any thoughts linked to that eating helps you become more aware of your eating habits. Recognising what is going on helps you feel in control and is a powerful way to start planning change. Keeping a food diary before you start to change your eating habits will also help you identify opportunities for cutting calories by substituting one food for another, cutting portion sizes of high-calorie foods or eating certain foods less often.

Simply write down every single item you eat or drink during the day and use this book to calculate the calories of each item. Then after a few days of eating normally, introduce some changes to your diet to achieve your daily calorie allowance. Remember to spread your daily calorie allowance fairly evenly throughout the day to prevent hunger. You'll find a template for a daily food and exercise diary on page 43.

Top Tip

If you only fill in your main food diary once a day, keep a pen and notepad with you to write down all those little extras you eat or drink during the day – that chocolate you ate in the office, the sliver of cheese you had while cooking dinner and the few chips you pinched from your husband's plate, for example! It's easy to forget the little things if they're not written down, but they can make the difference between success and failure.

QUESTION: Why are heavier people allowed more calories than those who have smaller amounts of weight to lose?

ANSWER: This confuses a lot of people but is easily explained. Someone who is 3 stone overweight, for example, is carrying the equivalent of 42 small packets of butter with them everywhere they go – up and down the stairs, to the local shops, into the kitchen. Obviously, it takes a lot more energy simply to move around when you're carrying that extra weight. As a consequence, the heavier you are, the more calories you need just to keep your weight steady. In turn, this means you'll lose weight on a higher calorie allowance. However, as you lose weight, you'll need to lower your calorie allowance slightly as you have less weight to carry around.

5. Control your portions

As well as making some smart food swaps to cut calories, it's likely you'll also need to reduce your serving sizes for some foods to help shift those pounds. Even 'healthy' foods such as brown rice, wholemeal bread, chicken, fish and low-fat dairy products contain calories so you may need to limit the amount you eat. When you first start out, weigh portions of foods like rice, pasta, cereal, cheese, butter, oil, meat, fish, and chicken rather than completing your food diary with a 'guesstimated' weight! That way you can calculate the calorie content accurately. Don't forget that drinks contain calories too, alcohol, milk, juices and sugary drinks all count.

6. Measure your success

Research has found that regular weight checks do help. Weighing yourself helps you assess how your eating and exercise habits affect your body weight. The important thing is to use the information in a positive way – to assess your progress - rather than as a stick to beat yourself up with. Remember that weight can fluctuate by a kilogram in a day, for example, due to fluid changes, premenstrually, after a big meal out, so weigh yourself at the same time of day and look at the trend over a week or two.

People who successfully lose weight and keep it off, also tend to continue weighing themselves at least once a week, and often daily (but not in an obsessive way), because they say it helps them stay 'on track'. Probably because they use it as an early warning system. People who weigh themselves regularly (or regularly try on a tight fitting item of clothing) will notice quickly if they have gained a few pounds - and can take action to stop gaining more. Checking your weight less often can mean that you might discover one day that you gained more than you thought. That can be pretty discouraging, and it might trigger you to just give up.

Top Tip

Don't just focus on what the bathroom scales say either – keep a record of your vital statistics, too. Many people find it doubly encouraging to see the inches dropping off, as well as the pounds!

7. Stay motivated

Each time you lose half a stone, or reach your own small goal – celebrate! Treat yourself to a little luxury – something new to wear, a little pampering or some other (non-food) treat. It also helps replace the comfort you once got from food and allows you to take care of yourself in other ways. Trying on an item of clothing that used to be tight can also help to keep you feeling motivated. Make sure you keep in touch with your supporters, and if the going gets tough take another look at the *'Coping with Common Slimming Saboteurs' section on page 21*. Once you've reviewed how well you've done, use this book to set yourself a new daily calorie allowance based on your new weight to help you lose the next half stone *(see point 3 - page 28 - Calculate your calorie allowance)*.

8. Keep it off

What you do to stay slim is just as important as what you did to get slim. Quite simply, if you return to your old ways, you are likely to return to your old weight. The great thing about calorie counting is that you will learn so much about what you eat, and make so many important changes to your eating and drinking habits, that you'll probably find it difficult to go back to your old ways – and won't want to anyway. It's still a good idea to weigh yourself at least once a week to keep a check on your weight. The key is to deal with any extra pounds immediately, rather than waiting until you have a stone to lose *(see page 30)*. Simply go back to counting calories for as long as it takes to shift those pounds and enjoy the new slim you. Page 25 has more information about how successful slimmers keep it off.

QUESTION: Do I need to stick to exactly the same number of calories each day or is it OK to have a lower calorie intake during the week and slightly more at the weekend?

ANSWER: The key to losing weight is to take in fewer calories than you need for as long as it takes to reach your target, aiming for a loss of no more than 2lb (1kg) a week. In general, most nutrition experts recommend a daily calorie allowance. However, it's just as valid to use other periods of time such as weeks. If you prefer, simply multiply your daily allowance by seven to work out a weekly calorie allowance and then allocate more calories to some days than others. For example, a daily allowance of 1,500 calories is equivalent to 10,500 calories a week. This means you could have 1,300 calories a day during the week and 2,000 calories a day on Saturday and Sunday.

Healthy Eating Made Easy

Juliette Kellow BSc RD

HEALTHY EATING doesn't just mean eating salads and smoothies. Eating healthily means we're positively encouraged to eat a wide range of foods, including some of our favourites – it's just a question of making sure we don't eat high fat, high sugar or highly processed foods too often.

Eating a healthy diet, together with taking regular exercise and not smoking, has huge benefits to our health, both in the short and long term. As well as helping us to lose or maintain our weight, a healthy diet can boost energy levels, keep our immune system strong and give us healthy skin, nails and hair. Meanwhile, eating well throughout life also means we're far less likely to suffer from health problems such as constipation, anaemia and tooth decay, or set ourselves up for serious conditions in later life such as obesity, heart disease, stroke, diabetes, cancer or osteoporosis.

Fortunately, it couldn't be easier to eat a balanced diet. To start with, no single food provides all the calories and nutrients we need to stay healthy, so it's important to eat a variety of foods. Meanwhile, most nutrition experts also agree that mealtimes should be a pleasure rather than a penance. This means it's fine to eat small amounts of our favourite treats from time to time.

To help people eat healthily, the NHS recommends eating plenty of different foods from four main groups of foods and limiting the amount we eat from a smaller fifth group. Ultimately, we should eat more fruit, vegetables, starchy, fibre-rich foods and fresh products, and fewer fatty, sugary, salty and processed foods.

The following guidelines are all based on the healthy eating guidelines recommended by health professionals.

Bread, other cereals and potatoes

Eat these foods at each meal. They also make good snacks.

Foods in this group include bread, breakfast cereals, potatoes, rice, pasta, noodles, yams, oats and grains. Go for high-fibre varieties where available, such as wholegrain cereals, wholemeal bread and brown rice. These foods should fill roughly a third of your plate at mealtimes.

TYPICAL SERVING SIZES

• *2 slices bread in a sandwich or with a meal*

• *a tennis ball sized serving of pasta, potato, rice, noodles or couscous*

• *a bowl of porridge*

• *around 40g of breakfast cereal*

Fruit and vegetables

Eat at least five portions every day.

Foods in this group include all fruits and vegetables, including fresh, frozen, canned and dried products, and unsweetened fruit juice. Choose canned fruit in juice rather than syrup and go for veg canned in water without added salt or sugar.

TYPICAL PORTION SIZES

• *a piece of fruit eg: apple, banana, pear*

• *2 small fruits eg: satsumas, plums, apricots*

• *a bowl of fruit salad, canned or stewed fruit*

• *a small glass of unsweetened fruit juice*

• *a cereal bowl of salad*

• *3tbsp vegetables*

Milk, dairy and alternatives

Eat two or three servings a day.

Foods in this group include milk, cheese, yoghurt and fromage frais. Choose low-fat varieties where available such as skimmed milk, reduced-fat cheese and fat-free yoghurt.

TYPICAL SERVING SIZES

- *200ml milk*
- *a small pot of yoghurt or fromage frais*
- *a small matchbox-sized piece of cheese*

Meat, fish and alternatives

Eat two servings a day

Foods in this group include meat, poultry, fish, eggs, beans, nuts and seeds. Choose low-fat varieties where available such as extra-lean minced beef and skinless chicken and don't add extra fat or salt.

TYPICAL SERVING SIZES

- *a piece of meat, chicken or fish the size of a deck of cards*
- *1-2 eggs*
- *3 heaped tablespoons of beans*
- *a small handful of nuts or seeds*

Healthy Eating on a plate

A simple way to serve up both balance and healthy proportions is to fill one half of your plate with salad or vegetables and divide the other half between protein-rich meat, chicken, fish, eggs or beans, and healthy carbs (potatoes, rice, pasta, pulses, bread or noodles).

Fatty and sugary foods

Eat only small amounts of these foods

Foods in this group include oils, spreading fats, cream, mayonnaise, oily salad dressings, cakes, biscuits, puddings, crisps, savoury snacks, sugar, preserves, confectionery and sugary soft drinks.

TYPICAL SERVING SIZES:

- *a small packet of sweets or a small bar of chocolate*
- *a small slice of cake*
- *a couple of small biscuits*
- *1 level tbsp mayo, salad dressing or olive oil*
- *a small packet of crisps*

Useful Tools

Body Mass Index

The Body Mass Index (BMI) is the internationally accepted way of assessing how healthy our weight is for most people. It is calculated using height and weight. Use the BMI Chart to look up your BMI, and use this table to see which range you fall into.

BMI Under 18.5	Underweight
BMI 18.5-25	Healthy
BMI 25-30	Overweight
BMI 30-40	Obese
BMI Over 40	Severely Obese

This is what different BMI ranges mean.

- **Underweight:** you probably need to gain weight for your health's sake. Talk to your doctor if you have any concerns, or if you feel frightened about gaining weight.

- **Healthy weight:** you are a healthy weight, so aim to stay in this range (note that most people in this range tend to have a BMI between 20-25).

- **Overweight:** aim to lose some weight for your health's sake, or at least prevent further weight gain.

- **Obese:** your health is at risk and losing weight will benefit your health.

- **Severely obese:** your health is definitely at risk. You should visit your doctor for a health check. Losing weight will improve your health.

Please note that BMI is not as accurate for athletes or very muscular people (muscle weighs more than fat), as it can push them into a higher BMI category despite having a healthy level of body fat. It is also not accurate for women who are pregnant or breastfeeding, or people who are frail.

Body Mass Index Table

HEIGHT IN FEET / INCHES

	4'6	4'8	4'10	5'0	5'2	5'4	5'6	5'8	5'10	6'0	6'2	6'4	6'6	6'8	6'10
6st 7	22.0	20.5	19.1	17.8	16.7	15.7	14.7	13.9	13.1	12.4	11.7	11.1	10.6	10.0	9.5
7st 0	23.7	22.1	20.6	19.2	18.0	16.9	15.9	15.0	14.1	13.3	12.6	12.0	11.4	10.8	10.3
7st 7	25.4	23.6	22.0	20.6	19.3	18.1	17.0	16.0	15.1	14.3	13.5	12.8	12.2	11.6	11.0
8st 0	27.1	25.2	23.5	22.0	20.6	19.3	18.1	17.1	16.1	15.2	14.4	13.7	13.0	12.3	11.8
8st 7	28.8	26.8	25.0	23.3	21.8	20.5	19.3	18.2	17.1	16.2	15.3	14.5	13.8	13.1	12.5
9st 0	30.5	28.4	26.4	24.7	23.1	21.7	20.4	19.2	18.1	17.2	16.2	15.4	14.6	13.9	13.2
9st 7	32.2	29.9	27.9	26.1	24.4	22.9	21.5	20.3	19.2	18.1	17.1	16.2	15.4	14.7	14.0
10st 0	33.9	31.5	29.4	27.4	25.7	24.1	22.7	21.4	20.2	19.1	18.0	17.1	16.2	15.4	14.7
10st 7	35.6	33.1	30.8	28.8	27.0	25.3	23.8	22.4	21.2	20.0	18.9	18.0	17.0	16.2	15.4
11st 0	37.3	34.7	32.3	30.2	28.3	26.5	24.9	23.5	22.2	21.0	19.8	18.8	17.9	17.0	16.2
11st 7	39.0	36.2	33.8	31.6	29.6	27.7	26.1	24.6	23.2	21.9	20.7	19.7	18.7	17.8	16.9
12st 0	40.7	37.8	35.2	32.9	30.8	28.9	27.2	25.6	24.2	22.9	21.6	20.5	19.5	18.5	17.6
12st 7	42.3	39.4	36.7	34.3	32.1	30.1	28.3	26.7	25.2	23.8	22.5	21.4	20.3	19.3	18.4
13st 0	44.0	41.0	38.2	35.7	33.4	31.4	29.5	27.8	26.2	24.8	23.5	22.2	21.1	20.1	19.1
13st 7	45.7	42.5	39.6	37.0	34.7	32.6	30.6	28.8	27.2	25.7	24.4	23.1	21.9	20.8	19.8
14st 0	47.4	44.1	41.1	38.4	36.0	33.8	31.7	29.9	28.2	26.7	25.3	23.9	22.7	21.6	20.6
14st 7	49.1	45.7	42.6	39.8	37.3	35.0	32.9	31.0	29.2	27.6	26.2	24.8	23.5	22.4	21.3
15st 0	50.8	47.3	44.0	41.2	38.5	36.2	34.0	32.0	30.2	28.6	27.1	25.7	24.4	23.2	22.0
15st 7	52.5	48.8	45.5	42.5	39.8	37.4	35.2	33.1	31.2	29.5	28.0	26.5	25.2	23.9	22.8
16st 0	54.2	50.4	47.0	43.9	41.1	38.6	36.3	34.2	32.3	30.5	28.9	27.4	26.0	24.7	23.5
16st 7	55.9	52.0	48.5	45.3	42.4	39.8	37.4	35.2	33.3	31.4	29.8	28.2	26.8	25.5	24.2
17st 0	57.6	53.6	49.9	46.6	43.7	41.0	38.6	36.3	34.3	32.4	30.7	29.1	27.6	26.2	25.0
17st 7	59.3	55.1	51.4	48.0	45.0	42.2	39.7	37.4	35.3	33.3	31.6	29.9	28.4	27.0	25.7
18st 0	61.0	56.7	52.9	49.4	46.3	43.4	40.8	38.5	36.3	34.3	32.5	30.8	29.2	27.8	26.4
18st 7	62.7	58.3	54.3	50.8	47.5	44.6	42.0	39.5	37.3	35.3	33.4	31.6	30.0	28.6	27.2
19st 0	64.4	59.9	55.8	52.1	48.8	45.8	43.1	40.6	38.3	36.2	34.3	32.5	30.8	29.3	27.9
19st 7	66.1	61.4	57.3	53.5	50.1	47.0	44.2	41.7	39.3	37.2	35.2	33.3	31.7	30.1	28.6
20st 0	67.8	63.0	58.7	54.9	51.4	48.2	45.4	42.7	40.3	38.1	36.1	34.2	32.5	30.9	29.4
20st 7	69.4	64.6	60.2	56.3	52.7	49.4	46.5	43.8	41.3	39.1	37.0	35.1	33.3	31.6	30.1
21st 0	71.1	66.2	61.7	57.6	54.0	50.6	47.6	44.9	42.3	40.0	37.9	35.9	34.1	32.4	30.9
21st 7	72.8	67.7	63.1	59.0	55.3	51.9	48.8	45.9	43.3	41.0	38.8	36.8	34.9	33.2	31.6
22st 0	74.5	69.3	64.6	60.4	56.5	53.1	49.9	47.0	44.4	41.9	39.7	37.6	35.7	34.0	32.3
22st 7	76.2	70.9	66.1	61.7	57.8	54.3	51.0	48.1	45.4	42.9	40.6	38.5	36.5	34.7	33.1
23st 0	77.9	72.5	67.5	63.1	59.1	55.5	52.2	49.1	46.4	43.8	41.5	39.3	37.3	35.5	33.8
23st 7	79.6	74.0	69.0	64.5	60.4	56.7	53.3	50.2	47.4	44.8	42.4	40.2	38.2	36.3	34.5
24st 0	81.3	75.6	70.5	65.9	61.7	57.9	54.4	51.3	48.4	45.7	43.3	41.0	39.0	37.0	35.3
24st 7	83.0	77.2	71.9	67.2	63.0	59.1	55.6	52.3	49.4	46.7	44.2	41.9	39.8	37.8	36.0
25st 0	84.7	78.8	73.4	68.6	64.2	60.3	56.7	53.4	50.4	47.6	45.1	42.8	40.6	38.6	36.7
25st 7	86.4	80.3	74.9	70.0	65.5	61.5	57.8	54.5	51.4	48.6	46.0	43.6	41.4	39.4	37.5
26st 0	88.1	81.9	76.3	71.3	66.8	62.7	59.0	55.5	52.4	49.5	46.9	44.5	42.2	40.1	38.2
26st 7	89.8	83.5	77.8	72.7	68.1	63.9	60.1	56.6	53.4	50.5	47.8	45.3	43.0	40.9	38.9
27st 0	91.5	85.1	79.3	74.1	69.4	65.1	61.2	57.7	54.4	51.5	48.7	46.2	43.8	41.7	39.7
27st 7	93.2	86.6	80.8	75.5	70.7	66.3	62.4	58.7	55.4	52.4	49.6	47.0	44.7	42.4	40.4
28st 0	94.9	88.2	82.2	76.8	72.0	67.5	63.5	59.8	56.4	53.4	50.5	47.9	45.5	43.2	41.1
28st 7	96.5	89.8	83.7	78.2	73.2	68.7	64.6	60.9	57.5	54.3	51.4	48.7	46.3	44.0	41.9
29st 0	98.2	91.4	85.2	79.6	74.5	69.9	65.8	62.0	58.5	55.3	52.3	49.6	47.1	44.8	42.6
29st 7	99.9	92.9	86.6	80.9	75.8	71.1	66.9	63.0	59.5	56.2	53.2	50.5	47.9	45.5	43.3

WEIGHT IN STONES / LBS

Weight Chart

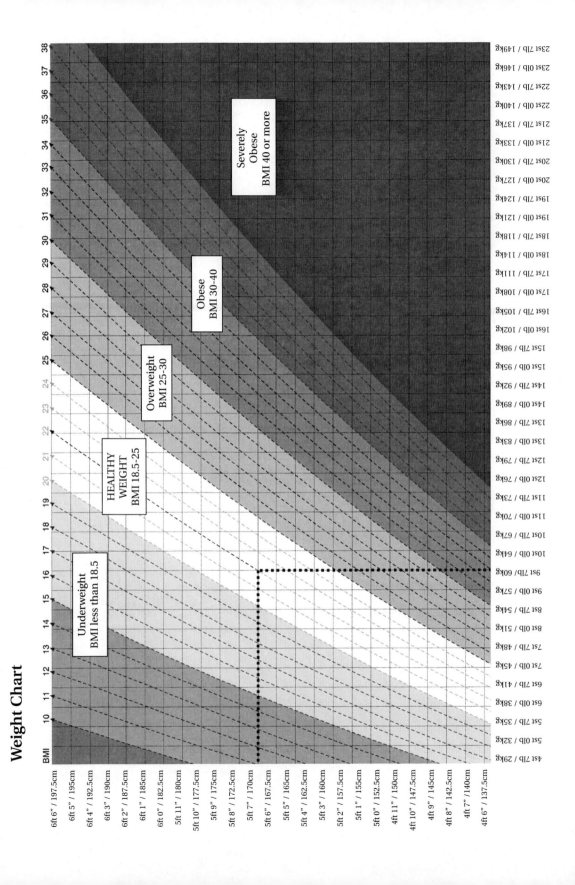

Calories Required to Maintain Weight
Adult Females

ACTIVITY LEVEL / AGE

WEIGHT IN STONES / LBS	VERY SEDENTARY			MODERATELY SEDENTARY			MODERATELY ACTIVE			VERY ACTIVE		
	<30	30-60	60+	<30	30-60	60+	<30	30-60	60+	<30	30-60	60+
7st 7	1425	1473	1304	1544	1596	1412	1781	1841	1630	2138	2210	1956
8st 0	1481	1504	1338	1605	1629	1450	1852	1880	1673	2222	2256	2008
8st 7	1537	1535	1373	1666	1663	1487	1922	1919	1716	2306	2302	2059
9st 0	1594	1566	1407	1726	1696	1524	1992	1957	1759	2391	2349	2111
9st 7	1650	1596	1442	1787	1729	1562	2062	1996	1802	2475	2395	2163
10st 0	1706	1627	1476	1848	1763	1599	2133	2034	1845	2559	2441	2214
10st 7	1762	1658	1511	1909	1796	1637	2203	2073	1888	2644	2487	2266
11st 0	1819	1689	1545	1970	1830	1674	2273	2111	1931	2728	2534	2318
11st 7	1875	1720	1580	2031	1863	1711	2344	2150	1975	2813	2580	2370
12st 0	1931	1751	1614	2092	1897	1749	2414	2188	2018	2897	2626	2421
12st 7	1987	1781	1648	2153	1930	1786	2484	2227	2061	2981	2672	2473
13st 0	2044	1812	1683	2214	1963	1823	2555	2266	2104	3066	2719	2525
13st 7	2100	1843	1717	2275	1997	1861	2625	2304	2147	3150	2765	2576
14st 0	2156	1874	1752	2336	2030	1898	2695	2343	2190	3234	2811	2628
14st 7	2212	1905	1786	2397	2064	1935	2766	2381	2233	3319	2858	2680
15st 0	2269	1936	1821	2458	2097	1973	2836	2420	2276	3403	2904	2732
15st 7	2325	1967	1855	2519	2130	2010	2906	2458	2319	3488	2950	2783
16st 0	2381	1997	1890	2580	2164	2047	2976	2497	2362	3572	2996	2835
16st 7	2437	2028	1924	2640	2197	2085	3047	2535	2405	3656	3043	2887
17st 0	2494	2059	1959	2701	2231	2122	3117	2574	2449	3741	3089	2938
17st 7	2550	2090	1993	2762	2264	2159	3187	2613	2492	3825	3135	2990
18st 0	2606	2121	2028	2823	2298	2197	3258	2651	2535	3909	3181	3042
18st 7	2662	2152	2062	2884	2331	2234	3328	2690	2578	3994	3228	3093
19st 0	2719	2182	2097	2945	2364	2271	3398	2728	2621	4078	3274	3145
19st 7	2775	2213	2131	3006	2398	2309	3469	2767	2664	4162	3320	3197
20st 0	2831	2244	2166	3067	2431	2346	3539	2805	2707	4247	3366	3249
20st 7	2887	2275	2200	3128	2465	2383	3609	2844	2750	4331	3413	3300
21st 0	2944	2306	2235	3189	2498	2421	3680	2882	2793	4416	3459	3352
21st 7	3000	2337	2269	3250	2531	2458	3750	2921	2836	4500	3505	3404
22st 0	3056	2368	2303	3311	2565	2495	3820	2960	2879	4584	3552	3455
22st 7	3112	2398	2338	3372	2598	2533	3890	2998	2923	4669	3598	3507
23st 0	3169	2429	2372	3433	2632	2570	3961	3037	2966	4753	3644	3559
23st 7	3225	2460	2407	3494	2665	2608	4031	3075	3009	4837	3690	3611
24st 0	3281	2491	2441	3554	2699	2645	4101	3114	3052	4922	3737	3662
24st 7	3337	2522	2476	3615	2732	2682	4172	3152	3095	5006	3783	3714
25st 0	3394	2553	2510	3676	2765	2720	4242	3191	3138	5091	3829	3766
25st 7	3450	2583	2545	3737	2799	2757	4312	3229	3181	5175	3875	3817
26st 0	3506	2614	2579	3798	2832	2794	4383	3268	3224	5259	3922	3869
26st 7	3562	2645	2614	3859	2866	2832	4453	3307	3267	5344	3968	3921
27st 0	3618	2676	2648	3920	2899	2869	4523	3345	3310	5428	4014	3973
27st 7	3675	2707	2683	3981	2932	2906	4594	3384	3353	5512	4060	4024
28st 0	3731	2738	2717	4042	2966	2944	4664	3422	3397	5597	4107	4076
28st 7	3787	2768	2752	4103	2999	2981	4734	3461	3440	5681	4153	4128

Calories Required to Maintain Weight
Adult Males

ACTIVITY LEVEL / AGE

WEIGHT IN STONES / LBS	VERY SEDENTARY			MODERATELY SEDENTARY			MODERATELY ACTIVE			VERY ACTIVE		
	<30	30-60	60+	<30	30-60	60+	<30	30-60	60+	<30	30-60	60+
9st 0	1856	1827	1502	2010	1979	1627	2320	2284	1878	2784	2741	2254
9st 7	1913	1871	1547	2072	2026	1676	2391	2338	1933	2870	2806	2320
10st 0	1970	1914	1591	2134	2074	1724	2463	2393	1989	2955	2871	2387
10st 7	2027	1958	1636	2196	2121	1772	2534	2447	2045	3041	2937	2454
11st 0	2084	2001	1680	2258	2168	1820	2605	2502	2100	3127	3002	2520
11st 7	2141	2045	1724	2320	2215	1868	2677	2556	2156	3212	3067	2587
12st 0	2199	2088	1769	2382	2262	1916	2748	2611	2211	3298	3133	2654
12st 7	2256	2132	1813	2444	2310	1965	2820	2665	2267	3384	3198	2720
13st 0	2313	2175	1858	2506	2357	2013	2891	2719	2322	3470	3263	2787
13st 7	2370	2219	1902	2568	2404	2061	2963	2774	2378	3555	3329	2854
14st 0	2427	2262	1947	2630	2451	2109	3034	2828	2434	3641	3394	2920
14st 7	2484	2306	1991	2691	2498	2157	3106	2883	2489	3727	3459	2987
15st 0	2542	2350	2036	2753	2545	2205	3177	2937	2545	3813	3525	3054
15st 7	2599	2393	2080	2815	2593	2253	3248	2992	2600	3898	3590	3120
16st 0	2656	2437	2125	2877	2640	2302	3320	3046	2656	3984	3655	3187
16st 7	2713	2480	2169	2939	2687	2350	3391	3100	2711	4070	3721	3254
17st 0	2770	2524	2213	3001	2734	2398	3463	3155	2767	4155	3786	3320
17st 7	2827	2567	2258	3063	2781	2446	3534	3209	2823	4241	3851	3387
18st 0	2884	2611	2302	3125	2828	2494	3606	3264	2878	4327	3917	3454
18st 7	2942	2654	2347	3187	2876	2542	3677	3318	2934	4413	3982	3520
19st 0	2999	2698	2391	3249	2923	2591	3749	3373	2989	4498	4047	3587
19st 7	3056	2741	2436	3311	2970	2639	3820	3427	3045	4584	4112	3654
20st 0	3113	2785	2480	3373	3017	2687	3891	3481	3100	4670	4178	3721
20st 7	3170	2829	2525	3434	3064	2735	3963	3536	3156	4756	4243	3787
21st 0	3227	2872	2569	3496	3112	2783	4034	3590	3211	4841	4308	3854
21st 7	3285	2916	2614	3558	3159	2831	4106	3645	3267	4927	4374	3921
22st 0	3342	2959	2658	3620	3206	2880	4177	3699	3323	5013	4439	3987
22st 7	3399	3003	2702	3682	3253	2928	4249	3754	3378	5098	4504	4054
23st 0	3456	3046	2747	3744	3300	2976	4320	3808	3434	5184	4570	4121
23st 7	3513	3090	2791	3806	3347	3024	4392	3862	3489	5270	4635	4187
24st 0	3570	3133	2836	3868	3395	3072	4463	3917	3545	5356	4700	4254
24st 7	3627	3177	2880	3930	3442	3120	4534	3971	3600	5441	4766	4321
25st 0	3685	3220	2925	3992	3489	3168	4606	4026	3656	5527	4831	4387
25st 7	3742	3264	2969	4054	3536	3217	4677	4080	3712	5613	4896	4454
26st 0	3799	3308	3014	4116	3583	3265	4749	4135	3767	5699	4962	4521
26st 7	3856	3351	3058	4177	3630	3313	4820	4189	3823	5784	5027	4587
27st 0	3913	3395	3103	4239	3678	3361	4892	4243	3878	5870	5092	4654
27st 7	3970	3438	3147	4301	3725	3409	4963	4298	3934	5956	5158	4721
28st 0	4028	3482	3191	4363	3772	3457	5035	4352	3989	6042	5223	4787
28st 7	4085	3525	3236	4425	3819	3506	5106	4407	4045	6127	5288	4854
29st 0	4142	3569	3280	4487	3866	3554	5177	4461	4101	6213	5354	4921
29st 7	4199	3612	3325	4549	3913	3602	5249	4516	4156	6299	5419	4987
30st 0	4256	3656	3369	4611	3961	3650	5320	4570	4212	6384	5484	5054

Calories Burned in Exercise

This table shows the approximate number of extra* calories that would be burned in a five minute period of exercise activity.

ACTIVITY	CALORIES BURNED IN 5 MINUTES	ACTIVITY	CALORIES BURNED IN 5 MINUTES
Aerobics, Low Impact	25	Situps, Continuous	17
Badminton, Recreational	17	Skiing, Moderate	30
Cross Trainer	30	Skipping, Moderate	30
Cycling, Recreational, 5mph	17	Squash Playing	39
Dancing, Modern, Moderate	13	Tennis Playing, Recreational	26
Fencing	24	Toning Exercises	17
Gardening, Weeding	19	Trampolining	17
Hill Walking, Up and Down, Recreational	22	Volleyball, Recreational	10
Jogging	30	Walking, Uphill, 15% Gradient, Moderate	43
Kick Boxing	30	Walking Up and Down Stairs, Moderate	34
Netball Playing	23	Walking, 4mph	24
Rebounding	18	Weight Training, Moderate	12
Roller Skating	30	Yoga	13
Rowing Machine, Moderate	30		
Running, 7.5mph	48		

*Extra calories are those in addition to your normal daily calorie needs.

My Personal Plan

Date:

Body Mass Index:

Weight:

Waist Measurement:

Height:

Body Fat % (if known)

10% Weight Loss Goal:

Current weight	16stone (224lb)	100kg
- 10% weight	1stone 8½lb (22½lb)	10kg
= 10% loss goal	14stone 5½lb (201½lb)	90kg

My smaller weight targets on the way to achieving my 10% goal will be:

_____ _____ _____ _____

Reasons why I want to lose weight:

Changes I will make to help me lose weight:
Diet:

Activity:

Potential saboteurs or barriers will be:

Ways I will overcome these:

My supporters will be:

I will monitor my progress by:

I will reward my progress with:
In the short term:

In the long term:

Food and Exercise Diary

Date: ___/___/___

Daily Calorie Allowance: [____] **(A)**

Food/Drink Consumed	Serving Size	Calories

You are aiming for your Calorie Balance (Box D) to be as close to zero as possible - ie. you consume the number of calories you need.

Your Daily Calorie Allowance (Box A) should be set to lose ½-2lb (¼-1kg) a week, or maintain weight, depending on your goals.

Total calories consumed [____] **(B)**

Exercise/Activity	No. mins	Calories

Daily Calorie Allowance (A) _plus_ Extra Calories used in Exercise (C) _minus_ Total Calories Consumed (B) _equals_ Calorie Balance (D)

Calories used in exercise [____] **(C)**

$$A + C - B = D$$

Calorie balance [____] **(D)**

You can also write down any comments or thoughts related to your eating if you want to.

Food Information

Nutritional Information

CALORIE AND FAT values are given per serving, plus calorie and nutrition values per 100g of product. This makes it easy to compare the proportions of fat, protein, carbohydrate and fibre in each food.

The values given are for uncooked, unprepared foods unless otherwise stated. Values are also for only the edible portion of the food unless otherwise stated. ie - weighed with bone.

Finding Foods

The Calorie, Carb & Fat Bible has an Eating Out section which is arranged alphabetically by brand. In the General Foods and Drinks A-Z most foods are grouped together by type, and then put in to alphabetical order. This makes it easy to compare different brands, and will help you to find lower calorie and/or fat alternatives where they are available.

This format also makes it easier to locate foods. Foods are categorised by their main characteristics so, for example, if it is bread, ciabatta or white sliced, you'll find it under "Bread".

Basic ingredients are highlighted to make them easier to find at a glance. You'll find all unbranded foods in bold - making the index easier to use, whether it's just an apple or all the components of a home cooked stew.

There are, however, some foods which are not so easy to categorise, especially combination foods like ready meals. The following pointers will help you to find your way around the book until you get to know it a little better.

FILLED ROLLS AND SANDWICHES - Bagels, baguettes, etc which are filled are listed as "Bagels (filled)" etc. Sandwiches are under "Sandwiches".

CURRIES - Popular types of curry, like Balti or Jalfrezi, are listed under their individual types. Unspecified or lesser known types are listed under their main ingredient.

BURGERS - All burgers from fast-food outlets are listed under "Burgers".

CHIPS & FRIES - Are listed separately, depending on the name of the particular brand. All other types of potato are listed under "Potatoes".

SWEETS & CHOCOLATES - Well-known brands, eg. Aero, Mars Bar, are listed under their brand names. Others are listed under "Chocolate" (for bars) and "Chocolates" (for individual sweets).

READY MEALS - Popular types of dishes are listed under their type, eg. "Chow Mein", "Casserole", "Hot Pot", etc. Others are listed by their main ingredient, eg. "Chicken With", "Chicken In", etc.

EATING OUT & FAST FOODS - By popular demand this edition has the major eating out and fast food brands listed separately, at the back of the book. They are alphabetised first by brand, then follow using the same format as the rest of the book, with calories provided per serving.

Serving Sizes

Many ready-meal type foods are given with calories for the full pack size, so that an individual serving can be worked out by estimating the proportion of the pack that has been consumed. For example, if you have eaten a quarter of a packaged pasta dish, divide the calorie value given for the whole pack by 4 to determine the number of calories you have consumed. Where serving sizes are not appropriate, or unknown, values are given per 100g and per 1oz/28g. Serving sizes vary greatly from person to person and, if you are trying to lose weight, it's important to be accurate – especially with high calorie foods such as those that contain a fair amount of fat, sugar, cream, cheese, alcohol etc.

Food Data

Nutrition information for basic average foods has been compiled by the Weight Loss Resources food data team using many sources of information to calculate the most accurate values possible. Some nutrition information for non-branded food records is from The Composition of Foods 6th Edition. Reproduced under licence from The Controller of Her Majesty's Stationary Office. Where basic data is present for ordinary foodstuffs such as 'raw carrots'; branded records are not included.

Nutrition information for branded goods is from details supplied by retailers and manufacturers, and researched by Weight Loss Resources staff. The Calorie Carb & Fat Bible contains data for over 1400 UK brands, including major supermarkets and fast food outlets.

The publishers gratefully acknowledge all the manufacturers and retailers who have provided information on their products. All product names, trademarks or registered trademarks belong to their respective owners and are used only for the purpose of identifying products.

Calorie & nutrition data for all food and drink items are typical values.

Caution
The information in The Calorie, Carb and Fat Bible is intended as an aid to weight loss and weight maintenance, and is not medical advice. If you suffer from, or think you may suffer from a medical condition you should consult your doctor before starting a weight loss and/or exercise regime. If you start exercising after a period of relative inactivity, you should start slowly and consult your doctor if you experience pain, distress or other symptoms.

Weights, Measures & Abbreviations

ABBREVIATIONS

kcal	kilocalories / calories
prot	protein
carb	carbohydrate
sm	small
med	medium
av	average
reg	regular
lge	large
tsp	teaspoon
tbsp	tablespoon
dtsp	dessertspoon
gf	gluten free

BRAND ABBREVIATIONS USED

ASDA	
Good for You	GFY
Chosen by You	CBY
Good & Counted	G&C
MARKS & SPENCER	M & S
Count on Us	COU
Balanced For You	BFY
MORRISONS	
Better For You	BFY
SAINSBURY'S	
Be Good to Yourself	BGTY
Way to Five	WTF
Taste the Difference	TTD
TESCO	
Healthy Eating	HE
Healthy Living	HL
Hearty Food Co	HFC
Light Choices	LC
WAITROSE	
Perfectly Balanced	PB
Cambridge Weight Plan	CWP

	Measure INFO/WEIGHT	per Measure KCAL	FAT	Nutrition Values per 100g / 100ml KCAL	PROT	CARB	FAT	FIBRE
ABSINTHE								
Average	*1 Pub Shot/35ml*	*127*	*0*	*363*	*0*	*38.8*	*0*	*0*
ACKEE								
Canned, Drained, Average	*1oz/28g*	*43*	*4.3*	*151*	*2.9*	*0.8*	*15.2*	*0*
ADVOCAAT								
Average	*1 Pub Shot/35ml*	*91*	*2.2*	*260*	*4.7*	*28.4*	*6.3*	*0*
AERO								
Creamy White Centre, Nestle*	1 Bar/46g	244	13.8	530	7.6	57.4	30	0
Honeycomb, Nestle*	1 Bar/40g	199	10	497	5.9	62.2	25	0
Milk Chocolate, Bubbles, Sharing Bag, Aero, Nestle*	1 Bag/113g	610	34.7	540	6.5	57.8	30.7	0
Milk, Giant, Bar, Nestle*	1 Bar/125g	674	38.6	539	6.6	57.7	30.9	2.2
Milk, Medium, Bar, Nestle*	1 Bar/43g	232	13.3	539	6.6	57.7	30.9	2.2
Milk, Snacksize, Bar, Nestle*	1 Bar/21g	110	6.5	537	6.6	55.9	31.9	2.2
Milk, Standard, Bar, Nestle*	1 Bar/31g	165	9.6	531	6.3	56.9	30.9	0.8
Minis, Nestle*	1 Bar/11g	57	3.2	518	6.8	58.1	28.7	0.8
Mint, Bubbles, Aero, Nestle*	1 Bubble/3g	16	0.9	533	4.4	62.7	29.1	0.8
Mint, Nestle*	1 Bar/41g	218	11.9	531	5.4	61.6	28.9	1.1
Mint, Snack Size, Nestle*	1 Bar/21g	112	6.7	548	7.7	55.3	32.8	0.9
Mint, Standard, Aero, Nestle*	1 Bar/43g	233	13.2	542	5.2	60.5	30.8	0.9
Orange Chocolate, Limited Edition, Aero, Nestle*	1 Bar/41g	221	12.3	539	5.1	61.4	29.9	0.9
Orange, Bubbles, Aero, Nestle*	1 Bubble/3g	16	0.9	538	5.4	60.5	30	1.4
Orange, Nestle*	6 Squares/22g	119	6.8	542	5.1	60.7	30.7	0.9
ALCOPOPS								
Smirnoff Apple Bite, Frozen, Smirnoff*	1 Pint/568ml	523	0	92	0	15	0	0
Smirnoff Ice, Frozen, Smirnoff*	1 Pint/568ml	511	0	90	0	15	0	0
Smirnoff Ice, Smirnoff*	1 Bottle/275ml	188	0	68	1.8	12	0	0
Smirnoff Lemon Sorbet, Frozen, Smirnoff*	1 Pint/568ml	517	0	91	0	15	0	0
Smirnoff Mango Sorbet, Frozen, Smirnoff*	1 Pint/568ml	511	0	90	0	15	0	0
Smirnoff Raspberry Sorbet, Frozen, Smirnoff*	1 Pint/568ml	517	0	91	0	15	0	0
ALFALFA SPROUTS								
Raw, Average	*1 Serving/33g*	*8*	*0.3*	*24*	*3*	*3*	*0.9*	*3*
ALLSPICE								
Ground, Schwartz*	1 Tsp/3g	11	0.1	358	6.1	74.3	4	0
ALMONDS								
Balls, Why Nut?*	1 Ball/6g	26	1.5	471	13.6	39.7	26.9	7.5
Blanched, Average	*1 Serving/100g*	*617*	*54.3*	*617*	*25.1*	*6.9*	*54.3*	*8.1*
Candied, Sugared	*1 Serving/100g*	*458*	*16.3*	*458*	*8.4*	*69.2*	*16.3*	*2.2*
Chocolate, Dark, Raspberry, Skinny Dipped*	1 Almond/2g	10	0.8	536	17.9	39.3	42.9	10.7
Flaked, Average	*1oz/28g*	*172*	*15.2*	*613*	*24.9*	*6.5*	*54.3*	*7.6*
Flaked, Toasted, Average	*1oz/28g*	*176*	*15.8*	*629*	*24.6*	*5.8*	*56.4*	*7.5*
Ground, Average	*1 Serving/10g*	*62*	*5.6*	*625*	*24*	*6.6*	*55.8*	*7.4*
Marcona, Average	*1 Serving/100g*	*608*	*53.7*	*608*	*22.1*	*13*	*53.7*	*9.7*
Moroccan Spiced, Mr Filbert's*	1 Pack/110g	684	54.1	622	22.4	17.1	49.2	10.4
Toasted, Average	*1oz/28g*	*178*	*15.8*	*634*	*25*	*6.6*	*56.4*	*6.6*
Whole, Average	*1 Serving/20g*	*122*	*11*	*612*	*23.4*	*6.9*	*54.8*	*8.4*
Yoghurt Coated, Holland & Barrett*	1 Pack/100g	536	37	536	10.9	45.3	37	2.8
ALOO								
Bombay, M&S*	½ Pack/114g	108	5.2	95	1.8	10.3	4.6	2.3
Saag, Canned, Tesco*	½ Can/200g	124	3.8	62	1.8	9.3	1.9	2
Saag, Gobi, Indian, Tesco*	1 Pack/225g	225	16.4	100	2.1	6.5	7.3	1.8
Saag, Gobi, Retail	*1 Serving/330g*	*314*	*22.8*	*95*	*2.2*	*7.1*	*6.9*	*1.4*
Saag, Gobi, Takeaway, Microwaved, Morrisons*	½ Pack/105g	88	3.6	84	2	9.5	3.4	3.9
Saag, Gobi, Tesco*	1 Serving/175g	166	8.9	95	2.1	9.5	5.1	1.9
Saag, Gobi, Waitrose*	½ Pack/150g	140	8.4	93	2	6.6	5.6	4.1

A

INFO/WEIGHT	Measure	per Measure		Nutrition Values per 100g / 100ml				
		KCAL	FAT	KCAL	PROT	CARB	FAT	FIBRE
ALOO								
Saag, Sainsbury's*	1 Pack/300g	300	19.2	100	1.8	7	6.4	3.4
Saag, Tesco*	1 Serving/200g	144	7	72	2.1	8	3.5	2
Tikki, Average	*1 Serving/25g*	*48*	*2*	*191*	*4.5*	*25.2*	*8*	*3.5*
AMARANTH								
Grain, Cooked	*1 Serving/100g*	*102*	*2*	*102*	*4*	*19*	*2*	*2*
Seed, Holland & Barrett*	1 Tbsp/15g	56	1	371	14	55	7	6.5
ANCHOVIES								
Fillets, in Extra Virgin Olive Oil, Drained, M&S*	¼ Jar/15g	30	1.4	210	26.4	3.7	9.9	0.1
Fillets, Tesco*	1 Serving/15g	34	2.1	226	25	0	14	0
in Oil, Canned, Drained	*1 Anchovy/4g*	*8*	*0.5*	*195*	*23.4*	*0*	*11.3*	*0*
Marinated, Sainsbury's*	¼ Pot/44g	78	4	177	22	2	9	0.1
Paste, Lusso Vita*	1 Tsp/5g	9	0.6	185	17.7	3.9	11	0
Paste, with Olive Oil, Admiral*	1 Tsp/5g	11	0.8	215	15.7	0	16.7	0
ANGEL DELIGHT								
Banana, Kraft*	1 Sachet/59g	280	12.3	474	2.3	69.3	20.9	0.3
Butterscotch, no Added Sugar, with Semi Skimmed, Kraft*	1 Portion/89g	97	4.1	109	3.8	13	4.6	0.5
Chocolate Flavour, Kraft*	1 Sachet/67g	305	12.1	455	3.7	69.5	18	0.4
Raspberry Flavour, no Added Sugar, Kraft*	1 Sachet/59g	292	15.3	495	4.8	59.5	26	0
Strawberry Flavour, Kraft*	1 Sachet/59g	286	12.4	485	2.5	71	21	0
Strawberry Flavour, no Added Sugar, Kraft*	1 Sachet/47g	230	12.5	490	4.8	59	26.5	0
Toffee Flavour, Kraft*	1 Sachet/59g	283	12.4	480	2.6	70	21	0
Vanilla Ice Cream Flavour, Kraft*	1 Sachet/59g	289	12.7	490	2.5	71.5	21.5	0
ANGEL HAIR								
Pasta, Dry	*1 Serving/50g*	*181*	*1.1*	*362*	*12.4*	*73.6*	*2.2*	*4.4*
ANTIPASTI								
in Oil, Grilled, Cucina, Aldi*	¼ Jar/43g	41	3.7	96	1.1	2.3	8.6	2.2
Mixed, in Olive Oil, Extra Virgin, Drained, M&S*	¼ Jar/40g	76	7	191	1.3	4.8	17.5	4.3
ANTIPASTO								
Artichoke, Sainsbury's*	1 Serving/50g	68	6.2	135	2	3.6	12.5	2.3
Coppa, from Selection Platter, TTD, Sainsbury's*	1 Serving/100g	255	17.1	255	25.2	0.1	17.1	0
Felino, from Selection Platter, TTD, Sainsbury's*	1 Serving/100g	349	24.9	349	31.1	0.1	24.9	0
Italian, Specially Selected, Aldi*	¼ Pack/30g	97	6.9	323	28	0	23	0
Mixed Mushroom, Sainsbury's*	¼ Pack/72g	70	6.5	97	2.7	1.4	9	3.7
Mixed Pepper, Sainsbury's*	½ Jar/140g	48	1.8	34	1.3	4.2	1.3	3.5
Mixed, Misto Cotto, Arrosto Erbe, Waitrose*	1 Slice/9g	11	0.4	129	22.2	0	4.4	0
Parma Ham, from Selection Platter, TTD, Sainsbury's*	1 Serving/100g	236	12.9	236	29.9	0.1	12.9	0
Parma, Salami Milano, Bresaola, Finest, Tesco*	¼ Pack/30g	104	7.9	345	26.4	0.5	26.3	0
Roasted Pepper, Drained, Tesco*	1 Jar /170g	128	9.4	75	0.9	5.5	5.5	4.1
Seafood, Drained, Sainsbury's*	½ Jar/84g	150	9.7	178	14.3	4.1	11.6	1.4
APPLES								
Cheddar, Boots*	1 Pack/70g	93	5	133	4.6	12	7.2	1.8
Bites, Average	*1 Pack/118g*	*58*	*0.1*	*49*	*0.3*	*11.6*	*0.1*	*2.2*
Braeburn, Average	*1 Apple/123g*	*58*	*0*	*47*	*0.3*	*12.9*	*0*	*2.9*
Cape, Tesco*	1 Apple/100g	50	0.1	50	0.4	11.8	0.1	1.8
Cooking, Baked with Sugar, Flesh Only, Average	*1 Serving/140g*	*104*	*0.1*	*74*	*0.5*	*19.2*	*0.1*	*1.7*
Cooking, Raw, Peeled, Average	*1oz/28g*	*10*	*0*	*35*	*0.3*	*8.9*	*0.1*	*1.6*
Cooking, Stewed with Sugar, Average	*1 Serving/140g*	*104*	*0.1*	*74*	*0.3*	*19.1*	*0.1*	*1.2*
Cooking, Stewed without Sugar, Average	*1 Serving/140g*	*46*	*0.1*	*33*	*0.3*	*8.1*	*0.1*	*1.5*
Cox, English, Average	*1 Apple/123g*	*53*	*0.1*	*43*	*0.4*	*10.2*	*0.1*	*1.8*
Discovery, Average	*1 Apple/182g*	*82*	*0.9*	*45*	*0.4*	*10.6*	*0.5*	*1*
Dried, Average	*1 Pack/250g*	*537*	*0.7*	*215*	*0.8*	*52.8*	*0.3*	*5.9*
Empire, Average	*1 Apple/120g*	*52*	*0.1*	*44*	*0.4*	*10.7*	*0.1*	*1.8*
Fuji	*1 Apple/132g*	*64*	*0.1*	*48*	*0.4*	*11.8*	*0.1*	*1.8*

	Measure INFO/WEIGHT	per Measure KCAL	FAT	Nutrition Values per 100g / 100ml KCAL	PROT	CARB	FAT	FIBRE
APPLES								
Gala, Average	**1 Apple/152g**	**66**	**0.2**	**43**	**0.3**	**10.4**	**0.1**	**1.4**
Golden Delicious, Average	**1 Med/102g**	**44**	**0.1**	**43**	**0.3**	**10.1**	**0.1**	**1.6**
Granny Smith, Average	**1 Sm/125g**	**56**	**0.1**	**45**	**0.3**	**10.7**	**0.1**	**1.8**
Green, Raw, Average	**1 Med/182g**	**86**	**0.2**	**48**	**0.4**	**11.3**	**0.1**	**1.8**
Jazz, Tesco*	1 Apple/133g	70	0.1	53	0.4	11.8	0.1	1.8
Kanzi, Tesco*	1 Apple/134g	71	0.1	53	0.4	11.8	0.1	1.8
Mackintosh, Red, Average	**1 Apple/165g**	**81**	**0.5**	**49**	**0.2**	**12.8**	**0.3**	**1.8**
Pink Lady, Average	**1 Apple/125g**	**56**	**0.1**	**45**	**0.4**	**10.6**	**0.1**	**1.9**
Pink Lady, Dried, M&S*	1 Pot/50g	101	0.1	202	2	45.3	0.2	5.3
Puree, Biona Organic*	1 Serving/100g	48	0.1	48	0.2	10.5	0.1	1.5
Red, Average	**1 Med/149g**	**71**	**0.2**	**48**	**0.3**	**11.8**	**0.1**	**2**
Sliced, Average	**1oz/28g**	**14**	**0**	**49**	**0.4**	**11.6**	**0.1**	**1.8**
APPLETISER*								
Juice Drink, Sparkling, Appletiser, Coca-Cola*	1 Glass/200ml	94	0	47	0	11	0	0.4
APRICOTS								
& Prunes, in Fruit Juice, Breakfast, Sainsbury's*	1 Pot/150g	134	0.2	89	1.1	21.2	0.1	0.7
Canned, in Syrup, Average	**1oz/28g**	**18**	**0**	**63**	**0.4**	**16.1**	**0.1**	**0.9**
Dried, Average	**1 Apricot/10g**	**17**	**0.1**	**171**	**3.6**	**37.4**	**0.5**	**6.3**
Dried, Soft, Average	**1 Serving/50g**	**104**	**0.2**	**208**	**2.4**	**48.5**	**0.4**	**5.2**
Golden Malatya, Dried, Snack On, Whitworths*	1 Serving/30g	53	0.2	178	4	36	0.6	6.3
Halves, in Fruit Juice, Average	**1 Can/221g**	**87**	**0.1**	**40**	**0.5**	**9.2**	**0.1**	**1**
Milk Chocolate Coated, Graze*	1 Pack/35g	158	8.6	450	6.1	55.9	24.7	5
Raw, Flesh Only, Average	**1 Apricot/37g**	**19**	**0.2**	**52**	**1.5**	**12**	**0.4**	**2.2**
Raw, Weighed with Stone, Average	**1 Apricot/40g**	**19**	**0.2**	**47**	**1.4**	**10.8**	**0.4**	**1.9**
Yoghurt Coated, Graze*	1 Pack/40g	176	9	441	3.4	58.6	22.4	0
AQUAFABA								
Average	**1 Tbsp/15ml**	**3**	**0**	**18**	**1**	**2.9**	**0.2**	**0**
ARANCINI								
Aubergine, Cauldron Foods*	1 Arancini/30g	63	2.8	211	5.6	24.9	9.2	3.2
Mozzarella Pecorino, World Cafe, Waitrose*	½ Pack/75g	223	10.9	314	8	34.8	15.3	2.5
ARCHERS*								
Aqua, Peach, Archers*	1 Bottle/275ml	206	0	75	0.3	7.7	0	0
Peach (Calculated Estimate), Archers*	1 Shot/35ml	91	0	260	0	0	0	0
Vea, Wildberry, Schnapps, Archers*	1 Bottle/275ml	124	0	45	0	5.8	0	0
ARTICHOKE								
Chargrilled, in Olive Oil, Cooks Ingredients, Waitrose*	1 Serving/30g	54	4.9	134	1.7	2.7	12.3	2.7
Chargrilled, Italian, Drained, Sainsbury's*	1/3 Tub/43g	40	2.7	92	3.1	2.8	6.1	6.5
Chargrilled, Italian, in Extra Virgin Olive Oil, Drained, M&S*	¼ Jar/35g	75	6.7	213	1.7	7.1	19.2	2.6
Chargrilled, Marinated with Garlic, Herbs, Tesco*	¼ Pot/35g	72	6.9	205	1.8	3.6	19.8	3
Fresh, Raw, Average	**1oz/28g**	**13**	**0**	**47**	**3.3**	**10.5**	**0.2**	**5.4**
Hearts, Canned, Drained, Average	**½ Can/117g**	**35**	**0.1**	**30**	**1.9**	**5.4**	**0**	**2.2**
Hearts, Marinated & Grilled, Waitrose*	1 Serving/50g	57	5	114	3	3	10	3
Hearts, Sliced with Extra Virgin Olive Oil, Waitrose*	1 Serving/40g	24	1.6	59	1.3	4.4	4	7
in Oil, Tesco*	1 Piece/15g	17	1.5	115	1.9	2.4	10	4
Marinated, Roasted, M&S*	1 Pack/200g	300	26.6	150	1.9	5	13.3	2.3
ASPARAGUS								
& Green Vegetables (Steamer Pouch), Waitrose*	½ Pack/125g	28	0.6	22	2.1	2.3	0.5	2.1
Boiled, in Salted Water, Average	**5 Spears/125g**	**16**	**0.5**	**12**	**1.6**	**0.7**	**0.4**	**0.7**
British with Butter, Tesco*	1 Serving/50g	26	2	52	2.6	1.6	4	2
Canned, Average	**1 Can/250g**	**41**	**0.4**	**16**	**2**	**1.8**	**0.2**	**1.4**
Trimmed, Raw, Average	**1 Serving/80g**	**20**	**0.4**	**24**	**2.9**	**1.9**	**0.6**	**1.7**
AUBERGINE								
Baby, Tesco*	1 Aubergine/50g	8	0.2	15	0.9	2.2	0.4	2.3

	Measure INFO/WEIGHT	per Measure KCAL	FAT	Nutrition Values per 100g / 100ml KCAL	PROT	CARB	FAT	FIBRE
AUBERGINE								
Baked Topped, M&S*	1 Serving/150g	165	11.6	110	2.4	7.4	7.7	0.9
Fried, Average	*1oz/28g*	*85*	*8.9*	*302*	*1.2*	*2.8*	*31.9*	*2.3*
Marinated & Grilled, Waitrose*	½ Pack/100g	106	10	106	1	3	10	2
Parmigiana, M&S*	1 Pack/350g	332	18.6	95	4.6	7.6	5.3	1.1
Raw, Fresh, Average	*1 Sm/250g*	*36*	*1*	*14*	*0.9*	*2.1*	*0.4*	*1.9*
Sliced, Chargrilled, Frozen, Oven Cooked, Tesco*	¼ Pack/78g	35	0.2	46	1.6	6.8	0.3	4.6
AVOCADO								
Flesh Only, Average	*1 Med/145g*	*276*	*28.3*	*190*	*1.9*	*1.9*	*19.5*	*3.4*
Smashed, Pure, Holy Moly*	¼ Pot/40g	64	6.4	160	2	9	16	7

	Measure INFO/WEIGHT	per Measure KCAL	FAT	Nutrition Values per 100g / 100ml KCAL	PROT	CARB	FAT	FIBRE
BACARDI*								
Diet Cola, Bacardi*	1 Bottle/275ml	85	0	31	0	1	0	0
37.5% Volume, Bacardi*	1 Pub Shot/35ml	72	0	207	0	0	0	0
40% Volume, Bacardi*	1 Pub Shot/35ml	78	0	222	0	0	0	0
Breezer, Apple, Half Sugar, Crisp, Bacardi*	1 Bottle/275ml	121	0	44	0	3.7	0	0
Breezer, Cranberry, Bacardi*	1 Bottle/275ml	154	0	56	0	7.1	0	0
Breezer, Lime, Bacardi*	1 Bottle/275ml	182	0	66	0	9.1	0	0
Breezer, Orange, Bacardi*	1 Bottle/275ml	179	0	65	0	8.2	0	0
Breezer, Raspberry, Half Sugar, Refreshing, Bacardi*	1 Bottle/275ml	99	0	36	0	3.3	0	0
Breezer, Watermelon, Bacardi*	1 Bottle/275ml	100	0	36	0	3.2	0	0
BACON								
Back, Dry Cured, Average	1 Rasher/31g	77	4.7	250	28.1	0.3	15.1	0.3
Back, Dry Fried or Grilled, Average	1 Rasher/25g	72	5.4	287	23.2	0	21.6	0
Back, Lean, Average	1 Rasher/33g	57	4	174	16.3	0.1	12	0.5
Back, Smoked, Average	1 Rasher/25g	66	5	265	20.9	0	19.9	0
Back, Smoked, Lean, Average	1 Rasher/25g	41	1.2	163	28.2	1.1	5	0.2
Back, Smoked, Rindless, Average	1 Rasher/25g	60	4.3	241	21	0.1	17.4	0
Back, Tendersweet, Average	1 Rasher/25g	63	3.6	250	29.8	0.4	14.4	0
Back, Unsmoked, Average	1 Rasher/32g	78	5.5	242	21.3	0.4	17.3	0
Back, Unsmoked, Rindless, Average	1 Rasher/23g	56	3.9	241	22.5	0	16.9	0
Bits, Average	1oz/28g	75	5.9	268	18.6	0.7	21.2	0.1
Chops, Average	1oz/28g	62	4.2	222	22.3	0	14.8	0
Collar Joint, Lean & Fat, Boiled	1oz/28g	91	7.6	325	20.4	0	27	0
Collar Joint, Lean & Fat, Raw	1oz/28g	81	7.4	290	13.3	0	26.3	0
Collar Joint, Lean Only, Boiled	1oz/28g	53	2.7	191	26	0	9.7	0
Fat Only, Cooked, Average	1oz/28g	194	20.4	692	9.3	0	72.8	0
Fat Only, Raw, Average	1oz/28g	209	22.7	747	4.8	0	80.9	0
Gammon Rasher, Lean Only, Grilled	1oz/28g	48	1.5	172	31.4	0	5.2	0
Lardons, Dry Cure, Finest, Tesco*	¼ Pack/45g	113	8.5	251	18.7	1.6	18.8	0.6
Lean Only, Fried, Average	1 Rasher/25g	83	5.6	332	32.8	0	22.3	0
Lean Only, Grilled, Average	1 Rasher/25g	73	4.7	292	30.5	0	18.9	0
Lean, Average	1 Rasher/33g	47	2.2	142	19.6	0.9	6.7	0.2
Loin Steaks, Grilled, Average	1 Serving/120g	229	11.6	191	25.9	0	9.7	0
Medallions, Average	1 Rasher/18g	27	0.6	151	29.4	0.9	3.3	0.1
Middle, Fried	1 Rasher/40g	140	11.4	350	23.4	0	28.5	0
Middle, Grilled	1 Rasher/40g	123	9.2	307	24.8	0	23.1	0
Middle, Raw	1 Rasher/43g	95	7.9	222	14	0	18.4	0
Rashers, Lean Only, Trimmed, Average	1 Rasher/20g	24	0.8	119	20.6	0	4	0
Rindless, Average	1 Rasher/20g	30	1.7	150	18.5	0	8.5	0
Smoked, Average	1 Rasher/28g	46	2.1	166	24.8	0.2	7.4	0
Smoked, Crispy, Cooked, Average	1 Serving/10g	46	2.7	460	53	2.1	26.9	0
Smoked, Diced, Frozen, Tesco*	1 Serving/50g	109	8	218	17	1.5	16	0
Smoked, Rindless, Average	1 Rasher/20g	21	0.6	106	19.8	0	3	0
Streaky, Cooked, Average	1 Rasher/20g	68	5.6	342	22.4	0.3	27.8	0
Vegetarian, Deli Style, Rashers, Quorn*	1 Rasher/15g	30	2.3	199	11.8	3	15.5	5
Vegetarian, Pieces, Bacon Style, Quorn*	1 Pack/100g	103	2.5	103	15	5	2.5	5
Vegetarian, Rashers	1 Rasher/16g	33	1.7	206	19.5	8.6	10.4	2.8
Vegetarian, Rashers, Cheatin', The Redwood Co*	1 Rasher/16g	32	1.2	196	25.9	7.3	7.3	0.5
Vegetarian, Rashers, Tesco*	1 Rasher/20g	41	2.2	203	22.5	3.3	11.1	3.9
Vegetarian, Smoky, Rashers, Sainsbury's*	2 Rashers/28g	87	6	309	24.6	2.2	21.6	3.3
Vegetarian, Streaky Style, Rashers, Tesco*	1 Rasher/8g	17	0.8	215	23.7	5	10.6	2.2
Vegetarian, Strips, Morningstar Farms*	1 Strip/8g	30	2.3	375	12.5	12.5	28.1	6.2
BAGUETTE								
Beef, Horseradish, Freshly Prepared, M&S*	1 Baguette/274g	795	31	290	12.1	37.2	11.3	2

B

B

	Measure INFO/WEIGHT	KCAL	FAT	KCAL	PROT	CARB	FAT	FIBRE
BAGUETTE								
Brie, Tomato, Rocket, Freshly Prepared, M&S*	1 Baguette/219g	570	21.7	260	10.3	33.2	9.9	1.9
Cheese, & Pickle, Fullfillers*	1 Baguette/280g	767	31.1	274	11.9	35.5	11.1	0
Cheese, Ham, Average	*1 Baguette/203g*	*593*	*20.8*	*292*	*14*	*35.9*	*10.3*	*1.4*
Cheese, Onion, Asda*	¼ Loaf/42g	154	7.4	366	12	39.8	17.6	1.3
Cheese, Tomato, Tesco*	1 Baguette/108g	243	8.3	225	9.7	29.3	7.7	1.8
Cheese, Mixed, & Spring Onion, Asda*	1 Pack/190g	629	34.8	331	9.5	32.1	18.3	1.3
Chicken, & Salad, Boots*	1 Baguette/132g	202	2.4	153	11	23	1.8	2
Chicken, & Stuffing, Hot, Sainsbury's*	1 Baguette/227g	543	16.3	239	13.7	29.6	7.2	0
Chicken, Salad, Asda*	1 Serving/158g	326	9.5	206	9	29	6	2.1
Chicken, Salad, Shapers, Boots*	1 Baguette/132g	222	2.6	168	11	27	2	1.5
Chicken, Tikka, Asda*	1 Pack/190g	439	17.9	231	10.4	32.8	9.4	1.3
Egg, Bacon, Tomato, Freshly Prepared, M&S*	1 Baguette/182g	455	17.3	250	12.9	28	9.5	1.7
Ham, & Turkey, Asda*	1 Baguette/360g	774	18.4	215	11.6	30.7	5.1	1.3
Ham, Cheese, Freshly Prepared, M&S*	1 Baguette/231g	555	11.3	240	13.4	35.9	4.9	2.4
Ham, Salad, with Mustard Mayonnaise, Sainsbury's*	1 Baguette/100g	412	15.9	412	17.6	49.6	15.9	0.1
Mozzarella, Tomato, & Pesto, Darwins Deli*	1 Serving/210g	531	20.4	253	11.7	29.7	9.7	0
Prawn Mayonnaise, Asda*	1 Pack/190g	399	9.3	210	9.1	32.5	4.9	1.3
Salmon, Smoked, Egg, Freshly Prepared	*1 Baguette/178g*	*455*	*17.3*	*255*	*13.7*	*28.4*	*9.7*	*1.6*
Steak, & Onion, Snack 'n' Go, Sainsbury's*	1 Baguette/177g	398	8.8	225	14.3	30.6	5	2.2
Tuna, Melt, Sainsbury's*	1 Serving/204g	373	8	183	11.3	25.8	3.9	0
BAILEYS*								
Almande, Dairy Free, Baileys*	1 Serving/25ml	10	0.2	38	0.6	3.1	0.8	0
Glide, Baileys*	1 Serving/200ml	212	2.4	106	0	18	1.2	0
Irish Cream, Original, Baileys*	1 Serving/50ml	164	6.5	327	3	25	13	0
BAKE								
Aubergine, Grain, Moroccan Inspired, Waitrose*	½ Pack/189g	151	8.3	80	1.3	6.9	4.4	3.7
Aubergine, Tomato, Mozzarella, Vegetarian, Tesco*	1 Pack/380g	257	10.5	71	3.6	5.9	2.9	3.2
Bean, Mexican, Georgia's Choice*	1 Bake/115g	266	12.9	231	4.3	28.9	11.2	3.8
Broccoli, & Cheese, Asda*	1 Bake/132g	269	15.4	204	5.3	19.3	11.7	2.5
Broccoli, & Cheese, M&S*	1 Pack/400g	480	31.2	120	6.5	5.4	7.8	1.6
Butternut Squash, & Mushroom, Roasted, BFY, M&S*	1 Pack/390g	339	10.5	87	6.1	8.4	2.7	2.1
Butternut Squash, Red Onion, Kale, Tesco*	½ Pack/121g	63	1.8	52	0.9	7.8	1.5	1.7
Cheese, Onion, Tesco*	1 Bake/110g	332	17	302	7.8	31.8	15.5	2.3
Chicken, & Mushroom, COU, M&S*	1 Serving/360g	324	8.3	90	7.3	10.3	2.3	1.1
Chicken, BBQ, Tesco*	1 Bake/131g	348	16	266	9.1	29.2	12.2	1.4
Chicken, Creamy, Puff Pastry, Sainsbury's*	1 Bake/126g	353	18.8	280	9.4	26.3	14.9	1.5
Cod, & Prawn, COU, M&S*	1 Pack/400g	320	8	80	6.5	8.8	2	1
Courgette, & Butternut Squash, Meat Free, Tesco*	1 Pack/375g	367	13.7	98	2.5	12.8	3.6	1.8
Courgette, & Tomato, Cauldron Foods*	1 Pack/285g	593	37	208	10	17	13	6.4
Fish, Three, Roast, Deluxe, Lidl*	1 Portion/300g	498	29.7	166	12.6	6.2	9.9	0.6
Haddock, Average	*1 Serving/400g*	*312*	*9.2*	*78*	*6.4*	*8*	*2.3*	*0.9*
Lentil, Spiced, Vegetarian, TTD, Sainsbury's*	1 Bake/132g	245	8.4	186	4.8	27.3	6.4	4.2
Mushroom, Leek, & Cheddar, CBY, Asda*	½ Pack/199g	181	8.8	91	3.7	8.1	4.4	1.9
Onion, & Potato, Roast, COU, M&S*	1 Pack/450g	338	5.8	75	1.9	13.6	1.3	1.5
Parsnip, & Mulled Red Onion Roast, Festive, M&S*	½ Pack/200g	256	9.4	128	2.9	16.9	4.7	3.3
Potato, & Vegetable, Co-Op*	1 Bake/340g	425	27.2	125	4	11	8	1
Potato, Cheese, & Leek, Aunt Bessie's*	½ Pack/275g	300	13.8	109	3.4	12.7	5	2.7
Potato, Cheese, & Onion, Roast, Asda*	½ Pack/200g	288	16	144	4.2	14	8	1.1
Potato, Cheese, & Onion, Tesco*	1 Pack/400g	376	19.6	94	2.4	10	4.9	1
Spinach, & Ricotta, As Consumed, M Kitchen, Morrisons*	1 Bake/128g	282	16	220	6.9	18.3	12.5	3.5
Steak, Puff Pastry, Sainsbury's*	1 Bake/126g	310	14.5	246	9.9	24.9	11.5	1.7
Vegetable, Mediterranean, Cooked, CBY, Asda*	1 Bake/120g	279	13.2	232	8.4	22.8	11	4.2
Vegetable, Tandoori, Cooked, Tesco*	¼ Pack/95g	70	2.6	74	2	8.7	2.8	3

	Measure INFO/WEIGHT	per Measure KCAL	FAT	Nutrition Values per 100g / 100ml KCAL	PROT	CARB	FAT	FIBRE
BAKING POWDER								
Average	**1 Tsp/2g**	**3**	**0**	**163**	**5.2**	**37.8**	**0**	**0**
BAKLAVA								
Average	**2 Pieces/50g**	**239**	**14.2**	**478**	**8**	**47.4**	**28.4**	**2.8**
BALTI								
Chick Pea & Spinach, Cauldron Foods*	1 Pack/400g	356	8	89	2.3	15.5	2	1
Chicken, & Mushroom, Tesco*	1 Serving/350g	326	10.5	93	12.3	4.2	3	0.7
Chicken, Asda*	1 Pack/400g	400	19.6	100	11	2.5	4.9	1.7
Chicken, M&S*	½ Pack/175g	245	15.2	140	13	2	8.7	1.7
Chicken, Morrisons*	1 Pack/350g	441	26.6	126	12.1	2.3	7.6	1.5
Chicken, Style, & Rice, Microwaved, Asda*	1 Pack/400g	498	19.9	125	3.8	15	5	2.3
Chicken, Tikka, Takeaway, Takeaway, Tesco*	1 Pack/385g	316	13.1	82	7.8	4.1	3.4	1.9
Chicken, with Pilau Rice, Asda*	1 Pack/504g	625	24.7	124	5	15	4.9	1.2
Chicken, with Pilau Rice, Weight Watchers*	1 Pack/329g	306	4.3	93	6.9	13.4	1.3	1.2
Lamb, Bhuna, Tesco*	1 Pack/400g	360	14.8	90	9.2	4.8	3.7	1.1
Prawn, Budgens*	1 Pack/350g	374	24.8	107	5.6	5.2	7.1	1.3
Vegetable, & Rice, Tesco*	1 Pack/450g	378	7.2	84	2	15.6	1.6	1.3
Vegetable, Asda*	½ Can/200g	206	12	103	2.2	10	6	2.5
Vegetable, Average	**1 Serving/200g**	**182**	**8.3**	**91**	**1.9**	**11.3**	**4.1**	**1.7**
Vegetable, CBY, Asda*	1 Pack/200g	190	11.6	95	2	7.7	5.8	2
Vegetable, GFY, Asda*	1 Pack/450g	324	4	72	1.9	14	0.9	1.5
BAMBOO SHOOTS								
Canned, Average	**1 Sm Can/120g**	**10**	**0.1**	**8**	**1**	**0.8**	**0.1**	**0.8**
in Water, Canned, Drained, M&S*	½ Can/60g	11	0.2	18	1.3	1.8	0.3	1.5
BANANA								
Chips, Average	**1oz/28g**	**143**	**8.8**	**511**	**1**	**59.9**	**31.4**	**1.7**
Green, Medium, Average	**1 Sm/101g**	**91**	**0**	**90**	**1**	**23**	**0**	**3**
Raw, Flesh Only, Average	**1 Med/118g**	**105**	**0.4**	**89**	**1.1**	**22.8**	**0.3**	**2.6**
Slices, Dried, Love Life, Waitrose*	1 Serving/25g	74	0.2	295	4.8	66.5	0.6	5.2
BARLEY								
Pot, Raw, Average	**1 Serving/60g**	**212**	**1.4**	**354**	**12.5**	**73.5**	**2.3**	**17.3**
Quick Cook, Wholefoods, Tesco*	1 Portion/83g	291	1.2	351	8	70.7	1.4	11.6
BARS								
All Bran, Apple, Kellogg's*	1 Bar/40g	158	7.6	395	8	48	19	5
All Bran, Honey Oat, Kellogg's*	1 Bar/27g	99	2.2	366	6	67	8	12
All Fruit, Frusli, Passion Fruit, Jordans*	1 Bar/30g	92	0.2	307	1.3	74	0.7	5
All Fruit, Frusli, Strawberry, Jordans*	1 Bar/30g	94	0.1	313	2.3	81.3	0.3	5
Almond, & Apricot, Weight Watchers*	1 Bar/34g	151	6.6	443	8.6	55.9	19.4	5.2
Almond, & Cranberry, Day Break, Atkins*	1 Bar/37g	137	5.9	371	37	23	16	15
Almond, Vanilla, Healthspan*	1 Bar/75g	301	10.5	401	10	52	14	0
Almond, Apricot, & Mango, M&S*	1 Bar/50g	205	7.4	410	9	60.2	14.8	5
Almond, Apricot, Yoghurt, Treat, M&S*	1 Bar/45g	195	9	433	6.2	55.2	19.9	4.2
Almond, Cashew Peanut, Eat Real*	1 Bar/40g	191	11.1	478	13.8	41.2	27.7	9.7
Almond, Crunch, Sweet & Salty, Advantage, Atkins*	1 Bar/40g	200	15	500	17.5	35	37.5	12.5
Almond, Kale, Protein, Ball, Bounce*	1 Ball/40g	176	8.4	440	22.5	43	21	0
Almond, Madagascan Vanilla, Kind*	1 Bar/40g	203	15.6	507	16	36	39	14
Almond, Marzipan, Dark & Milk Chocolate, M&S*	1 Bar/36g	171	8.4	474	6.9	57.4	23.2	4
Almond, Spirulina, Protein, Ball, Bounce*	1 Ball/40g	70	3.5	176	9	16.8	8.8	0
Almond, Sweet & Nutty, Nature Valley*	1 Bar/30g	143	6.9	475	10	54.3	23	5.4
Apollo, Morrisons*	1 Bar/38g	172	6.9	451	3.6	68.1	18	1.2
Apple, & Banana, Raw Fruit, The Foodie Market, Aldi*	1 Bar/30g	92	0.2	305	3	67	0.5	11
Apple, & Blackberry, Fruit Bake, McVitie's*	1 Bar/35g	124	2.5	354	2.7	73.8	7.2	1.2
Apple, & Blackberry, Fruit Bakes, Go Ahead, McVitie's*	1 Bar/35g	131	3	374	3.5	71.8	8.5	3.9
Apple, & Cinnamon, Breakfast Snack, Tesco*	1 Bar/38g	137	4.7	365	4.3	58.8	12.5	2

B

B

BARS

INFO/WEIGHT	Measure	per Measure		Nutrition Values per 100g / 100ml				
		KCAL	FAT	KCAL	PROT	CARB	FAT	FIBRE
Apple, & Raisin, Dorset Cereals*	1 Bar/30g	109	1.1	363	4	78.3	3.7	5.3
Apple, & Raisin, Harvest Cheweee, Quaker*	1 Bar/22g	89	2.6	405	5.5	68	12	3
Apple, & Raisin, Snack, Geobar, Traidcraft*	1 Bar/35g	127	1.7	362	3.3	76.4	4.8	2.3
Apple, & Raspberry, Chewy & Crisp, Tesco*	1 Bar/27g	123	5.3	456	3.4	66.8	19.5	2.8
Apple, & Sultana, Multigrain, Jordans*	1 Bar/40g	141	2.5	353	4.4	70	6.2	4.8
Apple, & Walnut, Food Bar, The Food Doctor*	1 Bar/35g	129	4.9	367	8.4	37.3	14	29.1
Apple, Sultana, Tesco*	1 Bar/30g	90	0.2	301	3	63.8	0.5	14.4
Apple, Fruit Bake, Go Ahead, McVitie's*	1 Bar/35g	124	2.5	354	2.7	73.8	7.2	1.2
Apple, Granola, McVitie's*	1 Bar/35g	128	3.4	366	6.6	63.1	9.7	4.3
Apple, Peanut, Almond, Goodness Knows*	1 Bar/34g	157	6.8	462	7.7	59.6	20	4.6
Apple, Pie, Baked, Weight Watchers*	1 Bar/27g	76	0.4	283	4.4	55.7	1.5	14.7
Apple, School, Fruit Bowl*	1 Bar/20g	67	0.7	337	1	72	3.6	7.1
Apricot, & Almond, Eat Natural*	1 Bar/50g	202	8.1	403	11.2	53.3	16.1	0
Apricot, & Almond, Truly Juicy, Raw Health*	1 Bar/45g	182	10.4	405	17	49	23	9
Apricot, & Almond, Yoghurt Coated, Eat Natural*	1 Bar/50g	233	13.1	476	6.6	49.7	26.7	5
Apricot, & Peach, Multigrain, BGTY, Sainsbury's*	1 Bar/25g	70	0.6	282	6.6	58.2	2.5	23.1
Apricot, Almond, Coconut, Harvest, Atkins*	1 Bar/40g	182	12.4	455	15	18.5	31	25
Apricot, Dried Fruit, Sunsweet*	1 Bar/33g	96	0	292	3.6	72.5	0.1	0
Apricot, Orange, Ginger, Juicy, Get Fruity*	1 Bar/35g	131	4.6	375	6.6	54	13	6.8
Banana, Mango Brazil, Cereal, Dove's Farm*	1 Bar/40g	196	4.6	490	6.5	63.3	11.5	5.3
Banana, Nut, Health Warrior*	1 Bar/25g	100	5	400	12	56	20	16
Beetroot, Cacao, Goodness, The Food Doctor*	1 Bar/40g	140	4.4	349	10	39	11	25
Beetroot, Walnut, Goodness, The Food Doctor*	1 Bar/40g	118	2.8	295	5.1	33.2	6.9	39.6
Berry, & Seed Oaty, Weight Watchers*	1 Bar/26g	87	2	333	10	46.8	7.5	19.3
Berry, Delight, GF, Nak'd*	1 Bar/35g	135	5.2	385	9	52	15	6
Berry, Mixed, Moist, Get Fruity*	1 Bar/35g	140	4.6	399	6	61	13	6.3
Berry, Mixed, Trek, Natural Balance Foods*	1 Bar/68g	204	1.5	300	15.6	56.5	2.2	6
Berry, Nut Free, Get Buzzing*	1 Bar/62g	173	8.7	279	3.2	50	14	2.9
Berry, Snack, Diet Chef Ltd*	1 Bar/27g	96	2.2	356	7.2	64	8.2	5.5
Biscuit, & Choco, Milk, Choceur, Aldi*	1 Bar/33g	174	9.6	526	7.9	59	29	1.3
Biscuit, & Choco, Orange, Choceur, Aldi*	1 Bar/33g	176	9.9	533	7.6	59	30	1.1
Biscuit, & Raisin, Reduced Fat, Tesco*	1 Bar/22g	90	2.8	410	4.9	69.5	12.5	1.8
Biscuit, Chocolate, Chunky, Belmont Biscuit Co, Aldi*	1 Bar/24g	126	6.7	526	6.6	61	28	1.8
Biscuit, Chocolate, Mint, Penguin, McVitie's*	1 Bar/25g	133	6.9	531	5.4	65	27.7	1.5
Biscuit, Chocolate, Orange, Penguin, McVitie's*	1 Bar/25g	133	6.9	531	5.4	65	27.7	1.5
Biscuit, Chocolate, Original, Penguin, McVitie's*	1 Bar/20g	106	5.6	515	5.1	61.4	27.1	2.4
Biscuit, Groovy, Aldi*	1 Bar/27g	123	5.3	457	4.9	64.2	19.7	1.8
Biscuit, Raisin Chocolate Hobnobs, Snack, McVitie's*	1 Bar/32g	132	3.9	420	5.5	71.1	12.5	3.6
Blue Riband, Double Choc, Nestle*	1 Bar/22g	113	5.6	513	4.8	66.4	25.3	1.1
Blueberry, & Almond, Goodness Knows*	1 Bar/34g	154	6.7	452	7.7	57	19.8	5.4
Blueberry, & Yoghurt Nougat, Shapers, Boots*	1 Bar/23g	85	3	369	1.8	76	13	1.7
Blueberry, Beond Organic, GF, Pulsin*	1 Bar/35g	166	6.7	475	8.7	46.8	19.2	4.9
Blueberry, Chocolate, Lean Protein, Nutramino*	1 Bar/60g	209	7.8	349	33	17	13	24
Blueberry, Fruit & Grain, Asda*	1 Bar/37g	124	2.6	335	4.1	64	7	3.9
Blueberry, Muffin, Fibre, Asda*	1 Bar/24g	86	2.3	359	3.6	54	9.5	22
Blueberry, Weight Watchers*	1 Bar/25g	91	1.8	365	4.5	74.9	7.4	2.2
Blueberry, Yoghurt & Honey, Altu*	1 Bar/40g	129	4.7	323	12.9	45.5	11.7	12
Brazil, Goji Chia, Protein Snack, High Five*	1 Bar/60g	292	16.2	487	20	37	27	8.1
Brazil, Sultanas, Almonds Hazelnuts, Eat Natural*	1 Bar/50g	227	11.3	454	11.2	40	22.6	5
Breakfast, Apple Crisp, Morning Start, Atkins*	1 Bar/37g	145	7.9	392	29.2	25.4	21.4	13.8
Breakfast, Blueberry, Free From, Sainsbury's*	1 Bar/35g	163	7.8	467	3.8	62.6	22.4	0.2
Breakfast, Cherry, Oats More, Nestle*	1 Bar/30g	109	2	363	6	70.2	6.5	3.6
Breakfast, Chocolate Chip, Crisp, Morning Start, Atkins*	1 Bar/37g	137	7	370	31.8	22.5	18.8	15

BARS

	Measure INFO/WEIGHT	per Measure KCAL	per Measure FAT	Nutrition Values per 100g / 100ml KCAL	PROT	CARB	FAT	FIBRE
Breakfast, Vitality, Fruit & Fibre, Asda*	1 Bar/29g	113	2.9	390	6	69	10	4.1
Breakfast, with Cranberries, Asda*	1 Bar/28g	105	1.4	376	6	77	4.9	3
Brownie, Chocolate, Fibre, Asda*	1 Bar/24g	89	2.9	369	5	49	12	23
Cacao, Almond, Energy Ball, Deliciously Ella*	1 Ball/40g	173	11.1	433	12.5	35.3	27.8	7.2
Cacao, Beond Organic, Pulsin*	1 Bar/35g	146	6.3	416	10.6	50.8	17.9	4.4
Cacao, Crunch, Natural Energy, Power Bar*	1 Bar/40g	156	3.8	391	8.3	65.5	9.4	5.7
Cacao, Mint, Protein, Organic, BodyMe*	1 Bar/60g	252	11.1	420	27	33.7	18.5	0
Cacao, Orange, Protein, Organic, BodyMe*	1 Bar/60g	251	11.1	419	26.8	34.4	18.5	5.4
Cacao, Raw Fruit & Nut, Wild Trail*	1 Bar/30g	115	3.3	383	8.6	56	11	11
Cappuccino, Intense, White, Dark, Milk Chocolate, M&S*	1 Bar/34g	211	16.3	620	5.2	40.7	47.8	3.1
Caramel, Crazy, Tesco*	1 Bar/40g	192	9.2	480	3.9	64	23	1
Caramel, Crisp, Go Ahead, McVitie's*	1 Bar/33g	141	4	428	4.8	75.1	12	0.8
Caramel, Crunch, Go Ahead, McVitie's*	1 Bar/24g	106	3.3	440	4.7	76.6	13.8	0.8
Caramel, Crunchy, Tesco*	1 Bar/21g	98	5.2	467	4.6	56	25	1.4
Caramel, Nougat, Soft, Shapers, Boots*	1 Bar/25g	86	2.5	343	2.9	60.4	10	0.6
Caramel, Nut Chew, Endulge, Atkins*	1 Bar/34g	130	2.7	382	5	5.9	8	6
Caramel, Salted, Protein, Ball, Bounce*	1 Ball/40g	170	7	425	1	30	17.5	25
Caramel, Salted, Protein, Diet Whey, PhD Nutrition*	1 Bar/60g	199	4.8	332	35	35	8	0
Caramel, Salted, Square, Fibre One*	1 Bar/24g	87	2.8	362	4	49.5	11.7	21.2
Caramel, Skinny Whip*	1 Bar/25g	96	2.3	384	3.6	64	9.2	15.2
Carrot, Cake, Fibre One*	1 Bar/25g	90	3.4	361	4.2	44	13.4	23.9
Cashew, & Cranberry, Eat Real*	1 Bar/40g	173	8.4	432	5.6	52.4	21	7.3
Cashew, Cookie, Raw Fruit & Nut, GF, Nak'd*	1 Bar/35g	143	8	410	10	46	23	5
Cashew, Crush, The Foodie Market, Aldi*	1 Bar/35g	158	8	451	12	46	23	7.6
Cashew, Sultana Pumpkin Seed, Eat Real*	1 Bar/40g	165	5.9	413	8.5	59.5	14.8	10.5
Cereal, & Apricot, Goodies, Organic, Organix*	1 Bar/30g	122	6.1	408	7.2	55.3	20.4	6.2
Cereal, & Milk, Nesquik, Nestle*	1 Bar/25g	108	3.7	433	6.2	68.5	14.9	1
Cereal, 3 Berries Cherries, Dorset Cereals*	1 Bar/35g	127	1.7	363	5.7	73.9	4.9	5.2
Cereal, 3 Fruit, Nuts Seeds, Dorset Cereals*	1 Bar/35g	136	3.6	389	7.4	66.6	10.3	6.2
Cereal, Apple & Raspberry, Chewy & Crisp, Tesco*	1 Bar/27g	123	5.3	456	3.3	66.7	19.6	3
Cereal, Apple Blackberry with Yoghurt, Alpen*	1 Bar/29g	117	3.1	404	5.4	71.8	10.6	5
Cereal, Apple Cinnamon, Boka*	1 Bar/30g	88	0.8	293	5.7	58	2.5	19
Cereal, Apple Cinnamon, Fruit 'n' Grain, Asda*	1 Bar/37g	131	2.6	353	4.5	68	7	2.9
Cereal, Apple Cinnamon, M&S*	1 Bar/24g	84	1.2	350	3.9	68.4	5.2	6.6
Cereal, Apple Cinnamon, Tesco*	1 Bar/38g	137	4.7	365	4.3	58.9	12.5	2.1
Cereal, Apple Raisin, Harvest, Quaker*	1 Bar/22g	87	2.5	396	5	70	11.5	4
Cereal, Apple Sultana, Light, Alpen*	1 Bar/20g	63	0.7	330	4.1	59.4	3.6	21.7
Cereal, Apple, Chewy, BGTY, Sainsbury's*	1 Bar/25g	85	0.5	340	4.8	76	2	2
Cereal, Apricot Yoghurt, COU, M&S*	1 Bar/21g	75	0.5	360	5.3	79.6	2.4	3.8
Cereal, Apricot, Almond, Yoghurt, Tesco*	1 Bar/35g	156	6.8	447	5.9	59.7	19.4	4.9
Cereal, Balance with Fruit, Sainsbury's*	1 Bar/25g	100	2.2	401	5.8	75.2	8.6	1.9
Cereal, Banana, Apricot, & Milk Chocolate, Eat Natural*	1 Bar/30g	108	2	362	3.7	71.8	6.7	4
Cereal, Banana, Value, Tesco*	1 Bar/21g	80	1.6	387	6	73.9	7.5	3.7
Cereal, Banoffee, Light, Alpen, Weetabix*	1 Bar/19g	66	1.3	346	4.7	54	7	24
Cereal, Banoffee, Vitality, Asda*	1 Bar/22g	73	0.6	331	6.5	69.6	2.9	13.5
Cereal, Brownie, COU, M&S*	1 Bar/21g	75	0.5	365	5.5	79.7	2.6	4.6
Cereal, Cheerios Milk Bar, Nestle*	1 Bar/22g	92	3	416	7.6	66.1	13.5	2
Cereal, Cherry Bakewell, Light, Alpen*	1 Bar/19g	65	1.1	341	5.1	56	5.6	23
Cereal, Chewy & Crisp with Choc Chips, Tesco*	1 Bar/27g	125	6.3	463	9.2	54	23.4	3.8
Cereal, Chewy & Crisp with Roasted Nuts, Tesco*	1 Bar/27g	127	6.2	471	9.3	57	22.9	2.5
Cereal, Chewy Chocolate Fudge, NUME, Morrisons*	1 Bar/21g	74	1.4	353	4.7	56.8	6.8	23
Cereal, Chewy Pomegranate, Vitality, Asda*	1 Bar/22g	76	0.6	346	4.1	69.3	2.8	13.4
Cereal, Chewy, BGTY, Sainsbury's*	1 Bar/25g	85	0.5	342	4.9	75.8	2.1	1.9

BARS

INFO/WEIGHT	Measure per Measure KCAL	FAT	Nutrition Values per 100g / 100ml KCAL	PROT	CARB	FAT	FIBRE
Cereal, Choc Chip Nut, Chewy Crisp, Sainsbury's*	1 Bar/27g	129	7	476	8.8	51.8	26	4.4
Cereal, Choc Chip, Brunch, Cadbury*	1 Bar/32g	140	5.3	445	6.1	64.5	17	4.8
Cereal, Choco Mallow, Boka*	1 Bar/30g	93	0.9	309	5.8	53	2.9	24
Cereal, Chocolate & Orange, Officially Low Fat, Fox's*	1 Bar/19g	54	0.4	286	5	61.6	2.3	17.5
Cereal, Chocolate Banana, Lidl*	1 Bar/25g	110	4	440	6.4	67.2	16	0
Cereal, Chocolate Crispy Rice, Organic, Dove's Farm*	1 Bar/35g	147	5.3	421	4.4	66.9	15.1	3
Cereal, Chocolate Fudge, Light, Alpen*	1 Bar/21g	71	1.3	342	4.9	55	6.5	22
Cereal, Chocolate Orange, Light, Alpen*	1 Bar/21g	71	1.2	339	4.8	56	5.5	23.1
Cereal, Chocolate Orange, Tesco*	1 Bar/22g	78	1.3	355	4.5	70.2	6	10.3
Cereal, Chocolate Raisin, Seeds of Change*	1 Bar/29g	107	2.3	370	5	69.6	7.9	3.7
Cereal, Chocolate Chip, Special Flake, Tesco*	1 Bar/21g	85	1.6	405	6.9	75.8	7.8	2.3
Cereal, Chocolate Chip, Special K, Kellogg's*	1 Bar/21g	84	1.5	401	9	76	7	1.5
Cereal, Chocolate, Fudge, Asda*	1 Bar/19g	66	1.3	347	4.5	53	6.9	28
Cereal, Chocolate, Dark, Le Noir, Orco*	1 Bar/21g	95	3.3	451	7.3	69.9	15.8	0
Cereal, Chocolate, Dark, with Ginger, Weight Watchers*	1 Bar/22g	82	1.5	371	4.5	67.1	6.8	11.9
Cereal, Chocolate, Geobar, Traidcraft*	1 Bar/32g	130	2.7	407	4.3	78.5	8.4	0
Cereal, Chocolate, Light Crispy, Sainsbury's*	1 Bar/24g	88	1.5	369	6	64	6.5	15
Cereal, Chocolate, Milk, Apricot, Value, Tesco*	1 Bar/22g	90	2.8	425	6.2	69.5	13.1	3.5
Cereal, Chocolate, Milk, Double, Special K, Kellogg's*	1 Bar/20g	79	1.8	396	9	66	9	10
Cereal, Chocolate, Milk, Double, Special K, Kellogg's*	1 Bar/20g	80	2	400	10	65	10	10
Cereal, Chocolate, Milk, Oaty, Weetabix*	1 Bar/23g	80	1.5	342	6.9	51.7	6.5	24.3
Cereal, Chocolate, Mint, Kellogg's*	1 Bar/22g	88	2.2	401	4.5	74	10	3.5
Cereal, Chocolate, Oats More, Nestle*	1 Bar/30g	118	3.2	395	6.8	68.3	10.5	3.4
Cereal, Cinnamon Grahams, Nestle*	1 Bar/25g	106	3.7	426	7.2	66.2	14.7	1.9
Cereal, Citrus Fruits, Light, Alpen*	1 Bar/21g	59	0.9	283	5.6	55.9	4.1	22.4
Cereal, Coconut, Original Crunchy, Jordans*	1 Bar/30g	141	6.8	470	6.5	60	22.7	6.2
Cereal, Cranberry Blackcurrant, LC, Tesco*	1 Bar/25g	75	0.7	295	4.4	62.7	2.9	21.9
Cereal, Cranberry Orange, BGTY, Sainsbury's*	1 Bar/26g	93	1.3	358	2.7	75.8	4.9	2.3
Cereal, Cranberry Orange, Brunch, Cadbury*	1 Bar/35g	154	5.6	440	5.9	67.7	15.9	0
Cereal, Cranberry Orange, Weight Watchers*	1 Bar/28g	102	1.1	365	4.5	77.6	4.1	2.3
Cereal, Cranberry Strawberry, Weight Watchers*	1 Bar/22g	69	1.2	314	6.4	51.8	5.4	16.8
Cereal, Cranberry Yoghurt, Harvest Morn, Aldi*	1 Bar/29g	117	2.6	403	6.5	71.9	9	4.1
Cereal, Cranberry, Raisin Nut, Shapers, Boots*	1 Bar/35g	140	4.4	400	7.1	65.7	12.6	3.7
Cereal, Crunchy Granola, Apple Crunch, Nature Valley*	1 Bar/21g	92	3.2	440	7.3	69	15	5.7
Cereal, Crunchy Granola, Ginger Nut, Nature Valley*	1 Bar/42g	189	7.1	451	7.9	64.2	16.9	2.3
Cereal, Crunchy Granola, Peanut Butter, Nature Valley*	1 Bar/21g	95	4	452	9.5	64.3	19	4.8
Cereal, Dark Chocolate, Cranberries, Special K*	1 Bar/27g	100	2.5	372	5.9	68	9.1	10
Cereal, Date, Beloved*	1 Bar/35g	133	3.3	379	6.7	64.1	9.4	5.7
Cereal, Double Chocolate, Light, Alpen, Weetabix*	1 Bar/19g	65	1.2	344	5	56	6.2	22
Cereal, Fig Prune, Eurodiet*	1 Bar/50g	162	5.8	324	30	31.5	11.6	7.5
Cereal, Fruit Fibre, Asda*	1 Bar/29g	111	2.8	390	6	69	10	4.1
Cereal, Fruit Fibre, You Count, Love Life, Waitrose*	1 Bar/25g	88	0.2	351	6	76.5	0.9	6.3
Cereal, Fruit Nut Break, Jordans*	1 Bar/37g	138	3.8	374	7	63.2	10.4	8.1
Cereal, Fruit Nut, Alpen*	1 Bar/28g	109	2.3	390	5.8	73	8.3	2.9
Cereal, Fruit Nut, Everyday Value, Tesco*	1 Bar/21g	78	1.2	373	5.2	72	5.9	5.5
Cereal, Fruit Nut, with Milk Chocolate, Alpen*	1 Bar/29g	123	3.8	425	6.4	70.5	13	2.2
Cereal, Fruit, Average	*1 Bar/34g*	*130*	*3.9*	*382*	*5.9*	*64.7*	*11.5*	*6.5*
Cereal, Fruity, Go, Soreen*	1 Bar/40g	143	1.8	358	6.8	72.6	4.5	0
Cereal, Frusli, Blueberry, Jordans*	1 Bar/30g	113	2.1	375	5.2	70.2	7.1	4.9
Cereal, Frusli, Cranberry Apple, Jordans*	1 Bar/30g	113	2.1	376	5.1	75.6	7.1	5
Cereal, Frusli, Raisin Hazelnut, Jordans*	1 Bar/30g	117	3.7	390	5.8	64.3	12.2	4.5
Cereal, Frusli, Red Berries, Jordans*	1 Bar/30g	112	2.2	374	4.8	75.1	7.2	5.4
Cereal, Granola, Alpen*	1 Bar/29g	119	3.1	410	5.9	72.4	10.7	0

BARS

INFO/WEIGHT	Measure	per Measure KCAL	per Measure FAT	Nutrition Values per 100g / 100ml KCAL	PROT	CARB	FAT	FIBRE
Cereal, Hazelnut, Brunch, Cadbury*	1 Bar/35g	160	7.4	460	7	60.5	21.4	2.2
Cereal, Milk Chocolate Chip, Chewy, Harvest Morn, Aldi*	1 Bar/22g	95	3.1	432	5.6	68	14	4.2
Cereal, Mixed Berry, Go Ahead, McVitie's*	1 Bar/35g	134	2.2	383	4.6	77.1	6.3	3.1
Cereal, Muesli Break, Breakfast in a Bar, Jordans*	1 Bar/46g	178	5	387	5.9	66.6	10.8	4.3
Cereal, Muesli, Apple, No Added Sugar, Crownfield, Lidl*	1 Bar/25g	96	2.8	386	6.3	67.9	11.2	6.7
Cereal, Multigrain, Peach Apricot, BGTY, Sainsbury's*	1 Bar/28g	77	0.6	274	6.4	57	2.3	24.2
Cereal, Nut & Seed, Organic, Green & Black's*	1 Bar/50g	258	16.3	516	8.4	47.2	32.6	10
Cereal, Nuts, Honey, Waitrose*	1 Bar/30g	145	7.8	483	26.3	33	26	0
Cereal, Nutty, Free From, Sainsbury's*	1 Bar/25g	114	5	454	6.8	61.8	20	2.3
Cereal, Oat Raisin, Basics, Sainsbury's*	1 Bar/25g	98	2.2	391	5.1	72.8	8.8	3.8
Cereal, Oat Raisin, Soft Oaties, Nutri-Grain, Kellogg's*	1 Bar/40g	173	6.4	432	6	66	16	3.5
Cereal, Oats Berries, Crunchy More, Nature Valley*	1 Bar/21g	95	3.5	453	7.4	64.6	16.9	6.1
Cereal, Oaty, Strawberry, Weetabix*	1 Bar/23g	69	1.4	299	6.2	54.7	6.1	24.5
Cereal, Oaty, Toffee Dazzler, Weetabix*	1 Bar/23g	80	1.5	348	6.2	54.9	6.7	21.5
Cereal, Peanut Butter Oat, Organic, Meridian Foods*	1 Bar/50g	204	9.2	407	12.6	50.9	18.4	5
Cereal, Raisin & Apricot, Weight Watchers*	1 Bar/28g	100	1.3	358	6.8	72.2	4.6	3.2
Cereal, Raisin & Nut Snack Bar, Benecol*	1 Bar/25g	98	2.8	390	3.9	68.5	11.1	2
Cereal, Raisin Coconut, Value, Tesco*	1 Bar/21g	84	2.4	400	5.5	67.2	11.6	5
Cereal, Raisin, Raisin, Cadbury*	1 Bar/35g	150	5.4	430	5.6	66.4	15.5	1.8
Cereal, Special Flake with Cranberries, Tesco*	1 Bar/23g	90	1.4	390	4.9	78.9	5.9	1.8
Cereal, Strawberry with Yoghurt, Alpen*	1 Bar/29g	120	2.9	415	4.8	75	10	2.7
Cereal, Strawberry, BGTY, Sainsbury's*	1 Bar/26g	100	1.2	385	3.8	82	4.6	5.2
Cereal, Strawberry, Fitness, Nestle*	1 Bar/24g	89	1.6	378	4.9	73.8	7	4.1
Cereal, Strawberry, Fruit 'n' Grain, Asda*	1 Bar/37g	126	2.6	340	4.2	65	7	4.5
Cereal, Strawberry, Value, Tesco*	1 Bar/21g	80	1.1	382	5.5	77.8	5.4	3.3
Cereal, Summer Fruits, Light, Alpen*	1 Bar/21g	70	0.9	334	4.4	58.7	4.1	22.4
Cereal, Toffee, Basics, Sainsbury's*	1 Bar/23g	92	1.9	398	4.8	75.8	8.4	2.5
Cereal, Very Berry, Weight Watchers*	1 Bar/27g	92	2.7	340	6.6	42.6	9.9	26.8
Cereal, White Chocolate Strawberry, Value, Tesco*	1 Bar/21g	85	1.7	405	6.2	76.2	8.1	2.4
Cereal, White Chocolate, Oaty, Weetabix*	1 Bar/23g	78	1.4	341	6.4	52.4	6.3	24.3
Cereal, Wholegrain, Choc Chunk, Special K, Kellogg's*	1 Bar/20g	78	1.9	388	7	62	9.6	14
Cherries, Almonds, a Yoghurt Coating, Eat Natural*	1 Bar/45g	200	9.5	444	6.6	58.8	21.1	3.6
Cherry, Crunch, Protein Flapjack, Trek*	1 Bar/56g	242	11.1	432	18.3	46	19.9	3.1
Chia, Apple Cinnamon, Health Warrior*	1 Bar/25g	100	5	400	12	56	20	16
Chia, Chocolate Peanut Butter, Health Warrior*	1 Bar/25g	100	1	400	12	52	4	16
Chia, Coffee, Health Warrior*	1 Bar/25g	100	5	400	12	52	20	12
Chia, Dark Chocolate Cherry, Health Warrior*	1 Bar/25g	100	5	400	12	56	20	16
Chia, Mango, Health Warrior*	1 Bar/25g	100	5	400	12	56	20	16
Chia, Vanilla, Protein, Organic, BodyMe*	1 Bar/60g	247	10.7	412	27.3	32.5	17.8	0
Choc Chip, Harvest Cheweee, Quaker*	1 Bar/22g	95	3.5	430	5.5	68	16	3.5
Chocolate Chip, & Hazelnut, Milk, Snack, Benecol*	1 Bar/25g	99	3.3	395	4.7	64.5	13.1	2.5
Chocolate Chip, Granola, Advantage, Atkins*	1 Bar/48g	200	8	417	35.4	37.5	16.7	12.5
Chocolate Chip, Muesli, Diet Chef Ltd*	1 Bar/50g	191	6	382	5.8	59.8	11.9	6.1
Chocolate Chip, Snack, Diet Chef Ltd*	1 Bar/27g	99	2.7	367	5.8	63.6	9.9	4.5
Chocolate, & Caramel, Rice Krispies Squares, Kellogg's*	1 Bar/36g	155	5	430	4.5	71	14	2
Chocolate, & Mint Crunch, Dark, Weight Watchers*	1 Bar/23g	85	3	371	2.7	48.7	13.1	23.7
Chocolate, & Orange, Crispy, Shapers, Boots*	1 Bar/22g	94	2.6	425	3.6	77	12	0.8
Chocolate, & Toffee, Free From, Sainsbury's*	1 Bar/30g	139	5.4	465	4.8	71	18	0.8
Chocolate, Honey, Nutricious, Healthspan*	1 Bar/75g	193	10.5	257	10	52	14	0
Chocolate, Raspberry, COU, M&S*	1 Bar/25g	90	0.7	360	5.4	78.2	2.7	3.2
Chocolate, Almond Fudge, Energy, Clif*	1 Bar/68g	252	6	370	13	56	8.8	7.4
Chocolate, Biscuit, with Caramel, Aldi*	1 Bar/21g	104	5.1	497	5.2	63.4	24.5	0.9
Chocolate, Brownie, Average	**1 Bar/68g**	**240**	**4**	**353**	**14.7**	**60.3**	**5.9**	**8.8**

BARS

INFO/WEIGHT	Measure	per Measure		Nutrition Values per 100g / 100ml				
		KCAL	FAT	KCAL	PROT	CARB	FAT	FIBRE
Chocolate, Brownie, Big Softies, to Go, Fox's*	1 Bar/25g	87	0.7	348	5.5	74.9	2.9	0
Chocolate, Brownie, Double, Protein, PhD Nutrition*	1 Bar/60g	199	5.2	332	33.3	31.7	8.7	0
Chocolate, Brownie, Essential, Waitrose*	1 Bar/26g	108	4.7	415	5.1	55.7	18.1	4.3
Chocolate, Caramel Whip, Weight Watchers*	1 Bar/25g	88	2.7	353	2.7	72.4	10.8	1
Chocolate, Caramel, Biscuit, Asda*	1 Bar/30g	150	8.3	508	8	56	28	2.5
Chocolate, Caramel, HiLo, Healthspan*	1 Bar/60g	193	6	322	33.3	23.3	10	0
Chocolate, Caramel, Nut Roll, Advantage, Atkins*	1 Bar/44g	170	12	386	18.2	43.2	27.3	18.2
Chocolate, Caramel, Protein, Battle Bites*	1 Bar/62g	227	8.7	366	32.3	25	14	0
Chocolate, Caramel, Wacko, Belmont, Aldi*	1 Bar/21g	102	4.6	485	5.3	65	22	1.7
Chocolate, Caramel, Weight Watchers*	1 Bar/20g	80	2.5	400	5	70	12.5	0
Chocolate, Coated, Orange Flavour, Milk, Energy, Boots*	1 Bar/70g	274	7	391	5.2	70	10	2.8
Chocolate, Coconut, Protein, Battle Bites*	1 Bar/62g	236	10.5	381	23.3	23.1	16.9	0
Chocolate, Cookie Caramel, Light Bites, Lighter Life*	1 Bar/30g	99	4.7	332	11.1	22.3	15.8	37.4
Chocolate, Cookie, Triple, Protein, PhD Nutrition*	1 Bar/60g	199	5	332	33.3	33.3	8.3	0
Chocolate, Cranberry, Dark, Organic, Biona*	1 Bar/40g	162	5.9	405	6.2	53.5	14.7	0
Chocolate, Crisp, Weight Watchers*	1 Bar/25g	92	2.6	369	5.4	75.1	10.2	0.8
Chocolate, Crisp, Weight Watchers*	1 Bar/25g	94	2.6	378	4.8	66.8	10.2	1.6
Chocolate, Crispy Wafer, Dark, Tasty Little Numbers*	1 Bar/20g	100	5.1	499	6.4	60.4	25.6	7
Chocolate, Crispy Wafer, Milk, Tasty Little Numbers*	1 Bar/20g	100	5	499	6.1	61.4	25.1	3
Chocolate, Crispy, Free From, Tesco*	1 Bar/30g	132	4.6	440	4.1	71.2	15.4	0.5
Chocolate, Dark, Almond, Nupo*	1 Bar/29g	99	2.8	343	11.2	41	9.8	27
Chocolate, Dark, Mint, HiLo, Healthspan *	1 Bar/60g	190	5.8	317	34	23	9.7	16
Chocolate, Dark, Chewy Delight, Special K, Kellogg's*	1 Bar/24g	97	3.4	404	4.5	57	14	17
Chocolate, Dark, Intense, The Dark One, M&S*	1 Bar/32g	180	10.9	564	9.6	53.1	34.2	2.5
Chocolate, Dark, Mint, Hi-Fi, Slimming World*	1 Bar/20g	70	1.8	351	4	54	8.8	20
Chocolate, Dark, Mint, Slimming World*	1 Bar/20g	70	1.8	351	4	54	8.8	20
Chocolate, Dark, Nuts, Sea Salt, Kind*	1 Bar/40g	199	15.2	498	14	39	38	18
Chocolate, Decadence, Atkins*	1 Bar/60g	233	12	388	30	27.3	20	9.8
Chocolate, Decadence, High Fibre, Musclefood*	1 Bar/42g	157	4.9	372	35.7	325	11.6	7.6
Chocolate, Double, Breakfast Snack, Tesco*	1 Bar/37g	144	6.4	385	5.3	52.7	17	3.3
Chocolate, Double, Caramel, Crunch, Atkins*	1 Bar/44g	160	9	364	22.7	50	20.4	25
Chocolate, Double, Dark, Zone Perfect*	1 Bar/45g	190	5.5	422	24.5	44.9	12.2	2
Chocolate, Fruit & Nut, M&S*	1 Bar/50g	235	12	470	6.5	57.1	24.1	2.5
Chocolate, Hazelnut, Atkins*	1 Bar/60g	227	10.2	378	32	29.1	17	9.8
Chocolate, Hazelnut, Day Break, Atkins*	1 Bar/40g	180	14	450	15	45	35	17.5
Chocolate, Healthy Meal, Herbalife*	1 Bar/56g	207	5.9	370	23.9	37.5	10.6	14.5
Chocolate, Honeycomb, Bunnycomb, Mini Moos*	1 Bar/25g	143	9.4	571	2.7	59.5	37.6	0
Chocolate, Juice Plus*	1 Bar/55g	210	6.4	382	24.8	39.4	11.6	10.2
Chocolate, Meal Replacement, Ultra Slim, Tesco*	1 Bar/60g	219	6.7	365	28.5	37.3	11.1	8.2
Chocolate, Milk White, Boohbah, M&S*	1 Bar/75g	405	24.2	540	7.9	54.7	32.3	1.2
Chocolate, Milk, Belgian, Sugar Free, Sweet' N Low*	1 Bar/42g	202	14.3	480	7.1	52.7	34.1	1.8
Chocolate, Milk, Chewy Delight, Special K, Kellogg's*	1 Bar/24g	95	3.1	397	5	57	13	17
Chocolate, Milk, Crispy, Endulge, Atkins*	1 Bar/30g	141	9.6	469	13	48	32	2
Chocolate, Milk, Meal Replacement, Shake that Weight*	1 Bar/35g	130	4.1	371	24.3	39.4	11.7	6
Chocolate, Milk, Swiss, M&S*	1 Bar/50g	285	18.4	570	0.2	51	36.8	2
Chocolate, Milkshake, Crisp, Weight Watchers*	1 Bar/21g	82	2.1	391	4.4	59.6	10	13.4
Chocolate, Mint, Club, Mcvitie's*	1 Bar/23g	117	6.1	510	5.7	61.2	26.4	2.3
Chocolate, Mint, Meal Replacement, Crunchy, CWP*	1 Bar/55g	215	7	391	27	42.7	12.8	5.6
Chocolate, Mint, Milk, Vitamin & Protein, Fulfil Nutrition*	1 Bar/55g	189	6.9	344	35.9	18.8	12.5	18.8
Chocolate, Mint, Whip, Weight Watchers*	1 Bar/20g	80	2	402	3.6	74	9.9	0.7
Chocolate, Orange, Montana*	1 Bar/25g	131	6.8	523	7	62.2	27.4	0
Chocolate, Original, Organic, Mini Moos*	1 Bar/20g	117	8	583	3	55.1	40	0
Chocolate, Peanut Butter, Atkins*	1 Bar/60g	250	14	417	26.7	38.3	23.3	20

BARS

	Measure INFO/WEIGHT	per Measure KCAL	FAT	Nutrition Values per 100g / 100ml KCAL	PROT	CARB	FAT	FIBRE
Chocolate, Peanut Butter, Smart, PhD Nutrition*	1 Bar/64g	239	10.2	373	31	38	16	1
Chocolate, Peanut, & Almond, Sweet & Salty, Nature Valley	1 Bar/30g	139	7.2	464	10.1	45.5	24	13
Chocolate, Peanut, Caramel, Shapers, Boots*	1 Bar/24g	96	4.1	401	6.6	42	17	28
Chocolate, Polar, Sainsbury's*	1 Bar/25g	133	7.2	533	5.5	63	28.6	1.2
Chocolate, Protein, Diet Chef Ltd*	1 Bar/60g	225	7.1	375	29.3	37.5	11.9	4.2
Chocolate, Racer, Dairyfine, Aldi*	1 Bar/38g	185	9.5	486	8.6	54	25	4.2
Chocolate, Raisin & Cereal, Morrisons*	1 Bar/30g	126	4.4	420	5.4	66.3	14.8	3.8
Chocolate, Sandwich, Rik & Rok*	1 Bar/22g	105	4.2	477	6.5	70	19	0
Chocolate, Sandwich, Seal, Aldi*	1 Bar/25g	131	7	523	5.5	60.6	28.1	3.1
Chocolate, Soya, Dairy Free, Free From, Sainsbury's*	1 Bar/50g	274	17.5	548	10.8	47.5	35	4.3
Chocolate, The Milk One, M&S*	1 Bar/32g	174	10.1	545	8.3	56	31.6	1.5
Chocolate, Titan, Aldi*	1 Bar/38g	169	6.8	444	3.5	66	18	0.5
Chocolate, Toffee Pecan, M&S*	1 Bar/36g	179	9.8	498	4.9	58.3	27.3	0.7
Chocolate, Triple, Atkins*	1 Bar/40g	160	9	400	30	42.5	22.5	12.5
Chocolate, Viennese, Sandwich, Fox's*	1 Biscuit/14g	76	4.4	542	6.9	57.4	31.6	1.6
Chocolate, Wafer, Blue Riband, 99 Calories, Nestle*	1 Bar/19g	99	4.7	514	5.5	66.5	24.6	2
Chocolate, Wafer, Caramel, Penguin, McVitie's*	1 Bar/21g	106	5.4	492	5.1	60.7	25.2	1.4
Chocolate, Whirls, Milk, Asda*	1 Bar/26g	116	4.2	447	3.7	72	16	0.8
Chocolate, White, Creamy, The White One, M&S*	1 Bar/32g	184	12	574	6.6	51.6	37.5	1.7
Chocolate, Wild Whippy, Tesco*	1 Bar/18g	78	2.8	447	3.7	72	16	0.8
Chocolix, Schar*	1 Bar/22g	101	3.9	463	3.6	70	18	4.2
Club, Fruit, Jacob's*	1 Bar/25g	124	6.2	496	5.6	62.2	25	2.3
Club, Milk Chocolate, Jacob's*	1 Bar/24g	123	6.3	511	5.8	62.6	26.4	2
Club, Mint, Jacob's*	1 Bar/24g	124	6.5	517	5.6	62.5	27.2	1.7
Club, Orange, Crunchies, McVitie's*	1 Bar/24g	115	6.1	481	5.1	59	25.7	1.4
Club, Orange, Jacob's*	1 Bar23g	117	6.1	509	5.7	61.8	26.5	2.3
Coco Pops, Milk, Kellogg's*	1 Bar/20g	85	2.6	423	7	70	13	1
Cocoa, & Hazelnut, Goodness, Go Ahead!*	1 Bar/30g	111	4	369	7.4	56	13.4	7.8
Cocoa, Brownie, Trek, The Natural Health Company*	1 Bar/68g	223	4.1	328	17	53	6	8
Cocoa, Coconut, Nak'd*	1 Bar/35g	133	5.5	379	5.9	50	15.7	7
Cocoa, Crunch, Nak'd*	1 Bar/30g	105	2.6	351	18.4	47.2	8.8	6.3
Cocoa, Delight, Wholefood, GF, Nak'd*	1 Bar/35g	135	5.3	386	9.4	49.4	15.1	6.8
Cocoa, Loco, Wildly Different, Nak'd*	1 Bar/30g	106	2.9	354	7.9	55.4	9.8	7.5
Cocoa, Mint, GF, Raw, Wholefood, Nak'd*	1 Bar/35g	135	5.3	386	9.4	49.4	15.1	6.8
Cocoa, Orange, GF, Nak'd*	1 Bar/35g	145	7	415	11	45.1	20	6.4
Cocoa, Twist, Nak'd*	1 Bar/30g	99	1.7	329	7	59.9	5.6	6
Coconut, & Apricot, Yoghurt Coated, Eat Natural*	1 Bar/45g	203	10.2	451	4.6	44.6	22.7	10.4
Coconut, & Chocolate, Vitamin & Protein, Fulfil Nutrition*	1 Bar/60g	207	8.5	344	34.4	19.6	14.1	18.7
Coconut, Almond, Cocoa, M&S*	1 Bar/30g	100	3.8	333	7.3	45.4	12.5	4.6
Coconut, Chocolate Crisp, Weight Watchers*	1 Bar/25g	89	2.6	356	3.6	71.2	10.4	3.2
Coconut, Crunch, Protein, Musclefood*	1 Bar/45g	171	6	379	33.4	32.4	13.3	7.6
Coconut, Cumin, Protein, Balls, Bounce*	1 Ball/40g	184	10	460	22.5	40	25	0
Coconut, Nutramino*	1 Bar/66g	290	14	439	30.3	33.3	21.2	2.9
Cookie, Apple Crumble, COU, M&S*	1 Bar/27g	90	0.7	335	5.8	72.6	2.6	2.3
Cookie, Oreo, Nabisco*	1 Bar/35g	180	10.2	514	2	66	29	0
Cookies Cream, Fit Crunch*	1 Bar/88g	380	16	432	34.1	30.7	18.2	9.1
Cookies Cream, Protein, Battle Bites*	1 Bar/62g	227	8.7	365	32	24	14	19.6
Cookies Cream, Protein, Musclefood*	1 Bar/42g	155	4.4	368	32.1	41.8	10.5	3.1
Corn Flakes, Chocolate Milk, Kellogg's*	1 Bar/40g	176	6.4	440	9	66	16	2
Cranberry, & Macadamia Porridge Oat, Stoats*	1 Bar/85g	385	22.9	453	6.9	71.8	26.9	5.9
Cranberry, & Raisin, Geobar, Traidcraft*	1 Bar/35g	131	2.8	374	3.7	72.6	8	2.3
Cranberry, & Raspberry, Multigrain, Jordans*	1 Bar/37g	135	2.4	364	4.8	71.3	6.6	4.8
Cranberry, & Roasted Almonds, Nutty, Chewy, Kellogg's*	1 Bar/35g	157	7	449	8.9	57.1	20	4.9

BARS

INFO/WEIGHT	Measure	per Measure KCAL	per Measure FAT	Nutrition Values per 100g / 100ml KCAL	PROT	CARB	FAT	FIBRE
Cranberry, Almond, Goodness Knows*	1 Bar/34g	153	6.7	451	7.5	56.8	19.8	6.1
Cranberry, Almond Macadamia, Kind*	1 Bar/40g	192	12	480	10	50	30	7.2
Cranberry, Crunchy, Meal Replacement, CWP*	1 Bar/55g	214	6.8	389	27.7	42.9	12.3	4.5
Crunchy Nut, Chocolate Peanut Crisp, Kellogg's*	1 Bar/35g	169	8.8	483	12	53	25	3.5
Crunchy Nut, Kellogg's*	1 Bar/30g	119	1.5	397	6	82	5	2.5
Date, & Fruit, Lyme Regis Foods*	1 Bar/42g	169	6.5	402	7.3	58.2	15.5	8.9
Date, & Peanut, Eat Real*	1 Bar/40g	155	4.6	387	7.8	59.7	11.5	6.3
Date, & Walnut, with Pumpkin Seeds, Eat Natural*	1 Bar/45g	218	9	434	9.1	46.6	18	4.5
Date, Cinnamon, Sticky, Grain, Eat Well, M&S*	1 Bar/45g	181	6.8	402	9.7	53	15.2	7.4
Date, Walnut, & Pumpkin Seed, Milk Chocolate, M&S*	1 Bar/40g	175	8.4	437	8	52	20.9	4.6
Digestive, Milk Chocolate, McVitie's*	1 Bar/23g	118	5.8	511	6.6	64.6	25.1	1.9
Digestive, Milk Chocolate, Tesco*	1 Bar/19g	96	4.9	506	6.8	61.6	25.8	2.4
Digestive, Milk Chocolate, Value, Tesco*	1 Bar/19g	96	4.9	505	6.6	61.8	25.8	3
Echo, Mint, Fox's*	1 Bar/25g	130	6.6	518	7.9	60.7	26.6	1.6
Energize, Berry Blast, Power Bar*	1 Bar/55g	199	2	362	10.9	70.8	3.7	2
Energy, Cocoa Brownie, Natural Balance Foods*	1 Bar/68g	216	4.1	318	17	51	6	0
Energy, Cool Mint, Chocolate, Clif*	1 Bar/68g	256	5	377	14.7	63.2	7.3	7.4
Energy, Ride, Power Bar*	1 Bar/55g	213	9.1	387	18.6	40.9	16.6	7.4
Fair Break, Traidcraft*	1 Bar/22g	116	6.2	528	6	63	28	0
Fig, & Mango, Wholesome, The Food Doctor*	1 Bar/35g	111	3.3	317	7.8	35.7	9.4	29.2
Flapjack, Apple Sultana, Organic, Dove's Farm*	1 Bar/40g	178	7.8	446	4.7	61.1	19.6	3.5
Flapjack, Buttery, Traditional, Organic, Dove's Farm*	1 Bar/40g	173	7.5	432	6.1	59.4	18.8	5.7
Flapjack, Cocoa, Raisin, Protein, Trek*	1 Bar/50g	222	10.7	444	18	43.1	21.4	4.2
Flapjack, Mixed Berry, Progain, Maxinutrition*	1 Bar/90g	324	7.2	360	26.5	50.1	8	2.6
Forest Fruit, & Raisin, LC, Tesco*	1 Bar/27g	95	0.7	350	4.5	76.8	2.7	3.6
Frosties, Milk, Kellogg's*	1 Bar/25g	102	2.8	408	7	71	11	1
Frosties, Snack Bar, Kellogg's*	1 Bar/25g	104	2.8	414	7	72	11	1
Fruit & Fibre, Coconut, Apricot, Oats, Spelt, Eat Natural*	1 Bar/40g	165	7	413	6.4	51.6	17.5	6.1
Fruit & Fibre, Plum, Peanut, Oats, Spelt, Eat Natural*	1 Bar/40g	173	7.8	432	10.1	51.1	19.4	6.4
Fruit Grain, Apple, Harvest Morn, Aldi*	1 Bar/37g	129	3	349	4.2	65	8	4.5
Fruit Grain, Strawberry, Harvest Morn, Aldi*	1 Bar/37g	130	2.6	349	4.2	65	7	4.5
Fruit Nut, Eat Natural*	1 Bar/50g	223	11.2	446	11.6	49.8	22.3	5.3
Fruit Nut, Milk Chocolate, Eat Real*	1 Bar/40g	196	11.7	490	8.1	46.3	29.3	9.3
Fruit Nut, Organic, Eat Natural*	1 Bar/50g	244	15.3	488	10.2	42.9	30.6	0
Fruit Nut, Yoghurt Coated, Eat Real*	1 Bar/40g	186	9.9	466	6.6	51.9	24.8	9.2
Fruit 'n' Fibre, Bakes with Sultanas, Kellogg's*	1 Bar/40g	146	5.2	365	4.5	58	13	9
Fruit 'n' Fibre, Kellogg's*	1 Bar/25g	95	2.2	380	5	71	9	5
Fruit, & Nut, Multigrain, Jordans*	1 Bar/40g	164	6.5	410	7	59.1	16.2	5.7
Fruit, & Yoghurt, Crunch, Meal Replacement, Slim Fast*	1 Bar/60g	218	6.8	364	25.4	26.9	11.3	18.7
Fruit, Mixed, Juice Plus*	1 Bar/55g	211	6.9	384	27.3	35.5	12.6	9.7
Fruit, Nut Seeds Cereal, Eat Well, M&S*	1 Bar/24g	88	2.6	365	6.1	60.8	10.9	6.9
Fruit, Zippy, Mini Chefs, Natco*	1 Bar/20g	60	0	300	1	70	0	5
Fudge, Brownie, Carb Killa, Grenade*	1 Bar/60g	215	8	359	38.9	22.6	13.3	11.3
Fudge, Mallow Delight, Whipple Scrumptious, Wonka*	1 Bar/38g	205	12	537	4.6	59.2	31.3	0.6
Fudge, Vanilla, Madagascan, Milk Chocolate Coated, M&S*	1 Bar/36g	174	8	484	3.6	67.1	22.2	0.9
Ginger, & Oat, Chocolate Covered, Snack, Waitrose*	1 Bar/27g	120	5	444	4.2	65	18.6	2.1
Ginger, Bread, GF, Nak'd*	1 Bar/35g	158	10.8	450	10	35	31	9.4
Ginger, Bread, Nak'd*	1 Bar/35g	157	10.7	450	10	35.4	30.8	9.4
Goji Berries, & Fax Seeds, Porridge Oat, Stoats*	1 Bar/85g	374	24.4	440	10.9	62.4	28.7	8.2
Golden Syrup, Morning, Oat So Simple, Quaker*	1 Bar/35g	142	3.5	407	8.2	67.6	10	6.8
Granola, Crunchy, Oats Chocolate, Nature Valley*	1 Bar/21g	98	4.1	464	8.3	59.8	19.8	7.1
Granola, Crunchy, Roasted Almond, Nature Valley*	1 Bar/42g	193	7.6	459	8.1	65.6	18.2	3.7
Granola, Kirkland*	1 Bar/24g	100	10.7	417	24.2	307.9	44.6	17.8

BARS

Measure INFO/WEIGHT		per Measure		Nutrition Values per 100g / 100ml				
		KCAL	FAT	KCAL	PROT	CARB	FAT	FIBRE
Granola, Maple Syrup, Crunchy, Harvest Morn, Aldi*	2 Bars/42g	189	6.7	450	8.2	65	16	5.9
Granola, Maple Syrup, Twin Pack, Tesco*	2 Bars/42g	204	9.4	485	6	64.7	22.3	4.1
Granola, Oats Hazlenuts, Nature Valley*	2 Bars/42g	195	8.4	465	8.4	58.9	20.1	7.5
Granola, Oats Honey, Crunchy, Harvest Morn, Aldi*	2 Bars/42g	191	6.7	455	8.2	66	16	6.2
Granola, Peanut Butter, Advantage, Atkins*	1 Bar/48g	210	11	438	29.2	39.6	22.9	10.4
Granola, Peanut Butter, Quaker*	1 Bar/28g	110	3.5	393	7.1	64.3	12.5	3.6
Granola, with Peanut Butter, Natco*	1 Bar/29g	129	4.1	445	10	69	14.1	5.5
Hazelnut, & Raisin, Energy Ball, Deliciously Ella*	1 Ball/40g	152	7.5	379	6.5	49.7	18.7	5.2
Hazelnut, Praline, Milk & Dark Chocolate, M&S*	1 Bar/36g	210	14.1	582	8.2	47.6	39.1	3.5
Healthy Meal, Herbalife*	1 Bar/56g	207	6	369	23.7	37.1	10.7	14.7
Hobnobs, Choc Golden Syrup, McVitie's*	1 Bar/31g	129	4	421	6.3	68.2	13.1	4.8
Honey Nut, Special K, Special K, Kellogg's*	1 Bar/22g	90	2	409	9.1	72.7	9.1	13.6
Honey Rice Crisp, Lower Fat, Go Ahead, McVitie's*	1 Bar/22g	90	2.2	411	3.9	75.8	10.2	1.1
Honey, & Almond, Crunchy, Original, Jordans*	1 Bar/30g	139	6.8	463	8.3	56.7	22.7	6.7
Honeycomb, Club, Jacob's*	1 Bar/23g	116	6	512	5.7	61.9	26.3	2.3
Jive, Chocolate, Caramel Shortcake Finger, Dairyfine, Aldi*	1 Twin Bar/42g	194	9.7	463	4.6	58	23	0.9
Lemon Drizzle, Nak'd*	1 Bar/35g	133	5.4	381	6.1	51.8	15.5	5.1
Luna, Chocolate Pecan Pie, Luna*	1 Bar/48g	180	4.5	375	20.8	50	9.4	2.1
Luna, Nutz Over Chocolate, Luna*	1 Bar/48g	180	4.5	375	20.8	50	9.4	2.1
Macadamia, & Coconut, Paleo, Aldi*	1 Bar/45g	212	12.2	470	7.6	43	27	11
Macadamia, & Fruit, Eat Natural*	1 Bar/50g	242	15.4	485	7.3	44.6	30.8	0
Macaroon, Lees*	1 Bar/70g	276	4.7	395	1.2	82.5	6.7	0
Malt Loaf, Soreen*	1 Bar/42g	124	1	295	8.2	57.8	2.3	5.1
Maple, & Pecan, Crunchy, Jordans*	1 Bar/33g	153	7.6	464	7.7	56.8	22.9	6.5
Maple, Glazed Pecan, Sea Salt, Kind*	1 Bar/40g	213	17.2	532	14	33	43	13
Marshmallow, Chewy, Rice Krispies Squares, Kellogg's*	1 Bar/28g	119	3.4	424	3	76	12	0.9
Mint, Crunch, Guilt Free Snacking, M&S*	1 Bar/24g	143	9.2	596	4.3	56.9	38.4	2.9
Mint, Double Take, Sainsbury's*	1 Bar/20g	107	6.2	534	7.2	56.9	30.8	1.3
Mudslide, Atkins*	1 Bar/48g	210	10	438	31.2	39.6	20.8	10.4
Muesli, & Seeds, Bountiful, Aldi*	1 Bar/30g	98	1.4	328	3	53	4.8	18
Muesli, Apricot & Almond, Carmen's*	1 Bar/45g	190	8.2	423	10.4	50.6	18.2	7.4
Muesli, Cherry & Milk, Sirius, Lidl*	1 Bar/25g	104	2.8	417	7.2	71.3	11.4	3.9
Muesli, Cookie Coach*	1 Bar/75g	289	8.3	385	6.8	65.1	11.1	0
Muesli, Fruit, Morning, Oat So Simple, Quaker*	1 Bar/35g	139	3.2	398	7.7	68.1	9.1	6.6
Muesli, Fruit, Special, Jordans*	1 Bar/40g	140	2.4	349	5	68.8	6	5
Muesli, Original, Diet Chef Ltd*	1 Bar/50g	199	6.9	398	6.1	59	13.8	6.4
Muesli, Peanut, No Added Sugar, Crownfield, Lidl*	1 Bar/25g	98	3.3	391	7.9	65.7	13.2	4.7
Muesli, Special, Jordans*	1 Bar/40g	152	4.8	379	6	61.6	12.1	5.8
Muesli, Yogurt Coated, Slim & Save*	1 Bar/45g	160	4.5	355	27.3	37.2	9.9	11
Muffin, Cadbury*	1 Bar/68g	274	17.3	403	5.6	38	25.4	0
Nine Bar, Mixed Seed with Hemp, Original, Wholebake*	1 Bar/40g	222	16.2	555	18.3	29.2	40.5	5.2
Nine Bar, Nutty, Wholebake*	1 Bar/50g	279	20.4	558	15.3	32.3	40.8	4.9
Noisettes Amandes, Special K, Kellogg's*	1 Bar/21g	83	2.1	397	8	66	10	7
Nougat, Cool Mint, Dark Chocolate, Shapers, Boots*	1 Bar/25g	81	3.1	324	2.4	48	12.4	1.2
Nougat, Summer Strawberry, Shapers, Boots*	1 Bar/23g	83	3	361	2.7	73	13	0.6
Nut, Absolute, Luxury, Jordans*	1 Bar/45g	251	18.6	557	12.7	33.3	41.4	7
Nut, Chewy & Crisp, Roasted, Sainsbury's*	1 Bar/27g	120	6.6	446	10.1	46.6	24.3	3.9
Nut, Dark Chocolate & Apricot, Natural, Nice & Natural*	1 Bar/35g	163	10.2	465	15.2	35.2	29.1	5.4
Nut, Feast, Mixed, Eat Natural*	1 Bar/50g	278	20.5	556	18.8	28	41	0
Nutri-Grain, Apple, Kellogg's*	1 Bar/37g	131	3.3	355	4	67	9	4
Nutri-Grain, Apple, Soft Fruity, Kellogg's*	1 Bar/37g	133	3	359	4	70.3	8.1	4
Nutri-Grain, Blackberry Apple, Kellogg's*	1 Bar/37g	131	3.3	355	4	67	9	4
Nutri-Grain, Blackberry Apple, Soft Fruity, Kellogg's*	1 Bar/37g	133	3	359	4	70.3	8.1	4

B

B

BARS

INFO/WEIGHT	Measure	per Measure		Nutrition Values per 100g / 100ml				
		KCAL	FAT	KCAL	PROT	CARB	FAT	FIBRE
Nutri-Grain, Blueberry, Kellogg's*	1 Bar/37g	133	3	359	3.5	69	8	3.5
Nutri-Grain, Blueberry, Soft Fruity, Kellogg's*	1 Bar/37g	133	3	359	4	70.3	8.1	4
Nutri-Grain, Chocolate Chip, Chewy, Kellogg's*	1 Bar/25g	103	3	413	4.5	73	12	2.5
Nutri-Grain, Crunchy Oat Granola, Choc Chip, Kellogg's*	1 Bar/40g	187	7.6	468	7	65	19	4.5
Nutri-Grain, Elevenses, Choc Chip Bakes, Kellogg's*	1 Bar/45g	179	5.8	397	4	66	13	2
Nutri-Grain, Elevenses, Ginger Bakes, Kellogg's*	1 Bar/45g	168	4	373	5	68	9	3
Nutri-Grain, Elevenses, Raisin Bakes, Kellogg's*	1 Bar/45g	168	4	374	4.5	68	9	2.5
Nutri-Grain, Oat Bakes, Cherry, Kellogg's*	1 Bar/50g	204	7	408	4.5	66	14	2.5
Nutri-Grain, Oat Bakes, Totally Oaty, Kellogg's*	1 Bar/50g	206	7.5	411	5	64	15	3
Nutri-Grain, Raspberry, Kellogg's*	1 Bar/37g	131	3.3	355	4	67	9	4
Nutri-Grain, Strawberry, Kellogg's*	1 Bar/37g	133	3	359	3.5	69	8	3.5
Nutri-Grain, Strawberry, Soft Fruity, Kellogg's*	1 Bar/37g	133	3	359	4	70.3	8.1	4
Nuts, & Berry, Weight Watchers*	1 Bar/24g	92	2.9	383	5.9	52.1	11.9	12.7
Nutty Crunch Surprise, Wonka*	1 Bar/37g	202	11.9	543	4.9	58.7	32.1	0.9
Nutty Nougat Caramel, Tesco*	1 Bar/40g	200	11.1	490	8.7	52.7	27.2	3.8
Oat, Original with Golden Syrup, Quaker*	1 Bar/38g	139	3.6	366	7.1	64.5	9.5	7.9
Oat, Quaker*	1 Bar/38g	137	3.4	360	6.8	64.5	8.8	8
Oats, Sweet Potato Orange, COU, M&S*	1 Bar/30g	111	3.9	369	7.2	53.4	12.9	5.2
Oaty with Cranberry Blueberry, Tesco*	1 Bar/38g	141	2.8	370	5.5	69	7.5	6.2
Oaty, Cranberry Cashew, Perkier*	1 Bar/40g	142	3.5	355	12	53	8.8	11
Oaty, Fruit Nut, Weight Watchers*	1 Bar/26g	90	2.4	345	10.5	42.4	9.2	25.5
Oaty, Strawberry Crusher, Weetabix*	1 Bar/23g	79	1.4	345	6.1	55.2	6.1	22.2
Orange, Crunch, Go Ahead, McVitie's*	1 Bar/23g	99	2.9	430	4.1	78	12.8	0.8
Original, Nut Free, Get Buzzing*	1 Bar/62g	248	12	400	6.8	51.6	19.4	3.7
Peach, & Apricot, Special K, Kellogg's*	1 Bar/23g	90	1.4	383	8	75	6	2.5
Peanut Butter, Breakfast, Bounce*	1 Bar/45g	168	7.2	374	22	27	16	16
Peanut Butter, Dark Chocolate, Specially Selected, Aldi*	1 Bar/40g	213	14.8	533	23	21	37	15
Peanut, & Banana, Protein, Meridian*	1 Bar/40g	173	9.5	432	17.4	34.8	23.8	4.8
Peanut, & Caramel Whip, Weight Watchers*	1 Bar/20g	76	2.7	381	4.4	73.7	13.7	1.2
Peanut, & Popcorn, Dark Chocolate Chunks, Eat Natural*	1 Bar/45g	204	9.9	453	10.7	50.6	21.9	5.2
Peanut, Dark Chocolate, Tesco*	1 Bar/35g	175	10.4	500	22.2	33	29.7	6
Peanut, Caramel, Payday, Hershey*	1 Bar/19g	88	4.8	462	13.5	51.9	25	3.8
Peanut, Mr Toms*	1 Bar/40g	210	13	525	20	42.5	32.5	2.5
Peanut, Raisin Chocolate, Weight Watchers*	1 Bar/25g	97	2.8	388	7.6	60	11.2	12.8
Peanut, Sweet Salty Nut, Nature Valley*	1 Bar/30g	143	7.8	478	12.3	43.1	26.1	11
Pecan, Apricot & Peach, M&S*	1 Bar/50g	255	17.8	510	9.3	38.2	35.5	4.9
Pecan, Pie, GF, Nak'd*	1 Bar/35g	156	10.3	477	7.6	36.4	31.4	8.9
Pineapple, Coconut, Goodness, The Food Doctor*	1 Bar/40g	150	5.2	376	6	48	13	19
Popcorn, Cranberry Yoghurt , Nature Valley*	1 Bar/20g	85	2.9	425	4.6	62.4	14.6	12.4
Popcorn, Peanut Butter, Fibre One*	1 Bar/21g	90	4.3	427	7.6	41.4	20.3	23.9
Protein, Apple Pie, GF, Quest*	1 Bar/60g	202	7.2	337	33	15	12	23
Protein, Banana Nut Muffin, GF, Quest*	1 Bar/60g	197	7.8	329	33	17	13	21
Protein, Banana, Hike, Aldi*	1 Bar/55g	169	0.8	306	20	45	1.5	18
Protein, Boysenberry Ripple, Whip'd, Aussie Bodies*	1 Bar/30g	94	2.8	313	30	4	9.3	14.7
Protein, Caramel Chaos, Carb Killa, Grenade*	1 Bar/60g	214	7.9	357	38.7	22.5	13.2	11.1
Protein, Caramel Peanut, My Bar Zero, Myprotein*	1 Bar/65g	211	7.2	325	31	6.2	11	37
Protein, Chocolate Banana, MuleBar*	1 Bar/65g	254	5.8	390	21	56	9	2
Protein, Chocolate Brownie, GF, Quest*	1 Bar/60g	191	7.2	318	33	12	12	25
Protein, Chocolate Chip Cookie Dough, GF, Quest*	1 Bar/60g	206	9	344	34	12	15	23
Protein, Chocolate Peanut Butter, GF, Quest*	1 Bar/60g	185	6.6	309	33	17	11	23
Protein, Chocolate Peanut, Musclefood*	1 Bar/42g	173	4	411	35.7	33	9.5	0
Protein, Chunky Peanut, Nutramino*	1 Bar/60g	236	10.8	393	35	35	18	1.3
Protein, Cinnamon Roll, GF, Quest*	1 Bar/60g	191	7.2	318	33	16	12	23

BARS

INFO/WEIGHT	Measure	per Measure		Nutrition Values per 100g / 100ml				
		KCAL	FAT	KCAL	PROT	CARB	FAT	FIBRE
Protein, Coconut Cashew, GF, Quest*	1 Bar/60g	202	8.4	337	33	14	14	23
Protein, Combat Crunch, MusclePharm*	1 Bar/63g	210	7	333	31.8	39.7	11.1	0
Protein, Cookies Cream, GF, Quest*	1 Bar/60g	209	9	349	35	12	15	23
Protein, Cookies Cream, My Bar Zero, Myprotein*	1 Bar/65g	202	6	311	32	6.5	9.2	37
Protein, Cranberry Kick, Chunks, Trek, Natural Balance*	1 Bar/60g	202	3.9	336	20.7	44	6.5	9
Protein, Double Chocolate Chunk, GF, Quest*	1 Bar/60g	191	7.8	318	33	18	13	21
Protein, Flapjack, Oat Crunch, Natural Balance Foods*	1 Bar/56g	249	12.9	444	18	43	23	3
Protein, Lemon Cream Pie, GF, Quest*	1 Bar/60g	181	6	302	33	16	10	23
Protein, Low Sugar, Chocolate, USN*	1 Bar/35g	116	4.2	332	31	30	12	13
Protein, Mint Chocolate Chunk, GF, Quest*	1 Bar/60g	209	9	348	33	11	15	24
Protein, Mixed Berry Bliss, GF, Quest*	1 Bar/60g	209	9	349	33	13	15	23
Protein, Peanut Blast, Natural Energy, Ball, Bounce*	1 Ball/49g	210	8	429	28.6	38.8	16.3	4.1
Protein, Peanut Butter Jelly, GF, Quest*	1 Bar/60g	217	10.2	361	33	13	17	21
Protein, Peanut Chewy Crisp, Chemical Protein Pro-Xs*	1 Bar/70g	243	5.2	347	42.9	5.5	7.5	12.5
Protein, Peanut Peak, Chunks, Trek, Natural Balance*	1 Bar/60g	232	7.9	386	20.9	42	13.2	7
Protein, Premium, Ball, Bounce*	1 Ball/49g	209	9	426	30.6	40.8	18.4	2
Protein, Pumpkin Pie, GF, Limited Edition, Quest*	1 Bar/60g	220	12	366	35	12	20	20
Protein, S'mores, GF, Quest*	1 Bar/60g	197	8.4	329	33	15	14	21
Protein, Strawberry Cheesecake, GF, Quest*	1 Bar/60g	188	6.6	314	33	17	11	22
Protein, Supreme Peanut, Musclefood*	1 Bar/44g	171	6.6	388	34.1	35.2	15	3.8
Protein, Toffee Triumph, Chunks, Trek, Natural Balance*	1 Bar/60g	213	6.4	355	21	39	10.7	11
Protein, Vanilla, Low Carb, Protein Plus, Power Bar*	1 Bar/35g	131	7.4	373	16	21.5	21	26.5
Protein, Whey, Sculptress, Maxitone*	1 Bar/60g	203	5.6	339	33.9	30.6	9.3	8.5
Protein, White Chocolate Raspberry, GF, Quest*	1 Bar/60g	215	9.6	358	33	13	16	23
Protin, Crispy Chocolate Brownie, Nutramino*	1 Bar/64g	268	10.9	418	31	39	17	0.5
Quinoa, Goji, Cranberry, Perkier*	1 Bar/35g	129	3.9	370	12.7	51.1	11.2	10.1
Raisin, & Oatmeal, Breakfast Snack, Tesco*	1 Bar/38g	133	4.4	355	5.6	56.8	11.7	2.8
Raisin, Munch, Tesco*	1 Bar/30g	126	4.4	420	5.4	66.3	14.8	3.8
Raspberry, & White Chocolate Crispie, Shapers, Boots*	1 Bar/24g	93	2	387	3.8	68	8.5	11
Raspberry, Baked, Asda*	1 Bar/27g	104	2.1	385	3.4	74.2	7.6	1.8
Raspberry, Cheesecake, Tesco*	1 Bar/90g	297	17.3	330	4.1	34.7	19.2	0.8
Raspberry, Crispy, Meal Replacement, Tesco*	1 Bar/60g	216	6.7	360	22.3	42.1	11.2	7.6
Raspberry, Pie, Weight Watchers*	1 Bar/40g	122	0.4	305	4.5	55.8	1	14.8
Rice Krispies, & Milk, Kellogg's*	1 Bar/20g	83	2.4	416	7	71	12	0.3
Rice Krispies, Snack, Kellogg's*	1 Bar/20g	83	2	415	7	70	10	0.5
Rice Krispies, Squares, Totally Chocolatey, Kellogg's*	1 Bar/36g	156	5.3	439	4.5	72	15	1.5
Rocky Road, M&S*	1 Bar/68g	330	18	486	4.1	56.7	26.5	1.9
Rocky Road, Rice Krispies Squares, Kellogg's*	1 Square/34g	143	3.7	420	4	76	11	1.5
Rocky Road, Romance Me, Hi-Fi, Slimming World*	1 Bar/20g	73	1.5	366	4.8	62.7	7.3	15.4
Sesame Snaps, Anglo-Dal*	1 Pack/30g	157	8.8	522	12.2	49.4	29.4	0
Sesame Snaps, in Chocolate, Anglo-Dal*	1 Pack/40g	211	11.9	527	9.3	55.6	29.7	0
Sesame Snaps, with Coconut, Anglo-Dal*	1 Pack/30g	155	8.8	517	9.7	52.9	29.5	0
Special K, Apple Pear, Kellogg's*	1 Bar/23g	92	1.8	400	8	73	8	2
Special K, Chocolate Chip, Kellogg's*	1 Bar/22g	90	1.6	401	9	76	7	1.5
Special K, Fruits of the Forest, Kellogg's*	1 Bar/22g	87	1.8	397	8	74	8	2.5
Special K, Mint Chocolate, Bliss, Special K, Kellogg's*	1 Bar/22g	88	2.2	401	4.5	74	10	3.5
Special K, Red Berry, Kellogg's*	1 Bar/23g	90	1.2	383	8	77	5	2
Strawberry, & Vanilla, Vitamin & Protein, Fulfil Nutrition*	1 Bar/60g	185	4.9	309	33.4	10.1	8.2	33.1
Strawberry, Fruit Bakes, Go Ahead, McVitie's*	1 Bar/35g	131	3	375	3.5	72	8.5	4
Strawberry, Fruit, Fruitina*	1 Bar/15g	43	0.2	289	1.9	61.9	1.1	12.2
Strawberry, Fruit, Sweet Vine, Aldi*	1 Bar/20g	67	0.8	334	1.2	73	3.9	1.7
Strawberry, Morning Shine, Atkins*	1 Bar/37g	145	8	392	28.9	24.9	21.6	14.1
Strawberry, Picked Pressed, Fruit Bowl*	1 Bar/19g	60	0.7	317	3.5	63	3.6	10

B

	Measure INFO/WEIGHT	per Measure KCAL	FAT	Nutrition Values per 100g / 100ml KCAL	PROT	CARB	FAT	FIBRE
BARS								
Strawberry, Scrumptious, Get Fruity*	1 Bar/35g	141	4.6	402	5.9	62	13	5.4
Strawberry, Shapers, Boots*	1 Bar/22g	75	2.4	343	2.5	77	11	0.9
Three Musketeer, Candy, Mars*	1 Bar/60g	260	8	430	3.3	76.2	13.2	1.7
Toffee, & Banana, Weight Watchers*	1 Bar/18g	67	0.7	372	6.1	77.2	3.9	1.7
Toffee, Chocolate, Snack, Skinny Whip*	1 Bar/25g	96	2.3	384	3.6	64	9.2	15.2
Toffee, Harvest Cheweee, Quaker*	1 Bar/22g	94	3.3	427	5	68	15	3
Toffee, Rich, Weight Watchers*	1 Bar/19g	68	1.7	358	2.6	51.6	9.1	30.1
Toffee, Sticky, Hi-Fi, Slimming World*	1 Bar/20g	69	2	343	4	51	9.9	17
Tracker, Breakfast, Banana, Mars*	1 Bar/37g	176	8.4	476	4.7	63.3	22.6	9.4
Tracker, Chocolate Chip, Mars*	1 Bar/37g	178	8.7	480	6.8	58	23.6	3.8
Tracker, Forest Fruits, Mars*	1 Bar/26g	123	5.8	474	4.6	64.1	22.2	0
Tracker, Roasted Nut, Mars*	1 Bar/26g	127	6.6	489	8.1	55	25.3	4.9
Trail, Big Berries, Alpen*	1 Bar/48g	180	2.7	376	6	61.9	5.7	4.3
Triple Dazzle, Wonka*	1 Bar/39g	195	10	504	5.9	61.9	25.9	0
Vanilla, Kubes, Tesco*	1 Bar/28g	107	1.8	381	6.8	72.1	6.5	3.6
Wafer, Chocolate, Coated, Milk, Value, Tesco*	1 Bar/24g	126	6.7	526	6.9	61.4	28.1	1.7
Wafer, Chocolate, Flavour Crisp, Carbolite*	1 Bar/25g	120	8.7	482	8.5	52.3	34.8	2
White Chocolate Chip, Harvest Cheweee, Quaker*	1 Bar/22g	94	3.4	425	6	67	15.5	3.5
White Chocolate, & Hazelnuts, Porridge Oat, Stoats*	1 Bar/85g	407	22.4	479	7.6	50.1	26.3	5.9
White Chocolate, Raspberry Matcha, M&S*	1 Bar/25g	147	9.9	588	5.2	52	39.7	0.8
White Chocolate, Cookie Dough, Fulfil Nutrition*	1 Bar/55g	195	7.2	355	38.6	20.2	13.2	14.2
White Chocolate, Crispy Wafer, Tasty Little Numbers*	1 Bar/20g	100	5.2	498	7	59	26	3
BASA								
Fillets, Chilli & Lemon Grass Butter Sauce, Birds Eye*	1 Fillet/140g	164	10.2	117	12	0.7	7.3	0
Fillets, in Tomato Chilli Sauce, Inspirations, Birds Eye*	1 Serving/147g	176	11.1	120	12	0.9	7.6	0.5
Fillets, Lemon & Herb, Tempura Battered, Gastro, Youngs*	1 Fillet/105g	116	3	110	20.8	0.5	2.8	0
Fillets, Lime, Chilli Coriander, Dusted, Gastro, Youngs*	1 Fillet/152g	288	13.9	189	15.6	11	9.1	0.4
Fillets, Mediterranean Marinated, Northern Catch, Aldi*	1 Fillet/128g	147	4.7	115	18	2.8	3.7	0.5
Fillets, Rocket, Basil & Parmesan Sauce, Gastro, Youngs*	1 Serving/136g	136	4.2	100	17.7	0.2	3.1	0.2
Fillets, Sea Salt & Cracked Black Pepper, Gastro, Youngs*	1 Fillet/151g	261	12.1	173	14.7	10.5	8	0.3
Fillets, Skinless Boneless, Aldi*	1 Fillet/120g	140	2.9	117	23.7	0.1	2.4	0
Fillets, Spicy Tomato & Chorizo Sauce, Gastro, Youngs*	1 Serving/133g	122	2.8	92	17.4	0.6	2.1	0.4
Fillets, Tempura Battered, Lemon & Herb, Gastro, Youngs*	1 Fillet/151g	279	14	185	14.2	10.6	9.3	1.1
Fillets, with Asian BBQ Sauce, The Saucy Fish Co.*	½ Pack/125g	124	2.1	99	17.8	4.2	1.7	0.1
BASIL								
Dried, Ground	*1 Tsp/1.4g*	*4*	*0.1*	*251*	*14.4*	*43.2*	*4*	*0*
Fresh, Average	*1 Tbsp/5g*	*2*	*0*	*40*	*3.1*	*5.1*	*0.8*	*0*
BATTER MIX								
for Yorkshire Puddings & Pancakes, Tesco*	1 Serving/17g	34	0.3	200	2.3	43.3	1.5	2.5
for Yorkshire Puddings, Baked, Aunt Bessie's*	1 Pudding/13g	48	1.1	356	9.8	34	8.1	2.3
Green's*	1 Bag/125g	296	9	237	8.7	34.3	7.2	0
Pancake, Buttermilk, Krusteaz*	3 Pancakes/16g	57	0.8	352	11.3	66	4.7	3.4
BAY LEAVES								
Dried, Average	*1 Tsp/0.6g*	*2*	*0.1*	*313*	*7.6*	*48.6*	*8.4*	*0*
BEAN SPROUTS								
Mung, Raw, Average	*1oz/28g*	*9*	*0.1*	*31*	*2.9*	*4*	*0.5*	*1.5*
Mung, Stir-Fried in Blended Oil, Average	*1 Serving/90g*	*65*	*5.5*	*72*	*1.9*	*2.5*	*6.1*	*0.9*
Raw, Average	*1 Serving/150g*	*55*	*2.6*	*37*	*2.2*	*3.2*	*1.8*	*1.2*
BEANS								
& Cheese, Combos, Fridge Raiders, GoGo's*	1 Serving/70g	297	21	424	26	9.8	30	4.5
& Meatballs, in Tomato Sauce, Sainsbury's*	½ Can/200g	216	7.2	108	5.5	13.3	3.6	2.6
Seeds, Steamer, Waitrose*	1 Bag/160g	213	7.7	133	9.4	8.1	4.8	9.9
Aduki, Cooked in Unsalted Water, Average	*1 Tbsp/30g*	*37*	*0.1*	*123*	*9.3*	*22.5*	*0.2*	*5.5*

BEANS

INFO/WEIGHT	Measure	per Measure		Nutrition Values per 100g / 100ml				
		KCAL	FAT	KCAL	PROT	CARB	FAT	FIBRE
Aduki, Dried, Raw	*1 Tbsp/30g*	*82*	*0.2*	*272*	*19.9*	*50.1*	*0.5*	*11.1*
Baked, & Sausage in Tomato Sauce, Smart Price, Asda*	½ Can/203g	256	12.2	126	5	13	6	0
Baked, Jumbo Sausages, Asda*	1 Can/405g	486	17	120	6.9	11.2	4.2	5
Baked, Sausage, Asda*	½ Can/203g	211	4	104	6.7	13	2	3.5
Baked, Sausages, Basics, Sainsbury's*	1 Serving/175g	149	2.6	85	4.8	13.1	1.5	2.6
Baked, Sausages, in Tomato Sauce, Sainsbury's*	1 Can/400g	480	16	120	6.2	12.9	4	3.5
Baked, Sausages, Meatfree, Sainsbury's*	1 Can/420g	500	16.8	119	8	12.6	4	2.7
Baked, Sausages, Value, Tesco*	½ Can/202g	232	7.1	115	5.6	15	3.5	2.8
Baked, Vegetarian Sausages, in Tomato Sauce, Asda*	½ Can/210g	204	4	97	7.4	12.5	1.9	8.4
Baked, Barbecue, Beanz, Heinz*	1 Can/390g	343	0.8	88	4.9	14.6	0.2	3.8
Baked, Cheesy Sausage, Meal For One, Iceland *	1 Pack/494g	721	30.6	146	6.4	14.3	6.2	3.7
Baked, Curried, Average	*½ Can/210g*	*203*	*1.9*	*96*	*4.8*	*17.2*	*0.9*	*3.6*
Baked, Curry, Beanz, Heinz*	1 Can/390g	382	1.2	98	4.8	17	0.3	4
Baked, Five, in Tomato Sauce, Heinz*	1 Can/415g	361	0.8	87	5.4	13.6	0.2	4.3
Baked, Giant, Sainsbury's*	½ Jar/110g	169	8.2	154	5.8	12.5	7.5	6.6
Baked, Gigantes, in Tomato Sauce, Odysea *	1 Jar/355g	593	29.1	167	5.8	14.1	8.2	0
Baked, in Tomato Sauce, Average	*1 Can/400g*	*318*	*1.6*	*80*	*4.6*	*13.9*	*0.4*	*3.7*
Baked, in Tomato Sauce, No Added Sugar, Red Salt, Asda*	½ Can/204g	149	1.2	73	4.5	9.9	0.6	4.8
Baked, in Tomato Sauce, Reduced Sugar Salt	*½ Can/210g*	*159*	*0.7*	*76*	*4.6*	*13.6*	*0.3*	*3.8*
Baked, in Tomato Sauce, Rich, Simply, M&S*	½ Can/205g	184	0.8	90	5.1	14.6	0.4	4
Baked, Mexican, Mean, Beanz, Heinz*	½ Can/208g	158	1	76	5	12.9	0.5	4
Baked, Peri Peri, Beanz, Heinz*	½ Can/195g	176	1.4	90	5.2	13.7	0.7	4.2
Baked, Smokey Bacon, Beanz, Heinz*	½ Can/195g	179	2.1	92	4.9	13.9	1.1	3.6
Baked, Sweet Chilli, Mean, Beanz, Heinz*	½ Can/195g	142	0.6	73	4.5	13	0.3	3.6
Baked, Virtually Fat Free, Heinz*	½ Can/207g	164	0.4	79	4.7	12.9	0.2	3.7
Baked, with Chicken Nuggets, Beanz, Heinz*	1 Can/200g	210	6.3	105	6.8	12.4	3.2	3.2
Baked, with Hidden Veg, Beanz, Heinz*	½ Can/208g	156	0.6	75	4.7	13.5	0.3	4.1
Baked, with HP Sauce, Beanz, Heinz*	½ Can/208g	158	0.6	76	4.8	13.7	0.3	3.9
Baked, with Lea Perrins Sauce, Beanz, Heinz*	1 Can/415g	303	0.8	73	4.8	13.1	0.2	3.8
Baked, with Sausages, Branston, Crosse & Blackwell*	½ Can/202g	233	6.5	115	6.9	12.2	3.2	5
Baked, with Spicy Meatballs, Beanz, Heinz*	1 Can/400g	372	9.6	93	5.8	12	2.4	2.9
Baked, with Vegan Burgers, Suma*	1 Can/400g	392	6.4	98	6.1	13	1.6	3.7
Baked, with Vegetable Sausages, Beanz, Heinz*	1 Sm Can/200g	210	7.2	105	6	12.2	3.6	2.9
Black, Cooked, Average	*1 Cup/172g*	*227*	*0.9*	*132*	*8.8*	*23.7*	*0.5*	*8.7*
Blackeye, Canned, Average	*1 Can/172g*	*206*	*1.3*	*120*	*8.4*	*19.8*	*0.8*	*3.3*
Blackeye, Dried, Raw	*1oz/28g*	*87*	*0.4*	*311*	*23.5*	*54.1*	*1.6*	*8.2*
Borlotti, Canned, Average	*1oz/28g*	*29*	*0.1*	*103*	*7.6*	*16.9*	*0.5*	*4.7*
Borlotti, Dried, Raw, Average	*1 Serving/100g*	*335*	*1.2*	*335*	*23*	*60*	*1.2*	*24.7*
Broad, Baby, Frozen, Simply, M&S*	1 Serving/80g	54	0.8	67	4.2	6.7	1	3.4
Broad, Canned, Drained, Average	*1 Can/195g*	*136*	*1.1*	*70*	*6.9*	*9.2*	*0.6*	*6.8*
Broad, Crispy, Wasabi Flavoured, Khao Shong*	1 Serving/30g	116	3	386	17	57	10	7
Broad, Dried, Raw, Average	*1oz/28g*	*69*	*0.6*	*245*	*26.1*	*32.5*	*2.1*	*27.6*
Broad, Fresh, without Pod, Boiled, Average	*1 Serving/80g*	*78*	*0.5*	*97*	*7.9*	*11.7*	*0.6*	*6.5*
Broad, Fried, Tesco*	½ Pack/40g	174	6.6	436	21.8	45.5	16.6	8.5
Broad, Frozen, Average	*1 Serving/80g*	*63*	*0.6*	*79*	*7.6*	*10.8*	*0.7*	*5.3*
Butter, Canned, Drained, Average	*1oz/28g*	*23*	*0.1*	*81*	*6*	*12.8*	*0.5*	*4.3*
Butter, Dried, Boiled, Average	*1oz/28g*	*30*	*0.2*	*106*	*7.2*	*18.6*	*0.6*	*5.2*
Butter, Dried, Raw, Average	*1oz/28g*	*81*	*0.5*	*290*	*19.1*	*52.9*	*1.7*	*16*
Butter, Frozen, Tesco*	1 Serving/80g	42	0.1	52	2.3	9.5	0.1	1.9
Cannellini, Canned, Drained, Average	*1 Portion/80g*	*75*	*0.4*	*94*	*8.7*	*15*	*0.5*	*5.7*
Cannellini, Dried, Tesco*	1 Serving/32g	83	0.3	260	24.8	37.4	0.8	20.9
Cannellini, with Chorizo & Red Peppers, Morrisons*	½ Pack/100g	155	10	155	6.9	9.2	10	2.8
Chilli, Canned, Average	*1 Can/420g*	*381*	*3.1*	*91*	*5.2*	*15.8*	*0.7*	*4.4*

B

BEANS

INFO/WEIGHT	Measure KCAL	FAT	KCAL	PROT	CARB	FAT	FIBRE
Dry Roasted, Mix, The Food Doctor*	1 Portion/25g	98	3.3	392	34	23.6	13.2	21.2
Edamame, Sainsbury's*	1 Serving/150g	212	9.6	141	12.3	6.8	6.4	4.2
Edamame, Shelled, Frozen, Mama San*	1 Serving/80g	130	6.1	163	13	10.6	7.6	9
Edamame, Shelled, Frozen, Yutaka*	1 Serving/80g	102	5	128	10.8	4.5	6.3	0
Edamame, Smokin', Mix, The Food Doctor*	1 Serving/30g	128	4.6	426	18.5	47.2	15.3	12.6
Edamame, with Soy Sauce, On the Go, Sainsbury's*	1 Pot/100g	119	5.8	119	11.4	20	5.8	6.5
Fajita Beanz, Heinz*	½ Can/196g	155	1.6	79	4	11.7	0.8	4.5
Fine, Trimmed, Boiled, Growers Selection, Asda*	1 Portion/76g	26	0.2	34	2.1	4	0.3	4.1
Flageolet, Canned, Average	*1 Can/265g*	*235*	*1.6*	*89*	*6.8*	*14*	*0.6*	*3.5*
Flageolet, Dried, Love Life, Waitrose*	1 Serving/50g	125	3.1	250	30.4	19.8	6.2	40.4
Four, Mix, Frozen, Tesco*	1 Serving/80g	83	0.3	103	8	8.4	0.4	17.1
French, Boiled, Average	*1 Serving/150g*	*38*	*0*	*25*	*2.3*	*3.8*	*0*	*3.7*
French, Canned, Average	*1oz/28g*	*5*	*0.1*	*17*	*1.3*	*2.7*	*0.2*	*1.9*
French, Raw	*1oz/28g*	*6*	*0.1*	*20*	*1.6*	*2.7*	*0.4*	*1.8*
Green, Cut, Average	*1oz/28g*	*7*	*0.1*	*24*	*1.7*	*3.6*	*0.2*	*2.7*
Green, Fine, Average	*1 Serving/75g*	*18*	*0.3*	*24*	*1.8*	*3.2*	*0.4*	*2.9*
Green, Sliced, Average	*1oz/28g*	*6*	*0.1*	*23*	*1.9*	*3.5*	*0.2*	*2.1*
Green, Sliced, Frozen, Average	*1 Serving/50g*	*13*	*0*	*26*	*1.8*	*4.4*	*0.1*	*4.1*
Green, Whole, Average	*1oz/28g*	*6*	*0.1*	*22*	*1.6*	*3*	*0.4*	*1.7*
Haricot, Canned, Average	*1 Can/400g*	*307*	*2*	*77*	*6.2*	*10.7*	*0.5*	*5.9*
Haricot, Dried, Boiled in Unsalted Water	*1oz/28g*	*27*	*0.1*	*95*	*6.6*	*17.2*	*0.5*	*6.1*
Haricot, Dried, Raw	*1 Serving/100g*	*286*	*1.6*	*286*	*22.4*	*49.7*	*1.6*	*17*
Keen Bean, Mix, Graze*	1 Punnet/31g	153	10.2	486	30.5	27.6	32.5	7.1
Kidney, Curried, Rajmah, Sohna *	½ Can/225g	217	1.1	97	3.7	17.6	0.5	1.4
Kidney, Red, Canned, Drained, Average	*½ Can/120g*	*115*	*0.7*	*96*	*7.4*	*20.7*	*0.5*	*5.5*
Kidney, Red, Dried, Boiled in Unsalted Water	*1oz/28g*	*29*	*0.1*	*103*	*8.4*	*17.4*	*0.5*	*6.7*
Kidney, Red, Dried, Raw	*1oz/28g*	*74*	*0.4*	*266*	*22.1*	*44.1*	*1.4*	*15.7*
Kidney, Red, in Chilli Sauce, Sainsbury's*	1 Can/420g	365	1.7	87	5.3	15.6	0.4	4.5
Kidney, White, Dry, Raw, Unico*	½ Cup/80g	270	0.9	338	22.5	61.2	1.1	21.2
Lupin, Avg *	1 Serving/80g	297	8	371	36	40	10	19
Mexican Style, Mix, Tinned, Asda*	1 Serving/81g	71	0.6	88	8.7	11.8	0.7	10.4
Mexican, Creationz, Heinz*	1 Can/390g	308	3.1	79	4	11.7	0.8	4.5
Mix, Great Fire Dragon, Graze*	1 Pack/25g	123	7	491	15	48.1	28.1	2.5
Mixed, Canned, Average	*1 Can/300g*	*300*	*3.5*	*100*	*6.8*	*15.6*	*1.2*	*4.1*
Mixed, in Mild Chilli Sauce, Sainsbury's*	1 Can/420g	328	1.3	78	4.9	13.8	0.3	3.7
Mixed, in Tomato Sauce, Canned, CBY, Asda*	½ Can/203g	196	1	97	5	15.8	0.5	4.6
Mixed, in Water, Canned, Drained, Sweet Harvest, Aldi*	½ Can/120g	125	0.6	104	7.5	12	0.5	11
Mixed, Spicy, Average	*1 Serving/140g*	*108*	*0.7*	*78*	*4.8*	*13.4*	*0.5*	*3.9*
Mixed, with Lentils, Waitrose*	1 Pack/300g	399	21.9	133	5.1	11.6	7.3	3.1
Mixed, with Passata, Tesco*	1 Can/300g	237	2.1	79	6	12.1	0.7	3.9
Mung, Whole, Dried, Boiled in Unsalted Water	*1oz/28g*	*25*	*0.1*	*91*	*7.6*	*15.3*	*0.4*	*3*
Mung, Whole, Dried, Raw	*1oz/28g*	*78*	*0.3*	*279*	*23.9*	*46.3*	*1.1*	*10*
Pinto, Dried, Boiled in Unsalted Water	*1oz/28g*	*38*	*0.2*	*137*	*8.9*	*23.9*	*0.7*	*0*
Pinto, Dried, Raw	*1oz/28g*	*92*	*0.4*	*327*	*21.1*	*57.1*	*1.6*	*14*
Pinto, in Water, Canned, Drained, Asda*	1 Can/175g	170	1	97	6.5	13	0.6	7.1
Red, Stewed, Canned, TamTad*	½ Can/150g	150	15	100	5.2	15	10	0
Refried, Average	*1 Serving/215g*	*162*	*1.5*	*76*	*4.6*	*12.7*	*0.7*	*1.8*
Refried, Mild, M&S*	1 Can/206g	194	1.2	94	5.9	14	0.6	4.4
Refried, Tesco*	¼ Can/100g	81	0.6	81	4.8	11.7	0.6	4.8
Runner, Average	*1 Serving/80g*	*15*	*0.3*	*19*	*1.3*	*2.8*	*0.4*	*2.2*
Six, Mix, Cooks' Ingredients, Waitrose*	¼ Pack/100g	77	0.4	77	4.2	11.8	0.4	4.5
Smoky Spicy Mighty, in a Tomato Sauce, Jamie Oliver*	½ Pouch/125g	154	6.8	123	5	11	5.4	4.6
Soya, Black, in Filtered Water, Nature Organic*	1 Serving/200g	240	6.4	120	8.8	14.2	3.2	6.2

	Measure INFO/WEIGHT	per Measure KCAL	FAT	Nutrition Values per 100g / 100ml KCAL	PROT	CARB	FAT	FIBRE
BEANS								
Soya, Dried, Average	1oz/28g	104	5.1	370	34.2	15.4	18.3	19.6
Soya, Dried, Boiled in Unsalted Water	1oz/28g	39	2	141	14	5.1	7.3	6.1
Soya, Shelled, Frozen, Raw, Average	1 Serving/80g	99	4.3	124	12.2	6.9	5.3	4.4
Tuscan, Beanz, Heinz*	½ Can/195g	178	3.3	91	4.9	12	1.7	4.1
Wasabi, Mix, Whitworths*	1 Serving/25g	108	3.4	430	30.9	40.1	13.7	10.7
White, Campo Largo, Lidl*	½ Jar/200g	180	1	90	7.1	11.2	0.5	0
BEEF								
Brisket, Boiled, Lean	1 Serving/100g	225	11	225	31.4	0	11	0
Brisket, Boiled, Lean Fat	1 Serving/100g	268	17.4	268	27.8	0	17.4	0
Brisket, Braised, Lean	1 Serving/100g	280	17.4	280	29	0	17.4	0
Brisket, Raw, Lean	1oz/28g	39	1.7	139	21.1	0	6.1	0
Brisket, Raw, Lean & Fat	1oz/28g	60	4.4	216	18.2	0	15.8	0
Carpaccio Del Lago, Dry Cured, Unearthed*	½ Pack/35g	41	0.5	116	26	0.5	1.4	0.5
Cheeks, Ox, Aberdeen Angus, Waitrose*	1 Serving/100g	123	4.6	123	22	0	4.6	0
Diced, Casserole, Lean, Average	1oz/28g	35	1.1	126	23	0	3.8	0
Escalope, Healthy Range, Average	1 Serving/170g	233	6.7	137	24.2	1.2	4	0.4
Flank, Pot-Roasted, Lean	1oz/28g	71	3.9	253	31.8	0	14	0
Flank, Pot-Roasted, Lean & Fat	1oz/28g	85	6.1	303	26.6	0	21.9	0
Flank, Raw, Lean	1oz/28g	49	2.6	175	22.7	0	9.3	0
Flank, Raw, Lean & Fat	1oz/28g	74	5.8	266	19.7	0	20.8	0
Fore Rib, Lean & Fat, Average	1oz/28g	40	1.8	144	21.7	0	6.2	0.2
Fore Rib, Raw, Lean	1oz/28g	41	1.8	145	21.5	0	6.5	0
Fore Rib, Roasted, Lean	1oz/28g	66	3.2	236	33.3	0	11.4	0
Fore Rib, Roasted, Lean & Fat	1oz/28g	84	5.7	300	29.1	0	20.4	0
Grill Steak, Average	1 Steak/170g	501	39.5	295	19.3	2.1	23.2	0.1
Grill Steak, Peppered, Average	1 Serving/172g	419	24.4	244	23.6	5.2	14.2	0.3
Joint, for Roasting, Average	1oz/28g	38	1	134	24.5	1.4	3.4	0.2
Joint, Sirloin, Roasted, Lean	1oz/28g	53	1.8	188	32.4	0	6.5	0
Joint, Sirloin, Roasted, Lean & Fat	1oz/28g	65	3.5	233	29.8	0	12.6	0
Mince, Cooked, Average	1 Serving/75g	214	15.3	286	24	0	20.3	0
Mince, Extra Lean, Raw, Average	1 Serving/100g	124	5	124	21.2	0.1	5	0
Mince, Extra Lean, Stewed	1oz/28g	50	2.4	177	24.7	0	8.7	0
Mince, Lean, Raw, Average	1oz/28g	48	2.8	172	20.8	0	10	0.1
Mince, Raw, Average	1oz/28g	68	5.1	242	19.6	0.2	18.1	0
Mince, Raw, Frozen, Average	1 Serving/100g	176	10	176	20.4	0	10	0
Mince, Steak, Extra Lean, Average	1oz/28g	37	1.6	131	20.5	0.4	5.6	0
Mince, Steak, Raw, Average	1 Serving/125g	318	25	254	17.2	0	20	0
Mince, Stewed	1oz/28g	59	3.8	209	21.8	0	13.5	0
Peppered, Sliced, Average	1 Slice/20g	26	1.1	129	18.2	1.3	5.6	1
Potted, Binghams*	1 Serving/30g	76	6.6	254	13.8	1	22	0.6
Potted, with a Kick of Mustard, M&S*	¼ Jar19g	36	2.5	192	17.4	0.3	13.2	1.3
Roast, Sliced, Average	1 Slice/35g	48	1.3	136	26.1	0.4	3.6	0.2
Roast, with Horseradish Dip, Tesco*	1 Pack/90g	155	7.3	173	20.9	3.7	8.1	1
Salt, Average	1 Serving/70g	80	1.7	114	21.7	1	2.5	0.1
Salted, Dried, Raw	1oz/28g	70	0.4	250	55.4	0	1.5	0
Silverside, Pot-Roasted, Lean	1oz/28g	54	1.8	193	34	0	6.3	0
Silverside, Pot-Roasted, Lean & Fat	1oz/28g	69	3.8	247	31	0	13.7	0
Silverside, Raw, Lean	1oz/28g	38	1.2	134	23.8	0	4.3	0
Silverside, Raw, Lean & Fat	1oz/28g	60	4.1	213	20.2	0	14.7	0
Silverside, Salted, Boiled, Lean	1oz/28g	52	1.9	184	30.4	0	6.9	0
Silverside, Salted, Boiled, Lean & Fat	1oz/28g	63	3.5	224	27.9	0	12.5	0
Silverside, Salted, Raw, Lean	1oz/28g	39	2	140	19.2	0	7	0
Silverside, Salted, Raw, Lean & Fat	1oz/28g	64	5	227	16.3	0	18	0

B

	Measure INFO/WEIGHT	per Measure		Nutrition Values per 100g / 100ml				
		KCAL	FAT	KCAL	PROT	CARB	FAT	FIBRE
BEEF								
Sliced, Cooked, From Supermarket, Average	*1 Slice/35g*	*47*	*1.2*	*135*	*23.6*	*2*	*3.5*	*0.5*
Steak, 8oz Rump Chips	*1 Serving/466g*	*870*	*41.1*	*187*	*10.7*	*16.2*	*8.8*	*0*
Steak, Braising, Braised, Lean	*1oz/28g*	*63*	*2.7*	*225*	*34.4*	*0*	*9.7*	*0*
Steak, Braising, Braised, Lean & Fat	*1oz/28g*	*69*	*3.6*	*246*	*32.9*	*0*	*12.7*	*0*
Steak, Braising, Lean, Raw, Average	*1oz/28g*	*40*	*1.4*	*144*	*24.8*	*0*	*5*	*0*
Steak, Braising, Raw, Lean & Fat	*1oz/28g*	*44*	*2.4*	*158*	*20.5*	*0*	*8.5*	*0*
Steak, Economy, Average	*1oz/28g*	*53*	*2.4*	*190*	*26.9*	*1.2*	*8.7*	*0.4*
Steak, Fillet, Cooked, Average	*1oz/28g*	*54*	*2.4*	*191*	*28.6*	*0*	*8.5*	*0*
Steak, Fillet, Lean, Average	*1oz/28g*	*42*	*2*	*150*	*21*	*0*	*7.3*	*0*
Steak, Fillet, Lean, Cooked, Average	*1oz/28g*	*52*	*2.2*	*186*	*28.6*	*0*	*8*	*0*
Steak, Frying, Average	*1 Steak/110g*	*128*	*2.7*	*116*	*23.7*	*0*	*2.5*	*0*
Steak, Ranch, with Garlic Butter, Finest, Tesco*	1 Steak/136g	199	6.9	146	24	0.9	5.1	0.5
Steak, Rump, Cooked, Average	*1oz/28g*	*69*	*4*	*246*	*29.1*	*0.5*	*14.1*	*0*
Steak, Rump, Grilled, Rare, Lean	*1 Steak/227g*	*381*	*15.6*	*168*	*26.5*	*0*	*6.9*	*0*
Steak, Rump, Lean, Cooked, Average	*1oz/28g*	*50*	*1.7*	*179*	*31*	*0*	*6.1*	*0*
Steak, Rump, Raw, Lean & Fat	*1oz/28g*	*49*	*2.8*	*174*	*20.7*	*0*	*10.1*	*0*
Steak, Rump, Raw, Lean, Average	*1 Steak/175g*	*219*	*7.2*	*125*	*22*	*0*	*4.1*	*0*
Steak, Sirloin, Fried, Rare, Lean	*1oz/28g*	*53*	*2.3*	*189*	*28.8*	*0*	*8.2*	*0*
Steak, Sirloin, Fried, Rare, Lean & Fat	*1oz/28g*	*65*	*3.9*	*231*	*26.5*	*0*	*13.9*	*0*
Steak, Sirloin, Grilled, Medium-Rare, Lean	*1oz/28g*	*49*	*2.2*	*176*	*26.6*	*0*	*7.7*	*0*
Steak, Sirloin, Grilled, Medium-Rare, Lean & Fat	*1oz/28g*	*59*	*3.5*	*211*	*24.6*	*0*	*12.5*	*0*
Steak, Sirloin, Grilled, Rare, Lean	*1oz/28g*	*46*	*1.9*	*166*	*26.4*	*0*	*6.7*	*0*
Steak, Sirloin, Grilled, Rare, Lean & Fat	*1oz/28g*	*60*	*3.6*	*216*	*25.1*	*0*	*12.8*	*0*
Steak, Sirloin, Grilled, Well-Done, Lean	*1oz/28g*	*63*	*2.8*	*225*	*33.9*	*0*	*9.9*	*0*
Steak, Sirloin, Grilled, Well-Done, Lean & Fat	*1oz/28g*	*71*	*4*	*254*	*31.5*	*0*	*14.3*	*0*
Steak, Sirloin, Raw, Lean & Fat	*1oz/28g*	*56*	*3.6*	*201*	*21.6*	*0*	*12.7*	*0*
Steak, Sirloin, Raw, Lean, Average	*1 Steak/150g*	*202*	*6.8*	*135*	*23.5*	*0*	*4.5*	*0*
Steaks, British, Louisiana Inspired, BBQ, Waitrose*	1 Steak/112g	197	6.3	176	28	3.1	5.6	0.7
Stewed Steak, Average	*1 Serving/220g*	*258*	*10.1*	*117*	*15.8*	*3.3*	*4.6*	*0*
Stewing Steak, Lean Fat, Raw, Average	*1 Serving/100g*	*136*	*4.3*	*136*	*24.2*	*0.1*	*4.3*	*0.1*
Stewing Steak, Raw, Lean	*1oz/28g*	*34*	*1*	*122*	*22.6*	*0*	*3.5*	*0*
Stewing Steak, Stewed, Lean	*1oz/28g*	*52*	*1.8*	*185*	*32*	*0*	*6.3*	*0*
Stewing Steak, Stewed, Lean & Fat	*1oz/28g*	*57*	*2.7*	*203*	*29.2*	*0*	*9.6*	*0*
Stir Fry Strips, Raw, Average	*1 Serving/125g*	*149*	*3.8*	*119*	*23*	*0*	*3*	*0.2*
Tongue, Raw, Average	*1 Serving/100g*	*224*	*16.1*	*224*	*14.9*	*3.7*	*16.1*	*0*
Topside, Lean Fat, Raw, Average	*1oz/28g*	*55*	*3.6*	*198*	*20.4*	*0*	*12.9*	*0*
Topside, Raw, Lean	*1oz/28g*	*32*	*0.8*	*116*	*23*	*0*	*2.7*	*0*
Vegetarian, Pieces, Beef Style, Quorn*	½ Pack/75g	69	1.7	92	13.5	4.5	2.2	5
Vegetarian, Slices, Peppered Style, Quorn*	¼ Pack/25g	29	0.5	115	14.5	7.6	2.1	4
Vegetarian, Steak Strips, Frozen, Quorn*	¼ Pack/75g	75	1.8	100	14.3	4.3	2.4	6
Vegetarian, Steaks, Peppered, Quorn*	1 Steak/98g	123	3.9	126	13.6	5.7	4	6.9
Wafer Thin Sliced, Cooked, Average	*1 Slice/10g*	*13*	*0.3*	*129*	*24.5*	*0.5*	*3.2*	*0.2*
BEEF &								
Black Bean Sauce, M&S*	½ Pack/175g	210	10.2	120	10.9	5.4	5.8	1.4
Black Bean with Rice, Weight Watchers*	1 Pack/320g	288	4.2	90	5	14.6	1.3	0.1
Onions with Gravy, Minced, Lean, Sainsbury's*	1 Sm Can/198g	285	13.9	144	17	3.1	7	0.2
Onions, Minced, Asda*	½ Can/196g	314	19.6	160	13	4.6	10	0.1
BEEF BOURGUIGNON								
Finest, Tesco*	½ Pack/300g	247	7.8	82	9.9	4.8	2.6	0.5
BEEF BRAISED								
Braised, Mash, Mini Meal, Tesco*	1 Pack/241g	251	9.2	104	6.5	10.5	3.8	1.1
Steak Mash, Tastes of Home, M Kitchen, Morrisons*	1 Meal/250g	209	6	87	6.4	9.1	2.5	1.1
Steak, Braised, & Mash, British, Meal for One, M&S*	1 Meal/450g	369	11.2	82	6.7	7.3	2.5	1.9

	Measure INFO/WEIGHT	per Measure KCAL	FAT	Nutrition Values per 100g / 100ml KCAL	PROT	CARB	FAT	FIBRE
BEEF BRAISED								
Steak, with Root Vegetable Crush, British, COU, M&S*	1 Pack/380g	243	3.8	64	7.1	5.9	1	1.4
Tender, Pub Specials, Birds Eye*	1 Pack/450g	243	3.6	54	5.5	6.1	0.8	1.8
BEEF CRISPY CHILLI								
Cantonese, Chilled, Sainsbury's*	1 Pack/250g	682	38.8	273	11.4	22.1	15.5	1.9
Tesco*	1 Pack/250g	472	17.2	189	10.8	21	6.9	0.5
BEEF DINNER								
British Classic, Serves 1, Classic, Sainsbury's*	1 Pack/400g	500	12.4	125	8.5	14.7	3.1	2.1
Roast with Trimmings	*1 Dinner/840g*	*1310*	*63*	*156*	*6.1*	*17.7*	*7.5*	*2.3*
Roast, Yorkshire Pudding, Potatoes, Veg, & Gravy, Iceland*	1 Pack/413g	429	5.4	104	6.2	15.8	1.3	2.4
BEEF IN								
Black Bean Sauce, CBY, Asda*	1 Pack/375g	368	12.4	98	8.5	8.2	3.3	0.8
Black Bean Sauce, Chinese Takeaway, Morrisons*	½ Pack/168g	234	11.3	139	10.3	8.3	6.7	2.3
Black Bean Sauce, Chinese, Tesco*	1 Pack/400g	396	12.4	99	9.1	8.7	3.1	0.5
Black Bean, Chinese Favourites Box, M&S*	½ Pack/120g	152	8.3	127	7.8	7.6	6.9	1.4
Black Pepper Sauce Egg Fried Rice, Tesco*	1 Pack/451g	622	24.8	138	7	15.2	5.5	1.2
Gravy, Roast, Birds Eye*	1 Pack/227g	177	3.9	78	13.4	2.2	1.7	0
Gravy, Sliced, Tesco*	1 Serving/200g	152	4.2	76	11.3	3.1	2.1	0.2
Rich Ale Gravy, Slow Cooked Brisket, COU, M&S*	1 Pack/350g	242	6.7	69	8.4	3.7	1.9	1.6
BEEF RAGU								
with Rigatoni Pasta, Chianti, Balanced for You, M&S*	1 Pack/400g	484	12.4	121	10.3	12.1	3.1	1.5
BEEF SZECHUAN								
Sizzling Hot Spicy, Oriental Express*	1 Pack/400g	380	7.6	95	6.4	13.2	1.9	2
BEEF WELLINGTON								
Average	*1 Serving/200g*	*530*	*33.3*	*265*	*12.4*	*17*	*16.6*	*1*
Extra Special, Asda*	1 Serving/218g	605	37.1	277	11	20	17	0.9
BEEF WITH								
Black Bean Sauce, Chilli, Sainsbury's*	1 Pack/300g	336	14.4	112	8.7	8.6	4.8	1
Black Bean Sauce, Rice Bowl, Uncle Ben's*	1 Pack/350g	368	4.9	105	5.6	17.4	1.4	0
Onion & Gravy, Minced, Princes*	1 Serving/200g	342	24.4	171	9.9	5.5	12.2	0
Oyster Sauce, Ooodles of Noodles, Oriental Express*	1 Pack/425g	378	5.5	89	4.9	14.2	1.3	1.5
Peppercorn Sauce, Steak, Just Cook, Sainsbury's*	½ Pack/128g	174	7.3	136	17.7	3.4	5.7	1.2
Steak, Rump with a Peppercorn Sauce, Waitrose*	½ Pack/180g	189	5.9	105	17.9	0.9	3.3	0.2
Steak, Rump, with Peppercorn Sauce, M&S*	½ Pack/213g	281	8.7	132	19.4	4.2	4.1	0.1
Vegetables & Gravy, Minced, Birds Eye*	1 Pack/178g	155	6.1	87	9.1	5.1	3.4	0.6
BEER								
Ale, 1698, Kentish Strong, Shepherd Neame*	1 Bottle/500ml	285	0	57	0.4	4.8	0	0
Ale, Bottled, Old Speckled Hen*	1 Bottle/330ml	124	0.3	38	0.2	1.8	0.1	0.2
Ale, Freeminer, Organic, Fairtrade, Co-Op*	1 Bottle/480ml	240	0.5	50	0.2	2.7	0.1	0
Ale, Gingerbread, Wychwood, Marstons PLC*	1 Bottle/500ml	304	0	61	0.3	3	0	0
Ale, Goliath, Wychwood, Marstons PLC*	1 Bottle/500ml	191	0	38	0.4	2.8	0	0
Ale, Honey Dew, Fullers*	1 Bottle/500ml	232	0	46	0	4.6	0	0
Ale, Hopped Bourbon, Cask, Innis & Gunn*	1 Bottle/330ml	201	0	61	0	4.9	0	0
Ale, Hopping Hare, Hall Woodhouse Ltd*	1 Bottle/500ml	189	0	38	0.4	3	0	0
Ale, Old Peculiar, Theakstons*	1 Serving/500ml	250	0	50	0	4.6	0	0
Ale, Old Speckled Hen*	1 Pint/568ml	185	0.6	32	0.2	1.6	0.1	0.2
Ale, Pale, Alcohol Free, Innis & Gunn*	1 Can/330ml	66	0	20	0.5	4.7	0	0
Ale, Pale, IPA, Greene King*	1 Pint/568ml	157	0.1	28	0.2	1.6	0	0.1
Ale, Pale, IPA, Innis & Gunn*	1 Bottle/330ml	162	0	49	0.3	4.6	0	0
Ale, Pale, IPA, TTD, Sainsbury's*	½ Bottle/250ml	128	0	51	0.5	4.4	0	0.5
Ale, Pale, Sierra Nevada*	1 Bottle/350g	175	0	50	0.4	4	0	0
Ale, Scarecrow, Wychwood, Marstons PLC*	1 Bottle/500ml	214	0	43	0.4	4.3	0	0
Ale, Wychcraft, Wychwood, Marstons PLC*	1 Bottle/500ml	210	0	42	0.3	4.2	0	0
Becks Blue Lemon, No Alcohol, Beck & Co*	1 Bottle/1196ml	275	0.1	23	0.2	6	0	0

	Measure INFO/WEIGHT	per Measure KCAL	per Measure FAT	Nutrition Values per 100g / 100ml KCAL	PROT	CARB	FAT	FIBRE
BEER								
Bitter, Average	*1 Can/440ml*	*141*	*0*	*32*	*0.3*	*2.3*	*0*	*0*
Bitter, Banks, Marstons PLC*	1 Pint/568ml	193	0.1	34	0.3	3.4	0	0
Bitter, Cask, Draught, London Pride, Fullers*	1 Pint/568ml	201	0	35	0	0	0	0
Bitter, Draught, Average	*1 Pint/568ml*	*182*	*0*	*32*	*0.3*	*2.3*	*0*	*0*
Bitter, Keg, Average	*1 Pint/568ml*	*176*	*0*	*31*	*0.3*	*2.3*	*0*	*0*
Bitter, Low Alcohol, Average	*1 Pint/568ml*	*74*	*0*	*13*	*0.2*	*2.1*	*0*	*0*
Bitter, Original, Tetley's*	1 Can/440ml	140	0	32	0.2	4.6	0	0
Bitter, Oxford Gold, Brakspear*	1 Bottle/500ml	161	0	32	0	0	0	0
Bitter, Strong, Broadside, Adnams*	1 Bottle/500ml	285	0	57	0	0	0	0
Brown Ale, Bottled, Average	*1 Bottle/330ml*	*99*	*0*	*30*	*0.3*	*3*	*0*	*0*
Brune, Leffe*	1 Bottle/330ml	184	0	56	0.5	11.3	0	0
Especial, Modelo*	1 Bottle/355ml	145	0	41	0	1.1	0	0
Guinness* Extra Stout, Bottled	1 Bottle/500ml	215	0	43	4	0	0	0
Guinness, Draught*	*1 Can/440ml*	*158*	*0.2*	*36*	*0.3*	*3*	*0*	*0*
Guinness, Stout*	*1 Pint/568ml*	*205*	*0*	*36*	*0.3*	*3*	*0*	*0*
Kilkenny, Diageo*	1 Pint/568ml	210	0	37	0.3	3	0	0
Low Calorie, Low Carb, Cobra*	1 Bottle/330ml	96	0	29	0.1	1.3	0	0
Mackeson, Stout	*1 Pint/568ml*	*205*	*0*	*36*	*0.4*	*4.6*	*0*	*0*
Mild, Draught, Average	*1 Pint/568ml*	*136*	*0*	*24*	*0.2*	*1.6*	*0*	*0*
Non Alcoholic, Zero, Cobra*	1 Bottle/330ml	79	0	24	0.8	2	0	0
Oak Aged, Original, Innis Gunn*	1 Bottle/330ml	182	0	55	0.3	4.7	0	0
Raspberry, Framboise, Lindemans*	1 Serving/355ml	185	0	52	0	8.8	0	0
Rum Finish, Oak Aged, Innis Gunn*	1 Bottle/330ml	188	0	57	0.3	4.8	0	0
Stout, Coopers*	1 Pint/375ml	191	0	51	0	2.9	0	0
Ultra, Michelob*	1 Bottle/275ml	88	0	32	0	0.9	0	0
Weissbier, Alcohol Free, Erdinger*	1 Bottle/500ml	125	0	25	0.4	5.3	0	0
Wheat, Tesco*	1 Bottle/500ml	155	0	31	0.5	0.4	0	0
BEETROOT								
Baby, Horseradish, Black Pepper, Finest, Tesco*	4 Beetroot/80g	77	0.3	96	2.3	18.5	0.4	4.4
Baby, Pickled, Average	*1 Beetroot/12g*	*5*	*0*	*37*	*1.7*	*7.2*	*0.1*	*1.2*
Cooked, Boiled, Drained, Average	*1 Serving/100g*	*44*	*0.2*	*44*	*1.7*	*10*	*0.2*	*2*
Golden, Spaghetti, Tesco*	½ Pack/125g	54	0.1	43	1.7	7.3	0.1	2.8
Grated, Tesco*	1 Serving/80g	34	0.1	42	1.7	7.2	0.1	2.8
Pickled, in Sweet Vinegar, Average	*1oz/28g*	*16*	*0*	*57*	*1.2*	*12.8*	*0.1*	*1.5*
Pickled, in Vinegar, Average	*1 Serving/50g*	*18*	*0*	*36*	*1.6*	*7.3*	*0.1*	*1.2*
Raw, Unprepared, Average	*1oz/28g*	*8*	*0*	*29*	*1.4*	*5.4*	*0.1*	*1.7*
Rosebud, M&S*	½ Pack/90g	45	0.3	50	1.9	8.9	0.3	3.2
Rosebud, Sweet Chilli Marinated, M&S*	1 Serving/80g	52	0.2	65	1.5	12.3	0.3	3.6
with Balsamic Vinaigrette, Side Salad, M&S*	1 Pack/225g	146	2.9	65	0.7	12.4	1.3	2.2
BERRIES								
Medley, Grapes, Strawberry, Blueberry, Blackberry, Tesco*	1/ 2 Pack/120g	67	0.2	56	0.6	12.2	0.2	1
Mixed, Strawberries, Raspberries & Blueberries, Tesco*	½ Pack/150g	102	0.4	68	0.7	14.5	0.3	2.4
Mixed, Summer Fruits, Frozen, Tesco*	1 Serving/80g	30	0.2	37	1.1	6.2	0.2	3.2
BHAJI								
Aubergine, & Potato, Fried in Vegetable Oil, Average	*1oz/28g*	*36*	*2.5*	*130*	*2*	*12*	*8.8*	*1.7*
Cabbage, & Pea, Fried in Vegetable Oil, Average	*1oz/28g*	*50*	*4.1*	*178*	*3.3*	*9.2*	*14.7*	*3.4*
Cauliflower, Fried in Vegetable Oil, Average	*1oz/28g*	*60*	*5.7*	*214*	*4*	*4*	*20.5*	*2*
Indian Snack Selection, Chef Select, Lidl*	1 Serving/50g	125	7.2	250	5.6	22.1	14.3	5.3
Kale, Calcutta, Oven baked, Mumbai Street Food, Iceland*	2 Bhajis/52g	163	10.7	316	7.2	23.1	20.7	4.2
Mushroom, Fried in Vegetable Oil, Average	*1oz/28g*	*46*	*4.5*	*166*	*1.7*	*4.4*	*16.1*	*1.3*
Okra, Bangladeshi, Fried in Butter Ghee, Average	*1oz/28g*	*27*	*1.8*	*95*	*2.5*	*7.6*	*6.4*	*3.2*
Onion, Fried in Vegetable Oil, Takeaway, Average	*1 Bhaji/70g*	*190*	*10.3*	*270*	*9.8*	*24.6*	*14.7*	*5.6*
Onion, Frozen, Tesco*	1 Bhaji/14g	28	1.4	203	6.3	20.1	9.8	4.5

	Measure INFO/WEIGHT	per Measure KCAL	per Measure FAT	Nutrition Values per 100g / 100ml KCAL	PROT	CARB	FAT	FIBRE
BHAJI								
Onion, Indian Starter Selection, M&S*	1 Bhaji/22g	57	3.7	260	5.7	19.3	17	3.5
Onion, Indian, Mini, Asda*	1 Bhaji/18g	33	1.8	186	4.9	19	10	6
Onion, M&S*	1 Bhaji/42g	100	5.3	237	5.1	24	12.6	3.5
Onion, Mini, Tesco*	1 Bhaji/23g	48	1.9	210	7.3	26.7	8.2	1.3
Onion, Tesco*	1 Bhaji/47g	85	4.9	181	5.7	16.2	10.4	4.3
Onion, Waitrose*	1 Bhaji/45g	124	9.4	276	4.7	17.5	20.8	2.5
Potato, & Onion, Fried in Vegetable Oil, Average	*1oz/28g*	*45*	*2.8*	*160*	*2.1*	*16.6*	*10.1*	*1.6*
Potato, Onion Mushroom, Fried, Average	*1oz/28g*	*58*	*4.9*	*208*	*2*	*12*	*17.5*	*1.5*
Potato, Spinach Cauliflower, Fried, Average	*1oz/28g*	*47*	*4.2*	*169*	*2.2*	*7.1*	*15.1*	*1.4*
Spinach, & Potato, Fried in Vegetable Oil, Average	*1oz/28g*	*53*	*3.9*	*191*	*3.7*	*13.4*	*14.1*	*2.3*
Spinach, Fried in Vegetable Oil, Average	*1oz/28g*	*23*	*1.9*	*83*	*3.3*	*2.6*	*6.8*	*2.4*
Vegetable, Fried in Vegetable Oil, Average	*1oz/28g*	*59*	*5.2*	*212*	*2.1*	*10.1*	*18.5*	*2.4*
BHUNA								
Chicken, Curry, Tesco*	1 Serving/300g	396	22.8	132	11.4	4.5	7.6	0.5
Chicken, Indian Takeaway, Tesco*	1 Pack/350g	438	27.6	125	8.3	4.6	7.9	2.2
Chicken, Tikka, Tesco*	1 Pack/350g	438	23.4	125	11.3	5	6.7	0.9
Chicken, with Naan Bread, Sharwood's*	1 Pack/375g	465	19.1	124	6.8	12.8	5.1	2.8
Chicken, with Rice, Ready Meal, Average	*1 Pack/350g*	*444*	*20.8*	*127*	*9.4*	*8.9*	*5.9*	*1.4*
Lamb, & Rice, Sainsbury's*	1 Pack/500g	619	26.5	124	7.4	11.6	5.3	2
Prawn, Co-Op*	1 Pack/400g	300	16	75	3	6	4	1
Prawn, King, M&S*	1 Pack/400g	308	15.2	77	6.7	3.3	3.8	1.5
Prawn, King, Morrisons*	1 Pack/350g	301	20.6	86	6.5	1.8	5.9	0.5
BILBERRIES								
Fresh, Raw	*1oz/28g*	*8*	*0.1*	*29*	*0.6*	*6.8*	*0.2*	*1.8*
BILTONG								
Average	*1 Serving/25g*	*64*	*1*	*256*	*50*	*0*	*4*	*0*
BIRYANI								
Chicken Tikka, Lentil Pilau, Fuller Longer, M&S*	1 Pack/400g	440	11.6	110	9.5	12	2.9	2.3
Chicken, Indian, Asda*	1 Pack/450g	778	22.5	173	9	23	5	0.7
Chicken, LC, Tesco*	1 Serving/450g	495	10.3	110	7	15	2.3	3.4
Chicken, Ready Meal, Average	*1 Pack/400g*	*521*	*17.1*	*130*	*7.5*	*15.2*	*4.3*	*1.6*
Chicken, Tikka, Ready Meal, Average	*1 Pack/400g*	*460*	*11.5*	*115*	*7.3*	*14.8*	*2.9*	*1.5*
Chicken, Vegetarian, Linda McCartney*	½ Pack/180g	300	11.7	167	8.6	17	6.5	3.3
Lamb, Average	*1 Serving/200g*	*390*	*19.4*	*195*	*7.3*	*20.9*	*9.7*	*0*
Lamb, HL, Tesco*	1 Pack/400g	560	17.6	140	5.1	19	4.4	3.1
Vegetable, Curry, Microwaved, Slimzone, Asda*	1 Pack/459g	395	2.3	86	3.3	16	0.5	2.9
Vegetable, HL, Tesco*	1 Pack/450g	454	9.4	101	2.7	17.9	2.1	1.6
Vegetable, Sainsbury's*	1 Serving/225g	328	17.8	146	2.4	16.3	7.9	1.1
Vegetable, Waitrose*	1 Pack/450g	521	19.8	116	2.4	14.9	4.4	3.6
Vegetarian, Chicken Style, Lunch Pot, Quorn*	1 Pot/300g	300	13	100	3.5	10.9	4.4	1.7
BISCUITS								
Breakfast, Fruit Seed, Weight Watchers *	2 Biscuits/36g	159	5.4	442	8	64.7	15.1	7.9
Abbey Crunch, McVitie's*	1 Biscuit/9g	43	1.6	477	6	72.8	17.9	2.5
Abernethy, Simmers*	1 Biscuit/12g	61	2.7	490	5.7	69.2	21.9	0
Ace Milk Chocolate, McVitie's*	1 Biscuit/24g	122	5.9	510	6.1	66.2	24.5	1.6
Aero, Nestle*	1 Bar/19g	99	5.4	534	6.4	59.4	29.4	2.1
Aero, Orange, Aero, Nestle*	1 Biscuit/19g	101	5.6	534	6	60.6	29.3	1.7
After Eight, Nestle*	1 Biscuit/5g	26	1.4	525	6.5	62.6	27.7	1.5
All Butter, M&S*	1 Biscuit/8g	42	2.1	505	5.8	63.1	25	2.2
All Butter, Tesco*	1 Biscuit/9g	44	2.1	486	6.3	63.5	23	1.9
Almond Chocolate, Biscotti, TTD, Sainsbury's*	1 Biscuit/30g	132	4.8	440	8.4	65.6	16	3.1
Almond Butter Thins, Extra Special, Asda*	1 Biscuit/4g	15	0.5	375	5	60	12.5	2.5
Almond Thins, Continental, Tesco*	1 Biscuit/3g	15	0.5	450	6.7	72.8	14.7	3.1

B

BISCUITS

INFO/WEIGHT	Measure	per Measure		Nutrition Values per 100g / 100ml				
		KCAL	FAT	KCAL	PROT	CARB	FAT	FIBRE
Almond Thins, Sainsbury's*	1 Biscuit/3g	13	0.3	430	7	80.3	9	1
Almond, Artisan Bakery, Extra Special, Asda*	1 Biscuit/19g	103	6.1	548	7.9	54.3	32.3	4.2
Almond, Thins, TTD, Sainsbury's*	1 Biscuit/4g	16	0.5	450	6.7	72.8	14.7	3.1
Amaretti, Average	*1 Biscuit/5g*	*22*	*0.8*	*434*	*8.1*	*66.4*	*15.4*	*2.8*
Amaretti, Doria*	1 Biscuit/4g	17	0.3	433	6	84.8	7.8	0
Amaretti, M&S*	1 Biscuit/6g	30	1.1	480	9.6	71.3	17.2	3.8
Amaretti, Sainsbury's*	1 Biscuit/6g	27	0.7	450	6.5	80.5	11.3	1.1
Amaretti, Soft, Arden Amici*	1 Biscuit/10g	47	2.5	470	13	46	25	5
Anzac, Bitesmart*	1 Biscuit/20g	84	4.6	420	5.1	46.8	23	0
Apple Blackberry, Oat Squares, Go Ahead, McVitie's*	1 Bar/40g	137	3.8	343	4.5	63.8	9.5	4.2
Apple Cinnamon Thins, Finest, Tesco*	1 Biscuit/5g	22	0.8	470	5.9	71.7	17.5	1.5
Apple Raisin, Slices, G&C, Asda*	1 Pack/29g	109	1.3	382	6	77	4.5	4.5
Apple Crumble, Officially Low Fat, Fox's*	1 Biscuit/23g	85	0.6	365	5.4	80.4	2.4	2.5
Apricot Yoghurt, Coupland's Bakeries*	1 Biscuit/30g	145	7.6	483	1.5	62.4	25.5	0
Apricot, Low Fat, M&S*	1 Biscuit/23g	79	1	343	6.1	69.6	4.4	7.8
Arrowroot, Thin, Crawfords*	1 Biscuit/7g	35	1.2	450	6.9	71.4	15.2	2.8
Baked Bites, Cheddar, Mini, Cathedral City*	1 Pack/22g	115	6.4	521	12.2	51.4	29.2	2.6
Belgian Chocolate Chip, Walkers Shortbread Ltd*	2 Biscuits/25g	124	6.1	494	5.1	63.3	24.5	2.2
Belgian Chocolate, Selection, Finest, Tesco*	1 Biscuit/10g	52	2.7	515	6	62	27	3
Belgian Chocolate, Thins, Extra Special, Asda*	1 Biscuit/9g	44	2	503	7	67	23	0.2
Belgian Milk Chocolate, M&S*	1 Biscuit/12g	60	2.5	490	6.2	70.1	20.3	2.5
Berry GI, Diet Chef Ltd*	1 Biscuit/20g	87	3.2	435	7	65.2	16.1	7.2
Billionaire, Salted Caramel, Squares, Moments, McVitie's*	1 Square/41g	194	10.4	473	3.8	56.6	25.4	1.3
Bisc & Twix, Master Foods*	1 Bar/27g	140	7.6	520	5.2	61.1	28.3	0
Biscbits, Honeycomb Crunch, Cadbury*	7 Pieces/25g	120	5.2	480	6	67.3	20.9	1.4
Biscotti, Almond, Kate's Cakes Ltd*	1 Biscotti/36g	137	5.5	381	8.8	51.7	15.4	3.1
Biscotti, Chocolate Chip, Kate's Cakes Ltd*	1 Biscotti/36g	134	4.6	372	6.5	57.9	12.7	2.7
Biscotti, Chocolate, Heinz*	1 Biscotti/20g	80	1.7	398	8.5	72	8.7	5.8
Biscuits, Digestive, Thins, Capuccino, Mcvitie's*	1 Biscuit/6g	31	1.5	508	6.9	64	24.2	3.1
Black Forest Gateau, Moments , Special K, Kellogg's*	2 Biscuits/25g	95	2.2	381	5.2	72	9	2.4
Blackcurrant with Wheat Bran, Bisca*	1 Biscuit/8g	32	0.9	420	6	72	12	5.5
Blueberry Vanilla, Oaty, Weight Watchers*	1 Biscuit/19g	86	3.3	452	7.3	62.1	17.6	8
Blueberry, Biscuit Moments, Special K, Kellogg's*	2 Biscuits/25g	99	2.3	394	4.5	73	9	1.5
Bn, Chocolate Flavour, McVitie's*	1 Biscuit/18g	83	3	460	6.6	71	16.7	2.6
Bn, Strawberry Flavour, McVitie's*	1 Biscuit/18g	71	1.2	395	5.6	78	6.8	0
Bn, Vanilla Flavour, McVitie's*	1 Biscuit/18g	85	3	470	5.9	74	16.6	1.2
Bourbon Creams, Asda*	1 Biscuit/14g	67	3.1	482	5	66	22	3.4
Bourbon Creams, Sainsbury's*	1 Biscuit/13g	60	2.4	476	5.7	70.4	19.1	1.7
Bourbon Creams, Tesco*	1 Biscuit/14g	66	2.9	486	5.6	66.2	21.4	3.4
Bourbon Creams, Value, Multipack, Tesco*	1 Biscuit/13g	62	2.9	494	5.9	68	22.8	1.7
Bourbon, Average	*1 Biscuit/13g*	*63*	*2.8*	*488*	*5.7*	*68.2*	*21.3*	*2.1*
Bourbon, Gluten Wheat Free, Lovemore*	1 Biscuit/15g	70	2.9	469	4.1	67.9	19.1	4.7
Bourbon, Trufree*	1 Biscuit/13g	61	2.8	486	7.5	62.6	22.6	1.1
Bournville, Cadbury*	1 Biscuit/16g	85	5	520	6	54.9	30.7	1.4
Brandy Snap, Askeys*	1 Basket/20g	98	4.3	490	1.9	72.7	21.3	0
Brandy Snaps, Average	*1 Biscuit/15g*	*69*	*2.2*	*460*	*2.7*	*79.8*	*14.4*	*0.5*
Breakfast, Apricot, Crunchy, Belvita*	1 Pack/50g	198	4.8	395	7.5	65	9.5	12
Breakfast, Blueberries, Soft Bakes, Belvita*	1 Biscuit/50g	194	6	388	5.5	63	12	7.5
Breakfast, Choc Chips, Crunchy, Belvita*	1 Pack/50g	208	6	415	8	63	12	12
Breakfast, Choc Chips, Soft Bakes, Belvita*	1 Pack/50g	202	7.5	405	5.7	61	15	6.9
Breakfast, Choco Hazlenut, Tops, Belvita*	1 Pack/50g	230	8	460	7.2	69	16	4.9
Breakfast, Chocolate Chip, Bakes, Genius*	1 Bake/28g	142	7.9	507	5.2	56	28.3	4
Breakfast, Cocoa, & Creamy Live Yoghurt, Belvita*	1 Pack/51g	228	7.6	450	7.5	68	15	4.4

BISCUITS

INFO/WEIGHT	Measure		per Measure		Nutrition Values per 100g / 100ml				
			KCAL	FAT	KCAL	PROT	CARB	FAT	FIBRE
Breakfast, Cocoa, Chocolate Chip, Belvita*	1 Pack/50g		220	7.5	440	7.8	66	15	7.1
Breakfast, Coconut Yoghurt, Sainsbury's*	2 Biscuits/46g		203	7.3	437	7.6	62.1	15.7	8.7
Breakfast, Cranberry Orange, High in Fibre, M&S*	2 Biscuits/30g		142	6.9	473	6.6	54.9	23	10
Breakfast, Forest Fruit, Belvita*	1 Pack/50g		225	8	450	7.5	68	16	4.6
Breakfast, Golden Grain, Soft Bakes, Belvita*	1 Pack/50g		192	6	385	5.9	63	12	6.7
Breakfast, Golden Oats, Belvita*	1 Pack/50g		220	7.5	440	7.7	67	15	5.7
Breakfast, Hazelnuts, Crunchy, Belvita*	1 Pack/50g		210	6	420	8.7	63	12	12
Breakfast, Honey Nuts, Belvita*	1 Pack/50g		228	7.5	455	7.6	69	15	4.4
Breakfast, Honey Oat, Eat Well, M&S*	2 Biscuits/20g		88	3	442	9	65.6	15	4.3
Breakfast, Milk Cereals, Belvita*	1 Pack/50g		220	7.2	440	7.9	67	14.5	6.5
Breakfast, Mixed Berry, Soft Bakes, Belvita*	1 Pack/50g		200	7	400	6	66	14	8
Breakfast, Original, All Bran, Kellogg's*	1 Pack/40g		176	8	440	8	49	20	16
Breakfast, Porridge Oats Blueberries , McVitie's*	1 Slice/20g		80	2.1	402	7.3	67.1	10.4	6.5
Breakfast, Porridge Oats, Oats & Honey, McVitie's*	4 Biscuits/50g		226	7	452	9.6	69.5	14	4.6
Breakfast, Porridge Oats, Raspberry & Yoghurt, Mcvities*	2 Biscuits/51g		248	10.8	487	9.1	63.5	21.1	3.2
Breakfast, Porridge Oats, Red Berries , McVitie's*	4 Biscuits/50g		226	6.9	452	9.6	71	13.8	5.1
Breakfast, Red Berries, Soft Bakes, Belvita*	1 Pack/50g		190	5.5	380	5.5	65	11	6.6
Breakfast, Strawberry, Tops, Belvita*	1 Pack/50g		208	5.5	415	6.6	72.5	11	4.2
Butter, Covered in Dark 70% Chocolate, Green & Black's*	1 Biscuit/12g		62	3.5	520	7.1	5.6	29.4	0.1
Butter, Crinkle Crunch, Fox's*	1 Biscuit/11g		50	1.9	460	5.8	69.8	17.5	2.4
Butter, Dark Chocolate, Momento, Aldi*	1 Biscuit/14g		69	3.2	491	6.2	63.5	22.6	4.2
Butter, Dark Chocolate, Tesco*	1 Biscuit/14g		72	3.7	511	6.9	58.3	26.7	4.9
Butter, Milk Chocolate, Tesco*	1 Biscuit/14g		71	3.6	508	7.8	61	25.4	2.2
Cadbury Creme Egg, Cadbury*	1 Biscuit/18g		80	3.7	435	5	58.3	20.1	1.3
Cafe Noir, with Coffee Flavour Icing, McVitie's*	1 Biscuit/6g		27	0.8	458	4.9	76	14	1.7
Cantucci, with Honey, Loyd Grossman*	1 Biscuit/7g		32	1.1	450	9.5	66.3	16.3	0.9
Cantuccini, with Almonds, Average	**1 Biscotti/30g**		**130**	**5**	**433**	**10**	**60**	**16.7**	**3.3**
Cantuccini, Sainsbury's*	1 Biscotti/8g		35	1.3	440	10.4	63.1	16.2	4.4
Caramac, Breakaway, Breakaway *	1 Biscuit/19g		100	5.2	524	6.5	61.7	27.4	1.9
Caramel Crunch, Go Ahead, McVitie's*	1 Bar/24g		106	3.3	440	4.7	76.6	13.8	0.8
Caramel Squares, Thorntons*	2 Biscuits/32g		150	6.4	470	6.2	65	20	2.4
Caramel, Treat Size, Asda*	1 Bar/21g		97	4.8	463	4.6	59	23	0.9
Caramelised, Biscoff, Lotus*	1 Biscuit/8g		38	1.5	484	4.9	72.7	19	1.3
Caramels, Milk Chocolate, McVitie's*	1 Serving/17g		81	3.6	478	5.6	65.8	21.4	2.3
Chcoolate Coated, GF, Chocoful, Prewett's*	1 Bar/20g		100	4.8	502	7.3	63.2	24	0
Cheese Melts, Carr's*	1 Biscuit/4g		21	1	493	10.8	59.6	22.9	2.5
Cheese Sandwich, Ritz*	1 Biscuit/9g		50	2.8	530	9.5	55	30.2	2
Cheese Savouries, Sainsbury's*	1 Serving/30g		159	9.4	531	11.3	50	31.3	2.1
Cheese, Chutney, Delicious, Boots*	1 Pack/134g		290	14.7	217	9	19	11	2.3
Cheese, Baked, Cheddars, Jacob's*	1 Cheddar/4g		20	1.2	525	10.8	47	31.8	2.9
Cherry Bakewell, Handfinished, M&S*	1 Biscuit/40g		200	9.7	495	5.9	62.1	24	0.5
Choc Chip, Paterson's*	1 Biscuit/17g		79	3.6	474	5.6	64	21.6	3.1
Chockas, Original, Fox's*	1 Biscuit/24g		85	1	355	1.1	10.4	4.2	0.4
Choco Caramel, Pick Up, Bar, Bahlsen*	1 Bar/28g		140	6.7	501	6	64	24	0
Choco Leibniz, Dark Chocolate, Bahlsen*	1 Biscuit/14g		69	3.6	493	6.8	59	26	5.1
Choco Leibniz, Milk, Bahlsen*	1 Biscuit/14g		72	3.6	515	7.9	63.4	25.5	2.4
Choco Leibniz, Orange Flavour, Bahlsen*	1 Biscuit/14g		70	3.7	504	7.9	58.5	26.4	0
Choco Leibniz, White, Bahlsen *	2 Biscuits/28g		142	7	508	5.1	65	25	0
Chocolate Coconut, Duchy Originals*	1 Biscuit/13g		68	4.3	543	6.3	52.1	34.4	2.6
Chocolate Hazelnut, Quirks, McVitie's*	1 Biscuit/13g		66	3.6	511	5	58.4	28	2.6
Chocolate Chip Peanut, Trufree*	1 Biscuit/11g		55	2.6	496	4	66	24	2
Chocolate Chip GI, Diet Chef Ltd*	1 Pack/20g		90	3.6	450	7.4	64.4	17.9	6.4
Chocolate Fingers, Milk, Cadbury*	1 Biscuit/6g		31	1.6	515	6.8	60.8	27.1	1.7

B

BISCUITS

INFO/WEIGHT	Measure	per Measure		Nutrition Values per 100g / 100ml				
		KCAL	FAT	KCAL	PROT	CARB	FAT	FIBRE
Chocolate Fingers, Milk, Extra Crunchy, Cadbury*	1 Biscuit/5g	25	1.2	505	6.6	66.2	23.6	0
Chocolate Fingers, Plain, Cadbury*	1 Biscuit/6g	30	1.6	508	6.2	60.6	26.8	0
Chocolate Fingers, Salted Peanut Crunch, Cadbury*	4 Fingers/21g	100	5.5	478	6.6	52.9	26.5	1.4
Chocolate Flavour, Taillefine, Lu*	1 Biscuit/8g	33	0.9	408	5.8	70.8	10.8	5.8
Chocolate Florentine, M&S*	1 Serving/39g	195	9.7	500	7.4	64.5	24.9	1.7
Chocolate Ginger, Organic, Duchy Originals*	1 Biscuit/12g	64	3.6	518	4.6	59.7	29	2.1
Chocolate Ginger, Thorntons*	1 Biscuit/19g	96	5.3	512	5.9	58.2	28.4	0
Chocolate Kimberley, Jacob's*	1 Biscuit/20g	86	3.4	428	3.9	64.4	17.2	1.1
Chocolate Mini Shorties, McVitie's*	1 Pack/25g	131	7.1	524	6	61.2	28.3	2
Chocolate Seville, Thorntons*	1 Biscuit/19g	97	5.3	512	5.7	59	28.1	0
Chocolate Toffee, Crunch, Moments, McVitie's*	1 Biscuit/17g	89	4.7	520	5.6	62.3	27.6	1.7
Chocolate Viennese, Fox's*	1 Biscuit/16g	85	4.9	530	6.7	56.6	30.7	1.7
Chocolate, Belgian Chocolate, Weight Watchers*	1 Biscuit/18g	87	4.1	481	7.1	61.8	22.8	4.5
Chocolate, Breakaway, Nestle*	1 Bar/19g	99	4.9	511	6.1	63.5	25.2	3
Chocolate, Chunky, Eat Me, Aldi*	1 Biscuit/24g	122	6	510	6	64	25	2.7
Chocolate, Fingers, Average	*1 Biscuit/6g*	*31*	*1.6*	*514*	*6.7*	*61.4*	*26.8*	*1.5*
Chocolate, Golden Crunch, Free From Milk, Tesco*	1 Biscuit/17g	85	4.9	510	4.2	57.2	29.4	4.6
Chocolate, Mint, Round, Tower Gate, Lidl*	1 Round/14g	74	4.1	529	4.3	60.7	29.3	0
Chocolinis, Milk Chocolate, Go Ahead, McVitie's*	1 Biscuit/12g	56	1.7	466	7.7	77.2	14	2
Chocolinis, Plain Chocolate, McVitie's*	1 Biscuit/12g	56	1.8	468	6.9	77	14.7	2.6
Christmas Shapes, Assorted, Sainsbury's*	1 Biscuit/15g	77	4.3	525	5.2	59	29.8	1.7
Classic, Creams, Fox's*	1 Biscuit/14g	72	3.6	516	4.4	65.2	25.8	1.7
Classic, Milk Chocolate, Fox's*	1 Biscuit/13g	67	3.1	517	6.1	64.9	24	1.6
Coconut Cream, Hill Biscuits Ltd*	1 Biscuit/12g	64	3	505	4.9	67	24	1.6
Coconut Crinkle, Sainsbury's*	1 Biscuit/11g	54	2.8	500	6.4	59.6	26.2	3.7
Coconut Crinkles, Fox's*	1 Biscuit/11g	53	2.5	487	5.2	63.8	22.6	3.7
Coconut Rings, Tesco*	1 Biscuit/9g	44	2	485	6.2	66.1	21.7	2.6
Coconut, Ring, Average	*1 Biscuit/9g*	*44*	*2*	*490*	*6.1*	*67.4*	*21.8*	*2.6*
Coffee, GF, Barkat*	2 Biscuits/15g	72	2.8	479	2	75	19	0
Cookies 'n Cream, Eat Me, Aldi*	1 Biscuit/12g	58	2.1	467	5.4	72	17	2.9
Cornish Fairings, Original, Furniss Of Cornwall*	1 Biscuit/17g	75	2.5	448	5.1	72.9	15.1	0
Cracked Black Pepper, Savoury, Weight Watchers*	1 Serving/16g	71	3.1	446	8.3	59.2	19.5	9.4
Cranberry Pumpkin Seed, BGTY, Sainsbury's*	1 Biscuit/17g	68	2.8	410	7.2	56.6	17.1	13.9
Cranberry Sunflower Seed, Oaty, Weight Watchers*	1 Biscuit/19g	87	3.7	457	7.9	58	19.3	10
Cranberry, Crispy Slices, LC, Tesco*	1 Biscuit/15g	54	0.6	370	6	76	3.9	5.5
Crinkles, Classics, Milk Chocolate, Fox's*	1 Biscuit/14g	67	3.1	487	5.7	65.2	22.7	2.7
Crispy Fruit Slices, Apple, Sultana, Go Ahead, McVitie's*	1 Slice/13g	50	0.9	388	5.4	74	7.1	2.9
Crispy Fruit Slices, Forest Fruit, Go Ahead, McVitie's*	1 Biscuit/13g	49	0.9	380	5.4	73.7	7	3
Crispy Slices, Raspberry, Go Ahead, McVitie's*	1 Slice/13g	50	0.9	385	5.3	74	7	2.8
Crispy Slices, Red Cherry, Go Ahead, McVitie's*	3 Slices/39g	147	2.7	380	5.5	73.9	7	2.9
Crunch Creams, Double Choc, Fox's*	1 Biscuit/15g	77	3.8	511	4.7	65	25	2.7
Crunchers, Salted, Savoury, Crackers, Sainsbury's*	1 Cracker/5g	22	1	448	6.1	59.4	20.4	1.4
Crunchie, Cadbury*	1 Biscuit/13g	64	3.1	495	4.8	65.7	23.6	0.9
Crunchy Caramel, Tesco*	1 Bar/21g	98	5.2	467	4.6	56	25	1.4
Custard Cream, Giant, Tesco*	1 Biscuit/90g	436	20.3	484	4.7	64.7	22.5	2.1
Custard Cream, Gluten Wheat Free, Lovemore*	1 Biscuit/15g	71	2.5	475	0	33	16.8	0
Custard Creams, 25% Less Fat, Sainsbury's*	1 Biscuit/13g	59	2.2	469	5.8	72.7	17.3	1.3
Custard Creams, 25% Less Fat, Tesco*	1 Biscuit/13g	59	2.2	473	5.8	72.2	17.9	1.2
Custard Creams, Asda*	1 Biscuit/12g	59	2.7	495	5	67	23	2
Custard Creams, BGTY, Sainsbury's*	1 Biscuit/12g	56	2.1	473	5.8	72.2	17.9	1.2
Custard Creams, Crawfords*	1 Biscuit/11g	57	2.7	517	5.9	69.2	24.1	1.5
Custard Creams, Everyday Value, Tesco*	1 Biscuit/13g	62	2.6	495	5.6	69.7	20.9	1.7
Custard Creams, Jacob's*	1 Biscuit/16g	77	3.3	481	5.3	68	20.9	1.6

BISCUITS

	Measure INFO/WEIGHT	per Measure		Nutrition Values per 100g / 100ml				
		KCAL	FAT	KCAL	PROT	CARB	FAT	FIBRE
Custard Creams, M&S*	1 Biscuit/13g	63	2.8	494	5.5	67.2	22	2.4
Custard Creams, Sainsbury's*	1 Biscuit/13g	67	3	514	5.5	70.4	23.4	1.6
Custard Creams, Smart Price, Asda*	1 Biscuit/13g	61	2.6	486	6	69	21	1.6
Custard Creams, Tesco*	1 Biscuit/12g	58	2.4	490	5.7	70.1	20.5	1.1
Custard Creams, Trufree*	1 Biscuit/12g	60	2.8	504	8.7	65	23	1
Custard Creams, Value, Tesco*	1 Biscuit/11g	51	1.6	450	7.2	72.5	14.3	3
Dark Chocolate All Butter, M&S*	1 Biscuit/15g	72	4.1	480	6.9	52.4	27.2	11.4
Dark Chocolate Ginger, M&S*	1 Biscuit/21g	105	5.7	505	5	58.8	27.6	4.2
Dark Chocolate Gingers, Border*	1 Biscuit/17g	74	3.4	445	4.4	61.4	20.1	2.9
Diet Fibre, Gullon*	2 Biscuits/16g	65	2.6	405	6.5	48.7	16.4	23
Digestive with Wheatgerm, Hovis*	1 Biscuit/12g	57	2.4	475	8.3	65	20	3.3
Digestive, 25% Less Fat, Asda*	1 Biscuit/16g	73	2.6	455	7.3	69.8	16.3	2.6
Digestive, 25% Less Fat, Tesco*	1 Biscuit/14g	65	2.3	462	7.3	71	16.5	3.8
Digestive, BGTY, Sainsbury's*	1 Biscuit/15g	70	2.6	468	7.4	71	17.2	3.8
Digestive, Caramels, Milk Chocolate, McVitie's*	1 Biscuit/17g	81	3.7	478	5.6	65.1	21.7	2.3
Digestive, Caramels, Plain Chocolate, McVitie's*	1 Biscuit/17g	82	3.8	481	5.7	65.5	22.1	2.1
Digestive, Chocolate	*1 Biscuit/17g*	*84*	*4.1*	*493*	*6.8*	*66.5*	*24.1*	*2.2*
Digestive, Chocolate Chip, Asda*	1 Biscuit/14g	68	3.2	491	6	65	23	2.9
Digestive, Chocolate, Free From, Co-Op*	1 Biscuit/11g	54	2.3	495	6.3	69	21	2.9
Digestive, Cracker Selection, Tesco*	1 Biscuit/12g	56	2.3	464	7.1	65.2	19.4	4.3
Digestive, Crawfords*	1 Biscuit/12g	58	2.4	484	7.1	68.8	20	3.4
Digestive, Creams, McVitie's*	1 Biscuit/12g	60	2.8	502	5.6	68.2	23	2.1
Digestive, Dark Chocolate, M&S*	1 Biscuit/17g	84	4.3	509	6.4	59.8	26.1	4.4
Digestive, Dark Chocolate, McVitie's*	1 Biscuit/17g	83	4.1	495	6	60.8	24.2	4.2
Digestive, Dark Chocolate, Thins, McVitie's*	1 Biscuit/6g	31	1.5	499	6	60.9	24.7	4.7
Digestive, Everyday Value, Tesco*	1 Biscuit/16g	80	3.4	490	6.7	66.5	21	3
Digestive, Fingers, Morrisons*	1 Finger/8g	39	1.8	482	6.8	63.6	22.2	3.2
Digestive, GF, Barkat*	1 Biscuit/15g	56	2.7	378	3.4	49.3	18.5	18.4
Digestive, GFY, Asda*	1 Biscuit/14g	65	2.4	461	6	71	17	3.6
Digestive, Gluten Wheat Free, Lovemore*	1 Biscuit/15g	55	2.7	378	3.4	49.3	18.5	18.4
Digestive, Happy Shopper*	1 Biscuit/13g	64	2.9	498	6.8	66.3	22.8	3.3
Digestive, High Fibre, Reduced Sugar, M&S*	1 Biscuit/13g	60	2.8	460	6.5	59.3	21.7	9.4
Digestive, Hovis*	1 Biscuit/6g	27	1.1	447	10.2	60	18.5	4.4
Digestive, Lemon & Ginger, McVitie's*	1 Biscuit/15g	72	3.1	480	6.7	66.7	20.7	2.7
Digestive, Light, McVitie's*	1 Biscuit/15g	66	2.1	444	7.3	69.5	14.3	3.6
Digestive, McVitie's*	1 Biscuit/15g	70	3.2	470	7.2	62.7	21.5	3.6
Digestive, Milk Chocolate Mint, McVitie's*	1 Biscuit/17g	81	3.9	487	6.7	62.6	23.4	2.9
Digestive, Milk Chocolate, 25% Reduced Fat, McVitie's*	1 Biscuit/17g	78	2.9	459	7.2	68.6	17.3	3.2
Digestive, Milk Chocolate, Basics, Sainsbury's*	1 Biscuit/14g	71	3.4	496	6.5	62.9	23.7	2.9
Digestive, Milk Chocolate, Cadbury*	1 Biscuit/16g	80	3.8	490	7.4	61.3	23.3	3.9
Digestive, Milk Chocolate, GFY, Asda*	1 Biscuit/17g	78	2.9	457	7	69	17	3.2
Digestive, Milk Chocolate, Homewheat, McVitie's*	1 Biscuit/17g	83	4.1	486	6	61.5	24	4
Digestive, Milk Chocolate, M&S*	1 Biscuit/17g	85	4.4	505	6.1	62.2	26	2.6
Digestive, Milk Chocolate, McVitie's*	1 Biscuit/17g	84	4	488	6.7	62.7	23.4	2.9
Digestive, Milk Chocolate, Mini, McVitie's*	1 Bag/25g	124	6.2	496	6.6	61.9	24.7	2.9
Digestive, Milk Chocolate, Mini, Tesco*	1 Pack/30g	153	8.1	510	6.6	59.8	27.1	1.8
Digestive, Milk Chocolate, Sainsbury's*	1 Biscuit/17g	87	6.3	511	6.9	65.9	36.8	2.5
Digestive, Milk Chocolate, Tesco*	1 Biscuit/17g	85	4.1	498	6.6	62.8	23.9	3.1
Digestive, Milk Chocolate, Thins, McVitie's*	1 Biscuit/6g	32	1.5	508	6.9	64.3	24.1	3.1
Digestive, Milk Chocolate, Trufree*	1 Biscuit/12g	63	3	521	4	70	25	2
Digestive, Munch Bites, McVitie's*	1 Pack/40g	205	10.2	512	6.5	64.5	25.5	2
Digestive, Oat, Weight Watchers*	1 Biscuit/11g	50	2.1	457	6	66.3	18.6	6.9
Digestive, Plain Chocolate, Asda*	1 Biscuit/17g	84	4	500	7	64	24	3.2

B

BISCUITS

	Measure INFO/WEIGHT	per Measure KCAL	FAT	KCAL	PROT	CARB	FAT	FIBRE
Digestive, Plain Chocolate, Tesco*	1 Biscuit/17g	85	4.1	499	6.2	63.5	24.4	2.8
Digestive, Plain Chocolate, Value, Tesco*	1 Biscuit/19g	97	4.9	510	6.4	61.5	26	2.9
Digestive, Plain, Average	*1 Biscuit/14g*	*67*	*2.9*	*480*	*7.1*	*65.6*	*20.5*	*3.5*
Digestive, Plain, M&S*	1 Biscuit/16g	80	3.9	490	6.5	62.7	23.8	3.3
Digestive, Reduced Fat, McVitie's*	1 Biscuit/15g	70	2.4	467	7.1	72.8	16.3	3.4
Digestive, Reduced Fat, Tesco*	1 Biscuit/16g	70	2.6	453	7	69.1	16.6	3.4
Digestive, Smart Price, Asda*	1 Biscuit/14g	67	2.9	465	6	65.3	20	3.1
Digestive, Sugar Free, Gullon*	1 Biscuit/13g	57	2.1	430	6.2	68	16	6.5
Digestive, Sweetmeal, Asda*	1 Biscuit/14g	68	3.1	499	7	66	23	3.5
Digestive, Sweetmeal, Sainsbury's*	1 Biscuit/13g	61	2.5	469	7.3	64.3	19.1	5.3
Digestive, Sweetmeal, Tesco*	1 Biscuit/18g	80	2.6	444	8.4	70	14.5	3.1
Digestive, Value, Tesco*	1 Biscuit/15g	74	3.4	490	6.9	64	22.4	3.3
Digestive, Whole Wheat, Organic, Dove's Farm*	1 Biscuit/13g	56	2.4	446	5.9	61.6	19.5	7.8
Digestives, Beastly Bakes, McVitie's*	1 Bake/40g	193	9.3	484	4.1	63.5	23.3	1.9
Digestives, Chocolate, Belmont Biscuit Co, Aldi*	1 Biscuit/17g	85	4	499	6.5	63.3	23.8	2.9
Digestives, Chocolate, Dark, McVitie's*	1 Biscuit/17g	83	4	495	6	60.8	24.2	4.2
Digestives, Double Chocolate, Mcvitie's*	1 Biscuit/17g	83	4.1	497	6.5	60.9	24.3	3.6
Double Choc Chip, Trufree*	1 Biscuit/11g	58	3	523	3	67	27	1.8
Extremely Chocolatey Mini Rings, M&S*	1 Biscuit/13g	67	3.5	515	7.4	60.2	27.2	1.9
Extremely Chocolatey Orange, M&S*	1 Biscuit/24g	120	6.2	510	7.5	59.9	26.5	2.7
Extremely Chocolatey, Dark Chocolate Rounds, M&S*	1 Biscuit/19g	97	5.6	510	6.2	55.7	29.3	6.3
Fig Roll, Tesco*	1 Biscuit/19g	70	1.6	375	4	69.3	8.8	3.1
Florentines, Decadent Dark Chocolate, Thomas J Fudge*	1 Florentine/19g	107	7.1	565	8	46.8	37.3	0
Florentines, Sainsbury's*	1 Florentine/8g	40	2.5	506	10	47.2	30.8	7
for Cheese, Oat Chive, Waitrose*	1 Biscuit/5.4g	26	1.2	483	10.8	57.5	22.4	4.1
Forest Fruit Slices, , Harvest Morn, Aldi*	1 Biscuit/14g	54	1	387	5.3	75	6.8	2.8
Forest Fruit, Yoghurt, Breaks, Go Ahead, McVitie's*	2 Slices/36g	144	3.6	402	5.4	72.6	10	2.2
Forest Fruits, Benefit Delights , Aldi*	2 Biscuits/25g	97	1.6	388	5	77	6.2	2.2
Fruit Spice Oat, Diet Chef Ltd*	2 Biscuits/20g	85	2.9	425	7.8	65.3	14.7	7.6
Fruit Bake, Organic, Tesco*	1 Biscuit/12g	53	2.1	453	7.5	65.1	18.1	5.6
Fruit Shortcake, McVitie's*	1 Biscuit/8g	37	1.5	462	5.6	65.9	18.9	3.1
Fruit Shortcake, Sainsbury's*	1 Biscuit/8g	39	1.6	483	5.9	69.6	20.1	2.1
Fruit Shortcake, Tesco*	1 Biscuit/9g	43	1.7	473	5.8	70.1	18.8	1.9
Fruit Slices, Apple, Raisin & Currant, Belmont, Aldi*	1 Biscuit/15g	57	1	379	7	72.8	6.4	1.3
Fruit, All Butter, Sainsbury's*	1 Biscuit/9g	45	2	477	5.6	66	21.2	1.9
Fruit, Oat, Gl, Diet Chef Ltd*	1 Biscuit/20g	85	2.9	425	7.8	65.3	14.7	7.6
Fruity Iced, Blue Parrot Cafe, Sainsbury's*	1 Pack/20g	83	1.4	415	6	82	7	1.1
Fruity Oat, Organic, Dove's Farm*	1 Biscuit/12g	53	2.1	453	7.5	65.1	18.1	5.6
Galettes, Chocolate Butter, Bonne Maman*	2 Biscuits/28g	146	7.6	521	7.1	61.1	27.1	3.6
Galettes, Lemon Poppy Seed, Butter, Bonne Maman*	2 Biscuits/28g	142	7.3	506	6.4	62	26	2
Garibaldi, Asda*	1 Biscuit/10g	39	0.9	375	4.7	68.5	9.1	2.2
Garibaldi, Sainsbury's*	1 Biscuit/9g	34	0.8	378	4.6	67.6	9.2	3.3
Garibaldi, Tesco*	1 Biscuit/10g	40	0.9	400	4.7	74	9.1	2.2
Ginger Crinkle Crunch, Fox's*	1 Biscuit/12g	50	1.4	435	4.7	75.3	12.5	1.6
Ginger Crinkle, Sainsbury's*	1 Biscuit/11g	53	2.5	486	6.2	63.8	22.9	2.9
Ginger Crunch Creams, Fox's*	1 Biscuit/15g	77	3.5	501	4.1	68	23	1.6
Ginger Crunch, Hand Baked, Border*	1 Biscuit/12g	54	2.3	470	4.7	71.4	20.4	0
Ginger Nuts, CBY, Asda*	1 Biscuit/10g	46	1.5	452	5.4	73.5	14.7	2.1
Ginger Nuts, McVitie's*	1 Biscuit/10g	46	1.5	452	5.4	73.5	14.7	2.1
Ginger Nuts, Tesco*	1 Biscuit/12g	54	1.9	457	5.9	71.9	15.7	2.4
Ginger Nuts, Value, Tesco*	1 Biscuit/12g	55	1.9	460	5.2	74.2	15.8	1.6
Ginger Snap, BGTY, Sainsbury's*	1 Biscuit/12g	51	1.2	427	6.5	78.2	9.8	1.8
Ginger Snap, Fox's*	1 Biscuit/8g	35	1	443	4.6	77.1	12.8	1.5

BISCUITS

	Measure INFO/WEIGHT	per Measure KCAL	FAT	Nutrition Values per 100g / 100ml KCAL	PROT	CARB	FAT	FIBRE
Ginger Snap, Sainsbury's*	1 Biscuit/10g	46	1.5	454	5.2	75	14.4	1.8
Ginger Snaps, Hand Baked, Ringtons *	1 Biscuit/15g	69	2.4	458	5	73.9	16.2	0
Ginger Snaps, Trufree*	1 Biscuit/11g	51	1.9	467	2.5	76	17	1.5
Ginger Thins, Anna's*	1 Biscuit/5g	24	1	480	6	70	20	2
Ginger Thins, Asda*	1 Biscuit/5g	23	0.8	462	6	73	16	1.9
Ginger, Belgian Dark Chocolate, Thins, Waitrose*	1 Biscuit/10g	48	2.2	481	6.2	61.2	22.5	4.6
Ginger, Snap, 35% Reduced Fat, Sainsbury's*	1 Biscuit/10g	42	0.9	421	6.8	77.1	9	2.4
Ginger, Traditional, Fox's*	1 Biscuit/8g	33	1	404	4.4	70.1	11.7	1.4
Ginger, Value, Morrisons*	1 Biscuit/12g	55	1.9	459	5.3	74	15.8	1.7
Gingerbread Man, Gluten Wheat Free, Lovemore*	1 Biscuit/37g	179	7.6	485	4.7	70.1	20.5	1.7
Gingerbread Shapes, Milk Chocolate, Favorina, Lidl*	1 Shape/28g	105	2.5	376	5.2	67.8	8.8	0
Gingernut	*1 Biscuit/11g*	*50*	*1.7*	*456*	*5.6*	*79.1*	*15.2*	*1.4*
Golden Crunch Creams, Fox's*	1 Biscuit/15g	75	3.8	515	4.7	64.8	26.3	1.2
Golden Crunch, Bronte*	1 Biscuit/15g	69	3.3	474	5.1	62.5	22.6	0
Golden Crunch, Go Ahead, McVitie's*	1 Biscuit/9g	38	0.9	419	7.7	75.2	9.7	2.1
Golden Crunch, Paterson's*	1 Biscuit/15g	69	3.3	474	5.1	62.5	22.6	4.8
Golden Shortie, Jacob's*	1 Biscuit/11g	54	2.6	492	6	64.9	23.2	0
Golden Syrup, McVitie's*	1 Biscuit/12g	63	3	508	5.1	67.3	24.2	2.2
Gouda Cheese, Chive, Buiteman*	1/3 Pack/25g	129	8	516	16	40	32	4
Gruyere Spinach Twists, Savoury, Ardens*	1 Twist/7g	33	1.4	466	13	56	20	5
Happy Faces, Jacob's*	1 Biscuit/16g	78	3.6	485	4.8	66.1	22.3	1.6
Hazelnut Crispies, Occasions, Sainsbury's*	1 Biscuit/7g	36	1.8	518	6	64.3	26.3	0
Hazelnut Meringue, Sainsbury's*	1 Biscuit/6g	24	1.4	404	5	43	23.5	1.1
Hobnobs, Chocolate Creams, McVitie's*	1 Biscuit/12g	60	3.1	503	6.7	60.3	26.1	4
Hobnobs, Light, 25% Reduced Fat, McVitie's*	1 Biscuit/14g	62	2.3	435	8.1	64.6	16.1	6.2
Hobnobs, McVitie's*	1 Biscuit/15g	72	3.2	473	7	61.8	20.7	5.4
Hobnobs, Milk Chocolate, McVitie's*	1 Biscuit/19g	92	4.5	479	6.8	60.7	23.3	4.5
Hobnobs, Milk Chocolate, Mini, McVitie's*	1 Pack/25g	121	5.9	483	6.6	61.3	23.5	4.4
Hobnobs, Plain Chocolate, McVitie's*	1 Biscuit/16g	81	3.9	498	6.7	63.3	24.3	4.2
Hobnobs, Vanilla Creams, McVitie's*	1 Biscuit/12g	60	3	501	6.1	62.3	25.2	3.6
Iced Gems, Jacob's*	1 Bag/25g	98	0.8	393	5	86.3	3.1	2
Iced, Shopkins*	1 Biscuit/10g	42	0.8	423	5.6	81	8.1	2.1
Jaffa Cakes, Asda*	1 Cake/12g	43	1	368	4.7	67.5	8.8	1.9
Jaffa Cakes, Belmont Biscuit Co, Aldi*	1 Biscuit/13g	52	1.3	400	3.7	72.8	10.2	1
Jaffa Cakes, Dark Chocolate, M&S*	1 Cake/11g	45	1.5	395	3.7	64.9	13.2	2.8
Jaffa Cakes, Dark Chocolate, Mini, M&S*	1 Cake/5g	20	0.8	410	3.9	62.8	15.8	1.9
Jaffa Cakes, Lemon Lime, McVitie's*	1 Cake/3g	12	0.3	357	4.9	65.2	8.1	2
Jaffa Cakes, Lunch Box, McVitie's*	1 Cake/7g	26	0.6	395	4.2	74.3	9	1.4
Jaffa Cakes, McVitie's*	1 Cake/12g	46	1	380	4.9	70.8	8	2.2
Jaffa Cakes, Mini Roll, McVitie's*	1 Cake/26g	99	2.7	374	3.5	67.1	10.1	2.3
Jaffa Cakes, Mini, Asda*	1 Cake/5g	21	0.8	412	3.9	63	16	1.9
Jaffa Cakes, Mini, Bags, McVitie's*	1 Cake/5g	20	0.7	396	4.2	65	13.1	3.5
Jaffa Cakes, Mini, Orange Pods, McVitie's*	1 Cake/40g	150	3.4	380	4.3	71.2	8.7	3.5
Jaffa Cakes, Plain Chocolate, Sainsbury's*	1 Cake/13g	50	1.1	384	4.4	73.3	8.1	1.3
Jaffa Cakes, Sainsbury's*	1 Cake/11g	41	1	373	4.3	69.3	8.8	2
Jaffa Cakes, Smart Price, Asda*	1 Cake/12g	43	1	374	4.3	69	9	2
Jaffa Cakes, Strawberry, McVitie's*	1 Cake/12g	45	1	375	4.9	69.8	8.1	2
Jaffa Cakes, Value, Tesco*	1 Cake/12g	45	1.1	388	4.7	70	9.4	2.2
Jam Cream, Belmont Biscuit Co, Aldi*	1 Biscuit/16g	78	3.6	490	5.9	65.8	22.3	1.2
Jam Creams, Jacob's*	1 Biscuit/15g	75	3.4	486	5	67.4	21.8	1.6
Jam Rings, Crawfords*	1 Biscuit/12g	56	2.1	470	5.5	73	17.2	1.9
Jam Sandwich Creams, M&S*	1 Biscuit/17g	80	3.7	485	5.7	64.5	22.6	1.8
Jam Sandwich Creams, Sainsbury's*	1 Biscuit/15g	75	3.4	488	4.9	65.6	22.4	2.2

BISCUITS

	Measure INFO/WEIGHT	per Measure KCAL	FAT	Nutrition Values per 100g / 100ml KCAL	PROT	CARB	FAT	FIBRE
Jam Sandwich Creams, Tesco*	1 Biscuit/15g	72	3.2	482	4.8	67.1	21.4	1.2
Jammie Dodgers, Minis, Lunchbox, Burton's*	1 Pack/20g	89	3	445	6	70	15.1	2.3
Jammie Dodgers, Original, Burton's*	1 Biscuit/18g	78	2.5	436	5.4	71.3	13.9	1.7
Jammy Wheels, GF, Prewett's*	1 Biscuit/24g	95	5.6	394	5	60.1	23.2	4.7
Jestives, Milk Chocolate, Cadbury*	1 Biscuit/17g	86	4.2	506	6.4	64.4	24.8	0
Key Lime Pie, Crunch Creams, Fox's*	1 Biscuit/16g	78	3.7	507	4.1	67.5	24.2	1.7
Kimberley, Bolands*	1 Biscuit/16g	72	1.7	449	5.1	82.6	10.9	1.4
Lebkuchen, Sainsbury's*	1 Biscuit/10g	39	0.8	400	5.7	76.1	8	1.3
Lemon Butter, Thins, Sainsbury's*	1 Biscuit/13g	65	3.5	515	5.3	60.7	27.9	2.2
Lemon Curd Sandwich, Fox's*	1 Biscuit/14g	69	3.3	494	4.7	66.2	23.4	1.3
Lemon Puff, Jacob's*	1 Biscuit/13g	69	4.1	533	4.3	58.8	31.2	2.8
Lemon Thins, Sainsbury's*	1 Biscuit/10g	47	1.7	468	5.6	72.3	17.3	1.7
Lemon, All Butter, Half Coated, Finest, Tesco*	1 Biscuit/17g	84	4.5	505	5.6	60.4	26.9	3.6
Lincoln, McVitie's*	1 Biscuit/8g	41	1.9	514	6.3	69	23.6	2
Lincoln, Sainsbury's*	1 Biscuit/8g	40	1.7	479	7.2	66.1	20.6	2.1
Malt, Basics, Sainsbury's*	1 Biscuit/8g	36	1.2	470	7.1	73.6	15.7	0
Malted Milk, Asda*	1 Biscuit/8g	39	1.8	490	7	66	22	2
Malted Milk, Average	**1 Biscuit/9g**	**42**	**1.9**	**490**	**7**	**65.6**	**22.2**	**1.8**
Malted Milk, Chocolate, Tesco*	1 Biscuit/10g	52	2.5	500	6.7	64.4	24	1.9
Malted Milk, Milk Chocolate, Asda*	1 Biscuit/11g	56	2.8	509	7	64	25	1.7
Malted Milk, Milk Chocolate, Sainsbury's*	1 Biscuit/11g	56	2.7	505	6.4	64.4	24.2	2.1
Malted Milk, Sainsbury's*	1 Biscuit/8g	40	1.8	488	7.1	65.5	21.9	2
Malted Milk, Tesco*	1 Biscuit/9g	44	1.9	495	6.6	66.8	21.8	2
Maple Leaf, M&S*	1 Biscuit/13g	50	1.9	395	5.1	59.8	14.8	2
Maria, Gullon*	1 Biscuit/6g	24	0.7	408	7	75	11	4.5
Marie, Crawfords*	1 Biscuit/7g	33	1.1	475	7.5	76.3	15.5	2.3
Melts, Sesame with Chive, Carr's*	1 Biscuit/5g	23	1.2	498	8.2	57.4	26.2	3.5
Mikado, Jacob's*	1 Biscuit/13g	53	1.6	397	4.2	67.7	12.1	2.5
Milk Chocolate Digestive, Everyday Value, Tesco*	1 Biscuit/17g	82	3.7	494	7.2	65.4	22.3	1.7
Milk Chocolate, All Butter, M&S*	1 Biscuit/14g	70	3.6	490	7.9	57.4	25.5	1.4
Milk Chocolate, Assortment, Cadbury*	1 Serving/10g	51	2.6	510	6.8	61	26.4	0
Milk Chocolate, Tesco*	1 Biscuit/25g	135	7.3	535	6.4	62.1	29	1.8
Mini Assortment, M&S*	1 Biscuit/3g	12	0.6	480	6.1	63.9	22.5	2.8
Mini Clotted Cream, Fosters Traditional Foods*	1 Biscuit/13g	66	3.6	507	5.4	59.5	27.4	0
Mint, Viscount*	1 Biscuit/13g	73	3.8	552	5.1	60.6	28.8	1.3
Mixed Berry, Oat Square, Go Ahead, McVitie's*	1 Bar/40g	137	3.7	342	4.6	64.4	9.2	4.2
Mixed Seed Honey, Oaty, Weight Watchers*	1 Biscuit/22g	106	5.1	482	9.2	59	23.2	4.9
Morning Coffee, Asda*	1 Biscuit/5g	22	0.7	455	8	72	15	2.4
Morning Coffee, Tesco*	1 Biscuit/5g	22	0.7	450	7.6	72.3	14.5	2.4
Nice Creams, Fox's*	1 Biscuit/13g	64	3	505	5	67	24	2
Nice, Asda*	1 Biscuit/8g	38	1.7	480	6	68	21	2.4
Nice, Average	**1 Biscuit/8g**	**36**	**1.6**	**484**	**6.3**	**67.3**	**21**	**2.5**
Nice, Belmont, Aldi*	1 Biscuit/8g	39	1.6	489	6.2	68.9	20.4	2.3
Nice, Fox's*	1 Biscuit/9g	39	1.7	450	6.3	62.4	19.4	5
Nice, Sainsbury's*	1 Biscuit/8g	41	2	498	5.8	63.2	23.9	3.5
Nice, Value, Multipack, Tesco*	1 Biscuit/8g	39	1.7	485	6.5	68	20.8	2.4
Oat & Wholemeal, Crawfords*	1 Biscuit/14g	67	3	482	7.7	64.2	21.6	4.8
Oat Chocolate Chip, Cadbury*	1 Biscuit/17g	80	3.9	485	6.9	60.2	23.9	4.2
Oat Walnut, M&S*	2 Biscuits/12g	59	3.1	492	10.8	54.2	25.8	2.5
Oat Wholemeal, Dbc Foodservice*	1 Biscuit/14g	67	3.1	466	7.1	60.8	21.7	5.5
Oat Bites, Caramelised Onion, Diet Chef Ltd*	1 Pack/23g	99	3.9	430	7.5	64.2	16.8	6
Oat Bites, Cheese, Diet Chef Ltd*	1 Pack/23g	99	3.6	430	15	57.4	15.8	4.9
Oat Bites, Chilli, Diet Chef Ltd*	1 Pack/23g	128	3.1	556	8.1	68.4	13.3	7.2

B

BISCUITS

	Measure INFO/WEIGHT	per Measure KCAL	FAT	Nutrition Values per 100g / 100ml KCAL	PROT	CARB	FAT	FIBRE
Oat Crisps, Orange, Swedish, Gille*	1 Biscuit/8g	40	2	500	4.7	63.8	25	0
Oat Crumbles, Border*	1 Biscuit/15g	66	3.1	443	5.3	58.9	20.7	1.8
Oat Crunch, M&S*	1 Biscuit/14g	65	2.7	450	7.8	62	18.7	6.1
Oat Crunch, Weight Watchers*	1 Biscuit/12g	52	2.1	448	7.4	65.2	17.8	6.1
Oat Digestives, Nairn's*	1 Biscuit/11g	50	2	437	12	57.8	17.5	7.8
Oat Digestives, TTD, Sainsbury's*	1 Biscuit/13g	56	2.3	448	9.8	56.4	18.5	8.5
Oat, Chocolate Chip, GF, Breaks, Nairn's*	1 Biscuit/10g	47	2	470	7.6	61.8	20.1	5.5
Oat, Stem Ginger, GF, Breaks, Nairn's*	1 Biscuit/10g	46	1.9	463	8.2	62.4	18.8	5.7
Oat, Beetroot, Nigella, Three Seed, Waitrose*	1 Biscuit/10g	48	2.4	481	11.9	50.7	23.9	7.7
Oat, Black Sesame Seaweed, 1, Waitrose*	1 Biscuit/5g	27	1.3	487	10.5	55.5	23.1	7.8
Oat, Fruit Spice, Nairn's*	1 Biscuit/10g	43	1.5	425	7.8	65.3	14.7	7.6
Oat, Mixed Berries, Nairn's*	1 Biscuit/10g	43	1.5	427	7.5	64.8	15.3	7.1
Oaten, Organic, Duchy Originals*	1 Biscuit/16g	71	2.7	441	9.8	62.3	16.9	5.3
Oatie Crumbles, CBY, Asda*	1 Biscuit/14g	68	2.9	483	6.6	65.6	20.6	4.5
Oaties, Belmont Biscuit Co, Aldi*	1 Biscuit/15g	71	3.1	475	7.8	66.7	20.4	3.3
Oaties, Oatland, Tesco*	1 Biscuit/15g	70	3.1	470	6.5	64.9	20.5	4.5
Oatmeal Crunch, Jacob's*	1 Biscuit/8g	37	1.5	458	6.8	65.9	18.6	3.6
Oatmeal, Asda*	1 Biscuit/12g	54	2.5	470	6	62	22	6
Oaty Thins, Rude Health*	1 Thin/6g	23	0.3	380	11.5	68.5	4.7	8.7
Oaty, 4 Seed, Rude Health*	1 Biscuit/13g	57	2.6	455	11.1	50.8	21	9.4
Orange Chocolate, Organic, Duchy Originals*	1 Biscuit/13g	64	3.5	509	5.5	60	28	3
Orange Sultana, Go Ahead, McVitie's*	1 Biscuit/15g	58	1.2	400	5.1	75.7	8.1	3
Oreo, Chocolate Cream, Thins, Mondelez*	4 Biscuits/24g	117	4.8	488	5.4	69	20	3.5
Oreo, Thins, Mondelez*	4 Biscuits/24g	118	5.1	490	4.8	69	21	2.6
Oreos, Choc o Brownie, Mondelez*	1 Biscuit/11g	52	2.1	473	5.7	67	19	3.8
Palmiers, Parmigiano, Green Pesto, Finest, Tesco*	1 Biscuit/5g	27	1.8	546	15.9	39.7	35.3	2.7
Parmesan Cheese, Sainsbury's*	1 Biscuit/3g	18	1	553	14.7	56.4	29.9	1.8
Party Rings, Iced, Fox's*	1 Biscuit/6g	29	0.9	459	5.1	75.8	15	0
Peanut Butter Cups, Mini, Hershey*	1 Cup/8g	44	2.4	564	10.3	56.4	30.8	2.6
Peanut Butter, American Style, Sainsbury's*	1 Biscuit/13g	63	2.9	504	5.2	68.7	23.1	2.2
Peppa Pig, Muddy Puddles, Peppa Pig*	1 Biscuit/24g	110	4.7	449	6	61.7	19.1	3.3
Petit Beurre, Stella Artois*	1 Biscuit/6g	26	0.9	440	9	73	15	0
Pink Wafers, Crawfords*	1 Biscuit/7g	36	1.9	521	2.5	68.6	26.5	1.1
Pink Wafers, Eat Me, Aldi*	1 Biscuit/8g	44	2.6	552	4.2	58.4	32.9	2.9
Pink Wafers, Sainsbury's*	1 Biscuit/8g	36	1.8	486	4.6	64.2	23.4	1.7
Puffin, Chocolate, Asda*	1 Biscuit/25g	133	7.2	533	5	63	29	1.2
Puffin, Orange, Asda*	1 Biscuit/25g	133	7.3	529	5	62	29	2.2
Raspberry Cream Viennese, Melts, Fox's*	1 Biscuit/16g	84	4.5	521	4	62.1	28.1	1.7
Raspberry, Yoghurt Breaks, Go Ahead, McVitie's*	1 Pack/35g	143	3.6	408	5.4	73.6	10.2	2.3
Redcurrant Puffs, Eat Well, M&S*	1 Biscuit/7g	32	1.4	470	5.6	67.7	19.8	2
Rich Shorties, Asda*	1 Biscuit/10g	50	2.3	486	6	66	22	2
Rich Tea, 25% Less Fat, Tesco*	1 Biscuit/10g	44	1.1	435	7.1	77	11	1.3
Rich Tea, Average	**1 Biscuit/10g**	**45**	**1.5**	**451**	**6.8**	**72.8**	**14.5**	**2.5**
Rich Tea, Basics, Sainsbury's*	1 Biscuit/8g	35	1.2	450	7.1	71.3	15.2	2.9
Rich Tea, Belmont Biscuit Co, Aldi*	1 Biscuit/8g	37	1.2	464	7.4	74	15	3.2
Rich Tea, CBY, Asda*	1 Biscuit/8g	34	1	447	7.2	72.9	13.4	3
Rich Tea, Classic, McVitie's*	1 Biscuit/8g	39	1.3	459	7	71.3	15.5	2.9
Rich Tea, Finger, Essential, Waitrose*	1 Biscuit/5g	22	0.7	450	7.2	72.5	14.3	3
Rich Tea, Finger, Tesco*	1 Finger/5g	23	0.7	451	7.4	72.9	14.4	2.3
Rich Tea, Fingers, Morrisons*	1 Finger/4g	22	0.7	550	10	90	17.5	5
Rich Tea, Light, McVitie's*	1 Biscuit/8g	36	0.9	436	7.6	75.3	10.7	3.1
Rich Tea, Plain Chocolate, Sainsbury's*	1 Biscuit/13g	65	3	497	6.6	66	23	2.6
Rich Tea, Sainsbury's*	1 Biscuit/8g	35	1	454	7.5	75.2	13.2	2

BISCUITS

	Measure INFO/WEIGHT	per Measure KCAL	FAT	Nutrition Values per 100g / 100ml KCAL	PROT	CARB	FAT	FIBRE
Rich Tea, Tesco*	1 Biscuit/10g	43	1.4	450	7.3	71.8	14.2	3.1
Rocky Road, Choccy, Cherry, Moments, McVitie's*	1 Slice/41g	193	8.9	470	4.2	63.6	21.6	2
Rocky, Chocolate & Caramel, Fox's*	1 Biscuit/21g	107	4.1	507	6.9	60.3	19.3	15.5
Rocky, Chocolate, Fox's*	1 Biscuit/21g	106	5.4	505	5.7	62.4	25.7	2.4
Rocky, Rounds, Caramel, Fox's*	1 Biscuit/15g	72	3.4	480	6.2	62.3	22.9	1.1
Rocky, Rounds, Chocolate, Fox's*	1 Biscuit/6g	31	1.7	517	7.2	58.5	28.3	1.6
Rosemary & Raisin, M&S*	1 Biscuit/7g	35	1.7	490	5.1	62.5	24.1	1.8
Rosemary Thyme, Oaten, Duchy Originals, Waitrose*	1 Biscuit/12g	58	2.7	467	8.5	56.8	21.5	6
Roundie, Caramel, Dairy Milk, Cadbury*	1 Biscuit/30g	158	8.7	528	6.3	59	29	2.3
Roundie, Milk Chocolate Covered Wafer, Cadbury*	1 Biscuit/30g	161	9.3	536	6.8	56	31	2.8
Safari Snacks, Belmont Biscuit Co, Aldi*	1 Bag/22g	108	4.8	492	6.4	65	22	2.8
Savoury Oat, with Thyme, Rick Stein*	1 Biscuit/10g	46	2.1	460	9.8	66.9	21.4	10.4
Savoury, Gluten, Wheat & Dairy Free, Sainsbury's*	1 Biscuit/17g	77	2.9	467	11.7	65.1	17.7	2.4
Savoury, Organic, M&S*	1 Biscuit/7g	28	1	395	7	58.4	14.6	8.7
Scotch Finger, Arnotts Australia*	1 Biscuit/18g	88	3.9	489	6.6	65.8	21.5	0
Scottish Sweet Oatie, Organic, Daylesford Organic*	1 Biscuit/23g	119	7.1	516	6.1	53.9	30.7	4.7
Sea Salt Black Pepper, for Cheese, TTD, Sainsbury's*	3 Biscuits/20g	93	4.3	484	8.8	60.1	22.4	3.8
Shortbread, All Butter, Fingers, Walkers Shortbread Ltd*	2 Fingers/48g	256	14.5	533	5.6	58.4	30.3	2.1
Shortcake with Real Milk Chocolate, Cadbury*	1 Biscuit/15g	75	3.5	500	6.3	65.8	23.5	0
Shortcake, Asda*	1 Biscuit/14g	73	3.6	518	5	66	26	2
Shortcake, Average	***1 Biscuit/11g***	***55***	***3***	***501***	***6.3***	***66.1***	***27.1***	***2.1***
Shortcake, Caramel, Mini, Festive, Thorntons*	1 Cake/14g	71	4.3	508	4	52.5	30.8	0.6
Shortcake, Caramel, Mini, Finest, Tesco*	1 Biscuit/15g	74	4.2	493	4.3	56.3	27.8	1
Shortcake, Caramel, Mini, Thorntons*	1 Biscuit/15g	71	4.6	492	4.8	46.3	31.9	0.6
Shortcake, Caramel, Squares, Tesco*	1 Square/54g	274	16.4	507	4.6	54.1	30.4	0.4
Shortcake, Chocolate Covered, Rounds, Galaxy, Mars*	1 Biscuit/16g	81	3.9	508	6.8	64.3	24.5	0
Shortcake, Crawfords*	1 Biscuit/10g	52	2.5	504	6.2	63.5	24.4	2.6
Shortcake, Dairy Milk Chocolate, Cadbury*	1 Bar/49g	252	13.5	515	7.5	59.2	27.5	0
Shortcake, Dutch, M&S*	1 Biscuit/17g	90	5.1	540	5.4	59	30.8	2.5
Shortcake, Fruit, Crawfords*	1 Biscuit/8g	34	1.5	419	5.4	55.9	19.3	2.4
Shortcake, Rounds, Value, Tesco*	1 Biscuit/22g	120	7	540	5.5	58.8	31.4	2.1
Shortcake, Sainsbury's*	1 Biscuit/11g	53	5.2	479	6.1	65.3	47.2	2.5
Shortcake, Snack, Cadbury*	2 Biscuits/15g	70	3.7	475	7	54.5	25	1.7
Shortcake, Value, Tesco*	1 Biscuit/10g	49	2.1	486	7.1	66.5	21.2	2.1
Shorties, Cadbury*	1 Biscuit/15g	77	3.6	511	6.5	67.3	24	0
Shorties, Fruit, Value, Tesco*	1 Serving/10g	46	1.7	457	5.7	69.3	17.4	3
Shorties, Rich Highland, Tesco*	1 Biscuit/10g	48	2.2	485	6.1	65.3	21.7	2.6
Shorties, Rich, Tesco*	1 Biscuit/10g	48	2.2	484	6.4	65.6	21.8	2
Shorties, Sainsbury's*	1 Biscuit/10g	50	2.2	500	6.4	69.8	21.8	2
Signature Collection, Cadbury*	1 Biscuit/15g	80	4.4	530	6.2	60.1	29.5	0
Snappy, Milk Chocolate Finger, Tesco*	2 Fingers/21g	113	6.1	528	6.5	60.8	28.3	2
Speculaas, Large, Hema*	1 Biscuit/23g	106	4.8	459	5.4	61.2	20.8	2.6
Spiced, German, Christmas, Favorina, Lidl*	1 Biscuit/10g	47	1.9	472	5.8	70.2	18.7	0
Spiced, Whole Wheat, Prodia*	1 Biscuit/5g	17	1	339	7.1	41.4	19.4	8.5
Sports, Fox's*	1 Biscuit/9g	41	1.7	483	6.7	67	20	2
Stem Ginger, Brakes*	1 Biscuit/13g	62	3.1	495	5.6	62.6	24.7	0
Stornoway, Water, Stag Bakeries Ltd*	1 Biscuit/9g	31	1.2	341	6.5	47.9	13.6	1.7
Strawberry, Biscuit Moments, Special K, Kellogg's*	2 Biscuits/25g	98	2	391	5	74	8	1.5
Strawberry, Cream Tease, McVitie's*	1 Biscuit/19g	97	4.8	510	4.8	65.9	25.2	1.2
Sugar Wafers, Vanilla, Flavoured, Triunfo*	1 Biscuit/10g	53	2.5	511	4.1	70.1	24.3	0.6
Sultana Cinnamon, Weight Watchers*	1 Biscuit/12g	51	1.7	441	4.3	72.3	15	3
Tangy Jaffa Viennese, Creations, Fox's*	1 Biscuit/17g	76	3.3	447	5	63.5	19.2	0.9
Tangy Stilton Wafers, Thomas J Fudge*	1 Wafer/3g	18	1.1	529	15.8	42.2	32.4	0

BISCUITS

	Measure INFO/WEIGHT	per Measure KCAL	FAT	Nutrition Values per 100g / 100ml KCAL	PROT	CARB	FAT	FIBRE
Tasties, Jam Cream, Sandwich, Mcvitie's*	1 Biscuit/15g	74	3.4	488	4.8	65.6	22.4	2.2
Taxi, McVitie's*	1 Biscuit/27g	134	6.9	504	4.2	63.3	26	0.7
Teddy Bear, Mini, M&S*	1 Biscuit/17g	80	3.8	475	5.4	62.6	22.7	3.2
The Oaty, Wheat Free, Rude Health*	1 Biscuit/12g	55	2.2	437	9	57.2	17.5	7.9
Toffee Apple Crumbles, Border Biscuits Ltd*	1 Biscuit/18g	77	3.7	427	5	56.7	20.4	2.3
Toffee Chip Crinkle Crunch, Fox's*	1 Biscuit/11g	51	2	460	4.6	69.6	18.2	0
Toffee Dodgers, Burton's*	1 Biscuit/18g	84	3.2	468	5.7	71.4	17.5	1.1
Tortina, Original, Milk Chocolate, Loacker*	1 Biscuit/21g	116	7.4	552	10	48	35	0
Tostada, Opey, Lidl*	1 Biscuit/6g	26	0.6	435	6.9	78.3	10.1	1.7
Treacle Crunch Creams, Fox's*	1 Biscuit/13g	65	3.2	502	4.5	65.3	24.8	1.4
Triple Chocolate, Caramel Shortcakes, Thorntons*	1 Bite/14g	62	3.2	445	4.6	54.8	22.7	0
Triple Chocolate, Fox's*	1 Biscuit/21g	100	5.2	478	5.7	57.3	25.1	2.5
Twix, Caramel Slice, McVitie's*	1 Slice/29g	142	7.8	491	4.5	57.3	26.8	1.4
Viennese Creams, Raspberry, M&S*	1 Biscuit/17g	90	4.9	520	4.6	60.4	28.6	1.3
Viennese Finger, Belmont Biscuit Co, Aldi*	1 Biscuit/16g	84	4.7	521	4.8	61	29	1.5
Viennese Whirl, Chocolate, Border*	1 Biscuit/19g	96	4.3	512	6.5	61.9	23.2	0
Viennese Whirl, Fox's*	1 Biscuit/25g	130	7	518	6.7	60.1	27.8	0
Viennese, Chocolate, Melts, Fox's*	1 Biscuit/12g	64	3.4	526	6.1	60.5	28.3	2.4
Viennese, Milk Chocolate, Thins, Tesco*	1 Biscuit/9g	48	2.7	533	5.1	59.7	30.1	1.5
Viennese, Sandwich, Chocolate, M&S*	1 Biscuit/15g	80	4.6	535	7.2	58	30.6	1.7
Viennese, with Milk Chocolate Filling	*1 Biscuit/15g*	*81*	*4.5*	*533*	*6.5*	*59.6*	*29.4*	*2.1*
Wafer, Vanilla, Loacker*	1 Pack/45g	231	12.6	514	7.5	58	28	0
Water, Asda*	1 Biscuit/6g	25	0.5	412	10	75	8	3.3
Water, Average	*1 Biscuit/6g*	*24*	*0.7*	*440*	*10.8*	*75.8*	*12.5*	*3.1*
Water, High Bake, Jacob's*	1 Biscuit/5g	22	0.4	414	10.5	76.4	7.4	3
Water, High Bake, Sainsbury's*	1 Biscuit/5g	21	0.4	412	9.8	76.3	7.5	3.2
Water, High Baked, Tesco*	1 Biscuit/5g	21	0.3	413	9.7	77.4	6.6	2.7
Water, Table, Carr's*	1 Biscuit/3g	14	0.3	417	10.1	74.7	7.6	4.2
Water, Table, Large, Carr's*	1 Biscuit/8g	31	0.6	408	9.9	73.1	7.5	4.1
Water, Table, Small, Carr's*	1 Biscuit/3g	14	0.3	406	10.1	80	7.6	4.2
Wheat, Fig, Plum, Cranberry, 1, Waitrose*	1 Biscuit/10g	40	1.2	399	9.3	62.6	11.8	3
White, Chocolate, Coated, Bakery Instore, Lidl*	1 Biscuit/8g	41	2	509	6	64	25	2
Wholemeal Brans, Fox's*	1 Biscuit/20g	90	4	451	8.5	58.8	20.2	7.5
Yoghurt Break, Blueberry, Go Ahead, McVitie's*	1 Slice/18g	72	1.8	401	5.5	72.1	10	2.2
Yoghurt Break, Plain, Go Ahead, McVitie's*	1 Slice/18g	72	2.1	394	6.5	66	11.5	3.3
Yoghurt Break, Red Cherry, Go Ahead, McVitie's*	1 Slice/18g	72	1.8	407	5.5	73.4	10.1	2.2
Yoghurt Break, Strawberry, Go Ahead, McVitie's*	1 Slice/18g	72	1.8	402	52	72.4	10.3	3.4
Yorkie, Nestle*	1 Biscuit/25g	128	6.7	510	6.7	60.4	26.8	1.3

BISON

Raw	*1oz/28g*	*31*	*0.5*	*109*	*21.6*	*0*	*1.8*	*0*

BITES

Blueberry Yoghurt Clusters, Mini, M&S*	1 Bite/13g	60	2.7	465	5	64.4	20.7	4.7
Blueberry, Lemon, Oat Squares, Superfood, Graze*	1 Bite/30g	136	7.5	454	5	53	25	4.8
Brownie, Chocolate, Tesco*	1 Bite/11g	43	1.6	394	5.3	58	15	30.7
Buttermilk, Quorn*	3 Bites/90g	163	3.3	181	12.3	22.1	3.7	4.8
Caramel Crisp Bite, Tesco*	1 Bite/11g	47	1.3	428	5	73.9	12.2	1.4
Caramel Crispy, Crunchy Tempting, Mini, Waitrose*	1 Bite/13g	54	1.7	412	4	69.9	12.7	1.2
Caramel Crispy, Extremely Chocolatey, Mini, M&S*	1 Bite/11g	50	2	455	4.7	68.2	17.9	2.8
Caramel Shortcake, Mini, Bakers Selection, Asda*	1 Bite/12g	60	3.1	499	5.6	60	26	1.4
Cheese & Garlic, M&S*	1 Bite/11g	40	3.1	350	8.3	17.2	27.3	5.8
Chicken, Kiev, Tesco*	1 Bite/18g	45	2.9	252	8.4	18.1	15.9	1.3
Chocolate Cornflake, Mini, M&S*	1 Bite/11.8g	55	2.4	470	6.2	66.3	20.1	3.6
Chocolate Orange, Mini, M&S*	1 Bite/22g	95	4.8	430	5.5	54.6	21.6	1.8

B

	Measure INFO/WEIGHT	per Measure KCAL	FAT	Nutrition Values per 100g / 100ml KCAL	PROT	CARB	FAT	FIBRE
BITES								
Chocolate, Double, Mini, M&S*	1 Bite/17g	82	4.1	469	5.8	57.2	23.6	2.1
Ciabatta, Garlic & Herb, Occasions, Sainsbury's*	1 Bite/12g	48	2.6	398	8.9	42.2	21.5	3.2
Cornflake Clusters, Chocolate, Mini, Holly Lane, Aldi*	1 Bite/10g	47	1.8	467	6.5	68	18	3.3
Extremely Chocolatey, Mini, M&S*	1 Bite/20g	90	4.9	450	5.7	52.4	24.6	1.6
Flapjack, Mini, M&S*	1 Bite/14g	64	3.1	458	6.1	56.7	21.9	5
Honeycomb Clusters, Rich Chocolatey, Mini, Waitrose*	1 Bite/11g	50	2	456	4.8	66.2	18.5	2.9
Jalapeno, Cream Cheese, Tesco*	1 Bite/20g	63	3.9	313	7.2	26.7	19.4	1.6
Millionaires, Tesco*	1 Bites/12g	60	3.4	500	5.1	55.6	28	2.5
Protein, Honey Seed, Oat Squares, Graze*	1 Square/30g	140	8.1	465	15	42	27	4.4
Rocky Road, Mini, M&S*	1 Bite/12g	50	1.6	410	5.2	66.9	13.3	2.5
Salted Caramel Popcorn, Mini, Extremely Indulgent, M&S*	1 Bite/9g	42	1.7	481	5.1	69.9	19.8	1.6
Spinach, Strong Roots*	3 Bites/75g	164	9.1	218	3.4	20.8	12.1	6.4
Tiffin, Chocolate, Belgian, Free From, Lazy Day Foods*	1 Tiffin/15g	73	4.5	488	3	52	30	3.5
BITTER LEMON								
Fever-Tree*	1 Glass/200ml	77	0	38	0	9.2	0	0
Low Calorie, Tesco*	1 Glass/200ml	6	0.2	3	0.1	0.3	0.1	0.1
Schweppes*	1 Glass/250ml	85	0	34	0	8.2	0	0
BLACK GRAM								
Urad Gram, Dried, Raw	*1oz/28g*	*77*	*0.4*	*275*	*24.9*	*40.8*	*1.4*	*0*
BLACK PUDDING								
Average, Uncooked	*1 Serving/40g*	*101*	*6*	*252*	*10.2*	*19*	*14.9*	*0.6*
BLACKBERRIES								
Fresh, Raw, Average	*1oz/28g*	*7*	*0.1*	*25*	*0.9*	*5.1*	*0.2*	*5.3*
Frozen, Average	*1 Serving/80g*	*37*	*0.1*	*46*	*0.9*	*9.6*	*0.2*	*5.3*
in Fruit Juice, Average	*½ Can/145g*	*52*	*0.3*	*36*	*0.6*	*7.9*	*0.2*	*1.3*
in Light Syrup, Canned, Tesco*	½ Can/145g	70	0.1	48	0.5	10.6	0.1	1.5
BLACKCURRANTS								
Dried, Graze*	1 Pack/30g	95	0.3	317	3.3	79	1	0
Fresh, Raw, Average	*1 Serving/80g*	*22*	*0*	*27*	*0.9*	*6.5*	*0*	*3.5*
in Fruit Juice, Average	*1 Serving/30g*	*11*	*0*	*38*	*0.6*	*8.6*	*0.2*	*2.4*
in Light Syrup, British, Canned, Tesco*	½ Can/145g	71	0.1	49	0.5	10.4	0.1	2.1
Stewed with Sugar	*1oz/28g*	*16*	*0*	*58*	*0.7*	*15*	*0*	*2.8*
Stewed without Sugar	*1oz/28g*	*7*	*0*	*24*	*0.8*	*5.6*	*0*	*3.1*
BLANCMANGE								
Chocolate Flavour, Made Up, Pearce Duff*	1 Serving/140g	137	5.6	98	3.3	12.3	4	0
Raspberry Flavour, Pearce Duff*	1 Serving/138g	123	2.5	89	3.1	15	1.8	0
Strawberry Flavour, Pearce Duff*	1 Serving/138g	123	2.5	89	3.1	15	1.8	0
Vanilla Flavour, Pearce Duff*	1 Serving/138g	123	2.5	89	3.1	15	1.8	0
BLUEBERRIES								
Chocolate Covered, Waitrose*	1 Serving/25g	120	5.6	481	4	65.6	22.4	3
Dried, Love Life, Waitrose*	1 Serving/30g	107	0.2	358	1.1	80.1	0.8	3.6
Frozen, Average	*1 Serving/80g*	*41*	*0.2*	*51*	*0.6*	*13.8*	*0.2*	*4.4*
Raw, Average	*50 Berries/68g*	*39*	*0.2*	*57*	*0.7*	*14.5*	*0.3*	*2.4*
BOAR								
Wild, Raw, Average	*1 Serving/200g*	*244*	*6.7*	*122*	*21.5*	*0*	*3.3*	*0*
BOILED SWEETS								
Average	*1 Sweet/7g*	*21*	*0*	*327*	*0*	*87.1*	*0*	*0*
Blackcurrant & Liquorice, Co-Op*	1 Sweet/8g	32	0.4	405	0.9	91	5	0
Cherry Drops, Bassett's*	1 Sweet/5g	18	0	390	0	98.1	0	0
Clear Fruits, Sainsbury's*	1 Sweet/7g	26	0	372	0.1	92.9	0	0
Fruit Drops, Co-Op*	1 Sweet/6g	24	0	395	0.2	98	0	0
Fruit Sherbets, Assorted, M&S*	1 Sweet/9g	35	0.4	405	0.3	91.6	4.3	0.1
Lockets, Mars*	1 Pack/43g	165	0	383	0	95.8	0	0

	Measure INFO/WEIGHT	per Measure KCAL	FAT	Nutrition Values per 100g / 100ml KCAL	PROT	CARB	FAT	FIBRE
BOILED SWEETS								
Mentho-Lyptus, Cherry, Sugar Free, Hall's*	1 Lozenge/4g	8	0	234	0	62.4	0	0
Mentho-Lyptus, Extra Strong, Hall's*	1 Lozenge/4g	14	0	389	0	96.9	0	0
Pear Drops, Bassett's*	1 Sweet/4g	16	0	390	0	96.4	0	0
Pear Drops, Sugar Free, Sula*	1 Sweet/3g	7	0	235	0.1	97	0.1	0
Soothers, Blackcurrant, Hall's*	1 Lozenge/5g	16	0	365	0	91.4	0	0
Soothers, Cherry, Hall's*	1 Pack/45g	165	0	365	0	91.3	0	0
Soothers, Strawberry Flavour, Hall's*	1 Sweet/5g	19	0	385	0	96	0	0
BOK CHOY								
Tesco*	1 Serving/100g	11	0.2	11	1	1.4	0.2	1.2
BOLOGNESE								
Courgetti, BGTY, Sainsbury's*	1 Pack/380g	224	6.8	59	5.9	4.1	1.8	1.4
Frozen, HFC, Tesco*	1 Pack/376g	376	9.3	100	5.1	13.7	2.5	1.4
Meatless, Granose*	1 Pack/400g	400	16	100	8	8	4	0
Pappardelle, Cooked, Stir Your Senses, Birds Eye*	1 Serving/350g	610	23	174	6.9	20.9	6.6	2.4
Pasta, Diet Chef Ltd*	1 Serving/300g	288	10.2	96	7.9	5.8	3.4	4.4
Spaghetti, Al Forno, Sainsbury's*	1 Pack/400g	460	19.6	115	7.8	10	4.9	1.1
Spaghetti, As Consumed, Savers, Morrisons*	1 Pack/300g	338	10.4	120	4.5	16.3	3.7	1.6
Spaghetti, BGTY, Sainsbury's*	1 Pack/400g	416	9.2	104	6.3	14.4	2.3	1.1
Spaghetti, CBY, Asda*	1 Pack/100g	108	2	108	6	15.6	2	2
Spaghetti, Cook*	1 Portion/390g	491	14.8	126	8.9	14.8	3.8	1.6
Spaghetti, Egg Pasta in Rich Beef Sauce, Waitrose*	1 Pack/400g	404	10.4	101	7.6	11.7	2.6	1
Spaghetti, Frozen, Tesco*	1 Pack/450g	472	9	105	5.8	15	2	1.8
Spaghetti, Hidden Veg, Heinz*	1 Can/400g	312	6.4	78	3.4	12.6	1.6	0.9
Spaghetti, HL, Tesco*	1 Pack/360g	342	7.2	95	6.4	12	2	1.6
Spaghetti, Italian, Chilled, Tesco*	1 Pack/400g	520	17.2	130	6.5	15.9	4.3	1.5
Spaghetti, Italian, Microwaved, Morrisons*	1 Pack/400g	398	9.1	101	6.5	12.7	2.3	1.6
Spaghetti, Italiano, Pro-Cuisine, Pro Cuisine*	1 Pack/600g	522	11.4	87	5.7	11.7	1.9	0
Spaghetti, Meal for One, M&S*	1 Pack/400g	612	31.6	153	7.4	12.3	7.9	1.6
Spaghetti, Ready to Cook, Musclefood*	1 Pack/371g	397	8.9	107	7.2	13.3	2.4	1.9
Spaghetti, Sainsbury's*	1 Pack/400g	525	18.8	131	6.1	16	4.7	2.2
Spaghetti, Serves 1, Basics, Sainsbury's*	1 Pack/300g	276	5.4	92	4.9	12.9	1.8	2.1
Spaghetti, Slow Cooked, TTD, Sainsbury's*	1 Pack/400g	561	27.3	148	8.8	10.8	7.2	2.5
Spaghetti, Weight Watchers*	1 Meal/320g	353	6.7	110	6.6	15.7	2.1	1
Tortellini, Beef, Rich, Italian, Giovanni Rana*	½ Pack/125g	222	9	178	7.6	20.6	7.2	4.1
Turkey, Microwaved, Slimzone, Asda*	1 Pack/419g	381	3.8	91	7.2	12	0.9	2.4
Vegetarian, M&S*	1 Pack/360g	360	12.6	100	4.5	12.5	3.5	2.1
Vegetarian, Spaghetti, Quorn*	1 Pack/300g	255	1.8	85	4.4	14.8	0.6	1.5
Vegetarian, Spaghetti, Sainsbury's*	½ Can/200g	132	2.4	66	3	9.9	1.2	1.8
BOMBAY MIX								
Average	**1oz/28g**	**141**	**9.2**	**503**	**18.8**	**35.1**	**32.9**	**6.2**
BON BONS								
Apple, Lemon & Strawberry, Co-Op*	¼ Bag/50g	202	2.5	405	1	88	5	0
Fruit, Bassett's*	1 Serving/7g	25	0	380	0.1	94.2	0	0
Lemon, Bassett's*	1 Sweet/7g	30	0.7	425	0	83.7	9.8	0
Mixed Fruit Flavour, Vimto, Tangerine Confectionery Ltd*	1 Sweet/5g	20	0.3	409	0.1	85.8	6.7	0.6
BOOST								
Standard Bar, Cadbury*	1 Bar/49g	250	13.8	515	5.8	58.6	28.5	1.5
Treat Size, Cadbury*	1 Bar/24g	130	7.4	535	5.3	59.6	30.5	0
BOUILLABAISSE								
Average	**1 Serving/400g**	**556**	**38.8**	**139**	**11.2**	**2**	**9.7**	**0.4**
BOUILLON								
Powder, Miso, Marigold*	1 Tsp/5g	12	0.5	248	7	34	9.3	1.4
Powder, Swiss Vegetable, Green Tub, Marigold*	1 Tsp/5g	12	0.4	245	10.1	30.1	8.5	0

	Measure INFO/WEIGHT	per Measure KCAL	FAT	Nutrition Values per 100g / 100ml KCAL	PROT	CARB	FAT	FIBRE
BOUNTY								
Dark, Mars*	1 Funsize/29g	141	7.9	493	3.6	55.8	27.5	0
Milk, Mars*	1 Funsize/29g	139	7.3	487	3.7	58.9	25.7	0
BOUQUET GARNI								
Handtied, Fresh, Asda*	1 Bunch/2.4g	11	0.2	455	8.3	69.4	7.9	31.6
BOURNVITA*								
Powder, Made Up with Semi-Skimmed Milk	*1 Mug/227ml*	*132*	*3.6*	*58*	*3.5*	*7.8*	*1.6*	*0*
Powder, Made Up with Whole Milk	*1 Mug/227ml*	*173*	*8.6*	*76*	*3.4*	*7.6*	*3.8*	*0*
BOVRIL*								
Beef Extract, Drink, Made Up with Water, Bovril*	1 Serving/12g	22	0.1	184	38.9	4.6	1.2	0
Chicken Savoury Drink, Bovril*	1 Serving/13g	16	0.2	129	9.7	19.4	1.4	2.1
BRANDY								
37.5% Volume, Average	*1 Pub Shot/35ml*	*72*	*0*	*207*	*0*	*0*	*0*	*0*
40% Volume, Average	*1 Pub Shot/35ml*	*78*	*0*	*224*	*0*	*0*	*0*	*0*
Cherry, Average	*1 Pub Shot/35ml*	*89*	*0*	*255*	*0*	*32.6*	*0*	*0*
BRAWN								
Average	*1 Serving/100g*	*153*	*11.5*	*153*	*12.4*	*0*	*11.5*	*0*
BRAZIL NUTS								
Average	*6 Whole/20g*	*136*	*13.7*	*682*	*15.3*	*2.8*	*68.4*	*5.4*
Milk Chocolate, Tesco*	1 Nut/8g	47	3.5	585	9.9	38	43.7	1.9
BREAD								
Ancient Grain, Pave, Bakery, Tesco*	1 Slice/80g	213	3.9	267	9.8	44.1	4.9	3.3
Apple Sourdough, Gail's*	1 Slice/50g	118	0.4	236	7.5	43.9	0.7	4.3
Apricot & Sesame Seed, Lifefibre*	1 Slice/43g	148	4.4	344	8.1	55	10.3	6.2
Arabic, El Amar Bakery*	1 Serving/110g	318	1.3	289	11.6	57.9	1.2	0
Bagel, 4 Everything, Finest, Tesco*	1 Bagel/100g	268	1.8	268	11.1	51.9	1.8	2.5
Bagel, Baked with Marmite, Marmite*	1 Bagel/85g	240	2.6	282	12.9	49.3	3.1	2.8
Bagel, Caramelised Onion & Poppyseed, Waitrose*	1 Bagel/86g	222	2.2	258	9.7	49.2	2.5	2.4
Bagel, Caramelised Onion Poppy Seed, Tesco*	1 Bagel/85g	221	2.1	260	10.9	47.6	2.5	3.8
Bagel, Cinnamon Raisin, Morrisons*	1 Bagel/85g	215	1.7	253	7.7	51.1	2	4.5
Bagel, Cinnamon Raisin, Tesco*	1 Bagel/85g	230	1.4	270	10.4	51.3	1.7	3.8
Bagel, Cranberry Orange, New York Bakery Co*	1 Bagel/90g	246	2.3	273	9.6	51	2.5	3.9
Bagel, Fruit & Spice, Sainsbury's*	1 Bagel/85g	234	1.8	275	9.7	54.3	2.1	3.8
Bagel, Fruit Fibre, Kingsmill*	1 Bagel/85g	225	1.2	265	9.8	50.8	1.4	5.2
Bagel, Granary, Bagel Factory*	1 Bagel/100g	288	2.1	288	11.9	57.4	2.1	4.5
Bagel, Mini, Sainsbury's*	1 Bagel/25g	67	0.4	268	11.2	52.4	1.6	2.8
Bagel, Multi Seed, BFree*	1 Bagel/80g	186	2	232	4.1	51.4	2.5	6.5
Bagel, Multi Seed, New York Bagel Co*	1 Bagel/90g	244	4.3	271	12.4	41.6	4.8	5.8
Bagel, Multigrain, Sainsbury's*	1 Bagel/113g	293	3.5	259	10	49.6	3.1	2
Bagel, Onion Poppy Seed, Average	*1 Bagel/85g*	*225*	*2.8*	*264*	*9*	*50.5*	*3.3*	*3.2*
Bagel, Onion, New York Bagel Co*	1 Bagel/85g	222	1.6	261	10.6	50.4	1.9	3.1
Bagel, Onion, Tesco*	1 Bagel/85g	233	2	274	10.5	52.4	2.4	1.9
Bagel, Original, Organic, New York Bagel Co*	1 Bagel/85g	220	1.2	259	9.3	52.2	1.4	4.1
Bagel, Plain	*1 Bagel/104g*	*290*	*2*	*279*	*10.6*	*53.8*	*1.9*	*2.9*
Bagel, Plain, Asda*	1 Bagel/85g	226	2	265	15	46	2.3	2.9
Bagel, Plain, Average	*1 Bagel/78g*	*202*	*1.5*	*259*	*10.1*	*50.4*	*1.9*	*3.1*
Bagel, Plain, Bagel Factory*	1 Bagel/150g	318	1.3	212	9.4	41.6	0.9	2.1
Bagel, Plain, Free From, Tesco*	1 Bagel/80g	215	5.5	270	3.4	47.7	6.9	4.7
Bagel, Plain, GFY, Asda*	1 Bagel/84g	218	1.8	259	10	50	2.1	1.8
Bagel, Plain, New York Bakery Co*	1 Bagel/90g	232	1.1	258	10.1	50.1	1.2	3.1
Bagel, Plain, Organic, Tesco*	1 Bagel/85g	216	2.3	254	9	48.4	2.7	3.6
Bagel, Plain, So Organic, Sainsbury's*	1 Bagel/85g	216	2.3	254	9	48.4	2.7	3.6
Bagel, Plain, Tesco*	1 Bagel/85g	225	1.3	265	9.3	52.2	1.5	2.7
Bagel, Red Onion, Chive, New York Bakery Co*	1 Bagel/90g	235	1	261	10.6	50.5	1.1	3.1

BREAD

INFO/WEIGHT	Measure	per Measure KCAL	FAT	Nutrition Values per 100g / 100ml KCAL	PROT	CARB	FAT	FIBRE
Bagel, Rye, Bagel Factory*	1 Bagel/85g	279	1.3	329	14.5	64.3	1.6	6.2
Bagel, Sesame Seed, Essential, Waitrose*	1 Bagel/85g	243	2.7	286	9.6	54.6	3.2	3.6
Bagel, Sesame Seed, GFY, Asda*	1 Bagel/84g	227	2.1	271	11	51	2.5	2.6
Bagel, Sesame, M&S*	1 Bagel/87g	240	2.8	275	10.2	51.2	3.2	2.1
Bagel, Sesame, New York Bakery*	1 Bagel/90g	242	2.5	269	10.7	47.8	2.8	4.5
Bagel, Thins, Plain, New York Bakery Co*	1 Thin/48g	133	0.6	277	9.4	55.8	1.2	2.7
Bagel, Thins, Seeded, Sliced, New York Bakery Co*	1 Thin/45g	129	1.5	286	10	52.1	3.4	3.9
Bagel, Thins, Sesame, Warburton's*	1 Thin/50g	130	1.7	260	10.1	46.8	3.4	3.6
Bagel, Wee Soda, Genesis Crafty*	1 Bagel/65g	148	2.5	227	6.9	41.3	3.9	2.9
Bagel, White, Asda*	1 Bagel/86g	227	2.7	264	10	49	3.1	0
Bagel, White, Original, Weight Watchers*	1 Bagel/67g	158	0.5	236	9.5	42.4	0.8	10.7
Bagel, Wholemeal, & White, Mini, New York Bakery Co*	1 Bagel/45g	114	1	254	10.8	45.2	2.2	5.1
Bagel, Wholemeal, Average	**1 Bagel/90g**	**235**	**2.7**	**261**	**12.7**	**44.6**	**3**	**7.7**
Bagel, Wholemeal, Multiseed, M&S*	1 Bagel/84g	215	5.6	255	13.1	35.4	6.6	8.3
Bagel, Wholemeal, New York Bagel Co*	1 Bagel/90g	225	2	250	10.9	42.8	2.2	7.7
Baguette, Bake At Home, Tesco*	½ Baguette/75g	216	0.9	289	8.6	59.1	1.2	3.5
Baguette, Budgens*	1 Baguette/125g	335	1.5	268	8.5	55.7	1.2	3.5
Baguette, Crusty Brown, M&S*	½ Loaf/71g	160	1.1	225	9.8	42.7	1.6	6.3
Baguette, French, Tesco*	1 Serving/60g	144	0.7	240	7.8	49.5	1.2	3.4
Baguette, Garlic, Slices, Frozen, CBY, Asda*	1 Slice/26g	92	4.7	355	8.2	38.3	18.1	2.8
Baguette, GF, Schnitzer*	½ Baguette/80g	186	6.2	233	4.7	30	7.8	12
Baguette, Granary, Co-Op*	1 Serving/60g	150	1.5	250	20	46	2.5	6
Baguette, Homebake, Half, Tesco*	1 Serving/75g	217	0.9	289	8.6	49.1	1.2	3.5
Baguette, Multiseed, Mini, GF, Fria*	1 Baguette/70g	203	6	290	3.5	47	8.5	6
Baguette, Part Baked, Classique, Deli France, Delifrance*	1 Pack/250g	745	3	298	9.8	54.8	1.2	2.7
Baguette, Part Baked, H.W. Nevill's*	½ Baguette/75g	216	0.9	289	8.6	59.1	1.2	3.5
Baguette, Part Baked, Half, Tesco*	½ Baguette/75g	216	0.9	289	8.6	59.1	1.2	3.5
Baguette, Paysanne, Stonebaked, Asda*	1/6 Loaf/46g	119	1.4	259	10	48	3	3.3
Baguette, Ready to Bake, Sainsbury's*	½ Baguette/62g	150	0.8	242	7.8	49.7	1.3	2.8
Baguette, Sourdough, la Brea Bakery*	1 Serving/60g	160	0.4	266	8.8	56.1	0.7	1.8
Baguette, White, Half, Crusty, M&S*	1 Baguette/162g	420	1.8	260	8.4	53.5	1.1	2.3
Baguette, White, Homebake, Tesco*	1 Baguette/150g	434	1.8	289	8.6	59.1	1.2	3.5
Baguette, White, Ready to Bake, Asda*	1 Serving/60g	168	1.1	280	10	56	1.8	2.6
Baguette, White, Sainsbury's*	1 Serving/50g	132	0.8	263	9.3	53.1	1.5	2.7
Baguette, Wholemeal, Part Baked, Asda*	½ Baguette/75g	176	1	235	8.2	47.7	1.3	3
Baguette, Wholemeal, Part Baked, Mini, Landgut*	½ Baguette/25g	56	0.2	223	7.5	46	1	0
Bakhar Khani, Mughal *	1 Bakhar/100g	220	8	220	3	28	8	1
Banana, with Dates Hazelnuts, Graze*	1 Slice/19g	59	2.7	309	4.8	38.7	14.4	2.7
Baps, Brown, Large, Asda*	1 Bap/58g	140	0.9	242	10	47	1.6	0
Baps, Brown, Large, G H Sheldon*	1 Bap/64g	169	4.3	264	5.3	47.5	6.7	4
Baps, Brown, Malted Grain, Large, Tesco*	1 Bap/93g	228	3.1	245	9.9	42.7	3.3	5.3
Baps, Cheese Topped, Baker's Soft, Tesco*	1 Bap/65g	176	3.3	268	10.8	43.5	5.1	2.6
Baps, Cheese Topped, Country Choice*	1 Bap/64g	194	5.6	303	12	43	8.8	2.5
Baps, Cheese Topped, G H Sheldon*	1 Roll/70g	197	5.8	282	12.4	38.6	8.3	1.4
Baps, Floured, M&S*	1 Bap/60g	168	3.7	280	11.5	46.8	6.2	2
Baps, Giant Malted, Sainsbury's*	1 Bap/109g	282	5.2	260	8.6	45.7	4.8	5.7
Baps, Malted, Large, Co-Op*	1 Bap/85g	208	2.6	245	10.2	44.3	3.1	5
Baps, Multigrain, Tesco*	1 Bap/98g	238	3.1	244	8.7	45.1	3.2	1.9
Baps, White Sandwich, Kingsmill*	1 Bap/80g	209	3.2	261	10.1	46.2	4	2.2
Baps, White, Average	**1 Bap/65g**	**167**	**2.3**	**257**	**9.5**	**47**	**3.5**	**1.9**
Baps, White, Floured, Waitrose*	1 Bap/60g	147	1.2	244	8	48.6	2	1.1
Baps, White, Giant, Sainsbury's*	1 Bap/86g	235	3.2	273	8.3	51.7	3.7	3.4
Baps, White, Giant, Waitrose*	1 Bap/104g	260	3.7	250	9.5	45	3.6	4.8

BRED

INFO/WEIGHT	Measure	per Measure		Nutrition Values per 100g / 100ml				
		KCAL	FAT	KCAL	PROT	CARB	FAT	FIBRE
Baps, White, Large, Tesco*	1 Bap/100g	250	1	250	9.2	49.7	1	2.6
Baps, White, Sliced, Large, Asda*	1 Bap/58g	148	1	255	10	50	1.7	0
Baps, White, Soft, Floured, M&S*	1 Bap/61g	175	3.4	285	11.5	46.6	5.5	2.8
Baps, White, Super Soft, The Bakery, M&S*	1 Roll/60g	161	2.8	268	8.4	46.6	4.7	3
Baps, White, Warburton's*	1 Bap/57g	144	2.5	252	9.8	43.4	4.3	2.7
Baps, Wholemeal, Brace's*	1 Bap/59g	137	2.6	234	10.5	42.5	4.4	4.3
Baps, Wholemeal, Country Oven*	1 Bap/40g	92	1.3	231	9.5	41	3.3	4.1
Baps, Wholemeal, Giant, Rathbones*	1 Bap/110g	230	2.1	209	9.4	39	1.9	8
Baps, Wholemeal, Giant, Sainsbury's*	1 Bap/86g	230	3.5	268	9.7	48.1	4.1	7.7
Baps, Wholemeal, Tesco*	1 Bap/46g	104	2.4	227	9.6	41.4	5.3	5.6
Baps, Wholemeal, Waitrose*	1 Bap/80g	191	3.4	238	12	34.8	4.2	6.7
Barmbrack, Irish, Rankin Selection*	1 Slice/48g	142	1.6	295	4.5	61.5	3.4	3.2
Best of Both, Farmhouse, Hovis*	1 Slice/44g	99	1.4	226	9.5	40	3.1	4.9
Best of Both, Med Sliced, Eat Well, M&S*	1 Slice/36g	83	0.8	229	9.4	41.2	2.2	3.5
Best of Both, Medium, Hovis*	1 Slice/38g	86	0.8	230	10.2	40.4	2.2	3.9
Best of Both, Thick Sliced, Hovis*	1 Slice/47g	108	1	230	10.2	40.4	2.2	3.9
Black Olive, Finest, Tesco*	1 Serving/72g	184	4.6	255	9.7	39.7	6.4	2.9
Bloomer, Brown, Slices, GF, Made Without Wheat, M&S*	1 Slice/53g	131	2.9	247	4.3	41.4	5.4	7.8
Bloomer, COU, M&S*	1 Slice/33g	78	0.5	235	9.5	45.5	1.5	3.6
Bloomer, Honey, Sunflower, Asda*	1 Slice/40g	110	2.5	274	9.5	42.8	6.2	4.5
Bloomer, Multi Seed, Organic, Sainsbury's*	1 Serving/60g	160	4.1	266	10.9	40.3	6.8	8.8
Bloomer, Multi Seed, Sliced, M&S*	1 Slice/54g	150	3.9	280	10.5	43.6	7.2	3.1
Bloomer, Multiseed, Average	***1 Slice/50g***	***120***	***2.4***	***240***	***11.8***	***37.2***	***4.9***	***7.7***
Bloomer, Multiseed, Finest, Tesco*	1 Slice/50g	145	3.8	290	9.8	40.2	7.6	7.4
Bloomer, Multiseed, TTD, Sainsbury's*	1 Slice/50g	119	1.8	239	12	39.7	3.6	8.8
Bloomer, Soft Grain, M&S*	1 Slice/34g	80	0.5	235	9.5	45.5	1.5	3.6
Bloomer, Sunflower Seeded, with Rye, TTD, Sainsbury's*	2 Med Slices/57g	181	6.9	317	12.6	36	12.1	6.8
Bloomer, White, Crusty, Bakery, Tesco*	1 Serving/100g	244	1.7	244	8.3	47.2	1.7	3.3
Bloomer, White, Sliced, Waitrose*	1 Slice/50g	130	0.9	259	8.5	52.1	1.8	2.6
Bloomer, Wholemeal, Organic, M&S*	1 Slice/50g	110	2.1	220	10.2	35.5	4.2	6.4
Both in One, Village Bakery, Aldi*	1 Slice/40g	95	1	237	8.5	43	2.5	4.3
Breadcakes, Big Brown, Morrisons*	1 Cake/63g	154	2.1	245	9	44.6	3.4	4.3
Brioche, Apple, Custard, Mini, Maitre Jean Pierre, Lidl*	1 Brioche/50g	148	4.3	296	6.8	48	8.6	4
Brioche, Buns, Burger, Sliced, St Pierre*	1 Bun/50g	164	4.1	328	9	53.3	8.2	2.5
Brioche, Burger Buns, Luxury, Specially Selected, Aldi*	1 Bun/50g	159	3.7	317	9.5	52	7.3	3.1
Brioche, Burger Buns, Signature, Morrisons*	1 Bun/55g	156	2.3	284	9.4	51	4.2	2.2
Brioche, Chocolate Custard, Rolls, Mini, Lidl*	1 Roll/50g	152	4.5	305	7	48	9	2
Brioche, Chocolate Chip, Brioche Pasquier*	1 Brioche/35g	132	5.6	376	7.7	49	16	2.8
Brioche, French Marble, with Vanilla, Bon Appetit, Aldi*	1 Serving/50g	132	3.4	264	6.6	42.6	6.7	1.8
Brioche, Loaf, Butter, Sainsbury's*	1/8 Loaf/50g	174	5.2	347	8	55	10.5	2.2
Brioche, Loaf, Finest, Tesco*	1 Serving/66g	242	9	367	7.4	52.9	13.6	1.9
Brioche, Loaf, Hand Plaited, Aldi*	1 Slice/50g	178	5.5	355	8.1	50	11	1.7
Brioche, Loaf, Sliced, Tesco*	2 Slices/42g	151	5	360	7.3	54.8	11.9	2
Brioche, Milk, Rolls, Brioche Pasquier*	1 Brioche/35g	127	4.4	364	8.8	53	12.6	1.5
Brioche, Raisin, Swirls, Sainsbury's*	1 Swirl/45g	130	3.4	288	6.9	47.3	7.5	2
Brioche, Rolls, Chocolate Chip, Morrisons*	1 Roll/35g	130	4.8	372	8.1	52.6	13.8	2.3
Brioche, Rolls, Chocolate Chip, Tesco*	1 Serving/35g	131	4.4	374	7.6	56.3	12.7	2.1
Brioche, Rolls, Sweet, GF, Schar*	1 Roll/50g	146	3.6	293	3.4	52	7.3	3
Brown, Bloomer, Organic, Bakery, Tesco*	1 Slice/80g	193	1.8	241	9	42.8	2.3	6.5
Brown, Ciabatta, Rolls, GF, Dietary Specials*	1 Roll/50g	137	4	274	5.8	36.9	8.1	8.9
Brown, Danish, Weight Watchers, Warburton's*	1 Slice/20g	48	0.4	233	10.3	40.7	1.8	6.2
Brown, Deli Sub, Roll, Asda*	1 Roll/60g	142	1.9	236	0	35	3.2	0
Brown, Farmhouse, GF, Newburn, Warburton's*	1 Slice/35g	82	1.9	234	7.8	35.8	5.4	5.7

BREAD

	Measure INFO/WEIGHT	KCAL	FAT	Nutrition Values per 100g / 100ml KCAL	PROT	CARB	FAT	FIBRE
Brown, Farmhouse, Linwoods*	1 Slice/25g	56	0.4	225	7.3	44.4	1.7	5.8
Brown, GF, Genius *	1 Slice/35g	97	4.7	277	6.7	42.2	13.3	9.5
Brown, Gluten & Wheat Free, Sliced	1 Slice/25g	56	1.3	224	3.4	41	5.2	9.4
Brown, Granary Malted, thick Sliced, Waitrose*	1 Slice/40g	95	0.9	238	9.4	44.8	2.3	5.1
Brown, High Fibre, Ormo*	1 Slice/24g	57	0.6	239	9.2	42.9	2.6	7.5
Brown, Irwin's Bakery*	1 Slice/64g	137	0.4	214	10.4	41.8	0.6	6.1
Brown, Kingsmill Gold, Seeds & Oats, Kingsmill*	1 Slice/45g	126	4.4	280	12.2	35.6	9.8	4.9
Brown, Malted, Average	*1 Thin Slice/25g*	*60*	*0.6*	*242*	*9.4*	*45.5*	*2.4*	*4.2*
Brown, Malted, Farmhouse Gold, Morrisons*	1 Slice/38g	94	0.5	248	8.2	49.6	1.4	3
Brown, Med Slice, Smart Price, Asda*	1 Slice/37g	77	0.6	210	8	41	1.6	6
Brown, Med Sliced	*1 Slice/34g*	*74*	*0.7*	*218*	*8.5*	*44.3*	*2*	*3.5*
Brown, Med Sliced, Asda*	1 Slice/36g	78	0.6	216	8	42	1.8	4.1
Brown, Med Sliced, Bettabuy, Morrisons*	1 Slice/31g	66	0.4	212	8.6	42	1.3	3.6
Brown, Med Sliced, Sainsbury's*	2 Slices/80g	187	2.3	234	11.9	36.7	2.9	6.6
Brown, Mixed Grain, Original, Vogel*	1 Slice/45g	102	0.6	227	9.8	47.1	1.2	6.4
Brown, Multi Grain, Wheat Free, GF	1 Slice/33g	76	1.7	229	5.1	40.8	5.1	5.6
Brown, Premium, Med Sliced, Warburton's*	1 Slice/24g	61	0.9	258	10.6	43.2	3.7	4.3
Brown, Sainsbury's*	1 Slice/34g	81	0.7	239	8.4	46.8	2.1	4.2
Brown, Sandwich Bread, GF, Udi's*	1 Slice/37g	79	1.1	216	5.2	39.2	2.9	6.3
Brown, Seeded, Dumpy, Low GI, Sasko*	1 Slice/55g	128	2.3	232	9.4	35	4.2	8
Brown, Seeded, Rolls, Free From, Tesco*	1 Roll/75g	167	5.5	222	6.7	28.8	7.3	7.4
Brown, Sliced, By Brennans, Weight Watchers*	1 Slice/20g	51	0.4	257	9.5	45.4	2.1	6.8
Brown, Sliced, Free From, Tesco*	1 Slice/42g	81	1.7	193	5.3	29.3	4	9.3
Brown, Slices, Chleb Wiejski, The Polish Bakery*	1 Slice/40g	93	0.6	233	5.7	51.1	1.5	6.5
Brown, Soda, M&S*	1 Slice/40g	92	1.4	229	9.2	43.6	3.6	4.9
Brown, Soft, Farmhouse , Warburton's*	1 Slice/42g	104	1.1	246	9.9	42.8	2.7	5.3
Brown, Sunflower Barley, Vogel*	1 Slice/42g	100	1.9	239	9.4	40.3	4.5	6.7
Brown, Thick Slice, Tesco*	1 Serving/50g	110	1.2	219	10.3	38.9	2.5	5.3
Brown, Thin Sliced, Sainsbury's*	1 Slice/29g	65	0.5	225	8.2	43.8	1.9	3.9
Brown, Toasted, Average	*1 Med Slice/24g*	*65*	*0.5*	*272*	*10.4*	*56.5*	*2.1*	*4.5*
Brown, Toastie, Thick Sliced, Kingsmill*	1 Slice/44g	101	1.4	230	9.5	40.5	3.3	4.7
Brown, Very Dark, Albert Heijn*	1 Slice/35g	84	1.4	240	12	35	4	7.4
Bruschettine, Italian, Toasted, Crosta Mollica*	1 Portion/11g	41	1.9	382	10.1	66.2	17.6	0
Buckwheat, Artisan*	1 Loaf/400g	736	7	184	6.1	38.1	1.8	4.3
Buns, Burger Seeded, Sliced, Warburton's*	1 Roll/60g	158	3.2	264	9	43.6	5.3	2.7
Buns, Burger, American Style, Sainsbury's*	1 Bun/50g	131	2.1	261	10.5	45.6	4.1	3.6
Buns, Burger, Cheese Onion Topped, Finest, Tesco*	1 Serving/105g	309	10	294	10.2	41.9	9.5	2.8
Buns, Burger, GF, Made Without Wheat, M&S*	1 Bun/80g	201	5	251	4.8	38.9	6.2	10.4
Buns, Burger, Giant, Sainsbury's*	1 Bun/95g	249	4.9	262	8.7	45.2	5.2	2.9
Buns, Burger, M&S*	1 Bun/58g	162	3.3	280	10.1	45.7	5.7	2.5
Buns, Burger, Sainsbury's*	1 Bun/56g	154	2.9	275	9.2	47.8	5.2	4.1
Buns, Burger, Seeded, Large, Tesco*	1 Bun/90g	240	3.2	267	9.5	47.7	3.6	2.9
Buns, Burger, Sesame, American Style, Sainsbury's*	1 Bun/60g	162	3.8	270	7.3	46.2	6.3	2.2
Buns, Burger, Sesame, Sliced, Tesco*	1 Bun/60g	168	4	280	7.9	47.3	6.6	2.1
Buns, White, Burger, Waitrose*	1 Serving/64g	169	2.5	264	10	47.2	3.9	2.7
Buns, White, Stay Fresh, Tesco*	1 Bun/56g	152	3.7	271	7.5	45.5	6.6	0
Butterbread, Nature's Own*	1 Slice/30g	70	0.6	231	11.5	46.2	1.9	0
Challah, Average	*1 Slice/50g*	*143*	*3.6*	*286*	*8.9*	*53.6*	*7.1*	*3.6*
Cheese, & Garlic, Pizza Style, Sainsbury's*	¼ Bread/63g	199	8.1	318	10.7	39.7	13	2.2
Cheese, & Garlic, Stonebaked, Morrisons*	¼ Bread/69g	228	9.9	331	10.9	39.5	14.4	1.9
Cheese, & Onion, Tear & Share, Sainsbury's*	¼ Bread/71g	202	6.6	285	9.8	40.6	9.3	1.9
Cheese, & Onion, Toastie, Warburton's*	1 Slice/42g	120	5.8	286	7.5	33.1	13.7	0
Cheese, & Tomato, Tear & Share, Sainsbury's*	¼ Bread/72g	211	9.5	293	8	35.7	13.2	1.5

B

BREAD

INFO/WEIGHT	Measure	per Measure		Nutrition Values per 100g / 100ml				
		KCAL	FAT	KCAL	PROT	CARB	FAT	FIBRE
Cheese, Morrisons*	1 Serving/96g	297	13.6	311	9.9	35.9	14.2	3
Cheese, Onion & Garlic, Tear & Share, Waitrose*	¼ Bread/112g	326	14.6	290	9.4	33.9	13	2.1
Cheese, Onion Mustard Seed, Cluster, Sainsbury's*	1 Cluster/100g	276	8.1	276	10	40.6	8.1	3.1
Cheese, Tear & Share, Tesco*	¼ Loaf/73g	225	7.8	310	8.8	44	10.7	0.8
Cheese, Three, Bloomer, Bakery, Tesco*	1 Slice/82g	214	5.3	261	13.1	36.7	6.4	2
Cheese, Topped, Baton, Bakery, Tesco*	½ Baton/100g	292	4.5	292	10.7	51.2	4.5	2
Cholla, Average	*1/10 Loaf/154g*	*421*	*14.3*	*274*	*6.9*	*40.8*	*9.3*	*1*
Ciabatta, Black Olive, Part Baked, Sainsbury's*	¼ Ciabatta/67g	172	2.5	257	8.8	46.8	3.8	2.4
Ciabatta, Finest, Tesco*	1/6 Ciabatta/45g	124	2.7	275	10.4	44.8	5.9	2.7
Ciabatta, Gluten Wheat Free, Average	*1 Slice/55g*	*136*	*1.6*	*248*	*2*	*52.4*	*2.9*	*4.2*
Ciabatta, Green Olive, Tesco*	¼ Ciabatta/70g	155	3.1	222	7.4	38.2	4.4	1.9
Ciabatta, Half, M&S*	1 Ciabatta/135g	354	5.5	262	10.3	48.1	4.1	2.1
Ciabatta, Half, Organic, Sainsbury's*	½ Ciabatta/63g	152	0.6	241	9.1	48.7	1	2.3
Ciabatta, Half, Part Baked, TTD, Sainsbury's*	¼ Pack/67g	173	3.3	257	8.6	44.6	4.9	3.5
Ciabatta, Half, Tesco*	1 Ciabatta/135g	351	4.7	260	8.9	47.7	3.5	2.2
Ciabatta, Italian Style, Waitrose*	1 Ciabatta/89g	231	1.2	260	10.7	51.2	1.4	2.2
Ciabatta, Loaf, Finest, Tesco*	1 Serving/45g	115	2.1	257	10.1	41.8	4.7	3.3
Ciabatta, Olive & Rosemary, Mini, Tesco*	1 Pack/75g	319	8.2	425	17.8	63	10.9	3.6
Ciabatta, Organic, Tesco*	1/3 Ciabatta/100g	240	3.6	240	8.7	43.2	3.6	2.4
Ciabatta, Part Baked, Half, Sainsbury's*	½ Ciabatta/67g	174	2.5	260	8.9	47.7	3.7	2.2
Ciabatta, Plain, Half, Two, Waitrose*	1 Roll/80g	248	5.8	310	10	51.3	7.2	2.2
Ciabatta, Plain, Tesco*	1 Serving/60g	166	3.1	277	9	47.4	5.1	2.5
Ciabatta, Ready to Bake, M&S*	1 Serving/150g	393	6.1	262	10.3	48.1	4.1	2.1
Ciabatta, Ready to Bake, Sainsbury's*	½ Ciabatta/66g	172	2.4	260	8.9	47.7	3.7	2.2
Ciabatta, Spicy Topped, Finest, Tesco*	1 Serving/73g	163	4	223	9.2	34	5.5	1.7
Ciabatta, Square, Bake at Home, Part Baked, Asda*	1 Roll/60g	157	2.1	262	8.4	49.1	3.5	2.1
Ciabatta, Stick, Organic, M&S*	1 Stick/140g	315	2	225	8.9	48.5	1.4	4.2
Ciabatta, Sun Dried Tomato Basil, Tesco*	¼ Ciabatta/75g	193	4.3	257	8.9	42.4	5.7	2.4
Ciabatta, Sweet Pepper, HE, Tesco*	1 Serving/50g	135	1.4	270	11.8	49.5	2.7	2.8
Ciabatta, Tomato & Basil, GFY, Asda*	1 Serving/55g	143	1.2	260	9	51	2.2	0
Ciabatta, Tomato & Mozzarella, Iceland*	1 Ciabatta/150g	374	15.2	249	10	29.6	10.1	3.3
Ciabatta, TTD, Sainsbury's*	¼ Pack/68g	185	4	274	10.4	44.8	5.9	2.7
Cinnamon, & Fruit Swirl, Genesis Crafty*	1 Slice/40g	133	4.1	332	6.8	53.8	10.2	0
Cinnamon, & Raisin, Toasty Loaf, Rankin*	1 Slice/40g	113	2	283	6.6	54.2	5	2.5
Cinnamon, Swirl, Asda*	1 Serving/25g	87	3.2	349	6	52	13	1.6
Cob, Cheese Chutney, Bakery, Tesco*	1 Slice/50g	124	2.2	249	11.3	39.7	4.4	2.5
Corn, Soft, Mexican, Discovery*	1 Tortilla/40g	119	2.8	297	7.4	51	7.1	2.3
Corn, Soft, Old El Paso*	1 Tortilla/42g	121	2	289	8.5	51.8	4.8	2.4
Corn, with Sunflower Seed Mixed Spice, Bakery, Tesco*	1 Slice/50g	131	2	262	9.9	45	4.1	2.6
Cottage Loaf, Stonebaked, Asda*	1 Serving/67g	155	0.9	232	10	45	1.3	3.2
Crostini, Olive Oil, TTD, Sainsbury's*	1 Roll/4g	16	0.3	409	11.4	72.2	8.3	3.3
Farina, Seeded, Crosta Mollica*	1 Pack/360g	878	9.4	244	9.5	43.4	2.6	4.1
Farl, Irish Soda, Irwin's Bakery*	1 Farl/150g	334	5.1	223	4	44	3.4	2.3
Farmhouse, Batch, Multiseed, Love Life, Waitrose*	1 Slice/50g	130	3.5	259	9.9	39.2	7	7.2
Farmhouse, Poppy Seed, Crusty, Loaf, M&S*	1 Slice/40g	104	1.3	260	9.4	47.6	3.3	2.3
Farmhouse, Soft Grained, Sliced, Warburton's*	1 Slice/42g	109	1.7	258	10.2	44.6	4	5
Farmhouse, Wholemeal, Average	*1 Slice/43g*	*94*	*1.4*	*219*	*10.7*	*36.2*	*3.3*	*7.3*
Farmhouse, with Oatmeal, Batch, Finest, Tesco*	1 Slice/44g	110	1.4	240	9.8	43.2	3.1	5.2
Ficelle, Mixed Olive, Waitrose*	1/5 Stick/50g	133	1.4	267	7.5	51.1	2.8	3.4
Fig, & Almond, BrÆ'¶derna Cartwright*	4 Slices/100g	267	7.5	267	9.2	39.7	7.5	0
Fig, & Hazelnut, Loaf, M&S*	1 Serving/100g	285	8.2	285	11	38.9	8.2	5.4
Flat, Italian, Piada Sfogliata, Italiamo, Lidl*	1 Piece/130g	402	12.5	309	7.9	45.9	9.6	2
Flatbread, Folded, Lge Plain, by, Sainsbury's*	1 Flatbread/65g	192	3.4	295	8.5	51.4	5.3	4.1

BREAD

INFO/WEIGHT	Measure KCAL	Measure FAT	KCAL	PROT	CARB	FAT	FIBRE
Flatbread, Garlic Herb, Tear Share, Sainsbury's*	¼ Bread/68g	201	6.3	297	10.9	42.5	9.3	3.7
Flatbread, Garlic, Cheese, Handcrafted, Tesco*	¼ Bread/58g	176	5.1	305	10.5	44.6	8.9	2.4
Flatbread, Garlic, BGTY, Sainsbury's*	¼ Bread/56g	177	5.7	316	9.6	46.6	10.1	2.7
Flatbread, Khobez, White, Dina Foods Ltd*	1 Bread/56g	158	0.6	282	10.5	57.5	1.1	3
Flatbread, Multi Seed, Tower Gate, Lidl*	1 Bread/8g	34	1.1	430	13.1	57.4	13.9	11.2
Flatbread, Multiseed, Folded, Tesco*	1 Flatbread/35g	107	2.4	305	10.4	47.8	6.8	5.3
Flatbread, Super Seeded, Folded, Village Bakery, Aldi*	1 Flatbread/35g	123	4.6	352	9.7	47	13	5.5
Flatbread, Tomato, Garlic, Sainsbury's*	1/3 Bread/73g	191	4.9	261	8.4	41.7	6.7	3.4
Flour, From Dinner Kit, Old El Paso*	1 Tortilla/42g	144	4.9	344	8.7	51.1	11.7	0
Flour, Soft, Discovery*	1 Tortilla/40g	119	2.8	298	8	49.6	7.1	2.4
Focaccia, Cherry Tomato, Basil Puglian Pesto, Graze*	1 Punnet/40g	120	6.5	301	7.2	31.6	16.2	3.2
Focaccia, Harissa Peperonata, Bake at Home, M&S*	1 Bun/114g	282	8.3	247	7.9	35.8	7.3	3.2
Focaccia, Onion & Herb, Tesco*	½ Pack/190g	547	23.8	288	8.7	35.2	12.5	3.7
Focaccia, Roast Cherry Tomato & Olive, GFY, Asda*	½ Pack/148g	350	6	237	9	41	4.1	2.8
Focaccia, Roasted Onion & Cheese, M&S*	1 Serving/89g	240	4.1	270	10.4	45.7	4.6	2.8
Focaccia, Rosemary Sea Salt, TTD, Sainsbury's*	1 Serving/50g	130	3.5	261	7.4	40.7	7	2.8
Focaccia, Rosemary, Sea Salt, Tesco*	1 Focaccia/50g	151	4.2	301	9.4	45.5	8.3	3.4
Focaccia, Tomato, Rosemary, TTD, Sainsbury's*	1 Serving/50g	118	3	236	6.9	37.1	6.1	2.7
French, Sliced, Parisian*	2 Slices/39g	100	1	256	5.1	48.7	2.6	0
French, Stick, Average	*1 Serving/60g*	*147*	*0.2*	*245*	*8.7*	*52.2*	*0.4*	*2.1*
Fresh Fibre, GF, Juvela*	1 Slice/29g	70	1.3	242	3.4	45	4.5	6.2
Fruit Loaf, & Cinnamon, Finest, Tesco*	1 Slice/37g	134	4.9	363	6.4	54.6	13.2	1.5
Fruit Loaf, Apple Cinnamon, Soreen*	1 Serving/10g	31	0.4	307	6.9	60.5	4.2	0
Fruit Loaf, Apple, M&S*	1 Slice/39g	100	0.6	255	8.5	51.9	1.5	3.3
Fruit Loaf, Banana, Soreen*	1 Slice/25g	76	1.2	305	7.2	55.6	5	4.4
Fruit Loaf, Cinnamon Raisin, Soreen*	1/8 Loaf/25g	77	1	308	7.7	54.1	4	4.1
Fruit Loaf, Fresh, Free From, Sainsbury's*	1 Slice/33g	93	2.5	279	3.2	45.5	7.5	8.1
Fruit Loaf, Fruity Five, Snack Pack, Soreen*	1 Pack/45g	148	4	329	7.1	54.9	9	2.7
Fruit Loaf, Luxury, Christmas, Soreen*	1 Serving/28g	85	0.6	303	4.5	66.6	2.1	0
Fruit Loaf, Mixed Berry, Weight Watchers*	1 Slice/34g	79	0.9	231	7.6	44.3	2.6	7.7
Fruit Loaf, Plum, Lincolnshire, Soreen*	1 Slice/25g	65	0.8	261	8.4	49.3	3.4	2.1
Fruit Loaf, Sliced, Bakers Selection, Asda*	1 Serving/36g	100	1.5	278	8.2	50	4.2	3.6
Fruit Loaf, Sliced, Sainsbury's*	1 Slice/40g	104	1.4	260	8.9	47.9	3.6	2.4
Fruit Loaf, Sliced, Tesco*	1 Slice/36g	101	1.3	281	7.9	52.6	3.6	3.2
Fruit Loaf, Sultana & Cherry, Sainsbury's*	1 Slice/50g	178	6.1	357	2.7	59	12.2	1.7
Fruit Loaf, Toffee Apple, Soreen*	1 Bar/30g	98	1.5	326	8	59.8	5.1	4.5
Fruit Loaf, Winter Spice, Soreen*	1 Slice/52g	155	1.5	299	7.3	63.8	2.8	5.2
Fruit, & Spice, Extra Thick, Sliced, Vogel*	2 Slices/120g	290	4.1	241	8.3	41.7	3.4	4.9
Fruit, Loaf, Banana, Lunchbox, Soreen*	1 Bar/30g	98	1.7	326	8.1	59.5	5.5	4.6
Fruit, Loaf, Toasted, Cafe Instore, Asda*	1 Slice/33g	89	1.2	269	8	51	3.7	2.9
Fruit, Raisin Swirl, Sun-Maid*	1 Slice/33g	95	1.9	287	8.3	50.4	5.8	2.6
Garlic, & Cheese, Slices, Tesco*	1 Slice/30g	114	5	380	11.7	43.9	16.8	2
Garlic, & Tomato, Pizza, Italiano, Tesco*	½ Bread/140g	405	15.1	289	7.5	40.5	10.8	2.5
Garlic, 30% Less Fat, Morrisons*	1 Serving/80g	231	7.4	289	7.9	43.8	9.2	2.7
Garlic, Average	*1 Serving/100g*	*327*	*13.8*	*327*	*8.1*	*43.7*	*13.8*	*1.4*
Garlic, Baguette, Average	*1 Slice/20g*	*66*	*2.8*	*330*	*7.8*	*43.1*	*14.2*	*1.8*
Garlic, Baguette, Everyday Essentials, Aldi*	¼ Baguette/43g	148	6.4	349	8.1	45	15	1.4
Garlic, Baguette, Extra Strong, Italiano, Tesco*	¼ Baguette/53g	178	8.7	340	7.9	39.8	16.6	2.8
Garlic, Baguette, Extra Strong, Sainsbury's*	½ Baguette/85g	278	12.6	327	8.4	40	14.8	3.4
Garlic, Baguette, Free From, Tesco*	¼ Baguette/39g	137	6.2	352	1.2	49.1	15.8	4.4
Garlic, Baguette, HFC, Tesco*	1 Serving/85g	325	18.9	383	6.7	38.2	22.2	1.7
Garlic, Baguette, Italian, Asda*	¼ Baguette/48g	173	9.5	364	7	39	20	3.4
Garlic, Baguette, Italiano, Tesco*	¼ Baguette/53g	186	9.9	355	6.9	39.2	18.8	2.4

BREAD

INFO/WEIGHT	Measure	per Measure KCAL	per Measure FAT	per 100g KCAL	PROT	CARB	FAT	FIBRE
Garlic, Baguette, LC, Tesco*	¼ Baguette/52g	130	2.9	250	7	42.2	5.5	2.4
Garlic, Baguette, M&S*	¼ Baguette/52g	172	8.2	330	6.8	38.6	15.8	2.9
Garlic, Baguette, Morrisons*	½ Baguette/95g	295	14.2	311	6.3	37.8	15	1.5
Garlic, Baguette, Sainsbury's*	½ Baguette/85g	342	16.3	403	8.9	48.6	19.2	2.3
Garlic, Baguette, Slices, Tesco*	1 Serving/60g	187	9.2	312	9.8	33.8	15.3	1.7
Garlic, Baguette, Value, Tesco*	½ Baguette/85g	270	11.1	318	8.1	42	13.1	2.3
Garlic, Baguette, Waitrose*	½ Baguette/85g	290	15.2	341	7.1	37.8	17.9	0
Garlic, Ciabatta, Herb Butter, Sainsbury's*	½ Ciabatta/105g	345	16.3	329	8.5	38.8	15.5	0
Garlic, Ciabatta, Finest, Tesco*	1 Serving/65g	205	8.9	316	8.1	40.1	13.7	2.4
Garlic, Ciabatta, Italiano, Tesco*	1 Ciabatta/65g	211	9.4	324	7.7	40.9	14.4	2.2
Garlic, Focaccia, & Rosemary, Sainsbury's*	¼ Focaccia/75g	219	7.4	292	8	43	9.8	2.8
Garlic, Focaccia, Herb, Italian Style, Morrisons*	1/6 Focaccia/76g	259	10.9	341	8.5	44.7	14.3	2.5
Garlic, Homebake, Tesco*	1 Serving/60g	209	12.3	348	7.1	33.7	20.5	1.5
Garlic, Italian Style Stone Baked, Morrisons*	½ Pack/115g	420	22	365	7.9	40.4	19.1	1.9
Garlic, Pizza Bread, Co-Op*	1 Pizza/240g	756	31.2	315	8	41	13	2
Garlic, Slices, 50 % Less Fat, Asda*	1 Slice/29g	75	1.1	262	7.9	47.1	3.9	3.2
Garlic, Slices, Asda*	1 Slice/27g	88	3.3	328	8	46.2	12.4	2.8
Garlic, Slices, BGTY, Sainsbury's*	1 Slice/32g	96	2.1	304	8.9	51	6.6	2.7
Garlic, Slices, Chilled, Sainsbury's*	1 Pack/368g	1369	60	372	9.1	47.3	16.3	3.2
Garlic, Slices, LC, Tesco*	1 Slice/30g	75	1.7	250	7.3	42.3	5.7	2.9
Garlic, Slices, Morrisons*	1 Slice/32g	109	4.1	341	8.5	46.9	12.9	1.7
Garlic, Stonebaked, M&S*	1 Loaf/85g	314	14.4	369	8.6	44.4	16.9	2.4
Garlic, with Cheese, Asda*	1 Slice/34g	130	6.1	382	11	44	18	0
GF, Loaf, Unsliced, Wellfoods*	2 Slices/100g	216	2.3	216	1.6	47.1	2.3	1.5
Giraffe, Sainsbury's*	1 Serving/50g	119	0.2	238	8.9	48.1	0.5	2.7
Grain, Three, Organic, Schneider Brot*	1 Slice/72g	142	1.6	199	5.3	34.5	2.3	9.3
Grained, Soft, Farmhouse, Warburton's*	1 Slice/42g	109	1.7	258	10.2	44.6	4	5
Grains, & Seeds, Tasty, Warburton's*	1 Slice/38g	100	1.6	264	10.6	45.6	4.3	5.2
Granary, Average	**1 Med Slice/35g**	**85**	**1**	**242**	**9.8**	**44**	**2.8**	**4.8**
Granary, Baps, Large, Asda*	1 Bap/64g	143	1.4	224	10	41	2.2	4.3
Granary, Country, Multiseeded, Hovis*	1 Slice/44g	104	1.1	236	10.6	39.8	2.4	6.8
Granary, M&S*	1 Slice/30g	75	0.9	250	9.5	46.4	3.1	3.2
Granary, Malted, Med Brown, Asda*	1 Slice/35g	81	0.9	231	9	43	2.6	3.3
Granary, Oatmeal, Hovis*	1 Slice/44g	104	0.9	236	9.2	45.3	2.1	3.1
Granary, Original, All Sizes, Hovis*	1 Thin Slice/33g	84	0.8	256	10.6	46.4	2.4	3.7
Granary, Seeded, Sunflower, Hovis*	1 Slice/44g	119	2.5	271	10.1	44.9	5.7	2.9
Granary, Thick Slice, COU, M&S*	1 Slice/25g	60	0.6	240	10.5	44.1	2.2	6
Granary, Thick, Sliced, 800g, Hovis*	1 Slice/44g	112	1	256	10.3	46.4	2.4	3.7
Granary, Waitrose*	1 Slice/40g	88	1	220	9.4	39.9	2.5	4.3
Granary, White, Hovis*	1 Slice/44g	102	1.5	233	9.7	40.8	3.5	5.6
Granary, White, Seeded, Med Sliced, Hovis*	1 Slice/44g	109	1.8	248	10.9	41.7	4.2	3.8
Granary, Wholemeal, Average	**1 Slice/35g**	**80**	**0.9**	**228**	**10.8**	**38.4**	**2.6**	**6.6**
Granary, Wholemeal, Seeded, Med Sliced, Hovis*	1 Slice/44g	104	1.1	237	10.6	39.8	2.4	6.8
Half Half, Medium, Warburton's*	1 Slice/40g	95	0.8	240	8.8	44.2	2	5
Half Half, Toastie, Warburton's*	1 Slice/47g	112	0.9	240	8.8	44.2	2	5
Herby, Basket, Snack, Graze*	1 Punnet/20g	101	5	503	8	61	25	3
Herby, Basket, Snack, Retail, Graze*	1 Punnet/18g	90	4.3	500	8.1	61	24	3.5
Hi Bran, M&S*	1 Slice/26g	55	0.8	210	12.6	32.5	3	6.3
Hi Fibre, Seed, Lifefibre*	1 Slice/35g	109	3.5	313	12.5	43.6	10.1	2.7
High Bran, Loaf, M&S*	2 Slices/62g	143	2.4	230	13.1	31.7	3.9	7.7
Irish, Barm Brack, Tesco*	1 Serving/75g	232	5.2	310	16	47.6	6.9	3
Irish, Brown Soda, Tesco*	1 Serving/50g	110	1.9	219	9.2	36.2	3.8	6.4
Irish, Cottage Wheaten, Loaf, Tesco*	1 Serving/50g	116	1.3	231	8.6	41.4	2.6	4.2

BREAD

	Measure INFO/WEIGHT	per Measure KCAL	FAT	Nutrition Values per 100g / 100ml KCAL	PROT	CARB	FAT	FIBRE
Jalapeno Chilli, Three Cheese, Bloomer, Bakery, Tesco*	1 Serving/82g	217	3.3	265	12	43.5	4.1	3
Juvela*	1 Slice/25g	60	0.8	240	3.3	50	3	1.7
Low Carb, Protein Rich, Carbzone*	1 Slice/50g	132	6.5	264	22	7.5	13	14
Low GI, Multiseed, Percy Ingle*	1 Med Slice/35g	99	3.1	283	0	0	8.9	6
Malt Loaf, Buttered, 2 Slices, Soreen*	1 Pack/45g	150	3.9	333	7.5	54.2	8.6	4.4
Malt Loaf, Apple, Lunchbox, Soreen*	1 Loaf/30g	92	1.3	307	7.7	57	4.5	4.4
Malt Loaf, Chocolatey, Soreen*	1/8 Loaf/28g	95	1.7	344	8	58.7	6.3	5.1
Malt Loaf, Family, Asda*	1 Serving/20g	54	0.3	270	8	56	1.5	5
Malt Loaf, Fruited, Sliced, Weight Watchers*	1 Slice/23g	68	0.4	294	8.9	60.2	1.9	3.6
Malt Loaf, Fruited, Weight Watchers*	1 Serving/23g	68	0.4	294	8.9	60.2	1.9	3.6
Malt Loaf, Fruity, Sliced, Soreen*	2 Slices/43g	129	1.3	300	8.2	58.2	3	3.9
Malt Loaf, Organic, Tesco*	1 Slice/28g	82	0.6	292	7.2	61.2	2	2.3
Malt Loaf, Original, Low Fat, Soreen*	1 Slice/22g	63	0.4	288	7.5	60	1.6	2
Malt Loaf, Tesco*	1 Slice/50g	146	1.4	291	8.6	58	2.7	4.8
Malted, & Seeded, Batch, Organic, Waitrose*	1 Slice/50g	118	2	236	10.9	39.5	3.9	6.2
Malted, Brown, Slice, BGTY, Sainsbury's*	1 Slice/22g	53	0.6	239	12.1	41.4	2.8	5.8
Malted, Brown, Thick Sliced, Organic, Tesco*	1 Slice/44g	111	0.9	249	8.9	48.8	2	3.5
Malted, Crusty, Sainsbury's*	1 Slice/42g	109	1.4	259	8.6	48.6	3.3	4.4
Malted, Danish, Weight Watchers, Warburton's*	1 Slice/20g	51	0.3	249	11.8	45.1	1.5	4.2
Malted, Farmhouse, Morrisons*	1 Serving/40g	94	0.7	235	9.1	45.6	1.8	4.7
Malted, Grain, Baton, Tesco*	¼ Baton/57g	143	0.5	251	10.5	47.6	0.9	5
Malted, Grain, Co-Op*	1 Slice/43g	99	0.9	230	8	46	2	3
Malted, Grain, Good As Gold, Kingsmill*	1 Slice/47g	114	1.2	243	9.5	45.4	2.6	4.2
Malted, Grain, Loaf, Bakery, Tesco*	1 Slice/40g	100	0.4	250	10.5	47.6	0.9	5
Malted, Grain, Loaf, Sliced, Bakery, Tesco*	1 Slice/50g	122	0.7	244	9.1	46.6	1.4	4.3
Malted, Oat, Duchy Originals*	1 Serving/80g	195	3	244	8.8	43.6	3.8	3.7
Malted, Wheat Loaf, Crusty, Finest, Tesco*	1 Slice/50g	115	0.8	230	9.8	44.2	1.5	4.4
Malted, Wheatgrain, Roberts Bakery*	1 Slice/30g	80	1	265	11	48	3.3	3.6
Mediterranean, Olive, Waitrose*	1 Slice/30g	82	2.8	273	7.4	40.1	9.2	4.9
Mediterranean, Style, M&S*	1/6 Loaf/48g	150	5.3	315	10.9	42.5	11.1	1.2
Mediterranean, Style, Stonebaked Tomato Batard, Tesco*	¼ Loaf/100g	256	3.1	256	9.8	45.5	3.1	3.5
Mixed Grain, Original, Sandwich, Vogel*	2 Slices/72g	144	1	201	9.7	34.7	1.4	4.5
Mixed Seed, Organic, Duchy Originals*	1 Slice/43g	114	3.4	269	10.9	39.1	8.1	5.3
Multigrain, Brennans*	1 Slice/40g	110	1.3	275	8.8	48	3.3	6.3
Multigrain, Brown, Farmhouse Baker's, M&S*	1 Slice/51g	115	2.8	225	13	31.2	5.4	5.1
Multigrain, Crusty, Finest, Tesco*	1 Slice/40g	98	1.4	245	9	44.7	3.4	5
Multigrain, GF, Sainsbury's*	1 Slice/17g	39	0.8	229	5.1	40.8	5	5.6
Multigrain, Med Sliced, Batch, Tesco*	1 Slice/50g	120	0.9	241	9.3	43.7	1.8	6.2
Multigrain, Sliced, Fresh And Easy*	1 Slice/40g	110	1	275	10	52.5	2.5	5
Multigrain, Soft Batch, Sainsbury's*	1 Slice/44g	106	2.9	242	11.3	34.5	6.5	5.6
Multigrain, Sunblest*	1 Slice/30g	76	0.8	254	9	47	2.5	4.5
Multigrain, Thick Sliced, Tesco*	1 Slice/50g	112	1.2	225	8.4	42.2	2.5	3.9
Multiseed, Farmhouse Batch, Finest, Tesco*	1 Slice/44g	108	1.9	245	9.9	40.4	4.4	7.5
Multiseed, Farmhouse, Finest, Tesco*	1 Slice /50g	135	3.8	270	12.5	37	7.7	5.8
Multiseed, Sliced, Free From, Tesco*	1 Slice/29g	85	3.4	294	6.7	34.8	11.8	10.7
Multiseeded, Bloomer, TTD, Sainsbury's*	1 Slice/50g	128	1.8	256	12	39.7	3.6	8.8
Naan, Asda*	1 Naan/130g	308	2.3	237	7.7	47.4	1.8	2.2
Naan, Average	*1 Naan/130g*	*344*	*5.6*	*264*	*8.3*	*48.5*	*4.3*	*2*
Naan, Bombay Brassiere, Sainsbury's*	1 Naan/140g	372	4.3	266	9.8	49.6	3.1	2.9
Naan, Chicken Tikka, Tandoori, Naanzza*	½ Naan/150g	337	9.6	225	10.9	30.7	6.4	1.3
Naan, Chilli Mango, Finest, Tesco*	½ Naan/90g	230	5.1	255	8.4	41.9	5.7	3.2
Naan, Fresh, BGTY, Sainsbury's*	1 Serving/150g	368	4.6	245	9.4	44.9	3.1	2.2
Naan, Garlic & Coriander, Free From, Tesco*	1 Naan/90g	215	6	240	5.1	38.7	6.7	4.9

BREAD

INFO/WEIGHT	Measure			Nutrition Values per 100g / 100ml				
		KCAL	FAT	KCAL	PROT	CARB	FAT	FIBRE
Naan, Garlic & Coriander, Tesco*	½ Naan/65g	169	3	261	7.6	45.9	4.6	3
Naan, Garlic & Coriander, TTD, Sainsbury's*	1 Naan/70g	219	8.4	313	7	44	12	2.9
Naan, Garlic Coriander, Heritage*	1 Naan/130g	344	4.7	265	7.5	49	3.6	2.7
Naan, Garlic Coriander, Mini, Asda*	1 Naan/110g	320	12.5	291	6.9	40.2	11.4	2.5
Naan, Garlic Coriander, Mini, Sainsbury's*	1 Naan/48g	147	3.4	307	8.3	51.2	7	3
Naan, Garlic Coriander, Mini, Sharwood's*	1 Naan/65g	196	4.2	302	8	51.5	6.5	2.8
Naan, Garlic Coriander, Mini, Tesco*	1 Naan/50g	130	2.3	261	7.6	45.9	4.6	3
Naan, Garlic Coriander, Mini, Weight Watchers*	1 Naan/40g	100	1	250	9.3	47.6	2.5	4.2
Naan, Garlic Coriander, Patak's*	1 Naan/127g	373	7.7	294	7.9	50.9	6.1	2.4
Naan, Garlic Coriander, Sainsbury's*	½ Naan/63g	167	2.5	264	8.1	47.3	4	3.4
Naan, Garlic Coriander, The Spice Tailor*	1 Naan/110g	366	12.1	333	8.5	49	11	2.2
Naan, Garlic Coriander, Weight Watchers*	1 Naan/60g	155	2.6	259	8.9	46	4.3	3.4
Naan, Garlic, Santosh*	1 Naan/100g	300	6	300	8	48	6	2
Naan, Indian Meal for One, BGTY, Sainsbury's*	1 Serving/45g	115	1.9	257	10.3	44.2	4.3	2.1
Naan, Indian Meal for Two, Sainsbury's*	1 Naan/125g	357	9.3	285	8.7	45.9	7.4	1.9
Naan, LC, Tesco*	1 Naan/71g	181	1.6	255	7.5	50.7	2.2	2.3
Naan, Mini, LC, Tesco*	1 Naan/65g	150	1.8	230	8.1	42.5	2.8	2.9
Naan, Ocado*	½ Naan/75g	194	1.7	258	8.4	48.3	2.3	5.3
Naan, Onion & Mint, M&S*	½ Naan/135g	351	11.7	260	8.9	35.8	8.7	2.5
Naan, Onion Bhaji, Sharwood's*	1 Pack/130g	378	9.9	291	7.3	48.4	7.6	2.2
Naan, Peshwari, Apple Coconut, Mini, Sharwood's*	1 Naan/65g	179	3.1	275	7.5	47.1	4.8	6.7
Naan, Peshwari, Flame Baked, Finest, Tesco*	½ Naan/75g	221	6.2	295	7.2	46.6	8.3	2.5
Naan, Peshwari, M&S*	1 Serving/127g	394	12.8	310	9.2	45.8	10.1	1.9
Naan, Peshwari, Mega, Asda*	1 Naan/220g	680	26.4	309	7.1	43.1	12	2.7
Naan, Peshwari, Mini, Bilash, Aldi*	1 Naan/58g	212	9.5	366	7	45.1	16.4	4.9
Naan, Peshwari, Sainsbury's*	1 Naan/166g	511	18.3	308	7.1	45.1	11	4.7
Naan, Peshwari, Sharwood's*	1 Naan/130g	334	6.9	257	7.2	45.1	5.3	2.5
Naan, Peshwari, Tesco*	1 Naan/215g	684	26.7	318	7.5	48.9	12.4	4.8
Naan, Plain, Average	**1 Naan/160g**	**437**	**10.5**	**273**	**8**	**45.7**	**6.5**	**2.1**
Naan, Plain, Finest, Tesco*	½ Naan/80g	206	4.1	257	8	43.2	5.1	3.1
Naan, Plain, Indian, Mini, Asda*	1 Naan/110g	329	12.6	299	6.6	42.2	11.5	2.1
Naan, Plain, Large, Sainsbury's*	½ Naan/70g	191	4.6	273	7.1	46.2	6.6	3
Naan, Plain, Mega, Indian Takeaway, Asda*	1 Naan/222g	572	8.4	258	7	49	3.8	2.5
Naan, Plain, Mini, Asda*	1 Naan/58g	156	2.7	269	8	49	4.6	2.3
Naan, Plain, Mini, BGTY, Sainsbury's*	1 Naan/50g	124	0.6	248	7.6	49.8	1.3	3.3
Naan, Plain, Mini, Weight Watchers*	1 Naan/44g	108	1.1	245	9.1	46.5	2.5	4.9
Naan, Plain, Sharwood's*	1 Naan/120g	326	8.9	272	8.5	42.9	7.4	2.4
Naan, Plain, Tesco*	1 Naan/150g	392	6.9	261	8.4	46.4	4.6	2.3
Naan, Plain, Value, Tesco*	1 Naan/135g	363	9.7	269	8.1	42.9	7.2	1.6
Naan, Santosh*	½ Naan/50g	150	3	300	8	48	6	2
Naan, Smart Price, Asda*	1 Naan/100g	233	1.9	233	8.7	45.3	1.9	2.8
Naan, Take Away, Tesco*	1 Naan/39g	97	1.3	248	8.7	45.6	3.4	1.7
Naan, Tandoori Baked, Waitrose*	1 Naan/140g	372	4.3	266	9.8	49.6	3.1	2.9
Naan, Tandoori, Sharwood's*	1 Naan/130g	330	6.5	254	7.3	45	5	2
Naan, Wholewheat, Santosh*	½ Naan/50g	150	3.5	300	8	40	7	4
Oatmeal, Farmhouse, Extra Special, Asda*	1 Slice/44g	102	1.1	231	11	41	2.6	6
Oatmeal, Farmhouse, Soft, M&S*	1 Slice/45g	110	2	245	11.1	39.5	4.4	5.2
Oatmeal, Farmhouse, Waitrose*	1 Slice/40g	110	2.1	276	9.4	47.9	5.2	4.6
Oatmeal, Sliced Loaf, Tesco*	1 Slice/50g	111	1.7	222	7.4	40.5	3.4	2.8
Olive, Waitrose*	1 Slice/28g	86	3	306	9	43.6	10.6	2
Oliven Ringbrot, Rewe*	1 Portion/100g	247	3.2	247	8.5	44.1	3.2	2.8
Onion, Roasted, M&S*	1 Slice/50g	125	1.6	250	9	46.7	3.3	2.1
Paleo, Almond, GF, Non GMO, Julian Bakery*	1 Slice/43g	60	3	140	16.3	14	7	11.6

BREAD

	Measure INFO/WEIGHT	per Measure KCAL	FAT	Nutrition Values per 100g / 100ml KCAL	PROT	CARB	FAT	FIBRE
Pane Pugliese, Italian, Toasting, Crosta Mollica*	1 Slice/69g	184	0.8	267	8.6	55.5	1.2	0.2
Pave, Walnut, Sainsbury's*	1 Serving/50g	140	4.8	280	9	40	9.5	3.5
Pave, Walnut, TTD, Sainsbury's*	1 Serving/50g	138	3.6	277	9.5	41.5	7.3	3.7
Petit Pain, Homebake, Mini, Tesco*	1 Roll/50g	144	0.6	289	8.6	59.1	1.2	3.5
Petit Pain, Mini, Homebake, Tesco*	1 Roll/45g	110	0.6	245	7.8	49.7	1.3	2.5
Petit Pain, Organic, Tesco*	1 Roll/100g	235	0.8	235	7.8	49.1	0.8	1.2
Petit Pain, Part Bake, Weight Watchers*	1 Roll/50g	111	0.4	223	6.8	43.5	0.9	6.8
Pitta, 159, Pride Valley*	1 Pitta/63g	159	1.2	252	10.1	51.2	1.9	2.6
Pitta, Brown, Organic, Waitrose*	1 Pitta/53g	124	0.5	234	8.5	43.9	1	7.4
Pitta, Free From, Sainsbury's*	1 Pitta/65g	164	2.5	252	4.1	50	3.9	2.9
Pitta, Garlic, Morrisons*	1 Pitta/60g	149	1.1	249	9.7	51.1	1.8	0
Pitta, Mediterranean Style, The Bakery, M&S*	1 Pitta/85g	247	3.7	291	6.7	54.9	4.3	2.8
Pitta, Pockets, Sainsbury's*	1 Pitta/75g	188	0.8	250	8.5	52	1	3.5
Pitta, Sd Tomato, Olive Oregano, Extra Special, Asda*	1 Pitta/75g	194	0.8	259	7.1	55.2	1.1	1.6
Pitta, Seeded, HL, Tesco*	1 Pitta/60g	153	3.6	255	10.8	39.4	6	12.8
Pitta, Spelt, Albert Heijn*	1 Pitta/80g	196	0.8	245	2.5	48	1	0
Pitta, White, Average	*1 Pitta/75g*	*191*	*1.1*	*255*	*9.2*	*50.8*	*1.5*	*2.7*
Pitta, White, Essential, Waitrose*	1 Pitta/60g	157	0.5	262	9	53.4	0.9	2.3
Pitta, White, Free From, Tesco*	1 Pitta/55g	140	1.2	255	6.5	52.6	2.1	5.5
Pitta, White, Greek Style, Asda*	1 Pitta/50g	126	1	253	8	51	1.9	0
Pitta, White, Large, Tesco*	1 Pitta/80g	220	0.8	275	9.4	54.9	1	4.5
Pitta, White, Mini, Sainsbury's*	1 Pitta/20g	54	0.2	268	8.8	54.6	1.2	2
Pitta, White, Mini, Tesco*	1 Pitta/30g	84	0.6	280	9.8	55.1	2.1	3.4
Pitta, White, Organic, Sainsbury's*	1 Pitta/59g	150	0.6	254	10.3	50.7	1.1	2.5
Pitta, White, Picnic, Waitrose*	1 Pitta/30g	75	0.4	249	10.3	49.3	1.2	3.5
Pitta, White, Sainsbury's*	1 Pitta/58g	160	0.7	275	9.8	54.7	1.2	3.1
Pitta, White, Soft, Sandwich, Warburton's*	½ Pitta/36g	81	0.9	228	9.8	41.4	2.6	1.8
Pitta, White, Speciality Breads, Waitrose*	1 Pitta/60g	149	0.7	249	10.3	49.3	1.2	3.5
Pitta, White, Tesco*	1 Pitta/58g	160	0.6	275	9.4	54.9	1	4.5
Pitta, White, Weight Watchers*	1 Pitta/45g	106	0.3	238	8.7	45.9	0.7	6.7
Pitta, Wholemeal with Extra Virgin Olive Oil, Tesco*	1 Pitta/60g	135	1.6	225	8.3	41.5	2.6	5.5
Pitta, Wholemeal, Acropolis, Lidl*	1 Pitta/57g	136	0.9	238	12	44	1.6	6
Pitta, Wholemeal, Asda*	1 Pitta/56g	133	0.9	238	12	44	1.6	6
Pitta, Wholemeal, Average	*1 Pitta/64g*	*154*	*1.1*	*241*	*11*	*45.8*	*1.7*	*6.4*
Pitta, Wholemeal, Essential, Waitrose*	1 Pitta/60g	159	0.7	264	9.7	50.1	1.2	7.2
Pitta, Wholemeal, Healthy Eating, Co-Op*	1 Pitta/63g	135	1.3	215	12	37	2	9
Pitta, Wholemeal, Hollyland Bakery*	1 Pitta/20g	48	0.3	242	13.1	43.7	1.6	6
Pitta, Wholemeal, M&S*	1 Pitta/60g	155	1.6	255	10	45	2.6	5.5
Pitta, Wholemeal, Mini, M&S*	1 Pitta/18g	44	0.4	247	10.3	45.8	2.5	5.6
Pitta, Wholemeal, Mini, Sainsbury's*	1 Pitta/30g	69	0.5	231	10	43.8	1.7	6.2
Pitta, Wholemeal, Mini, Tesco*	1 Pitta/30g	76	0.5	255	11.8	48.2	1.7	4.2
Pitta, Wholemeal, Sainsbury's*	1 Pitta/57g	154	0.9	271	10.9	49.7	1.5	7.4
Pitta, Wholemeal, Simple Versatile, As Sold, Tesco*	1 Pitta/58g	145	0.7	250	9.6	46.2	1.2	7.8
Pitta, Wholemeal, So Organic, Sainsbury's*	1 Pitta/60g	140	1	233	9.8	44.8	1.6	8.1
Pitta, Wholemeal, Tesco*	1 Pitta/58g	145	0.7	250	9.6	46.2	1.2	7.8
Pitta, Wholemeal, Waitrose*	1 Pitta/60g	145	0.5	242	12.4	46	0.9	3.1
Pitta, Wholemeal, Weight Watchers*	1 Pitta /46g	106	0.6	229	8.7	44.5	1.2	7.6
Potato, & Rosemary, M&S*	1 Serving/40g	108	2.7	270	9.4	42.2	6.8	2.3
Potato, Farls, Irish, Rankin Selection, Irwin's Bakery*	1 Farl/60g	110	2.2	184	2.3	34.4	3.6	2.5
Potato, Farls, M&S*	1 Farl/55g	79	0.2	144	4.2	33.8	0.4	4.7
Potato, Farls, Sunblest*	1 Farl/100g	156	0.9	156	3.8	33.2	0.9	1.9
Pumpernickel, Average	*1 Slice/50g*	*96*	*0.6*	*191*	*5.5*	*37.9*	*1.1*	*7.8*
Pumpernickel, Organic, Bavarian Pumpernickel*	1 Slice/50g	90	0.5	180	6	38	1	10

BREAD

INFO/WEIGHT	Measure INFO/WEIGHT	per Measure KCAL	per Measure FAT	Nutrition Values per 100g / 100ml KCAL	PROT	CARB	FAT	FIBRE
Pumpernickel, Organic, Biona*	1 Slice/80g	158	1.4	197	4.6	36	1.7	9.6
Pumpernickel, Rye, Kelderman*	1 Slice/50g	92	0.5	185	6	38	1	0
Pumpkin Seed, Chleb Dyniowy, The Polish Bakery*	1 Slice/40g	100	2	250	7.1	45.5	5.1	6.4
Pumpkin Seed, Raisin & Sunflower Seed, Sainsbury's*	1 Slice/30g	76	0.8	255	11.6	45.9	2.8	3.4
Pure Grain, Heart of Nature, Pure Nature*	1 Slice/55g	172	9.1	313	9.7	24.8	16.6	7.9
Pure Grain, with Prunes, Pure Nature*	1 Slice/50g	169	10.4	338	8	28.3	20.8	9
Raisin, & Pumpkin Seed, Organic, Tesco*	1 Slice/30g	76	1.7	253	9.7	40.6	5.8	3.8
Raisin, with Cinnamon, Warburton's*	1 Slice/36g	96	1.3	267	7.2	51.1	3.7	3.2
Rolls, American Style Deli, Tesco*	1 Roll/65g	162	2.2	249	7.8	46.8	3.4	1.6
Rolls, Ancient Grain, Tesco*	1 Roll/80g	231	6.7	289	14.7	34.4	8.4	8.6
Rolls, Best of Both, Hovis*	1 Roll/62g	148	2.9	239	9.8	39.7	4.6	5
Rolls, Brioche, Average	**1 Roll/49g**	**177**	**6.9**	**361**	**8.8**	**50.1**	**14.1**	**1.5**
Rolls, Brioche, Brialys*	1 Roll/35g	121	3.9	347	8.8	52.8	11.2	1.5
Rolls, Brioche, Butter, Tesco*	1 Serving/35g	120	3.7	344	8.5	52.9	10.5	2.2
Rolls, Brioche, Continental Classics*	1 Roll/35g	122	3.3	349	8.2	58.3	9.3	0
Rolls, Brioche, Finest, Tesco*	1 Roll/52g	207	11.6	398	10.8	38.3	22.4	2
Rolls, Brioche, French Milk, Bon Appetit, Aldi*	1 Roll/35g	116	2.7	330	8.3	56	7.8	2.2
Rolls, Brioche, Hot Dog, Specially Selected, Aldi*	1 Roll/45g	142	3.4	316	9.4	52	7.5	2
Rolls, Brioche, La Boulangere, Lidl*	1 Roll/35g	122	3.6	350	8.2	55.5	10.2	1.8
Rolls, Brioche, Plain Chocolate Chip, Sainsbury's*	1 Roll/35g	126	4.5	361	8	52.1	12.9	2.1
Rolls, Brioche, Sainsbury's*	1 Roll/35g	123	3.9	352	8.1	53.5	11.3	1.8
Rolls, Brioche, Tesco*	1 Roll/26g	92	2.9	349	8.5	54	11	0
Rolls, Brown, bake at Home, Aldi*	1 Roll/45g	131	1.5	291	10	52	3.3	5.8
Rolls, Brown, Carb Control, Tesco*	1 Roll/45g	98	2.7	218	20.5	20.7	5.9	10.7
Rolls, Brown, Ciabatta, Schar*	1 Roll/50g	138	4.1	274	5.8	40	8.1	8.9
Rolls, Brown, Crusty	**1 Roll/50g**	**128**	**1.4**	**255**	**10.3**	**50.4**	**2.8**	**3.5**
Rolls, Brown, Free From, Tesco*	1 Roll/65g	174	5.3	268	5.4	43.2	8.2	3.6
Rolls, Brown, Large, Asda*	1 Roll/57g	138	0.9	242	10	47	1.6	0
Rolls, Brown, M&S*	1 Roll/105g	242	6.4	230	9.2	37.3	6.1	4.4
Rolls, Brown, Malted Grain, Tesco*	1 Roll/58g	144	1.9	248	8.7	46.2	3.2	1.9
Rolls, Brown, Mini, M&S*	1 Roll/33g	80	2.5	245	9.8	35.5	7.6	3.8
Rolls, Brown, Morning, Farmfoods*	1 Roll/50g	134	1.8	269	12	47	3.7	4.2
Rolls, Brown, Old Fashioned, Waitrose*	1 Roll/63g	152	2.6	241	9.6	41.3	4.1	4.7
Rolls, Brown, Part Baked, Sunnyhills, Aldi*	1 Roll/50g	129	1.5	258	9.3	45.3	3	6.3
Rolls, Brown, Seeded, Organic, Sainsbury's*	1 Roll/70g	166	3.2	237	9.9	39.1	4.6	6.5
Rolls, Brown, Snack, Allinson*	1 Roll/44g	119	2.9	270	10.8	41.6	6.7	5.6
Rolls, Brown, Soft, Average	**1 Roll/50g**	**134**	**1.9**	**268**	**10**	**51.8**	**3.8**	**3.5**
Rolls, Brown, Soft, Organic, Sainsbury's*	1 Roll/70g	166	3.2	237	9.9	39.1	4.6	6.6
Rolls, Brown, Soft, Tesco*	1 Roll/50g	125	0.5	250	9.2	49.7	1	2.6
Rolls, Brown, Square, M&S*	1 Roll/105g	242	6.4	230	9.2	37.3	6.1	4.4
Rolls, Cheese Topped, Sandwich, Warburton's*	1 Roll/62g	168	4	270	12.1	40.7	6.5	2.6
Rolls, Cheese Topped, Village Green*	1 Roll/56g	159	4.1	284	13.1	41.2	7.4	4.8
Rolls, Chunky Cheese, Tesco*	1 Roll/80g	219	4.8	274	12.8	41.1	6	2
Rolls, Ciabatta, Cheese Topped, Mini, Finest, Tesco*	1 Roll/30g	85	2.4	282	11.5	40.9	8.1	3.8
Rolls, Ciabatta, Garlic, Asda*	1 Roll/93g	333	16.7	358	9	40	18	2.3
Rolls, Ciabatta, GF, Schar*	1 Roll/50g	112	1.3	219	3.7	41	2.6	8.7
Rolls, Ciabatta, Mini, Finest, Tesco*	1 Roll/30g	89	2	297	9.9	49.1	6.8	4.1
Rolls, Ciabatta, Sun Dried Tomato, Mini, Finest, Tesco*	1 Roll/30g	79	1.9	262	8.7	42.3	6.4	2.6
Rolls, Ciabatta, Tesco*	1 Roll/100g	295	5.6	295	9.2	50.5	5.6	3
Rolls, Country Grain, Mini, M&S*	1 Roll/31g	85	3	275	10.2	38.9	9.7	3.8
Rolls, Crisp, Original, Organic, Kallo*	1 Roll/9g	34	0.5	390	11	74	5.6	3
Rolls, Crusty, Booths*	1 Roll/50g	124	0.6	247	8.7	50.3	1.2	2.6

BREAD

INFO/WEIGHT	per Measure KCAL	FAT	Nutrition Values per 100g / 100ml KCAL	PROT	CARB	FAT	FIBRE
Rolls, Crusty, French, M&S*	1 Roll/65g	159	0.8	245	8.1	50.5	1.2	3.3
Rolls, Crusty, Part-Baked, Budgens*	1 Roll/50g	148	0.7	296	9.4	61.4	1.4	2.5
Rolls, Finger, Morrisons*	1 Roll/46g	119	0.8	259	10.7	50	1.8	2.3
Rolls, Finger, White, Sainsbury's*	1 Roll/40g	96	1	240	9	45.2	2.6	3.2
Rolls, Focaccia, Tesco*	1 Roll/75g	226	7	302	8.7	45.6	9.4	3.8
Rolls, GF, Antoinette Savill*	1 Roll/70g	157	1.5	224	1.9	48.8	2.2	1.5
Rolls, Granary Malted Wheatgrain, Soft, M&S*	1 Roll/80g	208	3.1	260	9.3	47.2	3.9	2.3
Rolls, Granary, Average	*1 Roll/70g*	*176*	*2.7*	*251*	*9.6*	*45.2*	*3.9*	*3.3*
Rolls, Granary, Bakers Premium, Tesco*	1 Roll/65g	158	0.8	243	9.9	47.8	1.3	2.3
Rolls, Granary, Homebake, Hovis*	1 Roll/75g	194	1.6	259	10.2	47.7	2.2	3.6
Rolls, Granary, Mini, Tesco*	1 Roll/34g	92	2.2	271	10	43.5	6.5	3.8
Rolls, Granary, Original, Hovis*	1 Roll/70g	180	2.9	257	10.7	44.3	4.1	5.3
Rolls, Granary, Waitrose*	1 Roll/59g	160	3.8	271	10	47.2	6.4	3.8
Rolls, Green Olive, M&S*	1 Roll/75g	210	4.5	280	11.2	44	6	1.8
Rolls, Half Half, Warburton's*	1 Roll/55g	144	2.5	261	10.4	42.7	4.5	4
Rolls, Hamburger, Gluten & Wheat Free	*1 Roll/55g*	*137*	*1.9*	*249*	*2*	*52.4*	*3.4*	*4*
Rolls, Heyford Wholemeal, Soft Grainy, Waitrose*	1 Roll/75g	164	1.3	219	11.2	36.7	1.7	5.8
Rolls, Hot Dog, Sliced, Asda*	1 Roll/84g	197	2.8	234	7	44	3.3	0
Rolls, Hot Dog, Tesco*	1 Roll/85g	200	2.8	235	7.3	44	3.3	1.9
Rolls, Hot Dog, Value, Tesco*	1 Roll/40g	93	0.8	232	8.7	45	1.9	2.2
Rolls, Hot Dog, White, Warburton's*	1 Roll/55g	142	2.1	259	8.8	46.4	3.9	1.6
Rolls, Low GI, Lidl*	1 Roll/60g	177	5.1	295	14	44.9	8.5	8.4
Rolls, Malted Grain, Sainsbury's*	1 Roll/68g	190	2.9	280	8.7	51.6	4.3	4.2
Rolls, Malted Grain, Submarine, M&S*	1 Roll/109g	300	4.7	275	8.9	53.6	4.3	3
Rolls, Malted Wheat, Sub, Organic, Tesco*	1 Serving/108g	279	4.4	258	10.1	45.2	4.1	4.8
Rolls, Malted, Whole Grain Rolls, Batched, Soft, M&S*	1 Roll/80g	180	3.6	225	7.8	38.5	4.5	3.1
Rolls, Mini Submarine, M&S*	1 Roll/23g	63	1.1	275	11.4	47.7	4.9	1.1
Rolls, Morning, Scottish, Warburton's*	1 Roll/50g	138	0.4	276	10.9	56.2	0.8	2.1
Rolls, Morning, Tesco*	1 Roll/48g	117	1.2	243	10.4	44.8	2.5	4.7
Rolls, Multi Seed, Free From, Free From, Tesco*	1 Roll/70g	214	8.3	305	5.4	44.2	11.8	6.3
Rolls, Multigrain, Pain Rustique, Homebake, Finest, Tesco*	1 Roll/60g	162	4.3	270	12.7	38.4	7.1	9.6
Rolls, Multigrain, Sub, Asda*	1 Sub/150g	357	6.3	238	0	0	4.2	0
Rolls, Multigrain, Torpedo, Sainsbury's*	1 Roll/112g	328	7.5	293	10.5	47.7	6.7	6.3
Rolls, Multiseed, Deli, Tesco*	1 Roll/65g	188	4.6	289	10.5	40.7	7.1	10.3
Rolls, Multiseed, Genius*	1 Roll/70g	209	7.8	299	3.9	40.6	11.2	10
Rolls, Nut Raisin, Bakery, Tesco*	1 Serving/120g	426	11.2	355	9	56.8	9.3	4
Rolls, Oatmeal, Co-Op*	1 Roll/70g	175	3.2	250	10.1	42.6	4.6	5.6
Rolls, Oatmeal, Ploughman's, GFY, Asda*	1 Roll/72g	181	3.2	252	10	43	4.4	3.9
Rolls, Oatmeal, Soft, M&S*	1 Roll/83g	224	3.9	270	12.3	43.4	4.7	3.4
Rolls, Panini, Sainsbury's*	1 Roll/90g	249	5.6	276	11	44.1	6.2	3
Rolls, Panini, White, Tesco*	1 Roll/85g	232	4.1	273	10.7	44.9	4.8	3.4
Rolls, Part Baked, Mini, Tesco*	1 Roll/50g	120	0.6	240	7.8	49.5	1.2	3.4
Rolls, Poppy Seeded Knot, Waitrose*	1 Roll/60g	169	3.2	282	10.3	48.3	5.3	2.2
Rolls, Pumpkin Seed, Lidl*	1 Roll/80g	271	9	339	15	42.5	11.2	3.8
Rolls, Rustic, Ready to Bake, Paul Hollywood*	1 Roll/75g	199	0.8	265	8.5	54.7	1	1.7
Rolls, Rye, Toasting, Good & Hot*	1 Roll/65g	143	0.7	220	7.3	44.6	1.1	7.1
Rolls, Scotch, Morning, Tesco*	1 Roll/50g	136	0.6	273	11.8	52	1.3	3.2
Rolls, Scottish Morning, Morrisons*	1 Roll/60g	157	1.3	261	11.3	51.4	2.2	2.4
Rolls, Seed Sensations, Deli, Hovis*	1 Roll/70g	184	6	263	10.3	36.5	8.5	10.6
Rolls, Seeded, Deli, Rowan Hill Bakery, Lidl*	1 Roll/75g	243	8.2	324	11.4	42.2	11	5.4
Rolls, Seeded, Mixed Mini Loaf Pack, M&S*	1 Roll/76g	220	7.3	290	10.6	39.7	9.6	4
Rolls, Seeded, Oval Bite, Gregg's *	1 Roll/79g	220	4.5	278	10.1	44.3	5.7	0
Rolls, Seeded, Sandwich, Warburton's*	1 Roll/77g	242	6.7	314	13.3	41.2	8.7	6

BREAD

INFO/WEIGHT	Measure	per Measure		Nutrition Values per 100g / 100ml				
		KCAL	FAT	KCAL	PROT	CARB	FAT	FIBRE
Rolls, Seeded, Soft, GF, Newburn, Warburton's*	1 Roll/65g	176	6.2	270	9	33.8	9.5	6.7
Rolls, Seeded, Three Seeds, Sandwich, Warburton's*	1 Roll/77g	242	6.7	314	13.3	41.2	8.7	6
Rolls, Snack, Mini, Tesco*	1 Roll/35g	95	2.1	271	19	43	6	4
Rolls, Soft, White, Rowan Hill Bakery, Lidl*	1 Roll/66g	157	1.6	238	8.5	44	2.5	2.8
Rolls, Soft, Wholemeal, Finger, M&S*	1 Roll/66g	145	1.3	220	12.6	38	2	5.8
Rolls, Stone Baked, Bakery Instore, Lidl*	1 Roll/100g	292	1.5	292	9.5	58.4	1.5	3.5
Rolls, Sub, White, Batch, Warburton's*	1 Roll/80g	215	3.5	269	11	45	4.4	2.4
Rolls, Sub, Wholemeal, Warburton's*	1 Roll/94g	231	4.1	246	10.9	40.6	4.4	6.3
Rolls, Submarine, Sainsbury's*	1 Roll/117g	305	4.6	261	9.1	47.4	3.9	2.4
Rolls, Sun Dried Tomato, Homebake, Tesco*	1 Roll/50g	123	1.5	246	11.3	44	3	0
Rolls, Sunflower Seed, Toasting, Good & Hot*	1 Roll/65g	162	3.2	250	8.5	41	5	8
Rolls, Tiger, Crusty, Baked by Us, Morrisons*	1 Roll/63g	143	1.8	227	6.3	46	2.9	2.5
Rolls, Tomato & Basil, Sub, COU, M&S*	1 Roll/33g	86	0.9	265	11	48.7	2.7	2.4
Rolls, Triple Seeded, Genius *	1 Roll/70g	209	7.8	299	3.9	40.6	11.2	10
Rolls, White with Mixed Seeds Bran, Wheatfield Bakery*	1 Roll/76g	190	3.9	250	8.5	41.6	5.1	6.1
Rolls, White, 4 Pack, Warburton's*	1 Roll/58g	145	2.5	253	9.7	42.6	4.3	2.4
Rolls, White, 50/50, Soft, Kingsmill*	1 Roll/63g	154	2.4	245	9.3	41.2	3.8	4.4
Rolls, White, BGTY, Sainsbury's*	1 Roll/50g	114	0.5	227	9.1	45.3	1	3
Rolls, White, Cheese Topped, Asda*	1 Roll/46g	121	2	264	10	46	4.4	2
Rolls, White, Cheese Topped, Sainsbury's*	1 Roll/75g	218	6.4	291	12.1	41.6	8.5	2
Rolls, White, Chunky, Hovis*	1 Roll/73g	173	2.4	237	9.4	41.7	3.3	2.5
Rolls, White, Crusty, Average	*1 Roll/50g*	*140*	*1.2*	*280*	*10.9*	*57.6*	*2.3*	*1.5*
Rolls, White, Crusty, Bakery, Tesco*	1 Roll/70g	193	0.6	276	9.3	56.7	0.8	2.6
Rolls, White, Crusty, Home Bake, Tesco*	1 Roll/69g	185	1	270	9.3	54.2	1.4	2.9
Rolls, White, Crusty, Morning, M&S*	1 Roll/65g	176	0.8	270	8.8	53.8	1.3	2.7
Rolls, White, Dinner, Village Bakery, Aldi*	1 Roll/70g	183	0.9	262	8.8	52	1.3	3
Rolls, White, Finest, Tesco*	1 Roll/80g	198	2	247	9.3	45.3	2.5	3
Rolls, White, Finger, Smart Price, Asda*	1 Roll/50g	121	0.8	242	9	48	1.6	2.1
Rolls, White, Finger, Tesco*	1 Roll/45g	112	0.4	250	9.2	49.7	1	2.6
Rolls, White, Finger, Value, Tesco*	1 Roll/50g	116	1	232	8.7	45	1.9	2.2
Rolls, White, Floured, Batch, Tesco*	1 Roll/76g	193	2.5	254	8.8	47.3	3.3	2.2
Rolls, White, Floury Batch, Sainsbury's*	1 Roll/68g	168	1.9	247	8.3	47.2	2.8	2.2
Rolls, White, Floury, Roberts Bakery*	1 Roll/63g	160	1.6	254	8.4	49.5	2.5	2
Rolls, White, Hot Dog, Jumbo, Sainsbury's*	1 Roll/85g	239	5.2	281	7.5	49.1	6.1	2.9
Rolls, White, Hot Dog, Tesco*	1 Roll/65g	162	0.6	250	9.2	49.7	1	2.6
Rolls, White, Hot Dog, Tesco*	1 Roll/70g	177	2.5	254	9	45.5	3.6	1.9
Rolls, White, Large, Warburton's*	1 Roll/88g	229	3.1	259	10.2	44.3	3.5	2.5
Rolls, White, Low Price, Sainsbury's*	1 Roll/44g	107	0.7	243	8.9	48.2	1.6	2.1
Rolls, White, Mini, Submarine, M&S*	1 Roll/30g	86	1.5	285	11.4	47.7	4.9	1.1
Rolls, White, Morning, Co-Op*	1 Roll/47g	134	1.4	285	12	53	3	2
Rolls, White, Old Fashioned, Waitrose*	1 Roll/64g	176	2.9	275	8.8	49.8	4.5	2.8
Rolls, White, Organic, Sainsbury's*	1 Roll/65g	170	2	262	8.7	49.9	3	1
Rolls, White, Part Baked, Morrisons*	1 Roll/75g	227	1	303	9.6	63	1.4	2.6
Rolls, White, Ploughman's, Sainsbury's*	1 Roll/65g	185	2.5	285	8.6	54.1	3.8	2.3
Rolls, White, Premium Soft, Rathbones*	1 Roll/65g	190	3.9	293	9.3	50.3	6	2.7
Rolls, White, Premium, Brown Hill Bakery*	1 Roll/74g	206	2.2	279	11	51.5	3	2.3
Rolls, White, Premium, Hovis*	1 Roll/70g	180	3.1	257	9.5	44.8	4.4	3
Rolls, White, Sandwich, Sliced, Warburton's*	1 Roll/55g	146	2.1	265	9.7	46.6	3.9	2.4
Rolls, White, Scottish, Tesco*	1 Roll/48g	117	1.2	243	10.4	44.8	2.5	4.7
Rolls, White, Seeded, Sainsbury's*	1 Roll/80g	217	4.7	271	10.9	43.4	5.9	4.8
Rolls, White, Seeded, Soft, M&S*	1 Roll/75g	214	4.3	285	11.7	46.2	5.7	2.8
Rolls, White, Sliced, Warburton's*	1 Roll/55g	146	2.2	265	9.7	46.6	3.9	2.4
Rolls, White, Snack, Bakery, Tesco*	1 Roll/100g	250	1	250	9.2	49.7	1	2.6

BREAD

	Measure INFO/WEIGHT			Nutrition Values per 100g / 100ml				
		KCAL	FAT	KCAL	PROT	CARB	FAT	FIBRE
Rolls, White, Snack, Sainsbury's*	1 Roll/67g	159	0.7	237	7.9	49.2	1	2.3
Rolls, White, Soft, Average	*1 Sm Roll/45g*	*114*	*1.5*	*253*	*9.2*	*46.5*	*3.3*	*2.2*
Rolls, White, Soft, COU, M&S*	1 Roll/37g	94	1	255	10.7	47.1	2.7	1.5
Rolls, White, Soft, Dietary Specials*	1 Roll/75g	130	2.9	172	2.2	29.8	3.8	4.7
Rolls, White, Soft, Farmhouse, TTD, Sainsbury's*	1 Slice/47g	111	0.8	235	8.1	45.4	1.7	2.9
Rolls, White, Soft, GF, Newburn Bakehouse, Warburton's*	1 Roll/65g	159	4	244	7.3	37.1	6.2	5.4
Rolls, White, Soft, Hovis*	1 Roll/70g	180	3.1	257	9.5	44.8	4.4	3
Rolls, White, Soft, M&S*	1 Roll/60g	150	1.9	250	10.3	45.2	3.1	2.7
Rolls, White, Soft, Morrisons*	1 Roll/42g	100	0.8	238	9.1	46.4	1.9	2.4
Rolls, White, Soft, Tesco*	1 Roll/55g	137	0.6	250	9.2	49.7	1	2.6
Rolls, White, Softgrain, GFY, Asda*	1 Roll/54g	128	1	237	9	46	1.9	2.9
Rolls, White, Split, Asda*	1 Roll/45g	113	1.5	251	10	45	3.4	2.8
Rolls, White, Submarine, M&S*	1 Roll/109g	300	5.4	275	11	47	5	1
Rolls, White, Super Soft, Bakers Selection, Asda*	1 Roll/64g	173	2.9	272	7.5	49	4.6	2.5
Rolls, White, Tesco*	1 Roll/65g	180	2.5	277	8.7	52	3.8	2.7
Rolls, White, Tesco*	1 Roll/30g	79	0.7	262	9.7	50.5	2.3	2.9
Rolls, Wholemeal	*1 Roll/45g*	*108*	*1.3*	*241*	*9*	*48.3*	*2.9*	*5.9*
Rolls, Wholemeal & White, Kingsmill*	1 Roll/60g	151	2.5	251	9.5	43.7	4.2	3.5
Rolls, Wholemeal with Cracked Wheat, Allinson*	1 Roll/58g	134	2.3	231	11	38	3.9	7
Rolls, Wholemeal, Asda*	1 Roll/58g	130	1.6	225	11	39	2.8	6
Rolls, Wholemeal, COU, M&S*	1 Roll/110g	226	3.1	205	11.3	33.4	2.8	7.1
Rolls, Wholemeal, Deli, Tesco*	1 Serving/65g	156	3.1	240	9	40.2	4.8	5.7
Rolls, Wholemeal, Finest, Tesco*	1 Roll/75g	182	2.6	243	11.3	39	3.4	5.9
Rolls, Wholemeal, Finger, Six, Bakers Selection, Asda*	1 Roll/49g	112	0.7	228	9.5	41	1.4	6.6
Rolls, Wholemeal, Floury Batch, Sainsbury's*	1 Roll/68g	152	2.3	223	9.9	37.8	3.4	6.5
Rolls, Wholemeal, Golden, Hovis*	1 Roll/50g	112	2	223	10.5	36.5	3.9	6.8
Rolls, Wholemeal, High Protein, High Fibre, Warburton's*	1 Roll/68g	156	2.9	229	14	30	4.2	7.7
Rolls, Wholemeal, HL, Tesco*	1 Roll/68g	155	1.4	230	10.4	41.3	2.1	6.6
Rolls, Wholemeal, Mini, Assorted, Waitrose*	1 Roll/35g	86	2.1	244	9.7	37.9	6	7.3
Rolls, Wholemeal, Morrisons*	1 Roll/67g	155	2.7	231	10.2	38.6	4	6.3
Rolls, Wholemeal, Oat Topped, Deli, Tesco*	1 Roll/65g	170	3.5	260	10.9	38.3	5.3	6.7
Rolls, Wholemeal, Oat Topped, Tesco*	1 Roll/65g	166	2.9	255	11.3	42.2	4.5	5.1
Rolls, Wholemeal, Oatbran, HL, Tesco*	1 Roll/56g	115	1.4	205	11.4	33.6	2.5	7.4
Rolls, Wholemeal, Old Fashioned, Waitrose*	1 Roll/57g	135	2.7	236	11.1	37.2	4.8	6.6
Rolls, Wholemeal, Organic, Sainsbury's*	1 Roll/66g	152	1.8	230	10.7	41	2.7	6.6
Rolls, Wholemeal, Organic, Tesco*	1 Roll/65g	177	4	273	10.3	44.1	6.2	5.5
Rolls, Wholemeal, Sainsbury's*	1 Roll/65g	153	2.1	236	10.7	40.8	3.3	7.4
Rolls, Wholemeal, Seeded, The Country Miller, Waitrose*	1 Roll/75g	190	7.7	255	13.6	26.9	10.3	7.6
Rolls, Wholemeal, Sliced, Hovis*	1 Roll/60g	150	3.5	250	10.6	38.7	5.9	6.8
Rolls, Wholemeal, Sliced, Sandwich, Warburton's*	1 Roll/56g	130	2.2	233	10.5	35.8	3.9	6.6
Rolls, Wholemeal, Soft, Average	*1 Roll/65g*	*151*	*2.7*	*233*	*10.8*	*37.3*	*4.1*	*6.3*
Rolls, Wholemeal, Soft, Batch Baked, Warburton's*	1 Roll/65g	158	2.1	245	10.7	37.3	3.2	6.1
Rolls, Wholemeal, Soft, Sainsbury's*	1 Roll/60g	133	2	221	9.9	37.8	3.4	6.5
Rolls, Wholemeal, Soft, Seeded, Sainsbury's*	1 Roll/75g	193	5.6	257	11.8	35.6	7.4	6.2
Rolls, Wholemeal, Submarine, Tesco*	1 Roll/100g	221	3.1	221	9.3	39	3.1	5.2
Rolls, Wholemeal, Submarine, Wheatfield Bakery*	1 Roll/100g	230	3.4	230	10.4	39	3.4	6.2
Rolls, Wholemeal, Sunflower & Honey, Sainsbury's*	1 Roll/100g	311	8.1	311	10.8	45.9	8.1	5.4
Rolls, Wholemeal, Super Soft, Bakers Selection, Asda*	1 Roll/65g	181	2.5	280	9.8	48	3.9	6.9
Rolls, Wholemeal, Tasty, Kingsmill*	1 Roll/68g	171	2.5	251	10.7	39.1	3.7	6.5
Rolls, Wholemeal, Tesco*	1 Roll/46g	115	1.8	250	10.9	41.8	4	7.5
Rolls, Wholemeal, The Best, Morrisons*	1 Roll/72g	174	2.1	242	10.5	39.7	2.9	7.6
Rolls, Wholemeal, Village Bakery, Aldi*	1 Roll/63g	144	0.9	228	10	40	1.5	5.3
Rolls, Wholmeal, Deli, Tesco*	1 Roll/65g	156	3.1	240	9	40.2	4.8	5.7

BREAD

INFO/WEIGHT	Measure KCAL	per Measure FAT	Nutrition Values per 100g / 100ml KCAL	PROT	CARB	FAT	FIBRE
Rolls, York Baps, Adkins Bakery*	1 Roll/100g	264	2.2	264	10.7	53.7	2.2	2.4
Roti, Tesco*	1 Bread/95g	256	5.2	269	8.4	46.4	5.5	3.2
Rye, & Flax, Organic, Profusion*	1 Slice/50g	120	4.4	241	20.1	14.4	8.9	11.4
Rye, Mixed Seed, Dark, Boule, Finest, Tesco*	1 Slice/35g	86	1.2	248	12.1	39.2	3.4	5.9
Rye, Artisan Bread Organic*	1 Slice/50g	80	0.7	160	5	28.4	1.4	7.1
Rye, Average	*1 Slice/25g*	*55*	*0.4*	*219*	*8.3*	*45.8*	*1.7*	*4.4*
Rye, Dark, Sliced, Trianon*	1 Slice/41g	74	0.6	180	6.5	35	1.5	0
Rye, German Style, Bolletje*	1 Slice/60g	114	1.2	190	6	35	2	9.5
Rye, German Style, Kelderman*	1 Slice/64g	122	1.3	190	6	35	2	9.5
Rye, German Style, Loaf, Bakery in Store, M&S*	2 Slices/50g	112	0.6	225	9.5	40.8	1.1	6.3
Rye, Half Wheat, The Polish Bakery, Tesco*	1 Slice/40g	93	0.6	233	5.7	51.1	1.5	6.6
Rye, Light, Finest, Tesco*	1 Slice/20g	47	0.4	237	10.4	44.3	2	3.7
Rye, Organic with Coriander, Village Bakery*	1 Slice/30g	63	0.8	209	4.9	49.9	2.7	8.5
Rye, Seeded, Organic, The Village Bakery*	1 Slice/50g	107	1.6	214	5	37.8	3.2	7.2
Rye, Sourdough, Part Baked, TTD, Sainsbury's*	1 Slice/30g	70	0.4	233	6.5	45	1.3	7.8
Rye, Swedish Style, Kelderman*	1 Slice/50g	92	1.6	185	7.2	31.5	3.2	4.3
Rye, Vitality, Organic, Biona*	1 Slice/71g	147	1.4	207	5.3	37	2	9.9
Rye, Whole Grain, Schneiderbrot*	1 Slice/50g	100	0.5	201	5.2	38.9	1	7.7
Rye, Wholegrain , Sliced, Rowan Hill Bakery, Lidl*	1 Slice/56g	118	1	210	5.8	38	1.8	9.3
Rye, Wholegrain, with Sunflower Seeds, Rowan Hill*	1 Slice/56g	126	2.6	225	6.3	35	4.6	9.3
Rye, Wholemeal with Sunflower Seeds, Organic, Biona*	1 Slice/72g	150	2.9	210	7	36	4	6
Rye, Wholemeal, Organic, House Of Westphalia*	1 Slice/71g	131	0.9	184	4.5	34.2	1.2	9.2
Rye, with Pumpkin Seed, Organic, Lindale*	1 Slice/71g	150	2.9	211	6.1	32.1	4.1	10.6
Rye, with Sprouted Seeds, Yeast Free, Biona Organic*	1 Slice/35g	71	0.7	204	5.3	36.6	2	9.9
Rye, with Sunflower Seeds, Organic, Schneider Brot*	1 Slice/72g	138	2.6	191	6.2	33.4	3.6	7.9
Rye, with Sunflower Seeds, Organic, Sunnyvale*	1 Slice/25g	50	1.6	198	5.1	30.3	6.3	7.9
Sandwich Thins, 50/50, Kingsmill*	1 Thin/40g	99	1.1	245	10	43	2.7	4.3
Sandwich Thins, Brown, Warburton's*	1 Thin/40g	100	1.1	252	9.9	45.2	2.8	3.5
Sandwich Thins, Seeded, Free From, Tesco*	1 Thin/50g	125	3.8	250	7.8	32.3	7.6	10.8
Sandwich Thins, Seeded, GF, Warburton's*	1 Thin/43g	122	3.5	284	6.5	43.1	8.1	6.5
Sandwich Thins, Seeded, Kingsmill*	1 Thin/40g	106	1.8	264	9.6	43.6	4.6	4.8
Sandwich Thins, White, CBY, Asda*	1 Thin/55g	141	2.2	257	9.3	44.3	4	3.1
Sandwich Thins, White, GF, Warburton's*	1 Thin/58g	143	3.7	247	6	38.7	6.3	5.7
Sandwich Thins, White, Kingsmill*	1 Thin/40g	99	1	248	9.4	45.6	2.5	2.9
Sandwich Thins, White, Warburton's*	1 Thin/40g	100	1.1	251	9	46.2	2.8	2.5
Sandwich Thins, Wholemeal, Good Inside, Hovis*	1 Thin/45g	114	2.3	254	11.1	37.5	5.2	7.1
Sandwich Thins, Wholemeal, Kingsmill*	1 Thin/41g	98	1.2	240	10.3	39.8	3	6.1
Sandwich Thins, Wholemeal, Protein & Fibre, Warburton's*	1 Thin/50g	121	2.8	241	14.7	29.6	5.5	7.3
Seeded, Batch, Finest, Tesco*	1 Slice/65g	168	4	259	9.3	41.8	6.1	6.1
Seeded, Deliciously, Lower Carb, Hovis*	1 Slice/36g	100	3	277	15.7	27.2	8.3	15.1
Seeded, Farmhouse, GF, Warburton's*	1 Slice/35g	92	3.2	262	8.7	33	9.1	6.5
Seeded, Farmhouse, Loaf, Extra Special, Asda*	1 Slice/44g	92	0.5	207	11	38	1.2	8
Seeded, Farmhouse, Organic, Cranks*	2 Slices/94g	232	3.5	247	10.1	39.9	3.7	6.9
Seeded, Farmhouse, Roberts Bakery*	1 Slice/37g	89	1.1	240	10.6	49	2.9	6.7
Seeded, Free From, Gluten, Wheat, & Milk, Tesco*	1 Slice/42g	95	3.7	227	7	25.7	8.8	8.7
Seeded, Free From, Tesco*	1 Slice/42g	90	3.3	214	6.4	24.8	7.9	9.2
Seeded, GF, Sandwich Thins, Free From, Waitrose*	1 Thin/50g	132	5.1	263	9.3	24.5	10.2	18
Seeded, Med Sliced, Average	*1 Slice/44g*	*116*	*2.9*	*262*	*11.3*	*38.6*	*6.5*	*5.6*
Seeded, Mighty, GF, Mini Loaf, Warburton's*	1 Slice/27g	75	2.9	277	7.7	33.5	10.9	7
Seeded, Multi, Loaf, Gluten & Wheat Free, Lovemore*	1 Serving/35g	102	4.3	291	0	3	12.3	0
Seeded, Rye, Loaf, la Brea Bakery*	1 Slice/55g	120	0.6	218	7	42.5	1	5.7
Seeded, Seriously, Gold, Kingsmill*	1 Slice/50g	136	3.4	272	10.9	41.6	6.9	6.4
Seeded, The Really Seeded One, Kingsmill*	1 Slice/44g	118	3.2	268	10.4	37.3	7.3	5.5

BREAD

INFO/WEIGHT	Measure	per Measure		Nutrition Values per 100g / 100ml				
		KCAL	FAT	KCAL	PROT	CARB	FAT	FIBRE
Seeded, Triple, Farmhouse, Loaf, GF, Genius*	1 Slice/36g	100	2.9	277	3.5	43.8	8	8
Seeds, Grains, 10, Allinson*	1 Slice/41g	120	3.9	292	11.9	37.6	9.4	4.8
Sesame Seed, la Brea Bakery*	1 Slice/35g	85	0.8	244	8.8	47.1	2.3	2
Soda	*1oz/28g*	*72*	*0.7*	*258*	*7.7*	*54.6*	*2.5*	*2.1*
Soda, Farls, M&S*	1 Farl/110g	267	3	243	9.6	50.1	2.7	2.3
Soda, Farls, Tesco*	1 Farl/142g	325	4.5	229	7.1	42.2	3.2	2.6
Soda, Fruit, M&S*	1 Slice/40g	105	1.9	260	5.9	51.3	4.6	2.5
Soda, M&S*	1 Slice/40g	82	0.6	205	8.7	39.2	1.6	4.2
Softgrain, Med Sliced, GFY, Asda*	1 Slice/35g	79	0.5	226	7	46	1.5	3.7
Softgrain, Mighty White*	1 Slice/36g	81	0.5	224	7.2	45.5	1.5	3.7
Sourdough, Average	*1 Slice/50g*	*144*	*0.9*	*289*	*11.8*	*56.4*	*1.8*	*2.4*
Sourdough, Loaf, Finest, Tesco*	1 Slice/33g	86	1.8	262	9.6	41.9	5.5	3.3
Sourdough, Rye, Bloomer, Tesco*	1 Slice/40g	97	0.5	243	8.3	47.2	1.2	4.9
Sourdough, Sandwich Thins, M&S*	1 Thin/50g	105	2.1	210	6.8	32	4.2	8.8
Sourdough, White, Cob, Free From, Tesco*	1 Slice/50g	92	1.4	184	5.1	31	2.7	7.4
Soy, & Linseed, 500g Loaf, Burgen*	1 Slice/42g	120	4.4	285	8.2	35.5	10.4	8.2
Soya, & Linseed, Vogel*	1 Slice/42g	95	2.1	227	11.7	34.1	4.9	6.8
Soya, Linseed, Sliced, Burgen *	1 Slice/44g	126	4.8	287	15.2	26.9	11	9.8
Spelt, & Seed, Sliced, Lifefibre*	1 Slice/42g	141	5.8	335	11.6	32.2	13.7	9.2
Spelt, Healthguard, T W Bakeries*	1 Slice/40g	80	0.7	201	6.2	36.5	1.7	7.2
Spinach, Goats Cheese, Twist, Waitrose*	1 Twist/45g	114	2.9	253	11.8	34.7	6.5	4.3
Sprouted Grain, Ezekiel *	1 Slice/34g	80	0.5	235	11.8	44.1	1.5	0.9
Sprouted Grain, Rolls, Finest, Tesco*	1 Roll/80g	209	3.3	262	8.4	45.5	4.1	4.5
Sprouted Spelt, with Raisins, Everfresh Bakery*	¼ Loaf/100g	230	1.9	230	9.2	43.9	1.9	6.6
Stoneground, Sm Loaf, Organic, Sainsbury's*	1 Slice/24g	50	0.5	208	10	37.9	2.1	7.9
Stoneground, Wholemeal, Thick, Love Life, Waitrose*	1 Slice/40g	86	1.1	214	10.1	36.5	2.8	7.9
Sundried Tomato, Pepper, Bloomer, Bakery, Tesco*	1 Slice/50g	132	1.5	266	9.9	47.3	3.1	4.5
Sunflower, & Honey, M&S*	1 Serving/67g	206	9	308	12.9	34	13.4	5.6
Sunflower, & Honey, Organic, Cranks*	1 Slice/30g	64	0.9	215	11.6	37.2	3	8.3
Sunflower, & Pumpkin Seed, So Organic, Sainsbury's*	1 Slice/30g	76	1.6	254	11.4	40	5.4	12.9
Sunflower, & Pumpkin, Cob, Sliced, Finest, Tesco*	1 Slice/40g	120	4.4	299	12.3	34.7	10.9	6.6
Sunflower, Bakers Selection, Asda*	1 Slice/60g	162	5.9	270	11.3	50	9.8	8.3
Sunflower, Multi-Grain, Allinson*	1 Slice/47g	113	2.2	240	9.8	39.6	4.7	3.9
Sunflower, Seed, Bolletje, Delhaize*	1 Slice/44g	106	3.1	240	7.5	35	7	6
Sunflower, Seed, Organic, Natural, Mestemacher*	1 Slice/75g	162	3	216	5.6	34.7	4	9.4
Superseeded, Sliced Loaf, Extra Special, Asda*	1 Slice/44g	135	4.4	306	12	38	10	6.3
Sweet Potato, with Pumpkin Sunflower Seeds, BFree*	1 Slice/40g	93	2.5	232	3.5	30.6	6.3	9.2
Tandoori, Rustic Marble, Graze*	1 Punnet/36g	117	5	324	8.7	41.2	13.8	4.8
Tiger, Artisan, Bloomer, GF, Warburton's*	2 Slices/100g	241	5.3	241	7.1	38.5	5.3	5.5
Tiger, Baton, Bakery, Tesco*	½ Baton/100g	288	2	288	9.1	57.4	2	2.2
Tiger, Loaf, Bloomer, Bakery, Tesco*	1 Slice/50g	133	1.6	266	8.4	49.2	3.2	3.2
Tiger, White, Warburton's*	1 Slice/40g	106	1.3	266	8.4	49.2	3.2	3.2
Toaster, White, Rathbones*	1 Slice/38g	92	0.5	243	9.1	48.6	1.3	2.3
Toastie Pockets, Brown, Easy Fill, Warburtons*	1 Pocket/55g	134	1.6	243	9.8	42.2	3	4.2
Tomato, & Chilli, BGTY, Sainsbury's*	¼ Bread/65g	155	3.1	238	11.9	36.9	4.7	2.8
Tomato, & Garlic, Italian Style, Morrisons*	½ Pack/155g	355	12.4	229	5.8	33.4	8	2.5
Tomato, & Herb, Tear & Share, Tesco*	¼ Pack/73g	164	3.2	226	6.3	40.2	4.4	2.1
Walnut, Waitrose*	1/8 Loaf/50g	170	7.6	339	10	40.6	15.2	5.9
Wheat	*1 Slice/25g*	*65*	*1*	*260*	*9.1*	*47.2*	*4.1*	*4.3*
Wheat, & Wholemeal Spelt, & Seeds, Love Life, Waitrose*	1 Slice/34g	88	2.6	267	10.5	33.5	7.9	9.9
Wheat, Golden, Warburton's*	1 Slice/40g	100	1	249	9.4	45.2	2.4	4.3
Wheat, Spelt, & Rye, Loaf, Baked by Us, Morrisons*	1 Serving/70g	165	1.4	236	11.3	39.9	2	6.6
Wheat, Tasty, Kingsmill*	1 Serving/38g	84	1.3	221	10.1	37.6	3.4	6.8

B

BREAD	Measure INFO/WEIGHT	per Measure KCAL	FAT	Nutrition Values per 100g / 100ml KCAL	PROT	CARB	FAT	FIBRE
Wheaten, Big Slice	**1 Slice/65g**	**139**	**1.7**	**214**	**7.5**	**40.2**	**2.6**	**3.6**
Wheaten, Loaf, Sliced, Genesis*	1 Slice/40g	86	1	214	7.5	40.2	2.6	3.6
Wheaten, Loaf, Sliced, No Added Sugar, Genesis Crafty*	1 Slice/40g	86	1	214	7.5	40.2	2.6	3.6
Wheaten, M&S*	1 Slice/33g	74	1.2	225	9.3	42.9	3.5	3.9
Wheaten, Sliced, Healthy, Irwin's Bakery*	1 Slice/40g	76	0.8	190	9	40.5	1.9	6.2
Wheatgerm, Hovis, Soft, Sliced, M&S*	1 Slice/23g	50	0.7	220	10.1	38.5	3	4.6
White, Average	**1 Slice/40g**	**94**	**0.8**	**235**	**8.4**	**49.3**	**1.9**	**1.5**
White, Batch Loaf, Extra Special, Asda*	1 Slice/47g	109	0.9	233	9	45	1.9	2.2
White, Batch, Warburton's*	1 Slice/42g	98	0.9	233	9.8	43.6	2.1	2.7
White, Ciabatta, Roll, GF, Dietary Specials*	1 Roll/50g	106	0.9	213	4.1	40.9	1.8	8.3
White, Classic, Med Sliced, Hovis*	1 Slice/38g	91	0.9	240	11.4	40.3	2.3	2.5
White, Commercially Prepared, Average	**1oz/28g**	**74**	**0.9**	**266**	**7.6**	**50.6**	**3.3**	**2.4**
White, Commercially Prepared, Toasted, Average	**1oz/28g**	**82**	**1.1**	**293**	**9**	**54.4**	**4**	**2.5**
White, Country Maid*	1 Slice/33g	76	0.7	229	8.5	44.1	2.1	3
White, Country, Sliced, Warburtons*	1 Slice/31g	72	0.7	233	9.1	43.1	2.2	2.2
White, Crusty, Farmhouse, Sliced, Bakery, Tesco*	1 Slice/40g	103	0.5	259	9.4	51.1	1.2	3.3
White, Crusty, Fresh, Finest, Tesco*	1 Slice/52g	130	1	250	8.6	48.5	1.9	2.4
White, Crusty, Gold, Kingsmill*	1 Slice/27g	70	0.8	258	9.4	48.5	2.9	2.7
White, Crusty, Hovis*	1 Slice/44g	103	1	233	8.8	44.3	2.2	2.1
White, Crusty, Premium, Warburton's*	1 Slice/31g	77	0.7	254	10.6	46.5	2.3	2.6
White, Crusty, Sliced Loaf, Tesco*	1 Slice/50g	127	0.6	254	9.2	50.1	1.2	3.2
White, Crusty, Sliced, Premium, Budgens*	1 Slice/50g	121	1.1	242	8.8	46.9	2.2	2.2
White, Crusty, Split Tin, Bakery, Tesco*	1 Slice/50g	134	0.8	268	9.4	52.6	1.5	3.3
White, Danish Style, Thick Sliced, Light, Tesco*	1 Slice/22g	55	0.6	255	9.4	47.3	2.9	2.7
White, Danish, Lighter, Warburton's*	1 Slice/26g	63	0.3	243	10.5	45.8	1.2	2.6
White, Danish, Soft & Light, Thick Cut, Asda*	1 Slice/26g	60	0.4	230	9	45	1.6	2.1
White, Danish, Soft, Weight Watchers, Warburton's*	1 Slice/21g	50	0.3	243	9.8	46.5	1.3	2.9
White, Danish, Thick Sliced, Tesco*	1 Slice/24g	60	0.6	250	9.7	47.4	2.3	2.9
White, Extra Thick Sliced, Kingsmill*	1 Slice/58g	135	1.4	232	8.8	43.8	2.4	2.8
White, Farmhouse Crusty, M&S*	1 Slice/34g	82	0.7	240	8.9	46.6	2.2	3
White, Farmhouse Gold Premium, Morrisons*	1 Slice/38g	90	0.5	236	8.9	47.4	1.2	2.2
White, Farmhouse, GF, Newburn, Warburton's*	1 Slice/35g	83	2.1	236	6.8	35.6	6.1	5.5
White, Farmhouse, Hovis*	1 Slice/44g	103	1	234	8.7	44.6	2.3	2.4
White, Farmhouse, Seeded, Waitrose*	1 Serving/75g	192	4.1	256	10.8	40.9	5.5	5.6
White, Farmhouse, Sliced, Bakery, Tesco*	1 Slice/44g	106	1	240	7.9	46	2.3	2
White, Farmhouse, Soft, 400g Loaf, Warburton's*	1 Slice/27g	66	0.7	245	10.1	43.7	2.6	2.8
White, Farmhouse, Soft, 800g Loaf, Warburton's*	1 Slice/43g	104	1.1	243	9	45	2.5	2.3
White, Fibre, Morrisons*	1 Slice/40g	96	0.7	240	8	48.4	1.7	0.3
White, Fresh, GF, Sliced, Juvela*	1 Slice/29g	64	0.7	221	3.8	44	2.4	4.7
White, Fried in Blended Oil	**1 Slice/28g**	**141**	**9**	**503**	**7.9**	**48.5**	**32.2**	**1.6**
White, Gluten Wheat Free, Free From, Sainsbury's*	1 Slice/89g	189	4.5	212	3.4	32.1	5.1	12.5
White, Gold Seeded, Kingsmill*	1 Slice/44g	108	2.5	245	9.7	38.8	5.7	3.5
White, Golden, Square Cut, M&S*	1 Slice/40g	85	0.8	215	8.9	40.7	2.1	6.1
White, Harvest Crust Premium, Ormo*	1 Slice/40g	92	0.6	229	9.4	47.4	1.5	2.7
White, Invisible Crust, Hovis*	1 Slice/40g	90	0.6	226	8.8	44.1	1.6	2.4
White, Loaf, Danish, Asda*	1 Serving/23g	53	0.5	236	9	45	2.2	2
White, Loaf, Gluten & Wheat Free, Lovemore*	1 Serving/35g	111	3.8	316	0	3.4	10.9	0
White, Loaf, Sliced, Finest, Tesco*	1 Slice/44g	103	0.6	236	8.6	45.5	1.3	4.1
White, Low Carb, Sliced, Tesco*	1 Slice/16g	35	0.4	211	11.3	36.4	2.2	6.9
White, Med Sliced, Average	**1 Slice/39g**	**93**	**0.6**	**238**	**7.5**	**48.5**	**1.6**	**1.8**
White, Med Sliced, Basics, Sainsbury's*	1 Slice/36g	83	0.5	231	8	46.4	1.5	2.1
White, Med Sliced, Brace's*	1 Slice/32g	75	0.4	235	9.5	46.6	1.2	2.6
White, Med Sliced, Great Everyday, Kingsmill*	1 Slice/40g	93	0.8	232	9	44.6	2	2.7

BREAD

INFO/WEIGHT	Measure	per Measure KCAL	FAT	Nutrition Values per 100g / 100ml KCAL	PROT	CARB	FAT	FIBRE
White, Med Sliced, Long Life, Asda*	1 Slice/36g	82	0.6	228	8	45	1.8	2.7
White, Med Sliced, Mother's Pride*	1 Slice/36g	82	0.6	229	8	45.6	1.6	3
White, Med Sliced, Sainsbury's*	1 Slice/36g	78	0.7	216	8.7	41.1	1.9	7.1
White, Med Sliced, Smart Price, Asda*	1 Slice/36g	81	0.5	226	7	46	1.5	2.8
White, Med Sliced, Stay Fresh, Tesco*	2 Slices/72g	172	1.6	240	8.3	45.8	2.2	2
White, Med Sliced, Superlife, Morrisons*	1 Slice/30g	79	1.2	263	9.6	47.4	3.9	2.5
White, Med Sliced, Tesco*	1 Slice/40g	96	0.9	239	8.1	45.6	2.2	2.3
White, Med Sliced, Value, Tesco*	1 Slice/36g	81	0.4	225	7.9	46.1	1	2.1
White, Medium, 400g Loaf, Warburton's*	1 Slice/24g	58	0.5	244	10.3	45.1	1.9	2.4
White, Medium, Round Top, Kingsmill*	1 Slice/42g	97	1	232	8.8	43.8	2.4	2.8
White, Medium, Sliced, H.W. Nevill's*	1 Slice/38g	90	0.8	238	8	45.3	2.2	2.7
White, Medium, Warburton's*	1 Slice/40g	98	0.8	244	9.1	46.4	2	2.3
White, Mega Thick, Roberts Bakery*	1 Slice/66g	154	1.2	233	8.3	46.2	1.8	2.2
White, Mighty, GF, Mini Loaf, Warburton's*	1 Slice/27g	67	1.8	249	6.7	37.9	6.5	5.8
White, Milk Roll, Warburton's*	1 Slice/18g	46	0.5	248	9.4	45	2.8	2.4
White, Multiseed, Farmhouse, Sliced, 400g, Waitrose*	1 Slice/33g	96	2.9	291	11.2	38.5	8.8	6.7
White, Multiseed, Med Sliced, Batch, Tesco*	1 Slice/50g	133	3	267	9.9	40.3	6.1	5.5
White, Old English, Warburton's*	1 Slice/40g	99	1.2	248	9.8	44.3	2.9	2.8
White, Organic, Bloomer, Bakery, Tesco*	1 Slice/40g	98	0.9	247	9.8	44.8	2.2	4.2
White, Organic, Sainsbury's*	1 Slice/36g	84	0.6	234	8.9	45.5	1.8	2.3
White, Plain, Scottish, Sunblest*	1 Slice/57g	133	1.5	233	10.1	42.3	2.6	2.8
White, Premium Farmhouse, Lidl*	1 Slice/44g	99	0.7	225	7.4	45.4	1.5	2.5
White, Premium, M&S*	1 Slice/40g	95	0.8	235	8.5	45.8	1.9	2.7
White, Rolls, GF, Promise*	1 Roll/60g	118	1.3	197	5	33.1	2.2	12.6
White, Sandwich, Bakery, Sainsbury's*	1 Slice/50g	121	0.3	242	10.3	49	0.6	2.9
White, Sandwich, Kingsmill*	1 Slice/42g	97	1	232	8.8	43.8	2.4	2.8
White, Scottish Plain, Medium, Mother's Pride*	1 Slice/50g	114	0.8	227	8.7	44.6	1.5	3
White, Sea Salt Black Pepper, Bloomer, Bakery, Tesco*	1 Slice/50g	131	0.8	262	10.1	50.4	1.6	3
White, Seeded, Batch, Loaf, Truly Irresistible, Co-Op*	1 Slice/47g	129	3.4	275	11.6	41.1	7.2	4.3
White, Seeds, Oats, Honey, TTD, Sainsbury's*	1 Slice/50g	154	5.4	308	12.1	36.7	10.9	7.1
White, Sliced, Free From, Tesco*	1 Slice/33g	91	1.7	278	2	52.1	5.3	7
White, Sliced, GF, Free From, Tesco*	1 Slice/42g	80	1.7	190	5.2	29.7	4	7.3
White, Sliced, Roberts Bakery*	1 Slice/35g	87	0.7	249	10	48	2.1	2.5
White, Sm Loaf, Classic, Hovis*	1 Slice/33g	75	0.8	228	11.4	40.3	2.3	6.5
White, Soft Batch, Sliced, Sainsbury's*	1 Slice/44g	102	0.8	232	8.2	45.4	1.9	2.3
White, Soft Crusty, M&S*	1 Slice/25g	64	0.6	256	9.3	49	2.5	2.4
White, Soft, Batch Loaf, Sliced, Tesco*	1 Slice/50g	116	1	233	7.5	46.1	2.1	2.1
White, Soft, Burger, Thins, Kingsmill*	1 Thin/44g	112	1.1	254	9.1	47	2.6	3
White, Soft, Extra Thick, Hovis*	1 Slice/67g	156	1.1	233	8.7	44.6	1.7	2.4
White, Soft, Gold, Kingsmill*	1 Slice/47g	112	1.5	239	8.2	44.5	3.1	2.7
White, Soft, M&S*	1 Slice/47g	105	0.8	225	7.3	46.1	1.7	2.4
White, Soft, Rolls, Genius*	1 Roll/70g	196	4.9	280	2	49.2	7	5.9
White, Soft, Sandwich, Loaf, BFree*	1 Slice/30g	60	0.3	200	7.7	35.7	1.1	8.4
White, Soft, Sliced, Hovis*	1 Slice/25g	58	0.6	234	8.7	44.6	2.3	2.4
White, Soft, Thick Sliced, Kingsmill*	1 Slice/44g	105	0.9	238	8	45.6	2	2.7
White, Sourdough, Country, Oval, la Brea Bakery*	1 Slice/60g	143	0.4	239	8.8	49.4	0.6	1.6
White, Sourdough, The Rustik Bakery*	1 Slice/35g	79	0.4	225	9.1	43	1.2	3.9
White, Sourdough, Waitrose*	1 Slice/50g	119	0.6	237	9	45.9	1.2	3.3
White, Square, Extra Thick Sliced, Hovis*	1 Slice/67g	155	1.3	231	8.5	44.7	2	2.6
White, Square, Med Sliced, Hovis*	1 Slice/40g	92	0.8	231	8.5	44.7	2	2.6
White, Square, Thick Sliced, Hovis*	1 Slice/50g	116	1	231	8.5	44.7	2	2.6
White, Super Grained, Farmhouse, Medium, Finest, Tesco*	1 Slice/44g	106	0.8	241	10.4	43.4	1.8	4.9

BREAD

	Measure INFO/WEIGHT	per Measure KCAL	FAT	Nutrition Values per 100g / 100ml KCAL	PROT	CARB	FAT	FIBRE
White, Superior English Quality, Thin Cut, Hovis*	1 Slice/73g	169	1.1	232	9.2	42.8	1.5	3.8
White, Thick Sliced, Bakers Gold, Asda*	1 Slice/44g	101	0.8	229	8	45	1.9	2.3
White, Thick Sliced, Brace's*	1 Slice/38g	90	0.5	235	9.5	46.6	1.2	2.6
White, Thick Sliced, Budgens*	1 Slice/40g	89	0.5	223	7.4	45.3	1.3	2.5
White, Thick Sliced, Fine Lady*	1 Slice/44g	113	0.5	254	7.8	53.1	1.2	2.3
White, Thick Sliced, Golden Sun, Lidl*	1 Slice/44g	100	0.7	228	7.5	46.1	1.5	2.4
White, Thick Sliced, Healthy, Warburton's*	1 Slice/38g	84	0.7	222	10.3	41.2	1.8	4.1
White, Thick Sliced, M&S*	1 Slice/42g	96	0.5	228	7.3	46.7	1.3	2.8
White, Thick Sliced, Organic, Tesco*	1 Slice/44g	108	0.9	245	8.5	46.8	2.1	3.1
White, Thick Sliced, Sainsbury's*	1 Slice/44g	95	0.8	216	8.7	41.1	1.9	7.1
White, Thick Sliced, Square Cut, Asda*	1 Slice/44g	101	0.7	230	8	46	1.5	2.1
White, Thick Sliced, Sunblest*	1 Slice/40g	91	0.6	228	8	45.7	1.5	2.8
White, Thick Sliced, Super Toastie, Morrisons*	1 Slice/50g	128	1.5	257	8.7	48.9	3	2.1
White, Thick Sliced, Tesco*	1 Slice/44g	106	0.7	240	8.2	47.8	1.5	3
White, Thick, So Organic, Sainsbury's*	1 Slice/44g	102	1	231	8.2	44.6	2.2	3.1
White, Thick, Super Soft, M&S*	1 Slice/48g	120	1.3	249	9	45.3	2.7	3.6
White, Thickest, Warburton's*	1 Slice/58g	137	1.2	239	9.9	43.8	2	2.6
White, Thin Sliced, Sainsbury's*	1 Slice/29g	66	0.4	228	7.1	46.4	1.5	2.8
White, Thin Sliced, Tesco*	1 Slice/30g	68	0.4	228	9.5	44.5	1.3	3.4
White, Toast, Gamle M̦lle*	1 Slice/32g	83	0.6	260	8	52	2	3
White, Toasted, Average	*1 Slice/33g*	*87*	*0.5*	*265*	*9.3*	*57.1*	*1.6*	*1.8*
White, Toastie, 400g Loaf, Warburton's*	1 Slice/29g	70	0.5	244	10.3	45.1	1.9	2.4
White, Toastie, GF, Genius*	1 Slice/33g	90	2	272	2.4	47	6.1	9.3
White, Toastie, Loved by Us, Co-Op*	1 Slice/50g	120	1.2	240	7.9	45.4	2.4	2.6
White, Toastie, Thick Cut, Hovis*	1 Slice/50g	115	1	230	8.5	44.8	2	2.5
White, Toastie, Thick, Love to Toast, Kingsmill*	1 Slice/50g	116	1	232	9	44.6	2	2.7
White, Toastie, Warburton's*	1 Slice/47g	116	0.9	244	9.1	46.4	2	2.3
White, Trio of Olive, Bloomer, Bakery, Tesco*	1 Serving/82g	199	4	243	6.8	41.3	4.9	3
White, Whole, Extra Thick, Kingsmill*	1 Slice/57g	130	1.4	228	9	42.3	2.5	4
White, Whole, Kingsmill*	1 Slice/38g	87	1	230	9	42.9	2.5	3.4
White, Wholesome, Loaf, Sainsbury's*	1 Serving/36g	81	0.7	224	9.4	42.5	1.8	4.4
White, Wholesome, Med Sliced, Asda*	1 Slice/35g	78	0.9	223	7	43	2.6	5
White, Wholesome, Thick Sliced, Tesco*	1 Serving/80g	177	1.5	221	10.5	40.5	1.9	4.8
Whole Seed, Cob, Crusty, Bakery, Tesco*	1 Slice/50g	179	6.1	359	13.7	45.7	12.3	5.2
Whole Seed, Loaf, Sliced, Tesco*	1 Slice/40g	109	2.9	272	10.9	38.4	7.2	5.3
Wholegrain, & Rye, Schneider Brot*	1 Slice/50g	98	0.6	197	5.9	36.6	1.2	8.2
Wholegrain, Oats, Warburton's*	1 Slice/40g	98	1.4	245	11.7	38.8	3.5	5.9
Wholegrain, Average	*1 Slice/44g*	*117*	*1.9*	*265*	*13.4*	*43.3*	*4.2*	*7.4*
Wholegrain, Batch, Finest, Tesco*	1 Slice/44g	112	1.2	254	9.8	47.7	2.7	4.2
Wholegrain, Brennans*	1 Slice/39g	79	0.6	203	9	40	1.5	4.9
Wholegrain, Med Sliced, Irish Pride*	1 Slice/38g	90	0.8	237	9.2	46.6	2.1	7.6
Wholegrain, Soft, M&S*	1 Slice/51g	115	2.8	225	13	31.2	5.4	8.2
Wholegrain, Toasted, Average	*1 Slice/40g*	*117*	*1.9*	*288*	*14.5*	*47.1*	*4.6*	*8.1*
Wholegrain, with Sunflower Seeds, Landgut*	1 Slice/83g	183	4.2	221	7	37	5	29
Wholemeal Oat, Loaf, Vogel*	1 Slice/42g	86	0.6	205	8.7	34.3	1.5	9.7
Wholemeal Tasty Spelt, Sliced, Hovis*	1 Slice/47g	108	1	230	11.1	38.4	2.1	6.7
Wholemeal Loaf, British Farmers, Hovis*	1 Slice/47g	108	1.3	229	10	37.9	2.8	6.8
Wholemeal Oatbran, Sliced, Tesco*	1 Slice/45g	90	0.7	200	10.1	35.3	1.6	7.4
Wholemeal, & Oat Flakes, Gold, Kingsmill*	1 Slice/47g	103	1.6	220	10	37.3	3.4	7
Wholemeal, Rye, Cob, Waitrose*	1 Slice/33g	80	0.7	242	11.7	40.5	2.1	6.9
Wholemeal, Rye, Farmhouse,, Extra Special, Asda*	1 Slice/50g	112	1.2	225	11	36	2.5	7.3
Wholemeal, 7 Seeded, Irwin's Bakery*	1 Slice/38g	90	2	237	9.5	33.4	5.2	9.4
Wholemeal, American Sandwich, Harry's*	1 Slice/43g	110	2.1	259	9	45	5	5

BREAD

INFO/WEIGHT	Measure	per Measure		Nutrition Values per 100g / 100ml				
		KCAL	FAT	KCAL	PROT	CARB	FAT	FIBRE
Wholemeal, Average	**1 Slice/40g**	**88**	**1**	**215**	**9.2**	**41.6**	**2.5**	**5.8**
Wholemeal, Baker`s Soft, Medium, Tesco*	1 Slice/40g	94	1.1	235	10.8	37.8	2.8	6.9
Wholemeal, Batch, Sliced, Organic, Duchy, Waitrose*	1 Slice/50g	121	1.2	242	10.2	41.8	2.3	6.8
Wholemeal, BGTY, Sainsbury's*	1 Slice/20g	41	0.2	207	12.6	36.8	1	7.3
Wholemeal, Brennans*	1 Slice/33g	78	1.4	236	11.2	38.4	4.2	7.7
Wholemeal, Brown, Med Sliced, 400g, Hovis*	1 Slice/29g	64	0.5	221	10	37.8	1.8	6.8
Wholemeal, COU, M&S*	1 Slice/21g	45	0.5	213	13.6	33.7	2.6	7
Wholemeal, Crusty, Finest, Tesco*	1 Slice/50g	103	0.8	206	10.8	37	1.7	6.9
Wholemeal, Crusty, Kingsmill*	1 Slice/42g	104	1.8	247	11.2	41.1	4.2	7
Wholemeal, Danish, BFY, Morrisons*	1 Slice/17g	39	0.3	228	11.2	47.9	1.8	6.2
Wholemeal, Economy, Sainsbury's*	1 Slice/28g	61	0.7	217	10.3	38.4	2.5	6.5
Wholemeal, Farmhouse, Bakery in Store, M&S*	1 Slice/35g	80	1	229	11.4	35.3	3	7.9
Wholemeal, Farmhouse, Hovis*	1 Slice/44g	91	1	207	11	36	2.2	7.1
Wholemeal, Farmhouse, Med Sliced, Waitrose*	1 Slice/36g	84	0.7	232	10.8	39.1	1.9	7.5
Wholemeal, Farmhouse, Rowan Hill Bakery, Lidl*	1 Slice/47g	102	0.7	218	10.3	37.8	1.4	6.3
Wholemeal, Farmhouse, Soft, Tesco*	1 Slice/44g	103	1.1	234	11.3	28.1	2.6	6.3
Wholemeal, Farmhouse, Thick Sliced, Waitrose*	1 Slice/44g	103	0.8	232	10.8	39.1	1.9	7.5
Wholemeal, Fh, Stoneground, Batch, Finest, Tesco*	1 Slice/50g	108	1.4	215	10.3	36.1	2.8	6.9
Wholemeal, Gold, Kingsmill*	1 Slice/44g	95	1.3	217	10.9	36.8	2.9	7
Wholemeal, Golden Crust, Ormo*	1 Slice/38g	83	0.8	218	10.4	36.1	2	7
Wholemeal, Golden Wheat, Kingsmill*	1 Slice/44g	97	1.3	221	10.9	37.8	2.9	6
Wholemeal, Healthy Range, Pat The Baker*	1 Slice/27g	58	0.5	215	10	36.4	1.8	6.6
Wholemeal, High Protein, High Fibre, Warburton's*	1 Slice/29g	66	1	227	13.5	32	3.3	7.8
Wholemeal, Light, Irish Pride*	1 Slice/28g	68	0.4	241	13.3	44.1	1.3	4.5
Wholemeal, Little Brown Loaf, Unsliced, Hovis*	1 Slice/40g	86	1.1	216	10	37.8	2.7	6.8
Wholemeal, Live Good, Hovis*	1 Slice/26g	67	0.4	258	10	46.9	1.5	6.9
Wholemeal, Loaf, 400g, Kingsmill*	1 Slice/29g	68	0.8	234	10.2	39	2.8	6.2
Wholemeal, Loaf, Sliced, Thick, 800g, Hovis*	1 Slice/47g	104	0.8	221	10	37.8	1.8	6.8
Wholemeal, Longer Life, Med Sliced, Sainsbury's*	1 Slice/35g	78	1.3	222	10.9	36.2	3.7	6.5
Wholemeal, Longer Life, Sainsbury's*	1 Slice/36g	85	1.2	237	10.7	41	3.4	6.2
Wholemeal, Longer Life, Thick Slice, Sainsbury's*	1 Slice/45g	101	1.6	224	10.6	37.4	3.6	5.9
Wholemeal, Lower Carb , Hovis*	1 Slice/36g	84	1.3	234	16	27	3.7	14.4
Wholemeal, Med Sliced, Great Everyday, Kingsmill*	1 Slice/40g	91	1.5	227	10.5	37.7	3.8	6.2
Wholemeal, Med Sliced, Little Big Loaf, Kingsmill*	1 Slice/39g	93	1.5	239	10.5	37.7	3.8	6.2
Wholemeal, Med Sliced, M&S*	1 Slice/40g	80	1.2	200	10.5	32.7	3.1	6.7
Wholemeal, Med Sliced, Morrisons*	1 Slice/33g	72	0.5	216	9.6	38	1.4	6.5
Wholemeal, Med Sliced, Organic, Tesco*	1 Slice/27g	55	0.7	209	9.2	37.2	2.8	6
Wholemeal, Med Sliced, Premium, Tesco*	1 Slice/36g	71	0.2	196	9.8	37.8	0.6	7.2
Wholemeal, Med Sliced, Roberts Bakery*	1 Slice/37g	86	0.6	233	10.9	38.1	1.5	6.6
Wholemeal, Med Sliced, Sainsbury's*	1 Slice/36g	77	0.9	214	10.3	37.8	2.4	7.4
Wholemeal, Med Sliced, The Village Bakery*	1 Slice/33g	69	0.7	209	9.8	38	2	6
Wholemeal, Med Sliced, Waitrose*	1 Slice/36g	76	0.9	213	10.1	37.6	2.4	7
Wholemeal, Medium, 400g Loaf, Warburton's*	1 Slice/24g	55	0.7	231	10.6	37.8	2.8	6.4
Wholemeal, Medium, 800g Loaf, Warburton's*	1 Slice/45g	103	1.3	231	10.6	37.8	2.8	6.4
Wholemeal, Medium, Sliced, Everyday Essentials, Aldi*	1 Slice/40g	85	0.7	213	10	36	1.7	6.3
Wholemeal, Medium, Sliced, H.W. Nevill's*	1 Slice/36g	83	0.9	231	9.6	39	2.5	7
Wholemeal, Multi Seeded, TTD, Sainsbury's*	1 Slice/47g	110	3.4	234	11.7	30.7	7.2	8.1
Wholemeal, Multigrain, Soft Batch, Sainsbury's*	1 Slice/44g	106	2.9	242	11.3	34.5	6.5	5.6
Wholemeal, Multiseed, Batch, So Organic, Sainsbury's*	1 Slice/30g	79	2.2	263	11.8	30.9	7.4	12.9
Wholemeal, Oat Topped, TTD, Sainsbury's*	1 Slice/47g	109	1.3	232	10	38.5	2.8	0.3
Wholemeal, Organic, Hovis*	1 Slice/44g	92	1.3	209	10.2	35.6	2.9	7.6
Wholemeal, Premium, Med Slice, M&S*	1 Slice/33g	65	1	200	10.5	32.9	3.1	6.7
Wholemeal, Premium, Thick Slice, M&S*	1 Slice/50g	95	1.5	190	9.8	30.8	3	6.4

	Measure INFO/WEIGHT	per Measure KCAL	FAT	Nutrition Values per 100g / 100ml KCAL	PROT	CARB	FAT	FIBRE

BREAD

	Measure INFO/WEIGHT	per Measure KCAL	FAT	KCAL	PROT	CARB	FAT	FIBRE
Wholemeal, Rustic, Tin, Tesco*	1 Slice/37g	92	1.3	249	12.2	44	3.5	3.1
Wholemeal, Sandwich Loaf, Brennans*	1 Slice/40g	88	0.7	221	9.8	38.5	1.7	8
Wholemeal, Seed Sensations, Hovis*	1 Slice/44g	109	2.5	249	11.9	31.4	5.6	12.4
Wholemeal, Seeded Batch, Truly Irresistible, Co-Op*	1 Slice/47g	115	1.9	245	11.5	36.2	4	6.6
Wholemeal, Seeded, Farmhouse, Rowan Hill Bakery, Lidl*	1 Slice/33g	84	2.1	256	12.4	32.7	6.3	9.4
Wholemeal, Seeded, Roll, Love Life, Waitrose*	1 Roll/72g	192	6.3	266	12.6	34.1	8.8	6.4
Wholemeal, Seeded, Rowan Hill Bakery, Lidl*	1 Slice/33g	86	1.9	261	12.7	34.9	5.8	9
Wholemeal, Seeded, Signature, Allinson*	1 Slice/46g	118	4	256	11.1	28.9	8.7	8.9
Wholemeal, Sliced, Loaf, Average	*1 Slice/40g*	*90*	*0.9*	*224*	*9.9*	*38.8*	*2.4*	*6.9*
Wholemeal, Sliced, McCambridge*	1 Slice/38g	90	0.7	237	7.9	44.7	1.8	0
Wholemeal, Sliced, Medium, Tesco*	1 Slice/40g	93	1.2	234	11.9	36.7	2.9	6.6
Wholemeal, Sliced, Organic, Harvestime*	1 Slice/44g	95	1.2	216	9	38.8	2.7	5.6
Wholemeal, Soft Crusty, M&S*	1 Slice/25g	58	0.8	230	11.4	39.1	3.1	6.5
Wholemeal, Soft, Multiseed, Farmhouse, TTD, Sainsbury's*	1 Slice/50g	140	4.4	280	12.1	33.4	8.8	9.3
Wholemeal, Soft, Thick, Rowan Hill Bakery, Lidl*	1 Slice/44g	104	1	236	9.7	41.1	2.3	5.8
Wholemeal, Square Cut, Thick Sliced, Asda*	1 Slice/44g	91	1	208	10	37	2.2	6
Wholemeal, Stoneground, Batch Baked, Warburton's*	1 Slice/45g	101	1.2	224	10.3	35.7	2.6	6.9
Wholemeal, Stoneground, Organic, Waitrose*	1 Sm Slice/25g	57	0.9	228	10.8	38.2	3.6	7.1
Wholemeal, Stoneground, Thick Sliced, Sainsbury's*	1 Slice/44g	92	0.8	210	10.2	37.9	1.9	7.8
Wholemeal, Supersoft, Eat Well, M&S*	1 Slice/33g	81	1.1	245	10.9	40	3.3	6.7
Wholemeal, Tasty, Medium, Kingsmill*	1 Slice/40g	93	1.1	233	10.2	38.6	2.8	6.3
Wholemeal, Tasty, Thick, Kingsmill*	1 Slice/44g	105	1.7	239	10.5	37.7	3.8	6.2
Wholemeal, The Champion, Batch, Allinson*	1 Slice/46g	108	1.3	234	11	37.8	2.9	6.1
Wholemeal, Thick Slice, Brennans*	1 Slice/27g	69	0.6	257	9.2	45.4	2.1	6.8
Wholemeal, Thick Sliced, Bakers Gold, Asda*	1 Slice/44g	99	1.4	225	12	37	3.2	6
Wholemeal, Thick Sliced, Great Everyday, Kingsmill*	1 Slice/44g	100	1.7	227	10.5	37.7	3.8	6.2
Wholemeal, Thick Sliced, Sainsbury's*	1 Slice/44g	103	1.3	234	11.9	36.7	2.9	6.6
Wholemeal, Thick Sliced, So Organic, Sainsbury's*	1 Slice/50g	120	1.6	239	9.6	39.3	3.2	7.2
Wholemeal, Thick Sliced, Stephenson's Bakery*	1 Slice/40g	84	0.8	209	10.7	37.3	1.9	6.2
Wholemeal, Thick Sliced, Tesco*	1 Slice/40g	96	1.1	240	9.5	40.9	2.7	6.8
Wholemeal, Thick Sliced, Waitrose*	1 Slice/44g	94	1.1	213	10.1	37.6	2.4	7
Wholemeal, Thick, Weight Watchers, Warburton's*	1 Slice/29g	72	0.8	250	9.2	43.6	2.9	6.5
Wholemeal, Toasted, Average	*1 Med Slice/26g*	*58*	*0.6*	*224*	*8.6*	*42.3*	*2.2*	*5.8*
Wholemeal, Toastie, Sliced, Tesco*	1 Slice/50g	116	1.4	234	11.9	36.7	2.9	6.6
Wholemeal, Unsliced, Organic, Dove's Farm*	1 Med Slice/35g	77	0.9	221	11.4	37.9	2.6	8.3
Wholemeal, with Rye, Rich Tasty, Warburton's*	1 Slice/45g	109	1.1	246	9.9	40.6	2.4	7.5
Wholemeal. Medium, Brace's*	1 Med Slice/32g	72	0.7	226	10.2	44.3	2.2	6
Wholesome, Five Seeded, GF, Genius*	1 Slice/36g	102	3.4	285	3.7	42.3	9.4	7.8
Wholesome, Vitality, GF, Schar*	1 Slice/32g	84	2.9	262	4.5	36	9.2	8.8
Wholewheat, 100%, Stoneground, Maxwell House*	1 Slice/27g	60	0.5	222	11.1	44.4	1.9	7.4
Wholewheat, Harvest	1 Serving/42g	90	1	214	7.1	45.2	2.4	7.1
Wholewheat, Nature's Own*	1 Slice/28g	66	1	236	14.3	39.3	3.6	10.7
Wholewheat, No Crusts, Harry's*	1 Slice/25g	58	1.1	233	8	40	4.5	5.5
Wholewheat, Soft, Trader Joe's*	1 Slice/37g	70	1	189	10.8	37.8	2.7	5.4
Wrap, Brown, Soft, Easy Roll, Warburton's*	1 Wrap/65g	190	2.9	292	12	49.3	4.5	3.2
Wrap, Half Half, Warburton's*	1 Wrap/41g	121	1.8	296	12.8	49.6	4.4	3.8
Wrap, Mediterranean Herb, Soft, Village Bakery, Aldi*	1 Wrap/64g	188	2.6	294	8	54.7	4.1	2
Wrap, Seeded, GF, Newburn Bakehouse, Warburton's*	1 Wrap/60g	178	4.5	297	5.5	48.1	7.5	7.4
Wrap, Tortilla, 8 Pack, Asda*	1 Tortilla/50g	143	3	286	8	50	6	1.9
Wrap, Tortilla, 8 Pack, LC, Tesco*	1 Tortilla/50g	135	1	270	7.1	53.2	2.1	3.5
Wrap, Tortilla, Ancient Grain, Blue Menu*	1 Tortilla/34g	100	2	294	8.8	50	5.9	5.9

BREAD

INFO/WEIGHT	Measure KCAL	FAT	Nutrition Values per 100g / 100ml KCAL	PROT	CARB	FAT	FIBRE
Wrap, Tortilla, Beetroot, Fibre Fest, Genius*	1 Wrap/40g	83	1.4	208	5.3	32	3.6	13
Wrap, Tortilla, Beetroot, GF, Warburton's*	1 Wrap/45g	131	2.6	292	4.6	52.2	5.8	6.4
Wrap, Tortilla, BGTY, Sainsbury's*	1 Tortilla/50g	136	1.4	271	7.9	53.7	2.7	1.9
Wrap, Tortilla, Both in One, Sunnyhills, Aldi*	1 Wrap/64g	184	2.9	287	8.1	52	4.5	3
Wrap, Tortilla, Bueno*	1 Tortilla/63g	171	3.6	272	6.9	48.2	5.7	2
Wrap, Tortilla, Deli, Multigrain, Mission Deli*	1 Tortilla/61g	202	6.1	330	7.9	50.5	10	3
Wrap, Tortilla, Flour, Soft, Mini, Stand n Stuff, Old El Paso*	1 Tortilla/12g	36	0.6	296	8.5	52.5	5.2	2.7
Wrap, Tortilla, Flour, Soft, Old El Paso*	1 Tortilla/41g	123	2.1	299	8.5	53.7	5.2	1.9
Wrap, Tortilla, Flour, Stand n Stuff, Old El Paso*	1 Tortilla/24g	71	1.2	296	8.5	52.5	5.2	2.7
Wrap, Tortilla, from Tex Mex Meal, Tesco*	2 Wraps/61g	190	4.7	310	8.5	50.4	7.6	1.6
Wrap, Tortilla, Garlic, Parsley, Sainsbury's*	1 Tortilla/60g	166	3.7	277	7.2	48	6.2	1.8
Wrap, Tortilla, GF, Lovemore*	1 Wrap/50g	150	4.2	299	1.8	48.1	8.3	4.1
Wrap, Tortilla, Healthy 'n' White, Wrap 'n' Roll, Discovery*	1 Tortilla/40g	161	3.5	288	8	49.7	6.3	2.6
Wrap, Tortilla, Large, Essential, Waitrose*	1 Tortilla/64g	190	3.7	297	7.2	52.5	5.8	3.1
Wrap, Tortilla, LC, Tesco*	1 Tortilla/64g	166	1.3	260	7.1	53.2	2.1	3.5
Wrap, Tortilla, Less Than 3% Fat, BGTY, Sainsbury's*	1 Tortilla/51g	128	1.1	250	7.8	50.1	2.2	2.9
Wrap, Tortilla, Low Carb, Carbzone*	1 Wrap/65g	182	8.4	280	18	10	13	26
Wrap, Tortilla, Low Carb, Gerry's Wraps*	1 Wrap/43g	142	3.7	330	6.9	30.3	8.6	31.9
Wrap, Tortilla, Low Fat, M&S*	1 Serving/180g	225	4	125	6.3	20.6	2.2	1.9
Wrap, Tortilla, Mediterranean Herb, Rowan Hill, Lidl*	1 Wrap/64g	178	2.2	278	7.3	53	3.5	2.5
Wrap, Tortilla, Mexican, Asda*	1 Tortilla/34g	100	2.8	295	7.9	47.2	8.3	3.9
Wrap, Tortilla, Morrisons*	1 Serving/60g	132	2.1	220	6.2	42	3.5	1.7
Wrap, Tortilla, Multiseed, Discovery*	1 Tortilla/57g	160	2.8	280	8.7	50.1	5	3.6
Wrap, Tortilla, Multiseed, Tesco*	1 Wrap/64g	186	4	290	8.6	47.6	6.3	4.4
Wrap, Tortilla, Organic, Sainsbury's*	1 Tortilla/56g	167	4.3	298	8.6	48.8	7.7	2.1
Wrap, Tortilla, Original, Mini, Mission Deli*	1 Wrap/31g	93	2	299	7.6	50.9	6.6	2.7
Wrap, Tortilla, Plain , Ocado*	1 Wrap/53g	154	4.4	291	6.7	45.7	8.4	3.1
Wrap, Tortilla, Plain, HL, Tesco*	1 Wrap/64g	182	3.2	284	8.2	49.7	5	3.7
Wrap, Tortilla, Plain, Mini, Morrisons*	1 Tortilla/34g	91	1.4	267	8.1	48.9	4	2.8
Wrap, Tortilla, Plain, Nannak*	1 Wrap/80g	134	3.5	167	8.9	62.2	4.4	0
Wrap, Tortilla, Plain, Ready to Eat, Sunnyhills, Aldi*	1 Wrap/64g	181	2.2	283	7.1	54.5	3.4	3
Wrap, Tortilla, Plain, Sainsbury's*	1 Wrap/64g	182	2.9	285	7.8	51.2	4.5	4.3
Wrap, Tortilla, Plain, Tesco*	1 Tortilla/64g	182	3.2	284	8.1	49.7	5	3.8
Wrap, Tortilla, Plain, Village Bakery, Aldi*	1 Wrap/65g	194	4.9	298	7.8	49.6	7.6	2.7
Wrap, Tortilla, Quinoa, Chia Seed, BFree*	1 Wrap/42g	105	2.4	250	7.6	36	5.7	11.4
Wrap, Tortilla, Rice, Mountain Bread*	1 Wrap/25g	68	0.3	272	10	53	1.3	2.6
Wrap, Tortilla, Seeded, Love Life, Waitrose*	1 Tortilla/64g	185	3.6	290	8.8	46.6	5.7	4.3
Wrap, Tortilla, Soft, M&S*	1 Wrap/64g	186	3.8	290	8	49.7	6	2.5
Wrap, Tortilla, Soft, Mini, Old El Paso*	1 Tortilla/25g	80	2.1	319	7.7	51	8.5	2.4
Wrap, Tortilla, Spicy Tomato, Morrisons*	1 Tortilla/55g	158	3.1	288	8.6	50.5	5.7	0.7
Wrap, Tortilla, Spicy Tomato, Tesco*	1 Tortilla/63g	175	3.5	278	7.8	49.2	5.6	2.4
Wrap, Tortilla, Super Seed, Protein, GF, Warburton's*	1 Wrap/45g	133	3	295	17	39	6.7	5.5
Wrap, Tortilla, Sweet Chilli, Mission Deli*	1 Wrap/62g	193	4.2	311	7.5	52.8	6.8	4.1
Wrap, Tortilla, Sweet Chilli, Tesco*	1 Wrap/64g	184	2.9	288	7.4	53.1	4.5	2.7
Wrap, Tortilla, Sweet Potato, GF, BFree*	1 Wrap/42g	95	0.9	227	4.6	41.7	2.2	11
Wrap, Tortilla, Tomato, Herb, Tesco*	1 Serving/63g	165	3.5	262	7.9	45.1	5.5	2.1
Wrap, Tortilla, Value, Tesco*	1 Wrap/47g	129	2.4	275	8.5	49.1	5	4.3
Wrap, Tortilla, Wheat White, Mini, Mission Deli*	1 Wrap/31g	93	2.1	299	7.5	50	6.9	3.6
Wrap, Tortilla, White, Bakers Selection, Asda*	1 Tortilla/62g	181	2.9	290	7.9	53	4.6	2.5
Wrap, Tortilla, White, GF, Warburton's*	1 Wrap/45g	138	2.6	306	3.9	57	5.8	5.3
Wrap, Tortilla, White, M&S*	1 Tortilla/64g	170	2.4	265	7.9	49	3.8	1.6
Wrap, Tortilla, White, Weight Watchers*	1 Wrap/50g	118	0.6	236	6.9	46.5	1.3	8.8
Wrap, Tortilla, Whole White, HL, Tesco*	1 Wrap/64g	182	1.7	284	8.5	54.1	2.7	4.5

	Measure INFO/WEIGHT	per Measure KCAL	FAT	Nutrition Values per 100g / 100ml KCAL	PROT	CARB	FAT	FIBRE

BREAD

Wrap, Tortilla, Whole 'n' White, Goodness, Kids, Tesco*	1 Wrap/27g	72	1.2	265	8.3	47.6	4.5	5.8
Wrap, Tortilla, Whole Wheat, Stand n Stuff, Old El Paso*	1 Tortilla/24g	71	1.2	294	8.9	50.3	5.2	6
Wrap, Tortilla, Whole, White, Mini, Kids, Sainsbury's*	1 Tortilla/26g	67	1.4	258	9.2	42.9	5.5	6.2
Wrap, Tortilla, Wholemeal , M&S*	1 Wrap/64g	160	2.4	250	11.2	42.5	3.8	6.5
Wrap, Tortilla, Wholemeal, Bakers Selection, Asda*	1 Wraps/63g	177	4.1	283	8	46	6.5	4
Wrap, Tortilla, Wholemeal, Discovery*	1 Wrap/40g	109	3.3	273	9.2	40.4	8.3	6.4
Wrap, Tortilla, Wholemeal, Mission Deli*	1 Wrap/60g	175	5	292	8.4	41.6	8.3	8.8
Wrap, White, Soft, Easy Roll, Warburton's*	1 Wrap/65g	192	2.8	296	11.7	51.6	4.3	2
Wrap, Wholegrain, GF, Mini, Warburton's*	1 Wrap/35g	101	2.3	288	9.2	44.7	6.6	6.7
Wrap, Wholemeal, High Protein & Fibre, Warburton's*	1 Wrap/68g	184	3.3	271	15	38.4	4.8	7.3

BREAD & BUTTER PUDDING

Average	*1 Serving/250g*	*400*	*19.5*	*160*	*6.2*	*17.5*	*7.8*	*0.3*
BGTY, Sainsbury's*	1 Serving/125g	126	2.9	101	6.3	13.4	2.3	5.4
Individual, M&S*	1 Pudding/130g	280	16.4	215	4.4	21.4	12.6	0.5
Low Fat, Individual, BGTY, Sainsbury's*	1 Pack/125g	125	2.9	100	6.3	13.4	2.3	5.4
Tesco*	½ Pack/198g	494	31.8	250	5	20.8	16.1	0.4

BREAD MIX

Brown, Sunflower, Sainsbury's*	1 Serving/60g	151	3.7	251	10	38.9	6.1	4
Ciabatta, Made Up with Water & Olive Oil, Wrights*	1 Slice/45g	113	1.8	251	10	43.6	4	1.8
Crusty White, Made Up, Tesco*	1 Slice/126g	316	2.3	251	9.4	49.3	1.8	2.5
Focaccia, Garlic & Herb, Asda*	1 Serving/125g	385	10	308	11	48	8	3.3
Italian Ciabatta, Sainsbury's*	1 Slice/45g	96	0.9	213	8.7	40	2	2.4
Mixed Grain, Sainsbury's*	1 Serving/45g	103	0.7	228	7.7	46	1.5	4.4
Multiseed, Baked, Sainsbury's*	1 Slice/44g	112	4.3	252	10.8	30.5	9.6	6.8
Pain De Compagne, Made Up, Francine*	2 Slices/100g	237	2.5	237	9.7	42.3	2.5	0
Parmesan Sun Dried Tomato, Made Up, Wrights*	1 Slice/45g	103	0.6	229	9.3	46	1.3	2.4
White Loaf, Asda*	1 Slice/60g	128	0.2	213	7.9	43	0.3	3.5
White, Premium, Dry Mix, Made Up, Wright's*	1 Avg Slice/45g	112	0.8	248	10.4	46.3	1.7	3
Wholemeal, CBY, Asda*	1 Slice/45g	93	0.3	207	9.6	37.5	0.6	6.5
Wholemeal, Hovis*	1 Serving/65g	148	3.1	227	10	35.8	4.8	6.8
Wholemeal, Made Up, M&S*	1 Loaf/600g	1410	14.4	235	11	42	2.4	5.3

BREADCRUMBS

Average	*1oz/28g*	*98*	*0.5*	*350*	*10.8*	*74.8*	*1.9*	*2.6*

BREADFRUIT

Raw	*1oz/28g*	*19*	*0.1*	*67*	*0.9*	*16.4*	*0.2*	*0*

BREADSTICKS

Asda*	1 Serving/5g	21	0.4	412	12	73	8	2.9
Bruschetta, Olive Rosemary, Graze*	1 Punnet/29g	138	7.5	480	13.4	53	26	4.1
Chive & Onion Twists, Tesco*	3 Twists/24g	115	5.3	480	11.6	57.6	22.1	2.2
Grissini, Black Olive, Crosta & Mollica*	1 Grissini/10g	41	0.9	410	10	69.7	9.4	3.2
Grissini, Italian, Sainsbury's*	1 Breadstick/5g	20	0.4	408	11.6	72.9	7.8	2.9
Grissini, Thin with Olive Oil, Forno Bianco*	1 Stick/5g	21	0.4	420	11	77	7.5	0
Grissini, Waitrose*	1 Breadstick/6g	25	0.4	397	12	72.5	6.2	3.1
Italian Original, Tesco*	1 Stick/5.5g	23	0.4	414	11.2	73.1	7.9	2.8
Mini, Sainsbury's*	4 Breadsticks/5g	20	0.4	404	15.6	68.7	7.4	4.8
Olive Oil Rosemary, Finest, Tesco*	2 Sticks/10g	42	1.2	427	13.9	64.4	12.6	4.1
Original, Italian, Tesco*	1 Stick/5.5g	23	0.4	410	11.6	72.9	7.8	2.9
Plain, You Count, Love Life, Waitrose*	1 Breadstick/5g	17	0.1	349	13.4	70.1	1.7	5.6
Rosemary, Asda*	1 Breadstick/7g	29	1	439	12	64	15	3.5
Sesame Seed Grissini, Sainsbury's*	1 Breadstick/6g	27	0.7	424	13.5	66.2	11	3.1
Sesame, Tesco*	3 Sticks/24g	113	4.6	469	15.3	57.2	19.3	2.6

BREAKFAST CEREAL

3 in One, Strawberry, Jordans*	1 Serving/50g	181	2.9	362	9.4	68	5.8	11.9

BREAKFAST CEREAL

INFO/WEIGHT	Measure		per Measure		Nutrition Values per 100g / 100ml				
			KCAL	FAT	KCAL	PROT	CARB	FAT	FIBRE
Advantage, Weetabix*	1 Serving/30g		105	0.7	350	10.2	72	2.4	9
All Bran, Asda*	1 Serving/40g		110	1.4	276	15	46	3.5	27
All Bran, Bran Flakes, & Fruit, Kellogg's*	1 Serving/40g		143	2.4	358	8	68	6	9
All Bran, Bran Flakes, Chocolate, Kellogg's*	1 Serving/30g		106	1.8	354	10	65	6	13
All Bran, Fruit 'n' Fibre, Kellogg's*	1 Serving/30g		114	1.8	380	8	69	6	9
All Bran, Fruitful, Kellogg's*	1 Serving/40g		136	3	340	12.5	57.5	7.5	0
All Bran, Golden Crunch, Kellogg's*	1 Serving/45g		182	5	405	8	62	11	13
All Bran, High Fibre, Morrisons*	1 Serving/40g		109	1.4	272	14.8	45.5	3.5	27
All Bran, Muesli, Cranberry Sultana, Kellogg's*	1 Serving/45g		158	2.5	350	10	58	5.5	14
All Bran, Original, High Fibre, Kellogg's*	1 Serving/40g		134	1.4	334	14	48	3.5	27
All Bran, Yoghurty Flakes, As Sold, Kellogg's*	1 Serving/30g		112	1.2	372	10	68	4	12
Almond, Oats More, Nestle*	1 Serving/40g		162	3.5	404	11	67	8.8	7
Almond, Pecan Cashew Muesli, Kellogg's*	1 Serving/45g		188	6.3	418	11	62	14	8
Alpen*, Crunchy Bran*	1 Serving/40g		120	1.9	299	11.8	52.3	4.7	24.8
Amaranth, Flakes, Organic, Gillian McKeith*	1 Serving/50g		198	2	396	10	80	4	3
Apple & Cinnamon Flakes, M&S*	1 Serving/30g		111	0.6	370	6	82.7	1.9	3.4
Apple & Cinnamon, Crisp, Sainsbury's*	1 Serving/50g		216	7.4	433	6.2	69.1	14.7	3.4
Apple Cinnamon Crisp, Tesco*	1 Serving/50g		217	6.6	433	8.7	67.1	13.1	6.1
Apple Cinnamon, Oat Fruit Breakfast, Quaker*	1 Sachet/200g		172	3.6	86	2.3	14	1.8	2.3
Apple Cinnamon, Quaker*	1 Sachet/38g		136	2.1	358	8	68	5.5	2.5
Apple Raisin, Additions, Weetabix*	2 Biscuits/43g		149	0.8	344	9.5	66	1.8	13
Apple, Spelt Chia, Ancient Legends, Kellogg's*	1 Serving/45g		171	2.1	380	10	70	4.7	8.6
Apricot Wheats, Harvest Morn, Aldi*	1 Serving/30g		101	0.4	337	7.6	72.3	1.4	8
Apricot Wheats, Whole Grain, Tesco*	1 Serving/40g		130	0.6	326	7.6	70.6	1.4	8
Balance, Sainsbury's*	1 Serving/30g		111	0.4	370	11.4	77.7	1.5	3.2
Banana & Toffee Crisp, Mornflake*	1 Serving/30g		133	4.8	443	5.7	68.8	16.1	5.4
Banana Mango, Oats Chia, The Chia Co*	1 Serving/45g		187	7	414	9.7	50.3	15.4	11.2
Banana, Papaya & Honey Oat, Crunchy, Waitrose*	1 Serving/40g		170	4.8	426	9.6	69.8	12	5.5
Benefit Flakes, Original, Harvest Morn, Aldi*	1 Serving/40g		154	0.5	384	12	80	1.3	2.2
Berry Granola, Rude Health*	1 Serving/40g		178	6.4	446	10	61	16	7
Bircher Mix, Almonds, Honey, Dorset Cereals*	1 Serving/30g		117	3.3	389	10	55	11	8.5
Bircher Muesli, Love Life, Waitrose*	1 Serving/45g		153	3.5	341	8.8	57.7	7.7	6.8
Biscuit, with Coconut Raisin, Additions, Weetabix*	2 Biscuits/43g		157	2.5	363	9.5	62	5.7	13
Biscuit, Baked with Golden Syrup, Weetabix*	2 Biscuits/44g		158	0.8	363	10.3	72	1.9	8.2
Biscuit, with Apple Raisin, Additions	*2 Biscuits/43g*		*149*	*0.8*	*344*	*9.5*	*66*	*1.8*	*13*
Bitesize Wheats, Crownfield, Lidl*	1 Serving/40g		142	0.8	356	10.6	67	1.9	14
Bitesize, Weetabix*	1 Serving/40g		135	0.8	338	11.5	68.4	2	10
Bixies, Wheat Biscuits, Wholegrain, Crownfield, Lidl*	2 Biscuits/40g		145	0.8	362	10.8	70.3	1.9	10
Blueberry Wheats, Tesco*	1 Serving/50g		168	0.8	336	7.5	71.6	1.5	8.5
Bran Crunch, Raisin, Kellogg's*	1 Pack/80g		280	1.5	350	6.2	83.8	1.9	7.5
Bran Flakes, Asda*	1 Serving/47g		157	1.5	333	11	65	3.2	14
Bran Flakes, Free From, Tesco*	1 Serving/30g		107	0.7	358	7.5	69.3	2.3	15
Bran Flakes, Harvest Home, Nestle*	1 Serving/30g		99	0.7	331	10.2	67.1	2.4	14.1
Bran Flakes, Honey Nut, Tesco*	1 Serving/40g		143	1.8	358	9.6	70	4.4	11
Bran Flakes, Kellogg's*	1 Serving/30g		108	1	359	12	63	3.2	15
Bran Flakes, Organic, Asda*	1 Serving/30g		99	0.7	330	10	67	2.4	14
Bran Flakes, Organic, Sainsbury's*	1 Serving/30g		100	0.7	332	10.2	67.4	2.4	14.1
Bran Flakes, Sultana Bran, Kellogg's*	1 Serving/40g		138	0.8	344	8	67	2	13
Bran Flakes, Sultana, Dry, Sainsbury's*	1 Serving/30g		98	0.6	325	8.3	68.6	1.9	12.1
Bran Flakes, Tesco*	1 Serving/30g		107	0.7	356	10.8	64.3	2.4	16.8
Bran Flakes, Wholegrain, Essential, Waitrose*	1 Serving/30g		107	0.7	356	10.8	64.7	2.4	16
Bran Flakes, Wholegrain, Sainsbury's*	1 Serving/30g		109	0.9	363	10.1	67.1	3	13.6
Bran, Natural, Sainsbury's*	1 Serving/30g		64	1.5	212	14.7	27	5	36

BREAKFAST CEREAL

INFO/WEIGHT	Measure	per Measure KCAL	per Measure FAT	Nutrition per 100g KCAL	PROT	CARB	FAT	FIBRE
Caribbean Crunch, Alpen*	1 Serving/40g	155	3.6	388	8.8	67.9	9	4.6
Cheerios, Chocolate, Dry, Nestle*	1 Serving/30g	115	1	384	8	73.4	3.5	2.2
Cheerios, Honey Nut, Nestle*	1 Serving/30g	112	1.1	374	7	78.3	3.7	5.2
Cheerios, Honey, Nestle*	1 Serving/50g	184	1.4	369	6.6	79.2	2.8	5.8
Cheerios, Low Sugar, As Sold, Nestle*	1 Serving/30g	120	2.3	399	11.1	67.4	7.6	8.5
Cheerios, Nestle*	1 Serving/30g	114	1.1	381	8.6	74.5	3.8	7.1
Cheerios, Oat Crisp, Nestle*	1 Portion/40g	154	2.1	385	11	70	5.2	8.5
Choc & Nut Crisp, Tesco*	1 Serving/40g	185	8	462	8.3	62.5	19.9	4.8
Choco Crackles, Morrisons*	1 Serving/30g	115	0.7	383	5.5	84.8	2.4	1.9
Choco Flakes, Asda*	1 Serving/50g	187	0.4	374	6	86	0.7	2.6
Choco Flakes, Kellogg's*	1 Serving/30g	114	0.9	380	5	84	3	2.5
Choco Hoops, Aldi*	1 Serving/30g	116	1.4	385	7	79.1	4.5	0
Choco Hoops, Asda*	1 Serving/40g	154	1.8	385	7	79	4.5	4
Choco Hoops, Tesco*	1 Serving/30g	116	1.2	385	7.5	75	4	8
Choco Snaps, Asda*	1 Serving/30g	115	0.7	382	5	85	2.4	1.9
Choco Squares, Asda*	1 Serving/30g	130	4.2	434	10	67	14	4
Chocolate Crisp, Minis, Weetabix*	1 Serving/36g	134	1.9	371	9	71.7	5.3	8.5
Chocolate Hoops, Average	*1 Serving/30g*	*116*	*1.3*	*386*	*7.2*	*79.3*	*4.4*	*3.4*
Chocolate Rice, Puffed, Average	*1 Serving/30g*	*117*	*1.2*	*389*	*5.7*	*81*	*4.1*	*3.2*
Chocolate Wheats, Kellogg's*	1 Serving/40g	148	3.6	369	10	62	9	12
Cinnamon Grahams, Nestle*	1 Serving/40g	164	3.9	411	4.7	76.1	9.8	4.2
Clusters, Honey, Nut, Harvest Morn, Aldi*	1 Serving/45g	200	6.3	445	9.6	68	14	5.6
Clusters, Nestle*	1 Serving/30g	113	1	377	9	74	3.4	7.9
Coco Pops, Crunchers, Kellogg's*	1 Serving/30g	114	1	380	7	81	3.5	3
Coco Pops, Kellogg's*	1 Serving/30g	115	0.6	382	6.3	84	1.9	3
Coco Rice, GF, Nestle*	1 Serving/30g	115	0.7	382	6.2	82	2.4	3.1
Coco Shreddies with 125ml Semi Skimmed Milk, Nestle*	1 Serving/40g	210	2.7	525	18	90.2	6.7	8.7
Coco Snaps, Value, Tesco*	1 Serving/30g	117	0.7	390	7	84.1	2.4	2.4
Coconut Wheat Flakes, Toasted, Dorset Cereals*	1 Serving/45g	171	3.6	381	8.2	54	8	8
Cookie Crunch, Nestle*	1 Serving/40g	154	1.1	385	4.6	85.3	2.8	1.8
Corn Flakes, Asda*	1 Serving/30g	111	0.2	370	7	84	0.7	3
Corn Flakes, Banana Crunch, Kellogg's*	1 Serving/40g	163	3.2	408	6	78	8	3
Corn Flakes, Crispy Nut, Asda*	1 Serving/30g	117	1.3	390	7	81	4.2	2.5
Corn Flakes, Hint of Honey, Kellogg's*	1 Serving/30g	113	0.2	377	6	87	0.6	2.5
Corn Flakes, Honey Nut & Cranberries, Sainsbury's*	1 Serving/40g	166	4	416	7.4	74.4	9.9	3.1
Corn Flakes, Honey Nut, Average	*1 Serving/30g*	*118*	*1.3*	*393*	*7*	*81.4*	*4.3*	*2.4*
Corn Flakes, Honey Nut, Harvest Home, Nestle*	1 Serving/30g	118	1.3	392	7.4	81.1	4.2	2.5
Corn Flakes, Kellogg's*	1 Serving/30g	113	0.3	378	7	84	0.9	3
Corn Flakes, Morrisons*	1 Serving/30g	111	0.2	371	7.3	83.8	0.7	3
Corn Flakes, Organic, Lima*	1 Serving/50g	178	0.5	355	8.3	77.7	1	6.4
Corn Flakes, Sainsbury's*	1 Serving/25g	93	0.2	371	7.3	83.8	0.7	3
Corn Flakes, Tesco*	1 Serving/30g	116	0.3	386	7.6	85.2	1.1	2.5
Corn Flakes, Value, Tesco*	1 Serving/30g	116	0.3	386	7.6	85.2	1.1	2.5
Cornflakes, Essential, Waitrose*	1 Serving/30g	116	0.3	385	7.4	84.8	1.1	3.1
Cornflakes, GF, Nestle*	1 Serving/30g	115	0.3	384	7.4	84.6	1.1	3.1
Cornflakes, Honey, GF, Nestle*	1 Serving/30g	114	0.2	381	5.6	86.2	0.8	3.5
Cornflakes, Simply, M&S*	1 Serving/30g	111	0.2	371	7.9	81.7	0.6	3.6
Country Crisp with Real Raspberries, Jordans*	1 Serving/50g	214	7.9	429	7.5	64.1	15.8	7.1
Country Crisp with Real Strawberries, Jordans*	1 Serving/50g	214	7.8	428	7.5	64.1	15.7	7.1
Country Crisp, Four Nut Combo, Jordans*	1 Serving/50g	240	12.4	480	8.9	55.4	24.7	6.9
Country Crisp, Wild About Berries, Jordans*	1 Serving/50g	222	7.8	443	7.5	68	15.7	5.7
Cranberry Wheats, Tesco*	1 Serving/50g	160	0.8	320	7.6	72	1.5	8
Cranberry Wheats, Whole Grain, Sainsbury's*	1 Serving/50g	162	0.7	325	7.3	70.9	1.4	7.7

BREAKFAST CEREAL

INFO/WEIGHT	Measure	per Measure KCAL	FAT	Nutrition Values per 100g / 100ml KCAL	PROT	CARB	FAT	FIBRE
Crispix Krispies, Kellogg's*	1 Serving/30g	110	0	367	6.7	86.7	0	0
Crispy Minis, Banana, Weetabix*	1 Serving/40g	156	2	389	9.3	72	4.9	9.7
Crispy Minis, Strawberry, Weetabix*	1 Serving/40g	150	0.9	375	9.4	74.1	2.3	10
Crispy Rice & Wheat Flakes, Asda*	1 Serving/50g	185	0.8	370	11	78	1.5	3.2
Crunchy Bran, Weetabix*	1 Serving/40g	140	1.4	350	11.9	57.6	3.6	20
Crunchy Choco, Crisp & Square, Tesco*	1 Serving/50g	212	7	423	8	66.3	14	6
Crunchy Nut, Clusters, Honey Nut, Kellogg's*	1 Serving/40g	161	2	402	6	82	5	2.5
Crunchy Nut, Clusters, Milk Chocolate Curls, Kellogg's*	1 Serving/40g	183	7.2	458	8	66	18	4
Crunchy Nut, Clusters, Peanut Butter, Kellogg's *	1 Serving/30g	146	7.5	488	14	49	25	5.5
Crunchy Nut, Clusters, Summer Berries, Kellogg's*	1 Serving/40g	176	6	439	8	68	15	5
Crunchy Nut, Corn Flakes, Kellogg's*	1 Serving/30g	118	1.2	392	6	83	4	2.5
Crunchy Nut, Oat Granola, with Chocolate, Kellogg's*	1 Serving/45g	224	11.2	497	8	57	25	6
Crunchy Nut, Red, Kellogg's*	1 Serving/40g	138	0.8	346	10	72	2	9
Crunchy Oat with Raisins, Almonds Fruit, Tesco*	1 Serving/50g	202	6.3	403	8.5	63.8	12.6	6.6
Crunchy Oat with Tropical Fruits, Tesco*	1 Serving/35g	146	4.8	417	7.8	65.3	13.8	6.1
Crunchy Oat, Golden Sun, Lidl*	1 Serving/50g	206	6.4	411	8.6	65	12.9	6.2
Crunchy Rice & Wheat Flakes, Co-Op*	1 Serving/30g	111	0.6	370	11	78	2	3
Curiously Cinnamon, Nestle*	1 Serving/30g	124	3	412	4.9	75.9	9.9	4.1
Fibre 1, Nestle*	1 Serving/40g	107	1	267	10.8	50.2	2.6	30.5
Fibre Flakes, GF, Organic, Dove's Farm*	1 Serving/30g	105	0.4	351	7.1	69.7	1.5	15
Fitnesse & Fruits, Nestle*	1 Serving/40g	148	0.4	370	6.6	83.4	1.1	3.4
Flakes & Grains, Exotic Fruit, BGTY, Sainsbury's*	1 Serving/30g	113	1.5	377	6.8	76.4	4.9	5.9
Flakes & Orchard Fruits, BGTY, Sainsbury's*	1 Serving/40g	154	0.5	385	13	80.6	1.2	4.5
Flakes Clusters, Tesco*	1 Serving/50g	220	8.5	440	11.2	55.4	17	10.5
Froot Loops, 30g, & 125ml Semi Skimmed, Kellogg's*	1 Serving/30g	176	3.5	587	23.3	100	11.7	3.3
Frosted Flakes, Sainsbury's*	1 Serving/30g	114	0.2	381	4.9	88	0.6	2
Frosted Flakes, Tesco*	1 Serving/30g	112	0.1	374	4.9	87.8	0.4	2.4
Frosted Wheats, Kellogg's*	1 Serving/30g	104	0.6	346	10	72	2	9
Frosties, Caramel, Kellogg's*	1 Serving/30g	113	0.2	377	5	88	0.6	2
Frosties, Kellogg's*	1 Serving/30g	112	0.2	375	4.5	87	0.6	2
Fruit & Fibre, Flakes, Waitrose*	1 Serving/40g	143	2.5	357	8.2	67.2	6.2	9.9
Fruit & Fibre, Morrisons*	1 Serving/30g	110	2.2	366	8.8	66.5	7.2	8.5
Fruit & Fibre, Value, Tesco*	1 Serving/40g	144	2.2	359	11.4	65.7	5.6	8
Fruit & Nut Crisp, Minis, Weetabix*	1 Serving/40g	148	1.6	371	9.9	69	4.1	9.3
Fruit Fibre, Asda*	1 Serving/40g	146	2.6	366	8.2	68.4	6.6	8.5
Fruit Fibre, Harvest Morn, Aldi*	1 Serving/30g	114	1.8	380	8.4	69	6.1	8
Fruit 'n' Fibre, Kellogg's*	1 Serving/40g	152	2.4	380	8	69	6	9
Fruit, Nuts Flakes, M&S*	1 Serving/30g	117	2.6	391	9.1	69.6	8.5	3.5
Golden Balls, Asda*	1 Serving/30g	112	0.4	374	5	85	1.5	1.5
Golden Grahams, Nestle*	1 Serving/30g	112	0.9	375	6	81	3	3.4
Golden Honey Puffs, Tesco*	1 Serving/30g	115	0.4	382	6.6	86.3	1.2	3
Golden Nuggets, Nestle*	1 Serving/40g	152	0.3	381	6.2	87.4	0.7	1.5
Golden Puffs, Sainsbury's*	1 Serving/28g	107	0.3	383	6.6	86.3	1.2	3
Granola	*1 Serving/45g*	*194*	*8.7*	*430*	*17.5*	*48.8*	*19.4*	*16.8*
Granola, 3 Seed, Oat, Wholegrain, M&S*	1 Serving/45g	217	9	483	16.1	50.8	20	7.7
Granola, 4 Nut, Flame Raisin, Wholegrain, M&S*	1 Serving/45g	206	8.3	458	10	59.5	18.5	6.5
Granola, 5 Ways, Honey, Almonds Seeds, Nutri Brex*	1 Serving/40g	165	5.9	413	12.4	54.1	14.7	7
Granola, Berry Orange, Wholegrain, M&S*	1 Serving/45g	178	4.3	396	8.5	65.5	9.6	6.7
Granola, Cherry Bakewell, 1, Waitrose*	1 Serving/40g	181	4.8	452	12	70	12	8
Granola, Chocolate, Dorset Cereals*	1 Serving/40g	206	12	515	8.8	47.2	30	10.5
Granola, Cranberry Honey Nut, Topper, Graze*	1 Punnet/35g	157	7.1	447	11	56.2	20.3	4
Granola, Crunchy Nut Glorious Oat, Kellogg's*	1 Serving/45g	212	9.4	470	7	61	21	4.5
Granola, Crunchy Oat, Raisin, Almond, Harvest Morn, Aldi*	1 Serving/40g	166	4.6	416	8.2	66.9	11.4	6.4

B

BREAKFAST CEREAL

Measure INFO/WEIGHT		per Measure		Nutrition Values per 100g / 100ml				
		KCAL	FAT	KCAL	PROT	CARB	FAT	FIBRE
Granola, Crunchy Oat, Tropical Fruits, Harvest Morn, Aldi*	1 Serving/40g	174	5.2	436	9.4	66	13	7.4
Granola, Fruit, Simply Sumptuous, Lidl*	1 Bowl/45g	198	8.1	440	10	56	18	7.1
Granola, Hazelnuts, & Pecans, Super Goodness, Quaker*	1 Serving/45g	187	5	416	9.6	67	11	8
Granola, High Protein, Lizi's*	1 Serving/40g	180	6.8	450	27	44	17	6.7
Granola, Honey, Dorset Cereals*	1 Serving/40g	204	12	511	13	44	30	7.4
Granola, Mango, Coconut, Wholegrain, M&S*	1 Serving/45g	196	6.7	435	10.5	61.3	14.8	7.4
Granola, Multigrain Nutty, Good & Balanced, Asda*	1 Serving/40g	178	7.6	444	12	52	19	7.6
Granola, Nut, Simply Nut, Dorset Cereals*	1 Serving/40g	200	10.8	500	11	48	27	8.3
Granola, Nuts, Pumpkin Seeds, & Fruit, Aldi*	1 Serving/45g	210	8.6	466	27	45	19	5
Granola, Oat Clusters, Apple & Cinnamon, Quaker*	1 Pack/48g	193	3.8	403	8	70.2	8	9.4
Granola, Oat, Golden Crunch, 30% Less Fat, Quaker*	1 Serving/45g	193	4.6	429	8.7	71.5	10.3	7.2
Granola, Oat, Simply Oat, Dorset Cereals*	1 Serving/40g	177	6.8	443	8.8	60	17	7.4
Granola, Organic, Lizi's, The GoodCarb Food Company*	1 Serving/50g	246	14	493	11.3	48.6	28.1	7.4
Granola, Original, Lizi's, The GoodCarb Food Company*	1 Serving/50g	248	14.6	496	10.9	46.2	29.3	10.6
Granola, Pink Apple Cinnamon, Diet Chef Ltd*	1 Pack/40g	193	10.7	483	10.1	49.3	26.8	11.2
Granola, Pumpkin & Sunflower, Super Goodness, Quaker*	1 Serving/45g	185	4.5	411	10	67	10	7.6
Granola, Quaker*	1 Serving/48g	210	7	438	10.4	72.9	14.6	6.2
Granola, Strawberries with Bio Yoghurt, Rumblers*	1 Pot/168g	267	9.7	159	4.3	22.4	5.8	1.1
Granola, Summer Fruits, Pomegranate Infused, M&S*	1 Serving/50g	200	6.4	400	8.6	63.2	12.7	5.8
Granola, Super Berry, Tesco*	1 Serving/45g	195	6	434	9.2	66	13.3	6.5
Granola, Super Fruity, Jordan's*	1 Serving/45g	194	5.6	431	9.5	66.6	12.4	7.5
Granola, Super Grains, Seeds, Tesco*	1 Serving/50g	225	7.8	450	10.7	63.1	15.6	7.3
Granola, Super Nutty, Aldi*	1 Serving/45g	217	9.9	483	11	56	22	7.2
Granola, Superfoods, Jordans*	1 Serving/50g	208	6.7	415	9	64.7	13.4	8.6
Granola, Tropical Twist, Paleo, Planet Organic*	1 Serving/35g	197	14.3	536	16	36	39	7.8
Granola, Very Berry, Asda*	1 Serving/45g	187	4.9	417	10	66	11	8
Grape Nuts, Kraft*	1 Serving/45g	158	0.9	350	10.9	81.9	2	11.9
Harvest Crunch, Nut, Quaker*	1 Serving/40g	184	7.8	459	8	62.5	19.5	6
Harvest Crunch, Real Red Berries, Quaker*	1 Serving/50g	224	8.5	447	7	66	17	4.5
Harvest Crunch, Soft Juicy Raisins, Quaker*	1 Serving/50g	221	8	442	6	67	16	4
Hawaiian Crunch, Asda*	1 Serving/50g	224	7.6	448	8	69.6	15.3	7
Hawaiian Crunch, Mornflake*	1 Serving/60g	247	7.4	411	8.1	66.8	12.4	6.8
High Bran, CBY, Asda*	1 Serving/40g	136	1.5	341	13.6	49.5	3.8	27.1
High Fibre Bran, Co-Op*	1 Serving/40g	110	1.6	275	15	46	4	27
High Fibre Bran, Sainsbury's*	1 Serving/40g	134	1.5	335	14.3	48.4	3.7	25.4
High Fruit Muesli, BGTY, Sainsbury's*	1 Serving/50g	164	1	328	6.7	71	1.9	6.6
Honey Nut Crisp, Mini, Weetabix*	1 Serving/40g	150	0.8	375	9.4	75.1	2	9.3
Honey Cheerios with 125ml Semi Skimmed Milk, Nestle*	1 Serving/30g	174	2.9	580	21	99.7	9.7	5.7
Honey Hoops, Harvest Morn, Aldi*	1 Serving/30g	117	1	389	6.5	81	3.4	4
Honey Loops, Kellogg's*	1 Serving/30g	110	0.9	367	8	77	3	6
Honey Numbers, Harvest Morn, Aldi*	1 Serving/30g	114	1	379	6.9	78.7	3.3	3.3
Honey Raisin & Almond, Crunchy, Waitrose*	1 Serving/40g	170	4.8	425	10.5	68.8	12	5.5
Honey, Crisp Minis, Weetabix*	1 Serving/40g	150	0.8	375	9.5	75	2	9.2
Honey, Oats More, Nestle*	1 Serving/30g	114	1.6	379	9.7	73.1	5.3	5.9
Hooplas, Sainsbury's*	1 Serving/30g	112	1.1	375	6.5	78.6	3.8	4.6
Hoops, Multigrain, Asda*	1 Serving/30g	113	1.2	376	6.5	78.4	4	4.6
Hoops, Multigrain, Tesco*	1 Serving/30g	112	1.1	375	6.5	78.6	3.8	4.6
Hoops, Mutigrain, Harvest Morn, Aldi*	1 Serving/30g	114	1	380	9	75	3.4	7.4
Hot Oat, Aldi*	1 Serving/40g	142	3.3	356	11.6	58.8	8.3	8.9
Hot Oats, Instant, Tesco*	1 Serving/30g	108	2.6	360	11.8	58.4	8.7	7.9
Instant Oats, Dry Weight	*1 Sachet/36g*	*129*	*3.1*	*359*	*11.5*	*59.1*	*8.5*	*8.3*
Just Right, Kellogg's*	1 Serving/40g	148	0.8	371	7	79	2	4.5
Kashi, Crunch, Seven Whole Grains, Original, Kellogg's*	1 Serving/40g	162	3.6	405	8	73	9	5

BREAKFAST CEREAL

	Measure INFO/WEIGHT	per Measure		Nutrition Values per 100g / 100ml				
		KCAL	FAT	KCAL	PROT	CARB	FAT	FIBRE
Krave, Chocolate Hazelnut, Kellogg's*	1 Serving/30g	136	4.8	452	7.2	68	16	3.4
Krave, Milk Chocolate, Kellogg's*	1 Serving/30g	134	4.5	445	7.1	69	15	3
Lion, Nestle*	1 Serving/40g	166	3.1	415	7.2	76.9	7.7	4.3
Luxury Muesli, Diet Chef Ltd*	1 Pack/40g	166	4.7	414	10.6	61	11.8	10.9
Malted Wheaties, CBY, Asda*	1 Serving/40g	146	0.8	366	10.3	72.7	1.9	8.2
Malted Wheats, Waitrose*	1 Serving/30g	110	0.6	365	10	72.7	1.9	8.5
Malties, Sainsbury's*	1 Serving/40g	137	1.2	343	10	69.2	2.9	10
Malty Flakes with Red Berries, Tesco*	1 Serving/30g	111	0.6	369	9.9	78.1	1.9	3.1
Malty Flakes, Tesco*	1 Serving/40g	148	0.6	371	11	78.4	1.5	4.3
Maple & Pecan Crisp, Sainsbury's*	1 Serving/50g	226	9.8	452	7.9	61.3	19.5	5.4
Maple & Pecan Crisp, Tesco*	1 Serving/50g	215	7.6	430	10.5	62.5	15.2	10.2
Maple & Pecan, Crisp, Asda*	1 Serving/30g	135	5.7	451	8	62	19	6
Millet Rice Oatbran Flakes, Nature's Path*	1 Serving/56g	204	3.2	365	11.3	67	5.8	10
Milo Duo, Nestle*	1 Serving/30g	116	1.7	386	8.2	75.6	5.6	4.9
Mini Wheats, Original, Frosted, Kellogg's*	1 Serving/30g	106	0.6	352	9.3	83.3	1.8	11.1
Minibix, Weetabix*	1 Serving/40g	134	1.5	335	8.8	71.2	3.8	8.1
Mixed Berry, Oats Chia, The Chia Co*	1 Serving/45g	188	7.2	417	10.6	47.1	16	12.7
Muesli Base, Wholesome, Waitrose*	1 Portion/50g	125	4.2	250	11.5	31.8	8.4	5
Muesli Mix, Perfect Start, Organic, The Food Doctor*	1 Serving/50g	196	7.1	392	12.1	55.5	14.2	7.1
Muesli, 4 Fruit, Almond Hazelnut, M&S*	1 Serving/45g	162	3.3	360	8.5	61.6	7.3	7.1
Muesli, 8 Fruit, Nut, Seed, Luxury, M&S*	1 Serving/45g	177	6.3	393	10.2	51.8	14	9.7
Muesli, Almonds Apricot, Toasted, Crisp, Eat Natural*	1 Serving/50g	206	7.5	412	9.2	44.6	15	6.6
Muesli, Base, Nature's Harvest*	1 Serving/50g	179	2.6	358	11	71.2	5.1	7.4
Muesli, Basics, Sainsbury's*	1 Serving/50g	178	2.6	355	11.2	61.5	5.1	9.2
Muesli, Berry, Cherry, Luscious, Dorset Cereals*	1 Serving/45g	149	0.9	332	7	67	2.1	8.3
Muesli, Carb Control, Tesco*	1 Serving/35g	154	9.3	439	25	25	26.6	13.8
Muesli, COU, M&S*	1 Serving/60g	201	1.5	335	7.6	70.2	2.5	8.1
Muesli, Creamy Tropical Fruit, Finest, Tesco*	1 Serving/80g	283	4.5	354	7.2	68.8	5.6	6.9
Muesli, Crunchy, Organic, Sainsbury's*	1 Serving/40g	168	5.8	420	10.6	62	14.4	9.2
Muesli, De Luxe, No Added Salt or Sugar, Sainsbury's*	1 Serving/40g	161	5.6	403	11.9	57.6	13.9	8.4
Muesli, Flahavans*	1 Serving/52g	187	2.8	360	10.4	72.1	5.3	5.5
Muesli, Fruit & Nut, 55%, Asda*	1 Serving/40g	151	5.6	378	9	54	14	7
Muesli, Fruit & Nut, COU, M&S*	1 Serving/40g	128	1.1	320	7.4	74.5	2.8	7.4
Muesli, Fruit & Nut, Luxury, Co-Op*	1 Serving/40g	150	4	375	8	64	10	6
Muesli, Fruit & Nut, Luxury, Lidl*	1 Serving/57g	205	5.6	360	8	60	9.8	7.5
Muesli, Fruit & Nut, Luxury, Simply Sumptuous, Lidl*	1 Serving/45g	179	6.2	398	8	57.6	13.8	5.8
Muesli, Fruit & Nut, Luxury, Waitrose*	1 Serving/40g	145	3.8	363	9	60.3	9.5	6.5
Muesli, Fruit & Nut, M&S*	1 Serving/40g	128	1.1	320	7.4	74.5	2.8	7.4
Muesli, Fruit & Nut, Organic, M&S*	1 Serving/50g	166	3	333	8.2	61.6	6	7.6
Muesli, Fruit & Nut, Tesco*	1 Serving/50g	190	5.6	380	8.4	60.3	11.3	5.3
Muesli, Fruit & Nut, Whole Wheat, Organic, Asda*	1 Serving/50g	172	3.5	343	10	60	7	7
Muesli, Fruit Fibre, M&S*	1 Serving/45g	171	4.7	380	8.7	59	10.4	7.6
Muesli, Fruit Nut, Essential, Waitrose*	1 Serving/45g	173	6.1	384	8.6	51.5	13.5	11
Muesli, Fruit Nut, Jordans*	1 Serving/50g	180	4.7	361	8	61.2	9.4	7.5
Muesli, Fruit Nut, Luxury, Sainsbury's*	1 Serving/50g	178	4.6	355	10.3	57.9	9.1	11.3
Muesli, Fruit Nut, Sainsbury's*	1 Serving/30g	114	3.1	379	9.5	58.7	10.3	6.9
Muesli, Fruit Nut & Seed, Organic, Dorset Cereals*	1 Serving/70g	251	6.9	358	10.8	56.6	9.8	8.4
Muesli, Fruit Sensation, M&S*	1 Serving/50g	158	1.5	315	6	66	3	7.4
Muesli, Fruit, Luxury, Weight Watchers*	1 Serving/40g	127	0.8	318	7.2	67.7	2	8.1
Muesli, Fruit, Nuts Seeds, Dorset Cereals*	1 Serving/70g	265	8	379	10.6	58.4	11.4	6.1
Muesli, Fruit, Sainsbury's*	1 Serving/40g	132	1.8	330	8.1	64.3	4.5	9.6
Muesli, Fruit, Waitrose*	1 Serving/30g	101	1.4	338	7.2	66.8	4.7	6.8
Muesli, GF, Nature's Harvest, Holland & Barrett*	1 Serving/60g	234	7.8	390	14.1	54.1	13	3.3

B

BREAKFAST CEREAL

INFO/WEIGHT	Measure	per Measure		Nutrition Values per 100g / 100ml				
		KCAL	FAT	KCAL	PROT	CARB	FAT	FIBRE
Muesli, Golden Sun, Lidl*	1 Serving/40g	144	3.9	360	8	60	9.8	7.5
Muesli, High Fibre, Neal's Yard*	1 Serving/50g	182	1	364	7.6	72.7	1.9	12.9
Muesli, High Fibre, You Count, Love Life, Waitrose*	1 Serving/45g	155	1.3	344	7.7	67.4	2.9	8.8
Muesli, HL, Tesco*	1 Serving/40g	126	0.9	315	7.6	64.3	2.3	7.5
Muesli, Light & Crispy, Jordans*	1 Serving/50g	172	2.5	343	7.7	66.7	5	9.5
Muesli, Lite n Natural, Saffola*	1 Serving/30g	114	1.6	381	10.2	78.7	5.5	6
Muesli, Luxury Fruit, Harvest Morn, Aldi*	1 Serving/50g	179	2.3	358	7.2	69	4.6	5.6
Muesli, Luxury, Finest, Tesco*	1 Serving/50g	197	6.6	394	8.3	60.8	13.1	5.4
Muesli, Luxury, Sainsbury's*	1 Serving/40g	144	4.3	359	8.5	57.1	10.7	7.7
Muesli, Natural, No Added Sugar or Salt, Jordans*	1 Serving/45g	161	2.2	357	9.5	63.7	5	9.7
Muesli, No Added Sugar Or Salt, Organic, Jordans*	1 Serving/50g	175	4.4	350	9.2	58.4	8.8	9.3
Muesli, No Added Sugar, Morrisons*	1 Serving/50g	166	2.6	331	11.2	64.7	5.1	6.3
Muesli, No Added Sugar, Waitrose*	1 Serving/40g	146	2.5	364	12	64.9	6.3	6.7
Muesli, Nuts Seeds , Tesco*	1 Serving/50g	195	5.5	390	10.9	57.2	11	9.2
Muesli, Nutty Crunch, Saffola*	1 Serving/30g	113	1.8	378	9	78.2	6	6.3
Muesli, Organic, Waitrose*	1 Serving/50g	188	0.8	375	10.3	59.6	1.6	8.3
Muesli, Original, Holland & Barrett*	1 Serving/30g	105	2.5	351	11.1	61.2	8.4	7.1
Muesli, Original, Raisins, Hazelnuts, & Almonds, Alpen*	1 Serving/40g	144	2.3	359	10.5	66.6	5.8	7.3
Muesli, Original, Simply, Hubbards*	1 Serving/50g	212	6.7	424	11.8	59.4	13.4	9.2
Muesli, Really Nutty, Dorset Cereals*	1 Serving/70g	253	6.1	362	9.8	61.1	8.7	6.3
Muesli, Really Nutty, Simply Sumptuous, Lidl*	1 Serving/45g	167	3.9	371	9.5	59.2	8.7	8.9
Muesli, Rich, Nature's Harvest*	1 Serving/40g	143	3.7	358	10	60.5	9.2	7.6
Muesli, Seriously Nutty, Mornflake*	1 Bowl/45g	202	10.1	449	14.5	43.4	22.5	7.6
Muesli, Simply Delicious, Dorset Cereals*	1 Serving/45g	160	3.3	356	9.9	58.1	7.4	8.9
Muesli, Simply Fruity, As Sold, Dorset Cereals*	1 Serving/45g	152	1.1	337	7.3	68	2.4	6.8
Muesli, Simply Sumptuous, Luxury Fruit, Lidl*	1 Serving/45g	154	1.5	343	6.5	68.7	3.3	6.2
Muesli, Six Nut, Finest, Tesco*	1 Serving/50g	224	9.6	448	14.2	50.2	19.3	8.4
Muesli, Special, Fruit, Jordans*	1 Serving/50g	162	1.4	323	6.6	68	2.7	8.4
Muesli, Special, Jordans*	1 Serving/50g	183	5.4	366	7.9	59.5	10.7	8.5
Muesli, Special, Luxury Fruit Nut, Goody*	1 Serving/50g	193	6.9	386	8	57.6	13.8	8
Muesli, Super Berry, Jordans*	1 Serving/50g	174	3.8	348	9	60.8	7.6	8.1
Muesli, Super High Fibre, Dorset Cereals*	1 Serving/70g	250	6.6	357	8	60.1	9.4	8.4
Muesli, Superfoods, Jordans*	1 Serving/50g	173	3.6	346	9.2	60.9	7.3	10.2
Muesli, Swiss Style with Fruit, Tesco*	1 Serving/40g	144	2.1	360	10.4	67.4	5.3	7.4
Muesli, Swiss Style, Bettabuy, Morrisons*	1 Serving/50g	170	2.5	340	11	62.8	5	9.4
Muesli, Swiss Style, Co-Op*	1 Serving/40g	148	2.4	370	11	67	6	6
Muesli, Swiss Style, No Added Salt or Sugar, Sainsbury's*	1 Serving/50g	178	3	357	10.9	64.9	6	6
Muesli, Swiss Style, No Added Salt or Sugar, Tesco*	1 Serving/50g	182	3.2	364	11	61	6.4	9.6
Muesli, Swiss Style, No Added Sugar or Salt, Asda*	1 Serving/50g	182	3.5	363	11	64	7	8
Muesli, Swiss Style, No Added Sugar, Lidl*	1 Serving/30g	111	1.8	371	10.9	64.5	6	7.8
Muesli, Swiss Style, Organic, Whole Earth*	1 Serving/50g	172	3.6	344	9.2	60.8	7.1	11.3
Muesli, Swiss Style, Smart Price, Asda*	1 Serving/60g	222	3.6	370	9	70	6	10
Muesli, Swiss Style, Tesco*	1 Serving/50g	189	3.1	378	10.4	67	6.2	6.4
Muesli, The Ultimate, Organic, Rude Health*	1 Serving/50g	163	4.5	326	10.8	50.5	9	12.3
Muesli, Toasted Spelt, Barley, Oat Flakes, Dorset Cereals*	1 Serving/40g	148	4.5	371	9.5	57.9	11.3	7.4
Muesli, Toasted, GF with Buckwheat, Eat Natural*	1 Serving/50g	230	11.4	461	11.7	53.2	22.8	2
Muesli, Tropical Fruit, Holland & Barrett*	1 Serving/60g	197	1.9	328	7.5	69.8	3.2	5.1
Muesli, Tropical Fruits, Jordans*	1 Serving/50g	164	1.4	329	6.9	68.7	2.9	7.1
Muesli, Tropical, Sainsbury's*	1 Serving/50g	182	3.4	365	6.5	69.4	6.8	6.4
Muesli, Tropical, Tesco*	1 Serving/50g	173	2.4	346	7.8	68.2	4.7	9.1
Muesli, Twelve Fruit & Nut, Sainsbury's*	1 Serving/50g	166	2.4	332	8.1	64.2	4.7	7.8
Muesli, Unsweetened, M&S*	1 Serving/40g	129	1.1	322	8.1	68	2.7	9.4
Muesli, Whole Wheat, Co-Op*	1 Serving/40g	140	2.8	350	11	61	7	7

BREAKFAST CEREAL

INFO/WEIGHT	Measure	per Measure KCAL	FAT	Nutrition Values per 100g / 100ml KCAL	PROT	CARB	FAT	FIBRE
Muesli, Whole Wheat, No Added Sugar Salt, Tesco*	1 Serving/40g	154	5	386	9.5	59.1	12.4	7.4
Muesli, Wholewheat, Asda*	1 Serving/45g	150	3.5	333	8	57.9	7.7	9.7
Muesli, with Berries, Swiss, Dry, Love Life, Waitrose*	1 Serving/45g	172	4.3	383	13.5	55.7	9.6	9.8
Muesli, with Toasted Nuts Seeds, Eat Natural*	1 Portion/50g	219	11.1	438	11.5	38.9	22.2	7.9
Multigrain Boulders, Tesco*	1 Serving/30g	112	0.4	375	8.2	82.3	1.3	3.6
Multigrain Flakes with Fruit Nuts, Aldi*	1 Serving/30g	108	0.7	360	7.5	77.1	2.4	4.5
Multigrain Flakes, with Fruit, Tesco*	1 Serving/40g	147	0.9	367	7.2	77.3	2.2	4.7
Multigrain Wheelies, CBY, Asda*	1 Serving/30g	115	1	384	8.9	76	3.5	6.5
Multigrain, Balanced Lifestyle, Aldi*	1 Serving/30g	108	0.7	360	7.5	77.1	2.4	4.5
Multigrain, Fitnesse, Nestle*	1 Serving/30g	109	0.4	363	8	79.8	1.3	5.1
Multigrain, Hoops, Average	*1 Serving/30g*	*112*	*1.1*	*374*	*6.6*	*77.4*	*3.6*	*6.1*
Museli, Premium, Lidl*	1 Bowl/45g	165	3.3	367	8.4	62.5	7.4	8.3
Nesquik, Chocolatey Corn Rice, Nestle*	1 Serving/30g	114	1.2	380	7.2	79.1	3.9	5.1
Nutri Brex, Biscuits, GF, Nutri Brex*	3 Biscuits/46g	174	1.7	378	12.3	70	3.6	6.8
Nutty Crunch, Alpen*	1 Serving/40g	159	4.5	398	10.7	63.6	11.2	6.5
Nutty Crunch, Deliciously, M&S*	1 Serving/50g	238	11.2	476	8.8	59.6	22.5	4.4
Oat & Bran Flakes, Sainsbury's*	1 Serving/30g	97	1.7	324	12.2	56	5.7	17.7
Oat Bran, Hodgson Mill*	1 Serving/40g	48	1.2	120	6	23	3	6
Oat Clusters, Triple Chocolate Crunch, M&S*	1 Serving/45g	212	8.9	471	8.5	61.9	19.8	5.6
Oat Crunchy, Blueberry Cranberry, Waitrose*	1 Serving/60g	259	9.1	432	8	65.9	15.2	8.5
Oat Granola, Quaker*	1 Serving/50g	206	4.4	411	8.6	73	8.8	5.2
Oat Granola, Raisin, Quaker*	1 Serving/45g	188	4.1	418	8	70.9	9.1	6.9
Oat Krunchies, Quaker*	1 Serving/30g	118	2.1	393	9.5	72	7	5.5
Oat Meal, Medium, Heart's Content, Mornflake*	1 Serving/30g	108	2.4	359	11	60.4	8.1	8.5
Oat, Crunchy, Sainsbury's*	1 Serving/50g	226	10.2	453	8.2	59.3	20.3	6.6
Oat, Raisin, Nut Honey, Crunchy, Dry, Sainsbury's*	1 Serving/50g	201	7	402	8.5	60.2	14.1	7.6
Oatbran Oatgerm, Prewett's*	1 Serving/30g	104	2.9	345	14.8	49.7	9.7	15.2
Oatbran 100%, Pure Simple, Mornflake*	1 Serving/40g	146	3.8	364	13.4	47.3	9.4	18.2
Oatbran Flakes, Nature's Path*	1 Serving/30g	124	1.4	414	8.7	83	4.7	6.7
Oatbran Flakes, Original, Mornflake*	1 Serving/40g	149	2.1	372	11.9	63.2	5.2	12.4
Oatbran Sprinkles, Mornflake*	1 Serving/40g	146	3.8	364	13.4	47.3	9.4	18.2
Oatbran, Original Pure, Mornflake*	1 Serving/30g	104	2.9	345	14.8	49.7	9.7	15.2
Oatbran, Very Berry, Flakes, Mornflake*	1 Serving/40g	149	2	372	11.7	63.8	5.1	12
Oatibix, Flakes, Weetabix*	1 Serving/50g	190	2.8	381	9.5	73.2	5.6	3.5
Oatibix, Original, Bitesize, Weetabix*	1 Serving/36g	133	2.4	370	10.6	66.5	6.8	10.1
Oatibix, Weetabix*	2 Biscuits/48g	189	3.8	394	12.5	64.3	8	7.3
Oatmeal, Coarse, Prewett's*	1 Serving/40g	137	4.2	343	14.3	47.6	10.6	16
Oatmeal, Instant, Cinnamon, Weight Control, Quaker*	1 Pack/45g	160	3	356	15.6	64.4	6.7	13.3
Oatmeal, Instant, Heart to Heart, Kashi*	1 Serving/43g	150	2	349	7	76.7	4.6	9.3
Oatmeal, Quick Oats, Dry, Quaker*	1 Serving/30g	114	2	380	14	66.7	6.7	10
Oatmeal, Raw	*1oz/28g*	*112*	*2.4*	*401*	*12.4*	*72.8*	*8.7*	*6.8*
Oats, Ginger Bread, Bench Press, Instant, Oomf*	1 Pot/75g	296	3.4	395	28.3	57.1	4.5	6.7
Oats, Golden Syrup Flavour, Instant, Hot, Waitrose*	1 Serving/39g	153	2.3	393	7.8	77.4	5.8	6
Oats, Jumbo, Organic, Waitrose*	1 Serving/50g	180	4	361	11	61.1	8.1	7.8
Oats, Original, Instant, Hot, Waitrose*	1 Sachet/27g	97	2.2	359	11	60.4	8.1	8.5
Oats, Pure, Free From, Sainsbury's*	1 Serving/40g	164	3.2	410	14.9	64	8	11
Oats, Strawberry Banana, Toasted, Crunch, White's*	1 Serving/40g	175	5.5	437	7.7	67.3	13.8	6.2
Oats, Superfast, Mornflake*	1 Serving/40g	147	3.4	367	12.1	56.1	8.4	9.1
Oats, Tesco*	1 Serving/40g	142	3.2	356	11	60	8	8
Oats, Wholegrain, Organic, Quaker*	1 Serving/25g	89	2	356	11	60	8	9
Optivita, Berry Oat Crisp, Kellogg's*	1 Serving/30g	107	1.5	357	10	68	5	9
Organic, Weetabix*	2 Biscuits/38g	134	0.7	358	11.5	68.6	2	10
Original, Crunchy, Tropical Fruits, Jordans*	1 Serving/50g	212	7.2	423	8.1	65.1	14.5	6.7

BREAKFAST CEREAL

INFO/WEIGHT	Measure	per Measure		Nutrition Values per 100g / 100ml				
		KCAL	FAT	KCAL	PROT	CARB	FAT	FIBRE
Perfect Balance, Weight Watchers*	1 Serving/30g	90	0.5	300	7.8	63.3	1.7	15.6
Pomegranate Raspberry, Wheats, Tesco*	1 Serving/45g	151	0.6	335	7.5	71.8	1.4	8.2
Porage Oats, Old Fashioned, Dry, Scotts*	1 Serving/40g	142	3.2	355	11	60	8	9
Porage Oats, Original, Dry, Scotts*	1 Serving/40g	149	3.2	372	11	60	8	9
Porage Oats, Original, So-Easy, Dry, Scotts*	1 Serving/30g	109	2.6	364	11	60	8.5	9
Porage Oats, Syrup Swirl, So-Easy, Dry, Scotts*	1 Sachet/37g	135	2.2	366	8	70	6	6.5
Porridge 5 Grain, 5 Seed, Rude Health*	1 Serving/50g	176	4.1	351	12.2	57.1	8.2	12.4
Porridge Oats, Bran, Co-Op*	1 Serving/40g	141	2.8	353	12.5	60	7	12
Porridge Oats, Co-Op*	1 Serving/40g	144	3.2	360	12	61	8	9
Porridge Oats, Dry Weight, Value, Tesco*	1 Serving/50g	180	4	359	11	60.4	8.1	8.5
Porridge Oats, Honey Flavour, Paw Ridge, Quaker*	1 Sachet/29g	103	2	361	9.6	64.7	7	7.9
Porridge Oats, Mornflake*	1 Serving/40g	147	3.4	367	12.1	56.1	8.4	9.1
Porridge Oats, Organic, Evernat*	1 Serving/40g	167	3.8	418	13	69	9.6	7.4
Porridge Oats, Organic, Kavanagh's, Aldi*	1 Serving/40g	148	2.1	370	12	64	5.3	8.6
Porridge Oats, Organic, Tesco*	1 Serving/50g	184	4.2	368	12.1	56.1	8.4	10
Porridge Oats, Original, Dry, Quaker*	1 Serving/45g	160	3.6	356	11	60	8	4
Porridge Oats, Original, Paw Ridge, Quaker*	1 Sachet/25g	89	2	356	11	60	8	9
Porridge Oats, Plain, Jumbo, Moma Foods*	1 Pot/40g	144	2.4	361	11.7	60.3	6	9.3
Porridge Oats, Rolled, Tesco*	1 Serving/50g	180	4	359	11	60.4	8.1	8.5
Porridge Oats, Scottish, Organic, Sainsbury's*	1 Serving/45g	172	2.2	383	10	74.4	5	7.9
Porridge Oats, Scottish, Tesco*	1 Serving/50g	180	4	359	11	60.4	8.1	8.5
Porridge Oats, Sprouted, Organic, Rude Health*	1 Serving/10g	38	0.6	375	16	64	6.5	10
Porridge Oats, with Bran, Scottish, Sainsbury's*	1 Serving/50g	190	2.5	380	9.6	74.1	5	10.3
Porridge Oats, with Grains Seeds, Tesco*	1 Serving/50g	198	5.6	395	12.1	56.5	11.1	10.5
Porridge Oats, with Oat Wheat Bran, HL, Tesco*	1 Sachet/30g	105	1.8	350	10.8	62.3	6.1	9.2
Porridge Oats, with Oatbran Wheatbran, Tesco*	1 Portion/50g	187	4.1	375	11	58.3	8.3	11.4
Porridge Oats, with Wheat Bran, Tesco*	1 Serving/50g	167	3.6	334	12.3	55	7.2	13
Porridge Oats, with Wheatbran, Essential, Waitrose*	1 Serving/50g	168	3.8	336	11.2	55.8	7.6	13
Porridge, 5 Grain, Seed, Organic, Harvest Morn, Aldi*	1 Serving/50g	190	5	380	12	55	10	11
Porridge, Apple Cinnamon, Express, Dry, Sainsbury's*	1 Sachet/36g	138	2.1	383	8.6	70.3	5.9	7.2
Porridge, Apple Cinnamon, Variety Box, Graze*	1 Bag/67g	240	3.4	356	8	68	5	10
Porridge, Apple Pear, Variety Box, Graze*	1 Bag/63g	226	3.7	359	9.4	65	5.9	11
Porridge, Apple, Sultana & Cinnamon, M&S*	1 Sachet/40g	144	3	360	10.3	62.3	7.5	8.6
Porridge, Banana, Ready Brek, Weetabix*	1 Serving/40g	146	2.6	365	8.9	68	6.4	6.7
Porridge, Berry Burst, Oat So Simple, Quaker*	1 Serving/39g	144	2.3	370	8	70	6	6.5
Porridge, Berry Burst, Wholegrain, Instant , M&S*	1 Pot/70g	252	3.3	360	12.6	62.7	4.7	8.4
Porridge, Blueberry, Cranberry, Guava, Made Up, Quaker*	1 Serving/35g	201	5.1	574	24.8	83.4	14.6	9.1
Porridge, Blueberry, Frozen, Tesco*	1 Pack/250g	202	4.4	81	3.5	12	1.8	1.7
Porridge, Caramel, Instant, Pot, Oat So Simple, Quaker*	1 Pot/57g	208	3.2	365	10.5	67.7	5.6	6.3
Porridge, Chocolate, Free From, Ocado*	1 Serving/45g	174	2.7	384	11	66	6	11
Porridge, Chocolate, Instant, Grasshopper*	1 Pot/60g	221	3	368	15	68.3	5	0
Porridge, Chocolate, Oatibix, Weetabix*	1 Pack/40g	149	3.9	372	9.9	61.3	9.7	6.2
Porridge, Chocolate, Ready Brek, Weetabix*	1 Serving/30g	114	2.4	380	10	63.6	8	7
Porridge, Coconut Date, Graze*	1 Punnet/45g	176	5.9	391	8	57	13	9
Porridge, Country Honey, Oat So Simple, Quaker*	1 Serving/36g	134	2.3	373	8.5	69	6.5	6
Porridge, Cranberry Raspberry, Fruity, Dorset Cereals*	1 Sachet/30g	99	1.8	330	10.2	58.7	6	12.3
Porridge, Flakes, Organic, Barkat*	1 Serving/30g	109	0.9	362	8.5	74.1	3	0
Porridge, Free From, Sainsbury's*	1 Serving/50g	174	1.5	348	8.6	72	3	3.4
Porridge, Fresh, Double Cream, & Demerara Sugar, M&S*	1 Pot/200g	254	15.2	127	4.3	9.7	7.6	1.3
Porridge, Fruit Nut, Fruity, Dorset Cereals*	1 Serving/70g	242	5.6	346	9.4	59	8	8.2
Porridge, GF, Oat So Simple, Quaker*	1 Sachet/35g	130	2.5	370	13.2	58.5	7.2	9.2
Porridge, Golden Honey, Oatibix, Weetabix*	1 Serving/40g	145	2.6	363	9.2	66.7	6.6	7
Porridge, Golden Syrup, Dry, Oat So Simple, Quaker*	1 Sachet/36g	137	2.2	380	8.4	68.7	6.2	6.8

BREAKFAST CEREAL

	Measure INFO/WEIGHT	per Measure KCAL	FAT	Nutrition Values per 100g / 100ml KCAL	PROT	CARB	FAT	FIBRE
Porridge, Golden Syrup, Instant, As Consumed, Slim Fast*	1 Sachet/29g	99	1.3	340	17.4	53.2	4.6	7.9
Porridge, Golden Syrup, Prepared, Oatilicious, Lidl*	1 Sachet/39g	140	1.5	358	8.8	69	3.9	6
Porridge, Honey & Vanilla, Express Pot, Quaker*	1 Pot/57g	213	2.9	374	15.1	64.1	5.1	5.5
Porridge, Instant, Sweet Cinnamon, Harvest Morn, Aldi*	1 Pot/57g	211	2.6	371	15	64	4.5	7.8
Porridge, Made with Semi Skimmed Milk, Waitrose*	1 Serving/50g	277	7.5	554	24.6	80.4	15	8.6
Porridge, Maple & Pecan, Oat So Simple, Quaker*	1 Pack/35g	132	2.3	376	8.4	66.6	6.5	8.8
Porridge, Maple Syrup Flavour, Pot, As Sold, M&S*	1 Pot/70g	260	2.6	371	11.6	70.7	3.7	4.3
Porridge, Maple, Pecan, Pot, Finest, Tesco*	1 Pot/210g	232	3.6	110	3.8	19.3	1.7	1.5
Porridge, Mixed Berries, Fruity, Dorset Cereals*	1 Serving/70g	243	4.2	347	10.8	62.6	6	7.9
Porridge, Morning Glory, Rude Health*	1 Bowl/50g	176	4.1	351	12.2	57.1	8.2	12.4
Porridge, Multigrain, Jordans*	1 Serving/40g	134	2.2	335	10.4	60.9	5.5	10
Porridge, Oat, Barley, Instant, M&S*	1 Pot/70g	257	4.3	367	11.4	62.2	6.1	9.4
Porridge, Oatmeal, Rude Health*	1 Serving/40g	152	2.6	380	10.2	66	6.4	7.6
Porridge, Oats, 100% Whole Grain, Rolled, Jumbo, Quaker*	1 Serving/40g	150	3.2	374	11	60	8	9
Porridge, Oats, 100% Whole Grain, Rolled, Quaker*	1 Portion/40g	150	3.2	374	11	60	8	9
Porridge, Oats, Apple Blueberry, Instant, Pot, Tesco*	1 Pot/205g	210	2.9	102	3.6	18.1	1.4	1.5
Porridge, Oats, Berry Cherry, Instant, Pot, Tesco*	1 Pot/225g	207	2.9	92	3.2	16.2	1.3	1.4
Porridge, Oats, Cinnamon, Instant, Pot, Tesco*	1 Pot/225g	212	3.2	94	3.3	16.4	1.4	1.4
Porridge, Oats, Dry, Smart Price, Asda*	1 Serving/50g	186	4	372	11	60	8	8
Porridge, Oats, Everyday Essentials, Aldi*	1 Portion/30g	118	2.3	392	11	66	7.7	7.1
Porridge, Oats, GF, Organic, Scottish, Alara *	1 Serving/40g	148	2.2	369	11.8	67.9	5.5	7.5
Porridge, Oats, Golden Syrup, Instant, Pot, Tesco*	1 Pot/55g	210	2.7	380	11.4	70	4.9	5.5
Porridge, Oats, Golden Syrup, Sainsbury's*	1 Sachet/39g	143	2.1	367	6.3	73.6	5.3	6.7
Porridge, Oats, Irish, Multi Seed, Flahavans*	1 Serving/40g	166	5.3	415	14	55.4	13.3	9
Porridge, Oats, No Added Sugar, Love Life, Waitrose*	1 Pot/60g	224	3.8	373	17.5	57.8	6.4	7.2
Porridge, Oats, Original, Instant, Pot, Tesco*	1 Pot/256g	208	3.3	81	3.1	13.5	1.3	1.6
Porridge, Oats, Twice the Fibre, M&S*	1 Portion/60g	230	3.5	384	10.4	62.6	5.9	19.5
Porridge, Oats, Whole, Chunky, Traditional, Jordans*	1 Serving/40g	143	2.7	358	6.7	63.6	6.8	7.9
Porridge, Original, Diet Chef Ltd*	1 Sachet/40g	157	2.5	392	12	67	6.3	9.8
Porridge, Original, Dry, Oat So Simple, Quaker*	1 Sachet/27g	100	2.1	370	11	58.9	7.7	10.5
Porridge, Original, Express, Sachet, Sainsbury's*	1 Pack/27g	100	2.2	370	11	58	8	10.8
Porridge, Original, Oatibix, Weetabix*	1 Sachet/30g	104	2.5	347	12.5	55.6	8.3	10.1
Porridge, Original, Pot, Made Up, Asda*	1 Pot/221g	199	2.7	90	3.3	16	1.2	2.1
Porridge, Original, Ready Brek, Weetabix*	1 Serving/40g	149	3.5	373	11.7	57.9	8.7	7.9
Porridge, Original, Simply, Sachet, Asda*	1 Sachet/27g	96	2.2	356	11	60	8	8
Porridge, Original, Super Goodness, Quaker*	1 Serving/31g	114	2.8	372	14.1	56.7	9.1	9.9
Porridge, Perfectly, Dorset Cereals*	1 Sachet/30g	107	2.5	356	11.8	58.2	8.4	11
Porridge, Plain, Instant, Quaker*	1 Serving/34g	124	2.9	364	11	60	8.5	9
Porridge, Raspberry & Cranberry, Made Up, Quaker*	1 Sachet/39g	217	5.6	564	26	81.6	14.6	9.4
Porridge, Ready Oats, CBY, Asda*	1 Serving/40g	149	3.5	374	12	58	8.7	7.9
Porridge, Red Berry, Instant, As Consumed, Slim Fast*	1 Sachet/29g	99	1.3	341	17.2	53.1	4.5	7.9
Porridge, Rice Buckwheat, Free From, Sainsbury's*	1 Serving/50g	179	0.4	358	6.8	81.1	0.7	1.4
Porridge, Scottish Oats, Frozen, Tesco*	1 Pack/251g	218	5.3	87	3.9	12.1	2.1	1.8
Porridge, Spelt, Sharpham Park*	1 Serving/50g	159	1.6	318	11.3	7	3.3	9.5
Porridge, Spiced Apple, Sultana, Oatibix, Weetabix*	1 Sachet/40g	138	2.3	345	9.7	65.4	5.7	8.5
Porridge, Superfoods, Jordans*	1 Serving/40g	145	3.6	362	10.4	59.8	9	8.3
Porridge, Vanilla Banana, Diet Chef Ltd*	1 Pack/40g	151	2.2	378	10.7	70.6	5.6	9.8
Porridge, with Blueberries, Cranberries, & Nuts, Alpen*	1 Sachet/40g	154	3.4	385	10.8	62.6	8.5	7.3
Porridge, with Cocao Nib, Diet Chef Ltd*	1 Pack/40g	164	3.5	410	10.9	67.3	8.8	9.5
Protein Crunch, Chocolate, Weetabix*	1 Serving/30g	114	1	379	20	64	3.2	7
Protein Crunch, Weetabix*	1 Serving/30g	114	0.8	379	20	66	2.5	6.1
Protein, Big Biscuit, Weetabix*	1 Biscuit/20g	72	0.4	360	19	62	1.9	9.6
Puffed Rice, Average	**1 Serving/30g**	**115**	**0.8**	**382**	**7.1**	**82.2**	**2.8**	**3**

B

BREAKFAST CEREAL

INFO/WEIGHT	Measure	per Measure KCAL	FAT	Nutrition Values per 100g / 100ml KCAL	PROT	CARB	FAT	FIBRE
Puffed Rice, Honey, Organic, Kallo*	1 Serving/25g	98	0.9	392	5	85	3.5	2.1
Puffed Rice, Organic, Natural, Kallo*	1 Bowl/25g	92	0.5	370	7	81	2	3
Puffed Rice, Wholegrain, Brown, Original, Organic, Kallo*	1 Serving/25g	95	0.8	380	8	80	3	9
Puffed Wheat, Quaker*	1 Serving/15g	49	0.2	328	15.3	62.4	1.3	5.6
Puffed Wheat, Tesco*	1 Serving/28g	104	0.9	373	13.9	72.2	3.2	5.7
Raisin & Almond, Crunchy, Jordans*	1 Serving/45g	186	5.7	412	9.9	61.6	12.6	6.6
Raisin Oats & More, & 125ml Semi Skimmed Milk, Nestle*	1 Serving/40g	207	3.9	518	19.8	88	9.8	6.2
Raisin Wheats, Kellogg's*	1 Serving/45g	104	0.6	345	9	69	2	9
Raisin, Bran Flakes, Asda*	1 Serving/50g	166	1.5	331	7	69	3	10
Raisin, Oats More, Nestle*	1 Serving/30g	112	1.4	373	8.9	73.7	4.7	5.8
Red Berries, Additions, Weetabix*	2 Biscuits/43g	152	0.8	350	9.8	67	1.9	13
Red Berries, Special K, Kellogg's*	1 Serving/30g	112	0.4	374	14	76	1.5	3
Red Berry, Almond, Luxury Crunch, Jordans*	1 Serving/40g	176	7.4	441	8.2	60.5	18.5	6.6
Rice & Wheat Flakes, Toasted, Love Life, Waitrose*	1 Serving/30g	115	0.4	382	11.7	79.7	1.3	2.2
Rice Krispies, Honey, Kellogg's*	1 Serving/30g	114	0.2	380	4	89	0.7	1
Rice Krispies, Kellogg's*	1 Serving/30g	115	0.3	383	6	87	1	1
Rice Krispies, Multi-Grain, Shapes, Kellogg's*	1 Serving/30g	111	0.8	370	8	77	2.5	8
Rice Pops, Blue Parrot Cafe, Sainsbury's*	1 Serving/30g	111	0.4	370	7.2	82.3	1.3	2.2
Rice Pops, GF, Nestle*	1 Serving/30g	116	0.4	385	7.5	85	1.2	1.5
Rice Pops, Organic, Dove's Farm*	1 Serving/30g	107	0.2	357	6.8	86.1	0.8	2
Rice Pops, Sainsbury's*	1 Serving/25g	98	0.4	391	6.7	87.1	1.4	1.7
Rice Snaps, Asda*	1 Serving/28g	105	0.4	376	7	84	1.3	1.5
Rice Snaps, Everyday Value, Tesco*	1 Serving/30g	115	0.3	380	7.5	84.5	0.9	1.4
Ricicles, Kellogg's*	1 Serving/30g	114	0.2	381	4.5	89	0.8	0.8
Right Balance, Morrisons*	1 Serving/50g	181	1.1	362	6.9	78.6	2.2	5.3
Shredded Wheat, Average	**2 Biscuits/45g**	**157**	**0.8**	**348**	**9**	**77**	**1.8**	**10**
Shredded Wheat, Bitesize, Nestle*	1 Serving/40g	148	0.9	369	11.8	69.6	2.2	11.8
Shredded Wheat, Fruitful, No Added Salt, Nestle*	1 Serving/40g	142	2	354	8.3	68.7	5.1	8.9
Shredded Wheat, Honey Nut, Nestle*	1 Serving/40g	151	2.6	378	11.2	68.8	6.5	9.4
Shreddies, Coco Orange Flavoured, Nestle*	1 Serving/40g	150	0.8	374	8.5	76.2	2	8.6
Shreddies, Coco, Nestle*	1 Serving/45g	161	0.9	358	8.4	76.5	2	8.6
Shreddies, Crunchy Cranberry & Oat Granola, Nestle*	1 Serving/45g	181	3.1	403	13	68	7	7.2
Shreddies, Frosted, Kellogg's*	1 Serving/50g	162	0.9	323	0.7	78.5	1.8	4.7
Shreddies, Frosted, Nestle*	1 Serving/45g	164	0.7	365	7.4	80.7	1.5	6.4
Shreddies, Frosted, Variety Pack, Nestle*	1 Pack/45g	163	0.6	363	6.7	81.1	1.3	6.8
Shreddies, Honey, Nestle*	1 Serving/45g	169	0.7	375	8.2	78.1	1.5	8.1
Shreddies, Malt Wheats, Tesco*	1 Serving/45g	169	0.9	375	10.3	73.8	2	8.2
Shreddies, Nestle*	1 Serving/45g	186	1	371	10	73.7	1.9	9.9
Smoothies, Strawberry, Quaker*	1 Sachet/29g	117	3.5	402	6.5	67	12	5.5
Special Flakes, Gluten, Wheat, & Milk, Free From, Tesco*	1 Serving/30g	115	0.6	382	6.5	83	2	3
Special Flakes, Honey, Oats, Almonds, Tesco*	1 Serving/30g	116	0.7	385	7.2	82.5	2.2	3.1
Special Flakes, Tesco*	1 Serving/20g	74	0.3	371	11	78.4	1.5	4.3
Special Flakes, with Red Berries, Crownfield, Lidl*	1 Serving/30g	113	0.5	377	6.5	81	1.6	6.4
Special K, Bliss, Creamy Berry Crunch, Kellogg's*	1 Serving/30g	114	0.8	379	13	76	2.5	2.5
Special K, Bliss, Strawberry & Chocolate, Kellogg's*	1 Serving/30g	115	0.9	383	13	76	3	2.5
Special K, Choco, Kellogg's*	1 Serving/40g	160	2.8	400	14	70	7	3.5
Special K, Clusters, Honey, Kellogg's*	1 Serving/45g	175	1.4	389	9	80	3	3.5
Special K, Kellogg's*	1 Serving/30g	114	0.4	379	14	76	1.5	2.5
Special K, Oats Honey, Kellogg's*	1 Serving/30g	114	0.9	381	9	77	3	5
Special K, Peach & Apricot, Kellogg's*	1 Serving/30g	112	0.3	373	14	77	1	2.5
Special K, Protein Plus, Kellogg's*	1 Serving/29g	100	3	345	34.5	31	10.3	17.2
Special K, Purple Berries, Kellogg's*	1 Serving/30g	112	0.3	374	13	77	1	3.5
Special K, Yoghurty, Kellogg's*	1 Serving/30g	115	0.9	383	14	75	3	2.5

B

INFO/WEIGHT	Measure	per Measure		Nutrition Values per 100g / 100ml				
		KCAL	FAT	KCAL	PROT	CARB	FAT	FIBRE

BREAKFAST CEREAL

	INFO/WEIGHT	KCAL	FAT	KCAL	PROT	CARB	FAT	FIBRE
Start, Kellogg's*	1 Serving/30g	117	1	390	8	79	3.5	5
Strawberry & Almond Crunch, M&S*	1 Serving/40g	186	7.4	465	8	66	18.6	4.9
Strawberry Crisp, Asda*	1 Serving/45g	194	7	431	8.1	64.7	15.5	5.9
Strawberry, Alpen*	1 Serving/40g	144	1.9	359	9.4	69.5	4.8	7.9
Sugar Puffs, Quaker*	1 Serving/30g	114	0.5	379	5.3	85.8	1.6	3.7
Sultana Bran, Co-Op*	1 Serving/40g	130	1.2	325	9	66	3	11
Sultana Bran, HL, Tesco*	1 Serving/30g	98	0.6	325	8.2	68	1.9	12
Sultana Bran, Morrisons*	1 Serving/30g	98	0.9	325	8.8	65.8	3	11.4
Sultana Bran, Waitrose*	1 Serving/30g	97	0.6	324	8.2	68.6	1.9	11.6
Toffee Crisp, Nestle*	1 Serving/30g	126	3	421	6.5	73.8	10	5
Vitality, Asda*	1 Serving/30g	111	0.4	370	11	78	1.5	3.2
Vitality, with Red Fruit, Asda*	1 Serving/30g	110	0.5	366	11	77	1.6	3.8
Weet Bix, Sanitarium*	2 Biscuits/30g	106	0.4	352	12	67	1.4	10.5
Weet-Bix, Blends, Multi-Grain, Sanitarium*	2 Biscuits/48g	185	2.1	385	10.7	70.2	4.4	8.9
Weetabix, Banana, Weetabix*	1 Serving/44g	157	0.9	357	10	70.4	2	9.8
Weetabix, Chocolate, Weetabix*	2 Biscuits/45g	166	1.8	368	10.1	67.9	4	10
Weetaflakes, Weetabix*	1 Serving/30g	102	0.4	340	8.9	72.9	1.4	11
Weetos, Chocolate, Weetabix*	1 Serving/30g	113	1.5	378	8.4	75.1	4.9	5.8
Wheat Biscuits, As Sold, Savers, Morrisons*	2 Biscuits/36g	127	0.6	353	10.8	67.6	1.8	11.6
Wheat Biscuits, Average	*2 Biscuits/38g*	*130*	*0.8*	*347*	*11.7*	*68.4*	*2.2*	*9.9*
Wheat Bisks, Banana, Mini, Asda*	1 Serving/50g	190	2.7	380	9.7	73.1	5.4	7.4
Wheat Bisks, Chocolate, Asda*	2 Biscuits/43g	158	1.5	367	10	69	3.4	10
Wheat Bisks, Harvest Morn, Aldi*	2 Biscuits/38g	136	0.8	358	11.5	68.6	2	10
Wheat Bisks, Wholegrain, M&S*	2 Biscuits/40g	141	0.7	353	10.9	68.1	1.7	10.7
Wheat Pillows, Wholegrain, Tesco*	1 Biscuit/45g	151	0.9	335	10.6	67.6	2.1	11.3
Wheat Shreds, Harvest Morn, Aldi*	2 Biscuits/45g	156	0.8	346	13	64	1.8	13
Wheats, Mini, Maple & Brown Sugar, Sainsbury's*	1 Serving/52g	99	0.5	190	4	44	1	5
Whole Wheat Biscuits, Organic, Dove's Farm*	1 Serving/30g	99	0.8	329	11	65	2.8	11
Wholegrain Hoops, Goldenvale, Aldi*	1 Serving/30g	111	0.8	371	6.9	74	2.6	10.7
Wholegrain, Apricot, Wheats, Sainsbury's*	1 Serving/45g	151	0.6	335	8	71.3	1.4	8.3
Wholegrain, Fruit Fibre, Sainsbury's*	1 Serving/40g	149	2.3	372	9.3	66.1	5.7	9.4
Wholegrain, Mini Wheats, Sainsbury's*	1 Serving/40g	144	0.7	359	11.8	68.2	1.8	11.2
Wholegrain, Minis, Weetabix*	1 Serving/40g	149	0.8	372	10.2	73.2	2	10
Wholegrain, Sultana Bran, Sainsbury's*	1 Serving/30g	98	0.6	325	8.3	68.6	1.9	12.1
Wholesome Crunch, Granola, Pecan Brazil Nut, Quaker*	1 Serving/45g	189	5	420	11.1	61.8	11.1	13.2
Wholesome Crunch, Granola, Goji Blueberry, Quaker*	1 Serving/45g	181	3.6	402	11	64.5	7.9	13.5
Yoghurt Raspberry, Crisp, Sainsbury's*	1 Serving/45g	191	6.7	424	7.5	65.2	14.8	6.4

BRESAOLA

	INFO/WEIGHT	KCAL	FAT	KCAL	PROT	CARB	FAT	FIBRE
Della Valtellina, Air Dried Beef, Deluxe, Lidl*	1 Pack/80g	130	2.4	163	33.5	0.5	3	0
Finest, Tesco*	1 Serving/35g	64	1.4	182	36	0.5	4	0

BROCCOLI

	INFO/WEIGHT	KCAL	FAT	KCAL	PROT	CARB	FAT	FIBRE
Cauliflower, Floret Mix, Fresh, Tesco*	1 Serving/80g	27	0.7	34	3.9	2.5	0.9	2.7
Green, Boiled, Average	*1 Serving/80g*	*19*	*0.6*	*24*	*3.1*	*1.1*	*0.8*	*2.3*
Green, Raw, Average	*1 Serving/80g*	*24*	*0.7*	*30*	*3.7*	*1.6*	*0.8*	*2.5*
Purple Sprouting, Boiled, Average	*1 Serving/80g*	*15*	*0.5*	*19*	*2.1*	*1.3*	*0.6*	*2.3*
Purple Sprouting, Raw	*1oz/28g*	*10*	*0.3*	*35*	*3.9*	*2.6*	*1.1*	*3.5*
Steamed, Average	*1 Serving/100g*	*24*	*0.8*	*24*	*3.1*	*1.1*	*0.8*	*2.3*
Tenderstem, Average	*1 Serving/80g*	*28*	*0.4*	*35*	*4.1*	*2.9*	*0.6*	*2.3*

BROWNIES

	INFO/WEIGHT	KCAL	FAT	KCAL	PROT	CARB	FAT	FIBRE
Average	*1 Brownie/60g*	*243*	*10.1*	*405*	*4.6*	*0*	*16.8*	*0*
Chocolate, Orange, Bites, Amaze, Cadbury*	1 Bite/14g	65	3.3	470	5.3	56.4	24.1	3.1
Chocolate, Average	*1 Serving/100g*	*446*	*22.3*	*446*	*5.9*	*55.6*	*22.3*	*2.2*
Chocolate, Chewy, M&S*	1 Brownie/29g	130	6	455	6.5	59.8	21.1	2

INFO/WEIGHT	Measure	per Measure		Nutrition Values per 100g / 100ml				
		KCAL	FAT	KCAL	PROT	CARB	FAT	FIBRE
BROWNIES								
Chocolate, Chunky, Belgian, M&S*	1 Brownie/55g	242	11.2	440	6.2	57.7	20.3	2.5
Chocolate, Double, Bites, Amaze, Cadbury*	1 Bite/14g	65	3.3	470	5.3	56.7	24.1	3.1
Chocolate, Double, Mini Bites, Sainsbury's*	1 Serving/18g	73	3.1	406	5.5	55.9	17.2	2.6
Chocolate, Fudge, Mini, Thorntons*	1 Bite/14g	61	2.8	435	5.6	57.4	20	0
Chocolate, Fudgy, M&S*	1 Brownie/87g	400	21.9	460	4.8	56.9	25.2	3
Chocolate, Mini Bites, Asda*	1 Brownie/15g	62	3	420	5	55	20	1.4
Chocolate, Orange, Organic, The Village Bakery*	1 Brownie/30g	126	6.7	421	5	50.5	22.2	0.9
Chocolate, Sainsbury's*	1 Brownie/60g	265	13.6	442	4.6	55	22.6	1.6
Chocolate, Slices, M&S*	1 Brownie/36g	158	8.7	440	5.3	51.1	24.1	1.3
Chocolate, Tray Bake, Tesco*	1 Brownie/37g	155	6.8	420	5.5	57.1	18.4	5.7
Chocolate, Waitrose*	1 Brownie/45g	192	8.9	426	6.3	55.6	19.8	2.7
Chocolate, Wheat GF, Mrs Crimble's*	1 Slice/48g	180	9.6	379	4.2	47.9	20.3	1.5
The Graze Brownie, Graze*	1 Portion/30g	110	5.4	368	7.1	50.5	17.9	3.8
BRUSCHETTA								
Cheese Tomato, Asda*	1 Bruschetta/38g	68	1.7	180	8.6	26	4.6	2.9
Garlic, Parsley, Valentina*	1 Bruschetta/10g	55	3.1	538	8.4	56.9	30.4	0
Pane Italia*	1 Serving/75g	367	18.8	489	12.4	53.6	25.1	1.4
Red Pepper & Onion, Brunchetta, Golden Vale*	1 Pack/90g	266	17.1	296	14.6	17	19	1.3
Soft Cheese & Cranberry, Brunchetta, Golden Vale*	1 Pack/95g	200	8.6	211	8.2	24.8	9	1.3
Toasted, Olive Oil & Sea Salt, Tesco*	1 Serving/30g	126	4.6	420	11.5	58.7	15.5	4.5
Topping, Tomato Basil, Spirit of Summer, M&S*	½ Jar/140g	99	4.9	71	1.6	6.6	3.5	3.2
BRUSSELS SPROUTS								
& Sweet Chestnuts, Asda*	1 Serving/100g	73	1.7	73	3.1	11	1.7	4.2
Boiled, Average	*1 Serving/80g*	*27*	*1*	*33*	*3*	*3*	*1.2*	*3.3*
Button, Raw, Average	*1 Serving/80g*	*28*	*1*	*36*	*3.3*	*2.8*	*1.3*	*3*
Canned, Drained	*1oz/28g*	*5*	*0.2*	*17*	*1.6*	*1.5*	*0.6*	*1.6*
Frozen, Morrisons*	1 Serving/200g	70	2.6	35	3.5	2.5	1.3	4.3
Raw, Average	*1 Serving/80g*	*28*	*0.8*	*35*	*3.3*	*3.1*	*1*	*2.9*
Red, Limited Selection, Waitrose*	1 Serving/80g	41	1.1	51	3.5	4.1	1.4	3.8
Steamed, Average	*1 Serving/100g*	*35*	*1.3*	*35*	*3.1*	*3.2*	*1.3*	*3.5*
with Chestnuts, Bacon, Tesco*	1 Serving/100g	151	6.6	151	4.7	14.4	6.6	7.7
BUBBLE & SQUEAK								
Tesco*	½ Pack/325g	256	3.7	79	1.5	14.7	1.1	1.9
Fried in Vegetable Oil	*1oz/28g*	*35*	*2.5*	*124*	*1.4*	*9.8*	*9.1*	*1.5*
BUCKWHEAT								
Average	*1oz/28g*	*102*	*0.4*	*364*	*8.1*	*84.9*	*1.5*	*2.1*
BUFFALO								
Mince, Raw, Lean, Abel Cole*	1 Serving/100g	95	0.7	95	21.7	0.4	0.7	0
Steak, Rump, Extra Lean, Pan Fried, Iceland*	1 Steak/125g	214	3.3	171	36.9	0.1	2.6	0.1
BULGUR WHEAT								
Dry Weight, Average	*1oz/28g*	*99*	*0.5*	*353*	*9.7*	*76.3*	*1.7*	*8*
Quinoa Rainbow Vegetables, As Prepared, Waitrose*	1 Pack/300g	372	11.4	124	3.1	17.6	3.8	3.6
with Chick Peas, Quinoa, Ready to Eat, Sainsbury's*	½ Pack/125g	239	4.1	191	7.7	30	3.3	4.7
BUNS								
Bath, Tesco*	1 Bun/80g	262	8.9	328	8	48.9	11.1	5.8
Belgian, Asda*	1 Bun/133g	464	19.9	350	4.8	49	15	2.2
Belgian, Co-Op*	1 Bun/118g	413	15.3	350	5	54	13	2
Belgian, Sainsbury's*	1 Bun/110g	398	11.3	362	6.1	61.3	10.3	1.9
Belgian, Tesco*	1 Bun/123g	438	15.7	356	5.2	54.9	12.8	2.2
Brioche, Burger, Genius*	1 Bun/70g	154	4.2	220	4.6	33	6	9.2
Chelsea	*1 Bun/78g*	*285*	*10.8*	*366*	*7.8*	*56.1*	*13.8*	*1.7*
Chelsea, Sainsbury's*	1 Bun/85g	239	4.4	281	6.9	51.6	5.2	2.9

BUNS

	Measure INFO/WEIGHT	per Measure		Nutrition Values per 100g / 100ml				
		KCAL	FAT	KCAL	PROT	CARB	FAT	FIBRE
Chelsea, Tesco*	1 Bun/85g	269	6.5	316	7.9	53.9	7.6	2.3
Choux, Caramel, Asda*	1 Bun/189g	745	51	394	4.3	33.5	27	1.3
Choux, Custard, M&S*	1 Bun/85g	234	18.7	275	4.2	15	22	0.3
Choux, Fresh Cream, Tesco*	1 Bun/95g	340	23.7	358	4.9	28.5	24.9	0.9
Choux, M&S*	1 Bun/78g	247	17.3	317	5.4	25.6	22.2	0.3
Cinnamon, Tear Share, Bakery, Tesco*	¼ Bun/108g	363	10.7	334	6.9	52.9	9.8	3.3
Currant	*1 Bun/60g*	*178*	*4.5*	*296*	*7.6*	*52.7*	*7.5*	*0*
Currant, Sainsbury's*	1 Bun/72g	197	3.7	274	7	50	5.1	2.8
Fruit, Waitrose*	1 Bun/54g	155	2.3	287	8.1	54	4.3	1.6
Hot Cross	*1 Bun/50g*	*156*	*3.5*	*312*	*7.4*	*58.5*	*7*	*1.7*
Hot Cross, 25% Reduced Fat, Asda*	1 Bun/61g	153	1.4	253	9	49	2.3	3
Hot Cross, Apple & Cinnamon, Large, Finest, Tesco*	1 Bun/117g	342	8.2	292	7.3	49.9	7	3.6
Hot Cross, Asda*	1 Bun/60g	190	3.8	317	10	55	6.3	3.3
Hot Cross, Best of Both, Hovis*	1 Bun/65g	185	4.3	285	9.1	47.3	6.6	4.4
Hot Cross, BGTY, Sainsbury's*	1 Bun/70g	189	1.8	270	6.7	53.7	2.6	2.4
Hot Cross, Bramley Apple Cinnamon, Waitrose*	1 Bun/70g	194	2.7	277	7.7	52.2	3.8	1.5
Hot Cross, Chocolate & Raisin, Mini, Tesco*	1 Bun/40g	127	4.4	318	8.1	47	10.9	2.8
Hot Cross, Chocolate Orange, Mini, M&S*	1 Bun/28g	86	2.3	307	8.2	48.2	8.2	3.9
Hot Cross, Chocolate, Mini, Sainsbury's*	1 Bun/39g	127	4.4	325	7.7	48.1	11.3	2.5
Hot Cross, Classics, M&S*	1 Bun/65g	159	1.2	245	8.5	49.1	1.8	2.2
Hot Cross, Co-Op*	1 Bun/60g	165	3.6	275	8	47	6	3
Hot Cross, Extra Fruit, Finest, Tesco*	1 Bun/80g	218	3.4	272	8.4	48.6	4.2	3.1
Hot Cross, Extra Spicy, M&S*	1 Bun/76g	175	1.4	230	8.6	44.1	1.9	4.2
Hot Cross, Golden Wholemeal, Sainsbury's*	1 Bun/65g	180	4	277	9.9	45.4	6.2	4.3
Hot Cross, HE, Tesco*	1 Bun/60g	155	1.5	258	8.6	50.3	2.5	2.6
Hot Cross, HL, Tesco*	1 Bun/70g	176	1.9	251	6.7	50.3	2.7	2.6
Hot Cross, Less Than 3% Fat, M&S*	1 Bun/70g	175	1.3	250	8.1	49.8	1.8	2.2
Hot Cross, Lightly Fruited, M&S*	1 Bun/64g	165	3.4	260	8.1	45.1	5.4	4.7
Hot Cross, Luxury, Cafe, M&S*	1 Bun/78g	199	3.1	255	8.6	46.2	4	2.1
Hot Cross, Luxury, Rowan Hill Bakery, Lidl*	1 Bun/75g	204	3.5	272	8.3	47	4.7	4
Hot Cross, Mini, M&S*	1 Bun/41g	110	1.4	265	7.8	51.4	3.4	3.7
Hot Cross, Mini, Tesco*	1 Bun/36g	99	2	274	7.9	48.1	5.5	2.7
Hot Cross, Morrisons*	1 Bun/72g	178	1.4	247	7.4	49.9	2	3.3
Hot Cross, Reduced Fat, GFY, Asda*	1 Bun/63g	156	1.6	248	8.4	47.9	2.5	3.7
Hot Cross, Reduced Fat, Waitrose*	1 Bun/67g	171	1.4	255	8.1	54.3	2.1	3.3
Hot Cross, Sticky Toffee, The Best, Morrisons*	1 Bun/77g	222	3.5	288	6.8	52.8	4.6	4
Hot Cross, Tesco*	1 Bun/70g	186	1.9	265	7.4	51.8	2.7	3.6
Hot Cross, The Village Bakery*	1 Bun/70g	178	1.5	254	7.2	50	2.2	2.9
Hot Cross, TTD, Sainsbury's*	1 Bun/75g	200	4.2	267	7.2	47	5.6	3.8
Hot Cross, White, Kingsmill*	1 Bun/70g	186	2.4	266	8.7	48	3.5	3.6
Hot Cross, White, LC, Tesco*	1 Bun/70g	185	1.4	260	8.3	50.3	1.9	3.8
Hot Cross, White, Sainsbury's*	1 Bun/70g	199	3.4	284	7.9	50.6	4.8	3.4
Hot Cross, White, Waitrose*	1 Bun/68g	174	2.1	258	8.1	49.5	3.1	3.9
Hot Cross, Wholemeal, Asda*	1 Bun/70g	182	4.2	262	9	43	6	6
Hot Cross, Wholemeal, Organic, Tesco*	1 Bun/55g	140	2.7	254	7.6	44.8	4.9	4.5
Hot Cross, Wholemeal, Waitrose*	1 Bun/64g	177	4.3	276	8.8	45.2	6.7	4.9
Hot Cross, You Count, Love Life, Waitrose*	1 Bun/70g	195	3.2	278	6.8	51.5	4.5	2.3
Iced Finger, Average	*1 Bun/40g*	*130*	*3.1*	*325*	*7.2*	*57*	*7.7*	*2.3*
Iced Finger, Coconut, Genesis Crafty*	1 Bun/64g	210	6.9	328	7.7	52.4	10.8	2.4
Iced Finger, Lemon, Aldi*	1 Bun/40g	130	3.4	325	6.4	55	8.5	2
Iced Finger, Sainsbury's*	1 Bun/40g	130	3.3	326	7	55.4	8.2	1.4
Iced Finger, Sticky, CBY, Asda*	1 Finger/40g	132	2.4	330	7.1	62	5.9	2.7
Iced Finger, Tesco*	1 Bun/40g	135	3.6	338	6.2	57.2	9	1.9

	Measure INFO/WEIGHT	per Measure KCAL	FAT	Nutrition Values per 100g / 100ml KCAL	PROT	CARB	FAT	FIBRE
BUNS								
Iced Lemon, Tesco*	1 Bun/48g	156	4.2	325	5.2	56.5	8.7	1.9
Iced, Filled with Raspberry Jam, M&S*	1 Bun/48g	155	3.2	320	6.4	58.9	6.6	1.9
Iced, Tesco*	1 Bun/35g	117	3.4	334	7	54.8	9.6	2.5
Marlborough, M&S*	1 Bun/71g	215	6.3	305	6.2	43.4	8.9	2.2
Raspberry, Iced, Aldi*	1 Bun/40g	133	3.6	332	6.5	55	9	2
Salted Caramel, Bakery, Tesco*	1 Serving/104g	344	7.6	331	7.7	58	7.3	1.1
Spiced, PB, Waitrose*	1 Bun/65g	177	2.2	272	8	52.3	3.4	2.9
Vanilla Iced, Soft, M&S*	1 Bun/39g	125	3.1	320	7.6	54.9	8	2.9
BURGERS								
American Style, Asda*	1 Burger/42g	156	10.8	374	25	10	26	1.1
American Style, Tesco*	1 Burger/125g	250	9.1	200	13	20.4	7.3	3.9
Aubergine, & Feta, Aromatic & Minty, Waitrose*	1 Burger/101g	238	12.9	235	5.2	22.3	12.7	5.3
BBQ, Gourmet, Flame Grilled, Rustlers*	1 Burger/215g	593	27.7	276	14.6	24.7	12.9	0
Bean, Chilli, Crisp & Spicy, Frozen, Cooked, Waitrose*	1 Burger/95g	226	8.3	238	5.8	31	8.7	6.1
Bean, Green, Vegan, My Best Veggie, Lidl*	1 Serving/100g	144	7.9	144	7.1	7.3	7.9	7.8
Bean, Mexican Style, Meat Free, Tesco*	1 Burger/106g	214	9.6	202	4.8	22	9.1	6.4
Bean, Mexican, Tomato Salsa, Love Life, Waitrose*	1 Burger/93g	255	14.3	274	6.5	24.3	15.4	6.1
Bean, Spicy Veg, with Chipotle Chilli, Good Life*	1 Burger/109g	219	9.6	201	5.2	22	8.8	6.4
Bean, Spicy, Ainsley Harriott*	1 Burger/200g	302	7.5	151	7.2	23.5	3.8	5.2
Bean, Spicy, BGTY, Sainsbury's*	1 Burger/113g	223	11.2	197	4.5	19.6	9.9	5.7
Bean, Spicy, Cauldron Foods*	1 Burger/88g	203	9.8	232	5.4	27.4	11.2	6.2
Bean, Spicy, in Herby Nacho Crumb, Morrisons*	1 Burger/102g	185	8.1	181	5.2	19.5	7.9	5.5
Bean, Spicy, Linda McCartney*	1 Burger/85g	190	9.5	223	4.3	26.2	11.2	2.9
Bean, Spicy, Quarter Pounder, Dalepak*	1 Burger/115g	237	12.5	206	4.6	22.3	10.9	2.6
Bean, Spicy, Quarter Pounder, Mae's Kitchen, Aldi*	1 Burger/105g	234	9.9	223	5.9	26	9.4	6.3
Bean, Sweetcorn & Roasted Red Pepper, Vegan, Tesco*	1 Burger/115g	201	8.4	175	4.8	19	7.3	7.2
Bean, Zesty, As Consumed, M Kitchen, Morrisons*	1 Burger/124g	207	8.1	167	4.7	18.4	6.5	7.9
Beef, Caramelised Red Onion, Steak, TTD, Sainsbury's*	1 Burger/133g	287	15.3	216	20.2	7.8	11.5	0.5
Beef, Mature Cheddar, Asda*	1 Burger/80g	178	10	223	21.5	6.2	12.5	0.5
Beef, Onion, Grilled, Asda*	1 Burger/81g	201	11.5	248	23.1	6.9	14.2	0.5
Beef, 100%, Average	**1 Burger/52g**	**148**	**11.6**	**286**	**20.5**	**0.6**	**22.3**	**0.1**
Beef, 100%, Birds Eye*	1 Burger/41g	120	10.2	292	17.3	0	24.8	0
Beef, 100%, Half Pounders, Sainsbury's*	1 Burger/148g	462	33.1	313	26	1.7	22.4	0.2
Beef, 100%, Organic, Waitrose*	1 Burger/57g	140	9.6	247	23.6	0	16.9	0
Beef, 100%, Pure, Ross*	1 Burger/56g	128	9.6	229	17.1	1.4	17.1	0
Beef, 100%, Quarter Pounders, Aldi*	1 Burger/114g	320	23.3	282	24.3	0.1	20.5	1.3
Beef, 100%, Quarter Pounders, Ross*	1 Burger/74g	222	18.8	301	16.8	1.1	25.5	0
Beef, 100%, Sainsbury's*	1 Burger/44g	133	10.4	302	21.4	0.9	23.6	0.9
Beef, 100%, with Seasoning, No Onion, Birds Eye*	1 Burger/41g	134	11.9	326	16.1	0.2	29	0
Beef, 30 Day Dry Aged Hereford, 1, Waitrose*	1 Burger/130g	300	17.7	231	24.1	2.7	13.6	0.6
Beef, 97%, Grilled, Heck*	1 Burger/113g	246	12.5	217	26.9	3.4	11	0
Beef, Aberdeen Angus, Asda*	1 Burger/112g	249	13.3	222	22.2	6.7	11.8	0.9
Beef, Aberdeen Angus, Fresh, Waitrose*	1 Burger/113g	269	21	238	16.4	1.2	18.6	0
Beef, Aberdeen Angus, Frozen, Waitrose*	1 Serving/57g	145	11.6	255	18.1	0	20.3	1.1
Beef, Aberdeen Angus, Gourmet, Finest, Tesco*	1 Burger/106g	258	15.8	243	25.2	2	14.9	0
Beef, Aberdeen Angus, M&S*	1 Burger/142g	298	18.9	210	18.3	4.1	13.3	0.1
Beef, Aberdeen Angus, Quarter Pounder, TTD, Sainsbury's*	1 Burger/69g	208	14.9	301	25.8	0.5	21.6	0.5
Beef, Aberdeen Angus, Scotch, Deluxe, Lidl*	1 Burger /170g	430	30.4	253	21.9	0.7	17.9	0.6
Beef, Aberdeen Angus, Virgin Trains*	1 Burger/240g	695	37.6	290	13.5	23.8	15.7	0
Beef, Asda*	1 Burger/114g	304	18.6	267	26.8	3.2	16.3	0.7
Beef, Barbecue, Tesco*	1 Burger/114g	295	22.7	260	15.6	3.5	20	0.5
Beef, BGTY, Sainsbury's*	1 Burger/110g	177	6	161	20.8	7.1	5.5	1.1
Beef, British, Cooked, Savers, Morrisons*	1 Burger/39g	79	4.2	203	0.3	7.2	10.7	0.5

BURGERS

	Measure INFO/WEIGHT	per Measure KCAL	FAT	Nutrition Values per 100g / 100ml KCAL	PROT	CARB	FAT	FIBRE
Beef, British, Grilled, Finest, Tesco*	1 Burger/95g	185	11.8	195	17.2	3.3	12.4	0.9
Beef, British, Organic, Waitrose*	1 Burger/85g	226	16.6	266	19	3.5	19.5	1
Beef, British, Waitrose*	1 Burger/113g	279	21	247	18.6	1.2	18.6	0
Beef, Caramelised Onion, Grilled, Finest, Tesco*	1 Burger/88g	196	11.4	223	19.1	7.4	12.9	0.5
Beef, Chargrill, Tesco*	1 Burger/114g	246	18.4	217	17	0.8	16.2	2.5
Beef, Cheese & Caramelised Onion Melt, Waitrose*	1 Burger/165g	378	26.6	229	14.2	6.9	16.1	0.5
Beef, Classic, Flame Grilled, Rustlers*	1 Burger/216g	613	31.9	284	16.1	20.6	14.8	0
Beef, Economy, Value, Tesco*	1 Burger/41g	105	5.9	255	21.6	8.5	14.5	0.3
Beef, Farmfoods*	1 Burger/50g	128	9.8	255	14.4	5.4	19.6	0.1
Beef, Filled with Gorgonzola, M&S*	1 Burger/167g	384	26.9	230	16.5	4.9	16.1	0.5
Beef, Flame Grilled, Feasters*	1 Burger/58g	164	13.5	282	19.3	2.6	23.2	0
Beef, Frozen, Butcher's Choice, Tesco*	1 Burger/41g	111	7.1	272	14.7	13.6	17.4	1.1
Beef, Frozen, Tesco*	1 Burger/44g	117	8.4	266	18.9	4.6	19.1	0
Beef, Giant, Chargrilled, Farmfoods*	1 Burger/170g	352	21.8	207	17.3	5.6	12.8	1.2
Beef, in a Bun, HE, Tesco*	1 Pack/189g	282	2.5	149	13.6	20.7	1.3	2.1
Beef, Morrisons*	1 Burger/57g	169	14.3	298	12.3	5.5	25.2	0.6
Beef, New York Style, Grilled, Tesco*	1 Burger/35g	80	5.2	229	18.6	5.7	14.9	0.6
Beef, Organic, M&S*	1 Burger/110g	239	17.6	217	18.2	0	16	0.2
Beef, Original, Best, Birds Eye*	1 Burger/46g	115	8.9	252	14.1	5.1	19.5	0.4
Beef, Original, with Onion, Grilled, Birds Eye*	1 Burger/38g	110	9.5	287	13.4	2.6	24.8	0.3
Beef, Quarter Pounder, Flame Grilled, Rustlers*	1 Burger/190g	505	25.1	266	13.6	22.4	13.2	0
Beef, Quarter Pounders, BGTY, Sainsbury's*	1 Burger/114g	188	9.3	166	16.9	6.1	8.2	1
Beef, Quarter Pounders, Chilled, Morrisons*	1 Burger/115g	228	13.9	198	17.2	4.4	12.1	0.2
Beef, Quarter Pounders, Farmfoods*	1 Burger/113g	289	22.1	256	14.4	5.4	19.6	0.1
Beef, Quarter Pounders, Flame Grilled, Tesco*	1 Burger/88g	246	20.4	280	13.1	4.8	23.2	0.8
Beef, Quarter Pounders, GF, Butchers Selection, Asda*	1 Burger/93g	210	13.1	225	16	8.5	14	0.5
Beef, Quarter Pounders, Morrisons*	1 Burger/114g	338	28.6	298	12.3	5.5	25.2	0.6
Beef, Quarter Pounders, Original, Birds Eye*	1 Burger/85g	251	21.2	296	15	2.7	25	0.5
Beef, Quarter Pounders, Reduced Fat, Tesco*	1 Burger/95g	171	12.4	180	14	1.8	13	0.8
Beef, Quarter Pounders, Scotch, Sainsbury's*	1 Burger/114g	255	15.4	225	22.2	3.5	13.6	0.5
Beef, Quarter Pounders, Scotch, The Best, Morrisons*	1 Burger/97g	223	13.9	230	21	4	14.3	0.5
Beef, Quarter Pounders, Steak Country, Lidl*	1 Burger/68g	188	15.1	276	16.3	2.4	22.2	0.1
Beef, Quarter Pounders, with Onion, BGTY, Sainsbury's*	1 Burger/83g	171	7.8	205	26.6	3.8	9.3	0.9
Beef, Quarter Pounders, with Onion, Birds Eye*	1 Burger/114g	286	22.1	252	14.1	5.1	19.5	0.4
Beef, Quarter Pounders, with Onion, Cooked, Birds Eye*	1 Burger/100g	230	16	230	16	5.9	16	0.4
Beef, Quarter Pounders, with Onion, Sainsbury's*	1 Burger/113g	306	22.4	271	18	5.1	19.8	1.5
Beef, Red Onion Cheese, Butchers Selection, Asda*	1 Burger/114g	243	13.7	213	21	5	12	0.5
Beef, Sainsbury's*	1 Burger/57g	152	9.1	267	29.6	1.3	15.9	1.5
Beef, Scotch, Ultimate, TTD, Sainsbury's*	1 Burger/119g	265	15.8	223	25.3	0.5	13.3	1
Beef, Steak, 5oz, As Sold, Birds Eye*	1 Burger/142g	476	41.2	335	17	1.4	29	0.5
Beef, Steak, British, Cooked, TTD, Sainsbury's*	1 Burger/93g	201	12	216	23.4	1.5	12.9	0.5
Beef, Steak, British, Tesco*	1 Burger/80g	184	10.9	230	24.8	2.2	13.6	0.1
Beef, Steak, Extra Lean, Musclefood*	1 Burger/113g	160	5.4	142	19.6	5.7	4.8	1.3
Beef, Steak, Full of Flavour, Finest, Tesco*	1 Burger/88g	265	18.7	302	26.4	0.5	21.3	1
Beef, Steak, Smoked Garlic, Finest, Tesco*	1 Burger/80g	178	12.6	223	18	2	15.8	0.5
Beef, Sweet Chilli, Skinniburger, Aldi*	1 Burger/113g	125	1	111	18.9	6.7	0.9	0
Beef, Sweetflame Red Chilli, Steak, TTD, Sainsbury's*	1 Burger/134g	245	11.5	183	21.6	4.2	8.6	1
Beef, Wagyu, Grilled, Specially Selected, Aldi*	1 Burger/150g	332	22.5	221	18	4	15	0.5
Beef, Wagyu, Specially Selected, Aldi*	1 Burger/150g	420	30	280	19	5.1	20	0.5
Beef, with Cheese Melt, COOK!, M&S*	1 Burger/182g	400	28.9	220	17.9	1.3	15.9	1.2
Beef, with Fresh Garden Herbs, Raw, TTD, Sainsbury's*	1 Burger/142g	280	14.8	197	21.5	4.4	10.4	1.3
Beef, with Herbs, Finest, Tesco*	1 Burger/105g	200	11.8	190	17.3	4.5	11.2	0.7
Beef, with Jalapeno Chilli, Finest, Tesco*	1 Burger /205g	379	22.3	185	17	3.4	10.9	0.4

BURGERS

	Measure INFO/WEIGHT	per Measure KCAL	FAT	Nutrition Values per 100g / 100ml KCAL	PROT	CARB	FAT	FIBRE
Beef, with Mediterranean Tomato Basil, M&S*	1 Burger/169g	304	18.6	180	15.7	5.1	11	1.4
Beef, with Onion, Sainsbury's*	1 Burger/42g	102	6.2	243	20.7	6.9	14.8	1
Beef, with Red Onion, Mustard, Finest, Tesco*	1 Burger/130g	308	24.2	237	17.2	0.2	18.6	2.6
Beef, with West Country Cheddar, TTD, Sainsbury's*	1 Burger/112g	252	13.7	225	26.4	2.3	12.2	0
Beetroot, & Root Vegetable, Vegetarian, Asda*	½ Pack/107g	158	8.8	148	3.7	11	8.2	7.2
Beetroot, Kale, Quinoa, Vegetarian, Tesco*	1 Burger/106g	140	5.2	132	3.1	15.8	4.9	6.1
Beetroot, Vegan, My Best Veggie, Lidl*	1 Burger/100g	69	0.1	69	5.2	8.5	0.1	6.5
Beetroot, Vegan, Vivera*	1 Burger/100g	87	1	87	5.1	11.5	1	6.1
Black Bean, Beetroot, Bean Supreme*	1 Burger/85g	108	3.6	127	5.7	13.8	4.2	5.7
Black Bean, Organic, Cauldron Foods*	1 Burger/88g	169	10.1	193	9.2	13.1	11.5	8.5
Cheese, & Spring Onion, Tesco*	1 Burger/87g	178	10.3	204	4.4	20	11.8	3.2
Cheese, Chips, Heat 'Em Up, Tesco*	1 Serving/220g	500	17.4	227	10	27.9	7.9	2.7
Cheese, Snax On The Go*	1 Burger/145g	375	14.8	258	14.2	26.6	10.2	1.7
Cheeseburger	*1 Serving/275g*	*706*	*29*	*257*	*13.7*	*25.6*	*10.6*	*1.8*
Cheeseburger, American, Tesco*	1 Burger/275g	660	26.3	240	13.6	24.9	9.6	1.6
Cheeseburger, Bacon with Bun, Chargrilled, Tesco*	1 Burger/265g	726	42.1	274	13	19.6	15.9	1
Cheeseburger, Double Decker, Rustlers*	1 Burger/237g	645	36.3	272	14.6	18	15.3	0
Cheeseburger, Micro Snack, Tesco*	1 Burger/115g	309	14.5	269	12.6	26.4	12.6	0
Cheeseburger, Quarter Pounder, Rustlers*	1 Burger/190g	505	25.1	266	13.6	22.4	13.2	0
Cheeseburger, Smart Price, Asda*	1 Burger/150g	374	14	249	13.3	28	9.3	1.4
Cheeseburger, Speedy Snacks*	1 Burger/147g	404	18.2	275	13.2	26.6	12.4	0
Cheeseburger, with Sesame Seed Bun, Tesco*	1 Burger/275g	644	32.2	234	12.2	20.1	11.7	2
Chicken, & Sweetcorn, Nacho, Asda*	½ Pack/144g	249	13	173	14	9	9	2.3
Chicken, Beef, Halal, Tahira*	1 Burger/65g	172	13	264	11	10	20	0
Chicken, Average	*1 Burger/46g*	*111*	*5.6*	*242*	*14.9*	*18.7*	*12.1*	*1*
Chicken, Breaded, Value, Tesco*	1 Burger/57g	165	10.8	290	10.5	19.2	19	1.4
Chicken, Cajun, Fillets, Birds Eye*	1 Pack/180g	275	8.8	153	21.5	5.8	4.9	0.3
Chicken, Cooked, Butcher's Choice, Sainsbury's*	1 Burger/97g	142	4.8	147	20	5.5	5	0.5
Chicken, Crunch & Fries, M&S*	1 Pack/425g	915	47.6	215	8.8	20.8	11.2	2.1
Chicken, Crunch Crumb, Tesco*	1 Burger/57g	161	10.8	282	12.3	15.6	18.9	0
Chicken, Fillets, Weight After Cooking, Birds Eye*	1 Burger/90g	126	4.1	140	20	5.1	4.6	0.2
Chicken, Fresh, Non Coated, Waitrose*	1 Burger/100g	141	4	141	16	10.4	4	0.9
Chicken, Golden Breadcrumbs, Frozen, Birds Eye*	1 Burger/56g	130	6.9	232	13.8	16.4	12.4	0.3
Chicken, Italia, Grilled, Heck*	1 Burger/114g	121	2.6	106	18.7	1.5	2.3	0
Chicken, Quarter Pounders, Birds Eye*	1 Burger/117g	280	16.1	239	13.5	15.2	13.8	0.6
Chicken, Sainsbury's*	1 Burger/46g	115	7	247	15.6	12.2	15.1	1.3
Chicken, Souther Fried, Microwavable, Snack'In, Iceland*	1 Pack/129g	321	7.5	249	11.8	36.4	5.8	1.8
Chicken, Southern Fried, Heat 'Em Up, Tesco*	1 Burger/111g	309	14.4	278	10	29	13	2.5
Chicken, Southern Fried, Sainsbury's*	1 Burger/52g	154	10.3	297	12.6	17.2	19.8	1.3
Chicken, Southern Fried, Snax On The Go*	1 Burger/132g	318	11.1	241	11.9	28.8	8.4	1.3
Chicken, Spar*	1 Burger/67g	163	7.5	244	16.1	20.8	11.2	1.5
Chicken, Speedy Snacks*	1 Burger/142g	354	12.9	249	10.3	30.4	9.1	0
Chicken, Style, Vegetarian, Quorn*	1 Burger/60g	122	5.1	205	12.1	16.5	8.6	6.6
Chicken, with Sesame Seed Bun, Breaded, Tesco*	1 Burger/205g	588	32.2	287	10.2	26.2	15.7	2.9
Chicken, Zesty, Grilled, Heck*	1 Burger/114g	165	2.2	145	25.2	8.1	1.9	0
Cod, Fish Fillet, Breaded, Birds Eye*	1 Burger/118g	241	8.6	204	13	21	7.3	1
Crocodile, Exotic Meat Feast, Kezie, Iceland*	1 Burger/110g	187	9.7	170	15.2	7.5	8.8	0
Economy, Smart Price, Asda*	1 Burger/49g	142	10.2	293	14	12	21	1.1
Falafel, Quinoa Fresh Cilantro, Fry's*	1 Burger/65g	128	5	197	7.8	19.8	7.7	8.8
Fish Fillet, Breaded, Tesco*	1 Burger/73g	148	6.3	203	12.5	18.2	8.6	1.5
Fish Fillet, Hot Spicy, Oven Baked, Birdseye*	1 Burger/116g	234	9	202	12.2	20.3	7.8	0.9
Goat's Cheese, Gourmet, as Sold, Heck*	1 Burger/114g	290	14.6	254	9	28.3	12.8	4.9
Hot & Spicy, Vegan, Quorn*	1 Burger/66g	118	2.6	179	10.9	23	4	3.7

BURGERS

	Measure INFO/WEIGHT	per Measure KCAL	FAT	Nutrition Values per 100g / 100ml KCAL	PROT	CARB	FAT	FIBRE
Kale, Quinoa, Vegetarian, Strong Roots*	1 Burger/75g	151	8.5	201	4.2	19.5	11.3	2.4
Lamb, Minted, Asda*	1 Burger/100g	234	14	234	22	4.9	14	0.3
Lamb, Minted, Average	*1 Burger/56g*	*125*	*7.4*	*223*	*20.6*	*5.5*	*13.2*	*0.2*
Lamb, Minted, Grilled, Specially Selected, Aldi*	1 Burger/92g	223	14.7	242	17	6.4	16	0.5
Lamb, Minted, Quarter Pounders, Asda*	1 Burger/114g	241	14	212	19.2	6.1	12.3	0
Lamb, Moroccan Spiced, Waitrose*	1 Burger/88g	215	13.2	245	16.9	10.5	15	0.1
Lamb, Quarter Pounder, Average	*1 Burger/113g*	*283*	*19.3*	*250*	*17.4*	*5.2*	*17.1*	*0.8*
Lamb, Quarter Pounders, Asda*	1 Burger/85g	213	13.9	251	20.9	5.2	16.3	0.9
Lamb, Quarter Pounders, Birds Eye*	1 Burger/112g	232	16.9	207	13.9	3.8	15.1	0.3
Lamb, Waitrose*	1 Burger/67g	99	4.7	148	15.7	5.4	7	0.9
Lentil, Beetroot, Veggie, M&S*	1 Burger/120g	191	5.9	159	12	13.4	4.9	6.8
Manhattan, Amy's Kitchen*	1 Burger/68g	88	2.9	129	3.8	18	4.2	1.8
Meat Free, Average	*¼ Pounder/113g*	*195*	*8.8*	*172*	*17.5*	*7.9*	*7.8*	*3*
Meat Free, Sainsbury's*	1 Burger/45g	67	1.8	149	19.1	6.4	4	5.6
Meat Free, Spicy, Bean Nacho, Cooked, Asda*	1 Burger/113g	247	9.6	218	5.3	27.7	8.5	4.7
Meat Free, Traditional, Fry's*	1 Burger/80g	119	4.5	148	14	7.4	5.6	6.2
Mushroom, & Spinach, Cooked, Love Veg, Sainsbury's*	1 Burger/97g	184	10.3	189	15.8	6.3	10.6	2.3
Mushroom, & Spinach, Grilled, Linda McCartney*	1 Burger/104g	188	7.8	181	13.6	11.3	7.5	6.9
Mushroom, & Wensleydale Cheese, Cauldron Foods*	1 Burger/87g	156	9.6	179	9	11	11	4
Mushroom, Cauldron Foods*	1 Burger/88g	125	5.5	143	5.5	16.1	6.3	2.6
Mushroom, Crunchy Quinoa, Parsley, Pepper, Tesco*	1 Burger/123g	230	4	188	8.1	25.8	3.3	11.2
Mushroom, Portobello, Creamy, Smoky, Waitrose*	1 Burger/120g	130	8.2	108	5	6	6.8	1.4
Ostrich, Quarter Pounder, Oslinc*	1 Burger/113g	132	1.5	117	22.9	3.5	1.3	1.1
Pork, Free Range, Waitrose*	1 Burger/115g	306	19.9	266	19.3	7.7	17.3	1
Pork, & Apple, Grilled, Finest, Tesco*	1 Burger/88g	251	18.4	285	14.3	9.6	20.9	1.2
Pork, & Apple, Quarter Pounder, Grilled, Asda*	1 Burger/80g	147	6.4	184	23.9	4.1	8	0.5
Pork, Chorizo, Quarter Pounders, Tesco*	1 Burger/88g	240	15.8	273	21.1	5.9	18	1.3
Pork, Chorizo Sliders, Cooked, TTD, Sainsbury's*	1 Burger/36g	134	8.5	377	17.2	22.3	23.8	2.2
Pork, Hog Roast, Waitrose*	1 Burger/190g	481	29.8	253	17.2	9.9	15.7	1.8
Pork, Pulled, Quarter Pounder, Grilled, Linda McCartney*	1 Burger/97g	150	4.5	154	16.1	11.1	4.6	2
Pork, Quarter Pounders, Birds Eye*	1 Burger/122g	292	23.2	239	13.9	3.2	19	0.2
Pumpkin, Spinach, Vegetarian, Strong Roots*	1 Burger/80g	162	7.5	202	3.9	24.6	9.3	2.3
Pumpkin, Sweet Potato, Vegetarian, Vivera*	1 Burger/99g	98	3	99	5.1	10.3	3	5.4
Quarter Pounder, Average	*1 Burger/113g*	*210*	*9.8*	*186*	*9.1*	*17.7*	*8.6*	*3.2*
Quarter Pounder, Beef Style, Sainsbury's*	1 Burger/114g	216	10.8	190	20	6	9.5	2.5
Quarter Pounder, Chargrilled, BGTY, Sainsbury's*	1 Burger/114g	184	6.3	161	20.8	7.1	5.5	1.1
Quarter Pounder, Chargrilled, Tesco*	1 Burger/114g	186	9.1	164	16	7	8	2.5
Quarter Pounder, Chilli, Asda*	1 Burger/88g	221	14	252	25	2	14	0
Quarter Pounder, Chilli, Farmfoods*	1 Burger/115g	285	23.3	248	13.5	2.9	20.3	0.9
Quarter Pounder, Chilli, Iceland*	1 Burger/84g	265	20.1	316	18.6	6.5	23.9	0.4
Quarter Pounder, Iceland*	1 Burger/83g	253	18.8	305	20.4	5.1	22.6	0.6
Quarter Pounder, Loved by Us, Co-Op*	1 Burger/114g	301	23.9	265	19	0.5	21	0
Quarter Pounder, Mexican Style, Quorn*	1 Burger/113g	180	6.3	159	18.3	8.9	5.6	3.8
Quarter Pounder, Mozzarella, Vegetarian, Linda McCartney*	1 Burger/98g	238	13.5	243	18.2	10.3	13.8	2.3
Quarter Pounder, Quorn*	1 Burger/114g	170	6.8	150	14.4	7.7	6	4
Quarter Pounder, Steak, Deluxe, Lidl*	1 Burger/98g	237	17.6	242	18	2.1	18	0
Quarter Pounder, with Cheese & Buns, Sainsbury's*	1 Burger/198g	471	22.8	238	15.6	19.1	11.5	1.4
Quarter Pounder, with Cheese, Flame Grilled, Feasters*	1 Burger/200g	550	19.8	275	17.2	22.1	9.9	0.9
Quarter Pounder, with Onion, Tesco*	1 Burger/88g	277	19.5	315	20.3	8.5	22.2	0.5
Quinoa, Sweet Potato, Lentil, Vegetarian, Sainsbury's*	1 Burger/88g	168	8.2	192	4.7	19.3	9.4	5.8
Salmon, Quarter Pounders, Tesco*	1 Burger/114g	145	2.7	128	15.9	10.6	2.4	1.2
Salmon, Smoky BBQ, The Grill, M&S*	1 Burger/90g	175	8.4	194	16.4	10.3	9.3	1.7
Salmon, Tesco*	1 Burger/100g	101	3	101	18.2	0.3	3	0

B

	Measure INFO/WEIGHT	per Measure KCAL	FAT	Nutrition Values per 100g / 100ml KCAL	PROT	CARB	FAT	FIBRE
BURGERS								
Steak, Peppered, M&S*	1 Burger/114g	310	24.4	272	18.8	0.8	21.4	0.7
Steak, Ribeye, Donald Russell*	1 Burger/200g	506	39.6	253	18.8	0	19.8	0
Steak, Rump, The Grill, M&S*	1 Burger/169g	330	20.6	195	18.7	2.6	12.2	1.1
Steak, Scotch, Quarter Pounder, Grilled, Deluxe, Lidl*	1 Burger/93g	236	16	254	21.5	3.3	17.2	0
Steak, with Cheese Melt, COOK!, M&S*	1 Burger/196g	480	35.7	245	18.4	2.3	18.2	0.2
Sweet Potato, & Blackbean, Coles*	1 Burger/125g	229	1.2	183	7.1	33	1	5.9
Sweet Potato, & Edamame, Meat Free, Morrisons*	1 Burger/88g	144	8	164	6.4	10.6	9.1	7.2
Sweet Potato, with Piri Piri Glaze, Frozen, Iceland*	1 Burger/140g	264	9.1	188	3.8	24.6	6.5	8.1
Sweetcorn, Chickpea, M&S*	1 Burger/120g	200	5.2	167	5.7	21.8	4.3	9.1
Turkey, Cheeseburgers, Tesco*	1 Burger/105g	252	14.8	240	15.4	12.8	14.1	1.3
Turkey, Crispy Crumb, Bernard Matthews*	1 Burger/60g	158	9.5	263	12.6	17.5	15.8	1.8
Turkey, Harvestland*	1 Burger/112g	179	9	160	23	1	8	0
Turkey, Sea Salt & Pepper, Butchers Selection, Asda*	1 Burger/96g	141	4.4	147	23	3.2	4.6	0.5
Vegan, Onion Bhaji, Frozen, As Consumed, Tesco*	1 Burger/117g	167	8.5	143	3.5	12.3	7.3	7.1
Vegan, Vivera*	1 Burger/100g	169	7.3	169	18.5	4.8	7.3	5
Vegeburger, Linda McCartney*	1 Burger/50g	62	1.4	124	15.8	10.7	2.9	5.8
Vegeburger, Retail, Grilled	**1oz/28g**	**55**	**3.1**	**196**	**16.6**	**8**	**11.1**	**4.2**
Vegetable, Average	**1 Burger/56g**	**100**	**4.5**	**179**	**4.4**	**22.4**	**8**	**2.3**
Vegetable, Captains, Birds Eye*	1 Burger/48g	96	4.2	200	4.7	25.5	8.8	2
Vegetable, Organic, Goodlife*	1 Burger/67g	114	3.9	170	3.2	26.3	5.8	2.6
Vegetable, Organic, Tesco*	1 Burger/90g	108	3.9	120	2.6	17.6	4.3	2.1
Vegetable, Quarter Pounders, Crisp & Golden, Waitrose*	1 Burger/113g	236	8.8	209	4.8	28.2	7.8	3.4
Vegetable, Quarter Pounders, Crunchy, Birds Eye*	1 Burger/114g	240	11.6	211	4.8	24.9	10.2	1.8
Vegetable, Quarter Pounders, Dalepak*	1 Burger/114g	227	9.6	200	4.8	26.3	8.5	1.8
Vegetable, Quarter Pounders, Meat Free, Vegan, Tesco*	1 Burger/106g	229	10.6	216	3.7	25.8	10	3.9
Vegetable, Spicy, Asda*	1 Burger/56g	108	6.2	193	3.4	20	11	0
Vegetable, Tesco*	2 Burgers/108g	178	5.9	165	2.9	23.7	5.5	4.9
Vegetarian, Flame Grilled, Linda McCartney*	1 Burger/60g	104	3.1	174	17.9	13.8	5.2	3.3
Vegetarian, Frozen, Grilled, Quorn*	1 Burger/50g	87	4	174	15.7	7.4	8.1	4.7
Vegetarian, Lamb, Style, Minted, Quorn*	1 Burger/80g	86	3.2	108	12	6	4	4
Vegetarian, Peri Peri, Frozen, Linda McCartney*	1 Burger/113g	251	9.7	222	20.8	14.7	8.6	4.1
Vegetarian, Quarter Pounders, Grilled, Linda McCartney*	1 Burger/105g	232	12.5	220	17.3	9.8	11.9	2.4
Vegetarian, Savoury, Cauldron Foods*	1 Burger/88g	145	8	166	108	7.9	9.2	2.4
Vegetarian, Sizzling, Quorn*	1 Burger/80g	123	4.8	154	18	7	6	3
Vegetarian, Smoked Chilli & Lime, Chef's Selection, Quorn*	1 Burger/90g	147	6.3	163	17	6.6	7	3
Venison, Sweet Onion, M&S*	1 Burger/142g	163	5	115	19.3	1.4	3.5	0.5
Venison, As Sold, Tesco*	1 Burger/113g	149	4	132	19.3	5.5	3.5	0.5
Venison, British Food, Sainsbury's*	1 Burger/64g	130	6.1	203	22.6	6	9.6	0.8
Venison, Finnebrogue Estate*	1 Burger/142g	170	7	120	19.9	4.2	4.9	0.5
Venison, Grilled, Extra Special, Asda*	2 Burgers/227g	331	8.2	146	21.5	5.3	3.6	3.2
Venison, Grilled, Tesco*	1 Burger/96g	149	4	155	22.8	6.2	4.2	0.5
Venison, Lightly Seasoned, As Consumed, Waitrose*	1 Burger/95g	159	6.2	168	23.8	3.3	6.6	0.1
Venison, Spirit of Summer, M&S*	1 Burger/90g	121	5.1	134	17.8	2.8	5.6	0.5
Zebra, Cooked, Kezie*	1 Burger/110g	160	3.8	145	25.3	2.2	3.5	0
BURRITO								
Beef	**1 Serving/225g**	**536**	**20.2**	**238**	**12**	**27**	**9**	**2.2**
Beef, Chilli, As Consumed, Morrisons*	½ Pack/200g	368	16	184	8.9	17.7	8	2.7
Beef, Chilli, Cooked, World Cafe, Waitrose*	½ Pack/87g	169	5.5	195	8.8	24.4	6.3	2.5
Beef, Chilli, with Sour Cream, Good to Go, Waitrose*	1 Pack/241g	431	12.8	179	7.5	23.7	5.3	3.2
Beef, Mix, Vegetarian, Linda McCartney*	1 Serving/200g	240	7.8	120	6.2	12.7	3.9	4.5
Beef, Spicy, Tex Mex, Tesco*	1 Burrito/192g	326	8.4	170	6.5	24.8	4.4	2.6
Black Bean, Chilli, Everdine*	1 Serving/450g	594	14.4	132	4.2	19.4	3.2	4.5
Chicken, On the Go, Sainsbury's*	1 Burrito/310g	511	15.5	165	8.1	21	5	2

	Measure INFO/WEIGHT	per Measure KCAL	FAT	Nutrition Values per 100g / 100ml KCAL	PROT	CARB	FAT	FIBRE
BURRITO								
Pork, Pulled, BBQ, Scratch, Waitrose*	½ Pack/404g	654	18.6	162	10.1	18.2	4.6	0
Veg Medley, Bowl, Musclefood*	1 Serving/435g	344	7.8	79	5.6	8.4	1.8	3.6
BUTTER								
Almond, 100%, Sainsbury's*	1 Tbsp/20g	128	10.9	639	29.3	4.3	54.4	7.6
Brandy, Average	*1 Serving/10g*	*56*	*3.8*	*556*	*0.2*	*46.2*	*38.4*	*0.1*
Cashew, Pip Nut*	1 Serving/15g	87	6.6	580	18	27	44	0
Coconut, Artisana*	2 Tbsp/32g	186	18	574	6.2	21.6	55.5	15.4
Creamery, Average	*1 Serving/10g*	*74*	*8.1*	*736*	*0.5*	*0.4*	*81.4*	*0*
Fresh, Average	*1 Thin Spread/7g*	*51*	*5.7*	*735*	*0.6*	*0.4*	*81.3*	*0*
Garlic, Crushed, Lurpak*	1 Serving/10g	69	7.5	692	1.3	3.7	75	0
Goat's, St Helen's Farm*	1 Thin Spread/7g	56	6.2	794	0.5	0	88	0
Granules, Butter Buds*	1 Tsp/1.4g	5	0.1	368	1.8	77.9	6.5	2.3
Nut, Cashew, with Peanuts, Sea Salt, M&S*	1 Tsp/5g	33	2.9	664	15.3	20.1	57.3	3.2
Reduced Fat, Fresh, Average	*1 Thin Spread/7g*	*26*	*2.8*	*368*	*2.3*	*1.2*	*39.4*	*0.2*
Salted, Average	*1 Thin Spread/7g*	*51*	*5.7*	*729*	*0.4*	*0.3*	*81.1*	*0*
Spreadable, Fresh, Average	*1 Thin Spread/7g*	*51*	*5.7*	*730*	*0.4*	*0.3*	*80.8*	*0*
Spreadable, Reduced Fat, Average	*1 Thin Spread/7g*	*38*	*4.2*	*540*	*0.5*	*0.5*	*60*	*0*
with Olive Oil, Lighter, Spreadable, Lurpak*	1 Thin Spread/7g	38	4.2	543	0.3	0.4	60	0
BUTTERMILK								
Average	*1 Mug/400ml*	*177*	*1.3*	*44*	*4.2*	*5.9*	*0.3*	*0*
BUTTERNUT SQUASH								
& Red Onion, Quick Roast, M&S*	1 Pack/340g	109	0.3	32	1	6	0.1	1.5
Sweet Potato, Lets Cook, Aldi*	1 Portion/100g	102	5.3	102	1.1	11	5.3	0
Chips, Crinkle Cut, Cooked, Sainsbury's*	½ Pack/95g	66	0.9	70	2.2	11.7	0.9	3.1
Frozen, Tesco*	1 Serving/80g	35	0.6	43	1.5	6.6	0.7	2.3
Fusilli, Tesco*	1 Pack/250g	98	0.2	39	1.1	7.7	0.1	1.6
Noodles, Ready Prepared, Sainsbury's*	½ Pack/152g	50	0.8	33	1.1	5.8	0.5	1.4
Spaghetti, Tesco*	1 Serving/80g	31	0.1	39	1.1	7.7	0.1	1.6
Squaffles, Cooked, Sainsbury's*	½ Pack/150g	102	2.6	68	1.7	10.4	1.7	2
Wedges, Moroccan Spiced, M&S*	½ Pack/200g	140	5.6	70	2.4	7.1	2.8	2.6
Winter, Boiled, Flesh Only	*1 Serving/80g*	*27*	*0.1*	*34*	*0.7*	*8.8*	*0.1*	*2.6*
Winter, Butternut, Baked, Average	*1 Serving/100g*	*32*	*0.1*	*32*	*0.9*	*7.4*	*0.1*	*1.4*
Winter, Butternut, Raw, Prepared, Average	*1 Serving/80g*	*29*	*0.1*	*36*	*1.1*	*8.3*	*0.1*	*1.6*
Winter, Butternut, Raw, Unprepared, Average	*1 Serving/80g*	*24*	*0.1*	*30*	*0.9*	*6.8*	*0.1*	*1.3*
BUTTONS								
Milk Chocolate, Asda*	1 Bag/70g	368	21	526	7	57	30	1.5
Milk Chocolate, Giant, Dairy Milk, Cadbury*	1 Button/2g	11	0.6	530	7.6	56.5	30.5	0.7
Milk Chocolate, M&S*	1 Pack/75g	375	19	500	8.6	59.8	25.3	1.9
Milk Chocolate, Tesco*	1 Bag/70g	359	19.3	513	7.1	59.1	27.6	2.1
Mixed, White Milk, Dairy Milk, Cadbury*	¼ Bag/28g	150	8.4	536	3.6	60.7	30	1.1
White Chocolate, Co-Op*	½ Pack/35g	186	9.8	530	7	64	28	0
White Chocolate, Dairy Milk, Cadbury*	1 Pack/32g	174	9.5	540	4.7	63	29.5	0
White Chocolate, Milkybar, Nestle*	1 Bag/30g	164	9.5	546	7.5	58.1	31.6	0
White Chocolate, Tesco*	1 Bag/70g	388	23.4	554	5.1	58	33.5	0

B

INFO/WEIGHT	Measure	per Measure		Nutrition Values per 100g / 100ml				
		KCAL	FAT	KCAL	PROT	CARB	FAT	FIBRE
CABBAGE								
& Leek, Crunchy Mix, Ready to Cook, Sainsbury's*	1 Serving/125g	34	0.6	27	1.9	3.7	0.5	2.6
Leek, Ready for Use, Cooked, Sainsbury's*	1 Bag/200g	68	1	34	1.5	4.9	0.5	3.2
Leek, Ready Sliced, Sainsbury's*	1 Pack/240g	53	1.2	22	1.1	2.2	0.5	2.1
Leek, Sliced, Tesco*	1/3 Pack/100g	32	0.6	32	2.1	3.4	0.6	2.6
Boiled, Average	*1 Serving/90g*	*14*	*0.3*	*15*	*1*	*2.2*	*0.3*	*1.7*
Creamed, Cooked, Sainsbury's*	½ Pack/150g	95	6.8	67	2	2.6	4.8	2.5
Greens, Trimmed, Average	*1oz/28g*	*8*	*0.1*	*28*	*2.9*	*3*	*0.5*	*3.4*
Raw, Average	*1 Serving/100g*	*21*	*0.4*	*21*	*1.3*	*3.2*	*0.4*	*1.8*
Red, Beetroot, Mash Direct*	1 Serving/88g	67	2.1	76	1.2	12.4	2.4	2.6
Red, Average	*1 Serving/90g*	*19*	*0.2*	*21*	*1*	*3.7*	*0.3*	*2.2*
Red, Braised with Red Wine, M&S*	½ Pack/150g	180	7.2	120	1.4	17.1	4.8	1
Red, Pickled, Average	*1 Serving/50g*	*13*	*0.1*	*26*	*0.9*	*4.6*	*0.2*	*1.6*
Red, Spiced, Steamer, Sainsbury's*	½ Pack/150g	105	3.3	70	1	10.5	2.2	2.9
Red, with Apple, Bramley, Aunt Bessie's*	1 Serving/125g	72	1.1	58	0.9	10	0.9	2.7
Red, with Apple, Bramley, British, Sainsbury's*	1 Pack/300g	213	1.5	71	1.2	14.9	0.5	2.3
Red, with Apple, Finest, Tesco*	½ Pack/150g	177	8.8	118	1.6	14.7	5.9	4.6
Savoy, Boiled in Salted Water, Average	*1 Serving/90g*	*15*	*0.4*	*17*	*1.1*	*2.2*	*0.5*	*2*
Savoy, Raw, Average	*1 Serving/90g*	*24*	*0.4*	*27*	*2.1*	*3.9*	*0.5*	*3.1*
Spring Greens, Boiled, Average	*1 Serving/80g*	*16*	*0.6*	*20*	*1.9*	*1.6*	*0.7*	*2.6*
Spring Greens, Raw, Average	*1 Serving/80g*	*22*	*0.7*	*28*	*2.5*	*2.6*	*0.8*	*2.9*
Steamed, Average	*1 Serving/100g*	*15*	*0.3*	*15*	*1*	*2.2*	*0.3*	*1.7*
Sweetheart, Raw	*1 Serving/100g*	*26*	*0.6*	*26*	*2.1*	*3.2*	*0.6*	*2.8*
White, Raw, Average	*1oz/28g*	*8*	*0.1*	*27*	*1.4*	*5*	*0.2*	*2.1*
CACAO								
Nibbles, Choc Go*	1 Pack/30g	137	8.8	456	9.6	24	29.5	28
Powder, Natural, 100%, Food Thoughts*	1 Tsp/5g	21	1	418	28.1	14.5	21	31
CAKE								
Almond, Slices, Mr Kipling*	1 Slice/35g	144	6.5	411	6	54.2	18.5	1.8
Almond, Slices, Sainsbury's*	1 Serving/27g	120	7.1	444	5.9	45.9	26.3	1.5
Almond, Slices, Weight Watchers*	1 Slice/26g	95	2.6	365	5.2	63.8	9.9	2.4
Angel, Average	*1 Slice/44g*	*175*	*7.9*	*397*	*4.2*	*54.9*	*17.9*	*0.8*
Angel, Layer, Tesco*	1 Serving/34g	130	5	387	5	57.8	14.8	1.1
Angel, Sainsbury's*	1/8 Cake/41g	171	8.1	417	4.1	55.7	19.8	0.8
Angel, Slices, Mr Kipling*	1 Slice/33g	145	6.1	431	3	63.4	18.2	0.6
Angel, Slices, Snap Packs, Mr Kipling*	1 Slice/34g	148	6.6	417	2.7	60.1	18.5	0.6
Angel, Slices, Tesco*	1 Slice/29g	117	5	407	3.8	57.9	17.4	1.6
Apple, & Blackcurrant, Crumble, Graze*	1 Punnet/33g	121	7.5	365	6.1	34.5	22.7	3.1
Apple, Bramley, & Blackberry Crumble, M&S*	1/8 Cake/56g	221	10	395	4.4	54.1	17.9	1.5
Apple, Crumble, Slices, Weight Watchers*	1 Slice/26g	90	2	346	4.5	64.8	7.7	2.3
Apple, Home Style, M&S*	1 Cake/54g	189	7.9	350	5.3	49.4	14.7	1.5
Apple, Slices, Delightful, Mr Kipling*	1 Slice/29g	92	1.1	317	4.4	66.2	3.9	1.3
Apple, Sticky Toffee, Finest, Tesco*	1 Slice/51g	247	9.2	487	3	52.7	18.1	0.6
Bakewell, Cherry, Co-Op*	1 Cake/47g	205	8	435	3.7	67.2	16.9	1.8
Bakewell, Cherry, Delightful, Mr Kipling*	1 Cake/45g	176	5.8	390	3.9	66.4	12.9	1.2
Bakewell, Cherry, M&S*	1 Cake/44g	185	7.8	420	4.5	61.7	17.7	1
Bakewell, Cherry, Mini, Sainsbury's*	1 Cake/27g	101	3.3	370	3.4	62.2	12	0.4
Bakewell, Cherry, Mr Kipling*	1 Cake/45g	193	8.3	428	3.9	61.3	18.5	1.4
Bakewell, Cherry, Slices, GFY, Asda*	1 Slice/29g	98	0.7	337	3.4	75.4	2.4	0.7
Bakewell, Cherry, Tesco*	1 Cake/39g	171	7.5	439	3.2	63.3	19.2	1.1
Bakewell, Cherry, Waitrose*	1 Cake/44g	184	8.5	419	3.8	57.4	19.3	2.1
Bakewell, Lemon, Average	*1 Cake/42g*	*173*	*6.4*	*411*	*3.7*	*64.6*	*15.2*	*1.3*
Bakewell, Lemon, CBY, Asda*	1 Cake/42g	181	7.3	432	3.8	64.4	17.4	1.4
Bakewell, Lemon, Mr Kipling*	1 Cake/43g	185	7.4	430	3.6	64.4	17.3	1

CAKE

	Measure INFO/WEIGHT	per Measure		Nutrition Values per 100g / 100ml				
		KCAL	FAT	KCAL	PROT	CARB	FAT	FIBRE
Bakewell, Slices, Mr Kipling*	1 Slice/35g	146	6.2	414	4.1	59.2	17.6	1
Bakewell, Slices, Weight Watchers*	1 Slice/26g	84	0.6	324	3.7	71	2.4	2
Bakewell, The Handmade Flapjack Company*	1 Cake/75g	311	17.1	415	4.5	47.4	22.8	0
Banana, Bread, Brilliant, Graze*	1 Cake/23g	72	3.6	312	5.2	40.4	15.6	3
Banana, Iced, Waitrose*	1/6 Cake/55g	190	5.9	345	4.2	58	10.7	2.7
Banana, Loaf, Tesco*	1 Slice/40g	152	6.9	380	5.3	50.3	17.2	1.6
Banana, Loaf, The Best, Morrisons*	1 Serving/75g	273	13.4	364	5.7	44.1	17.9	2
Banana, Loaf, Waitrose*	1 Slice/70g	236	7.5	337	5	55.2	10.7	1.7
Banana, with An Afternoon Tea Infusion, Graze*	1 Punnet/18g	55	2.5	307	5	39	14	3
Bara Brith, Tan Y Castell*	1 Serving/100g	261	1	261	4	58.8	1	1.5
Battenberg, Mini, Mr Kipling*	1 Cake/32g	128	3.2	399	3.8	72.9	10	1.2
Battenberg, Mr Kipling*	1 Serving/38g	161	4.6	421	5	73.3	12	1.6
Birthday, M&S*	1 Serving/60g	240	7.1	400	2.3	70.9	11.9	0.8
Birthday, Piece of Cake, M&S*	1 Serving/85g	395	24.4	465	4.3	39.7	28.7	0.9
Birthday, Present, Tesco*	1 Serving/79g	347	13.9	439	3.5	66.6	17.6	0.4
Butterfly, Mr Kipling*	1 Cake/29g	114	6.4	392	4.4	43.4	22.2	0.6
Caramel, Crunchy, Devondale*	1 Cake/80g	359	19.2	449	2.9	56.3	24	1.3
Caramel, Salted, The Best, Morrisons*	1/6 Cake/63g	262	12.2	416	3.9	56.2	19.4	0.5
Caramel, Shortcake, Slices, McVitie's*	1 Slice /32g	146	7.7	463	4.3	56.5	24.4	1.6
Caramel, Slices, M&S*	1 Slice/64g	304	16.1	475	4.9	60.4	25.2	2.6
Carrot, & Orange, Extra Special, Asda*	1/6 Cake/65g	240	11.7	369	4.7	47	18	0.9
Carrot, & Orange, Finest, Tesco*	1/8 Cake/50g	205	10.2	410	4.6	51.2	20.5	2.1
Carrot, & Orange, Waitrose*	1/6 Cake/47g	164	7.4	350	5.3	46.8	15.7	1.8
Carrot, & Walnut, Aldi*	¼ Cake/100g	409	23	409	5.1	44	23	2.2
Carrot, & Walnut, Layered, Asda*	1 Serving/42g	172	8	409	4.6	55	19	1
Carrot, & Walnut, Mini Classics, Mr Kipling*	1 Cake/39g	172	9.8	440	4.5	48.6	25.2	1
Carrot, Average	*1 Slice/56g*	*211*	*10.4*	*377*	*4.6*	*47.6*	*18.6*	*1.4*
Carrot, Entenmann's*	1 Serving/40g	156	8.2	391	4.1	47.4	20.5	1.5
Carrot, Free From, Finest, Tesco*	1 Slice/67g	288	17.7	429	3	43.3	26.3	3.5
Carrot, GF , Finest, Tesco*	1 Serving/50g	204	10.4	407	3.4	50.4	20.9	1.9
Carrot, Handmade, Delicious, Boots*	1 Slice/75g	292	13.5	389	4.1	53	18	1.4
Carrot, Iced, Tesco*	1 Serving/61g	246	12	404	3.1	53.7	19.6	1.6
Carrot, Lidl*	1/6 Cake/71g	280	13.7	394	4.7	48.9	19.3	3
Carrot, McVitie's*	1/9 of Cake/24g	87	3.5	360	4.8	52.8	14.4	2.3
Carrot, Mini, Weight Watchers*	1 Cake/31g	120	3.3	388	3.7	68.9	10.8	2.7
Carrot, Organic, Respect Organics*	1 Slice/45g	179	10.1	398	3.1	47.4	22.4	1.5
Carrot, Slices, Asda*	1 Slice/80g	302	13.2	377	3.4	53.8	16.5	1.7
Carrot, Slices, Inspirations, Mr Kipling*	1 Slice/34g	139	6.3	411	3.5	57.7	18.5	1.3
Carrot, Slices, Less Than 3% Fat, BGTY, Sainsbury's*	1 Slice/30g	94	0.8	313	3.4	68.7	2.7	2.4
Carrot, Slices, Weight Watchers*	1 Slice/27g	84	0.2	311	2.8	73	0.8	0.9
Carrot, Super, Graze*	1 Punnet/31g	102	4.9	330	4.1	46.5	15.7	3.5
Carrot, The Best, Morrisons*	1/6 Cake/64g	255	12.5	398	4.3	50	19.5	2.5
Carrot, TTD, Sainsbury's*	1 Slice/72g	287	13.7	398	4.5	51.1	19	2.5
Carrot, Wedge, Tesco*	1 Pack/175g	532	27.6	304	3.9	36.6	15.8	1.5
Carrot, with Cream Cheese Icing, On the Go, Sainsbury's*	1 Cake/64g	251	11.9	392	4.3	51.5	18.6	1
Cherry, Co-Op*	1/8 Cake/47g	190	8.5	405	4	57	18	0.8
Cherry, Linda Kearns*	1 Serving/100g	265	14.2	265	12.1	29.9	14.2	4.2
Cherry, M&S*	1 Serving/75g	285	9.5	380	5	60.6	12.7	0.8
Chocolate	*1oz/28g*	*128*	*7.4*	*456*	*7.4*	*50.4*	*26.4*	*1.7*
Chocolate Chip, Co-Op*	1/6 Cake/63g	275	16.9	440	5	44	27	0.5
Chocolate Chip, Slices, Mr Kipling*	1 Slice/25g	109	5.1	442	6.2	57.4	20.5	1.6
Chocolate Chip, The Cake Shop*	1 Cake/35g	178	11	508	4.7	50.2	31.5	1.1
Chocolate Slices, Mr Kipling*	1 Slice/32g	132	6	411	3.4	56.3	18.7	1.7

CAKE

INFO/WEIGHT	Measure	per Measure		Nutrition Values per 100g / 100ml				
		KCAL	FAT	KCAL	PROT	CARB	FAT	FIBRE
Chocolate, & Blood Orange, Bars, Lunchbox, Soreen*	1 Bar/30g	105	2.5	349	8.9	57.5	8.2	5.2
Chocolate, & Caramel Tiffin Bites, Gu*	1 Tiffin/35g	168	9.9	480	3.8	51.9	28.3	2.8
Chocolate, & Madeira, Marble Loaf, M&S*	1/6 Cake/88g	380	20.4	430	5	50	23.1	1
Chocolate, & Orange, Rolls, M&S*	1 Cake/60g	228	17	380	3.6	27	28.4	1.3
Chocolate, & Orange, Slices, GFY, Asda*	1 Serving/30g	95	0.8	315	3.2	70	2.5	1.3
Chocolate, Belgian, Waitrose*	1 Slice/55g	244	12.7	447	5.2	53.1	23.3	2
Chocolate, Birthday, Tesco*	1 Serving/54g	229	13.2	425	5.9	45.5	24.4	2.1
Chocolate, Box, Asda*	1 Serving/60g	263	13.8	439	5	53	23	0.7
Chocolate, Brownie, Devondale*	1 Cake/60g	246	12.9	410	4.4	51	21.5	2.1
Chocolate, Brownie, Fudge, Entenmann's*	1/8 Cake/55g	168	2.4	306	4	62.7	4.4	1.5
Chocolate, Caterpillar, Tesco*	1 Serving/54g	221	9.2	410	4.8	57.8	17.1	2.6
Chocolate, Celebration, Tesco *	1 Slice/61g	281	15.5	462	5.2	51.9	25.5	2.1
Chocolate, Crispy Clusters, Mini, Tesco*	1 Cluster/8g	37	1.5	470	7	67.8	18.7	2.5
Chocolate, Double, Ganache, M&S*	1/12 Cake/61g	281	16.8	460	5.9	46.1	27.6	2.5
Chocolate, Free From, Finest, Tesco*	1 Slice/64g	279	16.1	438	4.1	46.9	25.3	3.2
Chocolate, Fresh Cream, Flake, Cadbury*	1 Slice/54g	174	8.4	323	4.9	39.8	15.6	1.9
Chocolate, Fudge	*1 Serving/110g*	*415*	*19.1*	*377*	*4.4*	*50.4*	*17.4*	*1.4*
Chocolate, Fudge Slice, Waitrose*	1 Slice/60g	230	9.7	383	4.7	54.6	16.2	1.5
Chocolate, Fudge, & Vanilla Cream, M&S*	1/6 Cake/69g	310	17.9	450	5.2	49.8	26	1.3
Chocolate, Fudge, Alabama, Morrisons*	1/6 Cake/58g	195	6.4	337	4.5	55.1	11	2.3
Chocolate, Fudge, Belgian, TTD, Sainsbury's*	1 Avg Slice/66g	282	14.3	428	4.4	52.5	21.7	2.5
Chocolate, Fudge, Classics, M&S*	1 Serving/71g	195	7.5	275	2.8	42.8	10.6	1.1
Chocolate, Fudge, Hot, Frozen, Tesco*	1 Slice/75g	255	10.7	341	5.7	46	14.3	2.9
Chocolate, Happy Birthday, Tesco*	1 Serving/58g	241	13.2	415	4.7	46.9	22.7	2.9
Chocolate, Heaven, Extra Special, Asda*	1/6 Cake/66g	255	13.1	388	4	48	20	1
Chocolate, Iced, Tesco*	1 Serving/40g	158	6.3	395	4.7	58.5	15.8	1.8
Chocolate, Individual with Mini Eggs, Cadbury*	1 Cake/26g	119	6.1	455	4.6	57.5	23.1	1.3
Chocolate, Indulgence, Finest, Tesco*	1 Slice/51g	207	9.1	405	4.8	55.9	17.9	1.2
Chocolate, Large, Happy Birthday, Tesco*	1/14 Cake/63g	291	16	462	4.2	53.4	25.4	1.7
Chocolate, Log, Mini, Free From, Sainsbury's*	1 Slice/45g	202	10.8	450	5.6	51	24	3
Chocolate, Mini Roll, Bites, Tesco*	1 Bite/18g	78	3.6	435	6	58	19.8	1.9
Chocolate, Mousse, Galaxy, Mars*	1 Serving/71g	250	15.5	354	5.3	33	22	0
Chocolate, Orange, Sponge, Asda*	1 Serving/70g	298	18.2	425	4.9	42.9	26	3
Chocolate, Party, M&S*	1 Serving/61g	240	12.6	395	4.6	46.9	20.8	1.1
Chocolate, Party, Tesco*	1 Slice/62g	244	13.1	394	4.6	46.3	21.2	0.9
Chocolate, Rice Crispy, Knightsbridge, Lidl*	1 Cake/24g	88	4.2	368	3.9	48.7	17.5	0.1
Chocolate, Rich, Christmas, Tesco*	1 Slice/82g	300	13.5	367	7	47.5	16.5	1.6
Chocolate, Roll, Triple, Cadbury*	1 Serving/40g	165	6.7	410	4.3	60.1	16.6	1.5
Chocolate, Sainsbury's*	1 Serving/30g	118	5.6	395	4.1	52.6	18.5	1.3
Chocolate, Sensation, Sainsbury's*	1 Serving/92g	320	17.7	348	3.7	40	19.2	2.3
Chocolate, Sponge, Morrisons*	1 Serving/59g	179	7.6	303	4.4	42.5	12.8	0.7
Chocolate, Sponge, Tesco*	1 Serving/37g	129	3.6	358	5.1	60.8	10.1	1.7
Chocolate, Sponge, Victoria, Co-Op*	1 Slice/61g	201	9.8	330	5	42	16	1
Chocolate, The Best, Morrisons*	1/6 Cake/69g	294	15	426	4.3	52.5	21.7	1.5
Chocolate, The Handmade Flapjack Company*	1 Cake/75g	303	16.2	404	12.5	39.8	21.6	0
Chocolate, Thorntons*	1 Serving/87g	408	25.1	469	5.2	47.1	28.8	0.6
Chocolate, Triple Layer, Celebration, Tesco*	1/24 of cake/79g	345	18.8	430	5	47.7	23.4	2.8
Chocolate, Truffle, Mini, Finest, Tesco*	1 Cake/28g	125	6.6	448	5.9	52.9	23.7	0.3
Chocolate, with Butter Icing, Average	*1oz/28g*	*135*	*8.3*	*481*	*5.7*	*50.9*	*29.7*	*0*
Chorley, Asda*	1 Cake/60g	269	12.6	449	6	59	21	2.2
Christmas, Bites, M&S*	1 Bite/21g	75	1.7	359	4	66.5	8.3	1.1
Christmas, Connoisseur, M&S*	1 Slice/60g	216	5.5	360	4.1	64.7	9.2	3.3
Christmas, Fruit, Iced, Bar, Bakers Selection, Asda*	1 Serving/67g	233	5.3	349	3.8	64	7.9	2.5

CAKE

	Measure INFO/WEIGHT	per Measure KCAL	per Measure FAT	Nutrition Values per 100g / 100ml KCAL	PROT	CARB	FAT	FIBRE
Christmas, Iced Fruit, Decorative, Bakers Selection, Asda*	1/12 Cake/76g	276	8.3	365	4.6	62	11	1.4
Christmas, Iced Rich Fruit, Finest, Tesco*	1/8 Cake/50g	183	4.3	366	4.3	66.4	8.6	3.3
Christmas, Iced, Slices, Tesco*	1 Slice/45g	168	4.4	369	2.9	67.6	9.6	1.2
Christmas, Rich Fruit, Free From, Tesco*	1/12 Cake/75g	284	6.4	376	3	71	8.5	1.6
Christmas, Rich Fruit, Organic, Tesco*	1 Serving/76g	282	7.6	374	3.9	67.1	10	2
Christmas, Rich Fruit, Tesco*	1 Serving/75g	261	7.2	348	3.8	60.6	9.6	2.1
Christmas, Royal Iced, Waitrose*	1/6 Cake/75g	270	4.6	360	3.7	71.3	6.2	2
Christmas, Slices, Mr Kipling*	1 Slice/43g	159	3.8	368	3	68.4	8.8	1.4
Christmas, Top Iced, Rich Fruit , Essential, Waitrose*	1 Slice/75g	278	5.8	368	3.6	69.6	7.7	2.9
Coconut	*1 Slice/70g*	*304*	*16.7*	*434*	*6.7*	*51.2*	*23.8*	*2.5*
Coconut, & Raspberry, M&S*	1 Serving/52g	231	13.9	445	5	45.5	26.8	2.3
Coconut, Delight, Burton's*	1 Cake/21g	89	3.5	424	4	63	16.9	2
Coconut, Snowball, Bobby's*	1 Cake/18g	80	4	436	2.2	57.3	22.1	0
Coconut, Snowball, Tunnock's*	1 Cake/30g	134	6.2	446	4.2	56.7	20.8	3.6
Coconut, Sponge, Mini Classics, Mr Kipling*	1 Cake/38g	155	8.7	409	3.7	47	22.9	0.9
Coffee, & Walnut Slices, HE, Tesco*	1 Slice/23g	69	0.5	301	4.4	65.7	2.3	2.8
Coffee, & Walnut, Mrs Beeton's*	1 Slice/54g	219	13.5	405	3.7	41.4	25	0.3
Coffee, Walnut, Slices, Free From, Tesco*	1 Slice/38g	158	7.3	418	3.5	57.1	19.2	1.2
Coffee, Iced, M&S*	1 Slice/33g	135	6.5	410	4.4	54.5	19.6	1.6
Coffee, Iced, Tesco*	1 Slice/42g	164	6	391	4.4	60.4	14.2	1.9
Coffee, Sponge Roll, M&S*	1/6 Roll/42g	160	7.4	385	3.1	53.1	17.8	1.4
Coffee, The Best, Morrisons*	1/6 Cake/69g	296	13.5	429	3.8	59.1	19.5	0.8
Colin the Caterpillar, M&S*	1 Slice/60g	234	12.8	390	5.3	57.2	21.3	1.3
Cornflake, Average	*1 Cake/18g*	*83*	*3.7*	*464*	*5.2*	*64.6*	*20.4*	*2*
Cornflake, Bobby's*	1/6 Cake/45g	207	9.2	461	3.9	65.5	20.4	0
Cornflake, Chocolate Clusters, Asda*	1 Cake/14g	64	2.6	460	8.2	65.2	18.5	2.7
Cornflake, Chocolate, Mini Bites, Tesco*	1 Bite/14g	62	2.5	446	7.1	64.1	17.9	5.9
Country Farmhouse, Waitrose*	1 Serving/80g	308	12.1	385	4.7	57.5	15.1	1.4
Cream, Oysters, M&S*	1 Cake/72g	227	15.3	315	3.6	27.5	21.2	3
Cream, Slices, M&S*	1 Slice/80g	310	18.3	387	2.3	45.7	22.9	0.6
Date, & Walnut Loaf, Sainsbury's*	1/10 Slice/40g	148	8.2	371	6.7	40.1	20.4	1
Eccles, All Butter, M&S*	1 Cake/86g	345	14.8	400	4.5	57.4	17.2	3.2
Eccles, Fresh Baked	*1 Cake/45g*	*171*	*7.6*	*381*	*4.3*	*56.3*	*17*	*1.5*
Fairy, Average	*1 Cake/23g*	*96*	*4.6*	*416*	*5.1*	*53*	*20.2*	*1.5*
Fairy, Chocolate, Ms Mollys*	1 Cake/23g	95	4.9	413	4.2	49.7	21.4	2.5
Fairy, Iced, Average	*1 Cake/23g*	*91*	*3.4*	*394*	*4.2*	*60.8*	*14.8*	*0.9*
Fairy, Iced, Ms Mollys*	1 Cake/23g	96	4.6	416	4.3	54.3	19.8	1.4
Fairy, Lemon Iced, Average	*1 Cake/23g*	*90*	*3.1*	*393*	*4.4*	*63.2*	*13.6*	*1.1*
Fairy, Plain, Average	*1 Cake/23g*	*95*	*4.6*	*413*	*5.5*	*51.1*	*20.2*	*1.5*
Fairy, Plain, Sainsbury's*	1 Cake/20g	84	4.3	422	4.9	46.4	21.5	1.2
Fairy, Plain, Value, Tesco*	1 Cake/15g	52	1.3	348	5.3	62.4	8.6	0.9
Fairy, Smart Price, Asda*	1 Cake/15g	66	3.3	438	6	54	22	1
Fairy, Snowman, Christmas, Tesco*	1 Cake/24g	114	6.8	471	4.6	49.8	28.1	2.9
Fairy, Strawberry Iced, Tesco*	1 Cake/24g	94	3.2	392	4.9	62.9	13.4	1.4
Fairy, Vanilla Iced, Average, Tesco*	1 Cake/23g	89	2.8	388	4.4	65.1	12.2	1.2
Fairy, Victoria, Sainsbury's*	1 Cake/50g	218	10.8	436	3.7	56.1	21.5	1.3
Farmhouse, Slice, Weight Watchers*	1 Slice/23g	73	0.9	317	5.5	64.9	4	1.3
Flake, Cadbury*	1 Cake/20g	90	4.5	445	6.3	54.5	22.3	0
Fondant Fancies, Lemon, Waitrose*	1 Cake/40g	176	7.1	441	2.5	67.9	17.7	0.6
Fondant Fancies, Sainsbury's*	1 Cake/28g	103	2.5	373	2.7	69.7	9.1	0.7
Fondant, Dark Chocolate, Graze*	1 Pack/40g	157	5.8	393	3.5	66.2	14.5	0
Fondant, with Chocolate, Mini, Delhaize*	1 Cake Mini/20g	88	6.2	440	4.6	36.3	30.8	3.8
French Fancies, Average	*1 Cake/27g*	*100*	*2.5*	*371*	*2.7*	*69.6*	*9.1*	*0.8*

C

CAKE

INFO/WEIGHT	Measure	per Measure		Nutrition Values per 100g / 100ml				
		KCAL	FAT	KCAL	PROT	CARB	FAT	FIBRE
French Fancies, Lemon, Average	*1 Cake/28g*	*106*	*2.7*	*378*	*2.5*	*69.9*	*9.8*	*0.5*
French Fancies, Lemon, Mr Kipling*	1 Cake/28g	106	2.7	378	2.5	69.9	9.8	0.5
French Fancies, Mr Kipling*	1 Cake/28g	106	2.8	378	2.6	69.7	9.9	0.6
French Fancies, Strawberry, Mr Kipling*	1 Cake/28g	106	2.7	379	2.5	70.6	9.6	0.4
Fruit, Iced, Christmas Tree, Tesco*	½ Cake/75g	277	5.6	369	3.5	70.4	7.4	3.2
Fruit, Iced, Slices, Tesco*	1 Slice/50g	171	2.9	342	2.8	68	5.8	3.3
Fruit, Luxury, Fully Iced Slice, The Best, Morrisons*	1 Serving/50g	178	3.8	356	3.7	66.6	7.6	3.1
Fruit, Parisienne, Rich, Finest, Tesco*	1 Serving/69g	262	9.7	380	4.7	55.2	14.1	1.9
Fruit, Petit Cakes Aux Fruits, Bonne Maman*	1 Cake/30g	122	6.3	407	5.4	48	21	0
Fruit, Plain, Average	*1 Slice/90g*	*319*	*11.6*	*354*	*5.1*	*57.9*	*12.9*	*0*
Fruit, Rich, Average	*1 Slice/70g*	*225*	*8.8*	*322*	*4.9*	*50.7*	*12.5*	*1.7*
Fruit, Rich, Golden Bow, TTD, Sainsbury's*	1 Slice/85g	324	7.7	381	3.3	70.3	9	2.7
Fruit, Rich, Iced	*1 Slice/70g*	*249*	*8*	*356*	*4.1*	*62.7*	*11.4*	*1.7*
Fruit, Rich, Iced, Bar, Finest, Tesco*	1 Serving/100g	360	10.7	360	3.8	61.3	10.7	4.2
Fruit, Rich, Iced, Finest, Tesco*	1 Slice/57g	191	4.7	335	3.6	61.2	8.3	4.4
Fruit, Rich, Iced, Top, Sainsbury's*	1 Slice/75g	268	5.3	357	3	69.3	7.1	2.2
Fruit, Rich, M&S*	1 Serving/50g	158	3.2	315	3.1	60.9	6.5	4.3
Fruit, Rich, Slices, Free From, Sainsbury's*	1 Slice/40g	144	5	361	4.5	57.4	12.6	3.7
Fruit, Rich, Tesco*	1 Slice/67g	238	5.7	357	3.6	65.1	8.5	3
Fruit, Slices, Value, Tesco*	1 Slice/23g	84	4	372	4	48.7	17.7	1.3
Fudge, Brownie, The Handmade Flapjack Company*	1 Cake/75g	286	9.2	381	4.9	62.8	12.3	0
Genoa, Tesco*	1 Serving/44g	150	3.9	340	3.7	59.1	8.8	3.1
Ginger, & Syrup, Tesco*	1 Serving/32g	134	7	420	4.5	51.4	21.8	0.7
Ginger, Drizzle, Iced, Co-Op*	1/6 Cake/64g	226	7.7	350	3	58	12	1
Ginger, Jamaica, McVitie's*	1/9 Cake/26g	92	2.6	362	3.7	63.1	10.4	1.6
Ginger, Loaf , Stem, Waitrose*	1 Slice/35g	134	4.8	384	3.7	60.1	13.7	2.6
Ginger, Stem, Mrs Crimble's*	1 Slice/48g	153	1	319	2.5	71	2.1	3.2
Granola, Square, All Butter, Finest, Tesco*	1 Square/72g	322	16.1	447	7.8	50.7	22.4	5.9
Granola, Square, M&S*	1 Square/72g	330	18.1	464	7.9	49.3	25.5	5
Lemon, & Orange, Finest, Tesco*	1 Serving/53g	216	10.7	410	4.5	52.4	20.3	1.1
Lemon, Average	*1 Slice/81g*	*320*	*14.5*	*396*	*4.1*	*54.8*	*18*	*0.6*
Lemon, Buttercream & Lemon Curd, The Cake Shop*	1 Cake/28g	124	7.8	444	3.5	43.4	27.8	0.6
Lemon, Drizzle Cake, Asda*	1 Serving/50g	150	6	299	2.8	45	12	0.4
Lemon, Drizzle, Classic, M&S*	1 Serving/100g	333	13.6	333	4	47.5	13.6	2.2
Lemon, Drizzle, Finest, Tesco*	1 Slice/68g	266	11.2	391	3.6	56.3	16.5	1.6
Lemon, Drizzle, The Best, Morrisons*	1/6 Cake/72g	287	11.8	398	3.2	59.1	16.3	1.1
Lemon, Half Moon, Bobby's*	1/6 Cake/60g	244	11	406	4.1	55.7	18.4	0
Lemon, Loaf, M&S*	1 Slice/47g	190	8.8	400	2.1	55.8	18.6	0.6
Lemon, Madeira, Half Moon, Dan Cake*	1 Slice/50g	215	10	430	3.5	59	20	0
Lemon, Slices, Free From, Tesco*	1 Slice/38g	156	6.6	410	3	59.5	17.5	1
Lemon, Slices, Iced, Tesco*	1 Slice/29g	114	4.9	394	3	56.1	17.1	2
Lemon, Slices, Low Fat, Weight Watchers*	1 Slice/26g	79	0.5	303	3.1	68.1	2	2.2
Lemon, Slices, Mr Kipling*	1 Slice/33g	135	5.1	409	2.7	64.2	15.5	0.7
Lemon, Slices, Sainsbury's*	1 Slice/30g	130	6.3	432	4.1	56	20.9	1.7
Leo the Lion, Birthday, Asda*	1 Slice/81g	325	12.9	402	2.6	62	16	0.5
Madeira	*1 Slice/40g*	*157*	*6.8*	*393*	*5.4*	*58.4*	*16.9*	*0.9*
Madeira, All Butter, Sainsbury's*	1 Serving/30g	116	5.9	388	5.2	47.4	19.7	0.8
Madeira, Cherry, Tesco*	1 Serving/38g	135	4.2	357	4.6	58.9	11	1.8
Madeira, Iced, Sainsbury's*	1/8 Cake/47g	182	6.6	388	3.6	61.6	14.1	0.7
Madeira, Iced, Tesco*	1 Slice/40g	157	5.8	393	3.8	60.7	14.6	1.7
Madeira, Lemon Iced, Co-Op*	1 Cake/290g	1131	52.2	390	4	53	18	0.6
Madeira, Lemon Iced, Tesco*	1 Slice/40g	169	7.4	418	4.9	58.1	18.2	1.1
Madeira, Party, Sainsbury's*	1 Slice/75g	321	15.2	427	4.1	56.8	20.2	1.1

CAKE

INFO/WEIGHT	Measure	per Measure KCAL	FAT	Nutrition Values per 100g / 100ml KCAL	PROT	CARB	FAT	FIBRE
Madeira, Tesco*	1 Serving/37g	141	5.4	382	5.7	56.5	14.6	0.9
Madeleine, La, Bonne Maman*	1 Cake/25g	112	6.8	449	6.4	44	27	2.3
Madeleines, Chocolate, Mrs Crimble's*	1 Cake/28g	128	6.2	451	3.4	57	22	0
Madeleines, Classic, French, GF, Mrs Crimbles*	1 Cake/30g	136	7.8	453	4.7	49	26	0
Madeleines, Tesco*	1 Cake/25g	122	7.3	486	4.8	50.5	29.1	1.5
Manor House, Mr Kipling*	1 Serving/69g	277	13.8	400	5.3	49.7	20	1.4
Marble, Tesco*	1/8 Cake/45g	184	8.4	410	4.4	55.9	18.7	1.5
Mini Rolls, Cadbury*	1 Roll/27g	117	6.2	435	4.8	50.5	23	2.3
Mini Rolls, Chocolate, Average	*1 Cake/27g*	*122*	*6.2*	*453*	*4.8*	*56.9*	*22.9*	*0.9*
Mini Rolls, Chocolate, Tesco*	1 Roll/26g	117	5.6	450	5.6	57	21.5	3.3
Mini Rolls, Cola, Chocolate, Cadbury*	1 Roll/27g	115	6.1	435	4.8	50.4	23.1	2.3
Mini Rolls, Double Chocolate, Tesco*	1 Mini Roll/26g	117	5.6	451	5.6	57	21.5	3.3
Mini Rolls, Jaffa, Average	*1 Cake/29g*	*111*	*3.3*	*382*	*3.5*	*67.2*	*11.2*	*1.4*
Mini Rolls, Jam, Average	*1 Cake/29g*	*115*	*4.5*	*395*	*3.8*	*59.8*	*15.6*	*1.8*
Mini Rolls, Jammy Strawberry, Cadbury*	1 Cake/29g	119	4.8	411	4.9	59.8	16.5	0.5
Mini Rolls, Lemon, Average	*1 Cake/29g*	*125*	*5.8*	*430*	*4.8*	*58.6*	*19.9*	*0.9*
Mini Rolls, Mint, Cadbury*	1 Roll/27g	123	6.2	455	5	55.4	23.1	1.4
Mini Rolls, Raspberry Ripple , Cadbury*	1 Roll/27g	120	5.5	440	4.5	58.7	20.1	2
Mint Aero, Celebration, Nestle*	1 Slice/58g	232	11.8	400	4	49.7	20.3	1.7
Orange, & Cranberry, Mini Classics, Mr Kipling*	1 Cake/36g	164	7.3	455	4.5	42.2	20.2	0.7
Orange, Marmalade, M&S*	1 Slice/50g	195	9.2	390	3.6	53.2	18.3	1.8
Pandoro, Italian	*1/8 Cake/87g*	*357*	*18.2*	*408*	*7.1*	*47.2*	*20.8*	*1.6*
Panettone, Average	*1 Portion/90g*	*345*	*15.3*	*383*	*8*	*52*	*17*	*0*
Panettone, Classic, Sainsbury's*	1 Slice/63g	227	8.2	363	7.4	53.3	13.1	1.2
Panettone, Finest, Tesco*	1/8 Cake/93g	318	11.8	339	6.1	49.1	12.6	2.5
Panettone, Luxury, Christmas, Tesco*	1 Serving/83g	307	11.6	370	7	53.5	14	2.5
Panettone, Prosecco Maron Glace, TTD, Sainsbury's*	1 Slice/85g	328	14.6	386	6.6	50.1	17.2	2.2
Plum, & Ginger, Crumble, Graze*	1 Punnet/33g	119	9.1	361	6.2	35.1	27.6	3.3
Pumpkin, Patch, Cadbury*	1 Cake/31g	149	7.1	480	5.3	61.7	22.9	2.4
Punschrulle Punsch Roll, Delicato*	1 Roll/40g	173	8	433	5	59	20	0
Raisin, Fruit Slab, Basics, Sainsbury's*	1 Slice/50g	183	6.2	367	5.3	57.3	12.5	1.9
Raisin, Tesco*	1 Cake/38g	158	7.6	417	5.6	53.8	19.9	1.4
Raspberry, Rockin' Raspberry, Slices, Mr Kipling*	1 Slice/21g	85	4.2	397	4.3	50.6	19.5	1
Raspberry, Sponge, Value, Tesco*	1 Slice/39g	130	4.6	334	3.4	53.4	11.9	0.7
Red Velvet, Delicious, Boots*	1 Pack/65g	285	14.9	439	4.5	52	23	1.4
Red Velvet, The Best, Morrisons*	1/6 Cake/63g	277	13.2	440	3.7	58.8	20.9	0.8
Red Velvet, TTD, Sainsbury's*	1 Slice/71g	302	16	428	2.8	52.8	22.7	0.8
Rock	*1 Sm Cake/40g*	*158*	*6.6*	*396*	*5.4*	*60.5*	*16.4*	*1.5*
Rock, Tesco*	1 Serving/87g	311	8.4	357	7.4	60.1	9.7	1.6
Shrek Birthday, Tesco*	1/16 Cake/72g	248	8.8	344	3.3	64	12.2	0.5
Simnel Slices, Mr Kipling*	1 Slice/47g	177	5.9	379	2.9	63.4	12.6	1.2
Snowballs, Sainsbury's*	1 Snowball/18g	80	4.1	445	2.5	55.6	23	3.6
Snowballs, Tesco*	1 Snowball/18g	79	4	432	2.5	55.8	22.1	5.4
Sponge	*1 Slice/53g*	*243*	*13.9*	*459*	*6.4*	*52.4*	*26.3*	*0.9*
Sponge, Fatless	*1 Slice/53g*	*156*	*3.2*	*294*	*10.1*	*53*	*6.1*	*0.9*
Sponge, Fresh Cream Strawberry, Asda*	1/12 Cake/60g	170	6	284	4.6	44	10	1.1
Sponge, Jam Filled	*1 Slice/65g*	*196*	*3.2*	*302*	*4.2*	*64.2*	*4.9*	*1.8*
Sponge, Raspberry, Sandwich, Sainsbury's*	1 Slice/42g	159	6.3	383	3.8	57.4	15.1	0.9
Sponge, Roll, Chocolate, M&S*	¼ Cake/66g	251	12.1	380	3.9	50.5	18.4	1.8
Sponge, with Butter Icing	*1 Slice/65g*	*318*	*19.9*	*490*	*4.5*	*52.4*	*30.6*	*0.6*
St. Clements, Finest, Tesco*	1 Serving/49g	194	10.5	395	3.1	47.2	21.5	0.4
Stollen, Bites, Finest, Tesco*	1 Bite/17g	68	3.2	398	5	50.9	18.8	4.4
Stollen, Bites, Waitrose*	1 Bite/18g	71	3.1	395	4.6	54.5	17.1	2.2

CAKE

	Measure INFO/WEIGHT	per Measure KCAL	FAT	Nutrition Values per 100g / 100ml KCAL	PROT	CARB	FAT	FIBRE
Stollen, Chocolate Rum, Finest, Tesco*	1/8 Cake/68g	262	9.5	381	5.3	57	13.8	3.9
Stollen, Kuchenmeister*	1 Serving/80g	357	16	446	5	61.2	20	2.5
Stollen, Marzipan Butter, Mini, Favorina, Lidl*	1 Stollen/18g	81	4.2	452	9.5	49.2	23.3	0
Stollen, Marzipan, Marzipan, Finest, Favorina, Lidl*	1 Slice/50g	206	9.3	412	6.2	53.4	18.6	0
Stollen, Slices, Average	**1 Slice/42g**	**160**	**6.3**	**381**	**5.5**	**55.8**	**15**	**3.1**
Stollen, Slices, Finest, Tesco*	1 Slice/33g	130	5.8	394	5.2	52.5	17.6	2.5
Stollen, Slices, Waitrose*	1 Slices/35g	143	5.8	402	4.7	57.3	16.3	3.8
Strawberry, Milkshake, Slices, Mr Kipling*	1 Slice/34g	139	5.5	402	3.3	61.1	16	0.6
Strawberry, Sponge Roll, M&S*	1/6 Cake/49g	160	4.6	330	2.8	58	9.5	0.8
Sultana, & Cherry, Tesco*	1 Cake/37g	124	4	334	4.7	54.4	10.8	2.5
Sultana, Apple & Cranberry, 99% Fat Free, Trimlyne*	1/6 Cake/67g	130	0.6	195	4.6	45.5	0.9	3.3
Sultana, Fair Trade, Co-Op*	1/8 Cake/45g	155	4	345	5	60	9	1
Sultana, Fingerellas, Mrs Crimble's*	2 Cakes/25g	102	4	410	5.7	80	16	1.8
Swiss Roll, Average	**1oz/28g**	**77**	**1.2**	**276**	**7.2**	**55.5**	**4.4**	**0.8**
Swiss Roll, Butter Cream, M&S*	1/6 Roll/46g	162	4.3	354	2.9	63.9	9.5	0.5
Swiss Roll, Chocolate Flavour, Value, Tesco*	1 Slice/20g	79	3.9	394	5.5	49.2	19.5	1.4
Swiss Roll, Chocolate, Double, Tesco*	1 Slice/29g	104	2.3	361	2.5	69	8	1.3
Swiss Roll, Chocolate, Individual	**1 Roll/26g**	**88**	**2.9**	**337**	**4.3**	**58.1**	**11.3**	**0**
Swiss Roll, Chocolate, Lyons*	1 Serving/50g	190	9.6	379	4.3	47	19.3	0.9
Swiss Roll, Chocolate, M&S*	1 Serving/46g	168	11.1	365	4.6	32.6	24.2	1.2
Swiss Roll, Chocolate, Morrisons*	1/6 Roll/26g	103	4.9	401	4.4	56.4	18.9	3.1
Swiss Roll, Chocolate, Value, Tesco*	1 Serving/20g	81	3.7	404	5	54.1	18.7	2.1
Swiss Roll, Lemon, Tesco*	1 Slice/32g	118	3	371	3.7	67.4	9.4	1
Swiss Roll, Raspberry & Vanilla, Morrisons*	1 Serving/28g	98	2.7	350	4.2	61.8	9.5	0
Swiss Roll, Raspberry Jam, Mr Kipling*	1/6 Cake/52g	184	5.3	355	2.8	63	10.2	1
Swiss Roll, Raspberry, Average	**1 Slice/35g**	**107**	**1.2**	**305**	**3.8**	**64.8**	**3.5**	**0.6**
Swiss Roll, Raspberry, Lyons*	1 Roll/175g	485	2.4	277	5.2	60.6	1.4	0
Swiss Roll, Strawberry Cream, Tesco*	1 Slice/32g	113	2.5	353	3.5	66.6	7.8	1.4
Tea Loaf, Rowan Hill Bakery, Lidl*	1 Slice/50g	135	0.4	270	3.8	63.3	0.9	3.4
Tiffin, Chocolate, Sainsbury's*	1 Cake/61g	184	11.6	301	2.7	29.8	19	1.3
Toffee, & Pecan Slices, M&S*	1 Slice/36g	160	8.5	445	4.7	54	23.7	1.3
Toffee, Apple, McVitie's*	1 Slice/26g	95	2.9	363	3.8	61.5	11	1.6
Toffee, Fudge, Entenmann's*	1 Serving/65g	274	14.1	421	3.4	53	21.7	0.5
Toffee, Iced, Tesco*	1 Serving/35g	132	5.2	376	3.3	57.2	14.9	1.6
Toffee, Slices, BGTY, Sainsbury's*	1 Slice/27g	88	0.7	327	4.3	71.7	2.5	1.8
Toffee, Slices, Low Fat, Weight Watchers*	1 Slice/27g	80	0.7	297	4.2	63.9	2.6	3.2
Toffee, Temptation, Tesco*	1 Slice/67g	228	12.8	340	2.9	39.1	19.1	0.3
Toffee, Terror Whirls, Mr Kipling*	1 Whirl/28g	141	7.9	509	3.9	58.3	28.7	1.2
Toffee, The Handmade Flapjack Company*	1 Cake/75g	346	18.8	462	5.1	54	25.1	0
Toffee, Thorntons*	1/6 Cake/70g	302	16.8	431	4.6	49.2	24	0.8
Twinkie, Hostess*	1 Serving/77g	270	8.1	351	2.3	62.8	10.5	0
Vanilla, Sponge, Fresh Cream, Sainsbury's*	1 Slice/50g	152	5.1	304	7.5	45.6	10.2	0.4
Victoria Sandwich, Average	**1 Slice/68g**	**267**	**12.9**	**392**	**4.4**	**50.9**	**19**	**1**
Victoria Sandwich, Individual, M&S*	1 Pack/75g	299	13.1	399	3.6	55.8	17.5	1.8
Victoria Sponge, Free From, Finest, Tesco*	1 Slice/61g	238	11.8	393	2.9	51.3	19.4	0.8
Victoria Sponge, Fresh Cream, Value, Tesco*	1 Slice/60g	224	12.8	374	3.8	41.4	21.3	0.7
Victoria Sponge, Lemon, Co-Op*	1 Slice/42g	151	8	360	4	44	19	0.7
Victoria Sponge, Mini, Bobby's*	1 Cake/35g	164	9.6	469	4	51.3	27.5	0.2
Victoria Sponge, Mini, Mr Kipling*	1 Cake/36g	152	6.9	420	3.9	58.5	19	0.8
Victoria Sponge, Mini, Weight Watchers*	1 Cake/30g	103	2.5	343	5.7	57.2	8.3	8.4
Victoria Sponge, Tesco*	1 Pack/68g	280	12.1	412	3.5	59	17.8	0.9
Victoria Sponge, TTD, Sainsbury's*	1 Slice/57g	229	11	401	5	51.8	19.3	1.4
Victoria, Individual, On the Go, Sainsbury's*	1 Cake/57g	228	9.7	400	3.9	56.9	17.1	0

	Measure INFO/WEIGHT	per Measure		Nutrition Values per 100g / 100ml				
		KCAL	FAT	KCAL	PROT	CARB	FAT	FIBRE
CAKE								
Viennese, M&S*	1 Cake/51g	250	14.1	495	4.1	58.9	28	2.8
Viennese, Whirl, Average	*1 Cake/28g*	*131*	*6.9*	*467*	*4.1*	*56.7*	*24.8*	*1.1*
Viennese, Whirl, Chocolate, Mr Kipling*	1 Whirl/28g	134	7.8	484	4.6	53.1	28	2.1
Viennese, Whirl, Lemon, Mr Kipling*	1 Cake/28g	115	4.5	409	4.2	62.2	15.9	0.7
Viennese, Whirl, Mr Kipling*	1 Whirl/28g	140	8	498	3.8	55.4	28.5	2.2
Walnut, Sandwich, Sainsbury's*	1/8 Cake/48g	182	8.3	379	5.4	53.8	17.3	1.3
Walnut, Tesco*	1 Slice/40g	161	6.9	403	5.5	55.8	17.3	1.1
Wedding, Rich Fruit, with Cognac, Iced, Sainsbury's*	1 Slice/55g	212	5.5	385	3.8	68.9	10	2
Welsh, Average	*1oz/28g*	*121*	*5.5*	*431*	*5.6*	*61.8*	*19.6*	*1.5*
Yorkshire Parkin, Bakers Delight*	1oz/28g	111	4.1	395	5.1	60.3	14.8	1.5
CAKE BAR								
Blueberry, Trimlyne*	1 Cake/50g	142	1.1	283	3.9	64	2.2	2.2
Boost, Cadbury*	1 Bar/40g	190	10.8	475	5.3	52.8	26.9	1.1
Caramel, Tesco*	1 Cake/26g	103	4.9	395	5.1	50.8	19	8.2
Carrot, Tesco*	1 Bar/68g	239	12.6	351	4.7	41.4	18.5	2.4
Chocolate Orange, Go Ahead, McVitie's*	1 Cake/33g	109	2	330	4.3	64.9	6	1
Chocolate Chip, Average	*1 Cake/28g*	*428*	*21.6*	*428*	*6.3*	*51.9*	*21.6*	*1.6*
Chocolate Chip, Mr Kipling*	1 Bar/32g	151	8.4	472	5.3	53.5	26.3	1.2
Chocolate Chip, Sainsbury's*	1 Cake/25g	108	5.6	430	6.1	51.2	22.3	0.6
Chocolate Chip, Tesco*	1 Cake/30g	124	5.9	415	7	51.4	19.7	2.3
Chocolate Chip, Value, Tesco*	1 Cake/28g	115	5.5	410	6.3	52.2	19.5	1.7
Chocolate Dream, Go Ahead, McVitie's*	1 Bar/36g	141	4.8	391	4.6	63.2	13.4	0.9
Chocolate, Average	*1 Cake/28g*	*125*	*6.2*	*446*	*5.6*	*56.3*	*22.1*	*1.9*
Chocolate, Snack Cakes, Penguin, McVitie's*	1 Bar/24g	122	7.2	510	4.8	54.6	30.2	1.6
Chocolate, Squidgy, Minis, Soreen*	1 Cake/30g	99	1.8	330	9.2	59.5	6	3.4
Chocolate, Tesco*	1 Cake/30g	130	5.8	433	5.5	58.6	19.2	1.7
Cinder Toffee, Cadbury*	1 Cake Bar/32g	149	8.4	465	4.2	53.4	26.2	0.9
Double Chocolate, Free From, Sainsbury's*	1 Cake/50g	196	7.9	391	4.2	58.2	15.7	1
Double Chocolate, Free From, Tesco*	1 Serving/45g	190	9.1	425	4.2	55.6	20.3	4.1
Flake, Cadbury*	1 Cake/25g	120	6.2	470	4.8	56.5	24.4	1.9
Fudge, Cadbury*	1 Pack/52g	220	9.2	420	5.7	60.3	17.6	0
Galaxy, Salted Caramel, Festive, Galaxy, Mars*	1 Bar/26g	113	5.3	438	5.6	58.7	20.4	0
Golden Syrup, McVitie's*	1 Cake/33g	127	4.8	385	3.6	60.2	14.4	1.2
Jaffa Cakes, Spooky, McVitie's*	1 Bar/25g	96	3.5	390	3.2	62.1	14.2	2.7
Jaffa, McVitie's*	1 Bar/25g	96	3.5	395	3.1	62.9	14.5	2.5
Jamaica Ginger, McVitie's*	1 Cake/33g	128	4.9	388	3.5	60.2	14.7	1.2
Lemon Meringue, Indulgence, Weight Watchers*	1 Bar/24g	21	0.3	86	1.1	7.1	1.3	0
Milk Chocolate Orange, Crispy, Asda*	1 Bar/22g	91	2.2	413	4.8	75.6	10.2	2
Milk Chocolate Orange, Sandwich Bar, Lyons*	1 Bar/28g	142	8	516	5	62	29	0
Milk Chocolate, Cadbury*	1 Bar/25g	110	5.6	445	4.9	53.8	22.8	2.9
Milky Way, McVitie's*	1 Cake/26g	124	6.2	476	5.1	58.5	23.6	1.2
Rich Chocolate, Trimlyne*	1 Serving/40g	115	1.7	288	5.2	59.2	4.2	2.2
Toffee, Squidgy, Minis, Soreen*	1 Bar/30g	95	1.3	317	7.7	59.7	4.2	5.9
Vanilla, Raspberry, Mini Rolls, Ms Mollys*	1 Roll/20g	74	2.2	368	4.7	62	11	1.2
CAKE MIX								
Carrot Cake, Betty Crocker*	¼ Pack/125g	504	8.4	403	5.8	78.9	6.7	1.4
Cheesecake, Original, Made Up, Asda*	1/6 Cake/85g	228	10.2	268	4.1	36	12	1.4
Cheesecake, Tesco*	1 Serving/76g	199	7.9	262	4.1	38	10.4	1.6
Sponge, Value, Tesco*	1 Slice/55g	181	4.8	329	4.6	57.9	8.8	1.4
Yellow, Super Moist, Betty Crocker*	1 Cake/128g	517	9.5	404	3.3	81.6	7.4	1.1
CALLALOO								
Leaves, Raw, Unprepared	*1 Cup/28g*	*6*	*0.1*	*23*	*2.5*	*4*	*0.3*	*0*

C

	Measure INFO/WEIGHT	per Measure KCAL	FAT	Nutrition Values per 100g / 100ml KCAL	PROT	CARB	FAT	FIBRE
CALZONE								
Cream Cheese Pepperonata, Waitrose*	½ Pizza/165g	383	15.8	232	7	29.4	9.6	1.5
Ham Mushroom, Waitrose*	½ Pizza/145g	362	13.5	250	10	31.6	9.3	1.6
Speciale, Ristorante, Dr Oetker*	½ Pizza/145g	381	20.3	263	11	23	14	0
Three Cheese, Waitrose*	1 Pizza/265g	747	31.8	282	10.4	33	12	1.4
CANAPES								
Aegean Tomato, Finest, Tesco*	1 Canape/15g	45	2.2	300	7.2	34.3	14.7	2.1
Salmon Dill, Finest, Tesco*	1 Canape/15g	47	2.4	315	9.2	32.7	16.1	1.9
Smoked Salmon, Youngs*	1 Canape/10g	21	1.5	210	15.9	2	15.2	0.7
CANNELLONI								
Beef, As Prepared, Waitrose*	1 Pack/360g	501	26.7	139	6.2	11.5	7.4	1
Beef, Italian, Sainsbury's*	1 Pack/400g	498	26.2	124	5.9	10.5	6.6	1.6
Beef, Meal for One, M&S*	1 Pack/400g	572	30.8	143	6.7	10.7	7.7	2.1
Butternut Squash, with Spinach & Goats' Cheese, Tesco*	1 Pack/350g	490	29.4	140	5.1	10.7	8.4	1.9
Mushroom, Italian, Sainsbury's*	1 Pack/450g	598	31	133	5.2	12.5	6.9	0.5
Spinach Ricotta, Meal for One, M&S*	1 Pack/400g	412	17.2	103	4.8	10.2	4.3	2.2
Spinach Ricotta, Serves 1, BGTY, Sainsbury's*	1 Pack/400g	364	9.2	91	4.5	11.8	2.3	2.6
Spinach, & Ricotta, Fresh, Ready Meal, Average	*1 Serving/300g*	*393*	*22*	*131*	*5*	*10.8*	*7.4*	*1.2*
Spinach, & Ricotta, Low Fat, COU, M&S*	1 Pack/400g	340	7.6	85	4.8	11.4	1.9	1.7
Spinach, & Ricotta, Ready Meal, Average	*1 Serving/300g*	*426*	*22*	*142*	*5.6*	*13.3*	*7.3*	*1.4*
Spinach, & Ricotta, Sainsbury's*	1 Pack/400g	520	27.2	130	4.9	11.6	6.8	1.4
Tubes, Dry, Average	*1oz/28g*	*101*	*1*	*361*	*12.5*	*69.1*	*3.6*	*1.2*
Vegetarian, Tesco*	1 Pack/400g	552	34.4	138	5.3	9.8	8.6	1.5
CAPERS								
Caperberries, in Brine, Drained, Spirit of Summer, M&S*	¼ Jar/35g	7	0.2	20	1	0.3	0.5	5
Caperberries, Spanish, Waitrose*	1 Serving/55g	9	0.3	17	1.1	2.1	0.5	2.5
Capucine, in Brine, Sainsbury's*	1 Serving/15g	4	0.1	28	2	1.7	0.7	3.4
in Vinegar, Average	*1 Tsp/5g*	*2*	*0*	*34*	*1.7*	*3*	*0.6*	*0*
CAPONATA								
Antipasti, Made in Italy, M&S*	¼ Jar/66g	144	13.4	218	1.3	6.1	20.2	3.3
CAPPELLETTI								
Goats Cheese & Red Pesto, Waitrose*	½ Pack/125g	374	10.9	299	11.6	43.5	8.7	2.2
Parma Ham, Fresh, Waitrose*	½ Pack/125g	368	11.5	294	14.1	38.6	9.2	2.2
CAPRI SUN								
Orange	*1 Pouch/200ml*	*90*	*0*	*45*	*0*	*11*	*0*	*0*
Orange, 100%, Juice	*1 Pouch/200ml*	*75*	*0*	*38*	*0.5*	*9.2*	*0*	*0.1*
CARAMAC								
Nestle*	1 Bar/30g	174	11	571	5.9	55.5	36.1	0
CARAMBOLA								
Average	*1oz/28g*	*9*	*0.1*	*31*	*0.5*	*7.1*	*0.3*	*1.3*
CARAWAY								
Seeds, Schwartz*	1 Pack/38g	170	8.1	448	23.3	40.9	21.2	0
CARBONARA								
Chicken, & Bacon, Balanced for You, M&S*	1 Pack/375g	484	10.5	129	10.7	14.7	2.8	1.1
Chicken, Mushroom, & Ham, Spaghetti, Asda*	1 Pack/700g	686	14	98	10	10	2	1.5
Penne, Taste of Italy, Tesco*	½ Pack/400g	604	18.5	151	7.9	19	4.6	0.9
Spaghetti, COU, M&S*	1 Pack/330g	346	7.2	105	6.1	15.7	2.2	0.8
Spaghetti, Heated, HL, Tesco*	1 Pack/365g	372	5.1	102	6	16	1.4	0.8
Spaghetti, Italian Quisine, Microwaved, Aldi*	1 Pack/400g	669	33.4	174	7.1	16	8.7	1.5
Spaghetti, M&S*	1 Pack/400g	660	36	165	6.5	14.2	9	0.6
Spaghetti, M&S*	1 Pack/400g	560	27.2	140	5.2	14	6.8	0.9
Spaghetti, Ready Meal, Average	*1 Pack/400g*	*524*	*21.5*	*131*	*5.9*	*14.4*	*5.4*	*1.1*
Spaghetti, Tesco*	1 Pack/380g	338	4.9	89	5.4	13.4	1.3	1
Spaghetti, Waitrose*	1 Pack/383g	658	31.8	172	7	16.9	8.3	0.8

	Measure INFO/WEIGHT	per Measure		Nutrition Values per 100g / 100ml				
		KCAL	FAT	KCAL	PROT	CARB	FAT	FIBRE
CARBONARA								
Tagliatelle, PB, Waitrose*	1 Pack/350g	357	12.6	102	5.3	12.1	3.6	0.7
Tagliatelle, Ready Meal, Average	*1 Serving/400g*	*460*	*13.4*	*115*	*5.5*	*15.8*	*3.3*	*1*
Tagliatelle, TTD, Sainsbury's*	1 Pack/400g	658	31.1	167	7.3	15.7	7.9	1.9
CARDAMOM								
Black, Ground, Average	*1 Tsp/2g*	*6*	*0.1*	*311*	*10.8*	*68.5*	*6.7*	*28*
CAROB POWDER								
Average	*1 Tsp/2g*	*3*	*0*	*159*	*4.9*	*37*	*0.1*	*0*
CARP								
Fillet, Raw, Average	*1 Fillet/218g*	*244*	*10.2*	*112*	*17.5*	*0*	*4.7*	*0*
CARROT & SWEDE								
Diced, for Mashing, Average	*½ Pack/250g*	*58*	*0.7*	*23*	*0.6*	*4.7*	*0.3*	*1.9*
Mash, From Supermarket, Average	*1 Serving/150g*	*138*	*7.5*	*92*	*1.3*	*10.4*	*5*	*1.3*
Mash, Healthy Range, Average	*1 Serving/150g*	*98*	*4.2*	*66*	*1.3*	*8.6*	*2.8*	*2.1*
CARROTS								
& Peas, Sainsbury's*	1 Serving/200g	100	1	50	3.3	8.3	0.5	3.8
Houmous Dip, Tesco*	1 Pack/120g	96	4.9	80	1.9	7.1	4.1	3.6
Peas, Canned, in Water, Drained, Batchelors*	½ Can/108g	39	0.4	36	2.2	4.3	0.4	3.3
Baby, Canned, Average	*1 Can/195g*	*40*	*0.5*	*21*	*0.5*	*4.2*	*0.3*	*2.1*
Baby, Fresh, Average	*1 Serving/80g*	*28*	*0.1*	*35*	*0.6*	*8.2*	*0.1*	*2.9*
Batons, Fresh, Average	*½ Pack/150g*	*41*	*0.4*	*28*	*0.6*	*5.7*	*0.3*	*2.6*
Boiled, Average	*1oz/28g*	*6*	*0.1*	*22*	*0.6*	*4.4*	*0.4*	*2.3*
Canned, Average	*1oz/28g*	*6*	*0.1*	*20*	*0.5*	*4*	*0.2*	*1.9*
Chantenay, Cut, Frozen, Tesco*	1 Serving/80g	24	0.3	29	0.6	4.3	0.4	3.1
Chantenay, Wood Farm, Raw, Aldi*	1 Serving/80g	34	0.4	42	0.6	7.9	0.5	2.4
Raw, Scrubbed, Average	*1 Serving/80g*	*24*	*0.4*	*30*	*0.7*	*6*	*0.5*	*2.4*
Roasting, with Honey Ginger Glaze, Aunt Bessie's*	1 Serving/133g	80	4.1	60	0.7	6.1	3.1	2.5
Sliced, Canned, Average	*1 Serving/180g*	*36*	*0.2*	*20*	*0.7*	*4.1*	*0.1*	*1.5*
Sliced, Fresh, Average	*1 Serving/60g*	*17*	*0.2*	*28*	*0.7*	*5.7*	*0.3*	*2*
Whole, Raw, Peeled, Average	*1 Carrot/75g*	*21*	*0.2*	*29*	*0.6*	*6.4*	*0.3*	*2.2*
with Parsley & English Butter, M&S*	½ Pack/100g	65	3.9	65	0.6	7.1	3.9	2.4
CASHEW NUTS								
Cheese Flavour, Graze*	1 Pack/26g	140	10.8	540	15.3	35.7	41.5	0
Cracking Black Pepper, Graze*	1 Punnet/36g	216	16.6	600	19	26	46	4
Honey Glazed, Itsu*	1 Pack/30g	167	10.4	557	13.6	46.3	34.8	2.3
Mexican Chilli, Graze*	1 Pack/26g	140	10.8	539	14.3	34.9	41.6	0
Plain, Average	*½ Pack/25g*	*146*	*12.2*	*584*	*15.7*	*18.8*	*48.9*	*3.4*
Roasted Salted, Average	*1 Serving/50g*	*306*	*25.6*	*612*	*18.8*	*19.6*	*51.1*	*3.1*
Wasabi, Roasted, Vitasia, Lidl*	1 Serving/30g	185	14.6	616	17.5	25.6	48.6	0
CASSAVA								
Baked, Average	*1oz/28g*	*43*	*0.1*	*155*	*0.7*	*40.1*	*0.2*	*1.7*
Boiled in Unsalted Water, Average	*1oz/28g*	*36*	*0.1*	*130*	*0.5*	*33.5*	*0.2*	*1.4*
Gari, Average	*1oz/28g*	*100*	*0.1*	*358*	*1.3*	*92.9*	*0.5*	*0*
CASSEROLE								
Beef	*1 Serving/336g*	*490*	*23*	*146*	*16.3*	*4.6*	*6.8*	*0.6*
Beef, & Ale with Dumplings, Sainsbury's*	1 Pack/450g	711	32.8	158	7.7	15.4	7.3	0.6
Beef, & Ale with Mashed Potato, HL, Tesco*	1 Pack/450g	364	11.2	81	5.1	10.9	2.5	0.6
Beef, Ale, Average	*1 Serving/300g*	*251*	*6.8*	*84*	*9.4*	*6.5*	*2.2*	*1.3*
Beef, Red Wine, Average	*1 Serving/350g*	*290*	*7.3*	*83*	*7.2*	*8.2*	*2.1*	*1.5*
Beef, Meal for One, Tesco*	1 Pack/450g	425	18.9	94	3.6	10.6	4.2	1.7
Beef, with Dumplings, Ready Meal, Average	*1 Serving/350g*	*464*	*21.1*	*132*	*9.5*	*10.1*	*6*	*1.5*
Beef, with Herb Potatoes, Ready Meal, Average	*1 Serving/475g*	*504*	*17.1*	*106*	*6.8*	*11.5*	*3.6*	*1.6*
Chicken, & Asparagus, HL, Tesco*	1 Serving/450g	342	10.3	76	6.3	8.3	2.3	0.5
Chicken, & Dumpling, 548, Wiltshire Farm Foods*	1 Serving/440g	485	22.5	110	5.2	11	5.1	0.8

	Measure INFO/WEIGHT	per Measure KCAL	FAT	Nutrition Values per 100g / 100ml KCAL	PROT	CARB	FAT	FIBRE
CASSEROLE								
Chicken, & Dumplings, Sainsbury's*	1 Serving/450g	612	24.8	136	9.1	12	5.5	1.2
Chicken, & Vegetable, Ready Meal, Healthy Range	*1 Serving/330g*	*265*	*11.9*	*80*	*4.7*	*7.6*	*3.6*	*1.1*
Chicken, & White Wine, Ready Meal, Healthy Range	*1 Serving/300g*	*234*	*7.4*	*78*	*7.7*	*6.3*	*2.4*	*1.2*
Chicken, Vegetable, Tesco*	¼ Pack/240g	192	5	80	9.6	4.7	2.1	2.2
Chicken, Leek & Mushroom, Tesco*	1 Pack/350g	382	22	109	4.5	8.6	6.3	1
Chicken, with Dumplings, M&S*	½ Pack/227g	261	10	115	9.7	9	4.4	0.9
Lamb, & Rosemary, Eat Well, M&S*	1 Pack/380g	325	11	86	7.6	7	2.9	2.2
Lamb, Ready Meal, Healthy Range, Average	*1 Serving/300g*	*273*	*9.9*	*91*	*10.5*	*4.9*	*3.3*	*1*
Pork, Normandy Style, Finest, Tesco*	1 Pack/450g	405	21.6	90	7.6	4.1	4.8	2.3
Rabbit, Average	*1oz/28g*	*29*	*1.4*	*102*	*11.6*	*2.6*	*5.1*	*0.4*
Red Lentil Mixed Bean, Cook*	1 Portion/290g	258	7	89	4.7	12.1	2.4	3.9
Sausage, & Potato, M&S*	1 Serving/200g	190	11.8	95	3.3	7.5	5.9	0.9
Sausage, CBY, Asda*	1 Pot/400g	240	15.2	60	3.6	1.9	3.8	2.1
Sausage, Pork, Diet Chef Ltd*	1 Pack/300g	303	18.3	101	6.6	4.9	6.1	1.4
Sausage, with Root Vegetables, Mini's, Kirstys*	1 Pack/250g	210	9.8	84	4.4	6.1	3.9	3.7
Steak, & Mushroom, 214, Wiltshire Farm Foods*	1 Pack/360g	322	16.2	89	5	7.2	4.5	1.3
Steak, & Mushroom, Asda*	½ Pack/304g	411	30.4	135	7	4.2	10	0.3
Steak, Ale, Average	*1 Serving/275g*	*324*	*14.4*	*118*	*9*	*8.8*	*5.2*	*1*
Steak, Mushroom, Average	*1 Serving/275g*	*274*	*15.5*	*100*	*6.2*	*6*	*5.6*	*1*
Vegetable, Root, Kale, Waitrose*	1 Pack/357g	343	15	96	1.9	11.6	4.2	2.1
CASSEROLE MIX								
Beef & Ale, Colman's*	1 Pack/45g	144	0.9	320	9.2	66.3	2	2.3
Beef, Colman's*	1 Pack/40g	123	0.6	308	7.5	66	1.5	2.5
Beef, Recipe, Colman's*	1 Pack/42g	142	0.5	338	9.1	13.1	1.1	4
Beef, Recipe, Schwartz*	1 Pack/43g	123	0.9	287	7	56.6	2.1	6.6
Chicken Chasseur, Asda*	1 Pack/80g	273	0.8	341	9	74	1	1.4
Chicken, Authentic, Schwartz*	1 Serving/66g	210	0.7	318	14	62.1	1	2.1
Chicken, Recipe, As Sold, Colman's*	1 Pack/40g	131	1	328	6.2	68.2	2.6	3.1
Lamb, Authentic, Schwartz*	1 Pack/35g	116	1.2	332	7.7	68	3.3	1.3
Peppered Beef, Schwartz*	1 Pack/40g	129	2	323	7	62.9	4.9	7.3
Sausage, As Sold, Colman's*	1 Pack/39g	136	1	350	10	70	2.5	6
Sausage, Classic, Schwartz*	1 Pack/35g	96	0.9	275	12.4	50.1	2.7	14.9
CASSOULET								
Lamb, Spinach, High in Protein, Asda*	1 Pack/400g	340	10.4	85	7.2	4	2.6	4.5
CATFISH								
Cooked, Steamed, Weighed with Bone, Average	*1 Serving/100g*	*101*	*3.1*	*101*	*18.2*	*0*	*3.1*	*0.7*
Raw, Average	*1oz/28g*	*27*	*0.8*	*96*	*17.6*	*0*	*2.8*	*0*
CAULIFLOWER								
Bites, Buffalo, Tesco*	½ Pack/115g	163	7.5	142	2.6	16.5	6.5	3.7
Boiled, Average	*1 Serving/80g*	*22*	*0.7*	*28*	*2.9*	*2.1*	*0.9*	*1.6*
Cous Cous, Ready to Cook, As Sold, Morrisons*	1 Pack/330g	129	3	39	3.6	2.8	0.9	2.6
Raw, Average	*1 Serving/80g*	*25*	*0.7*	*31*	*3.2*	*2.7*	*0.8*	*1.6*
Rice, Nature's Pick, Aldi*	1 Pot/250g	85	2.2	34	2.9	2.1	0.9	2.7
Spiced, Roasted, Tesco*	½ Pack/70g	59	4.4	84	2.2	3.9	6.2	1.8
Steamed, Average	*1 Serving/100g*	*28*	*0.9*	*28*	*2.9*	*2.1*	*0.9*	*1.6*
CAULIFLOWER CHEESE								
& Bacon, Gastropub, M&S*	1 Pack/300g	318	21	106	6.3	4.5	7	1
Broccoli, Average	*1 Serving/200g*	*127*	*6.4*	*64*	*3.8*	*4.6*	*3.2*	*2*
Asda*	1 Pack/450g	486	36	108	4.6	4.3	8	1.5
Average	*1 Meal/400g*	*362*	*23.3*	*90*	*4.5*	*4.6*	*5.8*	*1.3*
BFY, Morrisons*	1 Pack/300g	231	12.3	77	4.5	5.4	4.1	1.2
Florets in a Cheese Sauce, As Prepared, Sainsbury's*	½ Pack/194g	149	7.7	77	4.8	4.3	4	2.2
Fresh, Oven Heated, Tesco*	½ Pack/170g	158	8.2	93	5.7	6.2	4.8	1.1

	Measure INFO/WEIGHT	per Measure KCAL	FAT	Nutrition Values per 100g / 100ml KCAL	PROT	CARB	FAT	FIBRE
CAULIFLOWER CHEESE								
Frozen, Iceland*	1 Serving/200g	190	12	95	4	5.5	6	1.6
Heated, Finest, Tesco*	½ Pack/168g	209	13.8	124	5.7	6.4	8.2	1.4
M&S*	½ Pack/225g	263	17.5	117	6.7	4.3	7.8	1.3
Made with Half Fat Cheese, HL, Tesco*	1 Pack/500g	285	13	57	6.5	2	2.6	2.2
Made with Semi-Skimmed Milk	*1oz/28g*	*28*	*1.8*	*100*	*6*	*5.2*	*6.4*	*1.3*
Made with Skimmed Milk	*1oz/28g*	*27*	*1.7*	*97*	*6*	*5.2*	*6*	*1.3*
Made with Whole Milk	*1oz/28g*	*29*	*1.9*	*105*	*6*	*5.2*	*6.9*	*1.3*
Morrisons*	½ Pack/225g	200	14.6	89	3.3	4.4	6.5	1
TTD, Sainsbury's*	¼ Pack/148g	169	11.1	114	5.1	5.8	7.5	1.3
with Wexford Mature Cheddar, M&S*	½ Pack/225g	263	17.6	117	6.7	4.3	7.8	1.3
CAVIAR								
Average	*1oz/28g*	*25*	*1.3*	*89*	*11.6*	*0.5*	*4.6*	*0*
CELERIAC								
Boiled in Salted Water, Average	*1oz/28g*	*5*	*0.1*	*18*	*0.9*	*1.9*	*0.4*	*3.2*
Raw, Average	*1 Serving/80g*	*17*	*0.3*	*21*	*1*	*1.9*	*0.4*	*3.2*
CELERY								
Boiled in Salted Water	*1 Serving/50g*	*4*	*0.2*	*8*	*0.5*	*0.8*	*0.3*	*1.2*
Raw, Trimmed, Average	1 Stalk/40g	3	0.1	7	0.5	0.9	0.2	1.1
CHAMPAGNE								
Average	*1 Glass/125ml*	*95*	*0*	*76*	*0.3*	*1.4*	*0*	*0*
CHANNA MASALA								
M&S*	1 Pack/225g	360	23.7	160	5.6	11.2	10.5	8.2
Waitrose*	1 Pack/300g	300	18.3	100	3.7	7.4	6.1	7.9
CHAPATIS								
Brown Wheat Flour, Waitrose*	1 Chapati/42g	128	3.4	305	8.6	49.4	8	4.6
Elephant Atta*	1 Chapati/45g	129	2.9	287	7.5	53.1	6.4	3.2
Indian Style, Asda*	1 Chapati/43g	95	0.4	221	8	45	1	2.9
Made with Fat	*1 Chapati/60g*	*197*	*7.7*	*328*	*8.1*	*48.3*	*12.8*	*0*
Made without Fat	*1 Chapati/55g*	*111*	*0.6*	*202*	*7.3*	*43.7*	*1*	*0*
Morrisons*	1 Chapati/40g	108	2.8	269	8.6	49.8	6.9	0
Plain, Original, Wrap, Patak's*	1 Chapati/42g	115	3.2	273	9.4	48.8	7.5	0
Wholemeal, Patak's*	1 Chapati/42g	130	4	310	11.2	44.9	9.5	9
CHARD								
Average	*1 Serving/80g*	*15*	*0.2*	*19*	*1.4*	*3.3*	*0.2*	*0.8*
Silverbeet, Fresh, Steamed	*1 Serving/100g*	*15*	*0*	*15*	*1.9*	*1.3*	*0*	*3.3*
Swiss, Boiled in Unsalted Water	*1oz/28g*	*6*	*0*	*20*	*1.9*	*4.1*	*0.1*	*2.1*
Swiss, Raw	*1oz/28g*	*5*	*0.1*	*17*	*1.7*	*3.4*	*0.2*	*1.5*
CHEDDARS								
Cheese & Ham, Baked, Mini, McVitie's*	1 Bag/30g	160	8.9	534	11	55.5	29.8	2
Cheese, Baked, Mini, Original, Jacobs*	1 Bag/25g	128	7.3	512	10.6	50.1	29.2	2.5
Chilli Beef, Baked, Mini, Jacob's*	1 Pack/50g	262	15	522	9	52.2	29.9	2.7
Mini, Average	*1 Bag/26g*	*134*	*7.8*	*516*	*11.2*	*50.8*	*29.9*	*2.4*
Red Leicester, Baked, Mini, Jacob's*	1 Pack/25g	132	7.9	530	8.7	50.2	31.8	2.5
Smokey BBQ, McVitie's*	1 Sm Pack/30g	155	8.9	516	9.3	52.8	29.8	2.6
Stilton, Baked, Mini, Jacob's*	1 Pack/25g	132	7.9	530	8.8	50.3	31.8	2.5
CHEESE								
Appenzeller, Extra, Strength 6, Waitrose*	1 Serving/30g	126	9.6	420	32	1	32	0
Appenzeller, Swiss, TTD, Sainsbury's*	1 Serving/30g	116	9.5	386	25.4	0	31.6	0
Babybel, Cheddar Variety, Mini, Fromageries Bel*	1 Cheese/20g	75	6.2	375	24	0	31	0
Babybel, Emmental, Fromageries Bel*	1 Serving/20g	63	4.9	316	23	1	24.5	0
Babybel, Goat's Variety, Mini, Fromageries Bel*	1 Cheese/20g	65	5.4	327	21	0	27	0
Babybel, Gouda Variety, Mini, Fromageries Bel*	1 Cheese/20g	68	5.6	340	22	0	28	0
Babybel, Light, Mini, Fromageries Bel*	1 Babybel/20g	42	2.4	208	25	0	12	0

C

CHEESE

INFO/WEIGHT Measure	per Measure KCAL	per Measure FAT	Nutrition Values per 100g / 100ml KCAL	PROT	CARB	FAT	FIBRE
Babybel, Original, Mini, Fromageries Bel*	1 Cheese/20g	61	4.8	304	22	0.1	24	0
Bavarian, Smoked with Ham, Sainsbury's*	1 Serving/30g	89	7.2	298	19.4	0.8	24.1	0
Bavarian, Smoked, Slices, Asda*	1 Slice/18g	50	4.1	277	17	0.4	23	0
Berthaut's, Epoisses, Strength 6, 1, Waitrose*	1 Serving/30g	86	7.2	285	17	1	23.7	0
Bites, Quattro Formaggi, Specially Selected, Aldi*	½ Pack/35g	185	10.5	528	20	44	30	3.1
Bleu D' Auvergne, Sainsbury's*	1 Serving/25g	84	6.6	335	22	2	26.5	0
Blue, Castello, Soft, Castello*	¼ Pack/37g	162	15.6	432	14	0.5	41.5	0
Blue, D'affinois, 1, Waitrose*	1 Serving/30g	126	12.3	421	12	1	41	0
Blue, French, CBY, Asda*	1 Serving/30g	90	7.4	301	20	0	24.5	0
Blue, Saint Agur*	1 Serving /30g	109	9.9	363	16	0.2	33	0
Blue, Savers, Morrisons*	1 Portion/30g	99	8.1	331	22	0.1	27	0
Blue, Sliced for Burger, Castello*	1 Slice/25g	100	9.2	400	17	0.5	37	0
Brie, Average	*1 Serving/25g*	*74*	*6*	*296*	*19.7*	*0.3*	*24*	*0*
Brie, Breaded, Bites, Frozen, Tesco*	1 Bite/17g	54	3.4	319	8.6	24.2	20.2	2.8
Brie, Reduced Fat, Average	*1 Serving/50g*	*99*	*5.7*	*198*	*23*	*0.8*	*11.4*	*0*
Caerphilly, Average	*1 Serving/50g*	*187*	*15.6*	*374*	*23*	*0.1*	*31.3*	*0*
Cambazola, Tesco*	1 Serving/30g	128	12.3	425	13.5	0.5	41	0
Camembert, Average	*1 Serving/50g*	*141*	*11.1*	*283*	*20.5*	*0.1*	*22.2*	*0*
Camembert, Breaded, Average	*1 Serving/90g*	*307*	*20.9*	*342*	*16.6*	*14.2*	*23.2*	*0.4*
Cantal, French, Sainsbury's*	1 Serving/30g	106	8.7	353	23	0.1	29	0
Cashel Blue, Waitrose*	1 Serving/28g	94	7.6	336	17.6	1.2	27.2	0
Cheddar, & Mozzarella, Spicy, Grated, Tesco*	1 Serving/40g	140	10.5	350	26	2.5	26.2	0
Cheddar, Walnut, Carron Lodge*	1 Serving/30g	118	8.8	392	22.8	9.1	29.4	1.6
Cheddar, Average	*1 Serving/30g*	*123*	*10.3*	*410*	*25*	*0.1*	*34.4*	*0*
Cheddar, Canadian, Average	*1 Serving/30g*	*123*	*10.3*	*409*	*25*	*0.1*	*34.3*	*0*
Cheddar, Davidstow, Mature, Average	*1 Serving/28g*	*115*	*9.6*	*410*	*25*	*0.1*	*34.4*	*0*
Cheddar, Extra Mature, Average	*1 Serving/30g*	*123*	*10.3*	*410*	*25.1*	*0.1*	*34.4*	*0*
Cheddar, Extra Mature, Slices, Tesco*	1 Slice/25g	104	8.7	416	25.4	0.1	34.9	0
Cheddar, Grated, Average	*1 Serving/50g*	*206*	*17.2*	*413*	*24.4*	*1.5*	*34.3*	*0*
Cheddar, Mature, Average	*1 Serving/30g*	*123*	*10.3*	*410*	*25*	*0.1*	*34.4*	*0*
Cheddar, Mature, Grated, Average	*1 Serving/28g*	*113*	*9.3*	*404*	*24.7*	*1.6*	*33.2*	*0*
Cheddar, Mature, Reduced Fat, Average	*1 Serving/25g*	*68*	*4.2*	*271*	*30*	*0.1*	*16.7*	*0*
Cheddar, Medium, Average	*1 Serving/30g*	*123*	*10.4*	*411*	*24.9*	*0.2*	*34.5*	*0*
Cheddar, Mild, Average	*1 Serving/30g*	*123*	*10.3*	*409*	*25*	*0.1*	*34.3*	*0*
Cheddar, Reduced Fat, Average	*1 Serving/30g*	*76*	*4.2*	*255*	*32.2*	*0.1*	*14*	*0*
Cheddar, Scotch Bonnet, Slices, Tesco*	1 Slice/28g	110	9	394	20.3	4.8	32.2	1.7
Cheddar, Smoked, Average	*1 Serving/30g*	*123*	*10.3*	*411*	*25.2*	*0.1*	*34.4*	*0*
Cheddar, Smoky, Mini Selection, Tesco*	1 Cheese/20g	81	6.8	406	25	0.1	34	0
Cheddar, West Country Farmhouse, Average	*1 Serving/28g*	*115*	*9.6*	*410*	*25*	*0.1*	*34.4*	*0*
Cheddar, Wexford, Average	*1 Serving/20g*	*82*	*6.9*	*410*	*25*	*0.1*	*34.4*	*0*
Cheddar, with Caramelised Onion, Sainsbury's*	1 Serving/28g	109	8.7	391	22.8	5.1	31	0
Cheddar, with Caramelised Onion, Tesco*	1 Serving/50g	183	14	366	21.4	7.1	28	0.4
Cheddar, with Onion & Chives, Davidson*	1 Serving/25g	100	8.3	400	24.3	0.6	33.3	0
Cheddar, with Pickled Onion Relish, Christmas, Tesco*	¼ Cheese/50g	191	15.5	382	23	2.7	31	0.1
Chedds, Bricks, Cathedral City, Dairy Crest Ltd*	1 Brick/18g	75	6.3	416	25.4	0.1	34.9	0
Chedds, Nibbles, Cathedral City, Dairy Crest Ltd*	1 Mini Bag/16g	67	5.6	416	25.4	0.1	34.9	0
Cheshire	*1oz/28g*	*106*	*8.8*	*379*	*24*	*0.1*	*31.4*	*0*
Chevre Pave D'affinois, Finest, Tesco*	1 Pack/150g	404	32.6	269	18.5	0	21.7	0
Cottage, Low Fat, 2% Fat, Natural, Average	*1 Serving/75g*	*68*	*1.4*	*90*	*13.7*	*3.6*	*1.9*	*0*
Cottage, Plain, Average	*1 Tbsp/20g*	*19*	*0.7*	*93*	*12*	*3.3*	*3.5*	*0.1*
Cottage, Plain, Reduced Fat, Average	*100g*	*85*	*1.9*	*85*	*12.3*	*4.4*	*1.9*	*0.1*
Cottage, Virtually Fat Free, Average	*1 Tbsp/20g*	*16*	*0.2*	*79*	*13*	*4.5*	*1*	*0*
Cottage, Whole Milk, Natural, Average	*1 Serving/75g*	*77*	*3.4*	*103*	*12.5*	*2.7*	*4.5*	*0*

C

CHEESE

	Measure INFO/WEIGHT	per Measure KCAL	FAT	Nutrition Values per 100g / 100ml KCAL	PROT	CARB	FAT	FIBRE
Cottage, with Black Pepper, HE, Tesco*	1 Pot/125g	101	2.2	81	12.1	4	1.8	0
Cottage, with Chives, Low Fat, Westacre*	1 Pot/100g	81	1.4	81	13.7	3.5	1.4	1.2
Cottage, with Chives, Virtually Fat free, Longley Farm*	½ Pot/125g	88	0.1	70	14.3	2.9	0.1	0
Cottage, with Cream, Lowicz*	1 Pack/150g	152	7.5	101	11	3	5	0
Cottage, with Cucumber & Mint, HE, Tesco*	½ Pot/125g	91	2.1	73	10.7	3.8	1.7	0.1
Cottage, with Grilled Pepper & Pesto, LC, Tesco*	1 Portion/60g	45	0.9	75	10.2	4.3	1.5	0.5
Cottage, with Mango & Pineapple, BGTY, Sainsbury's*	½ Pot/125g	112	0.9	90	10.7	10.4	0.7	0.2
Cottage, with Onion & Chive, GFY, Asda*	¼ Tub/75g	50	1	66	9.3	3.8	1.4	0.5
Cottage, with Onion & Chive, Iceland*	½ Pot/100g	81	1.3	81	8.5	8.9	1.3	0.3
Cottage, with Pineapple, 70% Less fat, CBY, Asda*	¼ Tub/75g	70	1	93	8.4	11.9	1.3	0
Cottage, with Pineapple, Fat Free, Tesco*	1 Serving/30g	22	0.1	73	8.8	8.6	0.4	0
Cottage, with Pineapple, GFY, Asda*	1 Pot/227g	193	2.3	85	9	10	1	0.5
Cottage, with Sweet Chilli, Red Pepper, CBY, Asda*	½ Tub/150g	118	2	79	9.9	7.1	1.3	0.3
Cottage, with Tomato & Cracked Black Pepper, Asda*	½ Pot/113g	86	2.4	76	10	3.1	2.1	1.3
Cottage, with Tuna & Sweetcorn, HL, Tesco*	1 Serving/150g	136	3.2	91	12.8	4.8	2.1	0.4
Cream, Average	*1 Portion/30g*	*132*	*14.2*	*439*	*3.1*	*0*	*47.4*	*0*
Cream, Garlic Herbs, Light, Boursin*	1 Portion/20g	26	1.8	131	8	4.5	9	0
Cream, Reduced Fat, Average	*1 Serving/20g*	*23*	*1.1*	*117*	*13*	*4*	*5.3*	*0.1*
Cream, with Onion & Chives, Morrisons*	1 Serving/20g	38	3	190	11	3	15	0
Cream, with Pineapple, Asda*	1 Serving/40g	77	5.2	193	8	11	13	0
Cream, with Red Peppers & Onion, GFY, Asda*	1 Serving/32g	42	1.9	130	13	6	6	0
Creme de Saint Agur, Saint Agur*	1 Serving/10g	28	2.5	285	13.5	2.3	24.7	0
Dairylea, Light, Slices, Kraft*	1 Slice/25g	44	1.9	177	16	8.2	7.6	1.6
Danish Blue, Average	*1 Serving/30g*	*106*	*8.7*	*352*	*20.8*	*0*	*29.1*	*0*
Demi Pont L'eveque, Finest, Tesco*	1 Serving/46g	138	10.6	301	21.1	0.4	23	0
Dolcelatte, Average	*1 Serving/30g*	*110*	*9.7*	*366*	*17.8*	*0.4*	*32.3*	*0.4*
Double Gloucester with Onion Chives, Sainsbury's*	1 Serving/30g	110	8.5	365	22.2	5.5	28.2	0
Double Gloucester, Average	*1 Serving/30g*	*121*	*10.2*	*404*	*24.5*	*0.1*	*34*	*0*
Double Gloucester, With Onion, Chives, Co-Op*	1 Serving/30g	122	9.9	407	23	3.2	33	0
Doux De Montagne, Average	*1 Serving/25g*	*88*	*7.1*	*352*	*22.9*	*1.5*	*28.3*	*0*
Edam, Average	*1 Serving/10g*	*33*	*2.5*	*326*	*25.3*	*0*	*24.9*	*0*
Edam, Dutch, Garlic & Herb Wedge, Asda*	1 Serving/60g	197	15	329	26	0	25	0
Edam, Reduced Fat, Average	*1 Serving/30g*	*69*	*3.3*	*230*	*32.4*	*0.1*	*11.1*	*0*
Edam, Slices, Average	*1 Slice/30g*	*96*	*7.2*	*320*	*25*	*0.4*	*24.1*	*0*
Emmental, Average	*1 Serving/10g*	*37*	*2.8*	*368*	*28.4*	*0*	*28.4*	*0*
Emmental, Light, Slices, President*	1 Slice/20g	60	3.6	298	34	0	18	0
Emmental, Spreadable, Low Low, Kerry*	1 Serving/20g	40	2.7	200	13	6.7	13.5	0
Feta, Apetina, Light, 10 % Fat, Arla*	1 Serving/30g	52	3	173	18.4	0.6	10.1	0
Feta, Average	*1 Serving/30g*	*79*	*6.4*	*262*	*16.3*	*1*	*21.5*	*0*
Feta, Lemon, Asda*	1 Serving/25g	76	6.8	302	13.2	1	27.2	0.6
Feta, Light, Greek, Salad, 40% Reduced Fat, Attis*	1 Portion/30g	51	3.6	170	20	0.6	12	0
Fondue, Original, Fromalp*	1 Pack/400g	888	68	222	15	2.5	17	0
Fondue, Swiss, Easy Cook, Tesco*	¼ Pack/100g	235	17	235	15.5	4	17	0
Fondue, Traditionnelle, Co-Op*	1 Serving/100g	409	34	409	26	0.9	34	0
Fontina, Average	*1 Serving/28g*	*109*	*9*	*389*	*25*	*0*	*32.1*	*0*
for Pizza, Grated	*1 Serving/50g*	*163*	*12.2*	*326*	*25*	*1.6*	*24.4*	*0*
Goats, Average	*1 Tsp/10g*	*26*	*2.1*	*262*	*13.8*	*3.8*	*21.2*	*0*
Goats, Breaded, Bites, Sainsbury's*	1 Bite/25g	84	6.2	337	13	15.1	25	0.8
Goats, Breaded, Cheese Emporium, Aldi*	1 Portion/25g	78	5.5	312	10.8	17.2	22	2
Goats, French, Mild, Average	*1 Serving/30g*	*49*	*3.5*	*163*	*11.2*	*3*	*11.8*	*0*
Goats, Premium, Average	*1 Serving/30g*	*98*	*7.8*	*327*	*20.5*	*0.6*	*26.1*	*0*
Goats, Soft, Average	*1 Serving/30g*	*79*	*6.3*	*262*	*16.7*	*1.8*	*20.8*	*0.5*
Goats, with Garlic & Chives, Welsh, Tesco*	1 Serving/32g	93	7.7	290	15.1	3.3	24.1	0.1

C

CHEESE

	Measure INFO/WEIGHT	per Measure KCAL	FAT	Nutrition Values per 100g / 100ml KCAL	PROT	CARB	FAT	FIBRE
Goats, with Herbs, Welsh, Sainsbury's*	1 Serving/30g	90	7.4	299	15.3	3.6	24.8	0.1
Gorgonzola, Average	*1 Serving/30g*	*100*	*8.1*	*334*	*20*	*0*	*27*	*0*
Gouda, Average	*1 Serving/30g*	*113*	*9.4*	*376*	*24*	*0*	*31.5*	*0*
Gran Padano, Reserva, Deluxe, Lidl*	1 Serving/10g	39	2.8	388	33	0	28.4	0
Grana Padano, Italian Cheese, Waitrose*	1 Serving/14g	54	4	388	33	0	28.4	0
Greek Style, for Salad, Weight Watchers*	1 Serving/30g	34	0.8	113	18	4.3	2.7	0
Greek Style, Salad Cheese, Everyday Value, Tesco*	1 Serving/30g	80	6.2	270	17.2	1.9	21	0
Gruyere	*1oz/28g*	*115*	*9.3*	*409*	*27.2*	*0*	*33.3*	*0*
Halloumi, Average	*1 Serving/80g*	*253*	*19.7*	*316*	*20.8*	*1.6*	*24.7*	*0*
Halloumi, Light Average	*1 Serving/100g*	*245*	*15.3*	*245*	*24.7*	*1.7*	*15.3*	*0*
Halloumi, Pesto, The Grill, M&S*	½ Pack/113g	318	23.6	283	19.8	3.2	21	1.1
Halum, Milky*	1 Serving/30g	70	7.6	234	21.8	0	25.5	0
Healthy Range, Average	*1 Slice/20g*	*39*	*2.1*	*197*	*20.6*	*5.2*	*10.4*	*0*
Healthy Range, Slices, Average	*1 Slice/25g*	*45*	*2.2*	*180*	*19.5*	*5.4*	*9*	*0*
Iberico, TTD, Sainsbury's*	1 Serving/30g	117	9.6	390	23.8	1	32.1	1
Italian, Grated, Average	*1 Serving/30g*	*144*	*10*	*481*	*44*	*1.1*	*33.4*	*0*
Jarlsberg, Slices, Average	*1 Slice/15g*	*54*	*4*	*360*	*27*	*0*	*27*	*0*
Kvarg, Raspberry, Lindahls, Nestle*	1 Pot/150g	90	0.3	60	11.3	3.4	0.2	0
Lactose Free, Arla*	1 Serving/30g	103	8.1	344	25.3	1	27	0
Lactose Free, Semi Hard, Lactofree, Arla*	1 Portion/30g	103	8.1	344	25.3	1	27	0
Lancashire	*1oz/28g*	*104*	*8.7*	*373*	*23.3*	*0.1*	*31*	*0*
Leerdammer, Lighter, Sliced, M&S*	1 Slice/23g	62	3.9	271	29.5	0.1	17	0
Leerdammer, Original, Sliced, Leerdammer*	1 Slice/20g	71	5.5	356	27	0.1	27.5	0
Manchego	*1 Serving/70g*	*340*	*30.8*	*485*	*22.2*	*0.1*	*44*	*0*
Marscapone, Lighter, Tesco*	½ Tub/125g	306	26.9	245	9.5	3	21.5	0
Mascarpone, 25% Less Fat, Sainsbury's*	1 Portion/30g	95	9	316	6.7	4.8	30	0
Mascarpone, Average	*1 Serving/30g*	*131*	*13.1*	*437*	*5.6*	*4.1*	*43.6*	*0*
Mature, Half Fat, Average	*1 Serving/25g*	*66*	*3.9*	*265*	*29.9*	*0.4*	*15.6*	*0.1*
Mild, Reduced Fat, Grated, Average	*1 Serving/30g*	*70*	*3.3*	*235*	*31.5*	*2.2*	*11.1*	*0*
Monterey Jack, Iga*	1 Serving/28g	110	9	393	25	0	32.1	0
Mozzarella, Average	*½ Ball/63g*	*172*	*12.9*	*275*	*21.2*	*1.2*	*20.6*	*0*
Mozzarella, Grated, Basics, Sainsbury's*	1 Serving/30g	98	7.5	327	26	2.5	25	0.5
Mozzarella, Lighter, BGTY, Sainsbury's*	1 Serving/30g	52	3.2	172	18.6	0.5	10.6	0
Mozzarella, Reduced Fat, Average	*½ Ball/63g*	*115*	*6.4*	*184*	*21.2*	*1*	*10.2*	*0*
Mozzarella, Sticks, Free From, Tesco*	2 Sticks/25g	75	4.5	301	15.3	18.6	18	1.7
Mozzarella, Sticks, Melting, Crispy Golden Crumb, M&S*	½ Pack/75g	269	18.1	359	18.2	16.4	24.1	1.8
Mozzarella, Sticks, Sainsbury's*	1 Stick/15g	53	3.2	356	15.5	23.2	21.8	2.4
Neufchctel, Soft, Average	*1 Serving/30g*	*76*	*6.9*	*253*	*9*	*3.6*	*23*	*0*
Norvegia, Sliced Light, Tine*	1 Slice/10g	27	1.6	272	32	0	16	0
Ossau-Iraty, Average	*1 Serving/30g*	*120*	*10.2*	*400*	*22.3*	*0.2*	*34*	*0*
Parlick Fell, Hard, Sheeps, Sainsbury's*	1 Serving/30g	112	8.9	372	20.8	4.1	29.6	2.9
Parmesan, Average	*1 Tbsp/10g*	*42*	*2.8*	*422*	*40*	*2*	*28.5*	*0*
Pecorino, Italian, Tesco*	1 Serving/30g	119	9.9	397	22	0	33	0
Pepper Jack, Sliced, Sargento*	1 Slice/21g	80	7	381	19	0	33.3	0
Poivre, Boursin*	1oz/28g	116	11.8	414	7	2	42	0
Port Salut, M&S*	1oz/28g	90	7.3	322	21	1	26	0
Provolone Piccante, Italiamo, Lidl*	1 Serving/30g	112	9	372	25	0.5	30	0.5
Quark, Average	*1 Serving/20g*	*13*	*0*	*66*	*11.9*	*4*	*0.2*	*0*
Quark, Soft, Fat Free, Tesco*	1 Serving/30g	18	0.1	63	11.5	3.5	0.2	0.5
Quark, Soft, Strawberry, Fat Free, Tesco*	1 Serving/30g	18	0	59	10.2	4.5	0	0.1
Quark, Soft, Tomato Basil, Tesco*	1 Serving/30g	18	0.2	60	9.9	4	0.5	0.2
Raclette, Richsmonts*	1 Slice/28g	100	8	357	25	0	28.6	0
Reblochon	*1 Serving/30g*	*95*	*8*	*318*	*19.7*	*0*	*26.6*	*0*

CHEESE

Measure INFO/WEIGHT	per Measure KCAL	per Measure FAT	Nutrition Values per 100g / 100ml KCAL	PROT	CARB	FAT	FIBRE
Red Hot Dutch, Deli, Morrisons*	1 Serving/30g	102	8.5	341	19.8	1.3	28.4	0.6
Red Leicester, Average	*1 Serving/30g*	*120*	*10.1*	*400*	*23.8*	*0.1*	*33.7*	*0*
Red Leicester, Reduced Fat, Average	*1 Serving/30g*	*78*	*4.6*	*261*	*30.2*	*0.1*	*15.4*	*0*
Red, Mozzarella, Grated, Low Low, Kerry*	1 Serving/30g	90	6.6	301	26	0.6	22	0
Ricotta, Average	*1 Serving/50g*	*67*	*4.8*	*134*	*9.3*	*2.9*	*9.5*	*0*
Roquefort, Average	*1oz/28g*	*105*	*9.2*	*375*	*19.7*	*0*	*32.9*	*0*
Rougette, Bavarian Red, Kaserei Champignon*	1 Serving/30g	129	12.9	429	14.3	0	42.9	0
Roule, French, Sainsbury's*	1 Serving/30g	96	9.2	321	8.5	3	30.5	0
Roule, Garlic & Parsley, Light, BGTY, Sainsbury's*	1 Serving/30g	51	3.2	171	16.4	2.6	10.6	0
Roule, Garlic, Herb, Lidl*	1 Serving/30g	90	8.4	301	7.3	5	28	0
Sage Derby	*1oz/28g*	*113*	*9.5*	*402*	*24.2*	*0.1*	*33.9*	*0*
Seriously Strong, Lighter, Spreadable, Mclelland*	1 Serving/30g	76	5.1	255	15.5	2.5	17	0
Shropshire, Blue, Average	*1 Serving/50g*	*196*	*17.1*	*391*	*21*	*0*	*34.2*	*0*
Slices, Average	*1 Slice/23g*	*82*	*6.6*	*358*	*24*	*0.8*	*28.6*	*0*
Slices, Caractere, Intense Nutty, Fol Epi*	1 Slice/22g	79	6.3	365	26	0.5	29	0
Slices, Lighter, Emporium Kids, Aldi*	1 Slice/25g	48	2.8	194	17	7.4	11	0.5
Slices, Red Leicester, Tesco*	1 Slice/30g	120	10.1	400	23.7	0	33.7	0
Slices, Smoked with Ham, Aldi*	1 Slice/21g	66	5.2	313	21	1	25	0.1
Soft, & Creamy with Onions & Garlic, GFY, Asda*	1 Serving/25g	32	1.5	126	13	5	6	0
Soft, & Smooth, Extra Light, HL, Tesco*	1 Serving/30g	39	1.8	130	14.2	3.7	6	0
Soft, 50% Lighter, NUME, Morrisons*	1 Serving/30g	51	3.8	169	9.7	4.2	12.5	0.5
Soft, Extra Light, Average	*1 Serving/20g*	*25*	*1.2*	*125*	*14.3*	*3.6*	*5.9*	*0.1*
Soft, Fruit & Rum Halo, Discover*	1 Serving/25g	104	8.5	414	8.6	11.7	34.1	0
Soft, Full Fat, Average	*1 Serving/50g*	*156*	*15.2*	*312*	*8.2*	*1.7*	*30.3*	*0*
Soft, Full Fat, Original, Lactose Free, Kraft*	1 Serving/30g	84	8.2	280	4.5	2.7	27.5	0.3
Soft, Full Fat, Simply, M&S*	1 Serving/30g	89	8.8	297	4.6	3.4	29.4	0.5
Soft, Garlic Herb, Extra Light, LC, Tesco*	1 Serving/38g	49	2.4	130	12.3	5.1	6.3	0.3
Soft, Garlic Herb, Roulade, M&S*	1 Portion/100g	295	27.3	295	7.8	4.1	27.3	1.3
Soft, Garlic Herbs, Light, Med Fat, Philadelphia*	1 Serving/20g	30	2.1	149	7.3	5.4	10.5	0.5
Soft, Greek Style, Philadelphia*	1 Serving/30g	34	2.1	114	7.7	4.3	7.1	0.2
Soft, Light, Average	*1 Tbsp/30g*	*54*	*3.9*	*179*	*12.1*	*3.2*	*13.1*	*0*
Soft, Med Fat, Average	*1 Serving/30g*	*62*	*5.4*	*207*	*8.4*	*3*	*17.9*	*0*
Soft, Mediterranean Herbs, Full Fat, Philadelphia*	1 Serving/30g	64	5.7	213	5	4.1	19	0.3
Soft, Pineapple Halo, Discover*	1 Serving/25g	101	8.2	404	7.2	16.6	32.6	1.2
Soft, Salmon Dill, Light, Med Fat, Philadelphia*	1 Serving/20g	28	2	142	7.3	5.1	10	0.5
Soft, Smoked Ham, Light, Med Fat, Philadelphia*	1 Serving/30g	48	3.6	160	6.9	5	12	0.3
Soft, Sweet Chilli, Light, Med Fat, Philadelphia*	1 Serving/20g	30	2	148	6.8	7.3	10	0.5
Soft, White, Lactofree, Arla*	1 Serving/30g	59	5	197	8.6	3	16.5	0
Soft, with Black Pepper, Light, Sainsbury's*	½ Pack/100g	205	16.5	205	11	3	16.5	0
Soft, with Chives, Light, Med Fat, Philadelphia*	1 Serving/20g	30	2.2	151	7.4	5.2	11	0.6
Soft, with Garlic & Herbs, Full Fat, Deli, Boursin*	1 Serving/28g	84	8.3	299	3.5	5	29.5	0
Soft, with Garlic Herbs, Light, Sainsbury's*	2 Servings/100g	157	11.4	157	10.6	3.1	11.4	0
Soft, with Onion & Chives, Lighter, Asda*	1 Serving/30g	32	1.3	105	11.6	4.5	4.3	0.2
Spreadable, Lighter, Squares, Mclelland*	1 Square/17g	33	2.4	192	14	2.5	14	0
Spreadable, Original, Squares, Mclelland*	1 Square/17g	41	3.4	244	13.4	2.6	20	0
Spreadable, Smokey, Mclelland*	1 Serving/30g	84	6.7	280	14	1	22.4	0
Stilton, Average	*1 Serving/30g*	*123*	*10.6*	*410*	*22.4*	*0.1*	*35.5*	*0*
Stilton, Blue, Average	*1 Serving/30g*	*124*	*10.7*	*412*	*22.8*	*0.1*	*35.7*	*0*
Stilton, White Apricot, M&S*	1oz/28g	94	6.5	337	13.8	18.5	23.1	0
Stilton, White with Cranberries, Tesco*	1 Serving/50g	184	14.8	368	15.8	9.5	29.7	0.7
Stilton, White with Mango Ginger, Tesco*	1/3 Pack/65g	228	14	350	13.1	25.8	21.6	0.6
Stilton, White, Average	*1oz/28g*	*101*	*8.8*	*362*	*19.9*	*0.1*	*31.3*	*0*
Substitute, Mozzarella Style, Grated, Value, Tesco*	1 Serving/40g	120	8.4	300	25	2.5	21.1	0

	Measure INFO/WEIGHT	per Measure KCAL	FAT	Nutrition Values per 100g / 100ml KCAL	PROT	CARB	FAT	FIBRE
CHEESE								
Sussex Slipcote, Soft, Creamy, High Weald Dairy*	1 Serving/25g	60	4.7	238	14	3	18.9	0.7
Taleggio D.o.p., Finest, Tesco*	1 Serving/30g	89	7.5	297	18	0	25	0
Twisted, Cheestrings*	1 String/20g	61	4.5	305	23	2.5	22.5	0
Ubriaco, Prosecco DOC, 1, Waitrose*	1 Serving/30g	127	10	422	29	1.9	33.2	0
Vacherin Badoz, Waitrose*	1 Serving/30g	87	7.2	289	17.6	0.7	24	0
Wedge, Leerdammer*	1 Serving/30g	107	8.2	356	27	0	27.5	0
Wedges, Camembert, Breaded, Morrisons*	1 Wedge/25g	88	5.6	352	15.1	22.9	22.2	2
Wensleydale, & Ginger, Truckle, Morrisons*	1 Truckle/90g	330	23.7	367	18	14	26.3	1.1
Wensleydale, Average	**1 Serving/25g**	**92**	**7.8**	**369**	**22.4**	**0.1**	**31**	**0**
Wensleydale, with Blueberries, M&S*	1 Portion/30g	111	7.9	370	18.7	13.4	26.4	0.9
Wensleydale, with Cranberries, Sainsbury's*	1 Serving/50g	180	13.9	359	20.7	6.4	27.8	0
CHEESE ALTERNATIVE								
Cheezly, Cream, Original Flavour, The Redwood Co*	1 Pack/113g	357	34.5	316	5.6	4.8	30.5	0
Cheezly, Feta Style in Oil, The Redwood Co*	1 Serving/25g	119	11.8	475	2.5	10.6	47	0
Cheezly, Mozzarella Style, The Redwood Co*	1 Portion/25g	69	6.4	274	5.4	5.9	25.4	1
Chive Garlic, Spread, Vegan, Go Veggie*	1 Mini Tub/37g	100	10	270	5.4	2.7	27	0
Hard, Italian Style, Free From, Tesco*	1 Serving/30g	92	5.9	306	1.2	29.5	19.6	3.6
Herbs Chives, Creamy Smooth, Tofutti*	1 Serving/18g	51	4.9	283	3.3	6.7	27	0
Mozzarella, Grated, Free From, Tesco*	1 Serving/30g	94	7.8	313	0	18.3	26	3.2
Mozzarella, Slices, Dairy Free	**1 Slice/19g**	**80**	**6**	**420**	**10.5**	**10.5**	**31.5**	**0**
Soft, Coconut Based, Garlic Herb, Free From, Sainsbury's*	1 Serving/30g	83	7.9	277	6.6	2.2	26.3	2.5
Soft, Coconut Based, Original, Free From, Sainsbury's*	1 Serving/30g	85	8	285	6.5	3.4	26.8	2
Soft, Cream Cheese, Koko*	1 Serving/30g	60	5.6	199	0.4	7.6	18.7	0.9
Vegetarian, Average	**1 Serving/30g**	**110**	**8.4**	**368**	**28.2**	**0**	**28.1**	**0**
CHEESE ON TOAST								
Average	**1 Slice/130g**	**494**	**34.2**	**380**	**13.8**	**23.8**	**26.3**	**0.7**
CHEESE PUFFS								
Average	**1 Bag/25g**	**129**	**7.4**	**517**	**7.8**	**54.8**	**29.5**	**1.5**
Cheeky, Tesco*	1 Bag/20g	108	7	542	6.7	50.2	34.9	0
Morrisons*	1 Bag/25g	136	8.7	542	6.7	50.2	34.9	1.1
Sainsbury's*	1 Pack/100g	530	32	530	9.1	51.4	32	1.9
Shapers, Boots*	1 Bag/16g	80	3.8	500	7.1	64	24	0.9
Value, Tesco*	1 Pack/16g	84	4.6	525	6.2	60	28.8	0.6
CHEESE SPREAD								
Average	**1 Serving/30g**	**76**	**6.4**	**254**	**9.4**	**5.9**	**21.4**	**0.1**
Cheese Ham, Primula*	1 Squeeze/25g	50	3.8	200	12.3	3.1	15	4.9
Dairylea, Light, Tub, Kraft*	1 Serving/30g	47	2.2	158	16.5	5.2	7.2	0
Dairylea, Tub, Kraft*	1 Serving/25g	60	4.9	240	11	5.3	19.5	0
Flavoured	**1oz/28g**	**72**	**5.7**	**258**	**14.2**	**4.4**	**20.5**	**0**
Healthy Range, Average	**1 Serving/30g**	**31**	**1**	**102**	**14.3**	**3.8**	**3.2**	**0.9**
with Chives, Primula*	1 Squeeze/25g	48	3.6	190	12.5	2.9	14.2	4.5
with Prawn, Primula*	1 Squeeze/25g	48	3.6	190	12.5	3.3	14.4	3.6
CHEESE STRAWS								
Cheddar, M&S*	1 Straw/11g	59	3.8	535	14.9	40.1	34.9	2.4
Cheese Twists, Tesco*	1 Twist/8g	40	2.1	507	13.8	52.1	26.4	2.8
Finest, Tesco*	1 Straw/7g	39	2.6	558	13.3	41.5	37.6	1.5
Homemade or Bakery, Average	**1 Straw/41g**	**173**	**12.6**	**422**	**12**	**24.2**	**30.7**	**0.7**
Selection, Sainsbury's*	1 Straw/7g	41	2.9	558	16.6	34.5	39.3	2.8
CHEESE TRIANGLES								
Average	**1 Triangle/14g**	**33**	**2.2**	**238**	**10.3**	**14.2**	**15.6**	**0.2**
Dairylea, Light, Kraft*	1 Triangle/18g	36	2.2	205	15.5	6.3	12.5	0
Light, Extra, The Laughing Cow, Fromageries Bel*	1 Triangle/18g	19	0.4	108	17	5.5	2	0
Light, with Blue Cheese, The Laughing Cow*	1 Triangle/16g	24	1.4	151	13	5.5	8.5	0

	Measure INFO/WEIGHT	per Measure KCAL	FAT	Nutrition Values per 100g / 100ml KCAL	PROT	CARB	FAT	FIBRE
CHEESE TRIANGLES								
Reduced Fat, Average	**1 Triangle/18g**	**27**	**1.2**	**154**	**15.4**	**7**	**7**	**0**
CHEESE TWISTS								
All Butter, M&S*	1 Pack/125g	625	33.4	500	14.2	50.2	26.7	3.2
Asda*	1 Twist/8g	42	2.4	500	14	48	28	5
Gruyere Poppy Seed, Truly Irresistible, Co-Op*	1 Twist/8g	42	2.4	520	13.2	48.8	30.1	2.5
Gruyere Poppy Seed, TTD, Sainsbury's*	1 Serving/8g	41	2.3	509	13.7	50.5	28	2.6
Gruyere, Poppy Seed, All Butter, Waitrose*	1 Twist/8g	40	2.2	505	12.7	48.2	28	4.8
Parmesan, All Butter, TTD, Sainsbury's*	1 Serving/8g	38	2	487	13.8	51	25.3	2.8
Pre Packed, Average	**1 Twist/8g**	**41**	**2.2**	**515**	**13.7**	**47.9**	**27.7**	**2.3**
CHEESECAKE								
After Noon, Mango Passionfruit, 3 Pack, Gu*	1 Portion/45g	155	11.3	345	3.4	26.5	25.2	0.4
American Red White Blueberry, Sainsbury's*	1/6 Cake/83g	264	15.4	318	3.8	35.1	18.5	0.4
Apple, & Cinnamon, Baked, M&S*	1 Serving/116g	390	22	335	3.7	39.7	18.9	2.1
Apricot, Co-Op*	1 Cake/100g	230	11	230	4	29	11	0.9
Apricot, HL, Tesco*	1 Pot/100g	179	2.3	179	4.9	34.7	2.3	1.6
Average	**1 Slice/115g**	**490**	**40.8**	**426**	**3.7**	**24.6**	**35.5**	**0.4**
Berry, Autumn, Waitrose*	1 Slice/92g	316	20.3	343	4.4	31.5	22.1	2
Berry, Red, Waitrose*	1 Slice/101g	350	22.5	346	4.6	31.3	22.2	1.4
Blackcurrant, Average	**1 Serving/90g**	**237**	**11.9**	**263**	**3.6**	**32.3**	**13.2**	**2.4**
Blackcurrant, Devonshire, McVitie's*	1/6 Cake/67g	193	11.5	288	3.8	29.7	17.1	1.7
Blackcurrant, Healthy Range, Average	**1 Serving/90g**	**182**	**4.7**	**203**	**4.7**	**33.6**	**5.3**	**2.1**
Blackcurrant, PB, Waitrose*	1/6 Cake/99g	212	3.6	214	4	39.6	3.6	2.4
Blackcurrant, Swirl, Heinz*	1/5 Cake/87g	241	13.4	277	4.1	30.3	15.4	3.6
Blackcurrant, Value, Tesco*	1 Serving/70g	174	8.6	248	2.8	31.4	12.3	1
Blackcurrant, Weight Watchers*	1 Cake/103g	191	2.9	185	4.6	35.4	2.8	3.5
Blueberry, & Lemon Flavour Wedges, Sainsbury's*	1 Serving/80g	262	16.9	327	5.1	29.2	21.1	1.2
Blueberry, & Vanilla, TTD, Sainsbury's*	1 Serving/95g	353	24.8	372	5.4	28.9	26.1	2.1
Blueberry, Gorgeous, Cooked, Aunt Bessie's*	1 Portion/75g	225	6.1	300	3.9	33.5	8.2	0.9
Caramel, Salted, Frozen, Tesco*	1 Serving/75g	241	10.6	321	6.5	41.5	14.1	0.9
Caramel, Salted, Mini, Iceland*	1 Cake/22g	85	4.7	380	3.2	44.5	20.9	0.6
Caramel, Swirl, Cadbury*	1 Slice/91g	373	23.5	410	6	40.1	25.8	0
Cherry, BGTY, Sainsbury's*	1 Serving/91g	181	3.9	199	4.6	35.5	4.3	0.5
Cherry, Healthy Range, Average	**1 Serving/90g**	**172**	**3**	**191**	**3.7**	**36.4**	**3.3**	**1.1**
Chocolate, & Hazlenut, Gold, Sara Lee*	1 Slice/65g	205	12.8	316	5.9	28.7	19.7	1.1
Chocolate, & Honeycomb, Slice, Sainsbury's*	1 Slice/98g	333	20.3	340	3.7	33.7	20.7	2.4
Chocolate, & Irish Cream Liqueur, Tesco*	1 Serving/93g	385	28	414	5	30.7	30.1	0.8
Chocolate, & Vanilla, Gu*	1 Pot/90g	379	27.1	421	4.1	34.6	30.1	1.6
Chocolate, & Vanilla, Reduced Fat, M&S*	1 Serving/114g	319	13.7	280	7	37.9	12	1.5
Chocolate, & Vanilla, Tesco*	1 Serving/90g	330	19.4	365	5.2	37.1	21.5	1.6
Chocolate, Average	**1 Serving/75g**	**265**	**15.7**	**353**	**5.7**	**35.6**	**20.9**	**1.9**
Chocolate, Belgian, M&S*	1 Slice/100g	385	23.9	385	5.3	39.2	23.9	2.5
Chocolate, Belgian, Milk, Specially Selected, Aldi*	1/6 Cake/93g	386	25.1	415	5	37	27	1.6
Chocolate, Belgian, Tesco*	1/6 Cake/90g	392	25.8	436	5.1	37.9	28.7	2.8
Chocolate, Double, Wedge, Sainsbury's*	1 Serving/75g	327	24.8	436	5.7	29	33	1.7
Chocolate, Orange, Aldi*	1/6 Pack/83g	262	16.6	316	4.4	29	20	1.1
Chocolate, Pure Indulgence, Thorntons*	1 Serving/75g	308	17.6	410	5.6	44.3	23.4	0.6
Chocolate, Slice, M&S*	1 Pack/100g	409	25.6	409	4.5	39.2	25.6	2.1
Chocolate, Truffle, HL, Tesco*	1 Slice/96g	250	13.2	260	10.3	23.7	13.8	6.5
Chocolate, Weight Watchers*	1 Cake/95g	143	3.8	151	7.5	20.7	4	0.7
Citrus, Good Choice, Mini, Iceland*	1 Cake/111g	198	4.7	178	3.5	31.6	4.2	0.4
Commercially Prepared	**1/6 Cake/80g**	**257**	**18**	**321**	**5.5**	**25.5**	**22.5**	**0.4**
Forest Fruits, Tesco*	1 Serving/74g	182	5.9	246	4.4	38.2	7.9	2.2
Fruit, Average	**1 Serving/75g**	**207**	**10.9**	**276**	**5.3**	**32.3**	**14.5**	**1.6**

CHEESECAKE

	Measure INFO/WEIGHT	per Measure KCAL	FAT	Nutrition Values per 100g / 100ml KCAL	PROT	CARB	FAT	FIBRE
Fudge, Tesco*	1 Serving/102g	384	23.6	376	4.6	37.5	23.1	0.5
Irish Cream, McVitie's*	¼ Slice/190g	616	36.9	324	4.4	33	19.4	0.4
Lemon, Asda*	1 Slice/90g	319	21.2	354	4.3	31.2	23.5	1.1
Lemon, Average	**1 Serving/90g**	**307**	**19.5**	**341**	**4.1**	**33**	**21.6**	**1.8**
Lemon, BGTY, Sainsbury's*	1/6 Cake/71g	142	2.7	200	4.4	37	3.8	0.5
Lemon, Creamy & Light, M&S*	1/6 Cake/68g	236	13.8	350	3.5	32.3	20.4	0.4
Lemon, Meringue, Tesco*	1 Slice/94g	352	25	375	3.8	30.1	26.6	0.3
Lemon, Sainsbury's*	1 Serving/180g	650	37.1	361	4	39.9	20.6	1.3
Lemon, Sicilian, Bella Italia*	1 Cake/109g	355	18.6	325	4.1	34.4	17	0.3
Lemon, Sicilian, Slices, Finest, Tesco*	1 Slice/100g	351	21	351	3	36.8	21	1.2
Lemon, Swirl, Asda*	1 Pack/125g	445	29.9	356	3.1	32.1	23.9	1.8
Lemon, Swirl, Individual, Sainsbury's*	1 Pot/125g	380	23	304	3	31.1	18.4	0.9
Lemon, Swirl, Ms Mollys*	1 Serving/75g	243	11.5	324	5.2	40.9	15.3	0.7
Lemon, Swirl, Sainsbury's*	1/6 Cake/95g	350	21	369	4.8	37.2	22.1	1
Lemon, Tesco*	1 Slice/93g	315	21	339	5.2	28.6	22.6	0.3
Lemon, Value, Tesco*	1 Serving/79g	221	11.8	281	4.3	32.2	15	4.2
Lemon, Zesty, M&S*	1/6 Cake/97g	325	18.9	335	4	38.7	19.5	2.6
Mandarin, Co-Op*	1 Slice/99g	297	16.8	300	4	32	17	0.3
Mandarin, GFY, Asda*	1/6 Cake/92g	178	4	194	3.6	35	4.4	1.2
Mandarin, Low Fat, Tesco*	1 Serving/70g	145	3.3	207	3.3	37	4.7	1.4
Mandarin, Morrisons*	1 Serving/135g	335	16.9	248	3.8	32.2	12.5	0.8
Mandarin, Weight Watchers*	1 Cake/103g	180	2.9	175	4.6	32.9	2.8	1.5
Mango, Passion Fruit, Baked, Weight Watchers, Heinz*	1 Dessert/85g	159	1.9	187	4.2	36.9	2.2	1
Millionaires, Toffee Chocolate, Thorntons*	1 Serving/94g	351	20.1	373	4.7	40	21.4	1
New York, Baked, The Ultimate, Entenmann's*	1 Cake/100g	347	21.3	347	4.2	35.7	21.3	0.9
New York, Baked, Waitrose*	1/12 Cake/83g	317	22.6	380	5.1	28.3	27.1	1.2
New York, Mini, Iceland*	1 Cake/22g	86	5.1	385	3.6	40.7	23	0.5
Pecan, Seriously Nutty, Waitrose*	1 Serving/91g	341	21	376	5.8	35.7	23.2	1
Praline, Asda*	1/8 Cake/62g	226	14.9	364	7	30	24	3.2
Raspberry, & Mascarpone, Best, Morrisons*	1 Cake/84g	257	14	306	3.9	34.8	16.7	1
Raspberry, & Strawberry, M&S*	1 Slice/105g	340	21.1	325	3.9	33.4	20.2	1.2
Raspberry, & Vanilla, Slices, M&S*	1 Slice/100g	300	17.5	300	4.4	30.4	17.5	1.7
Raspberry, BGTY, Sainsbury's*	1 Pot/95g	154	2.5	163	6.6	28.2	2.6	2.8
Raspberry, LC, Tesco*	1 Cake/95g	185	4.1	195	4.3	34.7	4.3	1.3
Raspberry, Rapture, Slices, Tesco*	1 Slice/110g	341	20.4	310	4.2	30.8	18.5	1.8
Raspberry, Ripple, Sainsbury's*	1 Portion/95g	355	21.8	373	4.5	37	22.9	0.9
Rhubarb, Crumble, Sainsbury's*	1 Serving/114g	268	10.6	235	3.1	34.8	9.3	2.4
Rocky Road, CBY, Asda*	1 Serving/75g	302	17.3	402	4.5	43.4	23.1	1.4
Sticky Toffee, Tesco*	1 Slice/66g	248	16	375	4	35.3	24.2	0.5
Strawberry, & Cream, Finest, Tesco*	1 Serving/104g	325	22.4	312	4.3	25.3	21.5	0.5
Strawberry, Rhubarb, Slice, M&S*	1 Pack/100g	377	23.8	377	4.3	35.7	23.8	1.3
Strawberry, Creamy, Weight Watchers*	1 Cake/105g	187	2.6	178	4.7	34.2	2.5	2.2
Strawberry, Devonshire, McVitie's*	1/6 Cake/66g	192	10.7	291	4.4	31.8	16.2	3.6
Strawberry, Finest, Tesco*	1 Slice/113g	383	25.1	339	4.8	30.1	22.2	0.9
Strawberry, Free From, Tesco*	1 Serving/77g	228	12.1	296	1.6	36.4	15.7	1.3
Strawberry, Fresh, M&S*	¼ Cake/125g	300	19.2	240	2.8	23.1	15.4	1.1
Strawberry, Frozen, Sainsbury's*	1/6 Cake/84g	277	14.2	332	4.3	40.4	17	2.3
Strawberry, Shortcake, Sara Lee*	1/6 Slice/68g	230	15.7	337	4.9	27.6	23	0.5
Strawberry, Swirl, Frozen, Ms Mollys*	1 Slice/75g	242	11.2	323	5.2	41.7	14.9	0.6
Summerfruit, GFY, Asda*	1/6 Cake/92g	175	3.8	191	3.7	34.5	4.2	1.4
Toffee, & Pecan, Wedge, Sainsbury's*	1 Serving/75g	296	21.8	395	5.4	28.1	29	3.1
Toffee, American Style, Asda*	1 Serving/75g	269	15.8	359	4.5	38	21	3.8
Toffee, Apple, Tesco*	1/6 Cake/80g	233	11	291	4	37.7	13.7	0.6

	Measure INFO/WEIGHT	per Measure KCAL	per Measure FAT	Nutrition Values per 100g / 100ml KCAL	PROT	CARB	FAT	FIBRE
CHEESECAKE								
Toffee, Asda*	1 Cake/87g	295	19.1	339	4.3	31	22	3.5
Toffee, Lidl*	1 Pot/100g	275	12.3	275	3	37.6	12.3	1
Toffee, M&S*	1 Serving/105g	357	22.6	340	5.2	37.2	21.5	0.9
Toffee, Mini, Asda*	1 Cake/20g	57	2.4	286	4.6	40	12	2.1
Toffee, Tesco*	1 Serving/100g	265	12.9	265	4.3	33.1	12.9	0.8
Vanilla	*1 Serving/100g*	*395*	*26.2*	*395*	*5.3*	*42.8*	*26.2*	*1.1*
Vanilla, & Chocolate, Baked, Slice, Sainsbury's*	1 Slice/90g	349	23	388	5.7	33.8	25.6	2.7
Vanilla, Berry, Weight Watchers*	1 Dessert/85g	156	3	184	3.6	34	3.5	1.8
Vanilla, Creamy, New York, Slices, Tesco*	1 Slice/90g	314	21.4	349	5.1	28.3	23.7	0.8
Vanilla, Madagascan, Finest, Tesco*	1 Serving/90g	319	19	354	5.7	35.1	21.1	0.7
Vanilla, Tesco*	1 Serving/115g	417	28.4	363	5.7	29.4	24.7	0.6
White Chocolate, Mixed Berry, Finest, Tesco*	1 Serving/70g	246	13.7	353	4.5	38.9	19.6	1.3
CHERRIES								
Black in Syrup, Average	*1 Serving/242g*	*160*	*0*	*66*	*0.6*	*16*	*0*	*0.7*
Black, Fresh, Average	*1 Serving/80g*	*41*	*0.1*	*51*	*0.9*	*11.5*	*0.1*	*1.6*
Black, in Kirsch, Drained, Opies*	1 Jar/250g	155	0.5	62	0.5	15	0.2	1.1
Dark, Sweet, Pitted, Frozen, Essential, Waitrose*	1 Serving/80g	44	0.1	55	0.9	11.5	0.1	2.1
Dried, Wholefoods, Tesco*	1 Serving/25g	86	0.2	345	1.9	81.6	0.8	4.6
Glace, Average	*1oz/28g*	*79*	*0*	*280*	*0.4*	*71.2*	*0.2*	*1.1*
Picota, Average	*1 Serving/80g*	*42*	*0.1*	*52*	*0.9*	*11.4*	*0.1*	*1.2*
Pitted, Dark, Sweet, Frozen, Tesco*	1 Serving/80g	53	0.2	66	1.1	13.9	0.2	2.1
Raw, Average	*1oz/28g*	*14*	*0*	*49*	*0.9*	*11.2*	*0.1*	*1.4*
Stewed with Sugar, Average	*1oz/28g*	*23*	*0*	*82*	*0.7*	*21*	*0.1*	*0.7*
Stewed without Sugar, Average	*1oz/28g*	*12*	*0*	*42*	*0.8*	*10.1*	*0.1*	*0.8*
CHERRYADE								
Barr's*	1 Serving/200ml	32	0	16	0	4	0	0
No Added Sugar, Morrisons*	1 Glass/250ml	2	0	1	0	0.1	0	0
Sugar Free, Tesco*	1 Glass/200ml	2	0	1	0	0	0	0
CHESTNUTS								
Average	*1 Serving/100g*	*174*	*2.3*	*174*	*2.9*	*31*	*2.3*	*8.9*
Candied, Marrons Glace, Wholefoods Online*	1 Piece/20g	65	0.2	325	0.8	76.4	0.8	4.8
Roasted, Peeled, Average	*1 Nut/10g*	*17*	*0.3*	*170*	*2*	*36.6*	*2.7*	*4.1*
CHEWING GUM								
Airwaves, Sugar Free, Wrigleys*	1 Pack/15g	23	0	155	0	62	0	0
Doublemint, Wrigleys*	1 Stick/3g	10	0	370	0	74.1	0	0
Extra, Cool Breeze, Wrigleys*	1 Piece/2g	3	0	153	0	64	0	0
Extra, Peppermint, Sugar Free, Wrigleys*	1 Piece/2g	3	0	155	0	39	0	0
Peppermint, Sugar Free, Active, Aldi*	2 Pieces/3g	4	0	146	0	61	0	0
Spearmint, Extra, Wrigleys*	1 Piece/1g	1	0	143	0	64.3	0	0
Spearmint, Wrigleys*	1 Piece/3g	9	0	295	0	73	0	0
Splash, Raspberry Peach, Trident*	1 Piece/2g	4	0	180	1.6	68.5	0.5	0
CHICK PEAS								
Canned, Drained, Average	*1 Can/240g*	*276*	*6*	*115*	*7.4*	*15.2*	*2.5*	*4.6*
Dried, Average	*1 Serving/100g*	*319*	*5.4*	*319*	*21.7*	*47.4*	*5.4*	*8*
Dried, Boiled, Average	*1 Serving/75g*	*85*	*1.7*	*114*	*7.3*	*16.4*	*2.2*	*2.6*
in Salted Water, Canned, Average	*1 Can/179g*	*204*	*5.2*	*114*	*7.2*	*14.9*	*2.9*	*4.1*
in Water, Canned, Average	*1 Can/250g*	*282*	*6.6*	*113*	*7.2*	*15.3*	*2.6*	*4.8*
CHICKEN								
Bites, Breaded, Sainsbury's*	1 Bite/22g	63	3.6	288	15.5	18.9	16.4	1.1
Bites, Hot Spicy, Tesco*	1 Pack/110g	143	1.8	130	18.9	9.6	1.6	2.5
Bites, Hot And Spicy, Fridge Raiders, Mattessons*	1 Bag/60g	131	7.3	218	21.1	5.4	12.2	1.1
Bites, Southern Fried, Fridge Raiders, Mattessons*	1 Bag/60g	133	8.5	221	18.8	4.2	14.2	0.8
Bites, Southern Fried, Tesco*	4 Bites/38g	93	5.2	247	17.8	11.9	13.8	1.9

CHICKEN

	Measure INFO/WEIGHT	per Measure KCAL	FAT	Nutrition Values per 100g / 100ml KCAL	PROT	CARB	FAT	FIBRE
Bites, Tikka, Average	1 Serving/50g	96	5.3	193	20.7	3.8	10.5	1.9
Breast, Chargrilled, Iceland*	1 Serving/80g	114	1.5	142	27.4	3.9	1.9	0
Breast, Chargrilled, Premium, Average	1 Piece/10g	13	0.3	134	25.9	0.6	2.6	0.3
Breast, Chargrilled, Sliced, Average	1 Slice/19g	24	0.5	124	24.4	0.5	2.7	0.4
Breast, Diced, Average	1 Serving/188g	242	4.4	129	26.9	0.1	2.4	0.1
Breast, Fillet, Pesto Breaded, Finest, Tesco*	½ Pack/151g	293	10.9	194	21.5	10.5	7.2	0.5
Breast, Fillets, Breaded, Average	1 Fillet/112g	246	11.6	220	17.6	14	10.4	1.3
Breast, Fillets, Breaded, Lemon & Pepper, Average	1 Fillet/89g	133	2	150	22	10.1	2.3	1.3
Breast, Fillets, Cajun, Average	1 Fillet/93g	124	2.6	134	23.6	3.5	2.8	0.3
Breast, Fillets, Chargrilled, Average	1 Serving/100g	120	1.1	120	27.3	0.3	1.1	0.3
Breast, Fillets, Korma Style, Average	1 Serving/100g	132	2.8	132	27.4	0.8	2.8	0.6
Breast, Fillets, Mini, Raw, Average	1oz/28g	34	0.4	121	26.9	0.2	1.5	0.1
Breast, Fillets, Organic, Average	1 Serving/150g	153	1.1	102	24	0	0.8	0
Breast, Fillets, Skinless Boneless, Raw, Average	1 Breast/100g	129	2	129	27.7	0	2	0
Breast, Grilled, Average	1 Breast/130g	174	2.8	134	29	0.1	2.2	0
Breast, in Breadcrumbs, GF, Sainsbury's*	1 Fillet/150g	294	12.6	196	18	11.5	8.4	1.3
Breast, Joint, Stuffing, Tesco*	1 Serving/128g	197	11.4	154	13.1	5	8.9	0.7
Breast, Meat Skin, Raw, Average	1 Serving/145g	249	13.4	172	20.8	0	9.2	0
Breast, Meat Skin, Weighed with Bone, Raw, Average	1oz/28g	39	2.1	138	16.7	0	7.4	0
Breast, Meat Only, Fried	1 Serving/50g	68	1.7	137	24.4	0.4	3.4	0
Breast, Morrisons*	½ Pack/180g	328	16.9	182	16.6	7.7	9.4	2
Breast, on a Stick, Chinese Marinated, Musclefood*	1 Pack/75g	93	1	124	21.9	5.9	1.3	0.8
Breast, On a Stick, Spicy Marinated, Musclefood*	1 Stick/75g	80	7.3	107	21.5	2.7	9.8	7.5
Breast, Pieces, BBQ, Sainsbury's*	½ Pack/70g	93	0.8	132	23.8	6.3	1.2	0.5
Breast, Pieces, Tikka, Average	1 Serving/100g	154	3.4	154	28.2	2.8	3.4	0.4
Breast, Roast, Sliced, From Supermarket, Average	1 Slice/13g	17	0.4	139	25	1.8	3.5	0.2
Breast, Roast, without Skin, Average	1oz/28g	41	1.3	146	24.8	1	4.6	0.2
Breast, Slices, Chargrill Style, Asda*	1 Slice/28g	31	0.6	112	22.7	0.8	2	0
Breast, Slices, Maple, Dulano, Lidl*	1 Slice/9g	10	0.2	111	20	3	2	0.5
Breast, Smoked, Sliced, Average	1 Slice/20g	22	0.5	110	20.7	0.9	2.6	0.1
Breast, Strips, Raw, Average	1 Serving/280g	358	5.7	128	27.1	0.4	2	0.3
Breast, Tandoori Style, Average	1 Serving/180g	237	6.8	132	22.3	2.3	3.8	1
Breast, Tikka, Sliced, Average	1oz/28g	34	0.5	120	24.9	2	1.7	0.6
Butter Basted, TTD, Sainsbury's*	1 Slice/30g	44	1.9	147	22.8	0	6.2	0.6
Chargrill, Sweet Sticky, As Sold, Birds Eye*	1 Grill/88g	148	7.2	168	17	6.6	8.2	0.5
Dippers, Battered, Tesco*	4 Dippers/78g	222	14	285	13.1	17.4	17.9	0.8
Dippers, Crispy, Average	5 Dippers/93g	231	14.3	249	13.2	14.4	15.4	0.6
Drumsticks, BBQ Flavour, Average	1 Serving/200g	348	16	174	22.6	3.1	8	0.4
Drumsticks, Breaded, Fried, Average	1oz/28g	66	3.9	237	18.7	9.4	13.9	0.6
Drumsticks, Chinese Style, Average	1 Serving/100g	178	8.1	178	22.6	3.6	8.1	0.7
Drumsticks, Meat & Skin, Weighed with Bone, Raw	1 Serving/133g	188	11	141	15.7	0.1	8.3	0
Drumsticks, Meat Only, Weighed with Bone, Raw	1 Serving/122g	159	9.3	130	14.4	0.1	7.6	0
Drumsticks, Meat Only, Weighed with Bone, Roast	1 Serving/100g	116	5.5	116	16	0.3	5.5	0.1
Drumsticks, with Skin, Average	1 Piece/125g	268	16.6	215	22.1	1.8	13.3	0.3
Escalope, Breaded, Average	1 Escalope/128g	361	21.6	282	13.4	19.1	16.9	0.7
Escalope, Plain, Breast, Average	1 Serving/100g	110	2.2	110	22.3	0.7	2.2	0.5
Fillets, Battered, Average	1 Fillet/90g	199	10.4	221	16.1	13.3	11.5	0.5
Fillets, Breaded, Average	1 Piece/98g	214	10.5	219	14.2	15.9	10.7	1.9
Fillets, Cajun, Ashfield Farm, Aldi*	1 Fillet/122g	161	3.3	132	26	0.7	2.7	0.5
Fillets, Chargrilled, Spicy, 5 Pack, Fridge Filler, Taste Inc*	1 Fillet/35g	51	1.4	147	24.6	3	4	0
Fillets, Chinese Style, Average	1oz/28g	37	0.5	132	24.4	4.6	1.8	0.5
Fillets, Honey & Mustard, Average	1 Serving/100g	138	3.7	138	18.4	7.5	3.7	0.8
Fillets, Hot & Spicy, Average	1oz/28g	58	3.1	206	16.4	10.5	11	1.1

CHICKEN

INFO/WEIGHT	Measure	per Measure		Nutrition Values per 100g / 100ml				
		KCAL	FAT	KCAL	PROT	CARB	FAT	FIBRE
Fillets, Lime & Coriander, Mini, Average	1 Fillet/42g	49	0.5	118	24.3	2.6	1.3	0.6
Fillets, Mini, Sweet Smokey, Eat Well, M&S*	½ Pack/60g	70	0.2	117	25.5	2.9	0.4	0.1
Fillets, Red Thai, Mini, Average	1oz/28g	36	0.6	128	21.7	5.4	2	0.6
Fillets, Southern Fried, Meat Only, Average	1 Piece/100g	222	12	222	16.4	12.2	12	1.1
Fillets, Sweet Chilli, Mini, Sainsbury's*	½ Pack/100g	119	1.1	119	21.8	5.4	1.1	0.9
Fillets, Tandoori Style, Mini, Average	1 Serving/100g	128	2	128	24.7	2.6	2	0.4
Fillets, Tikka, Average	1 Serving/100g	141	5	141	22.4	1.7	5	1.1
Fillets, Tikka, Mini, Average	1oz/28g	35	0.6	124	25.1	1.3	2.2	1.2
Fingers, Average	1 Serving/75g	188	9.9	250	13.7	18.8	13.2	1.2
Goujons, Breaded, Average	1 Serving/114g	293	17.1	258	15.8	15.2	15	1
Goujons, Breast, Fresh, Average	1oz/28g	36	0.5	127	28	0	1.6	0
Leg or Thigh, Hot Spicy, Average	1oz/28g	50	3	179	19.4	1	10.8	0.4
Leg Portion, Roast, weighed with Bone, without Skin	1 Portion/114g	175	11	153	30.9	0	9.6	0
Leg Portion, Roasted Dry, with Skin, without Bone	1 Portion/120g	188	11.8	156	16.7	0.2	9.8	0.2
Leg, Meat Only, Cooked, Stewed, Average	1 Serving/60g	111	4.8	185	26	0	8	0
Leg, Meat Only, Raw, Average	1oz/28g	34	1.1	120	20.1	0	3.8	0
Leg, Meat Only, Raw, Weighed with Skin & Bone	1oz/28g	21	0.7	76	12.8	0	2.4	0
Leg, Meat Only, Stewed with Bone Skin, Average	1oz/28g	31	1.4	111	15.8	0	4.8	0
Leg, with Skin, Raw, Average	1oz/28g	48	2.9	172	19.1	0	10.4	0
Leg, with Skin, Roasted, Weighed with Bone, Average	1oz/28g	47	3.3	166	15.3	0.1	11.6	0
Light Meat, Raw	1oz/28g	30	0.3	106	24	0	1.1	0
Light Meat, Roasted	1oz/28g	43	1	153	30.2	0	3.6	0
Meat & Skin Portions, Deep Fried, Average	1oz/28g	73	4.7	259	26.9	0	16.8	0
Meat & Skin, Roasted, Average	1oz/28g	60	3.9	216	22.6	0	14	0
Meat, Roasted, Average	1oz/28g	47	1.9	167	25	0	6.6	0
Mexican Chilli, Sliced, Eat Well, M&S*	1 Pack/130g	169	3.4	130	25.9	0.8	2.6	0.5
Mince, Average	1oz/28g	39	1.7	140	20.9	0.1	6	0.2
Nuggets, Battered, Average	1 Nugget/20g	50	2.9	251	13.5	16.9	14.4	0.9
Nuggets, Breaded, Average	1 Nugget/14g	37	2	263	14.8	19.8	13.8	1.9
Nuggets, Free From Gluten Wheat, Sainsbury's*	1 Nugget/19g	47	2.5	251	13.4	19.7	13.2	0.8
On a Stick, Chinese, Grabits*	1 Stick/55g	69	0.7	125	21.9	5.9	1.3	0.8
Pieces, Boneless, Breaded, Fried, From Restaurant	1 Piece/17g	51	3.3	301	17	14.4	19.4	0
Pieces, Flame Grilled, Waitrose*	1 Pack/130g	168	2.3	129	27.9	0.2	1.8	0.2
Poppers, Ready to Eat, Tesco*	1 Popper/10g	27	1.6	273	11.5	19.9	16.2	0.7
Roast, Chicken Style, Vegeroast, Realeat*	4 Slices/114g	211	10.2	186	23	3.2	9	1.5
Roll, Breast, Average	1 Slice/10g	17	1	167	16.1	3.2	10	0.2
Schnitzel, As Prepared, Easy to Cook, Waitrose*	½ Pack/99g	168	5.4	170	27	2.4	5.5	1.3
Skewers, Marinated, Asda*	1 Skewer/35g	50	0.4	142	24.9	8	1.2	0.9
Skewers, Yakitori, M&S*	1 Box/65g	125	4.5	192	20.9	11.2	6.9	0.6
Skin, Dry, Roasted or Grilled, Average	1 Serving/100g	501	46.1	501	21.5	0	46.1	0
Skin, Moist, Roasted or Grilled, Average	1 Serving/100g	452	42.6	452	17	0	42.6	0
Sliced, Cooked, Average	1 Slice/15g	18	0.4	118	22.4	1.6	2.4	0.1
Southern Fried, Popstars, Birds Eye*	¼ Pack/100g	272	14	272	17	19	14	1.1
Spatchcock, Poussin, Sainsbury's*	1 Serving/122g	168	6.6	138	21.1	0.1	5.4	0.2
Steaks, Average	1 Serving/100g	205	9.4	205	21.1	9	9.4	0.7
Strips or Tenders, Chinese Style, Average	1oz/28g	41	1.1	145	19.6	8	4.1	1
Strips, Mexican, Sliced, M&S*	½ Pack/70g	77	0.4	110	24.3	2.3	0.6	0.5
Thigh, Meat & Skin, Casseroled, Average	1oz/28g	65	4.6	233	21.5	0	16.3	0
Thigh, Meat Skin, Raw, Average	1 Serving/100g	218	14.7	218	21.4	0	14.7	0
Thigh, Meat Skin, Weighed with Bone, Raw, Average	1 Serving/100g	186	14.1	186	13.8	0.2	14.1	0
Thigh, Meat Only, Diced, Casseroled	1oz/28g	50	2.4	180	25.6	0	8.6	0
Thigh, Meat Only, Raw, Average	1 Thigh/90g	113	4.9	126	19.4	0	5.4	0

C

	Measure INFO/WEIGHT	per Measure KCAL	FAT	Nutrition Values per 100g / 100ml KCAL	PROT	CARB	FAT	FIBRE
CHICKEN								
Thigh, Roast, Average	*1 Serving/100g*	*238*	*15.6*	*238*	*23.8*	*0.4*	*15.6*	*0*
Thigh, Sweet Chilli, Oven Cooked, Sainsbury's*	¼ Pack/138g	293	18.4	213	19.1	3.9	13.4	0.5
Tikka, Mint Raita Dip, Tesco*	1 Pack/90g	171	9.4	190	19.8	3.9	10.4	0.9
Vegan, Slices, Deli Style, Quorn*	½ Pack/50g	47	1.2	94	11	4.1	2.3	6.2
Vegetarian, Chicken Style Pieces, Vivera*	1 Pack/175g	208	0.9	119	19.4	6.4	0.5	0
Vegetarian, Chicken Style, Strips, Meat Free, Fry's*	1 Serving/95g	226	12.3	238	20.4	10	13	5.6
Vegetarian, Dippers, Quorn*	4 Dippers/92g	195	8	212	11.1	21.2	8.7	2.4
Vegetarian, Fillets, Breaded, Mini, Quorn*	1 Fillet/30g	59	2.9	196	10.2	15	9.6	4.5
Vegetarian, Fillets, Crispy, Quorn*	1 Fillet/100g	192	8.5	192	12.5	14.2	8.5	4
Vegetarian, Fillets, Garlic Herb, Quorn*	1 Fillet/100g	208	9.8	208	13.9	16.1	9.8	4.1
Vegetarian, Nuggets, Crispy, Chicken Style, Quorn*	1 Nugget/17g	33	2	198	12	8	12	4.8
Vegetarian, Roast Style, Quorn*	1/5 Roast/91g	96	1.8	106	15	4.5	2	4.9
Vegetarian, Roast, Family, Frozen, Cooked, Quorn*	1 Serving/80g	91	2.2	114	16.7	3	2.7	5
Wafer Thin, Average	*1 Slice/10g*	*12*	*0.4*	*120*	*19*	*2.8*	*3.6*	*0.2*
Whole, Garlic Herb, Lidl*	3 Slices/150g	261	16.5	174	18	0.6	11	0.5
Whole, Roast, Average	*½ Chicken/685g*	*910*	*57.7*	*133*	*13.4*	*0.9*	*8.4*	*0.1*
Wing Quarter, Meat Only, Casseroled	*1oz/28g*	*46*	*1.8*	*164*	*26.9*	*0*	*6.3*	*0*
Wing, Breaded, Fried, Average	*1oz/28g*	*77*	*4.8*	*273*	*17.1*	*13*	*17.2*	*0.4*
Wing, Meat & Skin, Cooked, Average	*1oz/28g*	*67*	*4.4*	*241*	*23.3*	*1.9*	*15.6*	*0.3*
Wings, BBQ Flavour, Average	*3 Wings/150g*	*330*	*18.7*	*220*	*20.3*	*6.6*	*12.4*	*0.6*
Wings, Chinese Style, Average	*1oz/28g*	*72*	*4.3*	*256*	*24.2*	*5.1*	*15.5*	*0.6*
Wings, Hot & Spicy, Average	*1oz/28g*	*65*	*3.8*	*231*	*21.8*	*5.2*	*13.6*	*0.8*
Wings, Meat & Skin, Raw, Average	*1 Wing/150g*	*286*	*19.3*	*191*	*17.5*	*0*	*12.8*	*0*
CHICKEN &								
Black Bean Noodles, Sainsbury's*	1 Serving/130g	155	0.9	119	4.3	23.9	0.7	0.8
Black Bean Sauce, with Egg Fried Rice, Ready Meal	*1 Serving/400g*	*390*	*6.1*	*97*	*6.5*	*14.5*	*1.5*	*0.8*
Black Bean with Noodles, Tesco*	1 Pack/475g	470	7.6	99	7.6	13.6	1.6	0.2
Black Bean, Chinese Takeaway, Tesco*	1 Serving/200g	190	6.6	95	8.3	8	3.3	0.5
Cashew Nuts, Chinese, Ready Meal, Average	*1 Serving/400g*	*497*	*24*	*124*	*9.2*	*7.5*	*6*	*1.2*
Chorizo Paella, Go Cook, Asda*	½ Pack/475g	591	10.5	124	10.2	15.9	2.2	2.6
Fries, Southern Fried Style, Tesco*	1 Pack/500g	930	40	186	11.5	16	8	1.4
Gravy, COU, M&S*	1 Pack/300g	216	3.9	72	7.2	7.8	1.3	1.6
King Prawn Special Fried Rice, Finest, Tesco*	1 Pack/450g	734	32	163	7.7	17	7.1	0.7
Mushroom with Rice, Egg Fried, Average	*1 Serving/400g*	*421*	*10.1*	*105*	*6.3*	*14.4*	*2.5*	*0.8*
Pineapple, Chilled, Tesco*	1 Pack/350g	364	8.4	104	9.6	11.1	2.4	5.5
Roasted Potatoes, Spanish, Charlie Bigham's*	½ Pack/387g	479	25.9	124	7.2	9.8	6.7	0
CHICKEN ALFREDO								
Average	*1 Pack/400g*	*416*	*10*	*104*	*12.2*	*8.2*	*2.5*	*0.8*
CHICKEN ARRABIATA								
COU, M&S*	1 Meal/360g	396	6.5	110	8.4	14.5	1.8	1.3
Italian Kitchen, Tesco*	1 Pack/414g	492	11.6	119	8.3	14.2	2.8	1.8
Meal for One, M&S*	1 Pack/400g	528	20.8	132	7.9	12.5	5.2	1.9
CHICKEN BANG BANG								
Waitrose*	1 Pack/350g	368	17.2	105	9.4	5.9	4.9	1.2
CHICKEN BUTTER								
Mother, Microwaved, Mumbai Street Food, Iceland*	1 Meal/224g	397	23.8	177	9	11.1	10.6	0.8
with Rice, Average	*1 Serving/400g*	*561*	*27.6*	*140*	*10.6*	*8.9*	*6.9*	*1.4*
CHICKEN CANTONESE								
& Rice, Sizzler, Tesco*	1 Serving/450g	639	25.6	142	7.7	14.9	5.7	0.9
Breast, Fillets, Sainsbury's*	1 Serving/154g	168	2.3	109	20.3	3.6	1.5	0.6
Chinese, Tesco*	½ Pack/175g	196	6.5	112	10.3	9.4	3.7	0.4
Honey, Sesame, Sainsbury's*	1/3 Pack/135g	116	3.6	86	9.8	5.5	2.7	0.8

	Measure INFO/WEIGHT	per Measure KCAL	FAT	Nutrition Values per 100g / 100ml KCAL	PROT	CARB	FAT	FIBRE
CHICKEN CHAR SUI								
Shredded, Ready To Eat, Tesco*	½ Pack/65g	77	0.8	119	20.4	5.8	1.3	1
CHICKEN CHASSEUR								
Average	**1 Serving/400g**	**363**	**9.2**	**91**	**12.2**	**4.9**	**2.3**	**0.9**
Breast Fillets, Morrisons*	1 Pack/380g	384	11.4	101	15.7	2.9	3	0.8
Finest, Tesco*	½ Pack/200g	200	6.4	100	14.3	2.4	3.2	1.1
CHICKEN CHILLI								
Sweet, Battered, Chinese Favourites Box, M&S*	½ Pack/120g	220	4.9	183	11	24.9	4.1	1.1
Sweet, CBY, Asda*	½ Pack/170g	253	6.8	149	19.1	8.9	4	0.7
Sweet, Just Cook, Sainsbury's*	½ Pack/191g	200	1.3	105	15.2	9.4	0.7	0.5
Sweet, Pieces, Morrisons*	1 Pack/200g	282	5	141	25.5	4.1	2.5	0.5
Sweet, With Noodles, Ready Meal, Average	**1 Serving/400g**	**404**	**5.8**	**101**	**6.5**	**15.5**	**1.4**	**1.4**
CHICKEN CHINESE								
Balls, M&S*	1 Ball/16g	45	2.2	280	10.8	29.2	13.6	2.1
Stir Fry, Morrisons*	1 Serving/319g	341	5.4	107	5.7	17	1.7	1.5
with Ginger & Spring Onion, Tesco*	1 Serving/350g	299	10.1	85	7.6	7.3	2.9	0.6
CHICKEN DINNER								
Cooked, Eat Smart, Morrisons*	1 Pack/355g	245	4.3	69	8.2	4.4	1.2	4.1
Roast Potatoes, Peas, Carrots, & Stuffing, HFC, Tesco*	1 Pack/382g	368	9.1	96	9	8.8	2.4	2
Roast, Mini Meals, Tesco*	1 Pack/218g	234	7	108	6.9	12	3.2	1.7
Roast, Mini, As Consumed, Fresh Ideas, Morrisons*	½ Pack/209g	310	13.6	148	18.7	3.3	6.5	1
Roast, Serves 1, Sainsbury's*	1 Pack/373g	466	13.4	125	9.4	12.3	3.6	2.6
CHICKEN EN CROUTE								
Chef Select, Lidl*	½ Pack/206g	558	34.8	271	12.8	16.1	16.9	1.7
Just Cook, Sainsbury's*	1 Serving/180g	481	27.2	267	16.8	15.9	15.1	0.4
CHICKEN IN								
Barbeque Sauce, Breasts, COU, M&S*	1 Pack/350g	420	6.7	120	8.5	20.6	1.9	0.6
BBQ Sauce, Breast, Sainsbury's*	1 Serving/170g	199	1.2	117	14.5	13.1	0.7	1.3
Black Bean Sauce, Sainsbury's*	1 Pack/465g	484	7.9	104	5	17.3	1.7	0.3
Black Bean Sauce, Takeaway, Iceland*	1 Pack/375g	345	11.2	92	8.6	7	3	1.5
Black Bean Sauce, with Egg Fried Rice, Frozen, Tesco*	1 Pack/369g	464	14.1	126	8.3	13.9	3.8	1.3
Gravy, Breast, Sainsbury's*	1 Box/200g	124	1	62	11.8	2.9	0.5	0.2
Hunter's BBQ Sauce, Asda*	½ Pack /190g	348	14.1	183	19.1	10.3	7.4	0
Leek & Bacon Sauce, Chilled, Co-Op*	1 Pack/400g	460	20	115	15	2	5	0.2
Lemon Garlic Marinade, Thighs, Go Cook, Asda*	½ Pack/265g	493	30.2	186	19.7	1.2	11.4	0.8
Madeira Sauce with Mushrooms, Finest, Tesco*	½ Pack/200g	210	8.3	105	13.8	3	4.2	1
Mushroom, Sauce, Tesco*	1 Pack/370g	289	8	78	7.8	6.2	2.2	1.3
Oyster Sauce Mushrooms, Tesco*	1 Pack/350g	252	5.6	72	8	6.3	1.6	0.7
Reggae Reggae Sauce, Drumsticks, Levi Roots*	1 Serving/100g	165	7.3	165	21.5	3.4	7.3	0
Smoky BBQ Marinade, Breast, Fillets, Mini, CBY, Asda*	3 Fillets/150g	144	1.5	96	18.5	3.3	1	0
Sweet Chilli Sauce, Breast, Fresh Tastes, Asda*	½ Pack/180g	288	9	160	18.4	10.3	5	0.5
Tomato & Basil Sauce, Breast Fillets, Morrisons*	½ Pack/171g	231	7.5	135	21.3	2.5	4.4	1.4
Tomato & Basil Sauce, Breast, GFY, Asda*	1 Pack/392g	447	13.3	114	12	9	3.4	1.5
Tomato & Herb Sauce, Breasts, Tesco*	½ Pack/173g	155	2.4	90	15	3.6	1.4	0.5
White Wine & Tarragon Sauce, Breasts, Finest, Tesco*	½ Pack/200g	326	20.2	163	16.8	1.3	10.1	0
White Wine & Tarragon Sauce, Waitrose*	½ Pack/225g	281	17.3	125	10.7	3.1	7.7	0.3
CHICKEN LEMON								
Battered, Cantonese, Sainsbury's*	1 Pack/350g	560	19.6	160	10.7	16.6	5.6	0.9
Battered, Chinese Meal for Two, Tesco*	½ Serving/175g	294	13	168	6.6	18.8	7.4	2
Cantonese, Sainsbury's*	½ Pack/140g	218	8.8	156	11	13.9	6.3	0.6
COU, M&S*	1 Pack/150g	150	1.4	100	17.9	5.6	0.9	0.8
CHICKEN MADEIRA								
with Mushroom Rice, Finest, Tesco*	1 Pack/413g	570	16.9	138	9.9	14.5	4.1	1.5

C

	Measure INFO/WEIGHT	per Measure KCAL	FAT	Nutrition Values per 100g / 100ml KCAL	PROT	CARB	FAT	FIBRE
CHICKEN MOROCCAN								
Style, Sainsbury's*	½ Pack/269g	334	7	124	14.7	10.4	2.6	3.1
with Bulgur Wheat, Good & Balanced, Asda*	1 Pack/375g	365	3.4	98	7.4	13.3	0.9	3.4
with Cous Cous, GFY, Asda*	1 Serving/450g	414	5.8	92	8	12	1.3	0.8
CHICKEN PASANDA								
Sainsbury's*	1 Serving/200g	368	24.8	184	14.7	3.4	12.4	2.3
with Pilau Rice, HL, Tesco*	1 Pack/440g	466	11	106	5.7	15.2	2.5	0.9
CHICKEN STUFFED								
Breast with Mushrooms, HE, Tesco*	1 Serving/175g	152	3.2	87	16.3	1.5	1.8	0.2
with Moroccan Style Cous Cous, GFY, Asda*	½ Pack/180g	259	4.9	144	20	10	2.7	0
with Mushrooms, Finest, Tesco*	1 Serving/150g	177	7.6	118	15.9	2	5.1	0.6
CHICKEN SUPREME								
Breast, Sainsbury's*	1 Serving/187g	421	29.5	225	20.6	0.3	15.8	0.6
with Rice, Asda*	1 Pack/450g	616	31.5	137	15	3.4	7	1.1
with Rice, HE, Tesco*	1 Pack/400g	384	6.4	96	4.9	15.6	1.6	1.5
CHICKEN SZECHUAN								
Tesco*	1 Pack/350g	385	10.5	110	7.2	13.6	3	0.3
with Noodles, Sainsbury's*	1 Pack/450g	423	14	94	6	10.4	3.1	0.9
CHICKEN TANDOORI								
Basmati Rice, Aromatic, Asda*	1 Pack/380g	399	8	105	7.5	12	2.1	3.7
Spiced Rice, As Consumed, Eat Smart, Morrisons*	1 Pack/380g	416	4.8	113	7.8	16.1	1.3	2.8
Fresh Tastes, Asda*	1 Pack/400g	356	5.6	89	6.4	12.7	1.4	2.1
Masala Rice, HL, Tesco*	1 Serving/450g	410	7.6	91	6.6	12.9	1.7	0.6
Masala, Indian, Tesco*	1 Serving/350g	430	25.9	123	10.2	4	7.4	1.8
Masala, Sainsbury's*	1 Pack/400g	536	27.2	134	13.2	5	6.8	0.5
Royal, with Pilau Rice Aloo Gobi, Co-Op*	1 Pack/451g	591	26.6	131	7.4	12	5.9	0.5
Sizzler, Sainsbury's*	1 Pack/400g	536	29.2	134	12.8	4.3	7.3	1.7
Sizzler, Tesco*	1 Serving/175g	243	11.6	139	10	10	6.6	1
Steam Meal, As Consumed, Simply Bistro, Aldi*	1 Pack/400g	317	7.5	80	5.5	9.3	1.9	2.1
with Rice, City Kitchen, Tesco*	1 Pack/385g	597	21.2	155	6.7	19.6	5.5	1.8
with Vegetable Pilau Rice, HL, Tesco*	1 Pack/348g	400	9	115	8.4	14.1	2.6	1.9
CHICKEN TERIYAKI								
& Noodles, Asda*	½ Pack/340g	445	8.8	131	9	18	2.6	0.9
Japanese with Ramen Noodles, Sainsbury's*	1 Pack/450g	482	9.4	107	6.5	15.5	2.1	0.8
Noodles, HL, Tesco*	1 Pack/367g	282	1.8	77	6.4	10.5	0.5	2.3
CHICKEN TIKKA								
& Cous Cous, Boots*	1 Pack/160g	307	17.6	192	6.2	17	11	1.3
& Lemon Rice, Deli Meal, M&S*	1 Pack/360g	342	7.2	95	9.8	10.2	2	0.7
Coriander Rice, Weight Watchers*	1 Pack/400g	348	2.4	87	6.2	14.3	0.6	1.6
Rice, Toddler Meal, Annabel Karmel*	1 Pack/200g	204	3	102	6.1	15.6	1.5	1.4
Creamy, Breast, Tesco*	1 Breast/190g	215	10.4	113	15.1	0.7	5.5	0.8
Masala, Pilau Rice, Charlie Bigham's*	½ Pack/403g	737	43.9	183	6.9	15.3	10.9	0
Masala, with Rice, Weight Watchers*	1 Meal/320g	380	5.8	119	6.8	18.5	1.8	0.7
Takeaway	*1 Serving/350g*	*421*	*15*	*120*	*20.3*	*0*	*4.3*	*0.3*
with Basmati Rice, Weight Watchers*	1 Pack/380g	342	6.5	90	6.6	11.8	1.7	1.1
with Pilau Rice, GFY, Asda*	1 Pack/450g	382	2.7	85	7	13	0.6	1.8
CHICKEN WITH								
a Sea Salt & Black Pepper Crust, Breasts, Asda*	1 Serving/154g	186	4.3	121	19	5	2.8	0
a Sticky Honey & Chilli Sauce, Breast, Asda*	1 Serving/175g	247	5.6	141	20	8	3.2	0
Broccoli & Pesto Pasta, BGTY, Sainsbury's*	1 Pack/301g	328	5.1	109	10.3	13.2	1.7	2.5
Caesar Melt Prosciutto, Breast, M&S*	1 Pack/375g	488	18.8	130	19.6	1.3	5	1
Cous Cous, Lemon Herb, Finest, Tesco*	1 Pack/370g	492	18.5	133	10.5	11.5	5	0.9
Garlic Chilli Balti, Tesco*	1 Pack/400g	320	7.6	80	11	4.4	1.9	0.8
Honey Ginger Sauce, 125, Oakhouse Foods Ltd*	1 Dinner/365g	339	8	93	8.7	9.8	2.2	1.2

	Measure INFO/WEIGHT	per Measure		Nutrition Values per 100g / 100ml				
		KCAL	FAT	KCAL	PROT	CARB	FAT	FIBRE
CHICKEN WITH								
Leek Bacon, M&S*	½ Pack/183g	239	12.8	131	15.3	1.2	7	0.9
Leeks, White Wine Sauce, Finest, Tesco*	½ Pack/180g	258	10.3	143	20.9	1.5	5.7	1.2
Lime & Coriander, Easy, Waitrose*	½ Pack/168g	203	7.9	121	18.9	0.7	4.7	0.5
Lyonnaise Potatoes, M&S*	½ Pack/260g	286	8.1	110	12.6	8	3.1	0.9
Mushroom & Bacon, Fillets, M&S*	½ Pack/188g	225	11.2	120	15.5	0.5	6	1.7
Pork Stuffing, Breast, Roast, M&S*	1 Serving/100g	165	6.5	165	24.1	3	6.5	0
Rice, Jamaican Jerk, Healthier Choice, Co-Op*	1 Pack/406g	365	9.3	90	7.8	9.8	2.3	3.4
Sage Onion Stuffing, Breast, Roast, Sliced, M&S*	1 Slice/17g	27	1.1	165	24.1	3	6.5	0
Spring Vegetables, Chargrilled, COU, M&S*	1 Pack/414g	290	3.7	70	8.8	7.3	0.9	1.8
Stuffing, TTD, Sainsbury's*	1 Slice/34g	50	2	148	22.7	1.3	5.8	0.9
CHICORY								
Fresh, Raw, Average	*1 Head/150g*	*30*	*0.9*	*20*	*0.6*	*2.8*	*0.6*	*0.9*
CHILLI								
& Potato Wedges, Good Choice, Iceland*	1 Pack/400g	368	13.6	92	5.5	9.8	3.4	1.2
& Rice, Birds Eye*	1 Serving/285g	305	7.7	107	3.4	17.2	2.7	1
& Rice, GFY, Asda*	1 Pack/400g	352	1.6	88	5	16	0.4	1.8
& Wedges, BBQ, HL, Tesco*	1 Pack/420g	391	10.9	93	5.4	12.2	2.6	1.9
Potato Wedges, Sainsbury's*	1 Pack/371g	393	15.2	106	7.2	10.1	4.1	2.2
Rice, Morrisons*	1 Serving/500g	630	15.5	126	5.7	18.9	3.1	1.1
Wedges, GFY, Asda*	1 Pack/400g	364	10	91	7	10.1	2.5	2.5
Ancho, Paste, Waitrose*	1 Tbsp/15g	13	0.2	89	2.7	13.2	1.6	5.3
Bean, 3, Mexican, with Rice, Weight Watchers, Heinz*	1 Meal/400g	328	3.6	82	3	13.8	0.9	3.6
Bean, Mixed, Chipotle, with Wild Rice, Eat Well, M&S*	1 Pack/300g	312	5.7	104	3.9	15.9	1.9	3.9
Beef Mushrooms, GFY, Asda*	1 Pack/400g	364	6	91	9.1	10.2	1.5	1.2
Beef Potato Crush, Weight Watchers*	1 Pack/400g	232	6	58	5	5.9	1.5	3.4
Beef Rice Pot, Shapers, Boots*	1 Pot/301g	250	4.5	83	4	12	1.5	2.1
Beef with Rice, GFY, Asda*	1 Serving/402g	354	6	88	4.7	14	1.5	0.9
Beef with Rice, Sainsbury's*	1 Serving/300g	360	5.1	120	5.6	20.6	1.7	1.1
Beef, Rice, HL, Tesco*	1 Pack/370g	370	5.9	100	5	13.7	1.6	5.5
Beef, Rice, Tex Mex, Tesco*	1 Pack/440g	591	12.8	134	5.4	20.4	2.9	2.5
Beef, Asda*	½ Pack/200g	190	7.8	95	7	8	3.9	1.2
Beef, High Protein, Mexican Bean, Batchelors*	1 Pack/270g	228	4.1	84	4.7	11.3	1.5	3.4
Beef, Pulled, Cook*	1 Pack/320g	365	11.5	114	10.3	7.6	3.6	1.3
Con Carne Rice, Everyday, Value, Tesco*	1 Pack/400g	455	11.1	115	5	15.5	2.8	3.3
Con Carne Rice, Tex Mex, M Kitchen, Morrisons*	1 Pack/450g	580	22.9	129	0.5	14.9	5.1	0.5
Con Carne Sweetcorn Mash, Fuller Longer, M&S*	1 Pack/400g	380	13.2	95	8.5	7.4	3.3	3.9
Con Carne with Rice, GFY, Asda*	1 Serving/400g	456	6.4	114	6	19	1.6	0.9
Con Carne with Rice, Healthy Choice, Asda*	1 Pack/400g	412	8.4	103	6	15	2.1	0.9
Con Carne with Rice, Morrisons*	1 Pack/400g	328	5.2	82	5.3	12.2	1.3	1.4
Con Carne with Rice, Organic, Sainsbury's*	1 Pack/400g	472	10.8	118	5	18.5	2.7	1.8
Con Carne, Mexican Rice, Charlie Bigham's*	½ Pack/421g	589	25.2	140	7.2	14.1	6	0
Con Carne, Rice, Fiesta, Aldi*	1 Pack/450g	648	24.3	144	6.7	16	5.4	2.3
Con Carne, 2 Minute Meals, Sainsbury's*	1 Pouch/200g	146	3.2	73	6	8.6	1.6	2.7
Con Carne, Asda*	1 Can/392g	376	13.7	96	7	9	3.5	0
Con Carne, Baked Bean, Heinz*	1 Can/390g	324	5.8	83	7	10.3	1.5	2.8
Con Carne, Beef, Look What We Found*	1 Pack/250g	243	9.5	97	7.5	6.2	3.8	4.1
Con Carne, Canned, El Tequito, Lidl*	1 Serving/320g	365	10.2	114	7.1	14	3.2	0.5
Con Carne, Canned, Morrisons*	1 Can/392g	368	11.8	94	8.8	8	3	2.4
Con Carne, Canned, Sainsbury's*	½ Can/200g	162	4.2	81	6.6	8.9	2.1	2.5
Con Carne, Canned, Tesco*	½ Can/200g	220	11.4	110	7.8	6.4	5.7	4.7
Con Carne, Classic, Canned, Stagg*	½ Can/200g	260	10	130	7	13	5	4.5
Con Carne, Diet Chef Ltd*	1 Pack/300g	333	13.5	111	7.3	10.4	4.5	2.1
Con Carne, Dynamite Hot, Stagg*	1 Serving/250g	310	15.5	124	7.6	9.6	6.2	2.5

	Measure INFO/WEIGHT	KCAL	FAT	KCAL	PROT	CARB	FAT	FIBRE
CHILLI								
Con Carne, From Restaurant, Average	*1 Serving/253g*	*256*	*8.3*	*101*	*9.7*	*8.7*	*3.3*	*0*
Con Carne, Frozen, Co-Op*	1 Pack/340g	306	3.4	90	6	15	1	1
Con Carne, Heston from Waitrose, Waitrose*	½ Pack/300g	429	27	143	8.4	5.9	9	2.3
Con Carne, Homepride*	1 Can/390g	234	2.3	60	2.5	11.2	0.6	0
Con Carne, M&S*	1 Pack/285g	285	10.5	100	8.7	7.4	3.7	2
Con Carne, Recipe Mix, Colman's*	1 Pack/50g	158	1.2	316	10.4	62.9	2.5	6.8
Con Carne, with Brown Rice, Everdine*	1 Meal/450g	459	18.4	102	7.2	6.4	4.1	5.2
Con Carne, with Long Grain Rice, COU, M&S*	1 Pack/400g	388	7.6	97	5	13.9	1.9	2.1
Con Carne, with Rice, BGTY, Sainsbury's*	1 Pack/400g	392	8.3	99	6.3	12.5	2.1	2.2
Con Carne, with Rice, Classic, Co-Op*	1 Pack/400g	464	13.6	116	5.9	14	3.4	2.7
Con Carne, with Rice, Meal for One, M&S*	1 Pack/450g	536	12.2	119	5.5	18	2.7	0.5
Con Carne, with Rice, PB, Waitrose*	1 Pack/400g	404	7.2	101	5.8	15.3	1.8	1.7
Con Carne, with Rice, Weight Watchers*	1 Pack/300g	279	4.2	93	4.6	15.1	1.4	1.1
Con Veggie, Cook*	1 Portion/285g	194	4.3	68	5.9	7.8	1.5	0
Diced Beef,with Rice, 672, Wiltshire Farm Foods*	1 Portion/380g	328	9.2	86	5.5	10	2.4	1.6
Five Bean, Deliciously Ella*	½ Pack/200g	140	2	70	3.9	8.8	1	3.6
Five Bean, Mexican, Bol*	1 Pot/343g	340	7.9	99	3.7	14.3	2.3	2.9
Medium, Uncle Ben's*	1 Jar/500g	305	4	61	1.8	11.1	0.8	0
Mexican, Beanfeast, Batchelors*	1 Serving/65g	203	3.2	312	24.3	42.7	4.9	13.6
Minced Beef with Rice, Mini, CBY, Asda*	1 Pack/250g	308	9.8	123	5.3	15.8	3.9	1.7
Mixed Vegetable, Tesco*	1 Pack/400g	352	11.6	88	3.9	11	2.9	3.2
Red, Raw, Sainsbury's*	1 Avg Chilli/45g	14	0.2	30	1.8	4.2	0.5	1.5
sin Carne, Bio, Reichenhof*	1 Portion/200g	132	0.8	66	4.9	8.9	0.4	0
Speckled Lentil, with Parisienne Potatoes, Everdine*	1 Serving/450g	450	14.4	100	2.9	12.7	3.2	4.5
Steak Coriander Rice, Taste Mexico, M&S*	1 Pack/400g	532	15.2	133	7.1	16.4	3.8	2.4
Three Bean, Cauliflower Rice, Goodlife*	1 Pack/400g	276	8	69	3.8	5.8	2	6.5
Three Bean, Vegetable, Slimfree, Aldi*	1 Pack/500g	295	2.5	59	3.4	8.5	0.5	3.1
Three Bean, Diet Chef Ltd*	1 Pack/300g	195	2.7	65	4	10.3	0.9	3.6
Vegetable	*1oz/28g*	*16*	*0.2*	*57*	*3*	*10.8*	*0.6*	*2.6*
Vegetable & Rice, BGTY, Sainsbury's*	1 Pack/450g	410	5	91	3.5	16.7	1.1	3.5
Vegetable & Rice, HE, Tesco*	1 Pack/450g	392	5.4	87	2.8	16.1	1.2	1.5
Vegetable Garden, Stagg*	1 Can/400g	280	2	70	3.5	14	0.5	3
Vegetable, Canned, Heated, Asda*	½ Can/200g	158	1	79	3.2	14.1	0.5	2.5
Vegetable, Canned, Sainsbury's*	1 Can/400g	230	1.6	58	3.1	10.4	0.4	3.2
Vegetable, Canned, Tesco*	½ Can/200g	136	4.2	68	2.8	8.2	2.1	2.6
Vegetable, Diet Chef Ltd*	1 Pack/300g	258	4.8	86	3.4	14.5	1.6	4.4
Vegetable, Fast Diet Kitchen*	1 Pack/340g	194	1.4	57	3.6	12.2	0.4	4.8
Vegetable, Retail	*1oz/28g*	*20*	*0.6*	*70*	*4*	*9.4*	*2.1*	*0*
Vegetarian with Rice, Tesco*	1 Pack/500g	575	13	115	4	19	2.6	1.8
Vegetarian, Mexican, Chef's Selection, Quorn*	½ Pack/170g	143	4.3	84	6.6	6.5	2.5	4.5
Vegetarian, Soya Mince, Rice, Waitrose*	1 Pack/402g	442	8.4	110	5.4	14.9	2.1	5.4
Vegetarian, Tesco*	1 Pack/400g	340	3.2	85	4.4	15	0.8	2.1
Vegetarian, with Rice, Ready Meal, Average	*1 Serving/400g*	*434*	*6*	*108*	*3.8*	*20*	*1.5*	*1.3*
Veggie, Smoky, Jamie Oliver*	1 Serving/125g	111	2.6	89	4.6	10	2.1	5.1
CHILLI POWDER								
Average	*1 Tsp/4g*	*16*	*0.7*	*405*	*12.3*	*54.7*	*16.8*	*34.2*
CHIPS								
American Style, Oven, Co-Op*	1 Serving/150g	255	9	170	2	26	6	3
American Style, Thin, Oven, Tesco*	1 Serving/125g	210	8.1	168	2.7	24.6	6.5	2.1
Chip Shop, Fishnchickn*	1 Portion/311g	734	38.6	236	3.2	27.9	12.4	0
Chunky, M&S*	½ Pack/200g	292	7.6	146	2	24.7	3.8	2.6
Chunky Oven, Harry Ramsden's*	1 Serving/150g	184	5.4	123	2.8	19.9	3.6	1.6
Chunky, COU, M&S*	1 Serving/150g	158	2.4	105	2.1	20.5	1.6	2.3

CHIPS

INFO/WEIGHT	Measure	per Measure		Nutrition Values per 100g / 100ml				
		KCAL	FAT	KCAL	PROT	CARB	FAT	FIBRE
Chunky, Crisp Golden, Waitrose*	½ Pack/225g	259	7	115	2.1	17.7	3.1	3.9
Chunky, Gastropub, M&S*	1 Pack/400g	520	12.4	130	2.6	22.4	3.1	2.3
Chunky, Ready to Bake, M&S*	1 Serving/200g	310	8.4	155	2.2	26.8	4.2	2
Chunky, with Cornish Sea Salt, Finest, Tesco*	½ Pack/176g	294	6.2	167	2.7	29.6	3.5	2.8
Crinkle Cut, Frozen, Fried in Corn Oil	*1oz/28g*	*81*	*4.7*	*290*	*3.6*	*33.4*	*16.7*	*2.2*
Crinkle Cut, Homestyle, Tesco*	1 Serving/95g	168	4	177	2.5	30.5	4.2	3.5
Crinkle Cut, Oven Baked, Aunt Bessie's*	1 Serving/100g	206	9.2	206	2.9	28	9.2	3.2
Crinkle Cut, Oven, Asda*	1 Serving/100g	134	3.8	134	2	23	3.8	8
Family Fries, Oven, Tesco*	1 Serving/125g	164	4.6	131	2	22.4	3.7	1.8
Fine Cut, Frozen, Fried in Blended Oil	*1oz/28g*	*102*	*6*	*364*	*4.5*	*41.2*	*21.3*	*2.4*
Fine Cut, Frozen, Fried in Corn Oil	*1oz/28g*	*102*	*6*	*364*	*4.5*	*41.2*	*21.3*	*2.7*
Fried, Average	*1 Serving/130g*	*266*	*10.9*	*204*	*3.2*	*29.6*	*8.4*	*1.2*
Fried, Chip Shop, Average	*1 Small/100g*	*239*	*12.4*	*239*	*3.2*	*30.5*	*12.4*	*2.2*
Frites, M&S*	1 Pack/100g	185	7.1	185	2.2	26.5	7.1	3
Frozen, Crinkle Cut, Aunt Bessie's*	1 Serving/100g	163	7.3	163	3.1	21.3	7.3	2.2
Fry or Oven, Oven Cooked, Smart Price, Asda*	1 Serving/125g	192	4.3	153	2.1	26.9	3.4	3.3
Frying, Cooked in Sunflower Oil, Value, Tesco*	1 Portion/125g	172	4.9	138	2.5	23.1	3.9	1.6
Frying, Crinkle Cut, Tesco*	1 Serving/125g	161	4.1	129	2.6	22.2	3.3	1.9
Gourmet, Cornish Sea Salt, Oven Baked, McCain*	¼ Pack/100g	206	9.9	206	2	25.6	9.9	3
Home Chips, Straight, GF, Frozen, McCain*	1 Serving/100g	138	4.3	138	2	21.8	4.3	1.9
Homefries, Chunky, Weighed Baked, McCain*	1 Serving/100g	153	3.1	153	3.2	28	3.1	2.3
Homefries, Chunky, Weighed Frozen, McCain*	1 Serving/100g	123	2.5	123	2.5	22.6	2.5	1.6
Homefries, Crinkle Cut, Weighed Baked, McCain*	1 Serving/100g	176	5	176	2.6	30.1	5	2.3
Homefries, Crinkle Cut, Weighed Frozen, McCain*	1 Serving/100g	142	5.1	142	1.9	22.2	5.1	1.3
Homefries, Straight Cut, Weighed Baked, McCain*	1 Serving/100g	181	6.2	181	3.1	28.1	6.2	2.4
Homefries, Straight Cut, Weighed Frozen, McCain*	1 Serving/100g	134	4.6	134	2.2	21	4.6	1.7
Homemade, Fried in Blended Oil, Average	*1oz/28g*	*53*	*1.9*	*189*	*3.9*	*30.1*	*6.7*	*2.2*
Homemade, Fried in Corn Oil, Average	*1oz/28g*	*53*	*1.9*	*189*	*3.9*	*30.1*	*6.7*	*2.2*
Homemade, Fried in Dripping, Average	*1oz/28g*	*53*	*1.9*	*189*	*3.9*	*30.1*	*6.7*	*2.2*
Homestyle Oven, Sainsbury's*	1 Serving/125g	206	5.4	165	2.4	29.2	4.3	2.1
Homestyle, Frozen, Aunt Bessie's*	1 Serving/100g	124	3.5	124	2.4	20	3.5	1.9
Homestyle, Oven Cooked, Aunt Bessie's*	1 Serving/100g	191	7.8	191	3.1	27	7.8	2.9
Homestyle, Oven, Straight Cut, Tesco*	1 Serving/125g	218	5.1	174	2.1	30.9	4.1	2.5
Micro Chips, Crinkle Cut, Cooked, McCain*	1 Pack/100g	146	4	158	2.4	26	4.3	2.8
Micro Chips, Straight Cut, Cooked, McCain*	1 Pack/100g	163	4.8	163	2.3	27.7	4.8	2
Microwave, Cooked	*1oz/28g*	*62*	*2.7*	*221*	*3.6*	*32.1*	*9.6*	*2.9*
Oven, 5% Fat, Frozen, McCain*	1 Serving/200g	238	6	119	1.9	21	3	1.6
Oven, American Style, Champion*	1 Serving/200g	372	14.4	186	2.2	28.2	7.2	2
Oven, Best in the World, Iceland*	1 Serving/175g	332	11.7	190	3.4	28.9	6.7	3.5
Oven, Champion*	1 Pack/133g	210	6	158	2.5	27	4.5	0
Oven, Chunky Crispy, Tesco*	½ Pack/178g	304	10.5	171	2.9	24.9	5.9	3.5
Oven, Chunky, Extra Special, Asda*	1 Serving/125g	238	7	190	3.4	31.5	5.6	3.2
Oven, Cooked, Value, Tesco*	1 Serving/125g	308	9.8	246	4.5	39.5	7.8	2.9
Oven, Crinkle Cut, Frozen, Essential, Waitrose*	1 Serving/165g	225	6.4	136	2.7	22.6	3.9	1.7
Oven, Crinkle Cut, Sainsbury's*	1 Serving/165g	297	9.1	180	3.3	29.5	5.5	2.4
Oven, Frozen, Baked	*1 Portion/80g*	*130*	*3.4*	*162*	*3.2*	*29.8*	*4.2*	*2*
Oven, Frozen, Basics, Sainsbury's*	1 Serving/165g	249	8.1	151	3	23.6	4.9	2.9
Oven, Frozen, BGTY, Sainsbury's*	1 Serving/165g	226	4.6	137	2.9	25	2.8	2.7
Oven, Frozen, Value, Tesco*	1 Serving/125g	189	5.7	151	2.8	24.7	4.6	1.9
Oven, Homefries, McCain*	1 Serving/100g	134	4.6	134	2.2	21	4.6	1.7
Oven, Morrisons*	1 Serving/100g	134	3.9	134	2.4	22.2	3.9	0
Oven, Original, McCain*	1 Serving/100g	158	3.8	158	2.5	28.5	3.8	2.3
Oven, Steak Cut, Asda*	1 Serving/100g	153	4.1	153	2	27	4.1	2.5

C

INFO/WEIGHT	Measure	per Measure		Nutrition Values per 100g / 100ml				
		KCAL	FAT	KCAL	PROT	CARB	FAT	FIBRE

CHIPS

Oven, Steak Cut, Sainsbury's*	1 Serving/165g	266	7.8	161	2.6	27.1	4.7	2.8
Oven, Steak Cut, Waitrose*	1 Serving/165g	218	5.6	132	2.7	22.7	3.4	1.7
Oven, Steakhouse, Frozen, Tesco*	1 Serving/125g	165	4.2	132	2.7	22.7	3.4	1.7
Oven, Straight Cut, 5% Fat, Sainsbury's*	1 Serving/165g	280	8.1	170	3.4	28	4.9	2.5
Oven, Straight Cut, Asda*	1 Serving/100g	199	5	199	3.5	35	5	3
Oven, Straight Cut, BFY, Morrisons*	1 Serving/165g	249	5.8	151	2.8	27.1	3.5	2.1
Oven, Straight Cut, Reduced Fat, Tesco*	1 Serving/100g	127	3	127	2.3	22.7	3	2.1
Oven, Straight Cut, Waitrose*	1 Serving/165g	219	6.1	133	2	23	3.7	1.7
Oven, Sweet Potato, Cooked, Tesco*	¼ Pack/87g	153	4.8	175	3	26.2	5.5	4.5
Oven, Thick Cut, Frozen, Baked	*1oz/28g*	*44*	*1.2*	*157*	*3.2*	*27.9*	*4.4*	*1.8*
Oven, Thin Cut, American Style, Asda*	1 Serving/100g	240	10	240	3.4	34	10	3
Oven, Thin Fries, Morrisons*	1 Serving/100g	161	6.1	161	2.9	23.6	6.1	1.2
Potato, Lights, Reduced Fat, Lay's*	1 Serving/25g	118	5.5	470	7.5	60	22	5
Salt Pepper, Crinkle, Tesco*	1 Serving/112g	179	5.7	160	2.3	24.6	5.1	3.4
Steak Cut, Frying, Asda*	1 Serving/97g	181	6.8	187	2.9	28	7	2.8
Steak Cut, Oven, Tesco*	1 Serving/165g	233	6.4	141	2	24.4	3.9	2
Steakhouse, Fry, Tesco*	1 Serving/125g	278	15.1	222	3.1	25.2	12.1	2
Straight Cut, Frozen, Fried in Blended Oil	*1oz/28g*	*76*	*3.8*	*273*	*4.1*	*36*	*13.5*	*2.4*
Straight Cut, Frozen, Fried in Corn Oil	*1oz/28g*	*76*	*3.8*	*273*	*4.1*	*36*	*13.5*	*2.4*
Thick Cut, Frozen, Fried in Corn Oil, Average	*1oz/28g*	*66*	*2.9*	*234*	*3.6*	*34*	*10.2*	*2.4*
Tortilla, Lightly Salted, Everyday Value, Tesco*	1 Serving/25g	125	5.9	499	5.5	64.8	23.5	2.9
Triple Cooked, Finest, Tesco*	½ Pack/178g	262	6.8	147	2.6	24.1	3.8	3
Triple Cooked, Gastro, Frozen, McCain*	1 Serving/187g	379	22.2	203	1.9	21	11.9	2.2
Triple Cooked, Gastro, Oven Baked, McCain*	1 Serving/135g	379	20.5	281	2.9	31.6	15.2	3
Vegetable, Root, Ready to Roast, Tesco*	¼ Pack/125g	99	3.8	79	1.1	10.3	3	3.1
with Gravy, Mayflower*	1 Box/330g	403	19.2	122	1.8	15.8	5.8	1.4

CHIVES

Fresh, Average	*1 Tsp/2g*	*0*	*0*	*23*	*2.8*	*1.7*	*0.6*	*1.9*

CHOC ICES

Chocolate, Dark, Seriously Creamy, Waitrose*	1 Ice/82g	195	12.9	238	2.6	21.6	15.7	1.7
Chocolate, Real Milk, Sainsbury's*	1 Choc Ice/41g	126	8	311	3	29.9	19.8	0.6
Dark, Sainsbury's*	1 Choc Ice/44g	156	4.7	354	0	0	10.6	0
Dark, Tesco*	1 Choc Ice/43g	132	8.7	305	3.5	28	20	0.1
Everyday, Value, Tesco*	1 Choc Ice/31g	95	6.3	300	2.3	26.7	19.9	1
Neapolitan Chocolate, Co-Op*	1 Ice/62g	120	8.2	194	2	16.9	13.2	0.4
White Chocolate, Sainsbury's*	1 Ice/48g	140	8.9	292	3.8	27.3	18.6	0.1

CHOCOLATE

Advent Calendar, Dairy Milk, Cadbury*	1 Chocolate/4g	22	1.3	525	7.5	56.6	30.1	0.7
Advent Calendar, Maltesers, Mars*	1 Chocolate/4g	21	1.2	537	6.8	57.9	30.9	0
Advent Calendar, Sainsbury's*	1 Chocolate/4g	20	1.2	557	7.2	52.7	34.3	2.1
Advent Calendar, The Snowman, M&S*	1 Chocolate/4g	21	1.2	550	6.6	60.4	31	0
Almond Honey, Dairy Milk, Cadbury*	1 Sm Bar/54g	281	15.6	520	8	57.1	28.9	1
Alpine Milk , Milka*	1 Serving/25g	132	7.4	530	6.6	58.5	29.5	1.8
Baking, Belgian, Milk for Cakes, Luxury, Sainsbury's*	1 Chunk/8g	44	2.7	556	7.6	56.5	33.3	1.5
Bar, Animal, Nestle*	1 Bar/19g	97	5	513	5.8	63.6	26.1	0
Bar, Apricot & Raisin, Thorntons*	1 Bar/40g	185	10.9	462	8	46	27.3	3.5
Bar, Bliss Truffle, Cadbury*	1 Bar/40g	226	14.9	565	6.6	48.8	37.3	2.8
Bar, Bliss, Hazelnut Truffle, Cadbury*	1 Serving/100g	565	37.9	565	7.2	47.7	37.9	2.6
Bar, Bliss, Toffee Flavour Truffle, Cadbury*	2 Chunks/23g	128	8.1	555	6.9	51.6	35.3	1.6
Bar, Cappuccino, Thorntons*	1 Bar/38g	201	13.2	529	5.2	49.7	34.7	0.5
Bar, Chocolate Cream, Fry's*	1 Piece/10g	42	1.3	415	2.8	70.8	13.2	1.2
Bar, Cookies Cream, Hello, Lindt*	1 Square/10g	56	3.7	565	7	52	37	0
Bar, Dark Chocolate, Diabetic, Thorntons*	1 Bar/75g	345	26.8	460	5.4	28.5	35.8	8.1

CHOCOLATE

	Measure INFO/WEIGHT	per Measure KCAL	FAT	Nutrition Values per 100g / 100ml KCAL	PROT	CARB	FAT	FIBRE
Bar, Dark with Ginger, Thorntons*	1 Bar/90g	495	35.1	550	8	39	39	0
Bar, Dark, 60% Cocoa with Macadamia, Thorntons*	1 Bar/70g	183	12.8	523	6.5	42.3	36.5	12.6
Bar, Dark, Thorntons*	1 Sm Bar/48g	250	17.7	521	7.3	39.9	36.9	10.9
Bar, Deliciously, Free From, Sainsbury's*	1 Bar/35g	190	12.2	543	2.5	48.2	35	12.4
Bar, Extra Dark, 60% Cocoa, Lindor, Lindt*	1 Bar/150g	900	73.5	600	5	35	49	2
Bar, Free From, Asda*	1 Bar/35g	194	12.1	563	2.5	58	35	2.8
Bar, Hazel Nut Cashew, Dairy Milk, Cadbury*	3 Chunks/18g	96	6	540	8.8	50.6	33.5	1.8
Bar, Jazz Orange, Thorntons*	1 Bar/56g	304	18.1	543	6.8	55.7	32.3	1.2
Bar, Mandolin, Cadbury*	1 Bar/28g	139	4.6	495	3.5	66.5	16.5	0.6
Bar, Milk, Thorntons*	1 Sm Bar/50g	269	16	538	7.5	54.8	32	1
Bar, Truffle, M&S*	1 Bar/35g	168	11.4	480	5.9	41.7	32.5	8.3
Bar, Truffle, Orange, M&S*	1 Bar/33g	177	10.5	535	6.6	55.6	31.9	1.4
Bar, Twisted, Creme Egg, Cadbury*	1 Bar/45g	210	9.4	465	5.2	64.6	20.8	0.5
Bar, Viennese, Continental, Thorntons*	1 Bar/38g	206	13	542	4.2	54	34.2	0.8
Bar, White, Thorntons*	1 Bar/50g	274	15.6	547	6.5	59.5	31.3	0
Bars, Alpini, Continental, Thorntons*	1 Bar/36g	192	11.4	538	6.9	55.3	32	2.7
Bars, Baby Ruth, Candy, Nestl©*	1 Bar/60g	296	14.1	494	6.7	63.9	23.5	1.7
Bars, Bubbles, Galaxy, Mars*	1 Bar/31g	172	10.6	555	6.5	54.7	34.2	1.5
Bars, Chocolate, Pistacho, Lindt*	1 Bar/100g	585	40.6	585	7.1	48.2	40.6	0
Bars, Chocolate, Strawberry, Lindt*	1 Bar/100g	470	22.8	470	4.5	61.6	22.8	0
Bars, Milk Chocolate, Galaxy, Mars*	1 Bar/42g	229	13.6	546	6.7	56	32.4	1.5
Bars, Milk Chocolate, Gold, Lindt*	1 Bar/300g	1605	92.9	535	6.6	58.7	31	0
Bars, Milk Chocolate, Hazelnut, Gold, Lindt*	1 Bar/300g	1665	108.2	555	7.9	50.7	36.1	0
Bars, Milk Chocolate, Hazelnut, Lindt*	1 Bar/100g	570	38.8	570	8.5	47	38.8	0
Bars, Milk Chocolate, Lindt*	1 Bar/100g	622	47	622	4.6	44	47	0
Bars, Milk Chocolate, Raisin & Hazelnut, Lindt*	1 Bar/100g	530	31.6	530	3.1	54.7	31.6	0
Beans, Coffee, Dark, Solid, M&S*	1 Serving/10g	53	3.8	532	4.7	42.4	37.6	11.6
Bear, Lindt*	1 Bear/11g	60	3.6	572	7.5	57.7	34.6	0
Belgian Milk, TTD, Sainsbury's*	1 Piece/10g	55	3.5	549	9.6	48.3	35.3	2
Belgian, Kschocolat*	4 Pieces/40g	212	12.2	530	6	57.5	30.5	2.3
Belgian, Milk, Mini Eggs, M&S*	1 Egg/8g	43	2.5	535	7	55.8	31.7	2.7
Blueberry Intense, Excellence, Lindt*	1 Serving/40g	200	12.4	500	6	50	31	0
Bubbly Santa, M&S*	1 Santa/23g	124	7.3	540	7	55.8	31.7	2.7
Bubbly, Dairy Milk, Cadbury*	1 Bar/35g	185	10.5	525	7.7	56.9	29.7	0.7
Bunny, Easter, Mars*	1 Bunny/29g	155	9.2	535	6.2	56.2	31.7	0
Bunny, Lindt*	1 Bunny/11g	60	3.6	572	7.5	57.7	34.6	0
Buttons, Dairy Milk, Cadbury*	1 Pack/32g	170	9.7	525	7.7	56.7	29.9	0.7
Buttons, Maltesers, Mars*	1 Bag/32g	166	8.6	518	7.4	60	27	0
Cappuccino, Nestle*	1 Serving/20g	109	6.6	545	6.1	56	32.9	0
Caramel, Chunk, Dairy Milk, Cadbury*	1 Chunk/33g	158	7.6	480	5	63	23	0
Caramel, Dairy Milk, Cadbury*	1 Bar/45g	215	10.4	480	4.9	62.8	23.2	0.4
Caramel, Irresistibly Smooth, Lindor, Lindt*	1 Bar/100g	625	48	625	4.7	43	48	0
Chips, Dark, The Pantry, Aldi*	1 Serving/25g	126	6.5	505	3.8	60	26	6.1
Chips, Extra Dark, 63%, Guittard*	1/3 Cup/60g	280	19.8	467	6.7	53	33	13.3
Chocolat Noir, Lindt*	1/6 Bar/17g	87	5.4	510	6	50	32	0
Chocolate Favourites, Tesco*	½ Box/227g	1015	43.6	447	4.2	64.3	19.2	0.3
Chomp, Cadbury*	1 Bar/24g	112	4.8	465	3.3	67.9	20	0.2
Christmas Tree Decoration, Average	*1 Chocolate/12g*	**63**	**3.6**	**522**	**7.6**	**56.4**	**29.9**	**0.4**
Christmas Tree Decoration, Cadbury*	1 Piece/12g	60	3.4	525	7.6	56.2	29.9	0
Chunk Bar, Dairy Milk, Cadbury*	1 Chunk/7g	35	2	525	7.5	57	29.8	0.1
Chunky Hazelnut Bar, M&S*	1 Bar/52g	293	19.4	563	8.8	48.1	37.3	1.7
Clusters, Popping Candy, Tesco*	1 Cluster/9g	43	1.8	479	6.5	68.3	19.6	1.6
Coco Mylk, Raw, Bar, Ombar*	1 Bar/35g	208	15.9	594	6.8	43.9	45.5	8

CHOCOLATE

INFO/WEIGHT	Measure	per Measure		Nutrition Values per 100g / 100ml				
		KCAL	FAT	KCAL	PROT	CARB	FAT	FIBRE
Cocoa Fudge, Hotel Chocolat*	1 Bar/45g	170	6.3	378	1.8	62.1	13.9	2.1
Coconut, White, Excellence, Lindt*	1 Square/10g	61	4.4	610	6	48	44	0
Coins, Marzipan, Cherry , Favorina, Lidl*	1 Serving/30g	132	5.7	439	5.3	58	19	3.3
Coins, Marzipan, Plum, Madeira, Favorina, Lidl*	1 Serving/30g	131	6	437	5.4	53	20	4.9
Coins, Milk, Sainsbury's*	1 Coin/5g	26	1.4	502	5.5	58.8	27.1	2.5
Cool & Delicious, Dairy Milk, Cadbury*	1 Bar/21g	110	6.3	525	7.6	56.1	30.1	0
Counters, Galaxy, Mars*	4 Counters/10g	53	2.9	529	6.8	59.4	29.1	1.4
Crispello Double Choc, Cadbury*	1 Piece/10g	55	3.5	560	7	51	36	1.9
Crispies, Chunk, Dairy Milk, Cadbury*	1 Chunk/31g	158	8.5	510	7.6	58.6	27.4	0
Crispies, Dairy Milk, Cadbury*	1 Bar/49g	250	13.4	510	7.6	58.6	27.4	0
Crispy, Sainsbury's*	4 Squares/19g	99	5.4	521	9.1	56.9	28.5	2.1
Dairy Milk with Oreo, Dairy Milk, Cadbury*	3 Chunks/15g	85	5.4	560	6.1	53.5	35.5	0.7
Dairy Milk, Cadbury*	1 Bar/45g	242	13.6	534	7.3	57	30	2.1
Dairy Milk, Oreo, Mint, Dairy Milk, Cadbury*	3 Chunks/15g	84	5.2	557	5.9	54	35	1.5
Dairy Milk, Toffee Popcorn, Dairy Milk, Cadbury*	1 Bar/150g	765	39.8	510	7	59.5	26.5	1.7
Dark + Nibs, Artisan, Raw, Raw Halo Ltd*	1 Bar/35g	212	17.6	606	8.3	29.4	50.4	0
Dark + Sweet Orange, Artisan, Raw, Raw Halo Ltd*	1 Bar/33g	199	16.4	602	7.8	31.3	49.7	0
Dark with Chilli, Thorntons*	4 Squares/20g	107	7.9	533	7.2	36.3	39.5	10.4
Dark, Finest, 85% Cocoa, Moser Roth, Aldi*	1 Bar/25g	152	12.8	608	11	18	51	15
Dark, 60%, Amazonas, Lidl*	1 Square/13g	75	5.2	574	5.7	44	40	7.5
Dark, 70% Cocoa Solids, Extra Fine, Lindt*	1 Square/10g	54	4.1	537	8	33	41	12.2
Dark, 70% Cocoa Solids, Organic, Green & Black's*	1 Sm Bar/35g	193	14.4	551	9.3	36	41.1	11.5
Dark, 70% Cocoa Solids, Organic, Morrisons*	½ Bar/50g	266	20.6	531	7.9	31.6	41.1	11
Dark, 70%, with Raspberries, Divine Chocolate*	1 Square/5g	29	2.2	584	6.7	32.2	45	11.3
Dark, 70%, Velvet, Green & Black's*	1 Piece/10g	62	4.9	619	6.1	33	49	9.7
Dark, 75% Cacao, Rausch*	1 Row/31g	163	12.9	522	8.8	28.5	41.1	15
Dark, 85% Cocoa, Excellence, Lindt*	1 Serving/40g	212	18.4	530	11	19	46	16.3
Dark, 85% Cocoa, TTD, Sainsbury's*	1 Serving/25g	149	12.8	596	9.6	16.8	51.4	14.1
Dark, 99% Cocoa, Excellence, Lindt*	1 Serving/25g	142	12.5	567	13	8	50	20
Dark, Assorted Collection, Velvet, Green & Black's*	1 Piece/10g	61	4.8	612	5.8	35	48	9.2
Dark, Belgian, Extra Special, Asda*	2 Squares/20g	102	8	508	11	26	40	16
Dark, Belgian, Luxury Continental, Sainsbury's*	1 Bar/100g	490	38.7	490	11.1	24.2	38.7	7.4
Dark, Belgian, No Added Sugar, Chocologic*	4 Pieces/13g	58	4.7	432	5.3	18.7	34.8	34.8
Dark, Bournville, Classic, Cadbury*	1 Bar/45g	238	13.5	530	3.8	59.5	29.9	5.5
Dark, Chilli, Excellence, Lindt*	1 Serving/40g	202	12.8	506	5.4	49	32	0
Dark, Classic, Bourneville, Cadbury*	4 Squares/25g	125	6.8	505	4.7	58.8	27.3	2
Dark, Co-Op*	1 Bar/50g	252	14.5	505	4	57	29	6
Dark, Continental, Luxury, Tesco*	1 Bar/100g	571	37.8	571	11.3	46.5	37.8	0.1
Dark, Dominican Republic, 90%, 1, Waitrose*	1 Piece/10g	63	5.5	627	11	15	55	14
Dark, Fair Trade, Co-Op*	1 Bar/45g	214	13	475	4	49	29	6
Dark, Feuilles with Orange, Nestle*	1 Piece/8g	42	2.6	524	4.6	54.4	32	0
Dark, Goji, Cranberry Linseed, M&S*	1 Bar/28g	172	11.7	614	12	41.4	41.7	12.6
Dark, Hazelnut Crisp, Mini Bar, Mister Choc, Lidl*	1 Mini Bar/18g	102	6.8	566	7.7	46.2	37.9	4.4
Dark, Luxury Continental, Sainsbury's*	½ Bar/50g	252	20	504	10.7	25.5	40	16.1
Dark, Mint, Intense, Lindt*	1 Square/10g	53	3.2	529	5	51	32	0
Dark, No Added Sugar, Red*	½ Bar/50g	150	12.5	299	4	34	25	0
Dark, Orange Almond, Moser Roth, Aldi*	1 Serving/25g	133	8	532	5.9	51	32	7.9
Dark, Orange Almond, No Added Sugar, Red*	¼ Bar/25g	76	6.5	305	5	34	26	0
Dark, Orange, Velvet Fruit, Green & Black's*	8 Pieces/26g	127	7.3	490	4.1	52	28	7.9
Dark, Plain, Average	**1oz/28g**	**143**	**7.8**	**510**	**5**	**63.5**	**28**	**2.5**
Dark, Plain, Rich, Co-Op*	1 Bar/200g	1010	58	505	4	57	29	6
Dark, Pure, Artisan, Raw, Raw Halo Ltd*	1 Bar/33g	201	16.9	610	7.7	30.1	51.1	0
Dark, Raw Organic, Loving Earth*	1 Serving/20g	99	7.9	495	9.3	46.4	39.5	0

CHOCOLATE

INFO/WEIGHT	Measure KCAL	FAT	KCAL	PROT	CARB	FAT	FIBRE
Dark, Rich, Tesco*	1 Serving/20g	98	6.1	491	5.8	60	30.4	11.5
Dark, Seriously Rich, 65%, Waitrose*	1 Sm Bar/30g	169	11.6	562	8.2	40.3	38.6	10.4
Dark, Simply, Lidl*	3 Squares/20g	98	5.6	491	4.6	51	28	8.1
Dark, Smooth, Bar, Galaxy, Mars*	1 Bar/125g	651	42	521	6.2	48	33.6	9.3
Dark, Smooth, No Added Sugar, Sainsbury's*	1 Piece/10g	53	4.2	529	8.2	34.3	42.2	11
Dark, Special, Hershey*	1 Pack/41g	180	12	439	4.9	61	29.3	7.3
Dark, Tiddly Pot, Hotel Chocolat*	1 Serving/58g	311	22.4	537	13.9	30.5	38.7	8.7
Dark, Whole Nut, Tesco*	1 Serving/13g	67	4.5	539	6.1	48.3	35.7	6.5
Dark, with Almonds, Green & Black's*	1 Row/18g	112	9	622	9.2	29	50	9.4
Dark, with Coconut, Indian Ocean, 1, Waitrose*	1 Square/10g	60	4.5	599	6	39	45	7
Dark, with Mint, Velvet, Green & Black's*	1 Row/18g	111	8.8	619	6.1	33	49	9.7
Dark, with Orange, 70% , Ecuador *	1 Square/13g	70	4.9	537	7.3	36	38	11
Dark, with Orange, Lidl*	1 Square/13g	67	4.7	537	7.3	36	38	11
Dark, with Salted Almonds, Benugo*	1 Bar/25g	138	9.2	550	6.1	43.7	37	7
Dark, with Salted Caramel, Velvet, Green & Black's*	1 Row/18g	108	8.1	600	5.2	39	45	8.2
Dark, with Sea Salt, Velvet, Green & Black's*	1 Row/18g	111	8.8	616	6.1	33	49	9.7
Diet, Ritter Sport*	1 Square/6g	25	1.8	412	6	44	30	0
Double Blend, Nestle*	1 Rectangle/11g	61	3.6	553	7.3	55.9	33	0
Dream with Real Strawberries, Cadbury*	1 Bar/45g	250	14.9	555	4.5	59.6	33.1	0
Drops, Plain, Asda*	1 Serving/100g	489	29	489	7	50	29	10
Drops, Plain, Sainsbury's*	1 Serving/125g	638	34.5	510	5.3	60.1	27.6	4
Drops, White for Cooking Decorating, Sainsbury's*	1oz/28g	152	8.6	544	6.5	60.3	30.8	0
Egg n Spoon, Mousse Centre, Oreo Pieces, Cadbury*	1 Egg/34g	191	11.9	561	7.1	53	35	1.2
Egg, Caramel, Cadbury*	1 Egg/39g	187	9.5	480	4	60	24.5	0.4
Eggs, Milk, Raspberry, Favorina, Lidl*	1 Egg/19g	86	3.6	453	4.1	64.3	19.1	0
Elves, Magical, with Popping Candy, Cadbury*	1 Elf/15g	77	4.2	515	6.9	60	27.7	0
Espresso Coffee Kick, 5 Bars, M&S*	1 Bar/12g	77	5.5	644	5.5	46	46.2	11.3
Ferrero Rocher, Ferrero*	1 Chocolate/13g	75	5.3	603	8.2	44.4	42.7	0
Ferrero Rocher, Heart, Ferrero*	1 Chocolate/13g	75	5.3	603	8.2	44.4	42.7	0
Fingers, Milk, Mister Choc, Lidl*	1 Finger/18g	104	6.9	579	6.2	51.7	38.4	0.9
Football, Milk Chocolate, Thorntons*	1 Football/200g	1088	67	544	7.6	52.9	33.5	1
Freddo, Caramel, Dairy Milk, Cadbury*	1 Freddo/19g	93	4.7	490	5.5	60.5	24.8	0.5
Freddo, Dairy Milk, Cadbury*	1 Freddo/18g	95	5.4	530	7.5	57	29.8	0.7
Fruit & Nut, Belgian, Waitrose*	1 Serving/50g	254	14.6	508	8.6	54.6	29.2	3.4
Fruit & Nut, Dark, Tesco*	4 Squares/25g	124	7	494	5.8	54.8	27.9	6.5
Fruit Nut, Dairyfine, Aldi*	4 Squares/25g	131	8	525	8.1	50	32	4.2
Galaxy, Crispy, Galaxy, Mars*	1 Portion/20g	111	6.6	546	6.4	56.7	32.2	0
Ginger, Traidcraft*	1 Bar/50g	212	7.4	424	3.9	68.2	14.8	0
Golden Biscuit Crunch, Dairy Milk, Cadbury*	4 Chunks /25g	135	8.2	545	6.2	55.5	33	0.8
Golf Balls, Milk Chocolate, Lindt*	1 Pack/110g	619	39.5	563	6.5	53.6	35.9	0
Hazelnut Crunch, Choceur, Aldi*	1 Serving/40g	226	14.4	564	9.2	49.7	36	2.4
Kinder Maxi, Ferrero*	1 Bar/21g	116	7.1	550	10	51	34	0
Kinder Surprise, Ferrero*	1 Egg/20g	110	6.8	552	8.1	52.3	34.2	0
Kinder, Bar, Small, Ferrero*	1 Bar/13g	71	4.4	566	8.7	53.5	35	0
Kinder, Bueno Bar, Milk, Ferrero*	1 Bar/22g	123	8	575	9.2	49.5	37.3	2
Kinder, Bueno, Bar, White, Ferrero*	1 Piece/20g	111	7	571	8.8	52.6	35.9	1
Kinder, Riegel, Ferrero*	1 Bar/21g	117	7.1	558	10	53	34	0
King Size, Dairy Milk, Cadbury*	1 Serving/85g	446	25.2	525	7.6	56.4	29.7	0
Kitten, Milk Chocolate, Lindt*	1 Kitten/11g	60	3.6	572	7.5	57.7	34.6	0
Lait Intense, Experiences, Cote D'or*	3 Squares/100g	575	40	575	7.2	44.5	40	5
Light & Whippy, Bite Sized, Sainsbury's*	1 Bar/15g	66	2.4	439	3.3	69.7	16.3	0.1
Little Bars, Dairy Milk, Cadbury*	1 Bar/18g	96	5.4	534	7.3	57	30	2.1
Macadamia Nut, Excellence, Lindt*	1 Bar/100g	560	37	560	7	51	37	0

CHOCOLATE

Measure INFO/WEIGHT		per Measure		Nutrition Values per 100g / 100ml				
		KCAL	FAT	KCAL	PROT	CARB	FAT	FIBRE
Mandarin Gubinge, Mylk, Loving Earth*	2 Squares/8g	55	4.4	621	4.6	42.7	50	0
Mars, Bites, Mars*	4 Bites/20g	90	3.3	449	4.1	70.2	16.6	0
Matchmakers, Mint, Nestle*	1 Stick/4g	20	0.8	477	4.3	69.7	20.1	0.9
Matchmakers, Yummy Honeycomb, Nestle*	4 Sticks/15g	72	3.1	495	3.7	70.6	21.3	2.4
Medley, Dark, Biscuit Fudge, Dairy Milk, Cadbury*	1 Piece/9g	52	3.2	555	5.9	54.5	34	2
Milk for Baking, Value, Tesco*	½ Bar/50g	265	14.5	530	6.7	60	29	2.2
Milk with Biscuit Pieces, Asda*	2 Squares/14g	73	4.1	521	8	57	29	1.9
Milk with Crisped Rice, Dubble*	1 Bar/40g	211	11.8	528	6.4	59.6	29.4	0
Milk with Honey Almond Nougat, Swiss, Toblerone*	1 Piece/8g	42	2.4	525	5.4	59	29.5	2.2
Milk with Peanut Butter Filling, Ghirardelli*	1 Serving/45g	250	17	556	8.9	48.9	37.8	2.2
Milk with Raisins Hazelnuts, Green & Black's*	1 Bar/100g	556	36.9	556	9.2	46.8	36.9	3.2
Milk with Whole Almonds, Organic, Green & Black's*	1 Bar/100g	578	42.2	578	11.8	37.7	42.2	5.2
Milk, White, Alpine, Sweet Winter, Milka*	¼ Bar/25g	133	7.4	531	6.2	59.5	29.5	1.6
Milk, Average	*1oz/28g*	*146*	*8.6*	*520*	*7.7*	*56.9*	*30.7*	*0.8*
Milk, Bars, M&S*	1 Bar/40g	214	12.8	535	7.8	54	32	1.9
Milk, Belgian, 57%, Rebel Chocolate*	1 Sm Bar/30g	162	11.6	539	25	32.7	38.5	4.1
Milk, Belgian, No Added Sugar, Chocologic*	4 Squares/13g	64	4.8	484	7.9	33.7	36.2	17
Milk, Biscuit Sticks, Mikado, Kraft*	1 Stick/2.3g	11	0.5	475	7.8	67	19.8	3.1
Milk, Bubbly, Swiss, M&S*	1 Serving/40g	218	13.7	545	8	52	34.3	2.5
Milk, Creamy, Organic, Green & Black's*	6 Pieces/20g	110	7	560	9.1	50.3	35.5	1.6
Milk, Extra Au Lait, Milch Extra, Lindt*	½ Bar/50g	268	15.5	535	6.5	57	31	0
Milk, Extra Creamy, Excellence, Lindt*	1 Bar/100g	560	37.1	560	6	51.1	37.1	0
Milk, Extra Fine, Swiss, M&S*	1 Serving/25g	141	9.2	565	7.2	50.9	36.7	2.3
Milk, Fair Trade, Tesco*	1 Serving/45g	236	13.3	524	7.6	56.7	29.6	2
Milk, Figures, Hollow, Dairyfine, Aldi*	1 Serving/11g	58	3.2	523	5.5	59.9	29	3.1
Milk, Giant Buttons, M&S*	1 Button/8g	44	2.7	550	7.1	52.3	34.2	0.4
Milk, Hazelnut, Macadamia, No Added Sugar, Red*	¼ Bar/25g	96	7	382	8	41	28	0
Milk, Honey, Traidcraft*	1 Bar/50g	272	16.5	545	6	54	33	0
Milk, Italian, Low Sugar, Groder*	1 Serving/40g	199	14.6	498	6.9	51.2	36.5	1.9
Milk, Latte Macchiato, Mini Bar, Mister Choc, Lidl*	1 Mini Bar/18g	106	7.4	588	7.7	46.2	41.2	2.8
Milk, Lindor, Lindt*	1 Square/11g	68	5.2	615	4.7	43	47	0
Milk, Mini Bar, Mister Choc, Lidl*	1 Mini Bar/18g	103	6.6	571	7.1	51.1	36.8	2.8
Milk, Organic, Tesco*	1 Serving/25g	140	9.1	558	6.3	51.4	36.3	2.3
Milk, Ryelands*	4 Squares/29g	155	8.2	520	7.3	60.7	27.6	1.7
Milk, Sainsbury's*	4 Squares/25g	133	7.7	533	9.2	54.6	30.8	2.2
Milk, Salted Caramel, Godiva*	1 Square/10g	53	3	524	7.1	57	30	0
Milk, Salted Caramel, Thin, Organic, Green & Black's*	1 Square/12g	67	4.1	550	8.4	51.5	33.5	2.6
Milk, Santas, Tesco*	1 Bag/90g	433	21.8	481	4.5	61.4	24.2	1.4
Milk, Single Estate, Madagascan, 57%, Rebel Chocolate*	1 Sm Bar/30g	162	11.6	539	25	32.7	38.5	4.1
Milk, Single Origin, Colombian, 57%, Rebel Chocolate*	1 Sm Bar/30g	162	11.6	539	25	32.7	38.5	4.1
Milk, Smart Price, Asda*	1 Square/6g	32	1.9	536	8	54	32	1.8
Milk, Strawberry Yogurt, Mini Bar, Mister Choc, Lidl*	1 Mini Bar/18g	102	6.5	566	6	52.8	36.3	2.8
Milk, Swiss, Diabetic with Fruit Nuts, Boots*	½ Bar/21g	97	6.7	462	7	55	32	2.7
Milk, Swiss, Finest, Tesco*	2 Squares/20g	112	7	558	8.5	50.6	35.2	2.3
Milk, Tesco*	1 Serving/25g	133	7.7	533	9.5	54.7	30.7	2.2
Milk, Value, Tesco*	1/6 Bar/16g	83	4.5	520	6.8	60	28	2.3
Milk, Whole Nut, Tesco*	1 Serving/25g	129	8.4	517	8.7	53.4	33.8	9
Milk, Winnie the Pooh, Solid Shapes, M&S*	1 Chocolate/6g	32	1.9	540	8.1	54.1	32.4	1.3
Milk, with Melting Nut Filling, No Added Sugar, Red*	¼ Bar/28g	104	7.7	378	8	41	28	0
Milk, with Orange, Divine Chocolate*	1 Sm Bar/35g	189	11	541	6.2	57.3	31.4	1.7
Milky Bar, Giant Buttons, Mars*	1 Sweet/2g	11	0.6	546	7.5	57.7	31.6	0
Mini Bites, Chunky, Moments, Fox's*	1 Roll/20g	90	4.9	450	5.7	52.4	24.6	2.2
Mini Eggs, Belgian, Doubly Divine, Moser Roth, Aldi*	1 Egg/11g	57	3.2	516	6.2	55	29	4.5

CHOCOLATE

	Measure INFO/WEIGHT	per Measure KCAL	FAT	Nutrition Values per 100g / 100ml KCAL	PROT	CARB	FAT	FIBRE
Mini Eggs, Cadbury*	1 Egg/3g	16	0.7	495	4.6	69.5	21.5	1.3
Mini Eggs, Caramel, Cadbury*	1 Mini Egg/11g	55	2.9	485	5.7	59	25.7	0.4
Mini Eggs, Daim, Cadbury*	1 Egg/11g	60	3.4	535	6.9	56.5	30.5	1.8
Mini Eggs, Golden, Galaxy *	½ Bag/40g	207	10.8	518	6.6	61.3	27	0
Mini Eggs, Lindor, Lindt*	3 Eggs/15g	92	6.8	611	5.4	45	45	0
Mini Eggs, Oreo, Cadbury*	1 Egg/10g	58	3.7	565	5.9	53.5	36	1.3
Mini, Toblerone*	1 Serving/6g	32	1.8	525	5.6	57.5	30	3.5
Mint Chips, Dairy Milk, Cadbury*	1 Bar/49g	247	12.8	505	6.6	61.6	26.1	0.6
Mint Creme, Sainsbury's*	1 Serving/20g	93	4.9	467	2.8	62.7	24.5	2.1
Mint Crisps, M&S*	1 Mint/8g	40	2.4	494	5.4	54.8	29.6	3.1
Mint, Fondant Thins, Dark Chocolate, Sainsbury's*	1 Thin/10g	48	2	478	4.9	67.5	19.9	4.6
Mint, Waves, Choceur, Aldi*	7 Waves/25g	129	7	516	6.4	56	28	6
Mistletoe Kisses, Mars*	1 Pack /42g	209	11.5	498	5.3	57	27.3	0
Mountain Bar with Orange, Swiss, M&S*	½ Bar/50g	268	16.4	535	8	52.2	32.8	3.2
Mountain Bar, Swiss, M&S*	1 Bar/100g	555	35.3	555	6.5	55.2	35.3	0.2
Mylk, Crispies, Artisan, Raw, Raw Halo Ltd*	1 Bar/33g	183	13.4	555	6.7	41.4	40.7	0
Mylk, Mint Crisp, Artisan, Raw, Raw Halo Ltd*	1 Bar/33g	187	13.9	567	7	41.5	42	0
Mylk, Pure, Artisan, Raw, Raw Halo Ltd*	1 Bar/33g	205	17.8	621	6.4	29.1	53.8	0
Mylk, Salted Caramel, Artisan, Raw, Raw Halo Ltd*	1 Bar/32g	198	17.2	618	6.4	28.8	53.6	0
Natural Orange, Excellence, Lindt*	1 Bar/100g	560	37	560	7	50	37	0
Natural Vanilla, Excellence, Lindt*	1 Bar/100g	590	40	590	6	51	40	0
Nibs, Raw, Cacao, Organic, Navitas Naturals*	1 Serving/28g	130	12	464	14.3	35.7	42.9	32.1
Noir, Special, Frey*	1 Bar/35g	197	15.8	562	8	30	45	0
NutRageous, Reese's, Hershey*	1 Bar/51g	260	16	510	11.8	54.9	31.4	3.9
Nuts About Caramel, Cadbury*	1 Bar/55g	272	15.1	495	5.8	56.6	27.4	0
Nutty Caramel, Dairy Milk, Cadbury*	4 Squares/28g	155	9.9	550	6.9	51	35	1.2
Nutty Nougat, Bite Sized, Sainsbury's*	1 Bar/23g	111	5.5	481	7.6	59	23.8	0.6
Oange, Crunchball, Terry's*	1 Segment/9g	45	2.4	520	6.9	59.8	28.1	2
Old Jamaica, Bournville, Cadbury*	4 Chunks/23g	107	5.4	465	4.2	59.6	23.4	2
Orange Cream, Cadbury*	1 Bar/51g	217	7.9	425	2.6	68.6	15.4	0
Orange Cream, Fry's*	1 Bar/50g	210	6.8	420	2.8	72.3	13.7	0
Orange, Bar, Terry's*	1 Bar/40g	210	11.7	530	7.3	58	29.5	2.1
Orange, Dark, Terry's*	1 Segment/9g	45	2.6	511	4.3	57	29.3	6.2
Orange, Fair Trade, Divine Foods*	4 Squares/17g	92	5.4	541	6.5	57.7	31.5	0
Orange, Milk, Mini Segments, Minis, Terry's*	1 Segment/4g	21	1.1	520	5.8	59.5	28	2.4
Orange, Milk, Terry's*	1 Orange/157g	816	44	520	5.8	59.5	28	2.4
Orange, Plain, Terry's*	1 Orange/157g	801	43.2	510	5.2	55.5	27.5	7.6
Orange, Sainsbury's*	4 Squares/19g	100	5.8	531	9.2	54.3	30.7	2.2
Orange, Segsations, Terry's*	1 Segsation/8g	43	2.3	520	6.9	58.5	28.5	2.8
Orange, White, Terry's*	1 Segment/11g	61	3.4	535	6.3	60.9	29.4	0
Oreo, Bar, Dairy Milk, Cadbury*	1 Bar/41g	226	13.7	550	6	55	33.5	1.6
Oreo, Bites, Dairy Milk, Cadbury*	1 Serving/25g	138	8.2	551	5	57	33	1.5
Oreo, Peanut Butter, Dairy Milk, Cadbury*	1 Chunk/5g	28	1.8	558	5.9	54	35	1.5
Panna Cotta & Raspberry, M&S*	1 Bar/36g	190	12.1	528	4.7	51.4	33.6	0.3
Peanut Butter Cup, Big Cup, Reese's, Hershey*	1 Cup/39g	210	12	538	10.3	53.8	30.8	2.6
Peanut Butter Cup, Mini, Reeses, Hershey*	2 Mini Cups/7g	38	2.1	542	8.8	58.3	30.5	0
Peanut Butter Cup, Miniature, Reese's, Hershey*	1 Cup/9g	44	2.6	500	9.1	59.1	29.6	2.3
Peanut Butter Cup, Reese's, Hershey*	1 Cup/21g	105	6.5	500	11.9	57.1	31	5.9
Peanut Butter Cup, White, Mini, Reese's, Hershey*	5 Cups/39g	210	12	538	12.8	53.8	30.8	2.6
Peanut Butter Cups, Sugar Free, Reese's, Hershey*	1 Cup/11g	45	3.3	409	6.8	61.4	29.6	13.6
Peanut Caramel Crisp, Big Taste, Dairy Milk, Cadbury*	1 Chunk/12g	63	3.9	547	9.8	49	34	2.5
Pen Pals, Hotel Chocolat*	1 Animal/40g	235	16.4	588	7.5	46.2	40.9	1.5
Peppermint Cream, Fry's*	1 Bar/51g	217	7.9	425	2.6	68.8	15.4	0

CHOCOLATE

INFO/WEIGHT	Measure	per Measure KCAL	per Measure FAT	Nutrition Values per 100g / 100ml KCAL	PROT	CARB	FAT	FIBRE
Peppermint Patty, Hershey*	3 Patties/41g	160	3	390	2.4	80.5	7.3	0
Peppermint, Ritter Sport*	1 Bar/100g	483	26	483	3	60	26	0
Plain with Hazelnuts, Tesco*	4 Squares/25g	135	8.9	539	6.1	48.3	35.7	6.5
Plain, 50% Cocoa Solids Minimum, Tesco*	4 Squares/22g	115	6.2	523	7.4	60	28.1	1.8
Plain, 72% Cocoa Solids, Finest, Tesco*	1 Square/10g	60	4.4	603	7.7	44	44	3.7
Plain, Belgian, Organic, Waitrose*	1 Bar/100g	505	37.6	505	9.6	32	37.6	5.6
Plain, Belgian, TTD, Sainsbury's*	1 Piece/10g	57	4.7	570	7	29.3	47.2	10.2
Plain, Continental, Waitrose*	1 Square/4g	23	1.8	558	7.7	32.9	44	5.9
Plain, Dark, Fruit & Nut, Rich, Sainsbury's*	4 Squares/25g	122	7	489	5.2	53.9	27.9	5.7
Plain, Everyday Value, Tesco*	1 Square/4g	22	1.3	520	5.7	51	31	7
Plain, Fair Trade, Tesco*	1 Bar/40g	200	11.8	501	4.8	53.8	29.6	6.6
Plain, Whole Nut, Belgian, Waitrose*	4 Squares/25g	135	9.5	540	6.3	45.4	38	7.8
Plain, Wholenut, Sainsbury's*	1 Serving/25g	142	9	567	5.7	54.6	36.2	2.5
Plain, with Mint, Tesco*	2 Squares/20g	111	7	557	6.7	50.2	35.2	6.7
Planets, Mars*	1 Pack/37g	178	8.3	481	4.9	65.4	22.4	0
Praline, M&S*	1 Bar/34g	185	12	545	7.3	49.6	35.2	3.1
Probiotic, Bar, Ohso*	1 Bar/14g	72	5	514	5	47	36	15.5
Puddles, Hazelnut Flavour Filling, Dairy Milk, Cadbury*	¼ Bar/23g	114	6.2	505	6.3	57	27.5	0.9
Rafaello, Roche, Ferrero*	1 Sweet/10g	60	4.7	600	9.7	35.4	46.6	0
Reese's Pieces, Bite Size, Minis, Hershey*	11 Pieces/39g	200	12	513	7.7	59	30.8	2.6
Reese's, Fast Break, Candy Bar, Hershey*	1 Bar/56g	260	12	464	8.9	62.5	21.4	3.6
Reindeer, Lindt*	1 Reindeer/107g	588	35.3	550	7.2	55	33	0
Rocky Road, Clusters, Tesco*	1 Bite/11g	52	2.2	470	5.6	65.2	20.3	2.1
Salted Butterscotch, Milk, The Best, Morrisons*	2 Squares/20g	112	7.1	558	6.2	53.1	35.3	1.6
Shortcake, Snack Shots, Cadbury*	½ Bag/50g	260	14	520	5.8	60.4	27.9	2
Smooth Praline, Choceur, Aldi*	1 Square/5g	27	1.6	544	7.8	52	33	3.9
Snack Bar, Kinder*	1 Bar/21g	116	7.1	554	10	52	34	0
Snack Size, Dairy Milk, Cadbury*	1 Bar/30g	159	9	530	7.8	57.1	29.9	0
Snaps, Milk, Cadbury*	1 Snap/3g	15	0.8	505	6.3	60.5	27	1
Snickers, More Nuts, Snickers*	1 Bar/58g	299	17.3	515	10.1	52.8	29.8	0
Snowman, Mousse, Dairy Milk, Cadbury*	1 Snowman/29g	162	10.2	560	6.7	54.5	35	0.4
Tabasco, Spicy, Tabasco*	1 Bar/28g	152	9.2	542	4.7	53.4	32.8	7.1
Tasters, Dairy Milk, Cadbury*	1 Bag/45g	238	13.7	530	7.6	56.4	30.5	0
Taz Chocolate Bar, Cadbury*	1 Bar/25g	121	6	485	4.8	62	24	0
Teddy Bear, Milk Chocolate, Thorntons*	1 Teddy/250g	1358	83.8	543	7.6	52.6	33.5	1
Tiffin, Limited Edition, Dairy Milk, Cadbury*	6 Chunks/24g	120	6	502	6.7	60	25	2.1
Toffee, Wholenut, Big Taste, Dairy Milk, Cadbury*	4 Chunks/33g	184	11.9	557	6.3	51	36	1.8
Toffifee, Storck*	1 Sweet/8g	43	2.4	516	5.9	58.5	28.7	0
Treatsize, Dairy Milk, Cadbury*	1 Bar/14g	73	4.2	525	7.5	57	29.8	0.7
Truffles, Belgian, Flying Tiger*	1 Truffle/10g	56	3.8	562	3.8	49	38	0
Turkish Delight, Dairyfine, Aldi*	3 Squares/25g	119	6	475	3.4	62	24	0.5
Turkish Delight, Lge Bar, Dairy Milk, Cadbury*	1 Square/8g	35	1.6	470	5.6	63.2	21.4	0.5
Twirl, Bites, Cadbury*	1 Bite/2g	11	0.6	530	7.7	56.5	30.3	0.8
Ultimate, Bar, Waitrose*	1 Portion/60g	263	18.9	438	4.6	32.3	31.4	3.7
Vanilla, Nestle*	1 Whip/28g	137	6.6	493	5.4	63.2	23.9	1.3
Wafer, Bar, Time Out, Cadbury*	1 Bar/21g	111	6.1	527	6.7	60	29	2.1
Wafer, Dairy Milk, Cadbury*	1 Bar/46g	235	12.9	510	7.7	57	28	0
Whips, Double Chocolate, M&S*	1 Whip/29g	140	7.3	485	6.6	57.8	25.3	1
White with Honey Almond Nougat, Toblerone*	1 Serving/25g	132	7.2	530	6.2	60.5	29	0.2
White with Strawberries, Divine*	1 Piece/3g	16	0.9	534	7.6	59.9	29.3	0.1
White with Strawberry Pieces, Under 99 Cals, M&S*	1 Bar/16g	86	4.9	540	6.6	60.4	30.4	0.3
White, 44%, Rebel Chocolate*	1 Sm Bar/30g	173	11.5	576	28	31.5	38.4	0
White, Average	**1oz/28g**	**148**	**8.7**	**529**	**8**	**58.3**	**30.9**	**0**

	Measure INFO/WEIGHT	per Measure KCAL	FAT	Nutrition Values per 100g / 100ml KCAL	PROT	CARB	FAT	FIBRE
CHOCOLATE								
White, Creamy Vanilla, Green & Black's*	1 Sm Bar/35g	201	12.8	573	7.4	53.5	36.6	0.1
White, Creamy, Aldi*	1 Bar/40g	220	13.2	551	5.5	58	33	0
White, Creamy, Tesco*	1 Serving/25g	139	8.7	557	5.1	55.7	34.9	3.3
White, Crispy, Fair Trade, Co-Op*	½ Bar/50g	278	17.5	555	9	51	35	0.1
White, Nestle*	4 Pieces/40g	220	13	550	7.5	55	32.5	0
White, No Added Sugar, Belgian, Boots*	1 Serving/30g	146	10.8	488	6	47.8	36	7
White, Protein Crunchers, Yumm*	1 Bag/23g	96	4.6	417	23	43	20	0
White, Smart Price, Asda*	1 Serving/25g	137	8.2	549	7	56	33	0
White, Value, Tesco*	1 Serving/10g	55	3.1	548	4.7	62	31.2	0
Whole Nut, Dairy Milk, Cadbury*	1 Bar/49g	270	17.4	550	8.9	49.5	35.4	1.7
Whole Nut, Sainsbury's*	4 Chunks/25g	142	9.4	566	8.5	48.5	37.6	2.6
Whole Nut, Smart Price, Asda*	½ Bar/16g	92	6.2	562	8	47	38	3.3
Wildlife Bar, Cadbury*	1 Bar/21g	109	6.2	520	7.8	56.8	29.3	0
Wispa, Bitsa Wispa, Cadbury*	¼ Bag/43g	238	14.7	550	7.3	53	34	0.9
with Creme Egg, Dairy Milk, Cadbury*	1 Bar/45g	210	9.3	470	5.2	64.8	20.9	0.5
with Crunchie Bits, Dairy Milk, Cadbury*	1 Bar/200g	1000	48.8	500	6.2	63.3	24.4	0
with Shortcake Biscuit, Dairy Milk, Cadbury*	1 Square/6g	31	1.7	520	7.5	59	28	0
CHOCOLATE NUTS								
Peanuts, Assorted, Thorntons*	1 Bag/140g	785	57.1	561	13.8	34.8	40.8	3.6
Peanuts, Belgian Coated, M&S*	1 Serving/20g	109	7.6	545	14.7	35.6	38	5.8
Peanuts, Milk, Tesco*	1 Bag/227g	1221	86	538	17.5	31.8	37.9	4.4
CHOCOLATE RAISINS								
Assorted, Thorntons*	1 Bag/140g	601	27.6	429	4.2	58.8	19.7	2.9
Californian, Tesco*	½ Bag/57g	268	11.7	472	5.2	66.2	20.7	1.3
Co-Op*	½ Pack/50g	205	7.5	410	4	64	15	1
Milk Chocolate Coated, Average	*1 Serving/50g*	*207*	*7.7*	*415*	*4.4*	*64.6*	*15.4*	*2*
Milk, Asda*	1 Serving/28g	120	4.2	430	5.1	66.4	15.1	4.2
Milk, Tesco*	1 Lge Bag/227g	933	35	411	4.8	63.3	15.4	0.9
CHOCOLATE SPREAD								
Average	*1 Tsp/12g*	*68*	*4.5*	*569*	*4.1*	*57.1*	*37.6*	*0*
Hazelnut, Jim Jams*	1 Tbsp/15g	74	5.5	494	6.4	49.4	36.6	0
Hazelnut, Nutella, Ferrero*	1oz/28g	149	8.7	533	6.6	56.4	31	3.5
Hazelnut, Smooth, M&S*	1 Tbsp/15g	86	5.8	573	5.6	48	38.5	4.4
Hazelnut, Weight Watchers*	1 Serving/15g	50	1.8	333	4.7	45.3	12	12
Luxury, Atkins Potts*	1 Tbsp/25g	115	7.1	459	6.3	46.6	28.3	2
with Nuts	*1 Tsp/12g*	*66*	*4*	*549*	*6.2*	*60.5*	*33*	*0.8*
CHOCOLATES								
All Gold, Dark, Terry's*	1 Serving/30g	152	8.7	505	4	57.5	29	4.3
All Gold, Milk, Terry's*	1 Serving/30g	158	9.2	525	4.8	58	30.5	1.5
Almond Marzipan, Milk Chocolate, Thorntons*	1 Chocolate/13g	60	2.9	464	6.6	59.4	22.6	5.6
Almond Mocca Mousse, Thorntons*	1 Chocolate/14g	76	5.3	543	8.5	40.7	37.9	2.9
Alpini, Thorntons*	1 Chocolate/13g	70	4.2	538	7	54.6	32.3	2.3
Assortment, Occasions, Tesco*	1 Chocolate/15g	70	3.1	470	4.6	65.8	20.9	0.5
Bites, Galaxy, Mars*	1 Pack/40g	197	9.7	492	5	63	24.2	0.8
Bittermint, Bendicks*	1 Mint/18g	80	3	440	4.3	68.9	16.3	2.4
Cafe Au Lait, from Continental Selection, Thorntons*	1 Chocolate/16g	77	4	481	5.3	58.1	25	0.6
Cappuccino, from Continental Selection, Thorntons*	1 Chocolate/13g	70	4.7	538	5.9	48.5	36.2	0.8
Caramels, Sainsbury's*	1 Sweet/12g	57	2.6	490	3.5	69	22.2	0.2
Celebrations, Mars*	1 Sweet/8g	40	2	497	5.6	61.7	25	1.7
Champagne Truffles, Milk, The Best, Morrisons*	1 Truffle/12g	57	2.9	479	5.2	57.9	24.8	1.4
Cherishes, Belgian, Hamlet *	2 Chocolates/24g	105	3.8	438	2.5	62.1	15.9	0
Coconut, Lindor, Lindt*	1 Ball/13g	79	6	632	5.4	42	48	0
Coffee Cream, Average	*1 Chocolate/12g*	*54*	*2*	*446*	*3.3*	*70.4*	*17*	*2.4*

C

CHOCOLATES

	Measure INFO/WEIGHT	per Measure KCAL	per Measure FAT	Nutrition Values per 100g / 100ml KCAL	PROT	CARB	FAT	FIBRE
Coffee Creme, Dark, Thorntons*	1 Chocolate/13g	52	1.4	400	3	71.5	10.8	0.8
Coffee Creme, Milk, Thorntons*	1 Chocolate/13g	52	1.3	400	2.8	74.6	10	0.8
Continental, Belgian, Thorntons*	1 Chocolate/13g	67	3.9	514	5.8	53.5	30.3	2.9
Continental, Thorntons*	1 Chocolate/15g	76	4.4	506	5.6	54.5	29.3	2.7
Country Caramel, Milk, Thorntons*	1 Chocolate/9g	45	2.4	500	4.6	62.2	26.7	0
Dairy Box, Milk, Nestle*	1 Piece/11g	50	2.1	456	4.4	65.9	19.4	0.7
Dark, Elegant, Elizabeth Shaw*	1 Chocolate/8g	38	1.8	469	2.9	62.5	23.1	0
Dark, Rose Violet Creams	*1 Chocolate/13g*	*55*	*1.6*	*422*	*2.2*	*76.1*	*12.5*	*1.7*
Dark, Swiss Thins, Lindt*	1 Pack/125g	681	46.2	545	4.8	49.2	37	0
Eclipse, Truffle, Plain, Dark, Montezuma*	1 Truffle/16g	93	8.5	581	0.6	21.9	53.1	0
Filled, Average	*1 Chocolate/13g*	*58*	*2.8*	*447*	*4.9*	*62.9*	*21.3*	*1.3*
Fondant, Chocolate Coated, Usda Average*	1 Chocolate/11g	40	1	366	2.2	80.4	9.3	2.1
Heroes, Cadbury*	1 Sweet/8g	38	1.8	480	4.8	65.1	22.4	0.4
Italian Collection, Amaretto, M&S*	1 Chocolate/13g	60	3.1	480	4.4	59.7	25.1	2.3
Italian Collection, Favourites, M&S*	1 Chocolate/14g	74	4.7	530	5.7	50.4	33.7	1.6
Italian Collection, Panna Cotta, M&S*	1 Chocolate/13g	70	4.7	545	5.3	49.4	36.4	0.1
Lemon Selector In White Chocolate, Hotel Chocolat*	1 Sphere /5g	26	1.8	525	6	47.2	35.5	0
Liqueurs, Brandy, Asda*	1 Chocolate/8g	34	1.4	409	4	60	17	0.8
Liqueurs, Brandy, Favorina, Lidl*	1 Keg/12g	53	2.6	444	1.7	54.3	21.4	0
Liqueurs, Cherry, Mon Cheri, Ferrero*	1 Chocolate/11g	50	2.2	455	3	52.8	20.3	0
Liqueurs, Cognac Truffle, Thorntons*	1 Chocolate/14g	65	3.8	464	7.3	40	27.1	2.9
Liqueurs, Cointreau, Plain, Barrels	*1 Chocolate/10g*	*44*	*1.8*	*435*	*3.5*	*57*	*18*	*0*
Milk White, Penguins, Cocoa Loco*	1 Chocolate/11g	63	4.1	572	6.5	52.3	37.2	0
Milk Tray, Cadbury*	1 Chocolate/9g	47	2.4	495	4.7	61.5	25.8	0.7
Milk, Mini Eggs, Green & Black's*	1 Mini Egg/8g	42	2.7	562	8.6	48.3	35.5	3.8
Milk, Swiss Thins, Lindt*	1 Pack/125g	688	43.3	550	5.8	53.6	34.6	0
Mini Eggs, Mix, Cadbury*	1 Pack/276g	1419	74.5	514	1.6	60	27	1.6
Mini Eggs, with Soft White Truffle Centre, M&S*	1 Egg/6g	33	2	550	6.5	56.3	33.9	1.4
Mint Creams, Dark, Smooth Fragrant, Waitrose*	1 Sweet/10g	42	0.9	410	3	77.9	9.1	2.4
Mint Crisp, Bendicks*	1 Mint/8g	38	2.3	494	5.2	55	29.9	0
Mint Crisp, Dark, Elizabeth Shaw*	1 Chocolate/6g	27	1.2	458	1.9	68	20.7	0
Mint Crisp, Milk, Elizabeth Shaw*	1 Chocolate/6g	30	1.3	493	4	70.9	21.4	0
Mint Crisp, Thorntons*	1 Chocolate/7g	34	2.2	486	7.7	40	31.4	4.3
Mint, Collection, Thorntons*	¼ Sm Box16g	83	4.8	516	4.9	54	30	0
Mints, After Eight, Dark, Nestle*	1 Sweet/7g	32	0.9	461	5	63	12.9	2
Mints, After Eight, Orange, Nestle*	1 Sweet/7g	29	0.9	417	2.5	72.6	12.9	1.1
Mints, After Eight, Straws, Nestle*	1 Sweet/5g	24	1.4	526	5.1	56.6	31	4
Misshapes, Assorted, Cadbury*	1 Chocolate/8g	41	2.3	515	5.2	57.5	29.1	0
Moments, Thorntons*	1 Chocolate/7g	37	2	511	5.4	59.9	27.8	1.9
Neapolitans, No Added Sugar , Chocologic*	3 Chocolates/14g	66	5.1	472	8.8	27.8	36.2	22
Orange Cream, Average	*1 Chocolate/12g*	*53*	*2*	*440*	*3.2*	*69.3*	*16.7*	*0*
Orange Crisp, Elizabeth Shaw*	1 Chocolate/6g	29	1.3	478	2.9	68.2	21.5	0
Peppermint Cream, Average	*1 Chocolate/12g*	*50*	*1.4*	*418*	*1.9*	*76.4*	*11.4*	*1.6*
Praline, Coffee, Thorntons*	1 Chocolate/7g	37	2.4	529	7	47.1	34.3	2.9
Praline, Hazelnut, Thorntons*	1 Chocolate/5g	27	1.8	540	7	48	36	4
Praline, Marzipan, Thorntons*	1 Chocolate/14g	63	3	450	5.9	58.6	21.4	2.1
Praline, Roast Hazelnut, Thorntons*	1 Chocolate/13g	70	4.4	538	6	51.5	33.8	3.1
Quality Street, Nestle*	1 Sweet/9g	44	1.9	470	3.5	67.3	20.5	1.5
Roses, Cadbury*	1 Chocolate/9g	41	1.9	480	3.3	66	22.5	1.3
Sea Shells, Belgian, Guylian*	1 Shell/11g	62	3.8	550	7.6	52	34	0
Seashells, Belgian, Woolworths*	1 Box/63g	346	19.6	550	5.5	52.9	31.1	0
Seashells, Milk & White, Belgian, Waitrose*	1 Serving/15g	77	4.6	511	5	53.1	31	2.8
Stars, Mini Wishes, Truffle Centre, Cadbury*	1 Star/13g	70	4.1	540	6.9	55.6	31.8	1.3

CHOCOLATES

INFO/WEIGHT	KCAL	FAT	KCAL	PROT	CARB	FAT	FIBRE
Strawberries Cream, Thorntons*	1 Chocolate/12g	64	3.9	533	5.1	54.2	32.5	0.8
Swiss Tradition, De Luxe, Lindt*	1 Pack/250g	1388	90.7	555	6.3	51.9	36.3	0
Swiss Tradition, Mixed, Lindt*	1 Pack/392g	2215	149.4	565	6.1	49.8	38.1	0
Truffle Balls, Swiss Milk Chocolate, Waitrose*	1 Chocolate/13g	78	5.8	621	4.1	47	46	1.4
Truffle, Amaretto, Thorntons*	1 Chocolate/14g	66	3.6	471	5.5	55	25.7	2.9
Truffle, Belgian, Flaked, Tesco*	1 Truffle/14g	80	5.4	575	4.4	52.7	38.5	2.3
Truffle, Belgian Milk, Waitrose*	1 Truffle/14g	74	4.8	525	5.8	52.9	34.1	1.2
Truffle, Brandy, Thorntons*	1 Chocolate/14g	68	3.8	486	6.1	52.1	27.1	0.7
Truffle, Caramel, Thorntons*	1 Chocolate/14g	67	3.6	479	4.2	57.9	25.7	2.1
Truffle, Caramel Milk Chocolate, Aldi*	1 Truffle/12g	76	5.8	633	5.8	42.5	48.3	4.2
Truffle, Champagne, Premier, Thorntons*	1 Chocolate/17g	88	5.6	518	6.9	45.3	32.9	2.4
Truffle, Cherry, Thorntons*	1 Chocolate/14g	58	3	414	4.2	50.7	21.4	1.4
Truffle, Chocada, Blissed, Organic, Raw Health*	1 Pack/65g	232	11	357	7	48	17	12
Truffle, Continental Champagne, Thorntons*	1 Chocolate/16g	78	4.5	488	6.1	51.3	28	0.6
Truffle, Dark, Balls, Lindor, Lindt*	1 Ball/12g	76	6.2	630	3.4	38.5	51.4	0
Truffle, Filled, Swiss, Balls, Finest, Tesco*	3 Balls/37g	240	19	640	5	40.7	50.8	1.5
Truffle, French Cocoa Dusted, Sainsbury's*	1 Truffle/10g	57	4.5	570	4	37	45	0
Truffle, Hazelnut, Balls, Lindor, Lindt*	1 Ball/12g	76	6.1	632	5	39.1	50.6	0
Truffle, Hearts, Baileys*	1 Chocolate/15g	76	4.3	506	5.2	52.6	28.9	1.3
Truffle, Irish Milk Chocolate Cream, Elizabeth Shaw*	1 Chocolate/12g	57	2.7	477	3.9	63.4	22.8	0
Truffle, Lemon, White, Thorntons*	1 Chocolate/14g	63	3.5	450	4.6	64.3	25	0.7
Truffle, Milk Chocolate, Balls, Lindor, Lindt*	1 Ball/12g	75	5.6	623	4.9	44	47	2.8
Truffle, Mini Milk Chocolate Balls, Lindor, Lindt*	3 Balls/15g	90	7	600	6.7	40	46.7	0
Truffle, Rum, Thorntons*	1 Chocolate/13g	63	3.2	485	4.8	58.5	24.6	4.8
Truffle, Selection, Tesco*	1 Chocolate/14g	75	4.2	539	5.1	62	29.8	0.5
Truffle, Seville, Thorntons*	1 Chocolate/14g	76	4.7	543	7.1	53.6	33.6	1.4
Truffle, Thorntons*	1 Chocolate/7g	33	1.9	471	6	48.6	27.1	1.4
Truffle, Vanilla, Thorntons*	1 Chocolate/13g	64	3.5	492	4.8	57.7	26.9	1.5
Truffle, Viennese, Dark, Thorntons*	1 Chocolate/10g	53	3.6	530	5.9	47	36	3
Truffle, Viennese, Milk, Thorntons*	1 Chocolate/10g	56	3.6	560	4.9	54	36	0
Truffle, White Chocolate, Balls, Lindor, Lindt*	1 Ball/12g	76	5.9	636	3.7	45	49	0
Truffle, Rum, Average	*1 Truffle/11g*	*57*	*3.7*	*521*	*6.1*	*49.7*	*33.7*	*1.9*
Twilight, Dark with Mint, Terry's*	1 Chocolate/6g	33	1.9	530	3.1	59.5	30.5	4.2
Valentine, Thorntons*	1 Chocolate/11g	60	3.8	542	5.7	52	34.5	2.1
Winter Selection, Thorntons*	1 Chocolate/10g	51	3.1	506	6.2	51.3	30.6	3.8

CHOP SUEY

Chicken with Noodles, Sainsbury's*	1 Pack/300g	300	7.5	100	5.7	13.6	2.5	1.2
Vegetable, M&S*	½ Pack/150g	90	6.1	60	2	3.1	4.1	2.9

CHOW MEIN

Beef, Ready Meal, Average	*1 Serving/400g*	*422*	*12.2*	*106*	*6*	*13.4*	*3*	*1*
Beef, Sainsbury's*	1 Pack/450g	500	11.2	111	6.6	15.5	2.5	0.8
Chicken, & Vegetable, Fuller Longer, M&S*	1 Pack/380g	266	4.9	70	6.3	8.7	1.3	2.1
Chicken, Vegetable, COU, M&S*	1 Pack/380g	262	3.8	69	6.6	7.4	1	1.9
Chicken, Chinese Takeaway, Tesco*	1 Serving/350g	294	8.4	84	8.1	7.5	2.4	1.1
Chicken, Co-Op*	1 Pack/300g	270	9	90	8	9	3	0.9
Chicken, COU, M&S*	1 Pack/200g	170	5.4	85	5.9	9.5	2.7	1.4
Chicken, High Protein, Musclefood*	1 Pot/308g	293	5.9	95	9.8	9.4	1.9	0.7
Chicken, Less Than 3% Fat, BGTY, Sainsbury's*	1 Pack/400g	292	6.2	75	5.9	7.8	1.6	2.7
Chicken, Meal for Two, Meal Box, Tesco*	½ Pack/183g	221	4.8	120	9.4	13.7	2.6	2.2
Chicken, Microwaved, Slimzone, Asda*	1 Pack/475g	342	3.3	72	7.4	8.4	0.7	1.5
Chicken, Morrisons*	1 Pack/400g	368	9.2	92	5.8	13	2.3	1.1
Chicken, Noodle, Pot, Tesco*	1 Pack/262g	280	8.1	107	6.4	12.4	3.1	2
Chicken, Ready Meal, Average	*1 Serving/400g*	*375*	*9.4*	*94*	*6.5*	*11.5*	*2.4*	*1.2*

	Measure INFO/WEIGHT	per Measure		Nutrition Values per 100g / 100ml				
		KCAL	FAT	KCAL	PROT	CARB	FAT	FIBRE
CHOW MEIN								
Chicken, Serves 1, Sainsbury's*	1 Pack/450g	432	11.2	96	7.8	9.5	2.5	2.6
Chicken, Taste of China, Frozen, Tesco*	1 Pack/355g	361	4.3	102	7.5	14.6	1.2	1.2
Chicken, Taste of China, Tesco*	1 Pack/372g	398	11.5	107	8.7	10.3	3.1	1.6
Pork, PB, Waitrose*	½ Pack/310g	332	2.8	107	7.6	17.2	0.9	1.6
Prawn, Takeaway, Chinese	*1 Portion/550g*	*792*	*60*	*144*	*5.6*	*6.1*	*10.9*	*2.8*
Special, COU, M&S*	1 Pack/400g	400	15.2	100	6.6	10.3	3.8	1.4
Special, Ready Meal, Average	*1 Serving/400g*	*383*	*9.7*	*96*	*6.5*	*12.1*	*2.4*	*1*
Vegetable, Cantonese, Stir Fry, Sainsbury's*	¼ Pack/100g	85	3.8	85	2.2	10.6	3.8	1.2
Vegetable, Chinese Favourites Box, M&S*	½ Pack/100g	93	1.5	93	3.3	15.7	1.5	1.9
Vegetable, Ready Meal, Average	*1 Serving/400g*	*337*	*6.7*	*84*	*4.2*	*12.8*	*1.7*	*2*
Vegetable, Taste of China, Tesco*	½ Pack/120g	132	4.8	110	2.7	14.8	4	2
Vesta*	1 Pack/433g	594	17.3	137	4.8	20.4	4	3.3
CHRISTMAS PUDDING								
Alcohol Nut Free, Matthew Walker*	1 Pudding/100g	277	2.3	277	3.1	59.3	2.3	3.4
Alcohol Free, 450g, Sainsbury's*	1 Serving/114g	330	3.5	290	2.7	61.3	3.1	3.2
Average	*1oz/28g*	*81*	*2.7*	*291*	*4.6*	*49.5*	*9.7*	*1.3*
BGTY, Sainsbury's*	1 Serving/114g	302	2.8	266	2.8	58.2	2.5	4.6
Champagne, Luxury, Specially Selected, Aldi*	¼ Pudding/113g	346	8.4	306	3.5	54	7.4	5.1
Classic, Asda*	¼ Pudding/113g	362	6.2	319	2.7	63	5.5	3.4
Cognac Laced, 450g, TTD, Sainsbury's*	¼ Pudding/113g	341	10	303	2.8	51.3	8.9	3.1
Connoisseur, Holly Lane, Aldi*	1 Pudding/100g	303	4.9	303	2.3	61	4.9	3.6
Gluten Wheat Free, Finest, Tesco*	1 Pudding/100g	305	7.1	305	3.3	55.1	7.1	3.7
Hidden Clementine, Heston, Waitrose*	1 Serving/114g	352	7.7	310	2.9	57.8	6.8	3.1
Hidden Clementine, Matured, Finest, Tesco*	¼ Pudding/113g	351	8.5	309	3	55.6	7.5	3.5
Individual, 6 Month Matured, Sainsbury's*	1 Pudding/100g	309	5.3	309	2.4	60.8	5.3	4
Light Fruity, 450g, Sainsbury's*	¼ Pudding/113g	331	5.3	293	1.8	59.3	4.7	3.4
Luxury	*1 Serving/114g*	*416*	*18.8*	*365*	*2.5*	*48.6*	*16.4*	*1*
Luxury, Tesco*	¼ Pudding/114g	346	11	305	3.7	50.8	9.7	1.3
Matured, Finest, Tesco*	1 Serving/113g	340	8.3	300	3.2	54.1	7.3	2.5
Nut Free Alcohol Free, Tesco*	1 Serving/114g	395	7.6	347	2.2	68.2	6.7	2.6
Pear Calvados Pudding, Finest, Tesco*	1/8 Pudding/113g	330	5.7	291	3.3	56.8	5	2.9
Rich Fruit, Tesco*	1 Serving/114g	331	6.7	290	2.4	55	5.9	0
Sticky Toffee, Tesco*	¼ Pudding/114g	372	7.3	326	2.5	64.5	6.4	0.8
Ultimate, Finest, Tesco*	1 Serving/100g	285	7	285	3.7	51.6	7	4.7
Vintage, M&S*	1/8 Pudding/113g	335	6.4	295	2.6	59.8	5.6	1.4
CHUTNEY								
Albert's Victorian, Baxters*	1 Serving/25g	40	0.1	159	1.1	37.9	0.3	1.5
Apple & Pear, TTD, Sainsbury's*	1 Serving/20g	39	0.2	193	0.6	45	0.8	1.7
Apple Walnut, Waitrose*	1 Serving/20g	49	0.5	243	12	53.8	2.6	3.8
Apple, Pear, Spiced, M&S*	1 Tbsp/15g	34	0	230	0.8	55.5	0.2	1.6
Apricot, Sharwood's*	1 Tsp/16g	21	0	131	0.6	32	0.1	2.3
Bengal Spice Mango, Sharwood's*	1 Tsp/5g	12	0	236	0.5	58	0.2	1.2
Caramelised Onion, Sainsbury's*	1 Serving/25g	28	0.4	111	1.1	23.5	1.4	1.1
Caramelised Red Onion, Loyd Grossman*	1 Serving/10g	11	0	111	0.5	27.2	0	0.5
Caramelised Red Onion, Specially Selected, Aldi*	1 Serving/15g	31	0.1	208	1.1	50	0.5	1
Cheese Board, Cottage Delight Ltd*	1 Tbsp/15g	42	0.5	277	1	46.6	3.1	0
Cranberry & Caramelised Red Onion, Baxters*	1 Serving/20g	31	0	154	0.3	38	0.1	0.3
Fruit, Spiced, Baxters*	1 Tsp/16g	23	0	143	6	34.8	0.1	0
Fruit, Traditional, M&S*	1oz/28g	43	0.1	155	0.9	37.2	0.3	1.7
Indian Appetisers, Pot, Waitrose*	1 Pot/158g	330	2.2	209	1.8	47.3	1.4	1.8
Lime & Chilli, Geeta's*	1 Serving/25g	69	0.4	277	2	64	1.4	1.9
Mango & Apple, Sharwood's*	1oz/28g	65	0	233	0.4	57.6	0.1	1.1
Mango & Ginger, Baxters*	1 Jar/320g	598	0.6	187	5	45.7	0.2	0.9

	Measure INFO/WEIGHT	per Measure KCAL	FAT	Nutrition Values per 100g / 100ml KCAL	PROT	CARB	FAT	FIBRE
CHUTNEY								
Mango Chilli, Geeta's*	1 Serving/30g	74	0	246	0.5	60.7	0.1	0.2
Mango Mint, Cofresh*	1 Tbsp/20g	31	0.1	155	1.7	36.4	0.3	2
Mango with Hint of Chilli Ginger, Waitrose*	1 Serving/20g	52	0	259	0.5	64.2	0	0.7
Mango, Green Label, Sharwood's*	1 Tsp/10g	24	0	241	0.3	59.7	0.1	0.9
Mango, Hot Spicy, Waitrose*	1 Serving/20g	46	0.1	230	0.6	51.6	0.3	1.8
Mango, Premium, Geeta's*	1 Serving/50g	126	0.1	253	0.8	62	0.2	0.8
Mango, Spicy, Mild, M&S*	1 Tsp/5g	11	0.1	217	0.4	49.3	1.7	1.6
Mango, Spicy, Sainsbury's*	1 Tbsp/15g	33	0.1	222	0.5	53.8	0.5	1.9
Mango, Sweet	***1 Tsp/16g***	***30***	***0***	***189***	***0.7***	***48.3***	***0.1***	***0***
Mango, Tesco*	1 Serving/20g	45	0	224	0.4	55.5	0.1	1.3
Mango, Waitrose*	1 Serving/20g	43	0.3	215	1	49	1.5	2
Mixed Fruit	***1 Tsp/16g***	***25***	***0***	***155***	***0.6***	***39.7***	***0***	***0***
Onion, Vitasia, Lidl*	1 Tbsp/15g	40	0.1	266	0.9	63.1	0.9	0
Peach, Spicy, Waitrose*	1 Serving/20g	43	0.3	215	1	49	1.5	1.5
Ploughman's Plum, The English Provender Co.*	1 Tsp/10g	16	0	160	1.3	38.1	0.2	1.6
Ploughman's, M&S*	1 Tbsp/15g	22	0	150	0.8	34.6	0.3	2.9
Plum, Ploughman's, Tesco*	1 Tsp/5g	8	0	154	1	34.1	0.4	5.3
Red Onion & Sherry Vinegar, Sainsbury's*	1 Serving/10g	24	0.1	236	0.5	57.1	0.6	1.4
Spicy Fruit, Baxters*	1 Serving/15g	22	0	146	0.6	35.4	0.2	0
Spicy Onion, Organic, The English Provender Co.*	1 Serving/10g	24	0	245	1.2	59	0.5	3.5
Sticky Fig Balsamic Chutney, M&S*	1 Servin/25g	57	0.3	228	1.6	49.8	1.3	5.4
Sweet Mango, Patak's*	1 Tbsp/15g	39	0	259	0.3	67.4	0.1	0.7
Sweet Tomato & Chilli, The English Provender Co.*	1 Tsp/10g	19	0	189	0.9	46	0.2	1.7
Tomato	***1 Tsp/16g***	***20***	***0***	***128***	***1.2***	***31***	***0.2***	***1.3***
Tomato Chilli, Specially Selected, Aldi*	1 Tbsp/15g	21	0.1	138	12	32	0.5	1.3
Tomato Red Pepper, Baxters*	1 Jar/312g	512	1.2	164	2	38	0.4	1.5
Tomato, Baxters*	1 Tsp/12g	18	0	152	1.1	35.9	0.4	1
Tomato, Waitrose*	1 Pot/100g	195	0.3	195	1.3	46.8	0.3	0
CIDER								
Apple, Low Alcohol, Sainsbury's*	1 Glass/250ml	75	0.4	30	0.5	5.4	0.2	0
Basics, Sainsbury's*	1 Glass/250ml	200	0	80	0	0	0	0
Berry, Irish, Magner's*	1 Bottle/500ml	215	0	43	0	4.3	0	0
Cyder, Organic, Aspall*	1 Serving/200ml	120	0.2	60	0.1	3.1	0.1	0
Cyder, Perronelle's Blush, Aspall*	1 Serving/200ml	122	0.2	61	0.1	5.4	0.1	0.5
Cyder, Premier Cru, Aspall*	1 Serving/200ml	120	0	60	0	3.1	0	0
Cyder, Suffolk, Medium, Aspall*	1 Serving/200ml	134	0	67	0.1	4.4	0	0
Diamond White*	1fl oz/30ml	11	0	36	0	2.6	0	0
Dry, Average	***1 Pint/568ml***	***205***	***0***	***36***	***0***	***2.6***	***0***	***0***
Dry, Strongbow*	1 Bottle/375ml	161	0	43	0	3.4	0	0
Fruit, Mixed, Alcohol Free, Kopparberg*	1 Bottle/500ml	190	2.5	38	0.5	9.2	0.5	0
Gold, Thatchers*	1 Bottle/500ml	230	0	46	0	4.5	0	0
Light, Bulmers*	1 Can/500ml	140	0	28	0	0.8	0	0
Low Alcohol	***1 Pint/568ml***	***97***	***0***	***17***	***0***	***3.6***	***0***	***0***
Low Alcohol, M&S*	1 Serving/200ml	50	0	25	0	6.5	0	0
Low Alcohol, Sainsbury's*	1 Serving/200ml	62	0	31	0	6.4	0	0
Low Carb, Stowford*	1 Bottle/500ml	140	0	28	0	0.2	0	0
Magner's*	½ Pint/284ml	105	0	37	0	2	0	0
Mulled, Waitrose*	½ Pint/284ml	145	0	51	0	0	0	0
Nordic Berries, Alska*	1 Bottle/500ml	195	0	39	0	1.1	0	0
Organic, Westons*	1 Serving/200ml	96	0	48	0	3.1	0	0
Original, Bulmers*	1 Serving/250ml	105	0	42	0	4	0	0
Original, Gaymers*	1 Bottle/330ml	148	0	45	0	4.7	0	0
Pear, Bulmers*	1 Serving/200ml	86	0	43	0	3.6	0	0

C

INFO/WEIGHT	Measure	per Measure		Nutrition Values per 100g / 100ml				
		KCAL	FAT	KCAL	PROT	CARB	FAT	FIBRE

CIDER

Pear, Gaymers*	1 Bottle/330ml	168	0	51	0	6.2	0	0
Pear, Magner's*	1 Bottle/568ml	179	0	32	0	0	0	0
Pear, Non Alcoholic, Kopparberg*	1 Bottle/500ml	170	0.5	34	0	8.4	0.1	0
Raspberry, Light, Kopparberg*	1 Can/250ml	85	1.2	34	0.5	2.6	0.5	0
Scrumpy, Average	*1 Serving/200ml*	*93*	*0*	*46*	*0*	*2.3*	*0*	*0*
Scrumpy, Westons*	1 Serving/200ml	94	0	47	0	1.8	0	0
Strawberry Lime, Non Alcoholic, Kopparberg*	1 Bottle/500ml	205	2.5	41	0.5	10.1	0.5	0
Sweet, Average	*1 Pint/568ml*	*239*	*0*	*42*	*0*	*4.3*	*0*	*0*
Vintage	*1 Pint/568ml*	*574*	*0*	*101*	*0*	*7.3*	*0*	*0*

CINNAMON

Casahew Butter, Protein Balls, Graze*	1 Serving/30g	119	5.1	397	17	48	17	9.3
Ground, Average	*1 Tsp/3g*	*8*	*0.1*	*261*	*3.9*	*55.5*	*3.2*	*0*

CLAMS

in Brine, Average	*1oz/28g*	*22*	*0.2*	*79*	*16*	*2.4*	*0.6*	*0*
Raw, Average	*20 Sm/180g*	*133*	*1.7*	*74*	*12.8*	*2.6*	*1*	*0*

CLEMENTINES

Easy Peelers, Sainsbury's*	1 Fruit/60g	25	0.3	42	0.9	8.7	0.5	1.2
Raw, Weighed with Peel, Average	*1 Med/61g*	*22*	*0.1*	*35*	*0.6*	*9*	*0.1*	*1.3*
Raw, Weighed without Peel, Average	*1 Med/46g*	*22*	*0.1*	*47*	*0.8*	*12*	*0.2*	*1.7*

COCKLES

Boiled	*1 Cockle/4g*	*2*	*0*	*53*	*12*	*0*	*0.6*	*0*
Bottled in Vinegar, Drained	*1oz/28g*	*8*	*0.1*	*28*	*6.3*	*0*	*0.3*	*0*
in Parsley Oil, The Best, Morrisons*	½ Pack70g	91	5.2	129	9.6	5.9	7.4	0.4

COCKTAIL

Alcoholic, Juice Based, Average	*1 Glass/200ml*	*464*	*29.2*	*232*	*6.4*	*18.7*	*14.6*	*1.4*
Bloody Mary, Average	*1 Glass/250ml*	*86*	*0*	*42*	*0*	*2.3*	*0*	*0.6*
Bucks Fizz, Premixed, M&S*	1 Glass/250ml	152	0	61	0	9	0	0
Cosmo, Skinny Brands*	1 Can/250ml	90	0.2	36	0	1.3	0.1	0
Cosmopolitan, Canned, M&S*	1 Serving/200ml	456	0	228	0	22	0	0
Daiquiri, Strawberry, Frozen, Average	*1 Glass/250ml*	*132*	*0*	*53*	*0*	*14.1*	*0*	*0*
Grenadine, Orange Juice, Pineapple Juice	*1 Serving/200ml*	*158*	*0.3*	*79*	*0.5*	*19.2*	*0.1*	*0.2*
Long Island Iced Tea, Average	*1 Glass/250ml*	*282*	*0*	*113*	*0*	*13.6*	*0*	*0*
Mai Tai, Average	*1 Serving/200ml*	*209*	*0.1*	*105*	*0.2*	*13.9*	*0.1*	*0.1*
Margarita, Skinny Brands*	1 Can/250ml	90	0.2	36	0	1	0.1	0
Mixer, Appletini, Jordan's Skinny Mixes*	1 Serving/120ml	5	0	4	0	1.7	0	0
Mixer, Appletini, Skinny, Jordan's Skinny Mixes*	1 Serving/90ml	15	0	17	0	5.6	0	0
Mixer, Margarita, Jordan's Skinny Mixes*	1 Serving/120ml	5	0	4	0	1.7	0	0
Mixer, Margarita, Skinny, Jordan's Skinny Mixes*	1 Serving/90ml	15	0	17	0	5.6	0	0
Mixer, Mojito, Skinny, Jordan's Skinny Mixes*	1 Serving/90ml	15	0	17	0	4.4	0	0
Mixer, Peach Bellini, Skinny, Jordan's Skinny Mixes*	1 Serving/90ml	15	0	17	0	4.4	0	0
Mixer, Pina Colada, Jordan's Skinny Mixes*	1 Serving/120ml	30	0	25	0	5.8	0	0
Mixer, Pina Colada, Skinny, Jordan's Skinny Mixes*	1 Serving/90ml	15	0	17	0	4.4	0	0
Mojito, Canned, My Cocktail, Manchester Drinks Co.*	1 Can/250ml	150	0	60	0	9.1	0	0
Mojito, Skinny Brands*	1 Can/250ml	90	0.2	36	0	1.1	0.1	0
Pina Colada	*1 Glass/250ml*	*592*	*20*	*237*	*1*	*28*	*8*	*0*

COCOA

Nibs, Naturya*	1 Serving/10g	58	5	578	13	18.2	50.3	13.4

COCOA POWDER

Cadbury*	1 Tbsp/16g	52	3.3	322	23.1	10.5	20.8	0
Dark, Fine, Dr Oetker*	3 Tbsp/25g	89	5.2	357	20	8.9	21	28
Dry, Unsweetened, Average	*1 Tbsp/5g*	*11*	*0.7*	*229*	*19.6*	*54.3*	*13.7*	*33.2*
Organic, Green & Black's*	1 Tsp/4g	16	0.8	405	22	19	21	27

C

	Measure INFO/WEIGHT	per Measure KCAL	per Measure FAT	Nutrition Values per 100g / 100ml KCAL	PROT	CARB	FAT	FIBRE
COCONUT								
Creamed, Average	*1oz/28g*	*186*	*19.2*	*666*	*6*	*6.7*	*68.4*	*7*
Desiccated, Average	*1oz/28g*	*169*	*17.4*	*604*	*5.6*	*6.4*	*62*	*13.7*
Flaked, Neal's Yard*	1 Serving/30g	181	18.6	604	5.3	44.4	62	13.7
Flakes, Unsweetened, Dr Goerg*	1 Serving/100g	686	67	686	7	6	67	15.6
Fresh, Flesh Only, Average	*1oz/28g*	*69*	*7.1*	*246*	*2.2*	*2.6*	*25.2*	*5.1*
Ice, Average	*1oz/28g*	*104*	*3.6*	*371*	*1.7*	*66.7*	*12.7*	*2.6*
Water with Pineapple, Vita Coco*	1 Carton /330ml	82	0	25	0	6	0	0
Water, M&S*	1 Bottle/263ml	50	0.3	19	0.1	4.7	0.1	0.1
COD								
Baked, Average	*1oz/28g*	*27*	*0.3*	*96*	*21.4*	*0*	*1.2*	*0*
Beer Battered, Crispy, Finest, Tesco*	1 Portion/250g	575	35	230	12	13.4	14	1.3
Dried, Salted, Average	*1oz/28g*	*82*	*0.7*	*290*	*62.8*	*0*	*2.4*	*0*
Dried, Salted, Boiled, Average	*1oz/28g*	*32*	*0.2*	*115*	*27*	*0*	*0.7*	*0*
Fillet, in Batter, Large, Birds Eye*	1 Fillet/120g	276	15.6	230	11	17	13	0.5
Fillets, Battered, Average	*1 Fillet/125g*	*219*	*10.2*	*176*	*12.6*	*13*	*8.2*	*1*
Fillets, Battered, Chunky, Frozen, Tesco*	1 Fillet/116g	239	12.1	206	13.6	13.8	10.4	1.5
Fillets, Battered, Extra Large, Tesco*	½ Pack/178g	464	25.3	261	12.2	20.3	14.2	1.4
Fillets, Beer Battered, Jumbo, Frozen, Chip Shop, Youngs*	1 Fillet/136g	307	17.5	226	11.8	15.2	12.9	0.8
Fillets, Breaded, Average	*1 Fillet/125g*	*258*	*12.2*	*206*	*13*	*16.7*	*9.8*	*1*
Fillets, Breaded, Chunky, Average	*1 Piece/135g*	*204*	*8*	*151*	*13.7*	*10.9*	*5.9*	*1.4*
Fillets, Breaded, Large, Oven Baked, Youngs*	1 Fillet/117g	254	12.1	218	11.9	18.8	10.4	1
Fillets, Breaded, Light, Healthy Range, Average	*1 Fillet/135g*	*209*	*6.9*	*154*	*13.6*	*13.3*	*5.1*	*1.2*
Fillets, Broccoli Mornay, Cooked, Ocean Trader*	½ Pack/155g	142	5.4	92	12	2.4	3.5	1.2
Fillets, Cajun, Lemon, with Roasted Veggies, Hello Fresh*	1 Serving/605g	472	7.9	78	4.9	9.4	1.3	0
Fillets, Chunky, Average	*1 Fillet/198g*	*267*	*7.3*	*135*	*17.1*	*8.2*	*3.7*	*0.8*
Fillets, in Batter, Chunky, Inspirations, Birds Eye*	1 Fillet/142g	293	15	206	12	15.5	10.6	0.6
Fillets, Skin On, Frozen, Tesco*	1 Fillet/124g	97	0.9	78	18	0	0.7	0
Fillets, Skinless Boneless, Raw, Average	*1 Fillet/140g*	*137*	*2.4*	*98*	*17.8*	*0*	*1.8*	*0.4*
Fillets, Smoked, Average	*1 Serving/150g*	*152*	*2.4*	*101*	*21.6*	*0*	*1.6*	*0*
Fillets, Tempura, Battered, Crispy, Gastro, Youngs*	1 Fillet/131g	252	12.1	192	12.9	14.1	9.2	0.8
Fillets, with Tomato Basil Sauce, Simply Bake, Tesco*	1 Fillet/142g	170	8.1	120	15.2	1.8	5.7	0.1
Fillets,Beer Battered, Gastro, Youngs*	1 Fillet/119g	232	10.7	195	13.6	14.4	9	1.1
Loins, Average	*1 Serving/145g*	*116*	*1.2*	*80*	*17.9*	*0.1*	*0.8*	*0.2*
Mornay, Fillets, Sainsbury's*	1 Serving/153g	236	14.4	154	15.2	2.2	9.4	0.9
Mornay, Gratin, Cooked, Just Cook, Sainsbury's*	1 Pack/320g	518	32.2	185	13.3	6.9	11.5	0.5
Mornay, Nutritionally Balanced, M&S*	1 Pack/400g	320	10.4	80	6.8	7.2	2.6	1.6
Mornay, Sainsbury's*	1 Serving/180g	277	16.9	154	15.2	2.2	9.4	0.9
Mornay, with Mash Peas, HL, Tesco*	1 Pack/367g	337	9.2	92	7.7	8.6	2.5	2
Poached, Average	*1oz/28g*	*26*	*0.3*	*94*	*20.9*	*0*	*1.1*	*0*
Smoked, Raw, Average	*1oz/28g*	*22*	*0.2*	*78*	*18.1*	*0*	*0.6*	*0*
Steaks, Battered, Chip Shop Style, Average	*1 Serving/150g*	*321*	*18*	*214*	*12.5*	*14.3*	*12*	*1.1*
Steaks, in Butter Sauce, Youngs*	1 Serving/137g	111	3.2	81	9.8	5.1	2.3	0.2
Steamed, Average	*1oz/28g*	*23*	*0.3*	*83*	*18.6*	*0*	*0.9*	*0*
Thai Green, Steamer, Cook In, Co-Op*	½ Pack/169g	149	4.7	88	13	2.4	2.8	0.9
COD & CHIPS								
Peas, 240, Oakhouse Foods Ltd*	1 Meal/300g	510	18.6	170	6.4	22.3	6.2	2.2
Asda*	1 Serving/280g	450	14	161	8	21	5	1.1
COD IN								
Butter Sauce, Ross*	1 Serving/150g	126	5.8	84	9.1	3.2	3.9	0.1
Butter Sauce, Sainsbury's*	1 Serving/150g	198	13.5	132	10.6	2	9	0.1
Butter Sauce, Steaks, Birds Eye*	1 Pack/170g	185	9.4	109	9.8	5	5.5	0.1
Butter Sauce, Steaks, Frozen, Asda*	1 Pouch/152g	163	4	107	16	5	2.6	0.8
Butter Sauce, Steaks, Morrisons*	1 Steak/170g	153	5.6	90	10.9	4.1	3.3	0.4

C

	Measure INFO/WEIGHT	per Measure KCAL	FAT	Nutrition Values per 100g / 100ml KCAL	PROT	CARB	FAT	FIBRE
COD IN								
Butter Sauce, Tesco*	1 Pack/150g	123	5.4	82	9.4	2.9	3.6	0.5
Cheese Sauce, BGTY, Sainsbury's*	1 Serving/170g	144	4.1	85	12.8	3.1	2.4	0
Cheese Sauce, Pre Packed, Average	***1 Serving/150g***	***136***	***4.4***	***90***	***11.8***	***4.2***	***3***	***0***
Cheese Sauce, Steaks, Birds Eye*	1 Pack/182g	175	6.4	96	10.9	5.2	3.5	0.1
Cheese Sauce, with Broccoli, Lidl*	½ Pack/155g	143	5.4	92	12	2.4	3.5	1.2
Mushroom Sauce, BGTY, Sainsbury's*	1 Serving/170g	112	2.9	66	9.9	2.8	1.7	0.1
Parsley Sauce, COU, M&S*	1 Pack/185g	130	4.6	70	10.6	1.4	2.5	0.6
Parsley Sauce, Frozen, M&S*	1 Pack/184g	156	7.2	85	11.1	1.9	3.9	1
Parsley Sauce, Portions, Ocean Trader*	1 Serving/120g	112	4.7	93	9.4	4	3.9	0.1
Parsley Sauce, Pre Packed, Average	***1 Serving/150g***	***123***	***4.7***	***82***	***10.1***	***3.3***	***3.1***	***0.5***
Parsley Sauce, Skinless Boneless, Sainsbury's*	1 Portion/150g	162	9	108	11.3	2.2	6	0.5
Parsley Sauce, Steaks, Birds Eye*	1 Steak/172g	155	4.8	90	10.5	5.6	2.8	0.1
Parsley Sauce, with Mash, Peas, & Carrots, Sainsbury's*	1 Serving/375g	311	71.2	83	6.9	8.8	19	1.6
Red Pepper Sauce, SteamFresh, Birds Eye*	1 Serving/125g	115	2.4	92	14.4	4.7	1.9	0.3
Red Pepper Sauce, Sweet, Fillets, GFY, Asda*	½ Pack/170g	143	2.7	84	15	2.3	1.6	0.1
COD MEDITERRANEAN								
Everdine*	1 Serving/450g	414	18	92	6.8	5.4	4	3.9
PB, Waitrose*	1 Serving/370g	255	3.7	69	13.1	1.9	1	1.2
Style, Fillets, GFY, Asda*	1 Pack/397g	274	9.9	69	9	2.5	2.5	0.9
COD WITH								
a Mediterranean Pepper Sauce, Fillets, Waitrose*	1 Pack/370g	240	4.8	65	12.2	1.1	1.3	0.9
a Thai Crust, PB, Waitrose*	1 Pack/280g	249	7	89	15.1	1.6	2.5	0.6
Fish Pesto, Fillets, COOK!, M&S*	½ Pack/165g	210	5.1	127	16.4	8.4	3.1	4.2
Parma Ham Sardinian Chick Peas, M&S*	½ Pack/255g	268	12.5	105	9.8	5.3	4.9	0.5
Roasted Vegetables, M&S*	1 Serving/280g	238	10.6	85	8	4.9	3.8	1.7
Salsa & Rosemary Potatoes, BGTY, Sainsbury's*	1 Pack/450g	356	4	79	4.7	13.1	0.9	1.6
Sunblush Tomato Sauce, GFY, Asda*	½ Pack/177g	117	2.7	66	13	0.1	1.5	1
Sweet Chilli, COU, M&S*	1 Pack/400g	360	2	90	7.7	13.1	0.5	1.6
Tomato Sauce, Fillets, Asda*	1 Serving/181g	210	10.9	116	13	2.6	6	2.3
COFFEE								
Chicory, Breakfast Drink, Ricore, Nestle*	1 Tsp/5g	7	0	141	2.7	9.1	0	45.3
Azera, Barista Style Instant, Nescafe*	1 Serving/200ml	2	0	1	0.1	0	0	0
Azera, Latte, To Go, Nescafe*	1 Serving/307ml	89	2.5	29	1	4.4	0.8	0.3
Baileys, Pod, Made Up, Tassimo*	1 Mug/256g	82	3.8	32	0.3	3.8	1.5	0.1
Black, Average	***1 Mug/270ml***	***5***	***0***	***2***	***0.2***	***0.3***	***0***	***0***
Cafe Caramel, Cafe Range, Nescafe*	1 Sachet/17g	72	2.4	423	9.2	64.6	14.1	1.3
Cafe Hazelnut, Nescafe*	1 Sachet/17g	73	2.4	428	9.3	66	14.1	0
Cafe Irish Cream, Cafe Range, Nescafe*	1 Sachet/23g	98	3.2	425	8.2	65.2	14.1	1.2
Cafe Latte, Dry, Douwe Egberts*	1 Serving/12g	58	2.6	480	10	60	22	0
Cafe Latte, Instant, Made Up, Maxwell House*	1 Serving/13g	53	1.7	424	6.4	68	13.6	0
Cafe Latte, Vita Coco*	1 Carton/330g	132	3.3	40	1.7	6	1	0
Cafe Mocha, Cafe Range, Nescafe*	1 Sachet/22g	92	2.9	418	8.5	66.6	13.1	0
Cafe Vanilla, Latte, Cafe Range, Nescafe*	1 Sachet/19g	73	1.6	395	9.2	68.3	8.5	4.1
Caffe Latte, Pre Packed, Starbucks*	1 Cup/220ml	154	5.7	70	2.8	8.9	2.6	0
Cappuccino Ice, Made Up, Dolce Gusto, Nescafe*	1 Serving/240ml	111	2.8	46	1.8	7.2	1.2	0.2
Cappuccino, Cafe Mocha, Dry, Maxwell House*	1 Serving/23g	100	2.5	434	4.3	78.2	10.8	0
Cappuccino, Cafe Specials, Dry, M&S*	1 Serving/14g	55	1.6	395	14	59	11.5	0.7
Cappuccino, Cappio, Iced, Kenco*	1 Can/200ml	138	6	69	3	7	3	0
Cappuccino, Cappio, Kenco*	1 Sachet/18g	79	1.9	439	11.7	73.9	10.6	0.6
Cappuccino, Co-Op*	1 Serving/13g	55	2	440	16	64	16	8
Cappuccino, Decaff, Instant, Made Up, Nescafe*	1 Mug/200ml	68	2.3	34	1	5	1.2	0
Cappuccino, Decaff, Nescafe*	1 Sachet/16g	68	2.3	428	11.6	62.6	14.6	0
Cappuccino, Decaff, Unsweetened, Nescafe*	1 Sachet/16g	70	3.1	437	14.5	51.2	19.4	4.3

COFFEE

INFO/WEIGHT	Measure	per Measure		Nutrition Values per 100g / 100ml				
		KCAL	FAT	KCAL	PROT	CARB	FAT	FIBRE
Cappuccino, Dreamy, Cafe, Options*	1 Serving/30g	77	5.1	256	12.9	58.1	16.9	0
Cappuccino, Dry, Maxwell House*	1 Mug/15g	52	1.4	350	12	64	9.6	0.4
Cappuccino, Dry, Waitrose*	1 Sachet/13g	58	2.3	439	15.1	56	17.2	4.4
Cappuccino, for Filter Systems, Kenco*	1 Sachet/6g	22	0.8	375	19	44	13.5	0
Cappuccino, Iced, Cowbelle, Aldi*	1 Serving/250ml	169	4.5	68	3.3	9.6	1.8	0.3
Cappuccino, Instant, Aldi*	1 Sachet/13g	49	1.7	393	12.5	55.1	13.6	0
Cappuccino, Instant, Asda*	1 Sachet/15g	60	2.3	399	13	53	15.2	0.9
Cappuccino, Instant, Kenco*	1 Sachet/20g	80	2.8	401	13.5	55.7	13.8	0
Cappuccino, Instant, Made Up, Maxwell House*	1 Serving/280g	123	5.3	44	0.6	5.8	1.9	0
Cappuccino, Instant, Unsweetened, Douwe Egberts*	1 Serving/12g	48	1.9	400	11	53	16	0
Cappuccino, Italian, Nescafe*	1 Cup/150ml	60	2.9	40	1.2	4.4	1.9	0
Cappuccino, Light, Alcafe, Aldi*	1 Sachet/15g	4	0.1	27	1.6	4.5	0.5	0.5
Cappuccino, Low Sugar, Tesco*	1 Serving/13g	55	2.6	425	18.4	43.3	19.8	0.4
Cappuccino, M&S*	1 Serving/164g	66	2.6	40	1.5	4.4	1.6	0
Cappuccino, Made Up, Dolce Gusto, Nescafe*	1 Serving/240ml	84	3.7	35	1.6	4	1.5	0.3
Cappuccino, Original Mugsticks, Maxwell House*	1 Serving/18g	73	2.8	406	14.4	52.8	15.6	0
Cappuccino, Original, Sachets, Nescafe*	1 Sachet/18g	80	3.1	444	11.7	60.3	17.4	0
Cappuccino, Sainsbury's*	1 Serving/12g	49	1.9	411	14.9	52.9	15.5	0.4
Cappuccino, Semi Skimmed Milk, Average	*1 Serving/200ml*	*63*	*2.3*	*31*	*2.2*	*3.2*	*1.2*	*0*
Cappuccino, Sweetened, Instant, Alcafe, Aldi*	1 Sachet/135ml	61	1.6	45	0.5	8.2	1.2	0.4
Cappuccino, to Go, Original, Nescafe*	1 Serving/19g	84	3.3	444	11.7	60.3	17.4	0
Cappuccino, Unsweetened Taste, Maxwell House*	1 Serving/15g	65	2.9	434	17.4	47.6	19.3	0.3
Cappuccino, Unsweetened, Cappio, Kenco*	1 Serving/18g	73	1.8	406	12.2	66.7	10	0.6
Cappuccino, Unsweetened, Gold, Nescafe*	1 Sachet/14g	55	1.8	392	12.9	52.5	13	5.7
Capuccino, Alcafe, Aldi*	1 Sachet/135ml	61	1.6	45	0.5	8.2	1.2	0.4
Chococino, Made up, Dolce Gusto, Nescafe*	1 Serving/210g	147	5.4	70	2.3	9.4	2.6	0.7
Coconut, Caffe, Alpro*	1 Carton/250ml	88	2.8	35	0.2	5.2	1.1	0.9
Columbian, Nescafe*	1 Serving/2g	2	0	111	16.7	11.1	0	5.6
Compliment*	1 Serving/14ml	20	1.8	143	1.4	6.4	12.9	0
Dandelion, Symingtons*	1 Tsp/6g	19	0	320	2.8	79.3	0	0
Espresso, Instant, Nescafe*	1 Tsp/2g	2	0	118	7.8	3.1	0.2	34.1
Espresso, Made Up, Dolce Gusto, Nescafe*	1 Serving/60ml	1	0.1	2	0.1	0	0.2	0.3
Frappe Iced, Nestle*	1 Sachet/24g	92	1	384	15	72	4	0.5
Gold Blend, Decafefinated, Nescafe*	1 Tsp/5g	3	0	63	7	9	0.2	27
Gold Blend, Nescafe*	1 Cup 200ml/5g	3	0	63	7	9	0.2	27
Green Mountain, Breakfast, Keurig*	1 Serving/227ml	0	0	0	0.1	0	0	0
Hazlenut, Caffe, Alpro*	1 Serving/250ml	78	2.2	31	0.2	5.2	0.9	1
Ice Mocha Drink, Nescafe, Nestle*	1 Bottle/280ml	160	3.4	57	1.1	10.5	1.2	0
Iced, Latte Espresso, Cafetto*	1 Cup/250ml	148	3	59	3	9	1.2	0
Iced, Mocha, Jimmys Iced Coffee*	1 Carton/300g	138	3.6	46	2.3	6.6	1.2	0
Iced, Original, Jimmys Iced Coffee*	1 Carton/330ml	129	3.6	39	2.4	4.9	1.1	0
Iced, Skinny, Jimmys Iced Coffee*	1 Carton/330ml	99	0	30	2.6	4.8	0	0
Infusion, Avg with Semi-Skimmed Milk	*1 Cup/220ml*	*15*	*0.4*	*7*	*0.6*	*0.7*	*0.2*	*0*
Infusion, Avg with Single Cream	*1 Cup/220ml*	*31*	*2.6*	*14*	*0.4*	*0.3*	*1.2*	*0*
Instant, Alta Rica, Nescafe*	1 Tsp/2g	2	0	98	13.8	10	0.3	21
Instant, Decaffeinated, Nescafe*	1 Tsp/2g	2	0	101	14.9	10	0.2	8.4
Instant, Fine Blend, Nescafe*	1 Tsp/2g	1	0	63	7	9	0.2	27
Instant, Made with Skimmed Milk	*1 Serving/270ml*	*15*	*0*	*6*	*0.6*	*0.8*	*0*	*0*
Instant, Made with Water Semi Skimmed Milk	*1 Serving/350ml*	*24*	*0.7*	*7*	*0.4*	*0.5*	*0.2*	*0*
Instant, Made with Water, Whole Milk	*1 Cup/220ml*	*18*	*0.9*	*8*	*0.5*	*0.6*	*0.4*	*0*
Instant, Original, Nescafe*	1 Tsp/2g	1	0	63	7	9	0.2	27
Instant, with Skimmed Milk, Costa Rican, Kenco*	1 Mug/300ml	17	0.1	6	0.6	0.8	0	0
Irish Latte, Gold, Nescafe*	1 Mug/22g	90	2.2	411	8.3	70.6	9.9	2.6

C

	Measure INFO/WEIGHT	per Measure KCAL	FAT	Nutrition Values per 100g / 100ml KCAL	PROT	CARB	FAT	FIBRE
COFFEE								
Latte Macchiato, Made Up, Dolce Gusto, Nescafe*	1 Serving/220g	89	4.2	40	2	4.1	1.9	0.3
Latte, Cafe, M&S*	1 Serving/190g	142	5.3	75	4.3	8.3	2.8	0
Latte, Iced, M&S*	1 Bottle/300ml	186	3.6	62	2.9	9.8	1.2	0.5
Latte, Macchiato, Tassimo*	1 Cup/275ml	135	7.7	49	2.3	3.6	2.8	0
Latte, Nescafe*	1 Sachet/22g	110	6.3	498	14.5	45.7	28.5	0
Latte, No Sugar, In Cup, From Machine, Kenco*	1 Cup/4g	17	0.9	400	7.6	44	22	0
Latte, Skinny, Nescafe*	1 Sachet/20g	72	1.1	359	24.1	54.3	5.3	1.1
Latte, Soya, Caramel, Chilled, Alpro*	1 Serving/200ml	84	24	42	2.1	5.2	12	1.3
Macchiato, Caramel, Iced, Pre-made, Starbucks*	1 Cup/220ml	136	3.5	62	2.8	9.1	1.6	0
Macchiato, Latte, Classic, Tassimo*	1 Serving/295ml	90	6.1	31	0.3	2.4	2.1	0.2
Mocha, Double Chocolate, Gold, Nescafe*	1 Sachet/23g	93	2.3	403	9.4	66.3	9.8	5.1
Mocha, Made Up, Dolce Gusto, Nescafe*	1 Serving/210g	117	5.1	56	2.4	6.1	2.4	0.6
Mocha, Sainsbury's*	1 Serving/22g	84	3	383	14	51	13.7	1.3
Mocha, Skinny, Nescafe*	1 Sachet/21g	77	0.7	367	13.6	70.3	3.5	4.3
Skinny Cappuccino, Made Up, Dolce Gusto, Nescafe*	1 Mug/15g	49	0.1	337	33.3	48.8	0.9	2.3
COFFEE SUBSTITUTE								
Bambu, Vogel*	1 Tsp/3g	10	0	320	3.5	75.3	0.5	0
COFFEE WHITENER								
Creamer, Hazelnut, Fat Free, Coffee Mate, Nestle*	1 Tbsp/15ml	25	0	167	0	33.3	0	0
Light, Asda*	1 Serving/3g	13	0.4	433	0.9	78	13	0
Light, Tesco*	1 Tsp/3g	12	0.2	406	1	85.5	6.7	0
Original, Coffee Mate, Nestle*	1 Tsp/3.5g	19	1.2	547	2.4	56.7	34.4	0
Tesco*	1 Tsp/3g	16	0.9	533	1.2	61.3	31.4	0
Virtually Fat Free, Coffee Mate, Nestle*	1 Tsp/5g	10	0.2	200	1	42	3	0
COGNAC								
40% Volume	*1 Pub Shot/35ml*	*78*	*0*	*222*	*0*	*0*	*0*	*0*
COLA								
Average	*1 Can/330ml*	*135*	*0*	*41*	*0*	*10.9*	*0*	*0*
Coke, Cherry, Coca-Cola*	1 Bottle/500ml	225	0	45	0	11.2	0	0
Coke, Cherry, Zero, Coca-Cola*	1 Can/330ml	1	0	0	0	0	0	0
Coke, Diet with Cherry, Coca-Cola*	1 Bottle/500ml	5	0	1	0	0	0	0
Coke, Diet, Caffeine Free, Coca-Cola*	1 Can/330ml	1	0	0	0	0.1	0	0
Coke, Mango, Exotic, Diet, Coca-Cola*	1 Bottle/500ml	2	0	0	0	0	0	0
Coke, Vanilla, Coca-Cola*	1 Bottle/500ml	215	0	43	0	10.6	0	0
Coke, with Lemon, Diet, Coca-Cola*	1 Can/330ml	5	0	1	0	0	0	0
Coke, with Vanilla, Diet, Coca-Cola*	1 Glass/200ml	1	0	0	0	0.1	0	0
Curiosity, Fentiman's*	1 Bottle/275ml	129	0	47	0.1	11.6	0	0
Diet, Average	*1 Serving/200ml*	*1*	*0*	*1*	*0*	*0*	*0*	*0*
Pepsi Max, Ginger, Pepsi*	1 Can/250ml	1	0	0	0	0	0	0
Twist, Light, Pepsi*	1 Bottle/500ml	4	0	1	0	0.1	0	0
Zero, Caffeine Free, Coca-Cola*	1 Glass/200ml	0	0	0	0	0	0	0
Zero, Coca-Cola*	1 Can/330ml	1	0	0	0	0	0	0
COLESLAW								
Potato Salad, Baby, Finest, Tesco*	1 Serving/50g	105	9.6	210	1.4	7.2	19.2	1.4
Apple, Raisin Walnut, TTD, Sainsbury's*	1 Serving/75g	212	19.6	283	2.3	8	26.2	2.8
Basics, Sainsbury's*	1 Serving/25g	27	2.4	107	1	3.7	9.8	1.6
Beetroot, Apple, Pink Cabbage, Skinny Slaw, M&S*	1 Pack/225g	220	11.2	98	1.5	10.8	5	2
Cheese, Deli Style, Waitrose*	¼ Tub/75g	247	24.3	330	3.8	5.1	32.5	0.9
Cheese, M&S*	1 Serving/57g	185	19.1	325	4.2	2	33.5	1.7
Cheese, Sainsbury's*	1 Serving/75g	184	16.8	246	3.8	6.5	22.4	1.4
Coronation, Sainsbury's*	¼ Pot/75g	145	11.6	193	1	11.4	15.5	1.9
COU, M&S*	½ Pack/125g	75	3.4	60	1.3	7.4	2.7	1.7
Creamy, Asda*	1 Serving/25g	62	6	248	0.9	7	24	1.8

	Measure INFO/WEIGHT	per Measure KCAL	per Measure FAT	Nutrition Values per 100g / 100ml KCAL	PROT	CARB	FAT	FIBRE
COLESLAW								
Creamy, LC, Tesco*	1/3 Pot/100g	105	8.8	105	1.2	4.9	8.8	1.6
Creamy, Morrisons*	1 Serving/50g	112	10.9	224	0.7	5.4	21.8	1.5
Creamy, Tesco*	1 Serving/75g	142	13.4	190	1	5.5	17.8	1.5
Deli Salad, Tesco*	1 Serving/50g	91	8.5	183	0.9	5.5	17.1	1.6
Deli Style, M&S*	1 Serving/50g	103	9.6	206	1.6	5.5	19.1	2.7
Eastmans*	1 Serving/50g	87	8.2	174	0.9	4.9	16.4	1.5
Essential, Waitrose*	1 Tbsp/20g	50	4.9	248	0.8	5.4	24.6	1.2
From Restaurant, Average	*3/4 Cup/99g*	*147*	*11*	*148*	*1.5*	*12.9*	*11.1*	*0*
Fruit, Celery, Nut, Sainsbury's*	1 Serving/75g	143	11.6	191	2.1	96	15.5	2.4
Half Fat, Waitrose*	1 Serving/100g	38	2.7	38	0.6	2.9	2.7	1.2
Jalapeno, Sainsbury's*	1 Serving/75g	142	13.4	190	0.9	5.6	17.9	1.6
Luxury, Asda*	1 Serving/50g	108	10.5	217	0.9	6	21	0
Luxury, Lidl*	1 Serving/50g	102	9.7	203	0.9	5.9	19.4	0
Luxury, Rich Creamy, TTD, Sainsbury's*	1 Serving/50g	123	11.8	246	1.8	5.9	23.6	1.5
Premium, Co-Op*	1 Serving/50g	160	17	320	1	3	34	2
Rainbow, Finest, Tesco*	¼ Pack/84g	192	18.7	229	1.3	4.9	22.3	1.7
Red, Tesco*	½ Pack/70g	53	1	76	1	13.5	1.5	2.4
Reduced Fat, Average	*1 Tbsp/20g*	*23*	*1.9*	*113*	*1*	*6.4*	*9.3*	*2*
Reduced Fat, Co-Op*	1 Serving/50g	45	3.5	90	0.9	6	7	2
Reduced Fat, Essential, Waitrose*	1/6 Tub/50g	65	5.1	130	1.2	8.3	10.2	1.6
Reduced Fat, M&S*	½ Tub/112g	230	22.4	205	1.1	5.4	20	2.8
TTD, Sainsbury's*	¼ Med Pot/75g	185	17.7	246	1.8	5.9	23.6	1.5
with Reduced Calorie Dressing, Retail	*1 Serving/40g*	*27*	*1.8*	*67*	*0.9*	*6.1*	*4.5*	*1.4*
COLEY								
Portions, Raw, Average	*1 Serving/92g*	*65*	*0.6*	*71*	*15.9*	*0*	*0.6*	*0*
Steamed, Average	*1oz/28g*	*29*	*0.4*	*105*	*23.3*	*0*	*1.3*	*0*
CONCHIGLIE								
Cooked, Average	*1 Serving/185g*	*247*	*1.6*	*134*	*4.8*	*26.6*	*0.8*	*0.6*
Dry Weight, Average	*1 Serving/100g*	*352*	*1.7*	*352*	*12.5*	*71.6*	*1.7*	*2.6*
Shells, Dry, Average	*1 Serving/100g*	*346*	*1.5*	*346*	*12.3*	*70.4*	*1.5*	*3*
Whole Wheat, Dry Weight, Average	*1 Serving/75g*	*237*	*1.5*	*316*	*12.6*	*62*	*2*	*10.7*
CONCHIGLIONI								
Dry, Waitrose*	1 Serving/75g	256	1	341	12.5	69.8	1.3	3.7
CONSERVE								
Apricot, Average	*1 Tbsp/15g*	*37*	*0*	*244*	*0.5*	*59.3*	*0.2*	*1.5*
Apricot, Reduced Sugar, Streamline*	1 Tbsp/20g	37	0	184	0.5	45	0.2	0
Blackberry, Bramble, Gin, M&S*	1 Tsp/5g	12	0.1	233	0.8	54.2	1.1	1.4
Blackcurrant, Average	*1 Tbsp/15g*	*37*	*0*	*245*	*0.6*	*60*	*0.1*	*1.9*
Blueberry, M&S*	1 Tsp/8g	15	0	206	0.3	51.1	0.1	1.3
Cherry, Morello, Tart, Full Flavoured, M&S*	1 Tsp/5g	13	0	256	0.4	62.6	0.3	0.8
Hedgerow, TTD, Sainsbury's*	1 Tbsp/15g	41	0	276	0.5	68.2	0.1	0.5
Morello Cherry, Waitrose*	1 Tbsp/15g	39	0	258	0.4	64.2	0	1.4
Plum, TTD, Sainsbury's*	1 Tbsp/15g	44	0	295	0.3	73.1	0.1	0.5
Raspberry, Average	*1 Tbsp/15g*	*37*	*0.1*	*249*	*0.6*	*61*	*0.3*	*1.3*
Raspberry, Seedless, Smooth Sharp, M&S*	1 Tsp/5g	13	0	252	0.5	61.1	0.3	1.2
Red Cherry, TTD, Sainsbury's*	1 Tbsp/15g	43	0	283	0.4	70.2	0.1	0.5
Rhubarb & Ginger, M&S*	1 Tbsp/15g	29	0	194	0.3	47.9	0.1	1
Rhubarb, Raspberry, Rose, M&S*	1 Tsp/5g	12	0	248	0.4	59.3	0.9	0.4
CONSERVE								
Rhubarb, Tangy Aromatic, M&S*	1 Tsp/5g	13	0	253	0.4	61.2	0.3	1.7
Strawberry, Average	*1 Tbsp/15g*	*37*	*0*	*250*	*0.4*	*61.6*	*0.1*	*0.5*
CONSOMME								
Average	*1oz/28g*	*3*	*0*	*12*	*2.9*	*0.1*	*0*	*0*

	Measure INFO/WEIGHT	per Measure KCAL	FAT	Nutrition Values per 100g / 100ml KCAL	PROT	CARB	FAT	FIBRE
CONSOMME								
Beef, Canned, Sainsbury's*	1 Can/415g	46	0	11	2	0.7	0	0
Beef, Luxury, with Sherry, Baxters*	1 Can/415g	62	0	15	2.7	1	0	0
COOKIES								
All Butter, Almond, Italian Style, M&S*	1 Cookie/23g	120	6.4	515	6.7	59.4	27.6	3.6
All Butter, Ginger Bread, M&S*	1 Cookie/23g	102	5	445	4.3	57.5	21.8	2.4
All Butter, Italian Style Sorrento Lemon, M&S*	1 Cookie/24g	120	6.4	500	4.9	60.4	26.7	2.1
All Butter, Melting Moment, M&S*	1 Cookie/23g	110	6.4	470	4.5	51.5	27.5	3.4
All Butter, Sultana, TTD, Sainsbury's*	1 Biscuit/17g	79	3.8	476	5.4	62.7	22.6	2
Almond, Ose*	1 Cookie/10g	46	1.4	456	8.4	74	14	0
Apple & Raisin, Go Ahead, McVitie's*	1 Cookie/15g	66	1.9	443	5.3	76.8	12.7	3.4
Apple Crumble, M&S*	1 Cookie/26g	90	0.5	345	4.6	76.8	2	2.9
Apple Pie, The Biscuit Collection*	1 Cookie/19g	90	4.2	474	3.9	65	22.1	0
Big Milk Chocolate Chunk, Cookie Coach*	1 Cookie/35g	174	8.8	497	6.2	61.4	25.1	0
Bites, Weight Watchers*	1 Pack/21g	97	4	464	5.8	67	19.2	4.3
Bounty, Mars*	1 Cookie/46g	215	9.6	468	5.7	63.4	20.9	0
Brazil Nut, Organic, Traidcraft*	1 Cookie/17g	91	5.4	547	5.8	57.7	32.6	2.1
Brazil Nut, Prewett's*	1 Cookie/50g	122	7.4	244	2.6	25.2	14.8	1
Butter & Sultana, Sainsbury's*	1 Cookie/13g	61	2.6	473	4.5	68.4	20.1	1.6
Cherry Bakewell, COU, M&S*	1 Cookie/25g	90	0.6	355	6	77.2	2.5	3.4
Chia Coconut, with Afternoon Infusion, Graze*	1 Punnet/22g	118	6.9	528	5.8	53	31	5
Choc Chip Coconut, Maryland*	1 Cookie/10g	55	2.5	512	5.1	62.9	23.7	0
Choc Chip Hazelnut, Maryland*	1 Cookie/11g	55	2.7	513	6.3	65.3	25	0
Choc Chip 'n' Chunk, McVitie's*	1 Cookie/11g	55	2.9	498	5.8	59.2	26.4	3.5
Choc Chip, Bronte*	1 Cookie/17g	79	3.6	474	5.8	64	21.6	0
Choc Chip, Giant, Paterson's*	1 Cookie/60g	296	15.2	493	0.1	61.3	25.3	3.2
Choc Chip, Lyons*	1 Cookie/11g	57	2.7	499	5.2	68.3	23.4	1.7
Choc Chip, Mini, Good to Go, Waitrose*	1 Bag/25g	127	6.6	508	6	60.4	26.4	2.4
Choc Chip, Parkside*	1 Cookie/11g	56	2.7	495	5.3	64.5	23.7	0
Choc Chip, Reduced Fat, Maryland*	1 Cookie/11g	51	1.9	478	5.9	73	18	0
Choc Chunk & Hazelnut, Co-Op*	1 Cookie/17g	89	5.3	525	6	56	31	3
Choc Chunk, Fabulous Bakin' Boys*	1 Cookie/60g	270	12.6	450	5	59	21	3
Choc Chunk, Finest, Tesco*	1 Cookie/80g	355	14.1	445	5.7	65.3	17.7	1.8
Chocolate & Nut, Organic, Evernat*	1 Cookie/69g	337	15.6	489	7.2	64.1	22.6	0
Chocolate & Orange, COU, M&S*	1 Cookie/26g	90	0.7	350	5.7	77.2	2.6	3.2
Chocolate Orange, Bites, Go Ahead, McVitie's*	1 Pack/23g	98	2.4	427	6.9	74.1	10.5	4
Chocolate Chip Caramel, Bites, Maryland*	5 Biscuits/20g	103	5.3	513	5.7	61.8	26.4	3
Chocolate Chip Hazelnut, Extra Special, Asda*	1 Cookie/25g	130	8.1	516	6	51	32	2.5
Chocolate Chip, Asda*	1 Cookie/12g	57	2.9	497	5	63	25	2.6
Chocolate Chip, Average	***1 Cookie/10g***	***49***	***2.5***	***489***	***5.5***	***64.1***	***24.7***	***2.9***
Chocolate Chip, BGTY, Sainsbury's*	1 Cookie/17g	72	2	428	4.5	75.6	11.9	2.5
Chocolate Chip, Chips Ahoy*	1 Cookie/11g	55	2.8	500	6	65	25	3
Chocolate Chip, Co-Op*	1 Cookie/11g	55	2.6	500	5	65	24	1
Chocolate Chip, Dough, Otis Spunkmeyer*	1 Cookie/38g	160	8	421	5.3	60.5	21	2.6
Chocolate Chip, Free From, Sainsbury's*	1 Cookie/19g	93	4.6	498	6.5	61.4	24.4	3.3
Chocolate Chip, Free From, Tesco*	1 Cookie/12g	59	2.6	488	5.2	65.6	22	3.4
Chocolate Chip, GF, Organic, Dove's Farm*	1 Cookie/17g	77	3.1	451	4.3	66.9	18.5	0
Chocolate Chip, GFY, Asda*	1 Cookie/10g	48	2	463	5	68	19	3.5
Chocolate Chip, Gluten Wheat Free, Lovemore*	1 Cookie/17g	81	4.5	483	3.8	57.8	26.8	3.5
Chocolate Chip, Handbaked, Border*	1 Cookie/15g	72	3.4	480	5.9	67.4	22.6	0
Chocolate Chip, High Protein, Dr Zak's*	1 Cookie/60g	214	6.4	356	25	48	10.7	2.3
Chocolate Chip, Low Price, Sainsbury's*	1 Cookie/11g	54	2.3	500	7	70.1	21.3	2.5
Chocolate Chip, Lyons*	1 Cookie/12g	56	2.5	483	5.6	66.5	21.6	1.7
Chocolate Chip, M&S*	1 Cookie/12g	59	3	495	5.7	62.1	24.8	2.7

	Measure INFO/WEIGHT	per Measure		Nutrition Values per 100g / 100ml				
		KCAL	FAT	KCAL	PROT	CARB	FAT	FIBRE
COOKIES								
Chocolate Chip, Maryland*	1 Cookie/11g	53	2.5	487	5.4	63.8	22.6	3.5
Chocolate Chip, McVitie's*	1 Cookie/11g	54	2.8	496	5.8	60.2	25.8	3
Chocolate Chip, Mini, Bites, Tesco*	1 Cookie/13g	61	2.7	469	5.6	64.5	20.7	1.4
Chocolate Chip, Mini, McVitie's*	1 Bag/40g	196	9.2	491	5.5	65.1	23.1	2.8
Chocolate Chip, Morrisons*	1 Cookie/10g	52	2.5	502	5	66.2	24.1	1.3
Chocolate Chip, Organic, Sainsbury's*	1 Cookie/17g	89	4.9	530	5	61.8	29.2	0.3
Chocolate Chip, Organic, Tesco*	1 Cookie/17g	88	4.7	520	4	63.3	27.4	2.8
Chocolate Chip, Tesco*	1 Cookie/11g	54	2.7	493	5.8	61.2	24.3	3.2
Chocolate Chip, Value, Tesco*	1 Cookie/11g	56	2.9	512	4.8	64.8	26	1.6
Chocolate Chip, Weight Watchers*	1 Cookie/11g	49	1.9	443	7.6	65.4	17.2	4.6
Chocolate Chunk & Hazelnut, Tesco*	1 Cookie/22g	118	6.7	538	6.2	60.2	30.3	1.9
Chocolate Chunk & Hazelnut, TTD, Sainsbury's*	1 Biscuit/25g	132	7.7	527	6.7	54.2	30.8	3.3
Chocolate Chunk, All Butter, M&S*	1 Cookie/24g	120	6	500	5.2	62.4	25.2	2.9
Chocolate Chunk, Cadbury*	1 Cookie/22g	119	6.9	540	6.5	58	31.2	0
Chocolate Chunk, Devondale*	1 Cookie/65g	308	16.3	474	4.6	59.2	25.1	2.8
Chocolate Fruit & Nut, Extra Special, Asda*	1 Cookie/25g	125	7.1	509	6	56	29	2
Chocolate Orange, Half Coated, Finest, Tesco*	1 Cookie/22g	107	5.6	488	4.9	59.6	25.5	1.2
Chocolate Thin Crisp, Simply Food, M&S*	1 Pack/23g	100	2	435	4.4	78.3	8.7	4.4
Chocolate, Belgian, Extra Special, Asda*	1 Cookie/26g	138	8	535	6	58	31	2
Chocolate, Dark, Ginger, Free From, Finest, Tesco*	1 Cookie/19g	92	4.2	485	4.6	66	22	2.1
Chocolate, Double, Sainsbury's*	1 Cookie/45g	202	8.5	450	5.8	63.1	18.9	2
Chocolate, Double, Tesco*	1 Cookie/42g	187	8.1	447	5.8	60.8	19.4	3.2
Chocolate, Milk, Free From, Tesco*	1 Cookie/20g	100	6.1	500	5.6	50.4	30.7	4.1
Chocolate, Quadruple, Finest, Tesco*	1 Cookie/25g	128	6.9	512	6.3	58.3	27.5	3
Chocolate, Soft, American Style, Budgens*	1 Cookie/50g	216	9.3	431	5.1	60.8	18.6	2.2
Chocolate, Triple, Half Coated, Finest, Tesco*	1 Cookie/25g	131	7.3	525	5.7	58.7	29.3	2.3
Chocolate, Triple, High Protein, Dr Zak's*	1 Cookie/60g	210	6.1	350	25	46	10.1	3.3
Chocolate, Triple, Wheat, GF, Finest, Tesco*	1 Cookie/19g	97	5	508	5.8	60.4	26.2	3.5
Chunkie Extremely Chocolatey, Fox's*	1 Cookie/26g	130	6.8	506	6.2	61	26.3	2.6
Chunkie, Chocolatey, Extremely, Fox's*	1 Cookie/25g	129	6.3	509	5.6	63	25	2.6
Chunky Chocolate, Kate's Cakes Ltd*	1 Serving/100g	441	22	441	5.2	55.5	22	2.4
Cocoa, Organic, Bites, No Junk, Organix*	1 Bag/25g	105	3.2	421	7	69	13	5.5
Coconut & Raspberry, GF, Sainsbury's*	1 Cookie/20g	102	5.9	511	5.9	56	29.3	6.7
Coconut, Gluten-Free, Sainsbury's*	1 Cookie/20g	103	6.1	516	5.6	54.4	30.7	4.1
Cranberry & Orange, Finest, Tesco*	1 Cookie/26g	125	5.8	490	4.1	67.4	22.6	3.2
Cranberry & Orange, Go Ahead, McVitie's*	1 Cookie/17g	77	2.2	452	5.3	78	13.2	2.4
Crunchy Muesli, Mini, Shapers, Boots*	1 Pack/30g	134	4.5	448	6.7	71	15	1.8
Dairy Milk, with Chocolate Chunks, Dairy Milk, Cadbury*	1 Cookie/45g	210	9.3	467	6	63.6	20.6	1.4
Danish Butter, Tesco*	1 Cookie/26g	133	6.6	516	4.7	66.7	25.6	1.3
Dark Chocolate Chunk Ginger, The Best, Morrisons*	1 Cookie/25g	126	6.4	503	4.6	63.7	25.5	2.8
Dark Treacle, Weight Watchers*	1 Cookie/11g	49	1.7	423	5.2	66.7	15.1	1.7
Double Choc Chip, Giant, Paterson's*	1 Cookie/60g	293	15.2	489	0.3	61.3	25.3	3.7
Double Choc Chip, Mini, M&S*	1 Cookie/22g	108	5.2	490	5.3	63.6	23.7	1.8
Double Choc Chip, Tesco*	1 Cookie/11g	55	2.7	500	4.2	65.3	24.7	3
Double Choc Chip, Weight Watchers*	1 Biscuit/11g	49	1.9	443	7.6	65.4	17.2	4.6
Double Choc, Maryland*	1 Cookie/10g	51	2.6	510	5.2	64.4	25.7	0
Double Chocolate Nuts, Bens Cookie*	1 Cookie/85g	364	17.4	428	8.7	71.2	20.5	2.8
Double Chocolate Walnut, Soft, Tesco*	1 Cookie/25g	116	6.4	463	5.8	52.1	25.7	4.7
Double Chocolate Chip, Co-Op*	1 Cookie/17g	87	4.6	510	5	63	27	2
Double Chocolate Chip, Organic, Waitrose*	1 Cookie/18g	96	5.6	535	5.1	58.6	31	1.9
Double Chocolate Chip, Traidcraft*	1 Cookie/22g	114	5.9	520	5.8	64.1	26.7	2.4
Double Chocolate Chip, Treat Yourself, Spar*	1 Cookie/20g	94	5	470	5.5	56	25	2.5
Double Fudge Chocolate, Sugar Free, Murray*	1 Cookie/12g	47	2.3	400	5.7	65.7	20	5.7

COOKIES

INFO/WEIGHT	Measure	per Measure		Nutrition Values per 100g / 100ml				
		KCAL	FAT	KCAL	PROT	CARB	FAT	FIBRE
Eton Mess, Finest, Tesco*	1 Cookie/66g	281	9.7	426	5.1	67.6	14.7	1.4
Farmbake, Arnotts*	1 Cookie/13g	61	2.4	470	5	68.4	18.7	0
Finest White Chocolate Honeycomb, Bakery, Tesco*	1 Cookie/65g	290	11.2	446	5.3	67.1	17.2	0.9
Fortune, Average	*1 Cookie/8g*	*30*	*0.2*	*378*	*4.2*	*84*	*2.7*	*1.6*
Fruit Oat, Soft, Diet Chef Ltd*	1 Cookie45g	198	9.1	440	4.8	61.9	20.2	4.3
Fruit, Giant, Cookie Coach*	1 Cookie/60g	280	13.2	466	4.9	62	22	0
Fruity Shrewsbury, Giant, Paterson's*	1 Cookie/60g	298	15.2	496	4.8	62.6	25.4	1.7
Fudge Brownie American Cream, Sainsbury's*	1 Cookie/12g	60	2.8	499	4.8	67.9	23.2	2.2
Fudge Brownie, Maryland*	1 Cookie/11g	56	2.8	510	5.8	63	25	0
Ginger Brazil Nut, Organic, Dove's Farm*	1 Cookie/17g	79	3.5	464	5	65	20.5	4.8
Ginger Choc Chip, BGTY, Sainsbury's*	1 Cookie/17g	69	3.2	415	5.8	55.3	19	12.1
Ginger, GF, Barkat*	1 Cookie/17g	85	4.4	501	3.2	63.8	25.9	0
Ginger, Low Fat, M&S*	1 Cookie/23g	82	1	358	5.1	74.9	4.3	2.4
Gman, Gingerbread, GF, Barkat*	2 Biscuits/34g	167	9.3	490	15.8	49.5	27.3	6
Hazelnut Choc Chip 'n' Chunk, McVitie's*	1 Cookie/11g	55	3	505	6.1	57.8	27.7	3.5
Hazelnut, GF, Organic, Dove's Farm*	1 Cookie/17g	79	3.7	463	4.8	61.5	21.9	1.8
Honey, Lemon Ginger, Nothing Naughty*	1 Cookie/60g	246	9	410	2.9	64.4	15	0
Jaffa, Tesco*	1 Cookie/42g	175	5.9	417	4.8	66.9	14	1.9
Lemon Currant, Weight Watchers*	2 Cookies/19g	86	3.4	451	5.1	63.6	17.7	8.4
Lemon Meringue, COU, M&S*	1 Cookie/25g	89	0.6	355	5.6	77.6	2.6	3
Lemon Zest, GF, Organic, Dove's Farm*	1 Cookie/17g	80	3.1	473	3.3	73.7	18.3	0
Malteaser, Mars*	1 Cookie/46g	212	9.2	462	5.2	64.5	20	1.4
Mango Coconut, Tesco*	1 Cookie/20g	90	3.9	450	5.5	61	19.5	5.5
Maple Syrup, Pecan, Finest, Tesco*	1 Biscuit/25g	127	6.6	507	6.7	59.9	26.4	1.7
Milk Chocolate Chunk, Average	*1 Cookie/25g*	*129*	*6.9*	*515*	*6.6*	*60*	*27.6*	*1.6*
Milk Chocolate, Classic, Millie's Cookies*	1 Cookie/45g	190	10.2	422	5.1	49.3	22.7	1.3
Oat & Cranberry, BGTY, Sainsbury's*	1 Cookie/28g	126	5	449	6.8	65	18	5.1
Oat & Raisin, Health Matters*	1 Cookie/8g	33	0.7	414	7	76.6	8.8	3.3
Oat & Treacle, TTD, Sainsbury's*	1 Biscuit/25g	121	5.9	482	5.7	61.8	23.6	3.7
Oat Fruit, Kate's Cakes Ltd*	1 Serving/100g	418	18.2	418	4.2	59.5	18.2	3
Oat Raisin, GF, Prewett's*	1 Cookie18g	80	2.7	442	6.2	63	15	5.1
Oat Sultana, Free From, Sainsbury's*	1 Cookie/19g	87	3.7	462	6.2	62.6	19.8	4.2
Oat, Raisin, Free From, Finest, Tesco*	1 Cookie/19g	80	2.8	422	6.2	63	15	5.1
Oat, Giant Jumbo, Paterson's*	1 Cookie/60g	299	16.2	499	0.4	58.4	27	3.2
Oatflake & Honey, Organic, Sainsbury's*	1 Cookie/17g	82	3.6	480	6.3	66	21.2	2.6
Oatflake & Raisin, Waitrose*	1 Cookie/17g	80	3.8	469	5.8	61.7	22.1	4.7
Oatflake Treacle, TTD, Sainsbury's*	1 Cookie/25g	122	5.9	490	5.7	61.8	23.6	3.7
Oaties, Grandma Wilds*	1 Cookie/50g	254	12.4	507	5.1	66	24.9	0
Oatmeal, Chocolate Chip, Chewy, Dad's*	1 Cookie/15g	70	3	467	6.7	66.7	20	3.3
Oreo, Mini, Oreo*	1 Pack/25g	120	4.8	480	4.8	70	19.2	2.4
Oreo, Mint, Mondelez*	1 Biscuit/11g	53	2.2	479	5.2	69	20	3
Oreo, Nabisco*	1 Cookie/11g	52	2.3	471	5.9	70.6	20.6	2.9
Pecan & Maple, Mini, Bronte*	1 Pack/100g	509	27.3	509	5.4	60.3	27.3	1.6
Pineapple, Coconut White Chocolate, M&S*	1 Cookie/23g	119	5.7	518	5.1	56.7	24.9	2.9
Raisin & Cinnamon, Low Fat, M&S*	1 Cookie/22g	78	0.9	355	6.2	73	4.1	3.2
Red Velvet, Filled, Bakery, Tesco*	1 Cookie/42g	170	5.5	405	4.6	66.6	13.1	1.3
Rolo, Nestle*	1 Cookie/39g	178	7.4	456	5.4	64.8	19	2.2
Salted Caramel, High Protein, Dr Zak's*	1 Cookie/60g	211	5.6	351	25	50	9.3	1.7
Stem Ginger, Aldi*	1 Cookie/13g	58	2.4	463	3.6	68.5	19.4	0
Stem Ginger, All Butter, Deluxe, Lidl*	1 Biscuit/17g	80	3.6	468	5.1	62	21	5.4
Stem Ginger, Deluxe, Lidl*	1 Cookie/17g	80	3.6	468	5.1	62	21	5.4
Stem Ginger, Free From, Asda*	1 Biscuit/19g	89	3.6	467	3	69	19	4.1
Stem Ginger, Free From, Sainsbury's*	1 Cookie/19g	89	3.6	476	4.1	70.8	19	2.7

	Measure INFO/WEIGHT	per Measure KCAL	FAT	Nutrition Values per 100g / 100ml KCAL	PROT	CARB	FAT	FIBRE
COOKIES								
Stem Ginger, Kate's Cakes Ltd*	1 Serving/100g	376	11.7	376	5	62.7	11.7	1.7
Stem Ginger, Less Than 5% Fat, M&S*	1 Cookie/22g	79	0.9	360	6.2	73.9	4.3	3
Stem Ginger, Reduced Fat, Waitrose*	1 Cookie/17g	75	2.7	448	4.5	71	16.2	1.6
Stem Ginger, Tesco*	1 Cookie/20g	98	4.8	489	4.2	64	24	2
Stem Ginger, TTD, Sainsbury's*	1 Cookie/25g	124	6.2	496	4.9	62.3	24.7	2.2
Sticky Toffee, Finest, Tesco*	1 Cookie/63g	258	9.4	410	4.5	63.5	15	1.5
Sultana, All Butter, Reduced Fat, M&S*	1 Cookie/17g	70	2.4	420	4.9	68.6	14.2	2.6
Sultana, Deluxe, Lidl*	1 Biscuit/17g	77	3.2	453	5.3	64.7	18.8	2.9
Sultana, Soft & Chewy, Sainsbury's*	1 Cookie/25g	104	3.5	414	4.4	67.8	13.9	2.5
Toffee Popcorn, Butter Buds*	1 Cookie/40g	184	7.6	459	4.2	66.8	19	1.4
Toffee, Weight Watchers*	2 Cookies/152g	686	27.4	451	6.8	61.7	18	7.5
Treacle Oat, All Butter, Finest, Tesco*	1 Biscuit/20g	100	5	500	4.8	62.9	25	2.1
Triple Chocolate, Belgian, Bakery, Finest, Tesco*	1 Cookie/65g	310	14.9	478	6.1	60.1	23	2.9
Triple Chocolate, TTD, Sainsbury's*	1 Cookie/72g	344	16.5	478	5.8	61.2	22.9	2
White Chocolate & Cranberry, Devondale*	1 Cookie/65g	300	15.3	462	4.7	60.7	23.5	2.1
White Chocolate & Raspberry, McVitie's*	1 Cookie/17g	87	4.4	512	4.7	64.1	25.9	1.8
White Chocolate Cranberry, Kate's Cakes Ltd*	1 Serving/100g	389	13.4	389	4.7	62.3	13.4	2
White Chocolate Raspberry, Finest, Tesco*	1 Cookie/76g	304	9.6	400	5.2	66.3	12.6	2.4
White Chocolate, Cranberry, Free From, Finest, Tesco*	1 Cookie/19g	94	4.5	497	5.4	63.4	24	2.9
White Chocolate, Asda*	1 Cookie/54g	256	11.9	474	5	64	22	2.1
White Chocolate, Chunk, Average	*1 Cookie/25g*	*124*	*6.2*	*498*	*5.5*	*62.8*	*24.8*	*1*
White Chocolate, Maryland*	1 Cookie/10g	51	2.5	512	5.7	64	25	0
White Chocolate, TTD, Sainsbury's*	1 Cookie/25g	126	6.4	504	5.5	62.5	25.8	1.2
COQ AU VIN								
658, Oakhouse Foods Ltd*	1 Serving/400g	728	39.6	182	14	7.9	9.9	2.8
Diet Chef Ltd*	1 Pack/300g	285	13.2	95	7.7	6.1	4.4	2.2
Donald Russell*	1 Pack/250g	230	7.2	92	10.7	3.5	2.9	0.4
Finest, Tesco*	1 Serving/273g	251	9.8	92	14.3	0.7	3.6	1.8
M&S*	1 Serving/295g	398	22.7	135	14.2	1.5	7.7	1
Oven Cooked, TTD, Sainsbury's*	½ Pack/244g	337	17.1	138	15.2	3.1	7	1.1
Sainsbury's*	1 Pack/400g	484	17.6	121	16.8	3.5	4.4	0.2
CORDIAL								
Apple Mango, Hi Juice, As Prepared, Morrisons*	1 Serving/250ml	69	0	28	0	6.7	0	0.1
Blackcurrant, New Zealand Honey Co*	1 Serving/30ml	109	0.3	363	1	88	1	0
Cox's Apple Plum, Diluted, Bottle Green*	1 Serving/10ml	3	0	29	0	7.2	0	0
Elderflower, Made Up, Bottle Green*	1 Glass/200ml	46	0	23	0	5.6	0	0
Elderflower, Undiluted, Waitrose*	1 Serving/20ml	22	0	110	0	27.5	0	0
Lemon Lime, High Juice, M&S*	1 Glass/250ml	75	0	30	0	7	0	0
Lime Juice, Concentrated	*1 Serving/20ml*	*22*	*0*	*112*	*0.1*	*29.8*	*0*	*0*
Lime Juice, Diluted	*1 Glass/250ml*	*55*	*0*	*22*	*0*	*6*	*0*	*0*
Lime Juice, Waitrose*	1 Serving/20ml	21	0	104	10	23.7	0	0
Lime with Aromatic Bitters Ginger, Sainsbury's*	1 Serving/40ml	12	0.1	29	0	6.9	0.3	0.3
Lime, Crushed, Mint, Diluted, Robinson's*	1 Serving/200ml	34	0	17	0	4.1	0	0
Lime, Juice, Diluted, Rose's*	1 Serving/250ml	52	0	21	0	4.9	0	0
Lime, Sainsbury's*	1 Serving/50ml	14	0	27	0	6.2	0	0
Lime, Tesco*	1 Pint/74ml	8	0	11	0.2	0.5	0	0
Plum, Apple, Rosehip, Superfruit, Undiluted, Fiovana*	1 Serving/36ml	18	0	49	0	9.8	0	0
Pomegranate Elderflower, Bottle Green*	1 fl oz/30ml	9	0	30	0	7	0	0
CORIANDER								
Leaves, Dried, Average	*1oz/28g*	*78*	*1.3*	*279*	*21.8*	*41.7*	*4.8*	*0*
Leaves, Fresh, Average	*1 Bunch/20g*	*5*	*0.1*	*23*	*2.1*	*3.7*	*0.5*	*2.8*
CORN								
Baby, & Mange Tout, Eat Fresh, Tesco*	1 Serving/100g	31	0.2	31	2.9	3.3	0.2	2.1

C

	Measure INFO/WEIGHT	per Measure		Nutrition Values per 100g / 100ml				
		KCAL	FAT	KCAL	PROT	CARB	FAT	FIBRE
CORN								
Baby, Average	**1 Serving/80g**	**21**	**0.3**	**26**	**2.5**	**3.1**	**0.4**	**1.7**
Baby, Canned, Drained, Average	**1 Serving/80g**	**18**	**0.3**	**23**	**2.9**	**2**	**0.4**	**1.5**
Cobs, Boiled, Weighed with Cob, Average	**1 Ear/200g**	**78**	**1.7**	**39**	**1.5**	**6.8**	**0.8**	**0.8**
Cobs, with Butter, From Restaurant, Average	**1 Ear/146g**	**155**	**3.4**	**106**	**3.1**	**21.9**	**2.4**	**0**
Creamed Style, Green Giant*	1 Can/418g	238	2.1	57	1.2	11.9	0.5	3
CORN CAKES								
M&S*	½ Pack/85g	238	17	280	6.4	19.8	20	3.4
Organic, Kallo*	1 Cake/7g	26	0.1	383	7.6	83.6	1.1	7.2
Slightly Salted, Mrs Crimble's*	1 Pack/28g	104	0.9	380	7.9	80	3.4	5.4
Thick Slices, Orgran*	1 Cake/11g	42	0.4	385	13.2	79	3.7	14.2
with Chai Seeds, Kallo*	1 Cake/7g	27	0.2	389	8	81	2.4	0
CORN MEAL								
Yellow, Enriched Degerminated, Dry, Quaker*	1 Tbsp/9g	30	0.2	333	7.4	77.8	1.8	7.4
CORNED BEEF								
Average	**1 Slice/35g**	**75**	**4.3**	**214**	**25.9**	**0.7**	**12.2**	**0**
Lean, Healthy Range, Average	**1 Slice/30g**	**57**	**2.6**	**191**	**27**	**1**	**8.7**	**0**
Reduced Salt, Canned, Princes*	1 Can/340g	741	44.2	218	24.8	0.5	13	0
Sliced, Premium, Average	**1 Slice/31g**	**69**	**3.9**	**222**	**26.6**	**0.5**	**12.6**	**0**
CORNFLOUR								
Average	**1 Tsp/5g**	**18**	**0.1**	**355**	**0.6**	**86.9**	**1.2**	**0.1**
COULIS								
Passsion Fruit Mango, TTD, Sainsbury's*	1 Tbs/15ml	23	0.1	155	1.2	34.7	1	0.9
Raspberry, TTD, Sainsbury's*	1 Tbsp/15ml	25	0.1	165	0.4	39.1	0.6	1.4
COURGETTE								
Baby, Raw, Average	**1 Courgette/29g**	**6**	**0.1**	**22**	**2**	**2**	**0.5**	**1.2**
Courgetti, Italian, Tomato, Pot, Bol*	1 Pot/380g	441	18.2	116	2.5	15	4.8	1.4
Fried, Average	**1oz/28g**	**18**	**1.3**	**63**	**2.6**	**2.6**	**4.8**	**1.2**
Raw, Average	**1 Whole/224g**	**40**	**0.9**	**18**	**1.8**	**1.8**	**0.4**	**0.9**
Spaghetti, Waitrose*	½ Pack/80g	16	0.3	20	1.8	1.8	0.4	1.2
Spirals, Tomato, Basil, Vegetable Pot, Tesco*	1 Pot/230g	94	0.8	41	2.5	5.4	0.4	3
COUS COUS								
4 Grain, Unprepared, Artisan Grains*	1 Serving/100g	341	2.7	341	11.7	64.9	2.7	8
Cauliflower, & Broccoli, Waitrose*	½ Pack/110g	43	1	39	4	2.4	0.9	2.8
Citrus Kick, Cooked, Ainsley Harriott*	1 Serving/130g	182	1.6	140	4.3	27.9	1.2	2.4
Citrus Kick, Dry, Ainsley Harriott*	½ Sachet/50g	184	1.2	368	11.6	77	2.4	9.2
Cooked, Average	**1 Tbsp/15g**	**24**	**0.3**	**158**	**4.3**	**31.4**	**1.9**	**1.3**
Cooked, From Restaurant, Average	**1 Cup/157g**	**176**	**0.3**	**112**	**3.8**	**23.2**	**0.2**	**1.4**
Coriander & Lemon, Morrisons*	1 Serving/100g	159	3.4	159	4.4	27.7	3.4	1.4
Coriander Lemon, As Consumed, Sainsbury's*	½ Pack/140g	195	1	139	4.8	27.5	0.7	1.9
Dry, Average	**1 Serving/50g**	**178**	**0.7**	**356**	**13.7**	**72.8**	**1.5**	**2.6**
Fruity, Sainsbury's*	1 Portion/100g	194	4.5	194	4.4	33.2	4.5	1.7
Garlic, & Coriander, Dry, Waitrose*	1 Serving/70g	235	2.5	336	11.7	64.2	3.6	6.2
Giant, Tesco*	1 Pack/220g	350	14.4	160	4.1	20.7	6.6	1.2
Giant, with Butternut Squash, Feta, Co-Op*	1 Pack/218g	246	7.6	113	4.5	13.3	3.5	5.5
Harissa, Style, Savoury, Sainsbury's*	1 Serving/260g	434	12	167	4.7	26.8	4.6	1.3
Hot & Spicy, Flavour, Dry, Amazing Grains, Haldane's*	1 Serving/50g	182	2.1	365	12.5	67	4.2	3.1
Mint & Coriander, Flavour, Dry, Amazing Grains*	1 Sachet/99g	349	2.7	353	12.2	70	2.7	3.2
Moroccan, Medley, Ainsley Harriott*	½ Sachet/130g	178	2	137	5.4	25.4	1.5	2.2
Moroccan, Pot, Prepared, NutriPot*	1 Pot/322g	315	2.9	98	6.2	14.9	0.9	2.6
Moroccan, Style, Break, GFY, Asda*	1 Pack/150g	215	2.7	143	5.6	26.1	1.8	1.8
Moroccan, Style, Fruity, M&S*	1 Serving/200g	370	5.4	185	3.4	36.7	2.7	3.4
Moroccan, Style, Spiced, Meadow Fresh, Lidl*	1 Pack/280g	456	14.8	163	3	25	5.3	1.6
Moroccan, Style, TTD, Sainsbury's*	¼ Pot/100g	203	4.7	203	5.1	33.1	4.7	3.7

	Measure INFO/WEIGHT	per Measure KCAL	FAT	Nutrition Values per 100g / 100ml KCAL	PROT	CARB	FAT	FIBRE
COUS COUS								
Mushroom, Prepared, without Oil or Butter, Tesco*	½ Pack/140g	194	1.3	139	4.3	27.7	0.9	1.4
Pearl, Cooked, Artisan Grains*	1 Serving/100g	114	0.5	114	3.8	23	0.5	0.9
Pepper, Red & Yellow, Chargrilled, Tesco*	1 Pack/200g	212	3.6	106	4.6	17.8	1.8	0.5
Pepper, Red, & Chilli, Waitrose*	1 Pack/200g	344	13.8	172	4.5	23	6.9	1.3
Spice, Fusion, Lyttos*	1 Serving/100g	134	1.5	134	4.3	23.9	1.5	3.4
Spice, Sensation, Batchelors*	1 Pack/120g	163	1.1	136	4.7	26.3	0.9	1.8
Tomato, & Basil, Made Up, Tesco*	1 Serving/200g	348	16.6	174	3.9	21	8.3	3.4
Tomato, & Mediterranean Herb, Made Up, Co-Op*	½ Pack/138g	189	1.5	137	5.3	26	1.1	1.6
Tomato, & Onion, Dry Weight, Waitrose*	1 Pack/110g	376	4	342	12.6	64.9	3.6	5.1
Tomato, Mediterranean, GFY, Asda*	½ Pack/141g	192	1.3	136	5	27	0.9	1.7
Tomato, Sun Dried, CBY, Asda*	1 Pack/310g	515	12.1	166	4.6	26.2	3.9	4
Tomato, Sundried, & Garlic, Newgate, Lidl*	1 Serving/135g	181	1.5	134	4.5	25.7	1.1	1.7
Tomato, Tangy, Cooked, Ainsley Harriott*	1 Serving/133g	166	0.8	125	4.6	25.3	0.6	3.3
Tricolour, Unprepared, Artisan Grains*	1 Serving/100g	350	1	350	14	67	1	5
Vegetable, & Olive Oil, Chargrilled, Delphi*	½ Pot/75g	105	2.9	140	3.8	22.5	3.9	1.9
Vegetable, Chargrilled, Morrisons*	1 Serving/225g	227	5.4	101	3.3	16.5	2.4	1.3
Vegetable, Chargrilled, Smoky, Finest, Tesco*	½ Pack/125g	194	5.6	156	4.3	23.2	4.5	2.6
Vegetable, Roasted, Cooked, Ainsley Harriott*	1 Serving/130g	180	2	138	5.6	25.5	1.5	2.6
Vegetable, Roasted, Dry, Ainsley Harriott*	½ Sachet/50g	180	2	360	14.6	66.4	4	6.8
Vegetable, Roasted, Snack Salad Pot, HL, Tesco*	1 Pack/60g	213	2.4	355	15.1	64.6	4	4.2
Vegetable, Roasted, Waitrose*	1 Serving/200g	328	13.2	164	3.9	22	6.6	0.9
Vegetable, Spicy, GFY, Asda*	½ Pack/55g	71	0.6	129	4.7	25	1.1	2
Vegetable, Spicy, Morrisons*	1 Pack/110g	187	5.5	170	5.1	26.2	5	2.9
Vegetable, Sweet, CBY, Asda*	1 Serving/100g	120	0	120	2.9	14.8	0	0
Vegetable, Chargrilled, M&S*	1 Serving/200g	200	3	100	3.9	17.3	1.5	1.6
Wholewheat, Tesco*	1 Serving/50g	178	1	355	12	72	2	5
with Barrel Aged Feta, Toasted, Finest, Tesco*	½ Pack/90g	183	8.6	203	8.9	19.5	9.5	2.1
CRAB								
Blue, Soft Shelled, Raw, Average	*1 Crab/84g*	*73*	*0.9*	*87*	*18.1*	*0*	*1.1*	*0*
Boiled, Meat Only, Average	*1 Tbsp/40g*	*51*	*2.2*	*128*	*19.5*	*0*	*5.5*	*0*
Cornish 50/50, Seafood Eat It*	1 Pot/100g	144	5.8	144	21.6	1.2	5.8	0.5
Cornish Potted, Seafood Eat It*	1 Pack/100g	235	17.5	235	15	5.1	17.5	0.8
Dressed, Average	*1 Can/43g*	*66*	*3.4*	*154*	*16.8*	*4.1*	*7.9*	*0.2*
Meat in Brine, Average	*½ Can/60g*	*41*	*0.2*	*69*	*15.6*	*0.8*	*0.4*	*0.1*
Meat, Raw, Average	*1oz/28g*	*28*	*0.2*	*100*	*20.8*	*2.8*	*0.6*	*0*
CRAB CAKES								
Goan, M&S*	1 Pack/190g	228	7.6	120	8	12.9	4	1.8
Iceland*	1 Serving/18g	52	3.2	288	7.2	25.6	18	1.3
Shetland Isles, Dressed, TTD, Sainsbury's*	1 Cake/75g	130	8.3	174	12.4	6	11.1	0.5
Tesco*	1 Serving/130g	281	16	216	11	15.4	12.3	1.1
Thai Style, TTD, Sainsbury's*	1 Cake/141g	297	14.1	210	8.7	20.5	10	1.8
CRAB STICKS								
Average	*1 Stick/15g*	*14*	*0*	*94*	*9.1*	*13.9*	*0.3*	*0*
CRACKERBREAD								
Original, Ryvita*	1 Cracker/5g	20	0.2	390	10.5	77.5	3.7	2.5
Quinoa, Red, Sesame, Protein, Ryvita*	1 Slice/10g	37	0.5	368	20.7	53.2	4.9	14.1
Wholegrain, Ryvita*	1 Cracker/5g	19	0.2	379	11.3	70.9	3.9	7.3
CRACKERS								
All Butter, Cheese, Oat, Nibbles, Finest, Tesco*	1 Oat Nibble/7g	39	2.6	563	13.1	43.3	36.9	2.8
Ancient Grains Crackers, Kirkland*	3 Crackers/18g	90	4	500	11.1	66.7	22.2	0
Bath Oliver, Jacob's*	1 Cracker/12g	52	1.6	432	9.6	67.6	13.7	2.6
Bean Mix, Habas Tapas, Graze*	1 Punnet/30g	131	3.8	438	11.7	68.9	12.8	1.5
Beetroot, Seed, Finest, Tesco*	2 Crackers/15g	75	3.7	497	12.2	53.1	24.8	6.4

CRACKERS

INFO/WEIGHT	Measure	per Measure		Nutrition Values per 100g / 100ml				
		KCAL	FAT	KCAL	PROT	CARB	FAT	FIBRE
Black Olive, M&S*	1 Cracker/4g	20	1	485	8.3	59.4	23.5	4.3
Black Pepper for Cheese, Ryvita*	1 Cracker/7g	27	0.2	384	13.2	72.9	2.9	6.8
Bran, Jacob's*	1 Cracker/7g	32	1.3	454	9.7	62.8	18.2	3.2
Brooklyn Bites, Graze*	1 Punnet/29g	157	11.3	541	4.1	33	39	4
Buckwheat Chia, Rude Health*	1 Cracker/7g	29	0.7	388	14	56	8.8	15
Butter Puff, Sainsbury's*	1 Cracker/10g	54	2.7	523	10.4	60.7	26.5	2.5
Butter Puffs, Jacob's*	1 Cracker/11g	55	2.7	502	9.3	59	24.8	3.1
Caramelised Onion, Ciabatta, Jacob's*	1 Cracker/10g	43	1	426	12.5	68.6	10.3	4.3
Carrot Crunch, Sweet Smokey, Graze*	1 Punnet/28g	140	8.1	499	13	42	29	11
Charcoal, Wafer, Miller's Damsel*	1 Cracker/5g	21	0.7	420	13.8	59.5	13.9	0
Cheddar, Goldfish, Pepperidge Farm*	1 Pack/43g	200	7	465	11.6	65.1	16.3	2.3
Cheese Onion, Crispy, Bites, Ritz*	1 Bag/23g	109	4.8	474	7	63	21	2.7
Cheese onion, Triangles, Eat Well, M&S*	1 Bag/30g	128	3.3	425	9.8	69.4	11	4.7
Cheese Bites, Sour Cream Onion, Mrs Crimbles*	1 Pack/30g	125	4.6	416	15.9	54	15.2	2
Cheese Snack Mix, Christmas, M&S*	1 Serving/30g	133	4.2	442	9.9	67.2	14	4
Cheese Thins, Asda*	1 Cracker/4g	21	1.3	532	12	49	32	0
Cheese Thins, Cheddar, The Planet Snack Co*	1 Serving/30g	153	8.8	509	11.5	50.1	29.2	2.1
Cheese Thins, Co-Op*	1 Cracker/4g	21	1.3	530	12	49	32	3
Cheese Thins, Mini, Snack Rite*	1 Bag/30g	144	6.8	480	12.9	55.9	22.7	2.5
Cheese Thins, Tesco*	1 Biscuit/4g	20	1.2	543	11.3	47.5	33.7	2.5
Cheese Thins, Waitrose*	1 Cracker/4g	21	1.2	545	11.9	52.6	31.9	2.5
Cheese, Cheddar, Crispies, TTD, Sainsbury's*	1 Thin/4g	21	1.5	576	14.2	39	40.4	2.2
Cheese, Mini, Heinz*	1 Pack/25g	108	3.6	433	9.4	68.6	14.6	0.6
Cheese, Mini, Shapers, Boots*	1 Serving/23g	97	3.2	421	9.4	65	14	4.6
Cheese, Oat Bakes, Nairn's*	1 Bag/30g	130	4.7	432	15	57.4	15.8	1.3
Cheese, Ritz*	1 Cracker/4g	17	0.9	486	10.1	55.9	24.7	2.2
Chives, Jacob's*	1 Cracker/6g	28	1	457	9.5	67.5	16.5	2.7
Choice Grain, Jacob's*	1 Cracker/8g	32	1.1	427	9	65.5	14.3	5.4
Ciabatta, Sundried Tomato Basil, Jacobs*	1 Cracker/10g	42	1	424	12.4	68.5	10.2	4.3
Corn Thins, 97% Fat Free, Real Foods*	1 Cracker/6g	23	0.2	378	10.2	81.7	3	8.6
Corn Thins, Real Foods*	1 Serving/6g	22	0.2	378	10.2	81.7	3	8.6
Cream Cheese Onion Flavour, Bakefuls, Ritz*	1 Bag/23g	109	4.8	474	7	63	21	2.7
Cream, 45% Less Fat, Morrisons*	1 Cracker/8g	32	0.6	403	10.5	74.2	7.1	3.3
Cream, Aldi*	1 Cracker/8g	36	1.2	456	9.1	71.7	14.7	3
Cream, Asda*	1 Cracker/8g	35	1.2	443	10	67	15	0
Cream, Average	*1 Cracker/7g*	*31*	*1.1*	*440*	*9.5*	*68.3*	*16.3*	*2.2*
Cream, BFY, Morrisons*	1 Cracker/8g	32	0.6	406	10.9	74.4	7.2	2.8
Cream, BGTY, Sainsbury's*	1 Cracker/8g	32	0.6	400	10.9	71.7	7.7	3.1
Cream, Choice Grain, Jacob's*	1 Cracker/7g	30	0.9	400	9	64.5	11.8	7
Cream, Jacob's*	1 Cracker/8g	35	1.1	440	10	67.7	13.5	3.8
Cream, Light, Jacob's*	1 Cracker/8g	31	0.5	388	10.6	72.2	6.3	4.1
Cream, Lower Fat, Tesco*	1 Cracker/5g	20	0.3	393	11	72.4	6.6	3.1
Cream, Morrisons*	1 Cracker/8g	36	1.2	446	9.6	68.5	14.8	2.7
Cream, Reduced Fat, Tesco*	1 Cracker/8g	31	0.5	406	10.9	74.4	7.2	2.8
Cream, Roasted Onion, Jacob's*	1 Cracker/8g	35	1.2	441	10.2	66.8	14.8	2.9
Cream, Sainsbury's*	1 Cracker/8g	35	1.3	422	9.5	66.7	15.2	2.8
Cream, Sun Dried Tomato Flavour, Jacob's*	1 Cracker/8g	35	1.1	434	10.2	66.7	14	3
Cream, Tesco*	1 Cracker/8g	37	1.2	454	10.1	68.2	14.8	3.6
Crispy Cheese, M&S*	1 Cracker/4g	20	1	470	9.4	58.1	22.1	3
Crispy Chickpea, M&S*	¼ Pack/25g	99	1.4	396	17.6	67.8	5.5	2.5
Crispy, Salt Vinegar Flavour, Walkers*	1 Serving/30g	130	4.5	434	6.9	66	15	3.6
Crunchy Grain, Breaks, Ritz*	5 Crackers/33g	143	5.8	440	8.6	60	18	3.3
Cruskits, Arnotts*	2 Cruskits/12g	40	0.2	331	9	63.7	1.5	0

CRACKERS

INFO/WEIGHT	Measure	per Measure		Nutrition Values per 100g / 100ml				
		KCAL	FAT	KCAL	PROT	CARB	FAT	FIBRE
El Picante, Graze*	1 Punnet/25g	126	6.7	506	15	49	27	6
Extra Wheatgerm, Hovis*	1 Serving/6g	27	1.1	447	10.2	60	18.5	4.4
Flamed Baked, Traditional English, Water, Rakusen's*	1 Cracker/20g	79	1.1	394	8.6	75.8	5.5	3.3
Flatbread, Multigrain, Jacob's*	1 Cracker/10g	42	0.7	411	11	73.8	6.8	5.3
Flax, Pumpkin, Organic, Raw Health*	1 Cracker/12g	64	5	533	19	8	42	21
Garden Herbs, Jacob's*	1 Cracker/6g	28	1	457	9.5	67.5	16.5	2.7
Garlic Herb, Jacob's*	1 Cracker/10g	45	1.7	450	10	68.3	16.7	3.3
Garlic, CBY, Asda*	2 Biscuits/12g	58	2.6	483	7	63.3	21.5	4.2
Glutafin*	1 Serving/11g	52	2.2	470	2.4	70	20	0.7
Harvest Grain, Sainsbury's*	1 Cracker/6g	27	1.1	458	8.5	64.5	18.4	4.1
Herb & Onion, 99% Fat Free, Rakusen's*	1 Cracker/5g	18	0	360	9.1	82.6	1	3.9
Herb & Spice, Jacob's*	1 Cracker/6g	27	1	457	9.5	67.5	16.5	2.7
Herb Onion, Trufree*	1 Cracker/6g	25	0.7	418	2.5	75	12	10
Herbs & Spice Selection, Jacob's*	1 Cracker/6g	27	0.9	451	9.5	68	15.7	2.7
High Fibre, Dietary Specials*	1 Cracker/6g	23	0.6	391	2.1	60	11	17
Japanese Beef Teriyaki, Sensations, Walkers*	1 Serving/24g	118	6.3	490	1.4	62	26	3.5
Light & Crispy, Sainsbury's*	1 Cracker/11g	42	1.2	384	11.3	61	10.5	13
Lightly Salted, Crispy, Sainsbury's*	1 Cracker/5g	25	1.3	533	7.8	62.6	27.9	2.1
Lightly Salted, Italian, Jacob's*	1 Cracker/6g	26	0.8	429	10.3	67.6	13	2.9
Louisiana Wild Rice Beans, Graze*	1 Pack/30g	136	5.7	454	17	49	19	8.8
Matzos, Flame Baked, Rakusen's*	1 Cracker/21g	75	0.2	357	10	79	1	4.3
Matzos, Tea, Flamed Baked, Round, Rakusen's*	1 Cracker/5g	19	0	382	9.9	85.7	0.8	3.7
Mediterranean Tomato Herb, Oat Bakes, Nairn's*	1 Bag/30g	129	4.7	431	8.1	64.2	15.8	8.3
Mediterranean, Jacob's*	1 Cracker/6g	27	1	450	9.7	66.5	16.1	2.7
Melty, Sour Cream Onion Flavour, Walkers*	1 Serving/30g	148	6.6	493	7.3	65	22	2.8
Melty, Sweet Chilli Flavour, Walkers*	1 Serving/30g	147	6.6	490	7.5	64	22	2.8
Mix, Yaki Soba, Graze*	1 Punnet/32g	159	9.3	498	24	36	29	6
Mixed Seed, Multi Grain, Asda*	1 Cracker/6g	28	1.1	445	11	62	17	4.4
Multi Seed, Thins, Ryvita*	1 Thin/9g	39	1.3	434	16.4	56.2	14.1	8.1
Multi-grain, Aldi, Savour Bakes, Aldi*	1 Cracker/5g	20	0.8	404	8.3	55	16.8	5.1
Multigrain, Corn Thins, Real Foods*	1 Cracker/6g	23	0.2	388	10.9	71	3.7	10.3
Multigrain, Morrisons*	10 Crackers/20g	76	2.2	379	8.8	61.3	11	5.1
Multigrain, Tesco*	1 Cracker/5g	24	1	477	8.8	60.8	20.8	5.7
Naan, Multiseed, Tesco*	1 Cracker/3g	14	0.6	477	11.4	61.2	20	3.2
Naan, Tandoori, Tesco*	1 Cracker/2g	11	0.4	451	10.9	65.8	15.4	2.9
Oat Wheat, Weight Watchers*	4 Crackers/20g	74	0.5	370	10.5	75	2.5	4
Olive Oil & Oregano, Mediterreaneo, Jacob's*	1 Cracker/6g	25	0.7	412	12.4	65.5	11.2	6
Oriental, Asda*	1 Serving/30g	115	6	383	1.7	49	20	4.3
Original, Breaks, Ritz*	1 Cracker/6g	29	1.1	460	8.4	65	18	3.5
Passionately Pizza, Jacobites, Jacob's*	1 Pack/150g	708	38.1	472	5.7	55.3	25.4	1.7
Peanut, Wasabi, Graze*	1 Pack/26g	125	5.6	479	15.2	53.8	21.4	5.4
Pizza Flavour, Mini, Sainsbury's*	1 Serving/25g	113	4	454	7.6	68.7	15.9	2.7
Poppy & Sesame Seed, Sainsbury's*	1 Cracker/4g	20	1	482	9.5	57	23	4.2
Poppy Oat, Cracker Selection, TTD, Sainsbury's*	1 Cracker/4g	19	0.7	467	9.8	65	17.7	4.1
Ritz, Mini, Kraft*	1 Bag/25g	126	6	504	7.9	63	24	2
Ritz, Original, Jacob's*	1 Cracker/3g	17	1	509	6.9	55.6	28.8	2
Rosemary, CBY, Asda*	1 Cracker/6g	29	1.2	486	6.5	68.3	20.2	2.4
Rye Cakes, Lightly Salted, Ryvita*	1 Cake/6g	23	0.1	363	8.9	69.9	2	13.7
Rye Cakes, Multigrain, Ryvita*	1 Cake/7g	23	0.2	352	9.4	66.3	2.5	13.3
Rye, Organic, Dove's Farm*	1 Cracker/7g	28	1	393	7	58.4	14.6	8.7
Salada Original, Arnotts*	4 Crackers/16g	68	1.6	427	10.4	71.5	10	3.9
Salt & Black Pepper, Jacob's*	1 Cracker/6g	27	1	457	9.5	67.5	16.5	2.7
Salt Black Pepper, Eat Well, M&S*	1 Pack/25g	106	3.7	422	9.6	62.9	14.7	5.1

	Measure INFO/WEIGHT	per Measure KCAL	FAT	Nutrition Values per 100g / 100ml KCAL	PROT	CARB	FAT	FIBRE
CRACKERS								
Salt Pepper, Sainsbury's*	1 Cracker/6g	27	1.2	485	7.3	64.5	21.3	3
Salted, Ritz, Nabisco*	1 Cracker/3g	17	0.9	493	7	57.5	26.1	2.9
Sea Salt Vinegar Flavour, Bakefuls, Ritz*	1 Bag/23g	108	4.8	471	7	61	21	2.8
Seeds, Sea Salt, Snacks, Finn Crisp*	1 Serving/30g	111	2.4	371	12	53	8.1	19
Selection, Finest, Tesco*	1 Serving/30g	136	4.3	452	9.6	71	14.4	0
Sesame Poppy Thins, Tesco*	1 Cracker/4g	20	1	485	9.9	57.6	23.5	4.4
Smokehouse BBQ Crunch, Graze*	1 Box/31g	137	4.7	441	10	62	15	5.4
Sour Cream Garlic, Crostini, Mix, Graze*	1 Punnet/25g	133	8	531	15	44	32	4
Spicy Indonesian Vegetable, Waitrose*	1 Pack/60g	295	16.3	492	1.2	60.6	27.2	2.2
Spicy, Trufree*	1 Cracker/6g	25	0.8	412	3.8	70	13	12.5
Sweet Chilli, Oat Bakes, Nairn's*	1 Bag/30g	128	4	426	8.1	68.4	13.3	7.2
Sweet Chilli, Thins, Ryvita*	1 Thin/8g	31	0.1	382	12	77.5	1.5	5.2
Sweet Chilli, Thins, Savours, Jacob's*	1 Cracker/4g	21	0.9	472	8	62.3	21.2	3.6
Table, Schar*	5 Crackers/30g	138	3	460	6.7	80	10	3.3
Tarallini with Fennel Seeds, Crosta Mollica*	1 Cracker/4g	21	0.9	529	8.2	67.5	22	4.2
Thai Spicy Vegetable, Sainsbury's*	1 Pack/50g	231	10.4	462	7.2	61.5	20.8	2.6
The British Barbecue, Graze*	1 Punnet/25g	127	8	508	17.4	36.8	32.2	7.4
Tom Yum Yum, Graze*	1 Pack/23g	90	0.6	390	7.2	84.8	2.4	1.4
Tuc, Cheese Sandwich, Jacob's*	1 Cracker/14g	72	4.3	531	8.4	53.8	31.4	0
Tuc, Cheese, Mini, Jacobs*	¼ Pack/50g	242	11.5	485	9.2	59	23	2.4
Tuc, Jacob's*	1 Cracker/5g	25	1.4	518	6.9	54.2	29.9	2.6
Tuc, Mini with Sesame Seeds, Jacob's*	1 Biscuit/2g	10	0.5	523	9.7	63.1	25.8	3.9
Unsalted, Tops, Premium Plus, Impress*	1 Cracker/3g	13	0.3	448	10.3	75.9	10.3	0
Wasabi, Vitasia, Lidl*	1 Serving/30g	167	9.9	557	3.6	61.3	32.9	0
Wasapeas, Graze*	1 Pack/32g	128	2.5	406	14.8	65.2	7.8	7.1
Waterthins, Wafers, Philemon*	1 Crackers/2g	7	0.1	392	10.6	77.9	3.6	5
Wheat, Tesco*	6 Crackers/30g	139	5.6	464	11.2	60.2	18.8	4.6
Wheaten, M&S*	1 Cracker/4g	20	0.9	450	10.2	57	20.2	5
Whole Wheat, 100%, Oven Baked, Master Choice*	1 Cracker/4g	17	0.4	429	10	75	9.6	12.1
Wholemeal, Tesco*	1 Cracker/7g	29	1	414	9.4	60.6	14.9	10.4
Wholmeal, Organic, Nairn's*	1 Cracker/14g	58	2	413	9	61.4	14.6	8.7
CRANBERRIES								
& Raisins, Dried, Sweetened, Ocean Spray*	1 Serving/50g	163	0.2	326	0.1	80.3	0.5	4.6
Craisins, Dried, Reduced Sugar, Ocean Spray*	1 Serving/30g	75	0.3	250	0	82.5	0.9	25
Dried, Sweetened, Average	***1 Serving/10g***	***34***	***0.1***	***335***	***0.3***	***81.1***	***0.8***	***4.4***
Fresh, Raw, Average	***1oz/28g***	***4***	***0***	***15***	***0.4***	***3.4***	***0.1***	***3***
Frozen, Sainsbury's*	1 Portion/80g	18	0.1	22	0.4	3.4	0.1	3
CRAYFISH								
Raw	***1oz/28g***	***19***	***0.2***	***67***	***14.9***	***0***	***0.8***	***0***
Tails in Brine, Luxury, The Big Prawn Co*	½ Tub/90g	46	0.6	51	10.1	1	0.7	0
Tails, Chilli & Garlic, Asda*	1 Serving/140g	133	4.3	95	16	1.1	3.1	0.8
Whole, Dried, Noor Madina*	1 Pack/40g	27	1.5	68	5.7	0	3.7	0
CREAM								
Aerosol, Average	***1oz/28g***	***87***	***8.7***	***309***	***1.8***	***6.2***	***30.9***	***0***
Aerosol, Reduced Fat, Average	***1 Serving/55ml***	***33***	***3***	***60***	***0.6***	***2***	***5.4***	***0***
Brandy, Extra Thick, TTD, Sainsbury's*	1 Serving/30ml	131	12.3	436	1.4	10.4	40.8	0.5
Brandy, Pourable with Remy Martin*, Finest, Tesco*	½ Pot/125ml	460	35.5	368	2.7	19.8	28.4	0
Brandy, Really Thick, Finest, Tesco*	½ Pot/125ml	579	49.5	463	1.3	19.7	39.6	0
Brandy, Really Thick, Tesco*	1 Pot/250ml	1162	98.2	465	1.4	21.3	39.3	0
Chantilly, TTD, Sainsbury's*	2 Tbsp/30g	136	14	455	1.4	6.9	46.8	0
Clotted, Fresh, Average	***1 Serving/28g***	***162***	***17.5***	***579***	***1.6***	***2.3***	***62.7***	***0***
Coconut, Soya, Cuisine, Alpro*	1 Tbsp/15g	15	1.3	100	1.2	2.3	8.8	0
Double, Average	***1 Tbsp/15ml***	***68***	***7.3***	***452***	***1.6***	***2.4***	***48.4***	***0***

Measure
INFO/WEIGHT

per Measure
KCAL FAT

Nutrition Values per 100g / 100ml
KCAL PROT CARB FAT FIBRE

CREAM

	Measure INFO/WEIGHT	per Measure KCAL	FAT	100g KCAL	PROT	CARB	FAT	FIBRE
Double, Brandy, Waitrose*	1 Serving/30ml	138	12.4	460	1.3	14.4	41.4	0
Double, Channel Island, Cointreau, Waitrose*	1 Serving/30ml	129	11.4	431	1.3	15.3	38.2	0
Double, Reduced Fat, Average	*1 Serving/30g*	*73*	*7*	*243*	*2.7*	*5.6*	*23.3*	*0.1*
Extra Thick, with Baileys, Baileys*	1 fl oz/30ml	129	11.6	431	1.5	13.4	38.6	0
Goat's, Double, St Helen's Farm*	1 Tbsp/15g	67	7.2	449	1.7	2.6	48	0
Half Half, Dairyland*	2 Tbsp/30ml	40	3	133	3.3	6.7	10	0
Oat Alternative, Dairy Free, Oatly*	1 Carton/250ml	375	32.5	150	1	6	13	0.8
Real Dairy, Lighter, Spray, Tesco*	1 Spray/13g	29	2.4	221	2.5	11	18.6	0
Real Dairy, Spray, Tesco*	1 Portion/13g	44	4.4	338	2.2	5.9	34	0
Remy Martin, Channel Island, Waitrose*	1 Serving/30ml	135	12.8	450	1.5	9.7	42.8	0
Single, Average	*1 Tbsp/15ml*	*28*	*2.7*	*188*	*2.6*	*3.9*	*18*	*0.1*
Single, Extra Thick, Average	*1 Serving/38ml*	*72*	*6.9*	*192*	*2.7*	*4.1*	*18.4*	*0*
Single, Soya, Fresh, Plant Based, Cuisine, Alpro*	1 Tbsp/15g	18	1.5	122	2	4.5	10.2	0.4
Single, Soya, UHT, Plant Based, Cuisine, Alpro*	1 Tbsp/15g	25	2.5	169	2	1.6	16.8	0.3
Soured, Fresh, Average	*1 Tsp/5ml*	*10*	*0.9*	*191*	*2.7*	*3.9*	*18.4*	*0*
Soured, Reduced Fat, Average	*1 Tsp/5ml*	*6*	*0.4*	*119*	*5.2*	*6.7*	*8.6*	*0.4*
Strawberry, Light, Real Dairy, Uht, Anchor*	1 Serving/13g	25	2.1	198	2.6	8.7	17	0
Thick, Sterilised, Average	*1 Tbsp/15ml*	*35*	*3.5*	*233*	*2.6*	*3.6*	*23.1*	*0*
Uht, Double, Average	*1 Tbsp/15g*	*41*	*3.9*	*274*	*2.2*	*7.4*	*26.3*	*0*
Uht, Reduced Fat, Average	*1 Serving/25ml*	*16*	*1.4*	*62*	*0.6*	*2.2*	*5.6*	*0*
Uht, Single, Average	*1 Tbsp/15ml*	*29*	*2.8*	*194*	*2.6*	*4*	*18.8*	*0*
Whipping, Average	*1 Tbsp/15ml*	*52*	*5.5*	*348*	*2.1*	*3.2*	*36.4*	*0*

CREAM ALTERNATIVE

Single, Oatly*	½ Carton/125ml	188	16.2	150	1	6	13	0.7

CREAM SODA

American with Vanilla, Tesco*	1 Glass/313ml	75	0	24	0	5.9	0	0
Diet, Sainsbury's*	1 Serving/250ml	2	0	1	0	0	0	0
No Added Sugar, Sainsbury's*	1 Can/330ml	2	0.3	0	0.1	0.1	0.1	0.1
Shapers, Boots*	1 Bottle/300ml	3	0	1	0	0	0	0
Traditional Style, Tesco*	1 Can/330ml	139	0	42	0	10.4	0	0

CREME BRULEE

Average	*1 Serving/100g*	*313*	*26*	*313*	*3.8*	*15.7*	*26*	*0.2*
Dine in Dessert, M&S*	1 Dessert/89g	186	13.1	210	4.9	14.2	14.8	0.5
French, Pots, Tesco*	1 Pot/100g	324	26	324	4.3	18	26	0.5
Gastropub, M&S*	1 Brulee/84g	285	24.6	340	3.1	15.7	29.3	0.7
M&S*	1 Pot/100g	360	32.6	360	3.3	13	32.6	0
Nestle*	1 Serving/100g	305	25.6	305	4	14.6	25.6	0
Reduced Fat, M&S*	1 Serving/89g	186	13.1	210	4.9	14.2	14.8	0.5

CREME CARAMEL

Asda*	1 Pot/100g	113	2.6	113	2.4	20	2.6	0
Average	*1 Serving/128g*	*140*	*2.8*	*109*	*3*	*20.6*	*2.2*	*0*
La Laitiere*	1 Pot/100g	135	4	135	5	20	4	0
Lidl*	1 Pot/89g	79	0.7	89	2.3	18.1	0.8	0.1
Tesco*	1 Pot/100g	115	1.6	115	2.8	21.8	1.6	0

CREME EGG

Cadbury*	1 Egg/40g	177	6	440	3.2	73	15	0.4
Minis, Cadbury*	1 Egg/12g	50	1.9	435	4.2	67	16.5	0.5

CREME FRAICHE

Average	*1 Pot/295g*	*1067*	*112.2*	*362*	*2.2*	*2.6*	*38*	*0*
French, Smooth Tangy, Waitrose*	1 Serving/30g	116	12.3	386	2	2.3	41	0
Half Fat, Average	*1 Tbsp/15g*	*27*	*2.4*	*181*	*3.1*	*5.5*	*16.2*	*0*
Lemon & Rocket, Sainsbury's*	1 Serving/150g	188	17.2	125	2.2	3	11.5	0.5
Low Fat, Average	*1 Tbsp/30ml*	*43*	*3.6*	*143*	*3.3*	*5.6*	*12.1*	*0.1*

C

INFO/WEIGHT	Measure	per Measure KCAL	FAT	Nutrition Values per 100g / 100ml KCAL	PROT	CARB	FAT	FIBRE
CREME FRAICHE								
Oat, Creamy, Oatly*	1 Tbsp/15ml	26	2.2	175	1.1	9.2	15	1
CREPES								
Chocolate Filled, Tesco*	1 Crepe/32g	137	5.2	429	5.9	63.5	16.2	3
Galette, Buckwheat, Average	*1 Serving/100g*	*161*	*1.7*	*161*	*5.8*	*30.2*	*1.7*	*1*
Lobster, Finest, Tesco*	1 Serving/160g	250	10.2	156	10.7	14	6.4	1.2
Mushroom, M&S*	1 Pack/186g	195	4.5	105	5.7	17.1	2.4	2.5
CRISPBAKES								
Broccoli Leek, Asda*	1 Bake/132g	263	13.2	199	6.3	21	10	2
Bubble & Squeak, M&S*	1 Bake/47g	79	4.1	170	2.7	19.6	8.8	1.5
Cheddar Onion, Cooked, Free From, Tesco*	1 Bake/125g	291	15.1	232	7.1	22.8	12.1	2
Cheese & Onion, Tesco*	2 Bakes/116g	233	12.6	201	5.4	18.6	10.9	3.3
Cheese Onion, Cooked, Dalepak*	1 Bake/86g	192	8.8	223	4.9	26.9	10.2	1.7
Cheese Onion, Meat Free, Morrisons*	1 Bakes/136g	282	13.8	207	1.5	23.5	10.1	4.9
Cheese Onion, Ovenbaked, Iceland*	1 Crispbake/77g	145	5.3	189	4.8	25.9	6.9	2.3
Cheese, Spring Onion Chive, Sainsbury's*	1 Bake/107g	232	10.2	216	6.4	25.1	9.5	2.2
Chicken Mushroom, Sainsbury's*	1 Crispbake/85g	174	7.6	205	10.5	20.6	8.9	1.8
Dutch, Asda*	1 Bake/8g	31	0.3	388	14.7	74.9	3.3	4.2
Dutch, Co-Op*	1 Crispbake/10g	38	0.4	375	16	69.6	3.5	6.5
Dutch, HL, Tesco*	1 Bake/8g	30	0.2	385	14.7	74.9	2.7	4.2
Dutch, Sainsbury's*	1 Bake/10g	38	0.5	392	14.5	72.3	5	5.8
Dutch, Tesco*	1 Crispbake/10g	40	0.5	397	13.6	71.7	5.3	4.2
Ham Hock, Cheddar, Free From, Tesco*	1 Crispbake/125g	277	12.6	222	12.4	19.4	10.1	2.1
Mature Cheddar, Crispy Thins, TTD, Sainsbury's*	1 Thin/4g	21	1.5	581	14.2	38.3	40.6	2.8
Minced Beef, M&S*	1 Bake/113g	226	12.3	200	10	15.6	10.9	1.5
Roast Vegetable & Basil, Cauldron Foods*	1 Bake/115g	242	11	210	3.5	26	9.6	2.9
Vegetable, M&S*	1 Bake/114g	200	10.3	175	2.5	19.2	9	2.6
Vegetable, Sainsbury's*	1 Bake/114g	246	13	216	2	26.2	11.4	2
Vegetarian, Salmon Style, Dill, Quorn*	1 Crispbake/100g	182	6.6	182	7	22	6.6	3.5
CRISPBREAD								
3 Grain 3 Seed, Foodie Market, Aldi*	1 Crispbread/25g	109	4.2	436	15	52	17	8.8
3 Grain, Foodie Market, Aldi*	1 Crispbread/25g	113	4.7	461	15	49	19	10
3 Grains 3 Seeds, Organic, Dr Karg*	1 Crispbread/25g	114	4.8	455	16	50	19	9.9
3 Seed, Classic, Gourmet, Dr Karg*	1 Bread/25g	108	4.9	430	16.5	46.6	19.7	10.9
3 Seed, Organic, Gourmet	*1 Bread/25g*	*101*	*4.7*	*405*	*15.8*	*48.8*	*18.8*	*14.6*
Apple Cinnamon, Ryvita*	1 Crispbread/15g	54	0.2	356	7.2	72.5	1.6	11.8
Brown, Baked, Leksands*	1 Slice/13g	46	0.3	350	9	64	2.6	21
Chia Seed, Buckwheat, Protein, Ryvita*	1 Crispbread/10g	38	0.4	371	21.5	56.9	3.7	12
Chickpea, Mung Bean Chive, Easy Bean*	1 Crispbread/22g	93	4.1	422	12.8	50.6	18.6	6.9
Corn Thins, Sesame, Real Foods*	1 Thin/6g	23	0.2	384	10.7	69.9	3.4	10.2
Corn, Orgran*	1 Bread/5g	18	0.1	360	7.5	83	1.8	3
Cracked Black Pepper, Thins, Ryvita*	1 Slice/10g	35	0.2	344	8.8	66.6	1.6	14.5
Cream Cheese Chives, Minis, Ryvita*	1 Pack/30g	114	2.3	380	8.7	75.7	7.7	13
Crisp 'n' Light, Wasa*	1 Bread/7g	24	0.1	360	12	73	2.2	5.3
Dark Rye, Morrisons*	1 Bake/13g	39	0.4	300	11.5	61.5	3.1	16.9
Dark Rye, Ryvita*	1 Bread/10g	34	0.1	342	8.5	66.5	1.2	15.2
Fibre Plus, Wholegrain with Sesame, Wasa*	1 Bread/10g	35	0.7	350	13	47	7	24
Five Seed, Bites, Knacks, Peters Yard*	1 Portion/25g	99	2.3	397	14	69.6	9.2	10.3
Fruit Crunch, Ryvita*	1 Slice/15g	54	0.8	358	8.3	61.8	5.4	14.9
GF	*1 Serving/8g*	*25*	*0.1*	*331*	*6.4*	*72.9*	*1.5*	*0*
Hint of Chilli, Ryvita*	1 Slice/12g	42	0.2	349	8.6	66.6	1.9	16.8
Knacke, Trader Joe's*	1 Crispbread/25g	118	5.1	462	16	50	20	0
Mini, Sesame Linseed, Dr Karg*	1 Crispbread/3g	13	0.4	424	12.1	57.6	12.1	9.1
Mixed Grain, Jacobs*	1 Cracker/10g	41	1.3	436	9.1	66.7	13.9	4.2

CRISPBREAD	INFO/WEIGHT	Measure KCAL	FAT	Nutrition Values per 100g / 100ml KCAL	PROT	CARB	FAT	FIBRE
Multigrain, Deli, Ryvita*	1 Slice/11g	41	0.8	370	11.2	56	7.2	18.3
Multigrain, Ryvita*	1 Slice/11g	41	0.8	370	11.2	56	7.2	18.3
Original Rye, Thin, Finn Crisp*	1 Slice/6g	22	0.2	339	10	59	2.6	20
Original Rye, Wasa*	1 Bread/11g	35	0.2	315	9	67	1.4	14
Original, Ryvita*	1 Crispbread/10g	35	0.2	350	8.5	66.9	1.7	16.5
Poppyseed, Wasa*	1 Bread/13g	46	1	350	13	56	8	14
Provita*	1 Bread/6g	26	0.6	416	12.5	68.4	9.9	0
Pumpkin Seeds Oats, Rye, Deli, Ryvita*	1 Crispbread/12g	46	0.9	370	11.2	56	7.2	18.3
Pumpkin Seeds Oats, Ryvita*	1 Slice/13g	46	0.9	370	11.2	56	7.2	18.3
Rice Cracked Pepper, Orgran*	1 Bread/5g	18	0.1	388	8.4	81.9	1.8	2
Rice, Sakata*	1 Bread/25g	26	0.2	102	1.7	22	0.7	0.3
Roasted Onion, Organic, Dr Karg*	1 Bread/25g	98	3.7	390	15.8	48.5	14.8	12.9
Rosemary Apricot, Toasts, M&S*	1 Toast/8g	34	1.4	434	12.3	54.3	17.8	3.7
Rounds, Multigrain, Finn Crisp*	1 Bread/13g	41	0.8	330	13	56	6	18
Rounds, Wholegrain Wheat, Finn Crisp*	1 Bread/13g	45	0.7	360	11	66	5.9	10
Rustikal, Wasa*	1 Crispbread/15g	51	0.2	340	9	6.4	1.5	16
Rye, Original, Tesco*	1 Crispbread/9g	32	0.3	357	11.6	62.4	2.8	18
Salt Vinegar, Minis, Ryvita*	1 Pack/24g	90	1.9	376	8.2	74	7.8	11.4
Scan Bran, Slimming World*	1 Slice/10g	31	0.5	310	14.9	29	5.3	42.1
Seeded, Spelt, Organic, Dr Karg*	1 Bread/25g	108	4.5	430	17.2	44.4	18	11.2
Sesame Rye, Tesco*	1 Biscuit/9g	34	0.8	385	12.5	55.6	8.7	17.2
Sesame, Ryvita*	1 Bread/10g	37	0.7	373	10.5	58.3	7	17.5
Sesame, Savour Bakes, Aldi*	1 Crispbread/9g	31	0.5	344	10	57.8	5.6	15.6
Snacks, Cheese, Onion Chive Flavour, Quaker*	1 Pack/28g	118	2.5	420	8.3	76	9.1	2.4
Sour Cream Onion, Mini, The Foodie Market, Aldi*	1/6 Pack/25g	107	3.8	427	14	54	15	7.9
Sourdough, Original, Peter's Yard*	1 Crispbread/3g	11	0.1	381	12.9	68.3	4.1	9.5
Spelt, Cheese, Sunflower Seeds, Organic, Dr Karg*	1 Bread/25g	103	4.5	411	19.2	42.8	18.1	10.4
Spelt, Muesli, Organic, Dr Karg*	1 Bread/25g	94	2.8	375	14.2	54.4	11.2	10.6
Sport, Wasa*	1 Bread/15g	46	0.2	310	9	64	1.5	16
Sunflower Seeds Oats, Ryvita*	1 Bread/12g	46	1.1	384	9.7	58.4	9	15.3
Super Chia, GF, Semper*	1 Crispbread/14g	50	0.4	357	5.3	72	3.2	9.4
Sweet Chilli, Minis, Ryvita*	1 Pack/24g	90	1.8	376	8.5	75.9	7.4	10.3
Sweet Onion, Ryvita*	1 Crispbread/12g	43	0.2	356	9	70.6	1.4	12.6
Sweet Onion, Wholegrain Rye, Deli, Ryvita*	1 Crispbread/10g	37	0.1	365	9	70.6	1.4	12.6
Thin Crisps, Original Taste, Finn Crisp*	1 Bread/6g	20	0.2	320	11	63	2.4	19
Toasted Corn, Orgran*	1 Crispbread/15g	55	0.2	367	6.7	75.5	1.4	1.9
Trufree*	1 Bread/6g	22	0.1	370	6	82	2	1
Wheat, Morrisons*	1 Crispbread/8g	28	0.3	377	11.5	73.1	3.4	4.2
Whole Grain, Crispy, Thin, Kavli*	3 Breads/15g	50	0.3	333	10	70	1.7	12.7
Wholegrain, Classic Three Seed, Organic, Dr Karg*	1 Bread/25g	101	4.5	405	15.8	44.8	18	14.6
Wholemeal Rye, Organic, Kallo*	1 Bread/10g	31	0.2	314	9.7	65	1.7	15.4
Wholemeal, Light, Allinson*	1 Bread/5g	17	0.1	349	11.7	69.7	2.6	11
Wholemeal, Organic, Allinson*	1 Bread/5g	17	0.1	336	14.2	66	1.7	12.2
Wholemeal, Rye with Milk, Grafschafter*	1 Bread/9g	29	0.1	316	11.4	64	1.6	15
CRISPS								
Apple, Dried, Snapz*	1 Pack/15g	52	0	344	2	77	0	14.7
Apple, Eat Smart, Morrisons*	1 Pack/20g	68	0.1	338	1.9	75.3	0.7	11.4
Apple, Pure, Dusted with Cinnamon, Graze*	¼ Bag/13g	47	0	364	2	81	0	14
Apple, Thyme & Sage, M&S*	1 Bag/55g	253	13.4	460	5.5	55.3	24.3	6.1
Bacon, Crispies, Sainsbury's*	1 Bag/25g	117	5.7	468	19.9	45.8	22.8	4.8
Bacon, Pillows, Light, Shapers, Boots*	1 Pack/12g	44	0.3	367	3.7	83	2.3	4
Bacon, Rashers, BGTY, Sainsbury's*	1 Pack/10g	34	0.2	340	10.8	70.3	1.6	3.5
Bacon, Rashers, Blazin, Tesco*	1 Bag/25g	121	6.6	485	16.5	45.7	26.3	3.8

CRISPS

INFO/WEIGHT	Measure	per Measure KCAL	FAT	Nutrition Values per 100g / 100ml KCAL	PROT	CARB	FAT	FIBRE
Bacon, Rashers, COU, M&S*	1 Pack/20g	72	0.6	360	9.4	77.5	2.9	3.5
Bacon, Rashers, Iceland*	1 Bag/75g	330	13.2	440	8.3	61.9	17.6	2.9
Bacon, Rashers, Snackrite, Aldi*	1 Bag/18g	89	4.3	496	5.6	63	24	1.7
Bacon, Rice Bites, Asda*	1 Bag/30g	136	4.8	452	7	70	16	0.4
Bacon, Shapers, Boots*	1 Bag/23g	99	3.4	431	8	66	15	3
Bacon, Sizzler, Ridge Cut, McCoys*	1 Bag/32g	165	9.7	516	7.1	53.6	30.3	3.9
Bacon, Sizzler, Ridged, Snackrite, Aldi*	1 Pack/30g	160	9.3	532	7.2	55	31	3.9
Bacon, Smoky, BGTY, Sainsbury's*	1 Bag/25g	118	5.9	472	6.5	58.5	23.6	5.7
Bacon, Smoky, Golden Wonder*	1 Bag/25g	131	8.4	523	5.9	49.1	33.7	2
Bacon, Smoky, Select, Tesco*	1 Bag/25g	134	8.7	536	6.4	49	34.9	4.3
Bacon, Smoky, Snackrite, Aldi*	1 Bag/25g	130	7.2	522	6	57	29	3.3
Bacon, Smoky, Sunseed Oil, Walkers*	1 Bag/35g	183	11.4	530	6.5	51	33	4
Bacon, Smoky, Tayto*	1 Bag/35g	184	11.9	526	7.6	47.3	34	4.5
Bacon, Webs, Monster Munch*	1 Pack/15g	74	3.4	497	6.5	65.2	23.1	1.6
Baked Bean, Walkers*	1 Bag/35g	184	11.6	525	6.5	50	33	4
Baked, Average	*1 Bag/25g*	*93*	*1.5*	*374*	*6.5*	*73.5*	*5.9*	*5.8*
Barbecue, Corn Chips, Popchips*	1 Bag/17g	73	2.9	430	6	65	17	1.6
Barbecue, Handcooked, Tesco*	1 Bag/40g	187	10	468	6.6	53.8	25.1	5.2
Barbecue, Pop Outs, Passions, Aldi*	1 Pack/100g	422	13	422	5.8	69	13	3
Barbecue, Savoury Snacks, Weight Watchers*	1 Pack/22g	81	1.9	366	18.6	61	8.7	6.1
Barbecue, Snack Rite*	1 Bag/25g	131	8.3	524	5.1	51.3	33.2	0
Barbecue, Sticky, Oven Baked, Walkers*	1 Pack/25g	109	3.4	435	6.8	68.4	13.5	6.3
Barbecue, Sunseed Oil, Walkers*	1 Pack/33g	171	10.7	525	6.5	50	33	4
BBQ Rib, Crusti Croc, Lidl*	1 Bag/25g	132	8.2	527	6.4	50	32.6	4
BBQ Rib, Sunseed, Walkers*	1 Bag/25g	131	8.2	525	6.5	50	33	4
BBQ, Bangin', Mountain Chips, Muscle Moose*	1 Pack/23g	93	2.1	406	22	55	9.1	7.9
BBQ, Honey, Wholgrain, Snacks, M&S*	1 Serving/30g	146	7.5	485	7.8	57.6	24.9	5.2
BBQ, Southern Style, Bugles, Walkers*	1 Pack/20g	105	6	525	6.5	56	30	3.5
BBQ, Stackers, Snackrite, Aldi*	1 Serving/25g	134	8.5	538	3.1	53	34	4
Beef, & Horseradish, Hand Cooked, Deluxe, Lidl*	1 Pack/25g	121	6.8	484	7	50.5	27.1	5.1
Beef, & Horseradish, Roast, Tyrrells*	¼ Pack/38g	165	10.1	439	5.3	41.7	26.9	4.7
Beef, & Mustard, Roast, Thick Cut, Brannigans*	1 Bag/40g	203	12	507	7.6	51.7	30	3.7
Beef, & Onion Flavour, Average	*1 Bag/25g*	*131*	*8.3*	*524*	*6.5*	*50*	*33.1*	*4.3*
Beef, & Onion, Tayto*	1 Bag/35g	184	11.9	526	7.6	47.3	34	4.5
Beef, & Onion, Walkers*	1 Bag/33g	171	10.7	525	6.5	50	33	4
Beef, & Red Wine, Specially Selected, Aldi*	1 Serving/25g	130	7.3	519	5.1	59	29	2.5
Beef, Angus, & English Mustard, Furrows, Tyrrells*	1 Bag/40g	201	11.3	502	6.8	52.2	28.2	0
Beef, Barbecue, Select, Tesco*	1 Pack/25g	134	8.7	536	6.4	49.2	34.8	4.4
Beef, Chinese Sizzling, McCoys*	1 Bag/35g	178	10.6	506	6.9	51.8	30.2	4
Beef, Discos, KP Snacks*	1 Pack/28g	145	8.2	518	5.1	58.7	29.3	2.4
Beef, Roast, English, & Yorkshire Pudding, Walkers*	1 Bag/35g	180	11.3	522	6.6	50.4	32.7	4
Beef, Roast, KP Snacks*	1 Bag/25g	134	8.8	534	6.6	47.5	35.3	4.7
Beef, Roast, Monster Claws, Snackrite, Aldi*	1 Pack/17g	87	4.4	511	6.3	62	26	1.2
Beef, Space Raiders, KP Snacks*	1 Pack/13g	64	2.9	495	6.5	65.3	22.8	1
Beef, Squares, Walkers*	1 Bag/25g	105	4.5	420	6	59	18	4.6
Beefy, Smiths, Walkers*	1 Bag/25g	133	9.2	531	4.3	45.2	37	0
Beetroot, Chips, Crunchy, Apple Snapz*	1 Bag/20g	52	0.2	260	14.7	76	1	28
Beetroot, Eat Smart, Morrisons*	1 Pack/20g	63	0.1	313	15.1	52	0.4	20.5
Beetroot, Seasoned In Salt, Glennans*	1 Bag/27g	130	8.9	480	8.2	36	32.8	13.2
Beetroot, Vinaigrette, Eat Well, M&S*	1 Pack/30g	92	0.1	306	13.6	51.4	0.2	21.9
Big Snak, Crisp 'n Tasty Potato Chips, Herrs*	1 Pack/43g	212	12.1	494	7.1	56.5	28.2	3.6
Brussels Sprout, Walkers*	1 Bag/25g	126	6.7	504	6	57.2	26.8	4.4
Bugles, Cheese Flavour, Walkers*	1 Pack/30g	158	8.8	525	7	56.9	29.3	3

CRISPS

INFO/WEIGHT	Measure	per Measure		Nutrition Values per 100g / 100ml				
		KCAL	FAT	KCAL	PROT	CARB	FAT	FIBRE
Builders Breakfast, Walkers*	1 Sm Bag/25g	131	8.3	524	5.6	50.8	33.2	4
Butter, & Chive, COOU, M&S*	1 Bag/26g	95	0.5	365	7.7	77.3	1.9	4.6
Carrot, Eat Smart, Morrisons*	1 Pack/200g	63	0.3	316	5.5	61.9	1.3	17.2
Cheddar, & Bacon, Temptingly, Walkers*	1 Pack/32g	169	10	520	6.2	52.3	30.9	4.2
Cheddar, & Chive, Mature, Kettle Chips*	1 Serving/50g	239	12.7	478	8.1	54.4	25.4	5
Cheddar, & Chive, Mature, Tyrrells*	1 Serving/30g	134	6.9	447	6.9	53.7	23.1	2.4
Cheddar, & Onion, Crinkles, Walkers*	1 Pack/28g	150	9.3	538	6	51.5	33.3	3.5
Cheddar, & Onion, Hand Cooked, Aldi*	1 Pack/150g	753	41.8	502	7.7	54.9	27.9	4
Cheddar, & Red Onion Chutney, Sensations, Walkers*	1 Bag/40g	198	11.2	495	6.5	54	28	4.5
Cheddar, & Red Onion, Mature, Finest, Tesco*	1 Bag/40g	208	8.3	519	5.1	58.6	20.8	2.5
Cheddar, & Sour Cream, Extra Crunchy, Walkers*	1 Serving/30g	143	6.8	476	6.6	59.1	22.6	4.7
Cheddar, & Spring Onion, 35% Less Fat, Sainsbury's*	1 Pack/20g	93	4.2	463	6.3	62.4	20.9	0.9
Cheddar, Mature, Red Onion, Hand Cooked, M&S*	1 Pack/40g	206	11.7	515	7.8	52.5	29.2	5.6
Cheese & Onion, 30% Less Fat, Sainsbury's*	1 Pack/25g	115	5.4	459	7.5	58.1	21.8	5.4
Cheese & Onion, BGTY, Sainsbury's*	1 Bag/25g	120	6.2	479	7	57	24.8	5.7
Cheese & Onion, Crinkle Cut, Low Fat, Waitrose*	1 Bag/25g	122	5.8	490	7.7	62.6	23.2	4.7
Cheese & Onion, Flavour Crinkles, Shapers, Boots*	1 Bag/20g	96	4.8	482	6.6	60	24	4
Cheese & Onion, GFY, Asda*	1 Pack/26g	122	5.7	470	7	61	22	4.2
Cheese & Onion, KP Snacks*	1 Bag/25g	134	8.7	534	6.6	48.7	34.8	4.8
Cheese & Onion, M&S*	1 Bag/25g	134	8.9	535	5.5	48.8	35.5	5
Cheese & Onion, Max, Walkers*	1 Pack/50g	266	16.4	533	6.8	51	32.9	2.9
Cheese & Onion, Organic, Tesco*	1 Bag/25g	128	8.2	514	5.2	49.9	32.6	7
Cheese & Onion, Potato Heads, Walkers*	1 Pack/23g	108	5.3	470	6	60	23	5.5
Cheese & Onion, Red Onion, Extra Crunchy, Walkers*	1 Serving/30g	140	6.3	468	6.8	60.6	20.9	4.9
Cheese & Onion, Rings, Crunchy, Shapers, Boots*	1 Bag/15g	56	0.4	374	5.9	81	2.9	2
Cheese & Onion, Sainsbury's*	1 Bag/25g	132	8.7	527	4.6	48.8	34.8	3.9
Cheese & Onion, Sprinters*	1 Bag/25g	137	9.2	549	5.4	49.4	36.6	0
Cheese & Onion, Squares, Walkers*	1 Bag/25g	108	4.5	430	6.5	61	18	5.5
Cheese & Onion, Value, Tesco*	1 Bag/20g	108	7.2	541	6	48.3	36	4.8
Cheese Onion Flavour, Asda*	1 Bag/25g	130	7.8	519	5.6	53.6	31.4	3.7
Cheese Onion, Baked, Walkers*	1 Bag/32g	164	5.1	436	6.7	68.6	13.6	6.2
Cheese Onion, Crinkle, Seabrook*	1 Pack/32g	170	10.5	536	5.9	51.1	33.1	5.2
Cheese Onion, Discos, KP Snacks*	1 Pack/28g	146	8.2	520	5.1	59.1	29.3	2.5
Cheese Onion, Golden Wonder*	1 Bag/25g	129	7.9	516	5.8	52.4	31.5	3.8
Cheese Onion, Hand Cooked, Ten Acre*	1 Bag/40g	201	11.5	503	6.6	51.8	28.7	6.2
Cheese Onion, Lights, Walkers*	1 Bag/24g	113	5	470	7.5	62	21	5
Cheese Onion, Oven Baked, Asda*	1 Bag/25g	95	2	380	5.1	72	8	3.3
Cheese Onion, Oven Baked, Tesco*	1 Bag/25g	102	1.6	410	5.3	74.7	6.6	7.7
Cheese Onion, Pom Bear, Intersnack Ltd*	1 Bag/19g	95	5.3	498	3.8	58.1	27.8	3.2
Cheese Onion, Snackrite, Aldi*	1 Pack/25g	137	8.2	548	7.2	55	33	1.5
Cheese Onion, Sunseed Oil, Walkers*	1 Bag/33g	171	10.7	525	7	50	33	4
Cheese Onion, Tesco*	1 Pack/25g	135	8	535	5.4	54.8	31.8	3.2
Cheese Curls, Asda*	1 Pack/17g	87	4.9	511	3.8	59.7	28.6	1.7
Cheese Curls, Asda*	1 Bag/16g	87	5.3	541	3.6	57	33	1.7
Cheese Curls, Bobby's*	1 Bag/40g	225	14.8	563	7.6	50.1	36.9	0
Cheese Curls, Morrisons*	1 Bag/17g	95	6.1	557	3.1	54.8	35.6	2.6
Cheese Curls, Shapers, Boots*	1 Pack/14g	68	3.8	489	4.5	57	27	2.7
Cheese Curls, Sprinters*	1 Bag/14g	68	3.8	483	4.1	56.4	26.8	0
Cheese Curls, Tesco*	1 Bag/14g	75	4.5	520	4.5	54.4	31.1	1.9
Cheese Curls, Tesco*	1 Pack/17g	90	5.4	530	3.5	56	32	1.9
Cheese Curls, Weight Watchers*	1 Pack/20g	78	1.7	392	5	73.8	8.6	3.4
Cheese Puffs, Co-Op*	1 Bag/60g	321	20.4	535	3	54	34	2
Cheese Puffs, Weight Watchers*	1 Pack/18g	80	1.9	444	7.8	77.2	10.6	3.3

C

CRISPS

	Measure INFO/WEIGHT	per Measure KCAL	per Measure FAT	Nutrition Values per 100g / 100ml KCAL	PROT	CARB	FAT	FIBRE
Cheese Tasters, M&S*	1 Pack/30g	156	8.7	521	8.2	56.2	29	1
Cheese Twirls, Boulevard, Simply Delicious*	1 Pack/25g	138	8.8	550	12.1	46.7	35	0
Cheese, & Chives, Mature, Potato Chips, Tyrrells*	1 Bag/50g	261	14	522	6.1	56.5	27.9	0
Cheese, & Chives, Walkers*	1 Bag/33g	172	10.7	530	6.5	50	33	4.1
Cheese, Bites, Weight Watchers*	1 Pack/18g	73	1	406	13.9	71.1	5.6	2.2
Cheese, Heads, Walkers*	1 Bag/27g	128	6	475	10.8	58	22.3	2.8
Cheese, Moments, Smiths*	1 Pack/28g	148	9.2	530	8	50	33	2
Cheese, Space Raiders, KP Snacks*	1 Bag/16g	76	3.5	473	7.1	61.6	22	3.1
Chicken, & Thyme, Oven Roasted, Tesco*	1 Pack/150g	728	40.5	485	6.5	54	27	4.5
Chicken, Chargrilled, Crinkles, Shapers, Boots*	1 Bag/20g	96	4.8	482	6.6	60	24	4
Chicken, Chargrilled, Ridge Cut, McCoys*	1 Pack/32g	167	10	521	7	52.9	31.3	4
Chicken, Chargrilled, Ridged, Snackrite, Aldi*	1 Pack/30g	157	9	524	6.5	54	30	4
Chicken, Coronation, Walkers*	1 Bag/25g	131	8.2	525	6.5	50	33	4
Chicken, Firecracker, McCoys*	1 Bag/35g	177	10.3	506	6.2	54	29.5	4
Chicken, Roast	*1 Bag/25g*	*130*	*7.7*	*519*	*5.2*	*53.5*	*30.8*	*3.7*
Chicken, Roast, Select, Tesco*	1 Bag/25g	134	8.8	536	6.6	48.6	35	4.4
Chicken, Roast, Snack Rite*	1 Bag/25g	132	8.3	526	5.3	51.3	33.3	0
Chilli, & Lemon, Houmous Chips, Eat Real*	1 Serving/28g	126	4.8	449	6.5	68.4	17	4.5
Chilli, & Lemon, Lentil Chips, Eat Real*	1 Serrving/28g	130	5.4	466	9.3	66	19.5	3.2
Chilli, & Lemon, Walkers*	1 Pack/25g	131	8.2	525	6.3	51	33	3.8
Chilli, & Lime, Quinoa Chips, Eat Real*	1 Pack/30g	165	8.7	549	7	66.2	28.9	2.5
Chilli, Lime, Strong, Max, Walkers*	1 Pack/30g	160	9.9	532	6.6	50.9	32.9	3.1
Chilli, Lime, Thai, Oven Baked, Fusions, Walkers*	1 Bag/22g	96	3	435	6.7	68.3	13.5	6.4
Chilli, Cheese, Hummus Chips, Eat Real*	1 Pack/45g	213	10.4	474	6.5	57.2	23	5.8
Chilli, Haze, Chickpea Puffs, Organic, Hippeas*	1 Serving/22g	90	3.9	408	13.5	49.6	17.5	7.9
Chilli, Spiced, McCoys*	1 Bag/35g	175	10.1	500	6.1	54.2	28.8	4.2
Corn Chips, Fritos*	1 Pack/43g	240	15	565	4.7	56.5	35.3	0
Corn Snacks, Crispy, Bugles*	1 Bag/20g	102	5.6	508	4.8	60.7	28	1.4
Cream Cheese, & Chive, Waffles, Spar*	1 Pack/27g	132	6.8	488	4.2	60.7	25.3	1.3
Cream Cheese, & Onion, Crisp & Thin, Ritz*	1 Serving/30g	135	4.8	450	5.7	68	16	5.1
Creamy Dill, Houmous Chips, Eat Real*	1 Serving/28g	126	4.8	449	6.5	68.4	17	4.5
Creamy Dill, Lentil Chips, Eat Real*	1 Serving/28g	130	5.4	466	9.3	66	19.5	3.2
Crinkle Cut, Lower Fat, No Added Salt, Waitrose*	1 Bag/40g	193	10	483	6.5	58	25	3.9
Crunchy Sticks, Ready Salted, M&S*	1 Pack/75g	398	24.8	530	5.6	52.2	33	3.8
Crunchy Sticks, Ready Salted, Tesco*	1 Serving/25g	119	5.9	475	5.6	60.3	23.5	3
Crunchy Sticks, Salt Vinegar, Sainsbury's*	1 Bag/25g	118	6.1	474	5.9	58	24.3	2.4
Crunchy Sticks, Salt Vinegar, Value, Tesco*	1 Bag/22g	112	5.7	509	5	64	25.8	0.8
Duck & Hoisin, Crispy, Walkers*	1 Bag/25g	131	8.2	523	5.8	51.5	32.6	4
Fajita, Far Out, Chickpea Puffs, Organic, Hippeas*	1 Bag/22g	90	3.8	410	13.7	49.9	17.4	7.9
Four Cheese & Red Onion, Sensations, Walkers*	1 Bag/40g	194	10.8	485	6.5	54	27	4.5
Garlic Herbs Creme Fraiche, Kettle Chips*	1 Bag/50g	248	14.2	497	6	54.7	28.3	4.2
Guinness, Burts*	1 Bag/40g	206	11.5	514	5.1	58.6	28.8	2.5
Ham, & English Mustard Flavour, Real*	1 Bag/35g	176	9.9	502	6.2	53.9	28.2	4.2
Ham, & Mustard, Salty Dog*	1 Pack/40g	192	10.8	480	7.5	54.5	27.1	4.2
Ham, & Pickle, Smoked, Thick Cut, Brannigans*	1 Bag/40g	203	11.9	507	7	52.8	29.8	3.8
Ham, Canadian, Seabrook*	1 Pack/30g	159	9.8	531	5.7	50.9	32.7	5.1
Ham, Honey Roast, Hand Cooked, Finest, Tesco*	1 Serving/25g	130	7.3	515	5.1	58.6	28.8	2.5
Hot & Spicy Salami, Tesco*	1 Bag/50g	216	18	431	26.2	0.7	35.9	0
Jalapeno Cheddar, Quinoa Puffs, Eat Real*	1 Serving/28g	130	6.9	465	4.6	52.9	24.7	2.8
Jalapeno, Cheese, Strong, Max, Walkers*	1 Pack/30g	159	9.9	531	6.5	51	33	3.1
Lamb & Mint, Slow Roasted, Sensations, Walkers*	1 Bag/35g	170	9.4	485	6.5	54	27	4.5
Lant Chips, Ikea*	1 Serving/25g	126	6.9	505	8.3	55.9	27.6	4.5
Lentil Curls, Sour Cream, Chive, Tesco*	1 Pack/20g	90	3.1	448	11.3	64.1	15.6	3.3

CRISPS

	Measure INFO/WEIGHT	per Measure KCAL	FAT	Nutrition Values per 100g / 100ml KCAL	PROT	CARB	FAT	FIBRE
Marmite, Sunseed, Walkers*	1 Bag/33g	168	9.9	517	7.3	51.1	30.5	4.3
Mediterranean, Quinoa Puffs, Eat Real*	1 Pack/40g	212	12.4	531	5.9	54.8	31	4.4
Naked, Tyrrells*	1 Pack/150g	680	36.8	453	5.6	50.8	24.5	0
Olive Oil, Mozzarella Oregano, Walkers*	1 Serving/30g	152	8.7	505	6.5	54	29	4
Onion Rings, Corn Snacks, Average	*1 Bag/25g*	*122*	*6.1*	*486*	*5.8*	*60.9*	*24.2*	*2.7*
Onion Rings, M&S*	1 Pack/40g	186	8.6	465	5.2	62.1	21.5	4.3
Onion Rings, Tayto*	1 Pack/17g	82	4.1	484	3	63.4	24	2.4
Onion Rings, Tesco*	1 Serving/25g	129	6.8	515	6	61	27.1	1.7
Onion, Pickled, Golden Wonder*	1 Bag/25g	131	8.5	524	5.6	49	34	2
Onion, Pickled, Space Raiders, KP Snacks*	1 Bag/13g	64	2.9	495	6.5	65.3	22.8	1
Onion, Pickled, Sunseed, Walkers*	1 Bag/33g	171	10.7	525	6.5	50	33	4
Paprika, Corn Snacks, Shapers, Boots*	1 Pack/13g	64	3.5	494	8.7	54	27	2.2
Paprika, Hand Cooked, M&S*	1 Pack/40g	210	12.5	524	5.9	52.3	31.3	4.5
Paprika, Max, Walkers*	1 Bag/50g	265	16.3	530	6.5	51.2	32.6	3.1
Pastrami & Cheese, Crinkle, M&S*	1 Bag/25g	120	5.9	485	6.5	61	24	3.5
Pea Pinto Bean, Sticks, Off The Eaten Path*	1 Bag/23g	102	3.9	443	9.6	59	17	7.9
Peanut Puffs, Roasted, Ellert*	1 Serving/25g	125	6	500	13	56	24	4.1
Pear, Fruit, Nims*	1 Pack/22g	78	0.2	353	4	76	1	12
Pigs in Blankets, Walkers*	1 Bag/25g	126	6.7	504	6	56.8	26.8	4.4
Plain, Quinoa Chips, Eat Real*	1 Serving/30g	159	8.6	531	7.1	62.3	28.7	2.4
Popped, Crazy Hot, Ridges, Popchips*	1 Sm Pack/28g	118	4.2	420	6.7	60	15	4.1
Potato	*1oz/28g*	*148*	*9.6*	*530*	*5.7*	*53.3*	*34.2*	*5.3*
Potato Squares, Ready Salted, Sainsbury's*	1 Bag/50g	192	8	384	6.5	53.8	15.9	7.8
Potato Twirls, Sainsbury's*	1 Serving/50g	218	7.3	435	3	72.8	14.6	3.1
Potato Zoo, Crispy Potato Animals, Kids, Tesco*	1 Bag/30g	57	1.9	190	2.5	24.5	6.3	2.1
Potato, Baked, COU, M&S*	1 Bag/25g	88	0.6	350	8.5	76.4	2.3	5.7
Potato, Low Fat	*1oz/28g*	*128*	*6*	*458*	*6.6*	*63.5*	*21.5*	*5.9*
Potato, Tyrrells*	1 Pack/261g	1362	72.8	522	6.1	56.5	27.9	0
Prawn Cocktail, 30% Less Fat, Sainsbury's*	1 Pack/25g	118	5.9	470	6.3	58.9	23.6	5.7
Prawn Cocktail, Boots*	1 Pack/21g	99	4.6	470	6.8	60	22	4.3
Prawn Cocktail, Crusti Croc, Lidl*	1 Pack/25g	136	8.2	546	5.3	55.1	33	3.9
Prawn Cocktail, Flavour, Seabrook*	1 Bag/30g	163	10.1	544	5.7	49.2	33.7	4.5
Prawn Cocktail, Golden Wonder*	1 Bag/25g	131	7.7	521	5.3	53.9	30.8	3.5
Prawn Cocktail, Hand Cooked, M&S*	1 Pack/40g	205	11.5	512	7.1	54.4	28.7	3.8
Prawn Cocktail, Lites, Advantage, Tayto*	1 Pack/21g	96	4.1	455	5.3	65.1	19.3	3.8
Prawn Cocktail, Lites, Shapers, Boots*	1 Bag/21g	92	3.8	438	5.1	64	18	4.1
Prawn Cocktail, Snaktastic, Lidl*	1 Pack/25g	134	8	535	5.9	54	32	3.5
Prawn Cocktail, Spirals, Shapers, Boots*	1 Bag/15g	73	3.8	489	3.3	61	25	3
Prawn Cocktail, Sunseed Oil, Walkers*	1 Bag/33g	171	10.7	525	6.5	50	33	4
Prawn Cocktail, Tayto*	1 Bag/35g	185	12.3	526	7.5	46.6	35	4.5
Prawn Crackers, Tesco*	1 Pack/40g	220	13.3	550	2.2	60.4	33.2	0.6
Prawn, Melts, Snackrite, Aldi*	1 Pack/16g	78	4.5	504	0.6	59	29	0.6
Prawn, Spirals, Shapers, Boots*	1 Pack/100g	468	22	468	3.1	64	22	2.8
Pretzel, Salted, Original, Pretzel Crisps*	1 Serving/28g	100	0	357	7.1	85.7	0	3.6
Red Leicester & Spring Onion, Handcooked, M&S*	1 Pack/40g	194	10.6	485	6.8	55	26.4	5.1
Reggae Reggae, Grove Cut, Levi Roots*	1 Pack/40g	200	11.5	500	5.1	58.6	28.8	2.5
Ribe, Spare, Chinese, Walkers*	1 Bag/25g	131	8.2	525	6.5	50	33	4
Salt & Vinegar, Sea Salt, Handcooked, Real *	1 Bag/35g	179	10.2	512	5.6	54.6	29.2	4.2
Salt & Pepper, Black, Cracked, Hand Cooked, M&S*	1 Bag/40g	206	11.8	516	7.5	52.2	29.5	6
Salt & Pepper, Black, Handcooked, M&S*	1 Bag/40g	180	9.2	450	5.7	55	22.9	5.2
Salt & Pepper, Indian Black, Pipers Crisps*	1 Pack/40g	195	11.6	487	6.6	49.9	29	0
Salt & Peppercorn, Black, Delux, Lidl*	1 Pack/25g	123	6.1	492	6.4	57.2	24.4	4.8
Salt & Vinegar, Asda*	1 Bag/25g	130	8.5	522	6	48	34	4.2

CRISPS

INFO/WEIGHT	Measure	per Measure KCAL	FAT	Nutrition Values per 100g / 100ml KCAL	PROT	CARB	FAT	FIBRE
Salt & Vinegar, Balsamic, Cracker, Jacob's*	1 Serving/25g	118	4.8	470	5.2	67	19.3	2.4
Salt & Vinegar, Balsamic, Delux, Lidl*	1 Pack/25g	121	6.3	484	6	56.8	25.2	4.4
Salt & Vinegar, Balsamic, Handcooked, M&S*	1 Bag/40g	208	12.1	521	6.7	52.8	30.4	4.6
Salt & Vinegar, Balsamic, Kettle Chips*	1 Bag/40g	204	11.2	509	5.7	55.8	28.1	4.9
Salt & Vinegar, Chiplets, M&S*	1 Pack/50g	220	9.4	440	5.7	61.3	18.9	4.7
Salt & Vinegar, Cider Vinegar & Sea Salt, Tyrrells*	1 Pack/40g	192	9.8	481	7.2	60.1	24.6	2.4
Salt & Vinegar, Cider Vinegar, Crinkle Cut, Finest, Tesco*	¼ Pack/38g	186	10	495	6.7	54.6	26.7	4.5
Salt & Vinegar, Crinkle, M&S*	1 Pack/25g	120	5.9	485	6.5	61	24	3.5
Salt & Vinegar, Fries, COU, M&S*	1 Bag/25g	85	0.4	340	5	80	1.6	4
Salt & Vinegar, Golden Wonder*	1 Bag/25g	130	8.5	522	5.4	48.5	34	2
Salt & Vinegar, Lights, Walkers*	1 Bag/28g	133	6.2	475	7	62	22	4.5
Salt & Vinegar, M&S*	1 Bag/25g	131	8.6	525	5.4	48.8	34.5	4.6
Salt & Vinegar, Malt, Hunky Dorys*	1 Serving/25g	132	7.9	527	5.1	54.7	31.4	0
Salt & Vinegar, Malt, Ridge Cut, McCoys*	1 Bag/32g	169	9.9	529	6.5	54	31	3.9
Salt & Vinegar, Morrisons*	1 Bag/25g	129	7.8	515	4.9	53.9	31.1	3.6
Salt & Vinegar, Sainsbury's*	1 Bag/25g	130	8.8	522	4.1	46.9	35.3	3.9
Salt & Vinegar, Sea Salt, Cider Vinegar, TTD, Sainsbury's*	1/3 Pack/50g	245	14.3	489	5.5	52.7	28.5	6.1
Salt & Vinegar, Sea Salt, Crisp & Thin, Ritz*	1 Serving/30g	134	4.8	445	5.6	67	16	5.3
Salt & Vinegar, Snack Rite*	1 Bag/25g	127	8.2	508	4.7	48.1	33	0
Salt & Vinegar, Snaktastic, Lidl*	1 Pack/25g	130	7.8	520	5.6	52	31.2	3.6
Salt & Vinegar, Tayto*	1 Bag/35g	184	11.9	526	7.6	47.3	34	4.5
Salt Shake, Walkers*	1 Pack/24g	128	7.8	533	6.2	52.2	32.3	4.4
Salt Vinegar, Average	**1 Bag/25g**	**130**	**8.2**	**519**	**5.5**	**50.3**	**32.9**	**3.4**
Salt Vinegar, Baked, Walkers*	1 Pack/38g	150	3	400	6	73.5	8.1	4.6
Salt Vinegar, Crinkle Cut, Reduced Fat, Lidl*	1 Pack/25g	116	5.2	464	6.7	60.6	20.8	3.6
Salt Vinegar, Crinkle Cut, Seabrook*	1 Pack/25g	126	7.2	502	5.9	52.9	28.7	3.9
Salt Vinegar, Discos, KP Snacks*	1 Bag/28g	145	8.3	517	4.7	58.3	29.5	2.3
Salt Vinegar, Distinctively, Walkers*	1 Pack/33g	169	10	519	5.9	52.6	30.8	4.2
Salt Vinegar, Oven Baked, Asda*	1 Bag/25g	95	2	380	5.1	72	8	2.9
Salt Vinegar, Reduced Fat, Crinkle, M&S*	1 Pack/40g	183	7.7	457	6.8	61.9	19.2	4.5
Salt Vinegar, Spirals, Shapers, Boots*	1 Pack/15g	73	3.8	486	3	61	25	3.4
Salt Vinegar, Squares, Walkers*	1 Bag/28g	122	5	443	6.5	61	18	5.5
Salt Vinegar, Sunseed Oil, Walkers*	1 Bag/33g	171	10.7	525	6.5	50	33	4
Salt Vinegar, Thick Ridged, Snackrite, Aldi*	1 Bag/30g	159	9.3	529	5.8	55	31	3.4
Salt Vinegar, Vibes, Chickpea Puffs, Organic, Hippeas*	1 Pack/22g	90	3.8	408	12.7	50.4	17.2	7.1
Salt Your Own, Excluding Salt, Aldi*	1 Pack/24g	130	8.1	536	6	52.6	33.5	4.5
Salt Your Own, Sainsbury's*	1 Pack/24g	127	7.9	520	5	52.2	32.3	3.7
Salt Your Own, Snackrite, Aldi*	1 Pack/24g	130	8.1	536	6	52.6	33.5	4.5
Salted, 30% Less Fat, Sainsbury's*	1 Serving/25g	122	5.6	486	7.3	63.7	22.4	8.2
Salted, Average	**1 Bag/25g**	**127**	**7.4**	**508**	**6.1**	**53.4**	**29.7**	**4**
Salted, Baked, Walkers*	1 Pack/25g	104	2.1	417	6.2	76.2	8.3	4.8
Salted, Co-Op*	1 Bag/25g	131	8.5	525	6	51	34	3
Salted, Crinkle Cut, Lights, Snackrite, Aldi*	1 Bag/25g	122	5.8	486	7	61	23	3.7
Salted, Crushed Natural Sea Salt, Darling Spuds*	1 Bag/40g	195	12	488	5.6	53.4	30	4.5
Salted, Deep Ridge, Walkers*	1 Pack/28g	148	9	529	6.4	51.1	32.1	4.6
Salted, Everyday Value, Tesco*	1 Pack/18g	100	6.1	535	5	52.8	32.7	3.8
Salted, Golden Wonder*	1 Bag/25g	135	8.8	539	5.5	49.9	35.3	2
Salted, Lightly, Deluxe, Lidl*	1 Pack/25g	123	6.4	492	6.3	56	25.8	5.1
Salted, Lightly, Handcooked, Finest, Tesco*	1 Bag/40g	206	11.5	515	5.1	58.6	28.8	2.5
Salted, Lightly, Kettle Chips*	1 Serving/50g	256	15	513	5.8	51.5	30.1	6.5
Salted, Lightly, Potato Thins, LC, Tesco*	1 Pack/20g	72	0.4	360	5.1	79.5	2	4.2
Salted, Lights, Simply, Walkers*	1 Bag/24g	113	5.3	470	7	61	22	5
Salted, M&S*	1 Bag/25g	136	9.2	545	5.6	47.8	36.6	4.9

CRISPS

	Measure INFO/WEIGHT	per Measure KCAL	FAT	Nutrition Values per 100g / 100ml KCAL	PROT	CARB	FAT	FIBRE
Salted, Morrisons*	1 Bag/25g	134	8.7	536	4.9	50.9	34.8	4.3
Salted, Oven Baked, Tesco*	1 Bag/25g	95	1.9	380	4.4	73.1	7.7	8.4
Salted, Potato Chips, Tesco*	1 Bag/25g	136	8.3	544	6.4	52.4	33.2	4.4
Salted, Potato Rings, Sainsbury's*	1 Serving/50g	257	14.2	514	3.2	61.5	28.4	1.8
Salted, Reduced Fat, Crinkle, M&S*	1 Pack/40g	188	8.2	471	6.3	62.8	20.6	4.6
Salted, Reduced Fat, Tesco*	1 Pack/25g	114	6.2	456	6.3	52	24.7	5.9
Salted, Ridge Cut, McCoys*	1 Bag/32g	168	10.2	524	6.6	52.6	31.9	4.1
Salted, Sainsbury's*	1 Bag/25g	132	8.1	530	5	52.5	32.5	3.7
Salted, Sea, Anglesey Sea Salt, Red Sky*	1 Serving/40g	185	8.7	463	6.8	59.8	21.8	5
Salted, Sea, Crinkle Cut, Seabrook *	1 Bag/32g	165	10	517	5.7	53.7	31.1	0
Salted, Sea, Furrows, Tyrells*	1 Serving/30g	143	7.2	476	6.2	59.9	23.9	0
Salted, Sea, Hand Cooked, Specially Selected, Aldi*	¼ Lge Bag/38g	182	9	486	6.2	59	24	4.5
Salted, Sea, Houmous Chips, Eat Real*	1 Serving/28g	126	4.8	449	6.5	68.4	17	4.5
Salted, Sea, Lentil Chips, Eat Real*	1 Serving/28g	130	5.4	466	9.3	66	19.5	3.2
Salted, Sea, Lightly, Hand Cooked, English, Tyrrells*	1 Pack/25g	125	6.4	501	5.9	49	25.4	5.3
Salted, Sea, Lightly, Potato Chips, Hand Fried, Burts*	¼ Bag/50g	252	13.8	504	6.4	57.4	27.7	0
Salted, Sea, Lightly, Potato Chips, Tyrrells*	1 Pack/150g	740	38.1	493	7.7	58.9	25.4	2.6
Salted, Sea, Popchips*	1 Bag/23g	94	3.2	410	5.5	62	14	4.3
Salted, Sea, Potato, Mackies*	1 Pack/40g	200	10.8	499	7.4	55	27	4.5
Salted, Squares, Walkers*	1 Pack/25g	109	4.8	435	6.5	60	19	6
Salted, Sunseed Oil, Walkers*	1 Bag/33g	175	11.1	537	5.9	49.7	34.1	4.2
Salted, Tesco*	1 Bag/25g	140	8.5	545	5	55.4	33.2	1.8
Scampi, Smiths, Walkers*	1 Bag/27g	134	7	496	13	52.5	26	0
Seaveg ,Crispies, Original, Organic, Clearspring*	1 Pack/5g	28	1.8	550	25	33	36	20
Shells, Prawn Cocktail, Asda*	1 Bag/18g	90	5.3	501	4.6	54.9	29.2	6.2
Smoky Bacon Flavour, Average	*1 Bag/25g*	*132*	*8.4*	*527*	*6.2*	*49.7*	*33.7*	*3.2*
Sour Cream, & Chilli Lentil Curls, M&S*	1 Pack/60g	243	5.2	405	13.6	65.3	8.7	4.3
Sour Cream, & Chive Flavour, Average	*1 Bag/25g*	*127*	*7.7*	*508*	*6.8*	*50.7*	*30.9*	*4.6*
Sour Cream, & Chive, Baked, Walkers*	1 Pack/38g	148	3.2	395	7	73	8.5	5
Sour Cream, & Chive, Crinkle, Reduced Fat, M&S*	1 Bag/40g	187	8.1	468	6.7	62.2	20.3	4.6
Sour Cream, & Chives, Quinoa Chips, Eat Real*	1 Pack/30g	165	8.6	550	8	66.4	28.8	2.5
Sour Cream, & Onion, Corn Chips, Popchips*	1 Multipack/17g	72	2.9	422	6.5	65	17	1.9
Sour Cream, Chive, Hummus Chips, Eat Real*	1 Pack/45g	213	10.4	474	6.7	58	23	5.8
Sour Cream, Onion, Stackers, Snackrite, Aldi*	1 Serving/25g	139	9.2	557	3.1	52	37	2.8
Spicy, Mix Ups, Walkers*	¼ Pack/30g	148	7.2	492	6.4	60	24	3.6
Spring Onion, Tayto*	1 Bag/35g	184	11.9	526	7.6	47.3	34	4.5
Squirrel, Cajun, Walkers*	1 Bag/25g	130	8.2	522	5.8	51.2	32.7	4.2
Steak, Chargrilled, Max, Walkers*	1 Bag/55g	289	18.2	525	6.5	50	33	4
Steak, Flame Grilled, Argentinean, Walkers*	1 Bag/35g	182	11.3	520	6.5	50.7	32.4	4.2
Steak, Flame Grilled, Ridge Cut, McCoys*	1 Bag/47g	250	14.7	526	6.9	53	31	3.9
Steak, Flamed Grilled, Max, Walkers*	1 Pack/50g	266	16.4	533	6.5	51.6	32.8	2.8
Steak, T Bone, Bubble Chips, Roysters*	1 Pack/28g	151	8.9	540	5.5	55	32	2.6
Sunbites, Cheddar Caramelised Onion, Walkers*	1 Bag/25g	120	5.4	480	7.6	60.8	21.6	6.4
Sweet Smokin', Hippeas*	1 Pack/22g	90	3.8	411	13.2	51.1	17.4	7.3
Sweet Chilli, & Red Pepper, Potato Chips, Tyrrells*	¼ Pack/37g	180	9.2	481	7.9	59.7	24.5	2.4
Sweet Chilli, Average	*1 Bag/25g*	*115*	*5.6*	*461*	*5.1*	*59.9*	*22.6*	*4.6*
Sweet Chilli, Crinkle Cut, Finest, Tesco*	1 Serving/25g	124	6.6	497	7.5	54.5	26.6	4.9
Sweet Chilli, Hand Cooked, M&S*	1 Pack/40g	207	12.1	517	6.1	52.8	30.2	4.6
Sweet Chilli, Lentil, Curls, Bites, Kettle Chips*	1 Pack/22g	94	2.6	428	13.2	65	11.9	4
Sweet Chilli, Mountain Chips, Muscle Moose*	1 Pack/23g	93	2.1	405	22	55	9.1	8.4
Sweet Chilli, Thai, Lentil Waves, Burts*	1 Pack/20g	91	3.3	453	11.7	62.6	16.3	4.9
Sweet Chilli, Thai, Sensations, Walkers*	1 Bag/40g	194	10.4	485	6	57	26	4.2
Sweet Chilli, Thai, Velvet Crunch, King*	1 Pack/20g	81	1.9	404	1.6	77.5	9.7	2

C

CRISPS

Measure INFO/WEIGHT	per Measure KCAL	FAT	Nutrition Values per 100g / 100ml KCAL	PROT	CARB	FAT	FIBRE

CRISPS

	Measure INFO/WEIGHT	KCAL	FAT	KCAL	PROT	CARB	FAT	FIBRE
Sweet Potato, Lightly Salted, Baked, Kettle Chips*	1 Serving/20g	82	2.7	409	6.3	60	13.4	11.6
Tangy Toms, Red Mill*	1 Bag/15g	76	4.1	507	6	60	27.3	0.7
Thai Bites, Mild, Jacob's*	1 Bag/25g	93	0.8	373	6.9	79	3.3	1
Thai Curry, & Coriander, Tyrrells*	1 Pack/50g	261	14	522	6.1	56.5	27.9	5.4
Tomato Basil, Houmous Chips, Eat Real*	1 Serving/28g	126	4.8	449	6.5	68.4	17	4.5
Tomato Basil, Lentil Chips, Eat Real*	1 Serving/28g	130	5.4	466	9.3	66	19.5	3.2
Tomato Herbs, Baked Fusions, Snacks, Walkers*	1 Pack/22g	95	3	433	6.7	68.3	13.5	6.4
Tomato Ketchup, Golden Wonder*	1 Bag/25g	135	8	521	5.1	54	30.8	3.6
Turkey, & Stuffing, Walkers*	1 Bag/25g	126	6.8	504	6.4	56.4	27.2	4.4
Twirls, Salt Vinegar, Co-Op*	1 Bag/40g	170	8	425	5	57.5	20	5
Twirls, Salt Vinegar, Sainsbury's*	½ Bag/40g	167	5.6	418	3	70.1	14	3
Twirls, Salt Vinegar, Tesco*	1 Bag/80g	349	14	436	3.9	65.8	17.5	2.4
Unsalted, Seabrook*	1 Bag/30g	163	10.7	544	5.7	47.9	35.8	4.1
Vegetable, Average	*1 Bag/25g*	*118*	*7.4*	*470*	*4.1*	*46.5*	*29.6*	*12.1*
Vegetable, Crunchy, Asda*	½ Bag/50g	251	12	502	1.4	70	24	6
Vegetable, Finest, Tesco*	1 Serving/50g	203	12.8	406	5	39	25.5	14.6
Vegetable, Waitrose*	1 Pack/100g	490	35.2	490	4.7	38.5	35.2	13
Veggie Kale, Straws, Eat Real*	1 Bag/22g	109	5.6	497	3.1	65.1	25.5	2.8
Wasabi, Strong, Max, Walkers*	1 Pack/30g	160	9.9	534	6.3	51.7	32.9	2.9
Wheat Crunchies, Golden Wonder*	1 Pack/35g	172	8.7	491	11.1	55.9	24.8	0
Worcester Sauce, Sunseed Oil, Walkers*	1 Bag/33g	168	9.9	516	6.2	52	30.5	4.3

CRISPY PANCAKE

	Measure INFO/WEIGHT	KCAL	FAT	KCAL	PROT	CARB	FAT	FIBRE
Beef Bolognese, Findus*	1 Pancake/65g	104	2.6	160	6.5	25	4	1
Chicken, Bacon & Sweetcorn, Findus*	1 Pancake/63g	101	2.5	160	5.5	26	4	1.1
Minced Beef, As Consumed, Findus*	1 Pancake/115g	178	2.9	155	6.2	26	2.5	1.9
Three Cheeses, As Consumed, Findus*	2 Pancakes/107g	183	3.6	171	6.5	28	3.4	1.4

CROISSANT

	Measure INFO/WEIGHT	KCAL	FAT	KCAL	PROT	CARB	FAT	FIBRE
All Butter, Bakers Selection, Asda*	1 Croissant/40g	164	8.4	412	6.9	48	21	1.9
All Butter, Finest, Tesco*	1 Croissant/62g	258	14.3	415	7.9	42.9	23.1	1.9
All Butter, M&S*	1 Croissant/40g	179	10.8	447	10.1	40.1	27	1.6
All Butter, Mini, Sainsbury's*	1 Croissant/30g	126	7	420	8.1	42.9	23.4	2.6
All Butter, Reduced Fat, Tesco*	1 Croissant/52g	164	5.5	315	7.5	47.4	10.6	1.8
All Butter, Sainsbury's*	1 Croissant/44g	166	7.5	377	9	46.2	17	1.3
All Butter, Tesco*	1 Croissant/44g	168	7.5	383	9	47.2	17	2.6
Almond, Bakery, Tesco*	1 Crossant/84g	342	17.7	407	9.3	43.8	21	2.4
Asda*	1 Croissant/47g	190	9.9	405	9	45	21	0
Average	*1 Croissant/50g*	*180*	*10.2*	*360*	*8.3*	*38.3*	*20.3*	*1.6*
Butter, Bakery, Tesco*	1 Croissant/72g	285	13.7	396	9.3	46.1	19	1.6
Butter, Charentes, Waitrose*	1 Croissant/41g	176	9.7	430	8.7	44.2	23.8	2.4
Butter, Morrisons*	1 Croissant/44g	196	12.5	446	9.3	38.2	28.4	2
Cheese & Ham, Delice de France*	1 Serving/91g	225	12.3	247	7	24.4	13.5	2.5
Cheese Ham, Mini, Waitrose*	1 Croissant/17g	64	4.1	383	13.2	28.1	24.6	3
Chocolate Filled, All Butter, Finest, Tesco*	1 Croissant/75g	267	11.3	355	7.4	45.9	15.1	2.8
Flaky Pastry with a Plain Chocolate Filling, Tesco*	1 Croissant/83g	369	20.8	445	8.6	45	25.1	2.6
French Butter, You Count, Love Life, Waitrose*	1 Croissant/44g	168	7.4	382	9.8	46.4	16.8	3.1
Hazlenut, Waitrose*	1 Croissant/95g	466	29.9	490	8.3	41.6	31.5	3.6
Low Fat, M&S*	1 Croissant/49g	195	7.8	398	9.8	52.9	15.9	1.8
Mini, Lidl*	1 Croissant/30g	112	5	373	7.8	48	16.6	0
Reduced Fat, Asda*	1 Croissant/44g	159	6.5	361	9.7	47.2	14.8	2
TTD, Sainsbury's*	1 Croissant/60g	264	15.7	440	9.7	40.6	26.1	0
Wholesome, Sainsbury's*	1 Croissant/44g	192	12.1	436	8.8	38.3	27.5	4
with Cocoa Filling, Max, 7 Days*	1 Croissant/28g	128	7.8	456	6	44	28	0

	Measure INFO/WEIGHT	per Measure KCAL	FAT	Nutrition Values per 100g / 100ml KCAL	PROT	CARB	FAT	FIBRE
CROQUETTES								
Potato, Asda*	3 Croquettes/81g	144	5.7	177	2	26.5	7	2.2
Potato, Birds Eye*	1 Croquette/29g	44	1.7	152	2.6	22.6	5.7	1.2
Potato, Chunky, Aunt Bessie's*	3 Croquettes/119g	192	9.5	162	2.3	19	8	2.8
Potato, Cooked, Sainsbury's*	2 Croquettes73g	157	7.6	214	2.9	26	10.3	2.6
Potato, Fried in Blended Oil, Average	*1 Croquette/80g*	*171*	*10.5*	*214*	*3.7*	*21.6*	*13.1*	*1.3*
Potato, Frozen, HFC, Tesco*	1 Serving/128g	266	11.7	208	3.3	26.5	9.1	3.2
Potato, Tesco*	1 Croquette/40g	83	3.6	208	3.9	26.6	9.1	2
Potato, Waitrose*	1 Croquette/30g	47	2.4	157	3	17.9	8.1	1.5
Serrano Ham Manchego, World Cafe, Waitrose*	½ Pack/78g	238	14	305	8.4	26.1	18	2.6
CROSTINI								
with Goats Cheese Red Onion Chutney, Waitrose*	1 Crostini/17g	47	1.3	274	9.1	33.5	7.8	3.1
with Oregano, Crosta & Mollica*	1 Pack/150g	726	21.2	484	11.7	74.2	14.1	6.4
CROUTONS								
Fresh, M&S*	1 Serving/10g	53	3.3	530	11.4	50	32.8	3.2
Garlic, Waitrose*	1 Serving/40g	209	12	522	10.8	52.1	30	2.7
Herb, Sainsbury's*	1 Serving/15g	64	1.7	429	13.4	68.2	11.4	2.8
Lightly Sea Salted, Asda*	1 Serving/20g	83	1.9	414	12.9	69.7	9.3	4.3
Prepacked, Average	*1 Serving/15g*	*74*	*3.6*	*495*	*10.8*	*58.7*	*24*	*2.6*
Sun Dried Tomato, Sainsbury's*	¼ Pack/15g	75	3.8	497	11.7	55.2	25.5	2.5
CRUDITES								
Platter, Sainsbury's*	1 Pack/275g	96	0.8	35	1.4	6.6	0.3	1.6
Selection, Prepared, M&S*	1 Serving/250g	75	1	30	1.4	5.8	0.4	2
Vegetable Sticks, Average	*1 Serving/100g*	*24*	*0.2*	*24*	*0.7*	*4.5*	*0.2*	*1.9*
with Cheese Chive Dip, Tesco*	1 Pack/115g	132	10.5	115	1.6	5.9	9.1	1.5
CRUMBLE								
Almond, & Apricot, Devondale*	1 Cake/80g	314	13.2	392	3.6	57	16.5	9.8
Apple, & Blackberry, Asda*	1 Serving/175g	427	15.8	244	2.7	38	9	1.2
Apple, & Blackberry, Bramley, BGTY, Sainsbury's*	1 Crumble/120g	217	3.2	181	1.7	35.8	2.7	2.2
Apple, & Blackberry, Budgens*	1 Serving/240g	821	31.2	342	3.7	54	13	0.6
Apple, & Blackberry, M&S*	1 Serving/135g	398	15.1	295	3.5	44.9	11.2	1.6
Apple, & Blackberry, Sainsbury's*	1 Serving/110g	232	6.2	211	3	37.1	5.6	2.1
Apple, & Blackberry, Tesco*	1/6 Pie/90g	286	11.7	318	3	45.8	13	2.8
Apple, & Custard, Asda*	1 Serving/125g	250	8.8	200	2.3	32	7	0
Apple, & Toffee, Weight Watchers*	1 Pot/98g	190	4.5	194	1.6	36.6	4.6	0
Apple, Average	*1 Serving/240g*	*497*	*12*	*207*	*0.9*	*40.5*	*5*	*1.1*
Apple, Basics, Sainsbury's*	¼ Crumble/125g	235	4.9	188	1.7	36.5	3.9	1.2
Apple, Blackberry & Plum, Bramley, Finest, Tesco*	½ Pack/175g	396	14.9	226	2.6	33.5	8.5	2.6
Apple, Bramley, 2 Pots, Sainsbury's*	1 Pot/116g	303	9.5	261	2.6	43.2	8.2	2.1
Apple, Bramley, CBY, Asda*	1 Serving/100g	257	8.4	257	2.5	41.8	8.4	2.3
Apple, Bramley, Favourites, M&S*	1 Serving/140g	390	13.8	279	4.6	43.2	9.9	1.2
Apple, Bramley, M&S*	1 Serving/149g	387	13.7	260	4.3	40.3	9.2	1.1
Apple, Bramley, Tesco*	1/3 Pack/155g	378	14.9	244	2.8	36.7	9.6	1.8
Apple, Co-Op*	¼ Crumble/110g	270	7.7	245	2	43	7	2
Apple, Fresh, Chilled, Tesco*	¼ Pack/135g	342	11.2	253	3	40.6	8.3	1.8
Apple, Sainsbury's*	1 Crumble/565g	1034	32.8	183	2.3	30.5	5.8	2.9
Apple, Sara Lee*	1 Serving/200g	606	18	303	2.3	53.3	9	1.2
Apple, Slices, Frozen, Tesco*	1 Slice/54g	173	8	321	4.9	40.6	14.9	2.8
Apple, Toffee, As Consumed, Morrisons*	¼ Crumble/122g	326	11.4	267	1.9	42.9	9.3	2
Apple, Waitrose*	1 Serving/125g	310	2.9	248	2.2	54.5	2.3	1.2
Apple, with Custard, Green's*	1 Serving/79g	171	5.3	216	1.9	37	6.7	1.2
Apple, with Custard, Individual, Sainsbury's*	1 Pudding/120g	286	13.9	238	2	31.4	11.6	2.4
Apple, with Sultanas, Weight Watchers*	1 Dessert/110g	196	4.3	178	1.4	34.2	3.9	1.3
Blackcurrant, & Apple, Devondale*	1 Cake/80g	314	13.2	393	3.6	57	16.5	9.8

	Measure INFO/WEIGHT	KCAL	FAT	Nutrition Values per 100g / 100ml				
				KCAL	PROT	CARB	FAT	FIBRE
CRUMBLE								
Fruit	*1 Portion/170g*	*337*	*11.7*	*198*	*2*	*34*	*6.9*	*1.7*
Fruit, Wholemeal	*1oz/28g*	*54*	*2*	*193*	*2.6*	*31.7*	*7.1*	*2.7*
Fruit, with Custard	*1 Serving/270g*	*463*	*17.6*	*171*	*2.4*	*27*	*6.5*	*1.3*
Gooseberry, M&S*	1 Serving/133g	379	14.2	285	3.5	43.3	10.7	1.7
Plum, & Cherry, 775, Wiltshire Farm Foods*	1 Serving/120g	248	7.4	194	2.3	34	5.8	0
Rhubarb, Asda*	½ Crumble/200g	460	24	230	2.4	28	12	5
Rhubarb, Average	*1 Portion/150g*	*330*	*11.1*	*220*	*2.7*	*35.5*	*7.4*	*1.9*
Rhubarb, Devondale*	1 Cake/80g	316	13.2	395	3.5	57	16.5	9
Rhubarb, M&S*	1 Serving/133g	366	13.2	275	3.4	42.6	9.9	1.4
Rhubarb, Sainsbury's*	1 Serving/50g	112	2.8	224	3.1	40.4	5.6	1.8
Rhubarb, Tesco*	1 Serving/136g	318	10.6	234	3.6	36.1	7.8	2.5
Rhubarb, with Custard, Sainsbury's*	1 Serving/120g	288	13.9	240	2.4	31.4	11.6	2.3
CRUMBLE MIX								
Luxury, Tesco*	¼ Pack/55g	243	9	441	5.7	67.9	16.3	3.2
Topping, Sainsbury's*	1 Serving/47g	188	9.2	401	5.9	50.3	19.6	5.3
CRUMPETS								
Asda*	1 Crumpet/45g	85	0.4	188	6	39	0.9	2.1
Bakers Selection, Asda*	1 Crumpet/50g	106	0.6	211	6.7	42	1.2	2.7
Buttermilk, TTD, Sainsbury's*	1 Crumpet/52g	102	0.6	195	6.5	38.5	1.1	2.6
Co-Op*	1 Crumpet/40g	70	0.3	175	7	35	0.7	2
Essential, Waitrose*	1 Crumpet/52g	94	0.6	182	6.5	35.1	1.1	2.6
Golden Sun, Lidl*	1 Crumpet/43g	83	0.7	193	7.8	37.1	1.6	1.6
Morrisons*	1 Crumpet/40g	90	0.2	225	7.8	47.2	0.5	3.2
Premium, Sainsbury's*	1 Crumpet/50g	96	0.7	191	6.1	38.6	1.4	1.7
Rowan Hill Bakery, Lidl*	1 Crumpet/44g	78	0.5	178	5.5	34.5	1.2	0
Square, Tesco*	1 Crumpet/60g	101	0.5	168	6.3	33.8	0.8	2.7
Thins , Kingsmill*	1 Thin/27g	54	0.3	199	6.9	39.3	1.1	2.3
Toasted, Average	*1 Crumpet/40g*	*80*	*0.4*	*199*	*6.7*	*43.4*	*1*	*2*
Toasted, Tesco*	1 Crumpet/55g	106	0.6	193	5.8	39.1	1	2.2
Waitrose*	1 Crumpet/62g	116	0.7	188	6.3	37.9	1.2	2.1
Warburton's*	1 Crumpet/55g	97	0.4	176	6	35.3	0.8	1.9
Wholemeal, Bakers Selection, Asda*	1 Crumpet/50g	94	0.4	189	7.3	36	0.8	3.7
CRUNCHIE								
Blast, Cadbury*	1 Serving/42g	199	8.3	480	4.7	69.6	20.1	0.7
Cadbury*	1 Bar/40g	185	7.5	465	4	69.5	18.9	0.5
Nuggets, Cadbury*	1 Bag/125g	569	20.5	455	3.8	73.1	16.4	0
Treat Size, Cadbury*	1 Bar/17g	80	3.1	470	4	71.5	18.4	0
CUCUMBER								
Average	*1 Serving/80g*	*8*	*0.1*	*10*	*0.7*	*1.5*	*0.1*	*0.6*
Baby, Pickled, Always Fresh*	1 Serving/30g	14	0.1	47	2	8	0.3	0
Baby, Raw, Tesco*	2 Cucumbers/80g	12	0.5	16	1	1.2	0.6	0.7
Crunchies with a Yoghurt Mint Dip, Shapers, Boots*	1 Serving/110g	35	1	32	2.1	3.7	0.9	0.8
CUMIN								
Seeds, Whole, Average	*1 Tsp/2g*	*8*	*0.5*	*375*	*17.8*	*44.2*	*22.7*	*10.5*
CUPCAKES								
Assorted, Sainsbury's*	1 Cake/38g	130	2.3	341	2.2	69.3	6.1	0.4
Carrot, Average	*1 Cake/40g*	*157*	*8.6*	*392*	*3.6*	*45.4*	*21.6*	*0.6*
Celebration, Tesco*	1 Cupcake/61g	310	17.8	510	2.6	58.5	29.3	1
Chocolate Filled, Free From, Tesco*	1 Cupcake/52g	238	13.1	459	3.4	53.6	25.3	1.6
Chocolate Fudge, Party Pack, Tesco*	1 Cupcake/63g	300	17.5	476	4.2	50.7	27.8	3
Chocolate Iced, Chocolate Buttons, Party Selection, Tesco*	1 Cake/32g	144	7.6	450	4.4	54.1	23.6	1.5
Chocolate, Average	*1 Cake/40g*	*159*	*6.4*	*398*	*3.5*	*59.9*	*16*	*1.2*
Chocolate, BGTY, Sainsbury's*	1 Cake/38g	121	1.7	318	2.5	66.5	4.6	0.8

	Measure INFO/WEIGHT	per Measure KCAL	FAT	Nutrition Values per 100g / 100ml KCAL	PROT	CARB	FAT	FIBRE
CUPCAKES								
Chocolate, COU, M&S*	1 Cake/45g	130	1.3	290	4.6	62.2	2.8	4.3
Chocolate, Fabulous Bakin' Boys*	1 Cupcake/34g	152	8.1	448	4	54	24	1
Chocolate, GF, Genius *	1 Cupcake/63g	295	15.1	469	3.1	59.2	24	1.7
Chocolate, Lyons*	1 Cake/39g	125	1.8	321	2.4	67.5	4.6	0.8
Chocolate, Mini, Weight Watchers*	1 Cupcake/20g	87	4.3	426	6.1	52	21.1	1.8
Chocolate, Party Platter, Holly Lane, Aldi*	1 Cake/55g	268	16	487	3.1	53	29	1.4
Chocolate, Party Selection, Tesco*	1 Cake/47g	230	13.3	486	3.3	54.1	28	2.5
Cookies Cream, Secret Chocolate Centre, Tesco*	1 Cupcake/69g	335	20	485	2.7	52.2	29	1
Funcakes, Mini, Peppa Pig*	1 Cake/26g	104	5	400	3.2	53.5	19.1	0
Ginger, Christmas, Mini, Free From, Tesco*	1 Cupcake/22g	100	4.7	456	3.4	61.7	21.6	0.5
Iced Cupcake, Gluten Wheat Free, Lovemore*	1 Cake/33g	138	6.3	418	2.1	54.5	19	0.4
Jam Splatter, Tesco*	1 Cake/47g	221	10.2	470	2.3	65.6	21.8	0.5
Jelly Brain, Gruesome Gooey, Tesco*	1 Cupcake/84g	403	21.5	482	2.8	59.1	25.7	1.4
Lemon, Average	**1 Cake/40g**	**184**	**10.1**	**461**	**3**	**55.5**	**25.3**	**1.1**
Lemon, COU, M&S*	1 Cupcake/43g	130	0.9	305	3.3	68.1	2.1	2
Lemon, Healthy Option, Average	**1 Cake/40g**	**131**	**1.5**	**328**	**2.7**	**68.9**	**3.7**	**5.2**
Lemon, Mini, Weight Watchers*	1 Cupcake/17g	56	0.8	333	2.4	63.3	4.9	12.1
Pink Maggot, Gruesome Gooey, Tesco*	1 Cupcake/65g	303	15.3	468	2.4	60.7	23.6	1.3
Pink, M&S*	1 Cupcake/39g	160	3.3	410	2.5	81.3	8.5	0.6
Red Velvet, Party Pack, Tesco*	1 Cupcake/62g	308	17.5	497	2.5	56.8	28.3	2.6
Red Velvet, Tesco*	1 Cupcake/63g	308	16.6	490	3.1	59.3	26.4	1.2
Sponge Top, Individual, Tesco*	1 Cupcake/50g	220	10.5	443	3	59.5	21.1	1.3
Strawberry Cream, Party Pack, Tesco*	1 Cupcake/65g	316	17.8	486	2.5	56.8	27.3	1.8
Strawberry, Party Selection, Tesco*	1 Cake/46g	229	13.3	496	2	55.8	28.8	2.8
Toffee, Christmas, Mini, Free From, Tesco*	1 Cupcake/18g	82	4.1	460	3.6	59.4	23	0.5
Toffee, Thorntons*	1 Cupcake/80g	330	16	412	2.4	56	20	0
Unicorn, Tesco*	1 Cupcake/63g	316	17.6	502	3.2	58.6	28	1.1
Vanilla, Party Platter, Holly Lane, Aldi*	1 Cake/57g	282	16	494	2.6	56	28	2.1
Vanilla, Party Selection, Tesco*	1 Cake/46g	230	13.1	495	2.6	57.2	28.1	1.5
White Chocolate, Vanilla, Tesco*	1 Cupcake/76g	390	22.5	513	1.7	59.7	29.6	0.8
White Iced, with Sugar Strands, Party Selection, Tesco*	1 Cake/33g	142	6.7	430	4.2	57.1	20.2	1.4
CURACAO								
Average	**1 Pub Shot/35ml**	**109**	**0**	**311**	**0**	**28.3**	**0**	**0**
CURLY WURLY								
Cadbury*	1 Bar/26g	118	4.7	453	3.1	70	18	0.7
Squirlies, Cadbury*	1 Squirl/3g	13	0.5	442	3.5	69.2	17.3	0.8
CURRANTS								
Average	**1oz/28g**	**75**	**0.1**	**267**	**2.3**	**67.8**	**0.4**	**1.9**
CURRY								
Chips, Curry Sauce, Chipped Potatoes, Kershaws*	1 Serving/330g	391	8.2	118	10	14	2.5	2
Aubergine	**1oz/28g**	**33**	**2.8**	**118**	**1.4**	**6.2**	**10.1**	**1.5**
Aubergine, Masala, TTD, Sainsbury's*	½ Pack/115g	135	11.4	117	2.9	4.1	9.9	5.8
Beef, Sainsbury's*	1 Serving/400g	552	32.8	138	10.7	5.4	8.2	0.9
Beef, Thai, Finest, Tesco*	1 Serving/500g	770	29	154	9	16.5	5.8	1.2
Beef, with Rice, Iceland*,	1 Pack/500g	580	14.5	116	5	16.7	2.9	1.5
Beef, with Rice, Morrisons*	1 Serving/400g	480	20	120	6	12.6	5	0.6
Blackeye Bean, Gujerati	**1oz/28g**	**36**	**1.2**	**127**	**7.2**	**16.1**	**4.4**	**2.8**
Butternut Squash, with Long Grain Rice, Kirstys*	1 Meal/307g	338	16	110	1.7	13.2	5.2	1.9
Cabbage	**1oz/28g**	**23**	**1.4**	**82**	**1.9**	**8.1**	**5**	**2.1**
Cauliflower & Potato	**1oz/28g**	**17**	**0.7**	**59**	**3.4**	**6.6**	**2.4**	**1.8**
Cauliflower, & Chickpea, Lovely Vegetables, M&S*	1 Serving/390g	351	13.6	90	2.9	11.2	3.5	3.7
Chana Saag, Slimming World*	1 Pack/350g	256	4.9	73	4.4	7.3	1.4	6.8
Chennai Dhal, Chickpea, Mumbai Street Food, Iceland*	1 Meal/181g	174	8	96	4.3	8	4.4	4

C

	Measure INFO/WEIGHT	per Measure KCAL	FAT	Nutrition Values per 100g / 100ml KCAL	PROT	CARB	FAT	FIBRE
CURRY								
Chick Pea, Whole, Average	*1oz/28g*	*50*	*2.1*	*179*	*9.6*	*21.3*	*7.5*	*4.5*
Chick Pea, Whole, Basic, Average	*1oz/28g*	*30*	*1*	*108*	*6*	*14.2*	*3.6*	*3.3*
Chicken, Vegetable, Green Thai, with Rice, Tesco*	1 Serving/346g	339	3.5	98	6.1	15.8	1	0.9
Chicken, Butter, Rice, Taste of India, Tesco*	1 Pack/427g	624	29.9	146	6.4	12.8	7	3.1
Chicken, Butter, Takeaway, Tesco*	½ Pack/175g	224	13.3	128	7.9	6.4	7.6	1.2
Chicken, Chinese Style, Musclefood*	1 Serving/293g	264	5.3	90	14.9	3.4	1.8	0.5
Chicken, Chinese with Rice, Ready Meal, Average	*1 Serving/450g*	*490*	*11.5*	*109*	*7.2*	*14.1*	*2.6*	*1.3*
Chicken, Chinese, Meal for Two, Meal Box, Tesco*	½ Pack/163g	173	7.2	106	10.9	5.2	4.4	1
Chicken, Chinese, Morrisons*	1 Pack/340g	347	15.6	102	10.3	5	4.6	0.8
Chicken, Chinese, Sharwoods*	1 Pack/375g	420	10.1	112	5	16.1	2.7	1.5
Chicken, Chinese, Takeaway, Tesco*	½ Pack/182g	191	8.6	105	9.7	5.7	4.7	0.5
Chicken, Coconut, with Jasmine Rice, Tesco*	1 Pack/420g	482	8.8	115	7.1	16.7	2.1	0.4
Chicken, Dhansak, Kit, Musclefood*	1 Serving/506g	349	0.5	69	11.7	4.5	0.1	2.3
Chicken, Green Thai Style Sticky Rice, Asda*	1 Pack/450g	585	10.8	130	7	20	2.4	0.1
Chicken, Green Thai, Balanced for You, M&S*	1 Pack/395g	383	5.9	97	7.8	12.7	1.5	1
Chicken, Green Thai, Charlie Bigham's*	½ Pack/300g	342	21	114	8.7	4.8	7	0
Chicken, Green, Thai, Jasmine Rice, Sainsbury's*	½ Pack/188g	184	4.7	98	7.9	10.5	2.5	1.3
Chicken, Hot, Can, Tesco*	1 Can/418g	514	26.3	123	9.7	6.9	6.3	0.9
Chicken, Jamaican, with Rice, Well & Good, Co-Op*	1 Pack/350g	287	2.8	82	6.8	11	0.8	1.6
Chicken, Kashmiri, Waitrose*	1 Serving/400g	640	36.4	160	14.5	5	9.1	0.6
Chicken, Malaysian, Finest, Tesco*	1 Pack/375g	375	8.3	100	7.4	12.2	2.2	0.8
Chicken, Mild, Canned, Bilash, Aldi*	½ Can/200g	180	7.6	90	9.5	4.5	3.8	0.7
Chicken, Mild, Tinned, Sainsbury's*	1 Serving/200g	214	7	107	12.7	6.1	3.5	1.1
Chicken, Panang, Taste Thailand, Banquet Box, M&S*	½ Pack/115g	170	11.2	148	10.9	5.2	9.7	1.2
Chicken, Piri Piri, Cajun Rice, Asda*	1 Pack/380g	410	8.7	108	6.7	14	2.3	2.6
Chicken, Red Thai, with Jasmine Rice, Finest, Tesco*	1 Pack/413g	719	28.5	174	8.4	19.1	6.9	0.9
Chicken, Sweet Sour, Chinese, Tesco*	1 Pack/507g	684	21.8	135	6.6	16.7	4.3	1.6
Chicken, Thai Green, Curry Meal Box, Tesco*	½ Pack/162g	192	10	118	10.6	4.5	6.2	1.2
Chicken, Thai Green, Just Cook, Tesco*	1 Pack/304g	392	10.6	129	8.1	15.7	3.5	1.3
Chicken, Thai Green, Rice, Pot, Musclefood*	1 Serving/309g	272	2.2	88	10.8	8.8	0.7	1.8
Chicken, Thai Green, Taste of Thailand, Tesco*	½ Pack/223g	258	14.9	116	8.1	5.2	6.7	1.1
Chicken, Thai Red, Curry Meal Box, Tesco*	½ Pack/167g	195	10.3	117	10.1	4.8	6.2	1
Chicken, Thai Red, Takeaway, Tesco*	½ Pack/193g	233	13.1	121	8.9	5.7	6.8	0.5
Chicken, Thai, Green, & Jasmine Rice, Ready Meal	*1 Serving/450g*	*520*	*17.2*	*116*	*7.7*	*12.6*	*3.8*	*1.1*
Chicken, Thai, Green, No Rice, Average	*1 Serving/200g*	*174*	*7*	*87*	*8.2*	*5*	*3.5*	*1.4*
Chicken, Thai, Green, Taste Thailand, Banquet Box, M&S*	½ Pack/115g	155	11	135	8.9	2.7	9.6	1.1
Chicken, Thai, Red, & Jasmine Rice, Ready Meal	*1 Serving/450g*	*500*	*15.3*	*111*	*7.5*	*12.6*	*3.4*	*1*
Chicken, Thai, Red, & Rice, Ready Meal, Healthy	*1 Serving/400g*	*400*	*7.8*	*100*	*6.4*	*14*	*2*	*1*
Chicken, Thai, Red, & Sticky Rice, Ready Meal	*1 Serving/450g*	*527*	*15.7*	*117*	*6.7*	*14.2*	*3.5*	*1.7*
Chicken, Thai, Red, HE, Tesco*	1 Pack/380g	373	5	105	6.4	15.4	1.4	2.5
Chicken, Thai, Red, No Rice, Average	*1 Serving/200g*	*194*	*6.9*	*97*	*7.2*	*9*	*3.4*	*1.4*
Chicken, Tikka, Biryani, Tesco*	1 Pack/365g	599	13.9	164	10.2	20.7	3.8	3.5
Chicken, with Rice, Average	*1 Serving/400g*	*465*	*11*	*116*	*5.1*	*17.8*	*2.8*	*0.8*
Chicken, with Rice, Basics, Sainsbury's*	1 Pack/343g	477	9.3	139	6	21.7	2.7	1.7
Chicken, with Rice, Fresh, Co-Op*	1 Pack/300g	270	9	90	3	13	3	1
Chicken, with Rice, Fruity, HL, Tesco*	1 Pack/450g	495	5.4	110	6.5	18.2	1.2	1.2
Chicken, with Rice, Ready Meal, Average	*1 Serving/400g*	*446*	*10.5*	*112*	*5.2*	*16.8*	*2.6*	*1*
Chicken, Yellow Thai Style, HL, Tesco*	1 Pack/450g	504	12.2	112	9.3	12.6	2.7	0.5
Courgette, & Potato	*1oz/28g*	*24*	*1.5*	*86*	*1.9*	*8.7*	*5.2*	*1.2*
Dudhi, Kofta	*1oz/28g*	*32*	*2.1*	*113*	*2.6*	*9.4*	*7.4*	*2.8*
Fish, & Vegetable, Bangladeshi, Average	*1oz/28g*	*33*	*2.4*	*117*	*9.1*	*1.4*	*8.4*	*0.5*
Fish, Bangladeshi, Average	*1oz/28g*	*35*	*2.2*	*124*	*12.2*	*1.5*	*7.9*	*0.3*
Fish, Red Thai, Waitrose*	1 Pack/500g	275	11	55	5.2	3.7	2.2	1

CURRENT

INFO/WEIGHT	Measure	per Measure KCAL	FAT	Nutrition Values per 100g / 100ml KCAL	PROT	CARB	FAT	FIBRE
CURRY								
Fish, Thai Red, Snap Peas, Musclefood*	1 Pack/350g	315	6.3	90	7.1	11.1	1.8	0.8
Keralan, Sundown, Allplants*	½ Pack/380g	707	41.8	186	4.2	17	11	2.8
Lamb, & Potato, 385, Wiltshire Farm Foods*	1 Serving/210g	334	23	159	8.9	6.2	11	1.7
Lamb, Aromatic, Balanced for You, M&S*	1 Pack/380g	388	9.1	102	9	9.2	2.4	3.7
Lamb, Hot, M&S*	½ Can/213g	320	19.6	150	14.9	6	9.2	2.3
Lentil, Canned, Creationz, Heinz*	1 Can/390g	277	3.9	71	4	10.4	1	2.3
Mushroom, & Pea, Masala, Indian, Sainsbury's*	1 Pack/300g	264	14.7	88	3.3	5.2	4.9	5.1
Paneer, & Parsnip, Everdine*	1 Serving/450g	567	22.9	126	5.3	12.8	5.1	3.9
Paneer, & Sweet Potato, Kofte Biryani, Everdine*	1 Serving/450g	562	22.1	125	3.8	13.1	4.9	6.7
Paneer, Spiced Chilli, Bowl, Vegetarian, Indian, Waitrose*	1 Pack/300g	387	13.8	129	6.2	14.9	4.5	2.1
Pav Bhaji, Kohinoor*	1 Pack/300g	282	16.2	94	2.3	10.4	5.4	2.8
Potato & Pea	*1oz/28g*	*26*	*1.1*	*92*	*2.9*	*13*	*3.8*	*2.4*
Prawn, & Mushroom	*1oz/28g*	*47*	*4*	*168*	*7.3*	*2.5*	*14.4*	*1*
Prawn, Coconut & Lime, King, Sainsbury's*	½ Pack/351g	207	8.8	59	3.7	5.4	2.5	1
Prawn, Goan, King, M&S*	1 Pack/400g	680	44.4	170	5.1	11.6	11.1	1.5
Prawn, King, Taste Sri Lanka, M&S*	1 Pack/350g	413	23.4	118	6.3	7.3	6.7	1.6
Prawn, Malay, King, Waitrose*	1 Pack/350g	364	19.2	104	6.6	7.1	5.5	0.9
Prawn, Red Thai, King, City Kitchen, Tesco*	1 Pack/385g	460	14.4	119	4.5	16.7	3.7	1
Prawn, Red Thai, Sainsbury's*	1 Pack/300g	546	39.6	182	6.3	9.4	13.2	1.7
Prawn, Sri Lankan, Giraffe*	1 Pack/368g	497	24.3	135	4	13.8	6.6	2.1
Prawn, Takeaway, Average	*1 Serving/350g*	*410*	*29.8*	*117*	*8.2*	*2.2*	*8.5*	*2*
Prawn, with Rice, Basics, Sainsbury's*	1 Pack/331g	430	6.6	130	4.3	22.5	2	2.3
Prawn, with Rice, Frozen, Sainsbury's*	1 Pack/400g	552	7.6	138	3.9	26.4	1.9	2.1
Red Kidney Bean, Punjabi	*1oz/28g*	*30*	*1.6*	*106*	*4.7*	*10.1*	*5.6*	*3.8*
Red Thai, Vegetarian, Tesco*	1 Pack/429ml	588	21.9	137	5.4	17.3	5.1	1.6
Root, Ruby 7, Microwaved, Mumbai Street Food, Iceland*	1 Meal/224g	222	14.8	99	1.7	7.1	6.6	1.8
Salmon, Green, Waitrose*	1 Pack/401g	581	40.5	145	9.1	4.5	10.1	2.7
Sambar Mix, Lentil Vegetable, Fudco*	1 Box/100g	354	13.2	354	13.6	45.3	13.2	9.6
South Indian, Bowl, Tesco*	1 Pack/377g	351	11.1	93	4.3	11.5	2.9	1.8
Sri Lankan Sambar, Pot, Bol*	1 Pot/345g	310	8.6	90	5.3	9.4	2.5	4.4
Sri Lankan Veg, Weight Watchers*	1 Pack/380g	171	6.1	45	1.5	5.2	1.6	2
Sweet Potato, Slimfree, Aldi*	1 Pack/500g	250	3	50	2.3	6.5	0.6	4.8
Thai Green, Veggie, Organic, Pot, Clive's*	1 Pot/400g	268	14	67	2.1	5.6	3.5	0
Thai, Coconut, Veg Pot, Vegan, Bol*	1 Pot/345g	307	8.3	89	1.9	14.1	2.4	1.7
Vegetable, & Chickpea, Cook*	1 Serving/330g	224	6.3	68	3.2	7.9	1.9	3.3
Vegetable, Asda*	1 Pack/350g	329	21	94	1.9	8	6	1.9
Vegetable, Canned, Sainsbury's*	½ Can/200g	200	12.2	100	1.4	9.8	6.1	1.8
Vegetable, Canned, Tesco*	1 Can/400g	308	11.2	77	2	9.7	2.8	2.4
Vegetable, Diet Chef Ltd*	1 Pack/300g	153	3.6	51	2	8	1.2	2.1
Vegetable, Frozen, Mixed Vegetables, Average	*1oz/28g*	*25*	*1.7*	*88*	*2.5*	*6.9*	*6.1*	*0*
Vegetable, in Sweet Sauce, Average	*1 Serving/330g*	*162*	*6.9*	*49*	*1.4*	*6.7*	*2.1*	*1.3*
Vegetable, Indian Meal for One, Tesco*	1 Serving/200g	218	14.4	109	2	9	7.2	1.2
Vegetable, Indian, Canned, Tesco*	1 Can/400g	320	18	80	2	6.7	4.5	1.1
Vegetable, Indian, Sainsbury's*	½ Pack/200g	206	14.6	103	2.5	6.8	7.3	4.6
Vegetable, Indian, Tesco*	1 Serving/225g	257	17.8	114	2.1	8.6	7.9	1.6
Vegetable, LC, Tesco*	1 Pack/350g	350	4.2	100	2.3	19.4	1.2	1.5
Vegetable, Malay, Giraffe*	1 Pack/380g	471	36.1	124	2.2	6.2	9.5	2.4
Vegetable, Medium, Tesco*	1 Pack/350g	326	21.7	93	2.3	7.1	6.2	1.9
Vegetable, Mixed, Organic, Pure & Pronto*	1 Pack/400g	368	11.6	92	4.2	12.4	2.9	4.8
Vegetable, Pakistani, Average	*1oz/28g*	*17*	*0.7*	*60*	*2.2*	*8.7*	*2.6*	*2.2*
Vegetable, Red Thai, with Rice, Tesco*	1 Pack/385g	381	11.5	99	4.4	12.6	3	2.1
Vegetable, Sabzi Tarkari, Patak's*	1 Pack/400g	500	31.2	125	2.5	11.1	7.8	2.2
Vegetable, South Indian, Weight Watchers*	1 Pack/400g	256	7.6	64	2.7	7.9	1.9	2.4

INFO/WEIGHT	Measure	per Measure		Nutrition Values per 100g / 100ml				
		KCAL	FAT	KCAL	PROT	CARB	FAT	FIBRE

CURRY

Vegetable, South Indian, Weight Watchers, Heinz*	1 Pack/400g	256	7.6	64	2.7	7.9	1.9	2.4
Vegetable, Takeaway, Average	*1 Serving/330g*	*346*	*24.4*	*105*	*2.5*	*7.6*	*7.4*	*0*
Vegetable, Takeaway, Tesco*	1 Pack/385g	262	13.1	68	2.3	5.8	3.4	2.7
Vegetable, with Rice, Healthy Range, Average	*1 Serving/400g*	*351*	*4.6*	*88*	*2.3*	*16.8*	*1.1*	*1.9*
Vegetable, with Rice, Ready Meal, Average	*1 Serving/400g*	*408*	*12*	*102*	*3.3*	*16.4*	*3*	*0*
Vegetable, with Yoghurt, Average	*1oz/28g*	*17*	*1.1*	*62*	*2.6*	*4.6*	*4.1*	*1.4*
Vegetable, Yellow Thai, Sainsbury's*	1 Pack/400g	624	48.8	156	2.2	9.4	12.2	1.1

CURRY LEAVES

Fresh	*1oz/28g*	*23*	*0.3*	*81*	*6.6*	*11*	*1.1*	*0*

CURRY PASTE

Balti, Sharwood's*	¼ Pack/73g	328	28.7	453	5	19.2	39.6	3.1
Balti, Tomato & Coriander, Original, Patak's*	1 Tbsp/15g	58	5.1	388	4	14.6	34	3.7
Green Thai, Average	*1 Tsp/5g*	*6*	*0.4*	*128*	*2.1*	*11.7*	*7.9*	*3.1*
Jalfrezi, Patak's*	1 Serving/30g	96	8.1	320	3.7	14.2	26.9	5.6
Korma, Asda*	1 Tube/100g	338	23.5	338	5.1	26.6	23.5	1.2
Madras, Cumin Chilli, Hot, Patak's*	¼ Jar/70g	202	18.1	289	4.7	7.6	25.9	10.8
Madras, Pot, Patak's*	½ Pot/35g	98	8.1	279	4.4	7	23.1	0
Massaman, Thai, Pot, Blue Dragon*	½ Pot/25g	89	6.8	357	4.9	24	27	9.2
Medium, Asda*	1 Tsp/5g	18	1.6	364	5	14	32	5
Mild, Coriander Cumin, Original, Patak's*	1 Serving/35g	99	8.6	283	4.8	9.1	24.6	10.7
Red, Thai, Average	*1 Tsp/5g*	*7*	*0.5*	*132*	*2.3*	*9.5*	*9.1*	*3*
Rogan Josh, Tomato & Paprika, Patak's*	1 Serving/30g	119	11	397	4.1	12.7	36.7	5.9
Tandoori, Tamarind & Ginger, Patak's*	1 Serving/30g	33	0.5	110	3.1	20.4	1.8	2.6
Tikka Masala, Coriander & Lemon, Medium, Patak's*	1 Serving/30g	111	9.5	369	3.8	16.9	31.8	2.9
Tikka Masala, Spice, Patak's*	1 Tbsp/15g	40	3.4	270	3	7.8	22.9	6.8
Tom Yum, Thai Taste*	1 Tsp/13g	35	2	269	5.4	30.8	15.4	7.7
Yellow Thai, Tesco*	1 Tbsp/15g	15	0.6	100	1.9	13.6	4.1	4.9
Yellow, Thai, Barts*	1 Serving/30g	84	3.8	281	2.7	30.4	12.8	8.3

CURRY POWDER

Average	*1 Tsp/2g*	*6*	*0.3*	*325*	*12.7*	*41.8*	*13.8*	*0*

CUSTARD

Banana Flavour, Ambrosia*	1 Sm Pot/135g	139	3.9	103	2.9	16.1	2.9	0
Banana Flavour, Pot, Average	*1 Pot/135g*	*138*	*3.9*	*102*	*2.9*	*16*	*2.9*	*0*
Canned, Essential, Waitrose*	¼ Can/100g	101	3.2	101	2.7	15.3	3.2	0
Chocolate Flavour, Ambrosia*	1 Pot/150g	177	4.4	118	3	20	2.9	0.7
Chocolate Flavour, Pot, Average	*1 Pot/125g*	*138*	*3.4*	*111*	*3.1*	*18.2*	*2.7*	*0.6*
Instant, Just Add Water, Made Up, Weight Watchers*	1 Serving/145g	93	0.6	64	1.2	13.9	0.4	0.9
Instant, Mix, As Sold, Smart Price, Asda*	1 Pack/70g	204	2.7	291	2.6	61.3	3.9	0
Low Fat, Average	*1/3 Pot/141g*	*116*	*1.6*	*82*	*2.9*	*15*	*1.2*	*0*
Powder	*1 Tsp/5g*	*18*	*0*	*354*	*0.6*	*92*	*0.7*	*0.1*
Ready to Eat, Chocolate, Tesco*	1 Pot/150g	150	3.4	100	3.2	16.2	2.3	0.3
Ready to Eat. Low Fat, Pot, Tesco*	1 Pot/150g	132	2	88	3.2	15.9	1.3	0
Ready To Serve, Aldi*	¼ Pot/125g	152	7.2	122	2.7	15	5.8	0
Ready to Serve, Average	*1 Serving/50g*	*59*	*2.3*	*118*	*3.3*	*16.1*	*4.6*	*0.2*
Ready to Serve, Canned, Everyday Value, Tesco*	½ Can/192g	133	1.3	69	2.8	12.9	0.7	0
Salted Caramel Flavour, Morrisons*	½ Pot/150g	167	4.8	111	2.9	17.4	3.2	0.5
Soya, Vanilla, Dairy Free, Deliciously, Alpro*	1 Tbsp/15g	12	0.3	81	3	13.3	1.8	0.5
Toffee Flavour, Ambrosia*	1 Pot/150g	156	4.2	104	2.8	17	2.8	0
Vanilla Bean, Dollop*	1 Dollop/100g	127	3	127	20.2	27.7	3	0
Vanilla Flavour, Pot, Average	*1 Pot/125g*	*128*	*3.5*	*102*	*2.8*	*16.4*	*2.8*	*0*
Vanilla with Apple Crunch, Ambrosia*	1 Pack/193g	276	8.7	143	3.4	22.4	4.5	0.8
Vanilla, Low Fat, Fresh, Waitrose*	1/5 Pot/100g	104	2.4	104	3.5	17.1	2.4	0
Vanilla, Oat, Oatly*	¼ Pack/63g	97	6.2	155	1	15	10	0

	Measure INFO/WEIGHT	per Measure KCAL	FAT	Nutrition Values per 100g / 100ml KCAL	PROT	CARB	FAT	FIBRE
CUSTARD								
Vanilla, TTD, Sainsbury's*	1 Pot/150g	312	23.2	208	2.5	14.7	15.5	0.1
CUSTARD APPLE								
Cherimoya, Weighed without Skin Seeds, Average	*1 Serving/312g*	*234*	*2.1*	*75*	*1.6*	*17.7*	*0.7*	*3*
CUTLETS								
Nut, Goodlife*	1 Cutlet/88g	283	19.4	322	9.1	21.8	22	3.4
Nut, Meat Free, Tesco*	1 Nut Cutlet/82g	198	12.2	241	6.8	15.7	14.9	8.7
Nut, Retail, Fried in Vegetable Oil, Average	*1 Cutlet/90g*	*260*	*20.1*	*289*	*4.8*	*18.7*	*22.3*	*1.7*
Nut, Retail, Grilled, Average	*1 Cutlet/90g*	*191*	*11.7*	*212*	*5.1*	*19.9*	*13*	*1.8*
Vegetable & Nut, Asda*	1 Cutlet/88g	296	20.3	335	10	22	23	4.6
CUTTLEFISH								
Raw	*1oz/28g*	*16*	*0.2*	*56*	*12.7*	*0*	*0.6*	*0*

C

	Measure INFO/WEIGHT	per Measure KCAL	FAT	Nutrition Values per 100g / 100ml KCAL	PROT	CARB	FAT	FIBRE
DAB								
Raw	*1oz/28g*	*21*	*0.3*	*74*	*15.7*	*0*	*1.2*	*0*
DAIM								
Mondelez*	1 Bar/28g	148	8.7	530	2.9	59	31	1.2
DAIRYLEA DUNKERS								
with Jumbo Tubes, Kraft*	1 Pack/43g	108	5.1	255	9.1	27	12	0.9
with Ritz Crackers, Dairylea, Kraft*	1 Tub/46g	118	5.5	258	9.6	26	12	2.2
DAMSONS								
Raw, Weighed with Stones, Average	*1oz/28g*	*9*	*0*	*31*	*0.4*	*7.7*	*0*	*1.4*
Raw, Weighed without Stones, Average	*1oz/28g*	*11*	*0*	*38*	*0.5*	*9.6*	*0*	*1.8*
DANDELION & BURDOCK								
Barr*	1 Bottle/250ml	40	0	16	0	4	0	0
Fermented, Botanical, Fentiman's*	1 Bottle/275ml	130	0	47	0	11.6	0	0
Original, Ben Shaws*	1 Can/440ml	128	0	29	0	7	0	0
Slightly Sparkling, Fentiman's*	1 Serving/200ml	98	0	49	0	11.7	0	0
Sparkling, Diet, Morrisons*	1 Glass/200ml	2	0	1	0	0.3	0	0
DANISH PASTRY								
Apple & Cinnamon, Danish Twist, Entenmann's*	1 Serving/52g	150	1	288	5.6	62	1.9	1.5
Apple & Sultana, Tesco*	1 Pastry/72g	293	16.4	407	5.4	45	22.8	1.4
Apple Danish, Bakery, Waitrose*	1 Pastry/123g	400	22.2	325	5.1	35.7	18	2.4
Apple, Fresh Cream, Sainsbury's*	1 Pastry/67g	248	14.6	368	3.1	40.2	21.6	0.4
Average	*1 Pastry/110g*	*411*	*19.4*	*374*	*5.8*	*51.3*	*17.6*	*1.6*
Cherry Custard, Bar, Tesco*	1 Bar/350g	910	49	260	3.5	29.9	14	7.7
Custard, Bar, Sara Lee*	¼ Bar/100g	228	6.4	228	6.6	36.1	6.4	0.8
Fruit Bears Claw , Waitrose*	1 Pastry/97g	339	15.8	349	4.6	45	16.3	2
Fruit Filled, Average	*1 Pastry/94g*	*335*	*15.9*	*356*	*5.1*	*47.9*	*17*	*0*
Maple, Pecan, Plait, Frozen, Tesco*	1 Pastry/78g	348	22.8	447	5.6	39	29.3	2.7
Toasted Pecan, Danish Twist, Entenmann's*	1 Slice/48g	171	7.6	351	7	47.2	15.6	1.4
DATES								
Dried, Average	*1 Date/5g*	*13*	*0*	*266*	*2.8*	*64.1*	*0.4*	*4.1*
Dried, Medjool, Average	*1 Date/20g*	*56*	*0.1*	*279*	*2.2*	*69.3*	*0.3*	*4.3*
Fresh, Raw, Yellow, Average	*1 Date/20g*	*21*	*0*	*107*	*1.3*	*27.1*	*0.1*	*1.5*
Medjool, Stuffed with Walnuts, Tesco*	2 Dates/40g	98	2.3	245	4.4	44	5.7	3.4
Milk Chocolate Coated, Julian Graves*	1 Pack/200g	768	22.6	384	4.5	66	11.3	2.6
DELI FILLER								
Cheese Onion, Essential, Waitrose*	1 Pot/170g	692	64.8	407	10.8	4.5	38.1	1.5
Chicken Bacon, Co-Op*	1 Pack/200g	420	29.6	210	17.6	1	14.8	2.6
Chicken, Caesar Style, Sainsbury's*	1 Pack/80g	212	18.2	265	14	1	22.7	2.6
King Prawn & Avocado, M&S*	1 Pack/170g	425	38.8	250	9.5	1.4	22.8	0.5
Prawn & Mayonnaise, M&S*	1 Serving/60g	150	13.8	250	11.3	1	23	0.5
Prawn Cocktail, Eat Well, M&S*	½ Pot/85g	119	7.3	140	9.1	6.4	8.6	0.6
DESSERT								
After Dark, Black Forest, Gateaux, Gu*	1 Pot/85g	258	18.5	303	3	24.7	21.8	1.3
After Eight, Dark Chocolate Mint, Nestle*	1 Pot/70g	125	4.9	178	4.2	25.3	7	0
Apple Crumble, Sainsbury's*	1 Pot/136g	291	10.5	214	3.2	33	7.7	2.7
Banana Split	*1 Serving/175g*	*368*	*25.5*	*210*	*2.2*	*18*	*14.6*	*0.2*
Banoffee, Frozen, HL, Tesco*	1 Serving/60g	92	1.6	153	2.5	29.9	2.6	0.6
Banoffee, Layered, Sainsbury's*	1 Pot/115g	270	14.7	235	2.2	27.8	12.8	1
Banoffee, Pie, Frozen, Ed's Diner*	1 Dessert/98g	349	19.5	356	2.8	40.7	19.9	1
Banoffee, Sainsbury's*	1 Pot/140g	360	19.1	257	2.7	30.9	13.6	1.3
Banoffee, Weight Watchers*	1 Dessert/81g	170	3.6	210	4.9	37.7	4.4	1.4
Billionaire Bullion Bar, M&S*	1 Dessert/80g	353	22.5	441	5.4	41.2	28.1	0.7
Black Cherry, Dragana, Waitrose*	1 Pot/125g	236	11.4	189	2.1	24.7	9.1	0.5
Black Forest, LC, Tesco*	1 Pot/145g	188	2.3	130	3.2	25.8	1.6	0.9

D

DESSERT	Measure INFO/WEIGHT	per Measure KCAL	FAT	Nutrition Values per 100g / 100ml KCAL	PROT	CARB	FAT	FIBRE
Black Forest, Tesco*	1 Pot/100g	287	14.4	287	3.5	35.8	14.4	2.4
Blueberry, Muffin, Tesco*	1 Pot/91g	265	18.7	291	2	24.5	20.6	3
Butterscotch, Whip, Co-Op*	1 Pack/64g	241	0.1	377	0.6	93.4	0.1	0
Cafe Mocha, COU, M&S*	1 Dessert/115g	155	3.1	135	5.5	21.8	2.7	1
Candy Cane, Strawberries Cream, Tesco*	1 Serving/58g	134	9.6	232	1.9	18.8	16.6	0.1
Cappuccino, Italian, Co-Op*	1 Pack/90g	256	10.8	285	5	39	12	0.1
Caramel, Crunch, Weight Watchers*	1 Serving/89g	174	2.6	196	4.6	37.9	2.9	1.7
Caramel, Delights, Shape, Danone*	1 Pot/110g	109	2.5	99	3.3	16.3	2.3	0.1
Caramel, Pots Of Joy, Dairy Milk, Cadbury*	1 Pot/70g	150	7.3	215	2.5	27.1	10.5	0.1
Caramel, Soya, Creamy, Sweet, Alpro*	1 Pot/125g	106	2.2	85	3.2	13.7	1.8	0.5
Caramel, Soya, Dairy Free, Organic, Provamel*	1 Pot/125g	125	2.2	100	3	17.8	1.8	0.5
Chocolate & Caramel, Fix, Mullerlight, Muller*	1 Pot/80g	70	1.5	88	3	14.2	1.9	0
Chocolate, & Caramel, Semifreddo, Waitrose*	1 Slice/64g	217	12.3	342	3.4	37.4	19.4	2.1
Chocolate, & Summer Fruits, Specially Selected, Aldi*	1 Dessert/95g	277	16.2	292	1.8	32	17	2.7
Chocolate, Raspberry, Pots, Pudology*	1 Pot/50g	53	1.8	106	1.5	17	3.5	0
Chocolate, Banoffee, Gu*	1 Pot/85g	325	21.5	382	3.9	35	25.3	1
Chocolate, Brownie, Double, Weight Watchers*	1 Pot/86g	167	3.3	194	5.1	33.7	3.8	2.4
Chocolate, Brownie, M&S*	¼ Pack/144g	610	39.5	425	4.7	39.6	27.5	1
Chocolate, Buttons, Cadbury*	1 Pack/100g	275	14.5	275	5	30.5	14.5	0
Chocolate, Buttons, Milk, Cadbury*	1 Pot/100g	280	14.9	280	6.2	30.8	14.9	0
Chocolate, Cheeky & Saucy, Little Pots Au Chocolat, Gu*	1 Pot/45g	199	16.6	443	3.3	24.1	36.9	2.3
Chocolate, Creme, King Frais, Lidl*	1 Pot/125g	131	3.6	105	2.6	17	2.9	0
Chocolate, Dark, Soya, Alpro*	1 Pot/125g	118	2.9	94	3	14.7	2.3	1.4
Chocolate, Delights, Shape, Danone*	1 Pot/110g	109	2.4	99	3.3	16.3	2.2	0.6
Chocolate, Duetto, Weight Watchers*	1 Pot/85g	99	2.4	117	4.4	18.4	2.8	0
Chocolate, Everyday Value, Tesco*	1 Pot/100g	121	4	121	2.7	18.4	4	0.4
Chocolate, Fix, Mullerlight, Muller*	1 Pot/100g	94	1.9	94	3.2	15.2	1.9	0
Chocolate, Frappe, Skinny, COU, M&S*	1 Pot/100g	116	2.6	116	6.2	16.9	2.6	0.5
Chocolate, Fudge Brownie, Tesco*	1 Pot/125g	374	16.6	299	4.6	40.2	13.3	1.3
Chocolate, Hazelnut, Charolait, Aldi*	1 Serving/200g	270	11	135	3.3	18.1	5.5	0
Chocolate, Honeycomb Crisp, COU, M&S*	1 Serving/71g	110	2.1	155	4.6	27.6	2.9	1
Chocolate, Little Choc Pots, The Coconut Collaborative*	1 Pot/45g	105	6.5	234	2.2	23	14.4	1.5
Chocolate, Marshmallow, Weight Watchers*	1 Serving/50g	97	2.4	194	3.2	34.5	4.7	1.3
Chocolate, Milk, Pot, Love Something*	1 Pot/90g	395	31.5	439	3.4	26	35	0
Chocolate, Mint Torte, Weight Watchers*	1 Dessert/88g	174	4.1	198	4.7	34.3	4.7	5.2
Chocolate, Mousse Cake, Weight Watchers*	1 Dessert/75g	148	2.2	198	5.9	37.1	2.9	1
Chocolate, Muffin, LC, Tesco*	1 Pot/108g	140	2.4	130	4.3	22.6	2.2	1.3
Chocolate, Muffin, Skinny, Low Fat, COU, M&S*	1 Pot/110g	154	3.1	140	5.2	23.5	2.8	0.5
Chocolate, Muffin, Tesco*	1 Serving/104g	354	21.2	340	3.5	35.5	20.4	2.1
Chocolate, Muffin, Waitrose*	1 Serving/110g	138	3	126	5.2	20	2.7	0.4
Chocolate, Orange, Pots of Joy, Terry's*	1 Pot/70g	150	7.3	215	3.7	26	10.5	0.1
Chocolate, Pots Of Joy , Dairy Milk, Cadbury*	1 Pot /70g	158	8.2	225	4.2	25.6	11.7	0.1
Chocolate, Soya, Dairy Free, Organic, Provamel*	1 Pot/125g	111	3	89	3	13.6	2.4	1
Chocolate, Soya, Silky Smooth, Alpro*	1 Pot/125g	104	2.4	83	3	13	1.9	1.1
Chocolate, Toffee, Weight Watchers*	1 Dessert/89g	177	4	197	4.3	34.9	4.5	2.2
Chocolate, Weight Watchers*	1 Serving/82g	145	2.5	177	5.2	32.3	3	2.9
Chocolate, White Buttons, Pots of Joy, Cadbury*	1 Pot /70g	158	6.6	225	4.8	30.4	9.4	0
Chocolate, Fudge, Pot, Fabulous, Thorntons*	1 Pot /65g	168	10.4	258	5.5	22.7	16	0
Cookie Dough, Ed's Diner*	1 Dessert/100g	307	17	307	5	32.5	17	1.6
Creme Caramel, Sainsbury's*	1 Pot/100g	116	1.6	116	2.6	22.9	1.6	0
Custard, with Caramel, Layers, Ambrosia*	1 Pot/161g	183	4.7	114	2.5	19.6	2.9	0
Fudge, Cadbury*	1 Pot/90g	216	11.2	240	4.1	28.5	12.4	0
Galaxy, Mars*	1 Pot/75g	166	9.2	221	4.9	22.7	12.3	0

	Measure INFO/WEIGHT	per Measure KCAL	FAT	Nutrition Values per 100g / 100ml KCAL	PROT	CARB	FAT	FIBRE
DESSERT								
Gulabjam Indian, Waitrose*	1 Pot/180g	479	15.5	266	4.8	42.9	8.6	0.6
Jaffa Cake, COU, M&S*	1 Serving/120g	138	3.1	115	2.4	20.1	2.6	1
Jaffa, COU, M&S*	1 Pot/107g	155	4.9	145	3.4	22.4	4.6	0.5
Key Lime Pie	*1 Serving/125g*	*431*	*25*	*344*	*4.1*	*37.9*	*20*	*1.4*
Lemon, & Raspberry Semifreddo, Waitrose*	1 Slice/63g	193	12.3	305	1.9	30.4	19.4	0.5
Lemon, Yuzu, Pots, Pudology*	1 Pot/50g	45	1.6	89	0.5	15.9	3.2	0
Lemon, Meringue, Weight Watchers*	1 Pot/85g	161	0.4	189	2.4	43.1	0.5	0.6
Lemon, Mousse Cake, Weight Watchers*	1 Serving/90g	130	2.4	144	3.2	26.7	2.7	0.5
Lemon, Posset, Creamy, Pot, Love Something*	1 Pot/90g	290	22.5	322	1.4	23	25	0.1
Lemon, Sainsbury's*	1 Pot/115g	136	1.7	118	2.8	23.2	1.5	0.9
Lemon, Sicilian, & Raspberry, Buche, Finest, Tesco*	1 Slice/72g	155	10.3	215	3.8	17.1	14.3	1.3
Lemoncello, Italian, Co-Op*	1 Pot/90g	266	14.4	295	3	34	16	0.1
Mandarin, COU, M&S*	1 Serving/150g	195	5.7	130	1	22	3.8	0.1
Millionaire's Shortbread, M&S*	1 Dessert/120g	440	27.8	365	3.2	35.5	23.1	1
Mississippi Mud Pie	*1 Serving/125g*	*480*	*32*	*384*	*5.3*	*33.1*	*25.6*	*1.8*
Raspberry, Royale, Essential, Waitrose*	1 Pot/150g	216	10.6	144	1.1	18.9	7.1	0.5
Rolo, Nestle*	1 Pot/70g	170	8.3	243	3.3	30.8	11.9	0.5
Strawberry, & Raspberry, Charlotte, COU, M&S*	1 Pot/110g	153	1.2	139	2.1	29.7	1.1	1.1
Tiramisu	*1 Serving/150g*	*420*	*20.8*	*280*	*4.4*	*34*	*13.9*	*0.8*
Toffee, Cheesecake, Individual, Dessert Menu, Aldi*	1 Dessert/100g	266	12	266	2.5	36	12	0.5
Toffee, Fudge , Pot, Fabulous, Thorntons*	1 Pot/65g	178	10.5	274	4.8	27.3	16.1	0
Toffee, with Biscuit Pieces, Iced, Weight Watchers*	1 Pot/57g	93	2.7	163	2.7	26.2	4.8	0.2
Trifle, Chocolate, Cadbury*	1 Pot /90g	234	13.8	260	4.8	22.5	15.3	0
Vanilla, & Caramel, Little Desserts, Petits Filous, Yoplait*	1 Pot/50g	75	2.6	150	4.7	21	5.3	0.2
Vanilla, Choc Fudge, Non Dairy Soya, Frozen, Tofutti*	1 Tub/500ml	825	45	165	1.6	20	9	0.4
Vanilla, Soya, Dairy Free, Organic, Provamel*	1 Pot/125g	105	2.2	84	3.2	13.4	1.8	0.5
Vanilla, Soya, Heavenly Velvet, Alpro*	1 Pot/125g	106	2.4	85	3.2	13.6	1.9	0.5
Zabaglione	*1 Serving/100g*	*278*	*18.3*	*278*	*3.6*	*24.3*	*18.3*	*2.3*
DHAL								
Black Gram, Average	*1oz/28g*	*21*	*1*	*74*	*4.2*	*7*	*3.4*	*1.7*
Chick Pea	*1oz/28g*	*42*	*1.7*	*149*	*7.4*	*17.7*	*6.1*	*3.8*
Lentil, Red Masoor & Tomato with Butter, Average	*1oz/28g*	*26*	*1.4*	*94*	*4*	*9.7*	*4.9*	*0.9*
Lentil, Red Masoor & Vegetable, Average	*1oz/28g*	*31*	*1.1*	*110*	*5.8*	*14.7*	*3.8*	*1.8*
Lentil, Red Masoor with Vegetable Oil, Average	*1oz/28g*	*48*	*2.2*	*172*	*7.6*	*19.2*	*7.9*	*1.8*
Lentil, Red Masoor, Punjabi, Average	*1oz/28g*	*39*	*1.3*	*139*	*7.2*	*19.2*	*4.6*	*2*
Lentil, Red Masoorl & Mung Bean, Average	*1oz/28g*	*32*	*1.9*	*114*	*4.8*	*9.9*	*6.7*	*1.6*
Lentil, Tesco*	1 Serving/200g	248	13.2	124	5.1	10.6	6.6	2.5
Mung Bean, Bengali	*1oz/28g*	*20*	*0.9*	*73*	*4.2*	*7.4*	*3.3*	*1.7*
Mung Beans, Dried, Boiled in Unsalted Water	*1oz/28g*	*26*	*0.1*	*92*	*7.8*	*15.3*	*0.4*	*0*
Split Peas, Yellow, Chana, Asda*	1 Serving/275g	300	19.2	109	2.6	9	7	1.8
Tadkha, Rich Golden, Waitrose*	½ Pack/150g	172	8.3	114	6	10.9	5.5	5.5
Tarka, Asda*	½ Pack/150g	216	12	144	6	12	8	6
Tarka, M&S*	1 Serving/250g	235	8.8	94	4.3	9.4	3.5	3.7
Vegetable, Microwaved, Slimming World*	1 Pack/350g	259	2.1	74	5.4	8.3	0.6	7
DHANSAK								
Chicken with Bagara Rice, Waitrose*	1 Pack/450g	549	8.1	122	8.2	18.2	1.8	1.2
Vegetable, Curry, Microwaved, Slimzone, Asda*	1 Portion/459g	225	2.3	49	2.5	7.7	0.5	2.6
Vegetable, Sainsbury's*	1 Serving/200g	148	5.6	74	3.1	8.9	2.8	2.8
DILL								
Dried, Average	*1 Tsp/1g*	*3*	*0*	*253*	*19.9*	*42.2*	*4.4*	*13.6*
Fresh, Average	*1 Tbsp/3g*	*1*	*0*	*25*	*3.7*	*0.9*	*0.8*	*2.5*
DIP								
Aubergine, Fresh, Waitrose*	1 Serving/85g	159	12.8	187	2.5	10.5	15	1.7

D

DIP

	Measure INFO/WEIGHT	per Measure KCAL	FAT	Nutrition Values per 100g / 100ml KCAL	PROT	CARB	FAT	FIBRE
Baba Ganoush, Sabra*	1 Serving/75g	188	17.6	251	3.9	4.4	23.5	0
Bean, Mexican, Doritos, Walkers*	1 Tbsp/20g	18	0.7	89	2.7	12.1	3.3	2.4
Beetroot, & Sesame, Sainsbury's*	¼ Pot/45g	65	3.7	145	4.2	11.8	8.3	3.1
Beetroot, Mint, The Deli, Aldi*	¼ Pot/50g	66	3.8	131	3.5	10	7.6	4.2
Blue Cheese, Fresh, Sainsbury's*	1/5 Pot/34g	115	11.7	337	3.6	3.1	34.5	0.1
Butternut Squash, Cumin, Sainsbury's*	¼ Pot/45g	33	1.8	74	3.5	4.2	3.9	4
Caramel, Salted, for Mini Doughnuts, Tesco*	1 Dip/3g	11	0.3	386	2.9	68.7	11.1	0
Cheese & Chive, 50% Less Fat, Asda*	1 Pot/125g	261	21.5	209	4.5	9	17.2	0
Cheese & Chive, 50% Less Fat, Morrisons*	1 Serving/50g	86	6.4	172	8.8	5.2	12.7	0.2
Cheese & Chive, Mature Cheddar, Fresh, Waitrose*	½ Pot/85g	393	40.5	462	5.8	2.4	47.7	1.7
Cheese Chive, Asda*	1 Serving/43g	190	19.6	447	4.9	3.4	46	0
Cheese Chive, Tesco*	¼ Pack/50g	148	13.9	296	3.8	7.5	27.8	0.2
Chilli Cheese, Asda*	1 Serving/50g	131	11	262	8	8	22	1.1
Chilli, M&S*	1 Pot/35g	103	0.1	295	0.4	73.2	0.2	0.4
Endamame Pea, Waitrose*	¼ Pot/51g	85	5.9	166	6.3	8	11.6	2
Feta Cheese, Fresh, Tesco*	1oz/28g	81	7.1	288	6.8	7.9	25.5	0.7
Frijolemole, Cannellini Bean Chick Pea, Waitrose*	¼ Pot/50g	104	7.6	208	4.3	12.2	15.2	2.6
Garlic & Herb, Big Dipper, Morrisons*	¼ Pot/75g	278	28.1	370	1.3	6.9	37.5	0.4
Garlic & Herb, Reduced Fat, M&S*	1 Serving/10g	10	0.4	95	6	8.1	4	0.5
Garlic & Herb, Tesco*	¼ Pack/43g	257	27.8	604	0.9	3.2	65.4	0.3
Garlic Herb	*1 Serving/100g*	*584*	*62.4*	*584*	*1.4*	*4.1*	*62.4*	*0.2*
Garlic, Takeaway Pizza, Goodfella's*	1 Pot/18g	57	5.4	319	0.3	12	30	0
Guacamole, Tex-Mex Multipack Selection, Tesco*	½ Pot/53g	76	6.8	142	1.1	4	12.8	3
Indian Snack Selection, Vitasia, Lidl*	1 Serving/70g	122	7	175	1	19.7	10	1.2
Jalapeno, & Lime Hummus, with Coriander, Lisa's*	1 Serving/20g	47	2.8	235	7.3	21.5	13.9	6.9
Jalapeno, Chilli Cheese, Tex-Mex Selection, Tesco*	½ Pot/53g	147	13.6	276	4.7	6.6	25.6	0.3
Jalapeno, Greek Yoghurt, Skotidakis*	1 Tbsp/15g	25	1.8	167	6.7	13.3	11.7	0
Mint, Cucumber, Raita, Tesco*	1 Tbsp/15g	32	3	215	2.3	5.5	20.3	0.7
Moroccan, Spicy, BGTY, Sainsbury's*	½ Pot/85g	56	1.7	66	2.1	10	2	1.7
Nacho Cheese, Average	*1 Serving/50g*	*175*	*17.2*	*350*	*6.3*	*3.4*	*34.4*	*0.9*
Nacho Cheese, Doritos, Walkers*	1 Serving/40g	92	8.1	231	3.4	8.5	20.2	0.6
Nacho Cheese, Primula*	1 Serving/57g	144	14.2	253	2.7	3.6	24.9	2.1
Nacho Cheese, Sainsbury's*	1 Serving/50g	244	25.1	487	4.8	3.9	50.2	0
Nacho Cheese, Tex-Mex Multipack Selection, Tesco*	1 Tub/125g	619	62	495	5.9	5.8	49.6	0
Onion & Garlic, GFY, Asda*	1/5 Pot/34g	56	4.8	166	2.1	8	14	0.2
Onion & Garlic, HE, Tesco*	1 Pot/170g	345	29.9	203	3.3	7.9	17.6	0.1
Onion Garlic, Average	*1 Tbsp/15g*	*62*	*6.4*	*410*	*1.7*	*4.8*	*42.7*	*0.4*
Onion Garlic, HL, Tesco*	1 Serving/43g	80	7.2	188	2.5	6.3	17	0.1
Onion, Garlic, Classic Multipack Selection, Tesco*	1 Pot/129g	329	31.3	255	1.7	7.2	24.3	0.3
Onion, Garlic, The Deli, Aldi*	¼ Pot/50g	159	15.5	318	1.7	7.5	31	0.5
Pea, Mint, The Deli, Aldi*	¼ Pack/50g	52	3	103	3.3	6.4	6.1	4.4
Pea, Spinach, Tesco*	¼ Pot/46g	61	4	132	3.1	8.6	8.6	3.9
Pea, Yogurt Mint, Sainsbury's*	¼ Pack/50g	119	10.8	238	3.4	7.5	21.6	2.1
Peanut, Satay Selection, Occasions, Sainsbury's*	1 Serving/2g	4	0.2	186	7.1	13.8	11.4	1.1
Pecorino, Basil & Pine Nut, Fresh, Waitrose*	½ Pot/85g	338	33.7	398	5.1	5.1	39.7	0
Red Pepper, Sainsbury's*	1 Pot/100g	103	4	103	2.3	14.6	4	0
Red Pepper, Smoky, Gazpacho, Graze*	1 Punnet/23g	54	1.3	242	5.7	40.1	5.9	3.7
Red Pepper, The Deli, Aldi*	¼ Pot/50g	60	3	119	3.6	11	6	4
Salsa, Chunky Tomato, Tesco*	1 Pot/170g	68	2.2	40	1.1	5.9	1.3	1.1
Salsa, Chunky, Fresh, Sainsbury's*	1 Serving/100g	51	1.7	51	1.1	7.8	1.7	1.2
Salsa, Hot, Doritos, Walkers*	1 Jar/300g	99	0.3	33	1.1	6.4	0.1	0.9
Salsa, Hot, Snaktastic, Lidl*	1 Serving/50g	17	0.1	34	1.3	6.1	0.2	1.5
Salsa, Mango, Ginger & Chilli, Spiced, Weight Watchers*	1 Serving/56g	48	0.1	85	1	19.9	0.2	2.6

	Measure INFO/WEIGHT	per Measure KCAL	per Measure FAT	Nutrition Values per 100g / 100ml KCAL	PROT	CARB	FAT	FIBRE
DIP								
Salsa, Mild, Asda*	1 Portion/100g	47	0.3	47	1.4	8.7	0.3	1.8
Salsa, Mild, Doritos, Walkers*	1 Tbsp/30g	9	0.1	30	0.8	6	0.3	1.5
Sour Cream & Chive, BGTY, Sainsbury's*	1 Serving/170g	253	17.5	149	4.2	9.9	10.3	0.1
Sour Cream & Chive, Classic, Tesco*	¼ Pot/50g	124	11.9	249	2	6.6	23.8	0.2
Sour Cream & Chive, Doritos, Walkers*	1 Tbsp/20g	52	4.9	258	1.9	6.9	24.7	1.9
Sour Cream & Chive, Fresh, Tesco*	½ Pot/75g	305	31.8	407	2.1	4.1	42.4	0
Sour Cream & Chive, Half Fat, Waitrose*	½ Pot/85g	133	9.9	157	5.5	7.6	11.6	0.1
Sour Cream & Chive, Mexican Style, Morrisons*	¼ Pack/25g	68	7	274	2.2	3.4	27.9	0.4
Sour Cream & Chive, Morrisons*	1 Serving/100g	317	32.6	317	2.6	3.3	32.6	0
Sour Cream & Chive, Reduced Fat, Tesco*	¼ Pot/50g	80	6.1	159	4.2	7.9	12.2	0.2
Sour Cream & Chive, Sainsbury's*	1 Serving/50g	141	13.8	282	3.1	5.4	27.5	0.1
Sour Cream Chive, Average	**1 Tbsp/15g**	**48**	**4.8**	**317**	**3.2**	**4**	**32**	**0.3**
Sour Cream Chive, M&S*	½ Pack/57g	218	22.5	383	2.2	4.9	39.4	0.1
Sour Cream Chive, Primula*	1 Serving/57g	169	17.4	297	4.3	1.3	30.5	1
Sour Cream, Tesco*	1 Serving/38g	111	11.2	297	3.4	3.9	29.8	0.2
Soy, Gyoza Selection, Tesco*	1 Pot/30g	30	0.2	100	1.7	21.4	0.7	0.7
Sweet Chilli, Chinese Snack Selection, Morrisons*	½ Pot/20g	64	0	320	0.1	79.4	0.2	0.6
Sweet Chilli, Mango, Encona*	1 Tbsp/15ml	22	0.1	148	0.4	35.4	0.6	0
Sweet Chilli, Thai, Primula*	1 Serving/57g	126	0.1	221	0.6	54.4	0.1	0.2
Thousand Island, HL, Tesco*	1 Serving/31g	57	4.6	183	2.5	9.6	14.9	0.3
Thousand Island, M&S*	1oz/28g	69	6.2	245	2.1	9.4	22.2	0.7
Tortilla Chips, Cool Flavour, Big, Morrisons*	½ Pack/100g	453	22	453	6.4	57.4	22	8.1
Yoghurt & Cucumber, & Mint, Tesco*	1oz/28g	34	2	121	7	7.2	7.1	0.6
DOLMADES								
Stffed Vine Leaves, Delphi*	1 Dolma/30g	36	0.8	119	2.2	21.9	2.5	1.1
Stuffed with Rice, M&S*	1 Leaf/38g	40	1.6	105	2.6	14.2	4.1	1.2
DOPIAZA								
Chicken, M&S*	1 Pack/350g	402	21.4	115	11.5	3.7	6.1	2.5
Chicken, with Pilau Rice, Tesco*	1 Pack/400g	424	15.2	106	5.7	12.3	3.8	1.5
Mushroom, Retail	**1oz/28g**	**19**	**1.6**	**69**	**1.3**	**3.7**	**5.7**	**1.1**
Mushroom, Waitrose*	½ Pack/150g	81	4.6	54	2.2	4.3	3.1	2.3
DORITOS								
Chilli Heatwave, Walkers*	1 Bag/30g	148	7.6	495	6.3	57.3	25.3	6.7
Cool Original, Walkers*	1 Bag/40g	200	10.8	500	7.5	58	27	3
Cool Spice 3ds, Walkers*	1 Bag/24g	108	4.3	450	8	64	18	4.4
Dippas, Hint of Lime, Walkers*	1 Bag/35g	173	8.8	495	7	60	25	3.5
Dippas, Lightly Salted, Dipping Chips, Walkers*	1 Serving/25g	128	6.8	510	6.5	60	27	3
Lighly Salted, Corn Chips, Doritos*	1 Bag/30g	149	7.1	497	6.9	62.9	23.6	3.3
Tangy Cheese, Walkers*	1 Bag/40g	200	10.8	500	7	57	27	3
DOUBLE DECKER								
Dinky Deckers, Cadbury*	1 Piece/5g	22	0.8	456	4.2	71	17	1.5
Snack Size, Cadbury*	1 Bar/36g	165	7.4	465	4.8	64.5	20.9	0
DOUGH BALLS								
Garlic, Free From, Tesco*	3 Doughballs/42g	152	6.3	363	1.1	53.4	15	5
with Garlic Herb Butter, Aldi*	1 Ball/12g	45	2.2	365	7.7	46.7	18.2	1.8
with Garlic Butter Dip, Supermarlet, Pizza Express*	4 Balls/44g	137	1.3	311	10.8	59	3	2.5
DOUGHNUTS								
Chocolate, Bakery, Tesco*	1 Doughnut/66g	250	12.8	379	6.6	43.5	19.4	2.2
Chocolate, Iced, Ring, Bakery, Sainsbury's*	1 Doughnut/55g	212	10.3	386	6.3	47.4	18.8	1
Custard Filled, Average	**1 Doughnut/75g**	**268**	**14.2**	**358**	**6.2**	**43.3**	**19**	**0**
Custard, Sainsbury's*	1 Doughnut/70g	172	7.5	246	5.1	32.3	10.7	2.3
Custard, Tesco*	1 Doughnut/70g	199	7.4	284	6.8	39.5	10.6	1.8
Glazed, Bakery, Tesco*	1 Doughnut/52g	202	10.1	389	6.5	45.9	19.5	2

	Measure INFO/WEIGHT	per Measure		Nutrition Values per 100g / 100ml				
		KCAL	FAT	KCAL	PROT	CARB	FAT	FIBRE
DOUGHNUTS								
Glazed, Ring, Bakery, Sainsbury's*	1 Doughnut/62g	229	12	369	5.5	42.8	19.3	1.1
Jam, Bakery, Tesco*	1 Doughnut/70g	225	7.6	321	5.6	49.2	10.9	2
Jam, Filled, Average	*1 Doughnut/75g*	*252*	*10.9*	*336*	*5.7*	*48.8*	*14.5*	*0*
Jam, M&S*	1 Doughnut/49g	141	2	287	5	57.6	4	1.3
Mini, Ring, Bites, Sugar Coated, Simply Doughnuts*	1 Ring/12g	57	3.5	474	6.9	43	29	0
Mini, Sainsbury's*	1 Doughnut/14g	53	2.7	379	5.2	47.9	18.9	2.1
Oreo, CSM, UK LTD*	1 Doughnut/72g	326	19.5	453	5	46.8	27	1.1
Plain, Ring, Average	*1 Doughnut/60g*	*238*	*13*	*397*	*6.1*	*47.2*	*21.7*	*0*
Raspberry Jam, Sainsbury's*	1 Doughnut/58g	203	8.9	350	5.5	46.4	15.3	2.3
Ring, Iced, Average	*1 Doughnut/70g*	*268*	*12.2*	*383*	*4.8*	*55.1*	*17.5*	*0*
Ring, Sugar, Tesco*	1 Doughnut/56g	234	15.9	419	6.2	33.6	28.4	2.1
Selection, Bakers Selection, Asda*	1 Doughnut/75g	273	17.9	365	4.5	32	24	1.4
Strawberry, Iced, Ring, Bakery, Tesco*	1 Doughnut/58g	248	14.3	428	5.4	45.3	24.7	1.4
Strawberry, Iced, Ring, Mini, Bakery, Tesco*	1 Doughnut/15g	62	3.1	415	4.9	51.5	20.8	1.3
Sugar, Ring, Bakery, Sainsbury's*	1 Doughnut/51g	222	14	435	5.7	40.7	27.4	2.1
Vanilla, Bakery, Sainsbury's*	1 Doughnut/66g	248	12.9	376	6.1	42.7	19.6	2
Yum Yums, Glazed, Sweet, Waitrose*	1 Doughnut/45g	172	10	382	4	41.6	22.2	2
Yum Yums, M&S*	1 Doughnut/37g	155	8.9	420	4.9	45.7	23.9	1.6
DOVER SOLE								
Fillet, Raw, Average	*1oz/28g*	*25*	*0.5*	*89*	*18.1*	*0*	*1.8*	*0*
DR PEPPER*								
Coca-Cola*	1 Bottle/500ml	145	0	29	0	7.2	0	0
Zero, Coca-Cola*	1 Can/330ml	2	0	0	0	0	0	0
DRAGON FRUIT								
Raw, Edible Portion, Average	*1 Serving/100g*	*41*	*0.5*	*41*	*0.7*	*9.6*	*0.5*	*3.6*
DRAMBUIE								
39% Volume	*1 Pub Shot/35ml*	*125*	*0*	*358*	*0*	*23*	*0*	*0*
DREAM TOPPING								
Dry, Bird's*	1oz/28g	193	16.4	690	6.7	32.5	58.5	0.5
Sugar Free, Dry, Bird's*	1oz/28g	195	16.9	695	7.3	30.5	60.5	0.5
DRESSING								
French, Style, BGTY, Sainsbury's*	1 Tbsp/15ml	11	0.4	76	0.7	12.6	2.5	0.5
Aioli, Deli Style, Light, Praise*	1 Tbsp/20ml	76	7.1	380	5	15.5	35.5	0
Balsamic, & Olive Oil, Sainsbury's*	1 Serving/25ml	104	10.4	415	0.9	9.4	41.8	0.2
Balsamic, Bliss, Ainsley Harriott*	1 Tbsp/15g	41	3.2	272	0.8	19.3	21.1	0
Balsamic, Fig Glaze, Tesco*	1 Tbsp/15ml	31	0	208	1.4	47.9	0	0
Balsamic, Glaze, Odysea *	1 Tsp/5ml	9	0	171	0.5	40	0	0
Balsamic, Italian, Loyd Grossman*	1 Serving/10g	36	3.4	357	0.9	13.1	33.5	0.1
Balsamic, LC, Tesco*	1 Tbsp/14g	12	0.2	85	0.3	16.7	1.5	0.2
Balsamic, New, Sainsbury's*	1 Tbsp/15g	58	5.2	389	0.6	18.3	34.8	0.8
Balsamic, Oak Aged, TTD, Sainsbury's*	1 Tbsp/15ml	54	4.8	338	0.5	16.3	30	0.5
Balsamic, Raspberry Balsamic, GFY, Asda*	1 Tbsp/15ml	6	0.1	40	0.7	9.3	0.7	1.3
Balsamic, Raspberry, with Rosemary, Suzanne's*	1 Tbsp/15ml	22	0	148	1	48.1	0.1	0.5
Balsamic, Sweet, BGTY, Sainsbury's*	1 Tsp/5g	3	0	61	0.5	13.6	0.5	0.5
Balsamic, Sweet, Finest, Tesco*	1 Serving/10ml	16	0	155	0.4	36.9	0.1	0.4
Balsamic, Vinaigrette, Newman's Own*	1 Tbsp/15ml	56	5.7	372	0.1	7.2	38.2	0.5
Balsamic, Vinegar, Asda*	1 Tsp/5ml	7	0.2	146	0.5	27	4	0
Balsamic, Vinegar, Light, Kraft*	1 Serving/15ml	15	0.9	100	0.3	9.6	6.3	0.5
Balsamic, Vinegar, Morrisons*	1 Serving/15ml	17	0.2	111	0.1	22.9	1.6	0.1
Balsamic, Weight Watchers*	1 Serving/15ml	12	0.3	81	0.1	16	1.8	0.5
Blue Cheese, British, Specially Selected, Aldi*	1 Tbsp/15ml	60	6	403	2	9.3	40	0.9

DRESSING

INFO/WEIGHT	Measure	per Measure KCAL	per Measure FAT	Nutrition Values per 100g / 100ml KCAL	PROT	CARB	FAT	FIBRE
Blue Cheese, Hellmann's*	1 Tbsp/15g	69	7.1	459	0.7	6.3	47.2	1.1
Blue Cheese, Salad, Waitrose*	1 Serving/50g	265	25.2	530	2.1	17.3	50.3	4.1
Blue Cheese, True, Briannas*	2 Tbsp/30ml	120	11	400	3.3	16.7	36.7	0
Caesar, 95% Fat Free, Tesco*	1 Tsp/6g	5	0.2	88	4.1	8.9	3.7	0.3
Caesar, Asiago, Briannas*	1 Tbsp/15ml	70	7.5	467	3.3	3.3	50	0
Caesar, Chilled, Reduced Fat, Tesco*	1 Tsp/5ml	13	1.2	252	6.5	3.1	23.7	0.1
Caesar, Classic, Sainsbury's*	1 Tsp/5ml	22	2.3	442	2.7	4.6	45.9	0.5
Caesar, Creamy, M&S*	1 Tbsp/15ml	66	6.5	437	2.6	9.1	43.1	1
Caesar, Fat Free, Average	*1 Tsp/5g*	*4*	*0.2*	*84*	*4.6*	*11*	*4.1*	*0.2*
Caesar, Finest, Tesco*	1 Tbsp/15ml	72	7.6	477	1.9	2.8	50.9	0.2
Caesar, Fresh, Asda*	1 Dtsp/10ml	45	4.8	454	2.4	3.2	48	0
Caesar, Hellmann's*	1 Tsp/6g	30	3.1	499	2.5	4.5	51.7	0.3
Caesar, Just Add, M&S*	1 Tbsp/15ml	91	9.5	605	4.1	4	63.5	0.5
Caesar, LC, Tesco*	1 Serving/15g	9	0.2	60	1.5	9.5	1.5	0.5
Caesar, Less Than 3% Fat, BGTY, Sainsbury's*	1 Serving/20g	10	0.4	48	0.8	7	1.9	0.3
Caesar, Low Fat, Average	*1 Tsp/5g*	*4*	*0.1*	*77*	*2.3*	*11.1*	*2.6*	*0.2*
Caesar, Mary Berry*	1 Serving/100g	573	56.9	573	2.4	12.8	56.9	0.1
Caesar, Original, Cardini's*	1 Serving/10g	56	6	555	2.3	1.5	60	0.2
Caesar, Style, GFY, Asda*	1 Sachet/44ml	34	1	77	5	9	2.3	0
Caesar, Tesco*	1 Tbsp/15ml	65	6.8	435	0.9	5.4	45.1	0.3
Caesar, Waitrose*	1 Serving/15ml	72	7.6	479	4.5	0.9	50.8	0.2
Caesar, with Smoked Garlic, Hellmann's*	1 Tbsp/15ml	35	3.3	231	2	6.4	22	0
Chilli, Balsamic, Glaze, Jamie Oliver*	1 Tbsp/15ml	32	0	212	0.2	50	0	0
Cream Cheese & Chive, Creamy Ranch, Kraft*	1 Serving/15ml	31	2.6	205	1.2	11	17	0
Creme Fraiche, Salad, Kraft*	1 Tbsp/15ml	12	0.4	78	0.8	12.5	2.5	0
Cucumber, Mint, M&S*	1 Tbsp/15ml	46	3.9	305	0.7	16.7	26.1	0.1
French, Batts, Lidl*	2 Tbsp/30ml	95	8.7	317	1.7	12	29	0
French, Chilled, Tesco*	1 Tbsp/15ml	63	5.9	421	1.1	15.1	39.6	0
French, Classic, Fresh, M&S*	1 Serving/10ml	52	5.3	515	0.6	8.2	53.1	0.2
French, Classic, Sainsbury's*	1 Tbsp/15ml	71	7.4	473	1	5.7	49.6	0.5
French, Classics, M&S*	1 Tbsp/15ml	77	8	516	0.6	8.2	53.1	0.2
French, Finest, Tesco*	1 Tbsp/15g	56	5.8	370	0.4	5.1	38.7	1
French, Fresh, Organic, Sainsbury's*	1 Tbsp/15ml	45	4.6	301	0.4	5.5	31	0.4
French, Fresh, Sainsbury's*	1 Tbsp/15ml	64	6.7	429	0.6	6.6	44.6	0.6
French, LC, Tesco*	1 Tbsp/16g	8	0.3	50	0.8	7.6	1.6	1.1
French, Less Than 3% Fat, M&S*	1 Tbsp/15ml	10	0.4	68	0.7	11.5	2.6	0.7
French, Reduced Fat, M&S*	1 Tbsp/15g	10	0.4	70	0.7	11.5	2.8	0.7
French, Sainsbury's*	1 Tbsp/15ml	33	2.9	219	0.6	9.8	19.1	0.5
French, Salad, M&S*	1 Serving/25ml	156	16.8	625	0.5	3.8	67.3	0.1
French, Tesco*	1 Serving/25ml	110	11.2	441	0.7	7.2	44.9	0.2
French, Virtually Fat Free, Aldi*	1 Serving/10g	3	0	33	0.9	6.7	0.3	1.1
Garlic & Herb, Reduced Calorie, Hellmann's*	1 Tbsp/15ml	35	2.9	232	0.6	12.8	19.3	0.4
Garlic Herb, Tesco*	1 Tbsp/15g	32	3	210	0.9	5.8	20.2	0.8
Ginger, & Toasted Sesame, Naturally Righteous *	1 Serving/15ml	66	6.3	440	2.7	16	42	0
Herb, Garden, British, M&S*	1 Tbsp/15ml	38	3.2	251	0.9	12.7	21.5	1.5
Honey & Mustard, Dijon, Briannas*	1 Tbsp/15ml	65	6	433	0	20	40	0
Honey & Mustard, Dijon, Wholegrain, Loyd Grossman*	1oz/28g	93	8.9	331	1.2	9.9	31.8	1.3
Honey & Mustard, Light, Kraft*	1 Tbsp/15ml	19	0.7	126	1.2	19	4.6	1.1
Honey Mustard, BGTY, Sainsbury's*	1 Tbsp/15g	12	0.2	78	0.5	16.1	1.3	0.5
Honey Mustard, Finest, Tesco*	1 Serving/25ml	72	5.6	288	1.7	19.6	22.5	0.7
Honey Mustard, Fresh, M&S*	1 Serving/10ml	43	4.2	430	1.7	9.7	42.4	0.5
Honey Mustard, Hellmann's*	1 Serving/15ml	27	0.2	182	0.7	13.7	1.6	0.3
Honey Mustard, M&S*	1 Tbsp/15ml	64	6.4	427	1.7	9.7	42.4	0.6

DRESSING	Measure INFO/WEIGHT	per Measure KCAL	FAT	Nutrition Values per 100g / 100ml KCAL	PROT	CARB	FAT	FIBRE
Honey Mustard, Sainsbury's*	1 Serving/15ml	87	9	577	1.3	7.9	59.7	1.5
Honey Mustard, Tesco*	1 Tbsp/15ml	33	2.3	220	0.8	18.8	15.2	2.5
Honey, Orange Mustard, BGTY, Sainsbury's*	1 Tbsp/15ml	16	0.4	105	1.8	18.6	2.5	1.8
House, Classic, Salad, Hellmann's*	1 Tbsp/15ml	38	3.9	254	0.5	5.7	26	0
House, Light, Supermarket, Pizza Express*	1 Tbsp/15ml	45	4.5	300	0.7	4.3	30	0.3
House, Supermarket, Pizza Express*	1 Tbsp/15ml	62	6.6	415	0.7	3.3	44	0.3
Italian, Newman's Own*	1 Tbsp/15g	82	9	545	0.2	1	59.8	0
Italian, Salad, Essential, Waitrose*	1 Serving/15ml	62	6	414	0.3	12	40.4	0.5
Lemon & Cracked Black Pepper, GFY, Asda*	1 Tbsp/15g	9	0	57	0.2	14	0	0.3
Lemongrass, Ginger Lime, Waitrose*	1 Serving/5ml	27	2.9	544	1.2	5.6	57.3	0.5
Mary Berry*	1 Serving/15g	77	6.6	513	0.8	28.5	44	0.1
Oil & Lemon	*1 Tbsp/15g*	*97*	*10.6*	*647*	*0.3*	*2.8*	*70.6*	*0*
Passion Fruit, & Mango, HE, Tesco*	1 Tbsp/15ml	25	0.3	169	0.6	36.7	2.2	0.4
Ranch, Creamy, 95% Fat Free, Kraft*	1 Tsp/6ml	7	0.3	111	1.4	14.5	5	0.3
Stilton, Long Clawson, M&S*	1 Tbsp/15ml	64	6	427	5.3	11.5	39.7	1
Sweet Chilli, Coriander, Sainsbury's*	1 Tbsp/15ml	38	2.4	255	1.1	26.5	16	0.5
Thousand Island	*1 Tsp/6g*	*19*	*1.8*	*323*	*1.1*	*12.5*	*30.2*	*0.4*
Thousand Island, BGTY, Sainsbury's*	1 Serving/20g	19	1.4	95	0.4	7.3	7.2	0.5
Thousand Island, Eat Smart, Morrisons*	1 Tbsp/15ml	38	3.2	253	0	0	21.3	0
Thousand Island, Hellmann's*	1 Tbsp/15ml	36	3	238	1	14	20	0
Thousand Island, Reduced Calorie	*1 Tsp/6g*	*12*	*0.9*	*195*	*0.7*	*14.7*	*15.2*	*0*
Thousand Island, Tesco*	1 Tbsp/15g	55	4.7	360	1.1	19.5	30.5	0.3
Thousand Island, Walden Farms*	2 Tbsps/30ml	3	0	9	0	4.3	0	1
Tomato & Red Pepper, BGTY, Sainsbury's*	1 Serving/50ml	42	2.2	83	1.1	10	4.3	0.6
Yoghurt & Mint, PB, Waitrose*	1 Serving/100ml	130	2.6	130	4.6	22.1	2.6	0.7
Yoghurt Mint, Crucials*	1 Tbsp/15g	58	5.9	387	1.4	6.2	39.5	0.4
DRIED FRUIT								
Apricots, Soft, Alesto, Lidl*	1 Serving/30g	81	0.1	269	2	61.3	0.3	6.4
Fruity Biscuit Shot, Whitworths*	1 Pack/25g	93	2.1	372	2.8	69.2	8.4	4.5
Pineapple, Sweetened, Whitworths*	1 Bag/35g	122	0.1	350	0.4	86.3	0.2	0.5
Raisin Chocolate, Shot, Whitworths*	1 Pack/25g	91	2.3	364	4	63.2	9.2	5.6
Trail Mix, Kick Start, Wholefoods, Asda*	1 Serving/50g	194	10.2	387	10.9	40	20.4	10.7
DRIED FRUIT MIX								
5 Fruits, Ready to Eat, Sundora*	½ Pack/100g	233	0.4	233	1.6	58.4	0.4	6.8
Average	*1 Tbsp/25g*	*67*	*0.1*	*268*	*2.3*	*68.1*	*0.4*	*2.2*
Berry, Love Life, Waitrose*	1 Serving/30g	89	0.3	296	1.9	70	0.9	3
Garden of England, Graze*	1 Punnet/25g	70	0.2	280	1	71.2	0.7	5.6
Luxury, Co-Op*	1 Serving/40g	114	0.2	285	2	68	0.6	4
Scandinavian Forest, Graze*	1 Punnet/28g	79	0.2	282	2	71	0.6	8
Sultanas Raisins Cranberries, Dunnes*	1 Handful/15g	47	0.1	315	2	80.2	0.9	4.7
Sultanas, Currants, Raisins & Citrus Peel, Asda*	1 Serving/100g	283	0.5	283	2.6	67	0.5	1.7
Tesco*	1 Tbsp/25g	71	0.1	284	2.3	67.9	0.4	2.2
Tropical Sundae, Graze*	1 Punnet/29g	86	0.3	299	2.7	72.7	1	8.5
DRIFTER								
Nestle*	1 Finger/20g	99	4.3	484	4.1	68.9	20.9	1.2
DRINK MIX								
Spritz, Pink Grapefruit, Vodka, Kalosa Natural Spritz*	1 Bottle/275ml	99	0	36	0	0	0	0
DRINKING CHOCOLATE								
Made Up with Semi-Skimmed Milk, Average	*1 Mug/227ml*	*129*	*4.3*	*57*	*3.5*	*7*	*1.9*	*0.2*
Made Up with Skimmed Milk, Average	*1 Mug/227ml*	*100*	*1.1*	*44*	*3.5*	*7*	*0.5*	*0*
Made Up with Whole Milk, Average	*1 Mug/227ml*	*173*	*9.5*	*76*	*3.4*	*6.8*	*4.2*	*0.2*
Powder, Made Up with Skimmed Milk	*1 Mug/227ml*	*134*	*1.4*	*59*	*3.5*	*10.8*	*0.6*	*0*
Powder, Made Up with Whole Milk	*1 Mug/227ml*	*204*	*9.3*	*90*	*3.4*	*10.6*	*4.1*	*0*

D

	Measure INFO/WEIGHT	per Measure KCAL	FAT	Nutrition Values per 100g / 100ml KCAL	PROT	CARB	FAT	FIBRE
DRIPPING								
Beef	*1oz/28g*	*249*	*27.7*	*891*	*0*	*0*	*99*	*0*
DUCK								
Breast, Meat Only, Cooked, Average	*1oz/28g*	*48*	*2*	*172*	*25.3*	*1.8*	*7*	*0*
Breast, Meat Only, Raw, Average	*1 Serving/160g*	*206*	*6.8*	*128*	*22.6*	*0*	*4.2*	*0.2*
Breast, Roast, Blueberries, Everdine*	1 Serving/450g	436	18.4	97	6	7.7	4.1	2.9
Leg, Meat Skin, Average	*1oz/28g*	*80*	*5.6*	*286*	*17.2*	*0.5*	*20*	*0.4*
Raw, Meat Only, Weighed with Fat, Skin Bone	*1 Serving/100g*	*38*	*1.8*	*38*	*5.5*	*0*	*1.8*	*0*
Raw, Meat, Fat & Skin	*1oz/28g*	*109*	*10.4*	*388*	*13.1*	*0*	*37.3*	*0*
Roast, Duckling, Half, Irish, Crispy, Deluxe, Lidl*	1 Serving/50g	172	12.4	343	13.1	17.4	24.7	0
Roasted, Meat Only, Weighed with Fat, Skin Bone	*1 Serving/100g*	*41*	*2.2*	*41*	*5.3*	*0*	*2.2*	*0*
Roasted, Meat, Fat Skin	*1oz/28g*	*118*	*10.7*	*423*	*20*	*0*	*38.1*	*0*
Vegetarian, Shredded Hoisin, Cooked, Linda McCartney*	½ Pack/167g	317	12.9	190	22.1	5.9	7.7	3.9
DUCK AROMATIC								
Crispy, ¼, Hoisin Sauce & 6 Pancakes, Tesco*	1/6 Pack/40g	92	3.3	231	13.3	25.3	8.3	1
Crispy, ¼, Hoisin Sauce, Pancakes, M&S*	½ Pack/155g	290	12.1	187	10.5	18.1	7.8	1
Crispy, ½, Duck & Pancakes, M&S*	½ Pack/311g	590	26.7	190	13.9	14	8.6	2.1
Crispy, ½, Hoisin Sauce, & 12 Pancakes, Tesco*	3 Pancakes/106g	263	9.5	248	17.9	23.4	8.9	1
DUCK CANTONESE								
Style, Roast, Tesco*	1 Pack/300g	375	6.9	125	8.2	17.9	2.3	0.5
DUCK IN								
Chinese Barbecue, Wings, Sainsbury's*	1 Serving/175g	430	25	246	19.4	9.7	14.3	0
Filo Pastry, Christmas Trees, Iceland*	1 Tree/24g	63	2.4	267	9.6	32.8	10	3.6
Orange Sauce, Breast, Simply, Gressingham Foods*	½ Pack/175g	254	11.9	145	15.9	5.1	6.8	0.4
Orange Sauce, Roast, a L'Orange, M&S*	½ Pack/259g	482	26.9	186	16.2	6.5	10.4	0.8
Plum Sauce, with Egg Fried Rice, Serves 1, Sainsbury's*	1 Pack/450g	738	18.9	164	6.2	24	4.2	2.8
DUCK PEKING								
Crispy, Aromatic, Sainsbury's*	½ Pack/300g	1236	110.7	412	19.5	0.6	36.9	0.1
DUCK WITH								
Port Orange Sauce, Legs, Slow Cooked, M&S*	½ Pack/158g	265	16.9	168	14.8	3	10.7	0.5
Pancakes Hoisin Sauce, M&S*	1 Pack/80g	136	3.2	170	13	19.9	4	0.9
DUMPLINGS								
Average	*1oz/28g*	*58*	*3.3*	*208*	*2.8*	*24.5*	*11.7*	*0.9*
Berry, Sweet, Gyoza, Itsu*	3 Gyoza/40g	64	0.1	159	3.1	35	0.2	2
Chicken, Jalfrezi, Naan , Boxed*	1 Pack/374g	719	35.2	192	9.2	17	9.4	2.4
Chocolate, Banana, Gyoza, Itsu*	3 Gyoza/40g	138	5.7	341	5.9	46	14.1	2.8
Dim Sum, Assorted Stuffing, Steamed, Restaurant	*1 Serving/100g*	*230*	*8.2*	*230*	*7.9*	*32*	*8.2*	*3*
Dim Sum, Chicken, Asian Fusion, Waitrose*	1 Dumpling/20g	30	0.4	152	9.5	22.8	2.2	1.4
Dim Sum, Chicken, Steamed, Restaurant	*1 Serving/100g*	*230*	*5.9*	*230*	*7.5*	*37*	*5.9*	*2.1*
Dim Sum, Chinese, Deep Fried, Restaurant	*1 Serving/100g*	*430*	*23*	*430*	*4.9*	*50*	*23*	*1.8*
Dim Sum, From Restaurant, Average	*1 Piece/12g*	*50*	*2.4*	*433*	*28.9*	*31.3*	*20.4*	*0*
Dim Sum, Meat Dumpling, Deep Fried, Restaurant	*1 Serving/100g*	*340*	*16*	*340*	*4.9*	*43*	*16*	*1*
Dim Sum, Pork, Restaurant, Average	*1 Serving/100g*	*270*	*7.3*	*270*	*7.3*	*43*	*7.3*	*1.6*
Dim Sum, Prawn, Steamed, Eat Well, M&S*	1 Dim Sum/20g	28	0.2	138	6.7	25.1	1.1	0.6
Dim Sum, Steamed, Prawn, M&S*	6 Dim Sum/120g	222	3.2	185	1.1	39	2.7	1.5
Dim Sum, Vegetable & Meat, Pan Fried, Restaurant	*1 Serving/100g*	*280*	*13*	*280*	*6.4*	*34*	*13*	*3.7*
Dim Sum, Vegetable & Meat, Steamed, Restaurant	*1 Serving/100g*	*240*	*7.9*	*240*	*5.9*	*37*	*7.9*	*2.5*
Dim Sum, Wonton, Deep Fried, Restaurant	*1 Serving/100g*	*430*	*29*	*430*	*9.7*	*32*	*29*	*1.2*
Gyoza, Chicken, Frozen, Itsu*	5 Gyoza/100g	157	4.4	157	8.2	20	4.4	1.3
Gyoza, Pork, Itsu*	5 Gyoza/100g	185	6.6	185	8.1	22	6.6	2.1
Gyoza, Prawn, Pot, Itsu*	6 Gyoza/120g	188	7.1	157	5.2	20	5.9	2.3
Gyoza, Vegetable, in Broth, The City Kitchen*	1 Pack/355g	270	8.5	76	2.1	10.7	2.4	1.6
Gyoza, Vegetable, Pot, Itsu*	1 Gyoza/20g	31	0.7	158	8.2	21	3.7	3.1
Gyozas, Chicken, Microwaved, Iceland*	1 Gyozas/18g	31	0.5	176	8.3	28	2.7	3.3

D

DUMPLINGS

	Measure INFO/WEIGHT	per Measure KCAL	per Measure FAT	Nutrition Values per 100g / 100ml KCAL	PROT	CARB	FAT	FIBRE
Homestyle, Baked Weight, Frozen, Aunt Bessie's*	1 Dumpling/53g	177	7.9	337	5.4	47	15	3.5
Mix, Cooked as Directed, Aunt Bessie's*	2 Dumpling/53g	126	4.9	238	4.5	33	9.2	2.4
Pork & Garlic Chive, Waitrose*	1 Pack/115g	215	8.1	187	9.4	20.4	7	1.1
Prawn Sui Mai, Selection, M&S*	6 Sui Mai/120g	143	0.8	119	9.4	13.3	0.7	1.5
Prawn, Siu Mai, Chinese, M&S*	8 Dumpling/170g	170	2.9	100	7.8	13.1	1.7	1.3
Vegetable, Steamed, Bibigo*	1 Dumpling/28g	29	1.9	103	6.9	18.5	6.7	1.4

D

	Measure INFO/WEIGHT	per Measure KCAL	FAT	Nutrition Values per 100g / 100ml KCAL	PROT	CARB	FAT	FIBRE
EASTER EGG								
After Eight Giant Chocolate Egg, Nestle*	¼ Egg /50g	274	16.8	547	5.5	51.8	33.7	7.1
Buttons, Chocolate Egg Shell Only, Cadbury*	1 Sm Egg/100g	530	30.5	530	7.6	56.5	30.5	0.7
Caramel, Chocolate Egg Shell Only, Cadbury*	1 Lge Egg/343g	1801	102.9	525	7.5	56.8	30	0.7
Chick, Dairy Milk, Chocolate Egg Shell Only, Cadbury*	1 Egg/167g	877	50.1	525	7.5	56.8	30	0.7
Chocolate Egg Shell Only, Dairy Milk, Cadbury*	1 Lg Egg/343g	1818	104.6	530	7.6	56.5	30.5	0.7
Chocolate Orange, Terry's*	1 Egg/120g	636	36.6	530	7.4	57	30.5	2.4
Creme Egg, Chocolate Egg Shell Only, Cadbury*	1 Egg/178g	943	53.4	530	7.5	56.8	30	0.7
Crunchie, Cadbury*	1 Lge Egg/200g	1072	61.9	537	7.3	56	31	2.1
Dark Chocolate, 70%, Green & Black's*	1 Med Egg/160g	944	69	575	9.1	36.5	42	10
Disney, Nestle*	1 Egg/65g	342	18.9	526	6.3	59.7	29.1	0.6
Flake, Chocolate Egg Shell Only, Cadbury*	1 Lge Egg/200g	1074	62	537	7.3	56	31	2.1
Galaxy Ripple Indulgence, with Chocolate Egg, Mars*	1 Egg /198g	1045	57.4	528	7.1	58.9	29	1.6
Kit Kat, Chunky, Nestle*	1 Med Egg/107g	575	31.5	537	5.2	61.9	29.4	1.4
Milk Chocolate, Nestle*	½ Egg/42g	205	9.7	489	5	65.2	23.1	0.5
Milk Chocolate, Swiss, Hollow, M&S*	1 Egg/18g	100	6.3	555	6.7	53.2	34.8	2.5
Milky Bar, Nestle*	1 Egg/40g	182	6.9	454	4.2	70.8	17.2	0
Mint Collection, Dark, Thorntons*	¼ Egg/41g	215	13.4	531	6.3	47	33	0
Roses, Chocolate Egg Shell Only, Cadbury*	1 Egg/200g	1060	61	530	7.6	56.5	30.5	0.7
Smarties, Nestle*	¼ Egg/31g	160	8.4	526	5.2	63.3	27.7	1.3
Twirl, Chocolate Egg Shell Only, Cadbury*	1 Lge Egg/325g	1722	99.1	530	7.6	56.5	30.5	0.7
White Chocolate, Thorntons*	1 Egg/360g	1958	109.1	544	5.5	62.2	30.3	2.1
Wispa, Chocolate Egg Shell Only, Cadbury*	1 Lg Egg/313g	1643	93.9	525	7.5	56.8	30	0.7
ECLAIR								
Chocolate, 25% Less Fat, Sainsbury's*	1 Eclair/58g	171	9.3	295	6.8	31.1	16	1.2
Chocolate, Asda*	1 Eclair/33g	144	11	436	6.7	27.3	33.3	4.8
Chocolate, Belgian, Cream, Essential, Waitrose*	1 Eclair/39g	148	9.5	379	6.2	33	24.4	1.6
Chocolate, Belgian, Fresh Cream, Tesco*	1 Eclair/61g	233	15.4	382	7.3	30.6	25.3	1
Chocolate, Fresh Cream, M&S*	1 Eclair/44g	170	12.2	390	6.3	28.4	27.9	2
Chocolate, Fresh Cream, Sainsbury's*	1 Eclair/35g	130	8.3	372	6.5	32.2	23.8	1.5
Chocolate, Frozen, Free From, Tesco*	1 Eclair/25g	81	4.2	327	4.1	38.9	17	0.8
Chocolate, Frozen, Morrisons*	1 Eclair/31g	116	9.6	374	5	18.8	31	1.3
Chocolate, Mini, Iceland*	1 Eclair/12g	49	3.6	418	5.3	29.3	30.8	1
EEL								
Cooked or Smoked, Dry Heat, Average	**1 Serving/100g**	**236**	**15**	**236**	**23.6**	**0**	**15**	**0**
Jellied, Average	**1oz/28g**	**26**	**1.9**	**93**	**8**	**0**	**6.7**	**0**
Raw, Average	**1oz/28g**	**32**	**2.1**	**113**	**11.1**	**0**	**7.6**	**0**
EGG SUBSTITUTE								
Vegan Egg, Follow Your Heart*	1 Serving/10g	40	1.7	401	5	0	17	40
EGGS								
Spinach, Pot, Meadow Fresh, Lidl*	1 Pot/118g	138	6.8	117	10	1.3	5.8	0.8
Spinach, Protein Pot, Tesco*	1 Pot/100g	103	5.1	103	11.3	2.7	5.1	0.4
Araucana, Bluebell, Free Range, Finest, Tesco*	1 Egg/50g	66	4.5	131	12.6	0.1	9	0
Boiled, Peeled, Free Range, Musclefood*	1 Serving/53g	70	4.1	133	12.1	3.6	7.8	0
Dried, White, Average	**1 Tbsp/14g**	**41**	**0**	**295**	**73.8**	**0**	**0**	**0**
Dried, Whole, Average	**1oz/28g**	**159**	**11.6**	**568**	**48.4**	**0**	**41.6**	**0**
Duck, Boiled & Salted, Weight with Shell	**1 Egg/75g**	**148**	**11.6**	**198**	**14.6**	**0**	**15.5**	**0**
Duck, Whole, Raw, Weight with Shell	**1 Egg/75g**	**122**	**8.8**	**163**	**14.3**	**0**	**11.8**	**0**
Free Range, Large, Weight with Shell	**1 Egg/68g**	**97**	**6.8**	**143**	**12.6**	**0.8**	**9.9**	**0**
Fried in Veg Oil, Average	**1 Med/60g**	**107**	**8.3**	**179**	**13.6**	**0.7**	**13.9**	**0**
Fried, without Fat, Average	**1 Med/60g**	**104**	**7.6**	**174**	**15**	**0.7**	**12.7**	**0**
Goose, Whole, Fresh, Raw, Weight with Shell	**1 Egg/144g**	**232**	**16.6**	**161**	**12.1**	**1.2**	**11.5**	**0**
Large, Weight with Shell	**1 Egg/68g**	**97**	**6.8**	**143**	**12.6**	**0.8**	**9.9**	**0**
Medium, Boiled, Weight with Shell	**1 Egg/60g**	**86**	**6**	**143**	**12.6**	**0.8**	**9.9**	**0**

E

	Measure INFO/WEIGHT	per Measure KCAL	FAT	Nutrition Values per 100g / 100ml KCAL	PROT	CARB	FAT	FIBRE
EGGS								
Medium, Weight with Shell	**1 Egg/56g**	**71**	**5**	**143**	**12.6**	**0.8**	**9.9**	**0**
Poached, Weight with Shell	**1 Med/58g**	**83**	**5.8**	**143**	**12.6**	**0.8**	**9.9**	**0**
Quail, Whole, Raw, Weight with Shell	**1 Egg/13g**	**20**	**1.4**	**151**	**12.9**	**0.4**	**11.1**	**0**
Ready Scrambled, Easy Egg Co*	1 Pack/125g	144	9.9	115	7.9	2.9	7.9	0.5
Savoury, Bites, Mini, Sainsbury's*	1 Bite/12g	34	2.1	285	9.4	21.1	17.9	1.2
Savoury, Mini, Tesco*	1 Egg/20g	55	3.5	274	9.2	20.2	17.4	2.3
Savoury, Vegetarian, Mini, Quorn*	1 Egg/20g	51	2.3	257	15	21	11.5	4.6
Scotch, Asda*	1 Egg/114g	286	19.2	251	11.2	13.7	16.8	1.4
Scotch, Cumberland, Waitrose*	1 Egg/114g	243	14.3	214	13	12.1	12.6	1.6
Scotch, Finest, Tesco*	1 Egg/114g	280	20.1	247	11.6	10.4	17.7	1.1
Scotch, Free Range, Sainsbury's*	1 Egg/113g	284	19	252	12.4	12.5	16.9	2.5
Scotch, Lincolnshire, M&S*	1 Egg/114g	306	21.1	268	12	12.8	18.5	1.2
Scotch, Morrisons*	1 Egg/114g	286	19.1	251	11.2	13.7	16.8	1.4
Scotch, Retail	**1 Egg/120g**	**301**	**20.5**	**251**	**12**	**13.1**	**17.1**	**0**
Scrambled with Milk, Average	**1 Serving/100g**	**257**	**23.4**	**257**	**10.9**	**0.7**	**23.4**	**0**
Scrambled, 1 Minute, Musclefood*	1 Serving/125g	144	9.9	115	7.9	2.9	7.9	0.5
Scrambled, Average	**1 Serving/100g**	**160**	**11.6**	**160**	**13.8**	**0**	**11.6**	**0**
Turkey, Whole, Raw, Weight with Shell	**1 Egg/79g**	**135**	**9.6**	**171**	**13.7**	**1.2**	**12.2**	**0**
Very Large, Average, Weight with Shell	**1 Egg/78g**	**112**	**7.8**	**143**	**12.6**	**0.8**	**9.9**	**0**
White, Free Range, Liquid, Two Chicks*	3 Tbsp/45g	23	0	50	10.5	1	0	0
Whites Only, Raw, Average	**1 Lg Egg/33g**	**17**	**0.1**	**52**	**10.9**	**0.7**	**0.2**	**0**
Yolks, Raw	**1 Yolk/17g**	**55**	**4.5**	**322**	**15.9**	**3.6**	**26.5**	**0**
ELICHE								
Dry Weight, Buitoni*	1 Serving/80g	282	1.5	352	11.2	72.6	1.9	0
ELK								
Raw, Meat only	**1 Serving/100g**	**111**	**1.4**	**111**	**23**	**0**	**1.4**	**0**
Roasted, Meat only	**1 Serving/100g**	**146**	**1.9**	**146**	**30.2**	**0**	**1.9**	**0**
ENCHILADAS								
3 Bean, Ready Meal, Average	**1 Pack/400g**	**505**	**16.6**	**126**	**4.4**	**16.9**	**4.2**	**3.2**
Beef, LC, Tesco*	1 Pack/400g	440	11.2	110	5.4	13.4	2.8	3.1
Chicken, American, HL, Tesco*	1 Serving/240g	353	4.3	147	10.4	22.5	1.8	1.2
Chicken, Asda*	1 Serving/500g	690	30	138	10	17	6	1
Chicken, Average	**1 Serving/295g**	**483**	**18.8**	**164**	**11.6**	**16**	**6.4**	**1.7**
Chicken, Diner Specials, M&S*	½ Pack/227g	340	12	150	9.9	15.4	5.3	2
Chicken, in a Spicy Salsa & Bean Sauce, Asda*	½ Pack/212g	373	17	176	10	16	8	0
Chicken, PB, Waitrose*	1 Pack/450g	482	14.4	107	6.9	12.7	3.2	1.1
Chicken, Suiza, Smart Ones, Weight Watchers*	1 Pack/255g	290	5	114	4.3	18	2	1.2
Spicy, Three Bean, Cooked, CBY, Asda*	1 Pack/400g	466	15.9	117	4.4	13.7	4	4.1
Vegetable, & Bean, Eat Smart, Morrisons*	1 Pack/380g	475	9.9	125	4.7	20.7	2.6	3.2
Vegetable, Morrisons*	1 Pack/400g	468	18.4	117	4.5	14.4	4.6	1.8
with Cheese & Beef, From Restaurant	**1 Serving/295g**	**496**	**27.1**	**168**	**6.2**	**15.9**	**9.2**	**0**
with Cheese, From Restaurant	**1 Serving/163g**	**319**	**18.8**	**196**	**5.9**	**17.5**	**11.6**	**0**
ENDIVE								
Raw	**1oz/28g**	**2**	**0**	**8**	**1.1**	**0.6**	**0.1**	**1.3**
ENERGY DRINK								
Average	**1 Can/250ml**	**118**	**0**	**47**	**0**	**11.4**	**0**	**0**
Blue Bolt, Sainsbury's*	1 Can/250ml	124	0	49	0	11.3	0	0
Cherry, Lucozade*	1 Bottle/500ml	345	0	69	0	17.1	0	0
Citrus Blast, Soft Drink, Mountain Dew, Britvic*	1 Bottle/500ml	240	0	48	0	13	0	0
Citrus, Isotonic, Umbro*	1 Bottle/500ml	139	0	28	0	6.5	0	0
Isostar Sport, Isostar*	1 Glass/250ml	74	0	30	0	7	0	0
Juiced Berry, Relentless*	1 Can/500g	230	0	46	0	10.7	0	0
Juiced Orange Tropical Fruit, Relentless*	1 Can/500ml	220	0	44	0	10.7	0	0

	Measure INFO/WEIGHT	per Measure KCAL	FAT	Nutrition Values per 100g / 100ml KCAL	PROT	CARB	FAT	FIBRE
ENERGY DRINK								
KX, Sugar Free, Diet, Tesco*	1 Can/250ml	5	0	2	0	0	0	0
KX, Sugar Free, Tesco*	1 Can/250ml	8	0	3	0	0	0	0
Lemon, Active Sport, Tesco*	1 Bottle/500ml	135	0	27	0	6.5	0	0
Libertus, Blue, Sugar Free, Relentless*	1 Can/500ml	20	0	4	0	0	0	0
Mixed Berries, First Start, Rockstar*	1 Can/500ml	30	0	6	0.5	1.3	0	0
Monster*	1 Can/500ml	240	0	48	0	12	0	0
Orange, Active Sport, Tesco*	1 Bottle/500ml	135	0	27	0	6.5	0	0
Original, Rockstar*	1 Can/500ml	290	0	60	0.4	13.6	0	0
Powerade, Aqua+*	1 Bottle/500ml	80	0	16	0	3.7	0	0
Red Devil, Britvic*	1 Can/250ml	160	0	64	0.4	15.1	0	0
Red Rooster, Hi Energy Mixer, Cott Beverages Ltd*	1 Can/250ml	112	0	45	0.6	10.3	0	0
Red Thunder, Diet, Low Calorie, Aldi*	1 Can/250ml	5	0	2	0.1	0	0	0
Relentless, Original, Relentless*	1 Can/500ml	230	0	46	0	10.4	0	0
Relentless, Sugar Free, Coca-Cola*	1 Can/500ml	20	0	4	0	0	0	0
Revive, Cranberry with Acai, Light Sparkling, Lucozade*	1 Bottle/380ml	50	0	13	0	2.8	0	0
Simulation, Emerge, Aldi*	1 Can/105g	44	0.1	42	0	10	0.1	0.1
SoBe, Appleberry Burst, Britvic*	1 Can/250ml	135	0	54	0.4	12	0	0
Sparkling Orange, Dual Energy, Powerade*	1 Bottle/500ml	225	0	45	0	10.5	0	0
Sugar Free, Boost Drinks Ltd*	1 Can/250ml	5	0	2	0	0	0	0
Sugar Free, Diet, Mountain Dew, Britvic*	1 Can/440ml	3	0	1	0	0	0	0
Tropical, Emerge, Cott Beverages Ltd*	1 Can/250ml	115	0	46	0	10.7	0	0
Ultra Citron, Zero Calorie, Monster*	1 Can/500ml	9	0	2	0	1	0	0
Ultra Red, Zero Sugar Plus Calorie, Monster*	1 Can/500ml	15	0	3	0	0.9	0	0
Ultra Violet, Monster*	1 Can/500ml	15	0	3	0	1.4	0	0
Ultra, Zero Calorie, Monster*	1 Can/500ml	10	0	2	0	0.9	0	0
V, Frucor Beverages*	1 Can/250ml	112	0	45	0	11.2	0	0
ESCALOPE								
Vegetarian, Garlic Herb, Quorn*	1 Escalope/140g	293	16.5	209	8.9	16.9	11.8	3.8
Vegetarian, Garlic Mushroom, Creamy, Quorn*	1 Escalope/120g	259	12.3	216	10.4	18.8	10.3	3.7
Vegetarian, Gruyere Cheese, Quorn*	1 Escalope/110g	267	15.4	243	10	18	14	2.6
Vegetarian, Korma, Quorn*	1 Escalope/120g	270	15.6	225	7	20	13	3
Vegetarian, Lemon Black Pepper, Quorn*	1 Escalope/110g	256	12.9	233	9.6	20.5	11.7	2.1
Vegetarian, Mozzarella Pesto, Quorn*	1 Escalope/120g	271	15.6	226	10	15	13	4.5
Vegetarian, Turkey Style, Sage Onion, Quorn*	1 Escalope/100g	188	9.8	188	10	15	9.8	4.5

E

	Measure INFO/WEIGHT	per Measure KCAL	FAT	Nutrition Values per 100g / 100ml KCAL	PROT	CARB	FAT	FIBRE
FAGGOTS								
Pork, West Country Sauce, Six Pack, Cooked, Mr Brains*	2 Faggots/218g	190	4.8	87	6	10	2.2	0
FAJITA								
Beef, GFY, Asda*	½ Pack/208g	354	9.8	170	11	21	4.7	1.6
Chicken, Average	**1 Serving/240g**	**357**	**12.8**	**149**	**10.2**	**15**	**5.4**	**2.3**
Chicken, BGTY, Sainsbury's*	1 Pack/172g	256	4.3	149	10.8	20.9	2.5	1.7
Chicken, Co-Op*	1 Serving/230g	391	16.1	170	11	15	7	3
Chicken, COU, M&S*	1 Pack/230g	288	5.3	125	10	16.5	2.3	1.5
Chicken, Crispy, Old El Paso*	1 Fajita/70g	183	5.4	263	7.6	41	7.8	1.8
Chicken, Hoisin, with Crispy Wedges, Hello Fresh*	1 Serving/677g	724	11	107	7.8	15.4	1.6	0
Chicken, M&S*	1 Pack/230g	345	12.2	150	8.6	17.7	5.3	1
Chicken, Mexican, No Mayo, Foo-Go*	1 Pack/198g	360	11.1	182	9.6	23.3	5.6	2.4
Chicken, Mini, Tesco*	1 Fajita/18g	37	1.1	205	8.7	27.8	6.3	3.4
Chicken, Sainsbury's*	½ Pack/275g	396	14.6	144	9.5	14.5	5.3	1.9
Chicken, Salt Balanced, COU, M&S*	1 Pack/230g	253	5.3	110	9.5	13.2	2.3	1.7
Chicken, Smoky, Everdine*	1 Serving/450g	585	15.3	130	9.1	14.3	3.4	3.1
Chicken, Spicy, Meal Box, M&S*	½ Pack/238g	382	15.7	161	9	15.5	6.6	1.9
Chicken, Tesco*	½ Pack /275g	382	14.3	139	9.2	13.9	5.2	1.9
Meal Kit, Mexican StyleMade Up, CBY, Asda*	¼ Pack/120g	280	6.6	234	6	39	5.5	2.3
Meal Kit, Roasted Tomato, Pepper, Old El Paso*	1 Fajita/63g	143	2.5	227	6.6	40.1	3.9	2.7
Meal Kit, Sizzling, Smoky BBQ, As Sold, Old El Paso*	1 Fajita/63g	141	2.3	224	6.8	40	3.7	1.8
Meal Kit, Tesco*	1 Serving/100g	210	3.4	210	6.1	38.2	3.4	2.1
Vegetable	**1 Serving/275g**	**472**	**14.9**	**172**	**4.9**	**25.6**	**5.4**	**1.9**
Vegetable, Tesco*	1 Fajita/112g	133	5.6	119	4.2	14.3	5	1.1
Vegetarian, Meal Kit, Quorn*	½ Pack/214g	268	5.4	125	7	18.5	2.5	3.5
Vegetarian, Strips, Cooked, Quorn*	½ Pack/70g	81	1.1	115	14.8	9.3	1.6	2.4
FALAFEL								
Feta, Snack pot, Lovely Vegetables, M&S*	1 Pack/300g	270	13.2	90	4.4	8.5	4.4	5.2
Houmous, Snack Pot, Tesco*	1 Pack/106g	354	26.2	324	8.4	14.5	24	8.4
Tabbouleh, Co-Op*	1 Pack/250g	308	13.8	123	5.5	9.7	5.5	6.5
12 pack, Sainsbury's*	1 Falafel/17g	48	2.6	281	6.8	25.2	15.5	6.4
Asda*	½ Pack/50g	140	9.6	281	8.3	18.9	19.1	8.2
Authentic Mediterranean, Great Food*	1 Falafel/22g	56	2.6	253	9.1	29.9	11.7	4.1
Balls, Meat Free, Meat Free, Tesco*	3 Balls/67g	135	5.3	205	7.1	21.7	8.1	6.3
Beetroot, with Red Pepper, Chilli, Gosh*	4 Falafel/88g	150	6	170	5.4	25.1	6.8	6.4
Fresh Herb, M&S*	1 Falafel/18g	45	2.2	248	8.3	22.6	12	8.1
Fried in Vegetable Oil, Average	**1 Falafel/25g**	**45**	**2.8**	**179**	**6.4**	**15.6**	**11.2**	**3.4**
Gourmet, Meat Free, Vegideli, The Redwood Co*	1 Patty/17g	26	1.4	159	6.1	20.5	8.5	8.1
Herby Aromatic, Waitrose*	2 Falafels/38g	85	3.4	224	8.5	23.3	8.9	8.4
Mini, M&S*	1 Falafel/14g	43	2.5	310	7.9	28.1	18.4	2.6
Mini, Sainsbury's*	1 Serving/168g	499	29.6	297	8	26.8	17.6	3.2
Mix, Asda*	1 Pack/120g	313	15	261	6.4	30.8	12.5	2.6
Mix, Authentic, Al'fez*	1 Serving/100g	235	13.8	235	7.1	26.3	13.8	8.8
Mix, Organic, Quick Easy, Hale Hearty*	1 Pack/200g	646	11	323	19.2	43.8	5.5	10.7
Moroccan Chicken Butternut Squash, Asda*	1 Pack/400g	428	12	107	8.9	9.2	3	3.7
Moroccan Inspired, Tesco*	1 Falafel/25g	70	3	279	11	26.6	12	10.4
Moroccan, Gluten Milk Free, Free From, Morrisons*	1 Falafel/24g	63	2.4	263	5.8	34	10.1	6.4
Organic, Cauldron Foods*	1 Falafel/25g	51	2.4	203	8.4	20.3	9.8	7.2
Original, Mediterranean, Great Food*	1 Falafel/22g	69	4	316	9.2	32	18.3	6.6
Shawarma, Everdine*	1 Serving/450g	590	18.4	131	4.5	16.7	4.1	5
Sweet Potato, Ella's Kitchen*	1 Falafel/25g	23	0.3	93	3.6	18.8	1.1	0.8
Sweet Potato, Meat Free, Vegan, Tesco*	3 Falafels/62g	123	6.2	199	4.2	18.1	10	9.6
Sweet Potato, with Houmous, On the Go, Sainsbury's*	1 Pack/250g	332	11.2	133	5.7	15.5	4.5	3.9
Vegetarian, Organic, Waitrose*	1 Felafel/25g	55	2.6	220	8	23.3	10.5	7.6

F

	Measure INFO/WEIGHT	per Measure KCAL	per Measure FAT	Nutrition Values per 100g / 100ml KCAL	PROT	CARB	FAT	FIBRE
FANTA								
Fruit Twist, Coca-Cola*	1 Serving/250ml	65	0	26	0	6.4	0	0
Icy Lemon, Coca-Cola*	1 Can/330ml	112	0	34	0	8.3	0	0
Icy Lemon, Zero, Coca-Cola*	1 Can/330ml	7	0	2	0	0.2	0	0
Lemon, Coca-Cola*	1 Can/330ml	165	0	50	0	12	0	0
Light, Coca-Cola*	1 Glass/250ml	5	0	2	0	0.5	0	0
Orange, Coca-Cola*	1 Can/330ml	63	0	19	0	4.6	0	0
Orange, Zero, Coca-Cola*	1 Can/330ml	11	0	3	0	0.5	0	0
Peach, Singapore, Coca-Cola*	1 Bottle/500ml	230	0	46	0	11	0	0
Red Fruits, Coca-Cola*	1 Serving/100ml	37	0	37	0	9	0	0
Summer Fruits, Z, Coca-Cola*	1fl oz/30ml	1	0	3	0	0.6	0	0
FARFALLE								
Bows, Dry, Average	**1 Serving/75g**	**265**	**1.4**	**353**	**11.4**	**72.6**	**1.9**	**1.9**
Salmon, Hot Smoked, Slimming World*	1 Pack/550g	605	12.1	110	6	15.3	2.2	2.4
FAT								
Duck, Sainsbury's*	1 Serving/15g	135	15	900	0.5	0.5	100	0.5
Goose, Sainsbury's*	1 Serving/15g	135	14.9	897	0.5	0.7	99.3	0.5
Vegetable, Pure, Trex*	1 Tbsp/12g	108	12	900	0	0	100	0
FENNEL								
Florence, Boiled in Salted Water	**1oz/28g**	**3**	**0.1**	**11**	**0.9**	**1.5**	**0.2**	**2.3**
Florence, Raw, Unprepared, Average	**1 Bulb/250g**	**24**	**0.4**	**10**	**0.7**	**1.4**	**0.2**	**1.9**
Florence, Steamed	**1 Serving/80g**	**9**	**0.2**	**11**	**9**	**1.5**	**0.2**	**2.3**
FENUGREEK								
Leaves, Raw, Fresh, Average	**10g**	**4**	**0**	**35**	**4.6**	**4.8**	**0.2**	**1.1**
FETTUCCINE								
Chicken Roasted Pepper, Love Life, Waitrose*	1 Pack/375g	329	5.7	92	6.3	12.1	1.6	1.9
Dry Weight, Buitoni*	1 Serving/90g	326	1.5	362	12.2	74.4	1.7	0
Edamame Mung Bean, Explore Asian*	¼ Pack/50g	168	2.1	335	47.2	16.8	4.2	20.6
Slim Pasta, Eat Water*	½ Pack/100g	9	0	9	0.2	0	0	4
with Tomato Mushroom, Easy Cook, Napolina*	1 Pack/120g	461	8.6	384	11.8	67.9	7.2	0
FIG ROLLS								
Asda*	1 Biscuit/19g	71	1.7	372	4.8	68	9	0
Jacob's*	1 Biscuit/17g	66	1.5	386	3.4	72.2	8.6	3
Sainsbury's*	1 Biscuit/19g	67	1.6	360	4.3	64.5	8.7	3.4
FIGS								
Almond Stuffed, Kounos*	3 Figs/34g	99	22.2	291	2.2	63.9	65.3	0.2
Dried, Average	**1 Fig/14g**	**32**	**0.1**	**232**	**3.6**	**53.2**	**1.1**	**8.6**
Dried, with Honey, Intermarche *	4 Figs/30g	80	0.4	268	3.2	57.1	1.2	8.4
Raw, Fresh, Average	**1 Fig/35g**	**16**	**0.1**	**45**	**1.3**	**9.8**	**0.2**	**1.5**
FISH								
Balls, Gefilte, M&S*	1 Pack/200g	280	7.8	140	14.1	11.9	3.9	1
Char, Arctic, Whole, Raw	**1 Serving/100g**	**137**	**6**	**137**	**20.8**	**0**	**6**	**0**
Chargrills, Sun Ripened Tomato, Basil, Birds Eye*	1 Chargrill/163g	127	2.5	75	14	1.4	1.5	0.5
Fillet, Battered Or Breaded, & Fried, From Restaurant	**1 Portion/256g**	**594**	**31.5**	**232**	**14.7**	**17**	**12.3**	**0.5**
Fillets in Parsley Sauce, Light & Easy, Youngs*	1 Pack/224g	139	4.3	62	8.4	2.8	1.9	1.4
Fillets, Breaded, GF, Captain Birds Eye, Birds Eye*	1 Fillet/125g	299	16.3	239	12	18	13	1.1
Fillets, Crispy, Sweet Chilli, Oven Baked, Gastro, Youngs*	1 Fillet/144g	311	13.4	216	12.3	20.3	9.3	0.9
Fillets, Dinner, Meal for One, Youngs*	1 Pack/378g	340	11	90	6	9.1	2.9	1.5
Fillets, Lemon & Pepper, Youngs*	1 Fillet/130g	283	16.7	218	10.3	15.3	12.9	4.3
Fillets, Lime Chilli, Fish Fusions, Birds Eye*	1 Portion/160g	270	10.1	169	15	12.9	6.3	0.5
Garlic Herb, Inspirations, Birds Eye*	½ Pack/160g	254	9.8	159	14	11.8	6.1	0.4
Goujons, Asda*	1 Serving/125g	240	8	192	12.8	20.8	6.4	0.2
Goujons, Vegetarian, Vivera*	1 Goujon/35g	87	3.5	248	13	25	10	2.7
Grouper	**1 Serving/100g**	**92**	**1**	**92**	**19.4**	**0**	**1**	**0**

F

	Measure INFO/WEIGHT	per Measure KCAL	FAT	Nutrition Values per 100g / 100ml KCAL	PROT	CARB	FAT	FIBRE
FISH								
Medley, SteamFresh, Birds Eye*	1 Bag/170g	170	6.3	100	13	2.3	3.7	0.1
Melts with Tomato Mozzarella Filling, Birds Eye*	1 Fillet/100g	255	15	255	13	17	15	0.6
Pie Mix, Ocado*	1 Pack/320g	410	18.2	128	19	0	5.7	0
Pie Mix, Seasonal, Sainsbury's*	1 Pack/320g	480	28.2	150	17.7	0	8.8	0
Pouting, Fillets, Tesco*	1 Serving/100g	85	0.3	85	19.7	0.3	0.3	0
River Cobbler, Smoked, Tesco*	1 Fillet /165g	124	3.5	75	13.9	0	2.1	1.5
River Cobbler, Value, Tesco*	½ Pack/133g	133	5.3	100	15.1	0.1	4	0.1
Salted, Chinese, Steamed	*1oz/28g*	*43*	*0.6*	*155*	*33.9*	*0*	*2.2*	*0*
Steaks, in Butter Sauce, HFC, Tesco*	1 Pouch/130g	120	4.9	92	9.2	5.1	3.8	0.3
Sticks, Crunchy, Mrs. Paul's*	6 Sticks/95g	220	10	232	11.6	21	10.5	0
White, Battered, HFC, Tesco*	1 Fillet/118g	243	12.1	206	10.9	17.1	10.3	0.7
White, Breaded, HFC, Tesco*	1 Fillet/117g	278	13.1	238	12	21.7	11.2	1.1
White, Fillets, Frozen, Bay Fishmongers, Tesco*	1 Fillet/104g	77	0.6	74	17.2	0	0.6	0
White, Smoked, Average	*1 Serving/100g*	*108*	*0.9*	*108*	*23.4*	*0*	*0.9*	*0*
FISH & CHIPS								
Breaded, Budgens*	1 Pack/340g	544	18	160	8.6	19.3	5.3	1.5
Co-Op*	1 Pack/250g	388	15	155	6	18	6	2
Haddock, Chunky Chips, Mushy Peas, Gastropub, M&S*	1 Pack/425g	654	25.1	154	7.2	17	5.9	2.2
Mini Meal, 093, Wiltshire Farm Foods*	1 Serving/185g	255	8.3	138	6.9	17.7	4.5	2.8
Quinoa Coated, Everdine*	1 Serving/450g	405	16.2	90	6.9	5.7	3.6	3.6
Takeaway or Fast Food, Average	*1 Serving/469g*	*998*	*115.6*	*213*	*17.7*	*45.7*	*24.6*	*2.6*
Tesco*	1 Serving/300g	489	18.6	163	5.5	21.2	6.2	1.6
with Mushy Peas, Kershaws*	1 Pack/315g	450	18.3	143	6.4	16.4	5.8	1.6
FISH CAKES								
Battered, Extra Large, Oven Baked, Chip Shop, Youngs*	1 Cake/100g	209	10.6	210	7.5	20	10.7	1.6
Breaded, Oven Baked, Youngs*	2 Cakes/96g	184	8.7	192	8	18.9	9.1	1.2
Breaded, Sainsbury's*	1 Cake/42g	75	3.4	179	10	16.2	8.1	0.7
Bubbly Batter, Youngs*	1 Cake/44g	109	6.7	247	7.1	20.5	15.1	1.4
Cod, & Parsley, Waitrose*	1 Cake/85g	147	6.5	173	9.2	16.9	7.6	1.1
Cod, & Prawn, Red Thai, Ovenbaked, Extra Special, Asda*	1 Cake/147g	258	8.6	176	9.5	20	5.9	2.3
Cod, Chorizo, Aldi*	1 Cake/137g	266	11.5	194	11	18	8.4	1.3
Cod, As Consumed, Morrisons*	1 Cake/130g	221	9	170	9.5	17.2	6.9	0.8
Cod, Baked, (2 Pack), Tesco*	1 Cake/135g	255	9.9	189	9.1	21.1	7.3	3.2
Cod, Breaded, Lighthouse Bay, Lidl*	1 Cake/132g	224	8.4	170	9.7	17.5	6.4	1.6
Cod, Chunky, Breaded, Chilled, Youngs*	1 Cake/90g	192	11.5	213	9.5	14.9	12.8	1.2
Cod, Fillet, & Sweet Potato, Finest, Tesco*	1 Cake/136g	202	6.4	149	8.4	17.1	4.7	2.3
Cod, Fresh, Asda*	1 Cake/75g	164	8.2	219	7	23	11	1.6
Cod, HFC, Tesco*	2 Cakes/96g	173	6.7	181	8.6	20.2	7	1.4
Cod, Homemade, Average	*1 Cake/50g*	*120*	*8.3*	*241*	*9.3*	*14.4*	*16.6*	*0.7*
Cod, M&S*	1 Cake/85g	153	7.8	180	8.9	15.4	9.2	1.3
Cod, Mornay, Easy to Cook, Waitrose*	1 Cake/149g	248	9.4	166	10.6	16.2	6.3	1.4
Cod, Naked, Butternut Squash, Harissa, Co-Op*	1 Cake/150g	178	6.4	119	0.8	11	4.3	1.7
Fried in Blended Oil	*1 Cake/50g*	*109*	*6.7*	*218*	*8.6*	*16.8*	*13.4*	*0*
Frozen, Average	*1 Cake/85g*	*112*	*3.3*	*132*	*8.6*	*16.7*	*3.9*	*0*
Haddock, & Vintage Cheddar, Smoked, Saucy Fish Co*	1 Cake/135g	220	7.6	163	9.7	18	5.6	0.9
Haddock, in Breadcrumbs, Sainsbury's*	1 Cake/88g	158	6.2	179	10.8	18.2	7	1.4
Haddock, Melting, Cheddar & Leek, TTD, Sainsbury's*	1 Cake/138g	276	13.5	200	9.7	17.8	9.8	0.9
Haddock, Sainsbury's*	1 Cake/135g	253	10	188	10.8	18.7	7.4	1.5
Haddock, Smoked, Breaded, Asda*	1 Cake/90g	202	11.7	225	9	18	13	1.6
Haddock, Smoked, Extra Special, Asda*	1 Cake/115g	218	10.9	190	12.8	13.2	9.5	1.3
Haddock, Smoked, M&S*	1 Cake/85g	153	8	180	10.6	13.4	9.4	2.6
Prawn, Thai Style, Finest, Tesco*	1 Cake/135g	196	6.8	145	9.5	14.6	5	1.8

	Measure INFO/WEIGHT	per Measure KCAL	FAT	Nutrition Values per 100g / 100ml KCAL	PROT	CARB	FAT	FIBRE
FISH CAKES								
Salmon, & Dill, Waitrose*	1 Cake/85g	206	11.9	242	11.5	17.5	14	1.8
Salmon, & Hollandaise Sauce, Saucy Fish Co*	1 Cake/135g	270	13	200	9.2	19.2	9.6	1.4
Salmon, Broccoli, Morrisons*	1 Cake/110g	211	10.3	191	9	16.7	9.3	2.2
Salmon, Asda*	1 Cake/132g	266	11.9	202	11	18	9	1.5
Salmon, Coated in a Light Crispy Breadcrumb, Tesco*	1 Cake/90g	212	10.8	235	9.7	21	12	1.2
Salmon, Fillet & Spinach, Finest, Tesco*	1 Cake/133g	267	10.5	201	12.7	19.2	7.9	1
Salmon, Homemade, Average	*1 Cake/50g*	*136*	*9.8*	*273*	*10.4*	*14.4*	*19.7*	*0.7*
Salmon, M&S*	1 Cake/86g	180	10.9	210	9.1	15.1	12.7	1.7
Salmon, Melting Middle, Lochmuir, M&S*	1 Pack/290g	551	30.4	190	9.1	14.3	10.5	1.5
Salmon, Morrisons*	1 Cake/90g	241	11.8	268	10.1	27.6	13.1	1.5
Salmon, Sainsbury's*	1 Cake/88g	171	7.6	194	12.6	16.5	8.6	1.4
Salmon, Spinach Sicilian Lemon, Finest, Tesco*	1 Cake/145g	290	16.2	200	9.9	14.3	11.2	1.4
Salmon, Tesco*	1 Cake/90g	239	13.5	266	11.4	21.3	15	0
Smart Price, Asda*	1 Cake/42g	78	3.3	188	7	22	8	0.9
Thai, Frozen, Sainsbury's*	1 Cake/15g	28	1.1	187	21.3	9.3	7.3	0.7
Thai, Oriental Selection, Waitrose*	1 Cake/11g	18	0.3	161	17.8	15.8	3	1.5
Tuna, Lime Coriander, BGTY, Sainsbury's*	1 Cake/91g	200	10.7	220	10.7	17.7	11.8	2.6
Tuna, Sainsbury's*	1 Cake/90g	183	7.5	203	13.7	18.4	8.3	2.1
Value, Tesco*	1 Cake/42g	88	4.8	210	8.2	19.5	11.5	1.1
FISH FINGERS								
Chip Shop, Youngs*	1 Finger/30g	75	4.9	251	9.3	16.6	16.4	1.2
Chunky, Cooked, Tesco*	2 Fingers/98g	230	10	235	13.2	21.6	10.2	1.3
Cod, 100% Cod Fillet, Tesco*	1 Finger/30g	53	2.2	177	12.4	14.9	7.5	1.4
Cod, Fillet, Chunky, Finest, Tesco*	2 Fingers/115g	225	8.7	196	12.2	19.1	7.6	1
Cod, Fillets, Asda*	1 Finger/31g	66	3.1	214	13	18	10	0
Cod, Fillets, Chunky, M&S*	1 Finger/40g	70	2.4	175	12	17.2	6	1
Cod, Fillets, Essential, Waitrose*	1 Finger/51g	111	4.3	218	13.9	20.9	8.4	1.5
Cod, Fillets, Waitrose*	1 Finger/30g	55	2.2	183	11.9	16.9	7.5	0.7
Cod, Fried in Blended Oil, Average	*1 Finger/28g*	*67*	*3.9*	*238*	*13.2*	*15.5*	*14.1*	*0.6*
Cod, Frozen, Average	*1 Finger/28g*	*48*	*2.2*	*170*	*11.6*	*14.2*	*7.8*	*0.6*
Cod, Grilled, Average	*1 Finger/28g*	*56*	*2.5*	*200*	*14.3*	*16.6*	*8.9*	*0.7*
Cod, HFC, Tesco*	3 Fingers/70g	162	7.6	231	14.5	18.1	10.9	1.4
Cod, Morrisons*	1 Finger/30g	54	2.2	180	11.7	16.4	7.5	1.1
Cod, Sainsbury's*	1 Finger/28g	53	2.1	190	12.5	17.7	7.7	1
Cod, Youngs*	1 Finger/24g	50	2	209	13.3	19.8	8.3	0.8
Economy, Sainsbury's*	1 Finger/26g	51	2.2	198	12.6	17.7	8.5	1.3
Free From, Sainsbury's*	1 Finger/30g	56	2.3	188	11.4	18	7.8	0.7
Haddock, Chunky, Panko Breaded, Gastro, Youngs*	2 Fingers/78g	154	7	198	13.1	15.7	9	0.9
Haddock, Fillets, Asda*	1 Finger/30g	62	2.7	205	14	17	9	0
Haddock, in Crispy Batter, Birds Eye*	1 Finger/30g	56	2.3	188	14.3	15.1	7.8	0.7
Haddock, in Crunchy Crumb, Morrisons*	1 Finger/30g	57	2.4	190	13.1	16.3	8	1.1
Iceland*	1 Finger/23g	44	2	192	11.5	17.3	8.5	1.3
Plaice, Cider Battered, M&S*	½ Pack/140g	372	24.6	266	12.3	14.1	17.6	1.2
Pollock, Sainsbury's*	3 Fingers/85g	160	6.7	188	13	15.9	7.9	0.8
Salmon, Birds Eye*	1 Finger/28g	63	2.7	225	13.2	21.7	9.5	0.9
Vegetarian, Fish Style, Breaded, The Redwood Co*	1 Finger/36g	94	5.2	262	16.5	16	14.5	0
Vegetarian, Fishless, Vegan, Quorn*	1 Finger/20g	37	1.4	187	4.4	24.1	7.1	4.7
FISH IN								
Butter Sauce, Steaks, Ross*	1 Serving/140g	111	4	84	10.6	3.6	3	0.3
Butter Sauce, Steaks, Youngs*	1 Steak/140g	102	2.9	73	9.6	3.7	2.1	0.5
Parsley Sauce, Steaks, Ross*	1 Serving/150g	123	5.6	82	9.1	3.1	3.7	0.1
FIVE SPICE								
Powder, Sharwood's*	1 Tsp/2g	3	0.2	172	12.2	11.6	8.6	23.4

F

	Measure INFO/WEIGHT	per Measure KCAL	FAT	Nutrition Values per 100g / 100ml KCAL	PROT	CARB	FAT	FIBRE
FLAKE								
Dipped, Cadbury*	1 Bar/41g	215	12.5	530	7.6	56.1	30.8	0.8
Luxury, Cadbury*	1 Bar/45g	240	13.6	533	7.3	57.8	30.2	0
Praline, Cadbury*	1 Bar/38g	201	12.9	535	7.7	49.5	34.3	0
FLAN								
Cheese Potato, Hot, Tesco*	¼ Flan/100g	282	19.7	282	6	20	19.7	2.3
Chicken Smoked Bacon, Hot, Sainsbury's*	¼ Flan/100g	293	18.5	293	10.2	21.5	18.5	1.2
Mediterranean Vegetable, Co-Op*	¼ Flan/88g	188	10.5	215	4	22	12	3
Pastry with Fruit	*1oz/28g*	*33*	*1.2*	*118*	*1.4*	*19.3*	*4.4*	*0.7*
Sponge with Fruit	*1oz/28g*	*31*	*0.4*	*112*	*2.8*	*23.3*	*1.5*	*0.6*
FLAN CASE								
Sponge, Average	*1oz/28g*	*90*	*1.5*	*320*	*7*	*62.5*	*5.4*	*0.7*
FLAPJACK								
Lemon Curd, Graze*	1 Punnet/53g	248	12.7	468	6	60	24	6
7 Fruits, Graze*	1 Punnet/55g	223	10.5	406	5.1	54.9	19.1	4.3
All Butter, Sainsbury's*	1 Flapjack/35g	156	8	446	5.7	54.5	22.8	2.7
All Butter, Squares, M&S*	1 Flapjack/34g	150	7.2	441	6.2	56.2	21.2	4.4
All Butter, Topped with Caramel, Spar*	1 Bar/65g	292	12.9	449	5	60.5	19.9	3.8
Apple & Raspberry, Fox's*	1 Flapjack/26g	105	5	403	4.8	52.5	19.4	3.7
Apple Cinnamon, Graze*	1 Punnet/52g	236	12	453	5	54	23	5
Apricot & Raisin, Waitrose*	1 Flapjack/38g	143	4.2	376	4.7	64.3	11.1	5.8
Average	*1 Sm/50g*	*242*	*13.3*	*484*	*4.5*	*60.4*	*26.6*	*2.7*
Bites, Sainsbury's*	1 Bite/17g	74	3.4	435	5.3	56	20	4.8
Cappuccino, Blackfriars*	1 Flapjack/110g	481	27.5	437	5	61	25	0
Caramel Bake, The Handmade Flapjack Company*	1 Flapjack/90g	375	13	417	6	65.6	14.5	0
Cherry & Coconut, Blackfriars*	1 Flapjack/110g	490	23.1	445	5	58	21	0
Cherry & Sultana, Cookie Coach*	1 Pack/90g	373	15.6	414	6.2	58.2	17.3	0
Cherry Bakewell, Iced, Devondale*	1 Flapjack/95g	432	21.9	455	3.7	54	23.1	2.6
Chocolate Chip, Boots*	1 Flapjack/75g	313	11.2	417	5.6	65	15	3.5
Chocolate Chip, Devondale*	1 Flapjack/95g	434	24.7	457	4.3	49	26	3.6
Chocolate Dipped, M&S*	1 Flapjack/96g	442	21.5	460	6.1	61.3	22.4	3
Chocolate Special, The Handmade Flapjack Company*	1 Flapjack/90g	392	17.8	436	5.7	58.7	19.8	0
Chocolate, Belgian, M&S*	1 Bar/80g	372	19.8	465	5.5	52.9	24.7	4.6
Chunky Chocolate, M&S*	1 FlapJack/80g	348	15.1	435	5.8	59.9	18.9	2.2
Cinnamon, Norfolk Cake Co*	1 Serving/100g	424	20	424	6.6	50.7	20	0
Co-Op*	1 Flapjack/38g	175	9.4	465	5	54	25	4
Cranberry, Orange, Free From, Tesco*	1 Flapjack/30g	131	5.5	440	5.9	60.4	18.5	4.3
Cranberry, Apple Raisin, LC, Tesco*	1 Flapjack/30g	98	1.7	325	5.7	63.1	5.6	5.7
Dark Chocolate, Delectable , Thomas J Fudge*	1 Flapjack/36g	171	7.4	476	5.5	64.9	20.6	0
Fruity, M&S*	1 Flapjack/68g	287	11.7	422	5.5	59.3	17.2	4.1
Golden Oaty Fingers, Tesco*	1 Flapjack/34g	142	5.7	420	5.7	59.7	16.8	3.7
Golden Oaty, Fingers, Fabulous Bakin' Boys*	1 Finger/28g	130	6.8	464	4.5	60.2	24.3	3.1
Granola, Traybake, Tesco*	1 Serving/46g	202	9.5	440	7.1	54	20.6	5
Hobnobs, Milk Chocolate, McVitie's*	1 Flapjack/35g	155	6	443	5.8	64.2	17.2	4.2
Hobnobs, Toffee Apple, McVitie's*	1 Flapjack/46g	202	7.6	440	5.8	64	16.6	5.2
Honey, Norfolk Cake Co*	1 Serving/100g	425	20	425	6.5	50.8	20	0
Jaffa Cake, Graze*	1 Punnet/53g	242	12.7	457	6	53	24	5
Lemon Drizzle, Graze*	1 Punnet/53g	248	12.7	468	5.9	54	24	5.8
Lemon, Lively, Retail, Graze*	1 Slice/17g	80	4.1	468	5.9	54	24	5.8
M&S*	1 Flapjack/53g	228	10.1	430	6	59.1	19	3.5
Mince Pie, Graze*	1 Punnet/52g	234	10.9	450	4.9	63	21	6.3
Mini, Sainsbury's*	1 Slice/15g	65	2.9	431	5.6	59.3	19	2.7
Mixed Fruit, Fabulous Bakin' Boys*	1 Serving/90g	350	9.4	389	5.5	71	10.5	4
Oat, GF, Hale Hearty*	1 Cake/36g	165	9.1	457	6.8	55.1	25.2	8.9

F

	Measure INFO/WEIGHT	per Measure KCAL	per Measure FAT	Nutrition Values per 100g / 100ml KCAL	PROT	CARB	FAT	FIBRE
FLAPJACK								
Protein, Cocoa, Vanilla, Retail, Graze*	1 Flapjack/53g	248	13.3	467	17	47	25	5.4
Raspberry Preserve, The Handmade Flapjack Company*	1 Flapjack/90g	310	2.1	345	6.4	74.4	2.4	0
Slices, Free From, Tesco*	1 Flapjack/30g	132	5.8	442	6.2	59	19.3	4
Summer Berry, Graze*	1 Punnet/52g	230	10.9	442	5	56	21	5
Toffee, Finest, Tesco*	1 Flapjack/35g	156	6.7	446	4.9	63.6	19.1	1.3
Traybake, Ms Mollys*	1 Serving/45g	180	6.4	401	6.8	59.4	14.3	3.8
FLATBREAD								
Cheddar, Tomato, Cooked, Sainsbury's*	¼ Pack/56g	153	3.8	284	11.6	42.4	7	2.2
Cheddar, Mature, & Garlic, Finest, Tesco*	¼ Flatbread/66g	188	6.3	285	7.2	41.8	9.6	2.6
Cheese, Tomato, Tesco*	¼ Flatbread/54g	158	3.5	291	11.6	45.7	6.4	1.9
Chicken, & Mango, Spiced, Love Life, Waitrose*	1 Pack/174g	298	4.7	171	9.7	26.1	2.7	1.9
Chicken, Mango Salad, Sainsbury's*	1 Pack/100g	251	2.5	251	16.9	40.4	2.5	2.5
Chicken, BBQ, Improved, Shapers, Boots*	1 Pack/165g	268	3.8	162	10	25	2.3	1.4
Chicken, Cajun Style, GFY, Asda*	1 Wrap/176g	231	2.1	131	9	21	1.2	0.9
Chicken, Cajun, Greggs*	1 Pack/173g	309	6.2	179	9.8	26	3.6	0
Chicken, Chargrilled, COU, M&S*	1 Pack/163g	245	3.1	150	10.8	23	1.9	5.2
Chicken, Harissa, & Roasted Vegetable, M&S*	1 Pack/186g	342	4.8	184	10.7	19.7	2.6	0
Chicken, Italian, Improved, Shapers, Boots*	1 Pack/151g	263	6.8	174	11	22	4.5	1.8
Chicken, Mexican, Stonebaked, Finest, Tesco*	1 Pack/155g	280	5.1	180	11.7	25.1	3.3	1.6
Chicken, Moroccan, Shapers, Boots*	1 Pack/164g	289	2.1	176	9.8	30	1.3	2.2
Chicken, Peri Peri, Hot, Greggs*	1 Pack/148g	308	7.3	208	14	27	4.9	0
Chicken, Spicy, Shapers, Boots*	1 Pack/181g	292	4.5	161	11	23	2.5	0
Chicken, Tikka, BGTY, Sainsbury's*	1 Flatbread/186g	292	4.5	157	11.6	20.5	2.4	3.5
Chicken, Tikka, Shapers, Boots*	1 Pack/1734g	303	5.7	175	11	25	3.3	1.8
Chicken, with Mango Salsa, Jerk Style, Chargrilled, M&S*	1 Flatbread/200g	300	7.6	150	12.5	15.4	3.8	2.6
Crispy, Marmite*	2 Flatbreads/18g	79	2.7	441	20.1	57.4	15.1	0
Falafel, Greggs*	1 Pack/165g	361	9.1	219	5.9	35	5.5	0
Feta, COU, M&S*	1 Pack/180g	225	4	125	6.3	20.6	2.2	1.9
Feta, Salad, Boots*	1 Pack/158g	241	5.7	153	6.4	24	3.6	1.2
Goats Cheese, Butternut Squash, Beetroot, Tesco*	1 Pack/164g	378	13.6	231	5.9	31.8	8.3	2.6
Ham, & Emmental, Smoked, Fold, Delicious, Boots*	1 Fold/165g	394	16.5	239	12	24	10	3.6
Mexican, Spicy, Shapers, Boots*	1 Pack/190g	296	7.6	156	7	23	4	3.7
Plain, Thins, Deli Kitchen*	1 Flatbread/35g	103	1.9	295	8.5	51.4	5.3	4.1
Pork, Bramley Apple, Stuffing, Tesco Finest*	1 Pack/201g	385	4.8	192	8.1	33.8	2.4	1.9
Prawn, Tikka, King, Waitrose*	1 Pack/165g	257	3.3	156	9.4	25.1	2	1.5
Salami, Calabrese, Carlos, Aldi*	½ Pizza/181g	490	21.7	271	10	30	12	1.7
Village Lavash, Ulta Thin, Yeast Free, Dina Foods Ltd*	1 Flatbread/110g	289	1.1	263	11.2	52.3	1	4.6
FLAXSEED								
Golden, Ground, P H Foods*	1 Serving/10g	51	4.2	514	18.3	1.6	42.2	27.3
Milled, Organic, Linwoods*	1 Tsp/5g	25	2	508	22.1	3	40	23.7
Organic, Premium Ground, Prewett's*	1 Tbsp/15g	73	6	489	24	2	40	23
with Bio Cultures Vitamin D, Linwoods*	2 Tbsps/30g	144	11	481	17.9	6	36.6	28.4
FLOUR								
Arrowroot, Average	*1oz/28g*	*100*	*0*	*357*	*0.3*	*88.2*	*0.1*	*3.4*
Bread, White, Strong, Average	*1oz/28g*	*94*	*0.4*	*336*	*11.8*	*68.4*	*1.5*	*3.4*
Brown, Chapati, Average	*1 Tbsp/20g*	*67*	*0.2*	*333*	*11.5*	*73.7*	*1.2*	*0*
Brown, Wheat	*1oz/28g*	*90*	*0.5*	*323*	*12.6*	*68.5*	*1.8*	*6.4*
Chakki Wheat Atta, Whole Wheat, Pillsbury*	1 Portion/30g	98	0.5	327	12	65	1.7	0
Chick Pea	*1oz/28g*	*88*	*1.5*	*313*	*19.7*	*49.6*	*5.4*	*10.7*
Coconut, Average	*1 Serving/100g*	*344*	*13.6*	*344*	*18.2*	*15.4*	*13.6*	*43.8*
Coconut, Organic, Raw, Sevenhills Wholefoods*	1 Tbsp/15g	40	1.4	267	18.4	9.6	9.1	36.4
Millet	*1oz/28g*	*99*	*0.5*	*354*	*5.8*	*75.4*	*1.7*	*0*
Plain, Average	*1oz/28g*	*98*	*0.4*	*349*	*10.3*	*73.8*	*1.5*	*2.2*

	Measure INFO/WEIGHT	per Measure KCAL	FAT	Nutrition Values per 100g / 100ml KCAL	PROT	CARB	FAT	FIBRE
FLOUR								
Potato	*1oz/28g*	*92*	*0.3*	*328*	*9.1*	*75.6*	*0.9*	*5.7*
Rice	*1 Tsp/5g*	*18*	*0*	*366*	*6.4*	*80.1*	*0.8*	*2*
Soya, Low Fat, Average	*1oz/28g*	*99*	*2*	*352*	*45.3*	*28.2*	*7.2*	*13.5*
Speciality GF, Dove's Farm*	1 Serving/100g	353	1.8	353	4.7	85.2	1.8	2.7
Spelt, Average	*1 Serving/57g*	*216*	*1.7*	*381*	*14.3*	*74.5*	*3*	*6.4*
White, Average	*1oz/28g*	*89*	*0.3*	*319*	*9.8*	*66.8*	*1*	*2.9*
White, Chapati, Average	*1 Tbsp/20g*	*67*	*0.1*	*335*	*9.8*	*77.6*	*0.5*	*0*
White, Self Raising, Average	*1oz/28g*	*94*	*0.4*	*336*	*9.9*	*71.8*	*1.3*	*2.9*
White, Self Raising, Gluten Wheat Free, Dove's Farm*	1 Serving/100g	344	1	344	5.5	78.1	1	1.4
Wholemeal, Average	*1oz/28g*	*87*	*0.6*	*312*	*12.6*	*61.9*	*2.2*	*9*
FLYTE								
Snacksize, Mars*	1 Bar/23g	98	3.3	436	3.8	72.5	14.5	0
FOOL								
Apricot, Fruit, Tesco*	1 Pot/113g	200	12.7	177	2.6	16.4	11.2	0.3
Fruit, Average	*1 Pot/120g*	*196*	*11.2*	*163*	*1*	*20.2*	*9.3*	*1.2*
Gooseberry, BFY, Morrisons*	1 Pot/114g	99	3.9	87	3.4	10.7	3.4	0.4
Gooseberry, Fabulously Fruity, Sainsbury's*	1 Pot/113g	197	11.6	173	2.7	17.1	10.2	1.2
Gooseberry, Fruit, Co-Op*	1 Pot/114g	211	11.4	185	3	22	10	1
Gooseberry, Tesco*	1 Pot/112g	225	14.1	200	3	17.8	12.5	0.7
Lemon, Fruit, BGTY, Sainsbury's*	1 Pot/113g	94	3.8	83	3.4	9.7	3.4	0.3
Lemon, Signature, Morrisons*	1 Pot/114g	213	11.8	187	3	20	10.4	0.5
Raspberry, Fruit, Tesco*	1 Pot/113g	234	12.8	207	2.6	23.6	11.3	0.3
Rhubarb, Fruit, Waitrose*	1 Pot/114g	182	12.9	160	2.7	11.9	11.3	0.3
Rhubarb, Timberly, Fabulously Fruity, Sainsbury's*	1 Pot/113g	167	11.7	147	2.4	10.9	10.3	0.5
Strawberry, Fruit, BGTY, Sainsbury's*	1 Pot/120g	100	3.1	83	3.7	11.1	2.6	0.8
Strawberry, Fruit, Co-Op*	1 Pot/114g	188	10.3	165	2	18	9	0.8
FRANKFURTERS								
Average	*1 Sausage/42g*	*123*	*11.2*	*292*	*12*	*1.3*	*26.6*	*0*
Chicken, Halal, Tahira*	1 Sausage/34g	64	4.7	187	11.5	4.5	13.7	0
Vegetarian, Quorn*	1 Sausage/45g	92	6.3	205	13.5	4.5	14	3.5
Vegetarian, Tivall*	1 Sausage/30g	73	4.8	244	18	7	16	3
FRAZZLES								
Bacon, Smith's, Walkers*	1 Bag/23g	113	5.3	488	7.5	62	23	1.3
FREEKEH								
Greenwheat, Cooked, Artisan Grains*	1 Serving/100g	165	2	165	8.8	30.2	2	5.2
Wholegrain, Unprepared, Artisan Grains*	1 Serving/100g	347	4.3	347	18.5	63.5	4.3	10.9
FRENCH FRIES								
Cheese & Onion, Walkers*	1 Pack/22g	95	3.5	430	5	66	16	5
Ready Salted, Walkers*	1 Bag/21g	91	3.4	434	5	65	16	5
Salt & Vinegar, Walkers*	1 Bag/22g	95	3.5	430	5	66	16	5
Seasoned, Frozen, Ovenbaked, Asda*	1/6 Pack/125g	286	10.9	229	3.1	33	8.7	3
Worcester Sauce, Walkers*	1 Bag/22g	96	3.5	435	5	65	16	5
FRENCH TOAST								
Asda*	1 Toast/8g	30	0.4	381	10	74	5	4
Sainsbury's*	1 Toast/8g	31	0.5	382	10	72	6.6	5
FRIES								
Chips, From Restaurant, Average	*1 Serving/105g*	*294*	*16.3*	*280*	*3.3*	*34*	*15.5*	*2.1*
Criss Cross, Oven Baked, Iceland*	1 Serving/125g	324	14.1	259	3.5	33.7	11.3	4.4
Curly, Cajun, Weighed Frozen, McCain*	1 Portion/100g	156	8.7	156	1.6	17.7	8.7	1.8
Curly, Lightly Seasoned, McCain*	1 Serving/125g	239	10.8	191	2.3	25.1	8.6	2.4
Curly, Ovenbaked, Iceland*	1 Serving/100g	253	12.1	253	3.5	30.8	12.1	3.5
Curly, Southern Style, Tesco*	1 Serving/50g	95	2.8	189	2.6	29.6	5.6	4.9
Dirty, Cheesy, M&S*	½ Pack/250g	518	30	207	7	16.7	12	2

F

	Measure INFO/WEIGHT	per Measure KCAL	FAT	KCAL	PROT	CARB	FAT	FIBRE
FRIES								
Extra Chunky, Oven Baked, Homefries, McCain*	1 Serving/200g	306	6.2	153	3.2	28	3.1	2.3
Pizza, Cheesy, Loaded, Cheese & Tomato Sauce, M&S*	½ Pack/240g	372	16.3	155	5.2	17.2	6.8	2
Skin On, Crispy, McCain*	1 Serving/125g	222	7.8	178	2.4	27	6.2	2.6
Skin on, Ovenbaked, Iceland*	1/10 Bag/100g	204	6.9	204	3.3	30.6	6.9	3.2
Southern, Oven Baked, Frozen, McCain*	1oz/28g	52	2.4	185	2.5	23	8.6	2.7
Spicy, Peri Peri, Frozen Weight, McCain*	1/6 Bag/125g	244	11	195	2	25.5	8.8	2.9
Sweet Potato, Crispy, McCain*	1 Serving/125g	170	5.7	136	1.6	20.4	4.6	3.5
Sweet Potato, Iceland*	1 Serving/125g	252	9.9	202	1.9	28.4	7.9	4.7
Sweet Potato, Oven Baked, CBY, Asda*	1 Serving/125g	188	6.5	150	5.6	19	5.2	2.4
Sweet Potato, Prefried Frozen, Cooked, Sainsbury's*	1 Serving/125g	297	14.7	237	2.4	28.3	11.7	4.6
Sweet Potato, Ready to Roast, Cooked, Sainsbury's*	½ Pack/116g	201	8.3	174	2.1	23.7	7.2	3.2
Sweet Potato, Season Savour, Oven Baked, McCain*	1 Pot/275g	605	20.1	220	3	33	7.3	5.3
Sweet Potato, Slims Kitchen *	1 Bowl/340g	578	25.5	170	1.5	22	7.5	0
FRISPS								
Tangy Salt & Vinegar, KP Snacks*	1 Bag/30g	160	10	532	5	52.6	33.5	2.9
Tasty Cheese & Onion, KP Snacks*	1 Bag/28g	150	9.4	537	5.5	53.2	33.6	3.2
FRITTATA								
Spinach Courgette, Meat Free, Tesco*	1 Frittata/120g	199	12.8	166	5.8	10.2	10.7	2.9
Vegetable, CBY, Asda*	1 Frittata/150g	183	7.8	122	6.2	12.1	5.2	1
Veggie, Ella's Kitchen*	1 Frittata/25g	24	1.3	95	6.5	6.2	5.1	0.9
FRITTERS								
Fritters, Hormel Foods*	1 Fritter/80g	221	14.5	276	10.2	18.1	18.1	2.2
Sweetcorn, Courgetti, Tesco*	1 Fritter/63g	89	3.4	142	2.5	18.5	5.5	4.1
Sweetcorn, Indian Platter, Tesco*	1 Fritter/12g	30	1.9	254	4.3	22.1	15.8	3.5
Sweetcorn, Tesco*	1 Fritter/25g	53	2.9	212	5.2	19.9	11.5	4.1
FROMAGE FRAIS								
0% Fat, Vitalinea, Danone*	1 Tbsp/28g	14	0	50	7.4	4.7	0.1	0
Apricot, Creamfields*	1 Pot/50g	41	0.4	83	6.9	11.7	0.9	0.1
Apricot, Summer Fruit, Layered, Weight Watchers*	1 Pot/90g	44	0.1	49	5.6	6	0.1	0.2
Blackberry, Berry Fruits, Layered, Weight Watchers*	1 Pot/100g	49	0.2	49	5.5	5.7	0.2	0.4
Cherry, 0% Fat, Vitalinea, Danone*	1 Serving/150g	88	0.2	59	6.1	8	0.2	1.6
Fabby, Loved By Kids, M&S*	1 Pot/43g	45	1.6	105	6.2	12.3	3.7	0
Fat Free, Average	*1 Pot/60g*	*35*	*0.1*	*58*	*7.7*	*6.8*	*0.2*	*0*
Kids, Yeo Valley*	1 Serving/90g	111	4.8	123	6.6	12.6	5.3	0
Munch Bunch, Nestle*	1 Pot/42g	44	1.3	105	6.7	12.6	3	0
Peach, BGTY, Sainsbury's*	1 Pot/100g	53	0.2	53	7.2	5.5	0.2	0.5
Peach, Summer Fruit, Layered, Weight Watchers*	1 Pot/90g	44	0.1	49	5.6	6	0.1	0.3
Plain, Average	*1oz/28g*	*32*	*2*	*113*	*6.8*	*5.7*	*7.1*	*0*
Raspberry, Berry Fruits, Layered, Weight Watchers*	1 Pot/90g	44	0.1	49	5.6	5.9	0.1	0.4
Raspberry, Creamfields*	1 Pot/50g	40	0.4	80	6.9	11.2	0.8	0.2
Raspberry, Little Stars, Muller*	1 Pot/60g	66	2.4	110	5	12.7	4	0.4
Raspberry, Organic, Yeo Valley*	1 Pot/100g	127	6.5	127	6.1	11.1	6.5	0.4
Raspberry, Value, Tesco*	1 Serving/60g	56	0.8	93	7.2	13.5	1.3	0
Strawberry Cheesecake, Dessert Selection, Sainsbury's*	1 Pot/90g	95	2.2	106	5.8	15.3	2.5	0.1
Strawberry Tart, Sainsbury's*	1 Pot/100g	54	0.2	54	7.6	5.5	0.2	1.1
Strawberry, 99.9% Fat Free, Onken*	1 Serving/50g	46	0	91	6.9	15.3	0.1	0
Strawberry, Creamfields*	1 Pot/50g	41	0.4	81	6.9	11.3	0.9	0.2
Strawberry, GFY, Asda*	1 Pot/100g	58	0.2	58	6	8	0.2	0
Strawberry, HE, Tesco*	1 Pot/100g	54	0.2	54	6.2	6.8	0.2	0.1
Strawberry, Langley Farm*	1 Pot/125g	189	9.8	151	7	13.3	7.8	0
Strawberry, Organic, Yeo Valley*	1 Pot/90g	116	5.4	129	6.3	12.5	6	0.2
Strawberry, Petits Filous, Yoplait*	1 Pot/50g	52	1.4	104	6.7	12.6	2.9	0.2
Strawberry, Pouches, Fruit King, Milbona, Lidl*	1 Pouch/80g	90	2.4	112	6.4	14.9	3	0.5

	Measure INFO/WEIGHT	per Measure		Nutrition Values per 100g / 100ml				
		KCAL	FAT	KCAL	PROT	CARB	FAT	FIBRE
FROMAGE FRAIS								
Strawberry, Thomas the Tank Engine, Yoplait*	1 Pot/50g	50	0.6	101	6.8	15.4	1.3	0
Strawberry, Value, Tesco*	1 Pot/60g	55	0.8	92	7.2	13	1.3	0
Toffee & Pecan Pie, Smooth & Creamy, Tesco*	1 Pot/100g	148	6.8	148	6.9	14.8	6.8	0.2
Vanilla, Danone*	1 Serving/200g	274	8.2	137	5.3	19.6	4.1	0
Wildlife, Strawberry, Raspberry Or Peach, Yoplait*	1 Pot/50g	46	0.6	93	7.1	13.2	1.3	0.2
with Fruit, Average	*1 Avg Pot/90g*	*74*	*2.2*	*83*	*6.1*	*9*	*2.5*	*0.8*
with Fruit, Healthy Range, Average	*1 Avg Pot/90g*	*40*	*0.1*	*45*	*5.8*	*5.1*	*0.2*	*0.3*
FROZEN YOGHURT								
Black Cherry, M&S*	1 Pot/125g	164	1.4	131	3.1	27.1	1.1	0.5
Cherry Garcia, Low Fat, Ben & Jerry's*	1 Serving/100g	143	2.4	143	3	26	2.4	1
Chocmoo, Yoomoo*	1 Serving/100g	142	1.7	142	3.5	26	1.7	4.1
Chocolate, Average	*1 Portion/100g*	*120*	*1.9*	*120*	*4.3*	*22*	*1.9*	*2.1*
Chocolate, Belgian, Calorie Controlled, Love Life, Waitrose*	1/5 Pot/100g	89	1.7	89	4.3	14	1.7	0.3
Chocolate, Pinkberry*	1 Sm Pot/140g	168	2.1	120	5	23	1.5	2
Chocolate, Snog*	1 Serving/100g	109	1.6	109	4.5	19.9	1.6	1.7
Coconut, Pinkberry*	1 Sm Pot/140g	196	0	140	4	30	0	0
Frae*	1 Sm/83ml	56	0	67	2.4	12	0	0
Green Tea, Pinkberry*	1 Sm Pot/100g	110	0	110	4	25	0	0
Mango, Pinkberry*	1 Sm Cup/140g	140	0	100	3	23	0	0
Mango, Snowconut, The Coconut Collaborative*	1 Serving/200ml	372	15	186	1.8	21	7.5	1
Nakedmoo, Yoomoo*	1 Serving/125g	168	2	134	3.3	24.5	1.6	4.1
Natural, Average	*1 Portion/100g*	*101*	*0.8*	*101*	*3.8*	*19.9*	*0.8*	*0.9*
Original, Pinkberry*	1 Sm Pot/140g	140	0	100	3	21	0	0
Passionfruit, Pinkberry*	1 Sm Pot/140g	140	0	100	3	22	0	0
Peanut Butter, Pinkberry*	1 Sm Pot/140g	238	9.8	170	7	23	7	1
Phish Food, Lower Fat, Ben & Jerry's*	½ Pot/211g	464	10.6	220	4	40	5	1.5
Pomegranate, Pinkberry*	1 Sm Pot/140g	168	0	120	3	26	0	0
Pumpkin, Pinkberry*	1 Sm Pot/140g	154	0	110	3	23	0	0
Raspberry Snowconut, The Coconut Collaborative*	1 Serving/200ml	378	15	189	1.8	21.2	7.5	1.2
Raspberry, Handmade Farmhouse, Sainsbury's*	1 Serving/100g	132	3.8	132	2.7	21.8	3.8	2.2
Salted Caramel, Pinkberry*	1 Sm Pot/140g	168	0	120	4	26	0	0
Strawberry Cheesecake, Low Fat, Ben & Jerry's*	1 Serving/100g	170	3	170	4	31	3	1
Strawberry, Average	*1 Portion/100g*	*114*	*2.2*	*114*	*2.6*	*21.2*	*2.2*	*0.5*
Strawberry, Lolly, Yoomoo *	1 Lolly/57g	73	0.8	128	2.8	25.5	1.4	0.5
Strawberry, Tesco*	1 Pot/60g	82	1.3	136	2.6	26.5	2.2	0.8
Tropical, Lolly, Yoomoo *	1 Lolly/57g	74	0.8	130	2.9	26.1	1.4	0.6
Vanilla, Less Than 5% Fat, Tesco*	1 Pot/120g	179	2.9	149	8.1	23.8	2.4	0.7
FRUIT								
Apple, Apricot, Strawberry, Pots, Aldi*	1 Pot/100g	55	0.9	55	0.5	10	0.9	1.9
Apple, Pineapple Grape, Ready to Eat, Sainsbury's*	1 Pack/180g	94	0.2	52	0.5	8.3	0.1	1.3
Apples & Grape, Snack Pack, Goodness for Kids, Tesco*	1 Pack/80g	44	0.1	55	0.3	12.3	0.1	2.6
Bananas Berries, Eat Well, M&S*	1 Pack/160g	96	0.3	60	0.9	13.1	0.2	1
Berry Medley, Freshly Prepared, M&S*	1 Pack/180g	90	0.4	50	0.7	10.9	0.2	2.9
Fabulous Fruity Fingers, Melon Mango, M&S*	1 Pack/240g	96	0.5	40	0.6	8.2	0.2	1
Fingers, Melon Pineapple, Sainsbury's*	1 Pack/240g	74	0.2	31	0.5	6.5	0.1	0.8
Mango, Pineapple, & Orange Melon, Fingers, M&S*	½ Pack/120g	54	0.2	45	0.6	9.1	0.2	2.3
Melon Grape Pot, Co-Op*	1 Pot/130g	39	0.1	30	0.6	6.9	0.1	0.7
Mixed, Fresh, Tesco*	1 Pack/200g	70	0.4	35	0.8	7.4	0.2	1.4
Mixed, Pieces, in Orange Jelly, Fruitini, Del Monte*	1 Can/140g	94	0.1	67	0.3	15.8	0.1	0
Orchard, Frozen, British, Delicious Colourful, Waitrose*	½ Pack/150g	60	0.2	40	0.6	7.7	0.1	2.7
Peach Pieces in Fruit Juice, Tesco*	1 Pot/125g	60	0	48	0.4	11.7	0	1
Peach, Nectarine, Slices, Frozen, Sainsbury's*	1 Serving/80g	34	0.4	42	1.2	8.1	0.5	1.8
Peach, Slices, Frozen, Sainsbury's*	1 Serving/80g	30	0	37	1	7.6	0	1.5

F

	Measure INFO/WEIGHT	per Measure KCAL	per Measure FAT	Nutrition Values per 100g / 100ml KCAL	PROT	CARB	FAT	FIBRE
FRUIT								
Pear, Plum, Figs, Blackberries, Waitrose*	1 Serving/80g	34	0.2	43	0	9.4	0.2	2.1
Pineapple Fingers, Snack Pack, Goodness for Kids, Tesco*	1 Pack/70g	31	0.1	44	0.4	10.1	0.2	2
Pink Lady Apple Grape, Snack Pack, On The Go, Tesco*	1 Pack/80g	44	0.1	55	0.3	12.3	0.1	2.6
Summer Berries, M&S*	1 Pack/160g	80	0.3	50	0.7	10	0.2	3
Tropical in Juice, Dole*	1 Pot/113g	59	0	52	0.3	14.2	0	1.8
FRUIT & NUT MIX								
Bounty Hunter, Graze*	1 Punnet/31g	147	8.3	474	4	54.4	26.8	5.6
Chocolate, On the Go, Sainsbury's*	1 Serving/30g	109	3.1	363	5.1	60.1	10.2	5.1
Daily Vigour Mix, Waitrose*	1 Pack/50g	265	18.8	530	14.6	30	37.6	6.4
Honeycomb Crunch, Graze*	1 Punnet/40g	181	9.7	446	9	50	24	4
Marvellous Macaroon, Graze*	1 Punnet/28g	157	10.9	562	11	41	39	6
Nuts Raisins, Mixed, Natural, Love Life, Waitrose*	1 Serving/50g	258	16.4	515	16.5	38.4	32.8	7.2
Salted Caramel, Nibbles, N'akd*	1 Bag/40g	138	4.7	345	6.6	56.1	11.8	3.3
Strawberry Milkshake, Graze*	1 Pack/39g	148	3.9	380	2	72	10	2
Trail Mix, Average	*1oz/28g*	*121*	*8*	*432*	*9.1*	*37.2*	*28.5*	*4.3*
Unsalted, Tesco*	1 Serving/25g	112	4.6	449	12.6	58.1	18.5	12.2
FRUIT COCKTAIL								
Fresh & Ready, Sainsbury's*	1 Pack/300g	117	0.3	39	0.6	9	0.1	1.2
in Apple Juice, Asda*	1/3 Can/80g	40	0.1	50	0.3	12	0.1	1.6
in Fruit Juice, Heinz*	1 Pot/125g	78	0	62	0.5	15	0	1
in Fruit Juice, Sainsbury's*	1 Serving/198g	97	0.2	49	0.3	11.9	0.1	1.3
in Fruit Juice, Waitrose*	1 Can/142g	71	0	50	0.4	12	0	1
in Juice, Del Monte*	1 Can/415g	203	0.4	49	0.4	11.2	0.1	0
in Light Syrup, Princes*	1 Serving/206g	64	0	31	0.4	7.3	0	1
in Light Syrup, Sainsbury's*	½ Can/125g	72	0.1	58	0.4	14	0.1	1.3
in Light Syrup, Valfrutta*	1 Serving/206g	95	0	46	0.2	11.4	0	1.5
in Syrup, Morrisons*	½ Can/205g	129	0.2	63	0.3	14.9	0.1	0
in Syrup, Smart Price, Asda*	1 Can/411g	173	0.4	42	0.3	10	0.1	1.6
Tropical, Canned, Asda*	½ Can/200g	120	0	60	0	15	0	1.6
FRUIT COMPOTE								
Vanilla Sponge, Weight Watchers*	1 Pack/140g	202	2.9	144	2.2	29	2.1	1.8
Apple, Strawberry & Blackberry, Organic, Yeo Valley*	½ Pot/112g	73	0.1	65	0.5	15.5	0.1	1.9
Apricot & Prune, Yeo Valley*	1 Pot/225g	207	0.2	92	0.6	22.3	0.1	1.6
Blackcurrant, Cassis, British, TTD, Sainsbury's*	1 Tbsp/35g	52	0.4	147	1.8	31	1.2	2.7
HE, Tesco*	1 Pot/140g	113	0.3	81	0.9	19.1	0.2	1.6
Orchard Fruits, GFY, Asda*	1 Pot/180g	113	0.2	63	0.5	15	0.1	0
Spiced, Tesco*	1 Serving/112g	122	0.6	109	1.7	24.4	0.5	3.1
Strawberry & Raspberry, M&S*	1 Serving/80g	72	0.1	90	0.7	23.5	0.1	2.3
Summerfruit, M&S*	¼ Pot/125g	119	0.8	95	0.9	22.7	0.6	0.8
FRUIT FLAKES								
Blackcurrant with Yoghurt Coating, Fruit Bowl*	1 Bag/21g	95	4	453	1.3	69	19	3.9
Raspberry with Yoghurt Coating, Fruit Bowl*	1 Serving/21g	95	4	453	1.3	69	19	3.9
Strawberry with Yoghurt Coating, Fruit Bowl*	1 Serving/21g	95	4	453	1.3	69	19	3.9
FRUIT GUMS								
Fruit Salad, Tesco*	6 Sweets/30g	100	0.2	335	8.3	73.4	0.5	0.3
Rowntree's*	1 Tube/49g	170	0.1	344	4.8	81.3	0.2	0
Sugar Free, Sainsbury's*	1 Serving/30g	63	0.1	209	7.7	71.3	0.2	0.1
FRUIT MIX								
Apple, Strawberry, Pot, Market Street , Morrisons*	1 Serving/125g	61	0.6	49	0.6	9.8	0.5	1.2
Blackforest, Berry Mix, Morrisons*	1 Serving/80g	38	0.1	47	0.9	9.3	0.1	2.4
Exotic, Frozen, Tesco*	1 Serving/80g	33	0	41	0.6	8.7	0	1.9
Pineapple, Melon, Mango, Tesco*	1 Pack/440g	242	0.9	55	1.1	11.4	0.2	1.3

	Measure INFO/WEIGHT	per Measure KCAL	FAT	Nutrition Values per 100g / 100ml KCAL	PROT	CARB	FAT	FIBRE
FRUIT MIX								
Plum, Berries, Eat Well, M&S*	1 Serving/100g	41	0.2	41	0.8	7.8	0.2	2.3
Plum, Pomegranate, Blueberry, Market Street, Morrisons*	1 Serving/80g	38	0.1	47	0.6	10	0.1	1.8
Red, Frozen, Crops*	3 Tbsp/80g	28	0.1	35	1	5.2	0.1	4.6
Sour Mango Tangtastic, Graze*	1 Pack/34g	110	0.2	323	1.3	79.8	0.6	2
Summer Fruits, British, Frozen, Waitrose*	1 Pack/380g	99	0.8	26	1	5.2	0.2	5.5
Summer Fruits, Frozen, Asda*	1 Serving/100g	28	0	28	0.9	6	0	2.5
Summer Fruits, Frozen, Sainsbury's*	1 Serving/80g	43	0.1	54	0.9	6.9	0.1	2
FRUIT PUREE								
Apple Blueberry, Organic, Clearspring*	1 Tub/100g	76	0.3	76	0.4	17.8	0.3	0
Apple Blueberry, Organix*	1 Pot/100g	54	0.6	54	0.4	11.6	0.6	2.5
Apple Peach, Organix*	1 Pot/100g	49	0.3	49	0.6	11	0.3	2.1
Apple, Kale Mango, Twist, Organic, Happy Squeeze*	1 Pouch/60g	40	0	67	0	15.6	0	1.1
Banana, Apple Apricot, Organix*	1 Pot/100g	68	0.4	68	0.8	15.4	0.4	2
FRUIT SALAD								
Apple, Orange, Pineapple Grape, Morrisons*	1 Serving/64g	40	0.1	62	0.8	13.1	0.1	2.6
Apple, Pineapple Grape, Sweet Tangy, Sainsbury's*	1 Pack/180g	70	0.2	39	0.5	8.3	0.1	1.3
Autumn, Fresh, M&S*	½ Pack/160g	64	0.2	40	0.7	9.4	0.1	2.9
Berry, Asda*	1 Pack/250g	122	0.2	49	0.6	10.9	0.1	0
Berry, Seasonal, Asda*	1 Pack/300g	93	0.3	31	0.6	7	0.1	2.1
Chunky in Fruit Juice, Canned, John West*	1 Can/411g	193	0.8	47	0.4	11	0.2	0.8
Citrus, Fresh, M&S*	½ Pack/225g	79	0.2	35	0.9	7.7	0.1	1.5
Classic, Fresh, Prepared, Sainsbury's*	1 Pack/320g	157	0.3	49	0.6	10.3	0.1	2
Classic, Ocado*	1 Pack/265g	130	0.3	49	0.7	12.1	0.1	1.2
Classic, Waitrose*	1 Pack/330g	162	0.7	49	0.8	10.4	0.2	1.2
Dried, M&S*	½ Pack/125g	269	0.5	215	1.8	51.4	0.4	5.9
Exotic with Melon, Mango, Kiwi Fruit Grapes, Asda*	1 Pot/300g	141	0.9	47	0.6	10.5	0.3	1.4
Exotic, Fresh, Tesco*	1 Serving/225g	86	0.4	38	0.7	8.4	0.2	1.5
Exotic, Fully Prepared, Sainsbury's*	1 Serving/200g	74	0.4	37	0.6	8.3	0.2	1.3
Exotic, Morrisons*	1 Serving/150g	78	0.3	52	0.6	12.2	0.2	0
Exotic, Waitrose*	1 Pack/300g	126	0.6	42	0.6	9.5	0.2	1.1
Fresh for You, Tesco*	1 Pack/160g	59	0.3	37	0.6	8.2	0.2	1.1
Fresh, Morrisons*	1 Tub/350g	150	0.4	43	0.7	9.9	0.1	0
Fresh, Tesco*	1 Pack/200g	84	0.4	42	0.7	9.3	0.2	1.5
Fresh, Washed, Ready to Eat, Tesco*	1 Pack/200g	92	0.2	46	0.7	10.6	0.1	1.6
Freshly Prepared, M&S*	1 Pack/350g	140	0.7	40	0.5	9.3	0.2	1
Fruit Crunch, Salad Bowl, M&S*	½ Pack/120g	174	4.1	145	3.1	25.5	3.4	0.6
Fruity Cocktail, M&S*	1 Serving/80g	33	0.1	41	0.6	8.5	0.1	1.7
Golden, Fresh, Asda*	1 Pot/147g	69	0.1	47	0.6	11	0.1	1.6
Grapefruit & Orange, Fresh, M&S*	1 Serving/250g	88	0.2	35	0.9	7.4	0.1	1.6
Green, M&S*	1 Pack/400g	200	0.8	50	0.6	10.9	0.2	1.2
Homemade, Unsweetened, Average	*1 Serving/140g*	*77*	*0.1*	*55*	*0.7*	*13.8*	*0.1*	*1.5*
Juicy Melon, Pineapple Grapes, Asda*	1 Pot/300g	111	0.3	37	0.5	8.4	0.1	0.9
Kiwi, Pineapple Grape, Fresh Tastes, Asda*	1 Pack/200g	106	0.6	53	0.6	11	0.3	1.8
Layered, Tropical Rainbow, Freshly Prepared, M&S*	1 Pack/375g	206	1.1	55	0.7	12.6	0.3	1.7
Mango, Kiwi, Blueberry & Pomegranate, Fresh, M&S*	1 Pack/350g	210	1	60	0.9	13.4	0.3	2.4
Mediterranean Style, Budgens*	1 Serving/250g	95	0.5	38	0.6	8.5	0.2	0.8
Melon & Red Grape, Freshly Prepared, M&S*	1 Pack/450g	158	0.4	35	0.5	8.4	0.1	0.7
Melon Mango, Shapers, Boots*	1 Pack/80g	29	0.1	36	0.6	7.8	0.1	1.2
Melon, Grape, Sainsbury's*	1 Pack/159g	59	0.8	37	0.6	7.8	0.5	1.2
Melon, Grape, Kiwi, Strawberry, Pomegranate, Tesco*	1 Pot/375g	172	0.8	46	0.8	9.6	0.2	1.2
Melon, Kiwi, Grapes Pomegranate Seeds, Morrisons*	1 Pack/400g	152	1.2	38	0.7	8.2	0.3	1.2
Melon, Kiwi, Strawberry, WTF, Sainsbury's*	1 Pack/245g	74	0.5	30	0.8	6.3	0.2	1.3
Melon, Pineapple Grapes, Fresh, Tesco*	1 Pack/300g	120	0.3	40	0.5	9.2	0.1	1

F

	Measure INFO/WEIGHT	per Measure KCAL	FAT	Nutrition Values per 100g / 100ml KCAL	PROT	CARB	FAT	FIBRE
FRUIT SALAD								
Mixed, Average	*1 Bowl/100g*	*42*	*0.2*	*42*	*0.6*	*9.4*	*0.2*	*1.5*
Mixed, Food to Go, M&S*	1 Pack/400g	400	1.2	100	0.9	23.3	0.3	2.8
Mixed, Fresh, Sainsbury's*	1 Pack/200g	84	0.4	42	0.7	9.4	0.2	1.9
Mixed, Tesco*	1 Pack/225g	86	0.4	38	0.7	8.3	0.2	1.3
Nectarine, Melon, Strawberry, Blueberry, Morrisons*	1 Pot/230g	78	0.5	34	0.9	6.7	0.2	1.1
Oranges, Apple, Pineapple Grapes, Fresh, Asda*	1 Pack/260g	120	0.3	46	0.6	10.5	0.1	2.1
Pineapple, Apple Strawberries, Tesco*	1 Pack/190g	80	0.2	42	0.4	9.8	0.1	1.4
Pineapple, Apple, Melon Grape, Shapers, Boots*	1 Serving/100g	49	0.1	49	0.4	10.5	0.1	1.2
Pineapple, Mango & Passion Fruit, Prepared, M&S*	1 Pack/400g	200	0.8	50	0.7	10.8	0.2	1.8
Pineapple, Mango, Apple Grape, Waitrose*	1 Pack/300g	186	0.6	62	0.5	14.7	0.2	1.7
Pineapple, Melon Grape, Eat Well, M&S*	1 Pot/120g	52	0.1	43	0.5	9.3	0.1	1.4
Pineapple, Melon, Kiwi Blueberry, Shapers, Boots*	1 Pack/179g	75	0.4	42	0.6	8.7	0.2	1.4
Pineapple, Melon, Mango, Apple, Kiwi, Blueberries, M&S*	1 Pack/185g	87	0.6	47	0.6	9.7	0.3	1.7
Pineapple, Strawberry, Grape Carrot, M&S*	1 Pack/240g	101	1	42	0.6	8.3	0.4	1.4
Plum, Blackberries, Fig, Tesco*	1 Pot/260g	109	0.5	42	0.8	8.2	0.2	2.5
Plum, Blackberry, Seasonal Opal Apple, Tesco*	1 Pack/105g	51	0.3	49	0.6	9.8	0.3	2.1
Rainbow Layers, Tesco*	1 Pack/270g	122	0.5	45	0.5	9.8	0.2	1.1
Rainbow, Asda*	1 Pack/350g	140	1	40	0.6	8.8	0.3	1.4
Rainbow, Fresh, Tesco*	1 Tub/270g	105	0.5	39	0.5	8.8	0.2	0.9
Seasonal Melon Grapes, Asda*	½ Pack/200g	66	1	33	0.5	7.5	0.5	0.4
Seasonal, Fresh, Asda*	1 Pack/125g	55	0.1	44	0.5	10.4	0.1	1.2
Seasonal, M&S*	1 Serving/200g	100	0.4	50	0.5	11.8	0.2	2.1
Sharing, Fresh Tastes, Asda*	1 Pack/450g	220	0.9	49	0.4	10.4	0.2	0
Strawberry Blueberry, Asda*	1 Pack/240g	86	0.2	36	0.9	7	0.1	1.5
Summer, Red, Fresh, M&S*	1 Pack/400g	160	0.8	40	0	10	0.2	1.2
Summer, Sainsbury's*	1 Pack/240g	84	0.5	35	0.7	7.8	0.2	1.3
Sunshine, Fresh, M&S*	1 Serving/200g	70	0.2	35	0	8.3	0.1	1.3
Tropical in Light Syrup, Passion Fruit Juice, Tesco*	½ Can/216g	130	0.2	60	0.3	14.1	0.1	1.1
Tropical Mix, Tesco*	½ Pack/140g	71	0.3	51	0.5	11	0.2	1.5
Tropical, Fresh, Asda*	1 Pack/400g	164	0.8	41	0.7	9	0.2	1.8
Tropical, Fruit Snacks, Frozen, Sainsbury's*	1 Serving/175g	79	0.2	45	0.7	10.4	0.1	1.6
Tropical, Mixed, Canned, Drained, M&S*	½ Can/124g	82	0.1	66	0.3	15.8	0.1	1
Tropical, Tropical Harvest*	1 Serving/100g	52	0	52	0.3	12.8	0	1.4
Virgin Trains*	1 Serving/140g	56	0.2	40	0.4	10	0.1	0.8
FRUIT SHOOT								
Apple Blackcurrant, Robinson's*	1 Bottle/200ml	10	0	5	0.1	0.8	0	0
Apple, Low Sugar, Robinson's*	1 Bottle/200ml	14	0	7	0	1.2	0	0
FRUIT SPREAD								
Apricot, Pure, Organic, Whole Earth*	1 Serving/20g	33	0.1	167	0.8	40	0.4	0.9
Blackcurrant, Carb Check, Heinz*	1 Tbsp/15g	8	0	54	0.5	12.8	0.1	2.7
Cherries & Berries, Organic, Meridian Foods*	1 Tbsp/15g	16	0	109	0.5	26	0.3	1.1
Cherry Berry, Meridian Foods*	1 Serving/10g	14	0.1	138	0.7	33.7	0.6	3.2
Raspberry & Cranberry, No Added Sugar, Superjam*	1 Spread/10g	22	0	216	2.1	47	0.3	0
Raspberry, Weight Watchers*	1 Tsp/6g	7	0	111	0.4	27.1	0.1	0.9
Seville Orange, Weight Watchers*	1 Tsp/15g	17	0	111	0.2	27.5	0	0.3
FRUIT WINDERS								
Strawberry, Kellogg's*	1 Roll/17g	67	1.4	393	0.2	79	8	2
FU YUNG								
Chicken, Chinese Takeaway, Tesco*	1 Pack/350g	315	3.5	90	5.6	14.5	1	0.8
Egg, Average	*1oz/28g*	*67*	*5.8*	*239*	*9.9*	*2.2*	*20.6*	*1.3*
FUDGE								
All Butter, Finest, Tesco*	1 Sweet/10g	43	1.4	429	1.3	73.4	14.5	0
Butter Tablet, Thorntons*	1oz/28g	116	3.1	414	0.9	77.6	11.1	0

	Measure INFO/WEIGHT	per Measure KCAL	per Measure FAT	Nutrition Values per 100g / 100ml KCAL	PROT	CARB	FAT	FIBRE
FUDGE								
Butter, Milk, Thorntons*	1 Sweet/13g	60	2.5	462	3.7	68.5	19.2	0
Cadbury*	1 Bar/25g	118	4	445	2.5	74.5	15	0.5
Chocolate, Average	*1 Sweet/30g*	*132*	*4.1*	*441*	*3.3*	*81.1*	*13.7*	*0*
Chocolate, Thorntons*	1 Bag/100g	459	19.1	459	3.1	69	19.1	0.6
Chunks for Baking	*1 Serving/100g*	*428*	*12.2*	*428*	*1.7*	*77.2*	*12.2*	*0.6*
Clotted Cream, Sainsbury's*	1 Sweet/8g	35	0.9	430	1.9	81.5	10.7	0.7
Dairy, Co-Op*	1 Sweet/9g	39	1.2	430	2	76	13	0
Minis, Cadbury*	1 Piece/5g	23	0.9	455	2.6	73	17	0.7
Salted Caramel, Fudgelicious, Ryedale Farm*	1 Piece/9g	43	1.8	473	2.1	72	20	0
Vanilla, Bar, M&S*	1 Bar/43g	205	10	476	3.7	63	23.3	0.4
Vanilla, Julian Graves*	1 Serving/10g	41	1	407	1	78.9	9.7	0
Vanilla, Thorntons*	1 Bag/100g	465	21.9	465	1.8	65.9	21.9	0
FUSILLI								
Brown Rice, Fusilli, GF, Dove's Farm*	1 Serving/30g	101	0.4	338	7.9	70.3	1.5	4.1
Cooked, Average	*1 Serving/210g*	*248*	*1.4*	*118*	*4.2*	*23.8*	*0.6*	*1.2*
Dry, Average	*1 Serving/90g*	*316*	*1.4*	*352*	*12.3*	*72*	*1.6*	*2.2*
Fresh, Cooked, Average	*1 Serving/200g*	*329*	*3.6*	*164*	*6.4*	*30.6*	*1.8*	*1.8*
Fresh, Dry, Average	*1 Serving/75g*	*208*	*2*	*277*	*10.9*	*53.4*	*2.7*	*2.1*
Fusilloni, TTD, Sainsbury's*	1 Serving/90g	321	1.5	357	12.3	73.1	1.7	2.5
GF, Cooked, Free From, Sainsbury's*	1 Serving/200g	340	2.4	170	3.3	36	1.2	0.9
Green Pea Quinoa, Pasta, GF, Dry, Clearspring*	1 Serving/80g	277	2	346	21	56	2.5	7.2
Green Pea, Organic, Uncooked, Napolina*	1 Serving/75g	99	0.1	132	9.2	20.4	0.1	6.9
Red Lentil, Dry, Cook Italian*	1 Serving/80g	283	1.6	354	23	58	2	6
Tricolore, Dry, Average	*1 Serving/75g*	*264*	*1.3*	*351*	*12.2*	*71.8*	*1.7*	*2.7*
Whole Wheat, Dry Weight, Average	*1 Serving/90g*	*290*	*2.1*	*322*	*13.1*	*62.3*	*2.3*	*9*
Wholegrain Spelt, Cooked, Sainsbury's*	1 Serving/75g	120	0.8	160	6.2	30.3	1	2.6
FYBOGEL								
Lemon, Reckitt Benckiser*	1 Serving/4g	4	0	95	2.4	11.3	1.1	64.8
Orange, Reckitt Benckiser*	1 Serving/4g	5	0	106	2.4	12.7	1.1	64.4

F

	Measure INFO/WEIGHT	per Measure KCAL	FAT	Nutrition Values per 100g / 100ml KCAL	PROT	CARB	FAT	FIBRE
GALANGAL								
Raw, Root, Average	*100g*	*71*	*0.6*	*71*	*1.2*	*15.3*	*0.6*	*2.4*
GALAXY								
Amicelli, Mars*	1 Serving/13g	66	3.5	507	6.2	59.7	27.1	0
Bubbles Filled, Chocolate Egg, Galaxy, Mars*	1 Egg/28g	155	9.5	555	6.5	54.7	34.1	1.5
Caramel Crunch, Promises, Mars*	1 Bar/100g	540	31.8	540	6.1	57.5	31.8	0
Caramel, Mars*	1 Bar/49g	254	13	518	5.8	64.2	26.4	0
Cookie Crumble, Mars*	1 Bar/114g	627	37.6	550	6.2	56	33	1.9
Fruit & Hazelnut, Milk, Mars*	1 Bar/47g	235	13.2	501	7.1	55.2	28	0
Hazelnut, Mars*	1 Piece/6g	37	2.5	582	7.8	49.4	39.2	0
Hazelnut, Roast, Promises, Mars*	1 Bar/100g	544	32.9	544	6.4	55.6	32.9	0
Swirls, Mars*	1 Bag/150g	747	39.8	498	4.9	60.2	26.5	0
GAMMON								
Breaded, Average	*1oz/28g*	*34*	*0.9*	*120*	*22.5*	*1*	*3*	*0*
Dry Cured, Ready to Roast, M&S*	½ Joint/255g	255	3.8	100	20.5	0.5	1.5	0.5
Honey & Mustard, Average	*½ Pack/190g*	*294*	*13.5*	*155*	*19.1*	*3.6*	*7.1*	*0.1*
Joint, Boiled, Average	*1 Serving/60g*	*122*	*7.4*	*204*	*23.3*	*0*	*12.3*	*0*
Joint, Honey Glaze, Just Cook, Sainsbury's*	1/3 Pack/123g	242	12.8	197	23.4	2.1	10.4	0
Joint, Raw, Average	*1 Serving/100g*	*138*	*7.5*	*138*	*17.5*	*0*	*7.5*	*0*
Shank, in Honey Mustard, Tesco*	½ Pack/218g	390	12.6	179	25.7	5.5	5.8	0.9
Shank, with Maple, Balsamic, Finest, Tesco*	1 Pack/347g	587	15.3	169	25.5	6.6	4.4	0.5
Steaks, Healthy Range, Average	*1 Serving/110g*	*107*	*3.5*	*97*	*18*	*0.4*	*3.2*	*0.2*
Steaks, Honey Roast, Average	*1 Steak/100g*	*142*	*5.3*	*142*	*21.5*	*2.3*	*5.3*	*0*
Steaks, Smoked, Average	*1 Steak/110g*	*150*	*5.5*	*137*	*22.7*	*0.1*	*5*	*0.1*
Steaks, with Pineapple & Mango Salsa, Easy, Waitrose*	1 Steak/163g	239	11.6	146	14.1	6.5	7.1	0.5
Vegetarian, Roast, Quorn*	¼ Roast/100g	141	4.4	141	17.6	3.8	4.4	7.6
GAMMON &								
Cheese, Ovenbaked, CBY, Asda*	½ Pack/182g	253	9.8	139	17.8	4.5	5.4	0.5
GARAM MASALA								
Dry, Ground, Average	*1 Tbsp/15g*	*57*	*2.3*	*379*	*15.6*	*45.2*	*15.1*	*0*
GARLIC								
Black	*1 Clove/5g*	*13*	*0*	*264*	*13.3*	*53.3*	*0*	*20*
Powder, Average	*1 Tsp/3g*	*7*	*0*	*246*	*18.7*	*42.7*	*1.2*	*9.9*
Raw, Average	*1 Clove/3g*	*3*	*0*	*98*	*7.9*	*16.3*	*0.6*	*2.1*
Very Lazy, The English Provender Co.*	1 Tsp/3g	3	0	111	6	20.9	0.4	3
Wild	*1 Leaf/1g*	*0*	*0*	*23*	*2.8*	*1.7*	*0.6*	*1.9*
GARLIC PUREE								
Average	*1 Tbsp/18g*	*68*	*6*	*380*	*3.5*	*16.9*	*33.6*	*0*
in Vegetable Oil, GIA*	1 Tsp/5g	12	0.9	248	3.6	18.8	17.7	0
with Tomato, GIA*	10g	7	0.1	70	5.1	0.5	1.2	0
GATEAU								
Black Forest, 500g Size, Tesco*	1 Cake/500g	1125	55	225	4	27.1	11	1.8
Black Forest, Dome, Tesco*	1 Dome/600g	1626	68.4	271	4	37.4	11.4	1.6
Black Forest, Mini, Tesco*	1 Serving/55g	136	5.1	247	5.7	35.3	9.2	1
Black Forest, Sara Lee*	1 Serving/80g	221	9.8	276	3.6	37.9	12.3	1.2
Caramel, Salted, Dome, Frozen, Tesco*	1 Serving/78g	233	9.9	298	4.2	41.2	12.7	0.9
Caramel, Salted, Profiterole, Tesco*	1 Slice/88g	248	13.6	282	4.3	31	15.5	0.9
Chocolate Layer, M&S*	1 Serving/86g	278	15.7	323	4.2	35.9	18.3	0.9
Chocolate, & Vanilla, Ice Cream, Iceland*	1 Serving/130g	252	12.2	194	3.3	24.1	9.4	0.6
Chocolate, Double, Frozen, Tesco*	1/5 Gateau/70g	115	4.4	255	5.5	34.2	9.8	3.5
Chocolate, Rich, Tesco*	1 Slice/84g	210	8.6	251	5.1	32.9	10.2	3.4
Chocolate, Swirl, Tesco*	1 Serving/83g	230	13.3	277	3.8	29.3	16	0.2
Chocolate, Triple, Heinz*	¼ Cake/85g	209	9.5	245	5.1	31.2	11.1	2.4
Orange, & Lemon, Iceland*	1 Serving/90g	220	9.9	245	2.6	33.8	11	0.3

	Measure INFO/WEIGHT	per Measure KCAL	FAT	Nutrition Values per 100g / 100ml KCAL	PROT	CARB	FAT	FIBRE
GATEAU								
Strawberry, Co-Op*	1 Serving/77g	222	12.9	288	5.1	29.2	16.7	1
Strawberry, Double, Sara Lee*	1/8 Cake/199g	533	24.3	268	3.2	36.2	12.2	0.6
Strawberry, Frozen, Tesco*	1 Serving/75g	144	6.2	192	2.6	26.3	8.3	0.7
Swiss, Cadbury*	1/6 Gateau/60g	228	10.1	380	5.2	52	16.8	0.9
GELATINE								
Average	*1 Tsp/3g*	*10*	*0*	*338*	*84.4*	*0*	*0*	*0*
GHEE								
Butter	*1oz/28g*	*251*	*27.9*	*898*	*0*	*0*	*99.8*	*0*
Vegetable	*1oz/28g*	*251*	*27.8*	*895*	*0*	*0*	*99.4*	*0*
GHERKINS								
Pickled, Average	*1 Gherkin/36g*	*4*	*0*	*12*	*0.8*	*2.1*	*0.1*	*1*
GIN								
Diet Tonic, Can, Greenalls*	1 Can/250ml	95	0	38	0	0	0	0
Tonic, Canned, Ready to Drink, M&S*	1 Can/250ml	175	0.8	70	0.2	5.6	0.3	0.1
37.5% Volume	*1 Pub Shot/35ml*	*72*	*0*	*207*	*0*	*0*	*0*	*0*
40% Volume	*1 Pub Shot/35ml*	*78*	*0*	*224*	*0*	*0*	*0*	*0*
41% Volume	*1 Pub Shot/35ml*	*83*	*0*	*237*	*0*	*0*	*0*	*0*
Average, 43%	*1 Serving/25ml*	*60*	*0*	*241*	*0*	*0*	*0*	*0*
Gordons & Schweppes Slimline Tonic, Canned, Diageo*	1 Can/250ml	75	0	30	0	0	0	0
Gordons & Schweppes Tonic, Canned, Diageo*	1 Can/250ml	152	0	61	0	6.2	0	0
GINGER								
Chopped, Frozen	*1 Serving/4g*	*2*	*0*	*51*	*1.8*	*8.1*	*0.8*	*2*
Chunks, Crystallised, Julian Graves*	1 Serving/10g	28	0	283	0.2	70.1	0.2	1.5
Ground, Average	*1 Tsp/2g*	*5*	*0.1*	*258*	*7.4*	*60*	*3.3*	*0*
Root, Raw, Pared, Average	*1 Tsp/2g*	*2*	*0*	*81*	*1.8*	*18*	*0.8*	*2*
Root, Raw, Unprepared, Average	*1 Tsp/2g*	*1*	*0*	*74*	*1.7*	*16.3*	*0.7*	*1.8*
Stem in Sugar Syrup, Sainsbury's*	1 Ball/10g	29	0	292	0.5	71.3	0.5	1.6
Very Lazy, The English Provender Co.*	1 Tsp/5g	3	0	52	0.7	10.9	0.8	0.8
GINGER ALE								
1870, Siver Spring*	1 Serving/100ml	18	0	18	0	4.2	0	0
American, Tesco*	1 Glass/250ml	58	0	23	0	5.5	0	0
Dry	*1 Glass/250ml*	*38*	*0*	*15*	*0*	*3.9*	*0*	*0*
Dry, Sainsbury's*	1 Glass/250ml	95	0.2	38	0.1	9.1	0.1	0.1
GINGER BEER								
Alcoholic, Crabbies*	1 Bottle/500ml	254	0	51	0	7.1	0	0
Classic, Schweppes*	1 Can/330ml	115	0	35	0	8.4	0	0
D G Old Jamaican*	1 Can/330ml	211	0	64	0	16	0	0
Diet, Crabbies*	1 Bottle/700ml	7	0	1	0	0	0	0
Light, Waitrose*	1 Glass/250ml	2	0.2	1	0	0	0.1	0.1
No Added Sugar, Canned, Tesco*	1 Can/330ml	3	0.3	1	0	0.1	0.1	0.1
Rhubarb, Sparkling, No Added Sugar, M&S*	1 Can/250ml	2	0.2	1	0.1	0.1	0.1	0.1
Scottish Raspberry, John Crabbie Co*	1 Serving/200ml	64	0	32	0	7.9	0	0
Tesco*	1 Serving/200ml	70	0.2	35	0.1	8.2	0.1	0
Traditional, Fentiman's*	1 Bottle/275ml	130	0	47	0	11.3	0	0
GINGER WINE								
Green Ginger Wine Scots Whisky, Crabbies*	1 Glass/125ml	192	0	153	14.3	14.3	0	0
Green, Crabbies*	1 Serving/125ml	202	0	162	0	21.8	0	0
GINGERBREAD								
Average	*1oz/28g*	*106*	*3.5*	*379*	*5.7*	*64.7*	*12.6*	*1.2*
GLYCERINE								
Average	*1 Tsp/5ml*	*22*	*0*	*440*	*0*	*100*	*0*	*0*
GNOCCHI								
Di Patate, Italfresco*	½ Pack/200g	296	0.4	148	3.3	33.2	0.2	0

G

	Measure INFO/WEIGHT	per Measure KCAL	FAT	Nutrition Values per 100g / 100ml KCAL	PROT	CARB	FAT	FIBRE
GNOCCHI								
Fresh, Cooked, Essential, Waitrose*	¼ Pack/134g	242	0.5	181	4.7	39	0.4	1
Fresh, Italian, Chilled, Sainsbury's*	½ Pack/250g	355	1.2	142	2.5	29.9	0.5	4
Potato, Quinoa, GF, Sottolestelle*	½ Pack/250g	385	0.5	154	1.6	36	0.2	1
Potato, Cooked, Average	*1 Serving/150g*	*200*	*0*	*133*	*0*	*33.2*	*0*	*0*
GOAT								
Meat, Uncooked	*1 Portion/100g*	*109*	*2.3*	*109*	*20*	*0*	*2.3*	*0*
GOJI BERRIES								
Average	*1 Serving/100g*	*287*	*0.7*	*287*	*6.6*	*65.1*	*0.7*	*6.8*
Dried, Tesco*	½ Pack/50g	181	0.9	362	14	70	1.8	5
GOOSE								
Leg with Skin, Fire Roasted	*1 Leg/174g*	*482*	*29.8*	*277*	*28.8*	*0*	*17.1*	*0*
Meat Skin, Roasted	*½ Goose/774g*	*2361*	*169.5*	*305*	*25.2*	*0*	*21.9*	*0*
Meat, Fat Skin, Raw	*1 Serving/125g*	*425*	*38.8*	*340*	*15.7*	*0*	*31*	*0*
Meat, Raw	*1 Portion/185g*	*298*	*13*	*161*	*23*	*0*	*7*	*0*
Meat, Roasted	*1 Portion/143g*	*340*	*18.1*	*238*	*29*	*0*	*12.7*	*0*
GOOSEBERRIES								
Dessert, Raw, Tops Tails Removed	*1oz/28g*	*11*	*0.1*	*40*	*0.7*	*9.2*	*0.3*	*2.4*
Stewed with Sugar	*25g*	*14*	*0.1*	*54*	*0.7*	*12.9*	*0.3*	*4.2*
Stewed without Sugar	*25g*	*4*	*0.1*	*16*	*0.9*	*2.5*	*0.3*	*4.4*
GOULASH								
Beef with Tagliatelle, COU, M&S*	1 Pack/360g	414	8.3	115	8.5	14.5	2.3	1
Beef, Average	*1 Serving/300g*	*310*	*9.5*	*103*	*8.1*	*10.4*	*3.2*	*0.9*
Beef, Finest, Tesco*	½ Pack/300g	297	9.3	99	11.6	6.2	3.1	0.6
GRAINS								
Curried, Coconut, Tesco*	½ Pack/150g	252	10.8	168	3.4	20.3	7.2	4.2
Rye, Uncooked	*1 Serving/100g*	*338*	*1.6*	*338*	*10.3*	*75.9*	*1.6*	*15.1*
Super, Garlic, Ginger, Tilda*	½ Pack/110g	183	6.6	166	4.6	22.6	6	1.6
Wheatberries, Kale, Sainsbury's*	½ Pack/150g	195	6.8	130	6.6	12	4.5	7.6
GRAPEFRUIT								
in Juice, Canned, Average	*1/3 Can/179g*	*82*	*0.1*	*46*	*0.5*	*10.6*	*0*	*0.4*
in Syrup, Average	*1oz/28g*	*19*	*0*	*69*	*0.5*	*16.8*	*0.1*	*0.5*
Raw, Flesh Only, Average	*½ Fruit/160g*	*48*	*0.2*	*30*	*0.8*	*6.8*	*0.1*	*1.3*
Raw, Weighed with Skin Seeds, Average	*1 Lge/340g*	*54*	*0.2*	*16*	*0.3*	*4*	*0*	*0.6*
Ruby Red in Juice, Average	*1 Serving/135g*	*54*	*0.1*	*40*	*0.6*	*9.4*	*0*	*0.5*
GRAPES								
Black, Seedless, Sable, TTD, Sainsbury's*	1 Serving/80g	56	0.4	70	0.5	15.4	0.5	0
Cotton Candy, 1, Waitrose*	1 Serving/80g	53	0.1	66	0.4	15.4	0.1	0.9
Cotton Candy, Black, Seedless, Finest, Tesco*	1 Portion/80g	53	0.1	66	0.4	15.4	0.1	0.7
Green, Average	*1 Grape/5g*	*3*	*0*	*62*	*0.4*	*15.2*	*0.1*	*0.7*
Red Green Selection, Average	*1 Grape/5g*	*3*	*0*	*62*	*0.4*	*15.2*	*0.1*	*0.8*
Red, Average	*1 Grape/5g*	*3*	*0*	*65*	*0.4*	*15.8*	*0.1*	*0.6*
Sable, 1, Waitrose*	1 Pack/400g	264	0.4	66	0.4	15.4	0.1	0.9
Sable, Finest, Tesco*	1 Serving/80g	53	0.1	66	0.4	15.4	0.1	0.7
Seedless, Red, Average	*1 Grape*	*4*	*0*	*74*	*0.6*	*17*	*0.3*	*0.6*
White, So Organic, Sainsbury's*	1 Serving/80g	53	0.4	67	0.7	15.2	0.5	0.7
GRAPPA								
Average	*1 Serving/30ml*	*85*	*0*	*283*	*0*	*6.7*	*0*	*0*
GRATIN								
Crab, & Lobster Mac & Cheese, Iceland*	1 Pot/100g	148	7.1	155	7.4	14	7.4	1.5
Haddock, Smoked, Frozen, Tesco*	1 Pot/90g	145	9.2	162	12.4	4.5	10.3	1.1
Leek, & Carrot, Findus*	1 Pack/400g	440	26	110	3.5	9.5	6.5	0
Potato, Spinach, M&S*	1 Serving/225g	259	16	115	2.9	9.1	7.1	1.3
Potato, Cheesy, Ovenbaked, Asda*	½ Pack/200g	179	8	90	1.7	11	4	1.4

G

	Measure INFO/WEIGHT	per Measure KCAL	FAT	Nutrition Values per 100g / 100ml KCAL	PROT	CARB	FAT	FIBRE
GRATIN								
Potato, Creamy, M&S*	½ Pack/225g	360	25	160	2.2	11.9	11.1	0.9
Potato, Dauphinoise, Finest, Tesco*	1 Gratin/107g	210	14.1	196	3.3	15	13.1	2
Vegetable, Root, Finest, Tesco*	½ Pack/214g	365	23.9	171	2.4	14	11.2	2
GRAVY								
Beef, Aunt Bessie's*	1 Serving/100g	73	5.3	73	1	5.3	5.3	0.5
Beef, Favourite, Granules, Made Up, Bisto*	1 Serving/50ml	13	0.5	26	0	4.2	1	0
Beef, Free From, Sainsbury's*	½ Pack/151g	47	1.5	31	1.5	4.1	1	0.2
Beef, Fresh, Sainsbury's*	1 Serving/83ml	47	2.7	56	2.4	4.5	3.2	0.6
Beef, Granules, Dry, Tesco*	1 Serving/6g	29	2.1	480	5.5	36.4	34.7	1.5
Beef, Granules, Made Up, Tesco*	1 Serving/140ml	48	3.6	35	0.3	2.6	2.5	0.1
Beef, Heat & Serve, Morrisons*	1 Serving/150g	27	0.4	18	0.3	3.9	0.3	0.5
Beef, Roast, Best in Glass Jar, Made Up, Bisto*	1 Serving/70ml	21	0.3	30	0.3	6.1	0.4	0
Beef, Roast, Traditional, Finest, Tesco*	¼ Pot/125g	68	3	54	2.4	5.5	2.4	0.3
Beef, with Winter Berry & Shallot, Made Up, Oxo*	1 Serving/105ml	24	0.3	23	0.6	4.3	0.3	0.1
Chicken, & Hint of Sage & Onion, Granules, Oxo*	1 Serving/30g	95	1.8	316	11.1	54.2	6.1	0.7
Chicken, & Turkey, Christmas, TTD, Sainsbury's*	¼ Pot/112g	66	1.7	59	6.9	4.2	1.5	0.5
Chicken, Finest, Tesco*	¼ Pouch/88ml	38	1.1	43	2.3	5.1	1.3	0
Chicken, Granules For, Dry Weight, Bisto*	1 Serving/20g	80	3.2	400	1.9	62.5	15.8	0.2
Chicken, Granules, Dry, Average	*1 Tsp/4g*	*17*	*0.9*	*428*	*4.5*	*49.4*	*23.6*	*1.2*
Chicken, Granules, Dry, Oxo*	1oz/28g	83	1.4	296	11.1	54.2	4.9	0.7
Chicken, Granules, Made Up, Average	*1 Serving/50ml*	*15*	*0.8*	*30*	*0.4*	*3.6*	*1.5*	*0.1*
Chicken, Granules, Made Up, Oxo*	1fl oz/30ml	5	0.1	18	0.7	3.3	0.3	0
Chicken, Granules, Made Up, Smart Price, Asda*	1 Serving/100ml	34	2.3	34	0.2	3	2.3	0.1
Chicken, Granules, Organic, Kallo*	1 Sachet/35g	121	0.8	345	1.6	79.1	2.3	0.4
Chicken, Rich Stock, Onions, Black Pepper, M&S*	½ Jar/168g	99	4.9	59	2	5.9	2.9	0.5
Granules, Dry, Bisto*	1 Serving/10g	38	1.6	384	3.1	56.4	16.2	1.5
Granules, Dry, Value, Tesco*	1oz/28g	111	5.2	397	3.2	54.4	18.5	1
Granules, Instant, Made Up	*1oz/28g*	*10*	*0.7*	*34*	*0.3*	*3*	*2.4*	*0*
Granules, Made Up, Oxo*	1 Serving/150ml	28	0.4	19	0.6	3.4	0.3	0
Instant, Made Up, BGTY, Sainsbury's*	1fl oz/30ml	10	0	32	0.3	7.4	0.1	0.1
Lamb, Fresh, M&S*	½ Pouch/75g	38	0.2	50	4.3	7.7	0.2	0.5
Lamb, Granules, As Prepared, Best, Bisto*	1 Serving/50ml	13	0.5	26	1	5.4	1	1
Lamb, Granules, Dry, Average	*1 Tsp/4g*	*14*	*0.3*	*344*	*10.8*	*56.2*	*8.4*	*2.8*
Lamb, Roast, Bisto*	1 Serving/20g	60	0.9	302	3.4	62.3	4.3	0
Meat, Granules, As Consumed, Quixo, Aldi*	1 Serving/70ml	24	1.6	34	0.5	3.1	2.3	0.5
Meat, Granules, Made Up, Asda*	1 Serving/100ml	38	2.4	38	0.6	4	2.4	0.1
Meat, Granules, Made Up, Sainsbury's*	1 Serving/100ml	37	2.4	37	0.4	3.5	2.4	0.1
Meat, Rich Beef Stock, Onions, Red Wine, M&S*	½ Jar/168g	89	4.7	53	1.7	5	2.8	0.7
Onion, Caramelised, Made Up, Bisto*	1 Serving/50ml	14	0.2	29	0.1	6.1	0.4	0.1
Onion, Fresh, Asda*	1/6 Pot/77g	30	1.6	39	1.7	3.3	2.1	0.4
Onion, Fresh, M&S*	¼ Pouch/75g	44	2.2	59	0.8	6.8	2.9	1
Onion, Granules For, Dry Weight, Bisto*	4 Tsp/20g	78	2.9	391	2.4	62.3	14.7	2.3
Onion, Granules, Made Up, Bisto*	1 Serving/50ml	14	0.3	28	0.2	5.6	0.6	0
Onion, Rich, M&S*	½ Pack/150g	60	1.8	40	2	5.9	1.2	0.3
Onion, Roast, Classic, Dry, Schwartz*	1 Pack/27g	85	1.1	315	8.8	61	4	4.6
Pork, & Sage, Roast, Classic, Dry, Schwartz*	1 Pack/25g	88	1.4	354	11.8	63.8	5.8	0
Pork, Best, Made Up, Bisto*	1 Serving/50ml	14	0.2	28	0.6	5.8	0.4	0
Pork, Roast, Best, in Glass Jar, Dry Weight, Bisto*	4 Tsp/20g	63	0.9	314	4.3	64.1	4.5	0
Powder, GF, Dry, Allergycare*	1 Tbsp/10g	26	0	260	0.3	63.8	0.4	0
Powder, Made Up, Sainsbury's*	1 Serving/100ml	15	0.1	15	0.4	3.2	0.1	0.1
Turkey, Finest, Tesco*	¼ Pouch/88ml	49	1.4	56	3.9	6.4	1.6	0
Turkey, Granules, Dry Weight, Bisto*	4 Tsp/20g	75	3.1	377	2.4	57.2	15.5	1
Turkey, Rich, Ready to Heat, Schwartz*	1 Pack/200g	62	2.4	31	1.9	3.1	1.2	0.5

G

	Measure INFO/WEIGHT	per Measure KCAL	FAT	Nutrition Values per 100g / 100ml KCAL	PROT	CARB	FAT	FIBRE
GRAVY								
Vegetable, Granules, Dry Weight, Bisto*	1 Tsp/4g	15	0.5	380	2.1	63	13.3	4.5
Vegetable, Granules, Dry, Oxo*	1oz/28g	88	1.4	316	8.4	59.5	4.9	0.9
Vegetable, Granules, Dry, Tesco*	½ Pint/20g	94	6.7	470	3.8	38.5	33.4	3.7
Vegetable, Granules, Made Up, Bisto*	1 Serving/50ml	14	0.2	28	0.2	5.6	0.4	0.2
Vegetarian, Granules, Dry Weight, Bisto*	1 Serving/28g	100	3.7	356	2.7	56	13.3	4.5
Vegetarian, Granules, Made Up, Sainsbury's*	1 Serving/50ml	16	1.1	32	0.2	2.8	2.2	0.8
Vegetarian, Powder, Organic, Marigold*	1 Serving/22g	79	1.7	361	10.6	61.5	7.7	1.3
GRILLS								
Grills, Tesco*	1 Grill/96g	236	13.7	246	5.6	22	14.3	3.2
GRITS								
Hominy, White, Enriched, Old Fashioned, Quaker*	¼ Cup/41g	140	0.5	341	7.3	78	1.2	4.9
GROUSE								
Meat Only, Roasted	*1oz/28g*	*36*	*0.6*	*128*	*27.6*	*0*	*2*	*0*
GUACAMOLE								
Average	*1 Tbsp/17g*	*33*	*3.3*	*194*	*1.6*	*3.4*	*19.2*	*2.4*
Avocado, Reduced Fat, The Fresh Dip Company*	1 Serving/113g	128	9.8	113	2.5	6.1	8.7	2.3
Dip, Tesco*	¼ Pot/41g	58	5.2	142	1.1	4	12.8	3
Reduced Fat Average	*1 Serving/100g*	*129*	*10.8*	*129*	*2.4*	*5.2*	*10.8*	*3*
Reduced Fat, Dip, BGTY, Sainsbury's*	¼ Pot/43g	62	5.7	146	1.3	2.9	13.5	4
Squeezy, Old El Paso*	1 Tbsp/15g	14	0.9	96	1.3	7.4	6.3	2.4
Style, Topping, Dip, Discovery*	1 Seving/37g	29	2.1	79	1.2	6	5.6	1.2
GUAVA								
Canned in Syrup	*1oz/28g*	*17*	*0*	*60*	*0.4*	*15.7*	*0*	*3*
Raw, Flesh Only, Average	*1 Fruit/55g*	*37*	*0.6*	*68*	*3*	*14*	*1*	*5*
GUINEA FOWL								
Boned & Stuffed, Fresh, Fayrefield Foods*	1 Serving/325g	650	39.3	200	19.1	3.3	12.1	0.5
Fresh, Free Range, Waitrose*	1 Portion/193g	258	11.9	134	19.5	0	6.2	0.3
GUMS								
American Hard, Sainsbury's*	1 Sweet/6g	22	0	360	0.1	90	0.1	0
American Hard, Tesco*	1 Serving/200g	646	0	323	0	80.8	0	0
Milk Bottles, Bassett's*	1 Pack/25g	88	0.4	353	6.2	78.3	1.6	0
Milk Bottles, Milk Flavour, Asda*	1 Pack/100g	369	2.3	369	7	80	2.3	0.4

G

	Measure INFO/WEIGHT	per Measure KCAL	FAT	Nutrition Values per 100g / 100ml KCAL	PROT	CARB	FAT	FIBRE
HADDOCK								
Parsley Sauce, Simply Steam, Microwaved, Youngs*	1 Pack/263g	179	2.6	68	7.7	6.4	1	1.2
Fillets, Battered, Average	*1oz/28g*	*64*	*3.4*	*228*	*13.4*	*16.3*	*12.2*	*1.1*
Fillets, in Breadcrumbs, Average	*1 Fillet/125g*	*253*	*12.4*	*203*	*13.5*	*14.9*	*9.9*	*1.2*
Fillets, in Lemon & Chive Butter Sauce, Birds Eye*	1 Portion/148g	190	11.3	128	14.6	0.4	7.6	0
Fillets, in Seeded Breadcrumbs, Waitrose*	1 Fillet/121g	278	12.8	230	15.6	16.8	10.6	2.5
Fillets, Raw, Average	*1 Fillet/140g*	*111*	*1.2*	*79*	*17.7*	*0.2*	*0.8*	*0*
Fillets, Smoked, Cooked, Average	*1 Pack/300g*	*337*	*7.7*	*112*	*21.9*	*0.4*	*2.6*	*0.1*
Fillets, Smoked, Raw, Average	*1 Pack/227g*	*190*	*1*	*84*	*19.9*	*0.1*	*0.4*	*0.2*
Florentine, with Garlic & Herb Potato, Gastropub, M&S*	1 Pack/370g	492	29.2	133	7.7	7.4	7.9	0.7
Flour, Fried in Blended Oil	*1oz/28g*	*39*	*1.1*	*138*	*21.1*	*4.5*	*4.1*	*0.2*
Goujons, Batter, Crispy, M&S*	1 Serving/100g	250	14.1	250	11.7	18.5	14.1	0.8
HAGGIS								
Traditional, Average	*1 Serving/454g*	*1119*	*66.5*	*246*	*12.4*	*17.2*	*14.6*	*1*
Vegetarian, Macsween*	1/3 Pack/151g	412	24.6	273	6	22.9	16.3	0
HAKE								
Fillets, in Breadcrumbs, Average	*1oz/28g*	*66*	*3.7*	*234*	*12.9*	*16*	*13.4*	*1*
Goujons, Average	*1 Serving/150g*	*345*	*17.8*	*230*	*12.4*	*18.6*	*11.9*	*1.3*
Raw, Average	*1oz/28g*	*28*	*0.6*	*100*	*20.1*	*0*	*2.2*	*0*
HALIBUT								
Cooked, Dry Heat, Average	*1oz/28g*	*38*	*1.1*	*135*	*24.6*	*0.4*	*4*	*0*
Raw	*1oz/28g*	*28*	*0.5*	*101*	*21.1*	*0*	*1.9*	*0*
with Roasted Pepper Sauce, Fillets, M&S*	1 Serving/145g	218	14.4	150	12.7	2.4	9.9	0.6
HALVA								
Average	*1oz/28g*	*107*	*3.7*	*381*	*1.8*	*68*	*13.2*	*0*
HAM								
Applewood Smoked, Average	*1 Slice/28g*	*31*	*0.8*	*112*	*21.2*	*0.6*	*2.8*	*0.2*
Baked, Average	*1 Slice/74g*	*98*	*3.7*	*133*	*21*	*1*	*5*	*0*
Black Forest, Slices, Dulano, Lidl*	1 Slice/11g	26	1.6	240	25	1	15	0.5
Boiled, Average	*1 Pack/113g*	*154*	*6.5*	*136*	*20.6*	*0.6*	*5.8*	*0*
Breaded, Average	*1 Slice/37g*	*57*	*2.3*	*155*	*23.1*	*1.8*	*6.3*	*1.6*
Breaded, Dry Cured, Average	*1 Slice/33g*	*47*	*1.8*	*142*	*22.2*	*1.4*	*5.4*	*0*
Brunswick, Average	*1 Slice/20g*	*32*	*1.8*	*160*	*19.5*	*0.6*	*8.8*	*0*
Cooked, Sliced, Average	*1 Slice/17g*	*18*	*0.5*	*109*	*19*	*1*	*3.2*	*0.1*
Crumbed, Sliced, Average	*1 Slice/28g*	*33*	*0.9*	*117*	*21.5*	*0.9*	*3.1*	*0*
Danish, Average	*1 Slice/11g*	*14*	*0.6*	*125*	*18.4*	*1*	*5.4*	*0*
Danish, Lean, Average	*1 Slice/15g*	*14*	*0.3*	*92*	*17.8*	*1*	*1.8*	*0*
Dry Cured, Average	*1 Slice/18g*	*26*	*1*	*144*	*22.4*	*1*	*5.6*	*0.2*
Extra Lean, Average	*1 Slice/11g*	*10*	*0.2*	*90*	*18*	*1.4*	*1.4*	*0*
Gammon, Breaded, Average	*1 Serving/25g*	*31*	*0.8*	*122*	*22*	*1.5*	*3.1*	*0*
Gammon, Dry Cured, Sliced, Average	*1 Slice/33g*	*43*	*1.4*	*131*	*22.9*	*0.4*	*4.2*	*0*
Gammon, Honey Roast, Average	*1 Serving/60g*	*81*	*2.8*	*134*	*22.4*	*0.4*	*4.8*	*0*
Gammon, Smoked, Average	*1 Slice/43g*	*59*	*2.1*	*137*	*22.3*	*0.7*	*4.9*	*0.2*
German Black Forest, Average	*½ Pack/35g*	*93*	*6*	*267*	*27.2*	*1.3*	*17*	*0.5*
Hock, Cooked, Shredded, Sainsbury's*	½ Pack55g	100	4.1	182	27.6	0.5	7.5	1
Hock, Pulled, M&S*	1 Pack/100g	165	6.5	165	26.5	0.1	6.5	0.1
Honey & Mustard, Average	*1oz/28g*	*39*	*1.2*	*140*	*20.8*	*4.6*	*4.3*	*0*
Honey Roast, Average	*1 Slice/20g*	*25*	*0.8*	*123*	*20.3*	*1.6*	*3.8*	*0.1*
Honey Roast, Dry Cured, Average	*1 Slice/33g*	*46*	*1.5*	*140*	*22.7*	*2.3*	*4.4*	*0.2*
Honey Roast, Lean, Average	*1 Serving/25g*	*28*	*0.8*	*111*	*18.2*	*2.7*	*3.1*	*0*
Honey Roast, Wafer Thin, Average	*1 Slice/10g*	*11*	*0.3*	*113*	*17.4*	*3.7*	*3.2*	*0.3*
Honey Roast, Wafer Thin, Premium, Average	*1 Slice/10g*	*15*	*0.6*	*149*	*22*	*1.6*	*6*	*0*
Jamon, Iberico de Bellota, Hand Carved, 1, Waitrose*	¼ Pack/16g	56	3.9	344	31.5	0.7	23.7	0.9
Joint, Cured, Roasted, Average	*1 Serving/100g*	*138*	*5.2*	*138*	*21.7*	*1*	*5.2*	*0.1*

H

INFO/WEIGHT	Measure	per Measure		Nutrition Values per 100g / 100ml				
		KCAL	FAT	KCAL	PROT	CARB	FAT	FIBRE

HAM

	INFO/WEIGHT	KCAL	FAT	KCAL	PROT	CARB	FAT	FIBRE
Joint, Roast, Christmas, Tesco*	1/6 Joint/167g	225	10.8	135	17.9	1.1	6.5	0
Lean, Average	*1 Slice/18g*	*19*	*0.4*	*104*	*19.5*	*1.1*	*2.4*	*0.3*
Oak Smoked, Average	*1 Slice/20g*	*26*	*0.9*	*130*	*21*	*1*	*4.7*	*0.3*
Parma, Average	*1 Slice/10g*	*21*	*1.1*	*213*	*29.3*	*0*	*10.6*	*0*
Parma, Premium, Average	*1 Slice/14g*	*36*	*2.3*	*258*	*27.9*	*0.3*	*16.1*	*0*
Peppered, Average	*1 Slice/12g*	*13*	*0.3*	*110*	*18.5*	*2*	*2.7*	*0*
Peppered, Dry Cured, Average	*1 Slice/31g*	*43*	*1.5*	*140*	*23.1*	*1.3*	*4.7*	*0.2*
Prosciutto, Average	*1 Slice/12g*	*27*	*1.5*	*226*	*28.7*	*0*	*12.4*	*0.4*
Pulled, in Mustard Sauce, BFY, M&S*	1 Pack/400g	304	10	76	6	6.9	2.5	0.9
Serrano, Average	*1 Slice/20g*	*46*	*2.4*	*230*	*30.5*	*0.4*	*11.8*	*0*
Smoked, Average	*1 Slice/18g*	*21*	*0.7*	*117*	*19.7*	*0.9*	*3.7*	*0*
Smoked, Dry Cured, Average	*1 Slice/28g*	*38*	*1.2*	*137*	*23*	*1.4*	*4.4*	*0.2*
Smoked, Wafer Thin, Average	*1 Serving/40g*	*41*	*1.2*	*102*	*17.7*	*1.2*	*2.9*	*0.2*
Sweet Smoky, Sliced, On the Go, Sainsbury's*	1 Pack/75g	113	2.3	151	28.3	1.9	3.1	1
Thick Cut, Average	*1 Slice/74g*	*94*	*2.9*	*127*	*22.4*	*0.6*	*3.9*	*0.1*
Tinned, Average	*½ Can/100g*	*136*	*8.8*	*136*	*12.2*	*2*	*8.8*	*0*
Tinned, Lean, Average	*½ Can/100g*	*94*	*2.3*	*94*	*18.1*	*0.2*	*2.3*	*0.4*
Vegetarian, Slices, Deli, Wafer Thin, Deli, Quorn*	1/3 Pack/60g	66	1.3	110	16	6.5	2.2	5.8
Vegetarian, Slices, Quorn*	¼ Pack/25g	30	0.5	122	16	6.5	2.2	5.8
Wafer Thin, Average	*1 Slice/10g*	*10*	*0.3*	*101*	*17.9*	*1.4*	*2.6*	*0.1*
Wiltshire, Average	*1oz/28g*	*41*	*1.7*	*148*	*23.1*	*0*	*6*	*0*
Wiltshire, Breaded, Average	*1oz/28g*	*41*	*1.4*	*145*	*23.9*	*1*	*5*	*0*

HARE

	INFO/WEIGHT	KCAL	FAT	KCAL	PROT	CARB	FAT	FIBRE
Raw, Lean Only, Average	*1oz/28g*	*35*	*1*	*125*	*23.5*	*0.2*	*3.5*	*0*
Stewed, Lean Only, Average	*1oz/28g*	*48*	*1.5*	*170*	*29.5*	*0.2*	*5.5*	*0*

HARIBO*

	INFO/WEIGHT	KCAL	FAT	KCAL	PROT	CARB	FAT	FIBRE
American Hard Gums, Haribo*	1 Pack/175g	630	3.3	360	0.3	85.5	1.9	0.2
Cola Bottles, Fizzy, Haribo*	1 Pack/175g	595	0.4	340	6.3	78.3	0.2	0.3
Cola Bottles, Haribo*	1 Pack/16g	56	0	348	7.7	78.9	0.2	0.3
Dolly Mixtures, Haribo*	1 Pack/175g	719	8.4	411	1.8	90.2	4.8	0.2
Fantasy Mix, Haribo*	1 Pack/100g	344	0.2	344	6.6	79	0.2	0.3
Fruitilicious, 30% Less Sugar, Haribo*	¼ Bag/30g	85	0.2	282	6.4	54	0.5	0
Gold Bears, Haribo*	1 Pack/100g	348	0.2	348	7.7	78.9	0.2	0.3
Happy Cherries, Haribo*	1 Serving/40g	139	0.1	348	7.7	78.9	0.2	0.3
Horror Mix, Haribo*	1 Pack/100g	344	0.2	344	6.6	79	0.2	0.3
Jelly Babies, Haribo*	1oz/28g	97	0.1	348	4.5	82.1	0.2	0.5
Jelly Beans, Haribo*	1 Pack/100g	379	0.2	379	0.6	93.8	0.2	0.1
Kiddies Super Mix, Haribo*	1 Pack/100g	344	0.2	344	6.6	79	0.2	0.3
Liquorice Favourites, Haribo*	1 Serving/40g	143	1.2	357	2.8	78.8	3	2.3
Liquorice with Stevia, Stevi-Lakritz, Haribo*	¼ Bag/25g	46	0	185	8.1	16	0.1	48.6
Magic Mix, Haribo*	1oz/28g	102	0.5	366	5.4	82	1.9	0.3
Maoam Stripes, Haribo*	1 Chew/7g	27	0.4	384	1.2	81.7	6.1	0.3
Mega Roulette, Haribo*	1oz/28g	97	0.1	348	7.7	78.9	0.2	0.3
Milky Mix, Haribo*	1 Pack/175g	607	0.4	347	7.1	79.6	0.2	0.4
Mint Imperials, Haribo*	1 Pack/175g	695	0.9	397	0.4	98.8	0.5	0.1
Pontefract Cakes, Haribo*	1 Serving/40g	118	0.1	296	5.3	68.2	0.2	0.5
Snakes, Haribo*	1 Snake/8g	28	0	348	7.7	78.9	0.2	0.3
Starmix, Haribo*	1 Pack/100g	344	0.2	344	6.6	79	0.2	0.3
Tangfastics, Haribo*	1 Pack/100g	359	2.3	359	6.3	78.3	2.3	0.5
Tropifruit, Haribo*	1oz/28g	97	0.1	348	4.5	82.1	0.2	0.5

HARISSA PASTE

	INFO/WEIGHT	KCAL	FAT	KCAL	PROT	CARB	FAT	FIBRE
Average	*1 Tsp/5g*	*6*	*0.3*	*123*	*2.9*	*12.9*	*6.7*	*2.8*

	Measure INFO/WEIGHT	per Measure KCAL	per Measure FAT	Nutrition Values per 100g / 100ml KCAL	PROT	CARB	FAT	FIBRE
HASH								
Beef, in Gravy, & Buttery Potato & Onion, Gastropub, M&S*	1 Pack/400g	432	16	108	9	8.1	4	1.7
Corned Beef, Homestyle, Hormel*	1 Can/400g	644	40.7	161	7.2	9.8	10.2	0.8
Steak, in London Porter Gravy, British, TTD, Sainsbury's*	1 Pack/400g	408	13.6	102	8.5	8.5	3.4	1.4
HASH BROWNS								
Homestyle, Aunt Bessie's*	2 Pieces/98g	182	9.2	186	1.6	23	9.4	1.9
Oven Baked, Weighed Cooked, McCain*	1 Piece/37g	64	2.4	170	1.8	24.9	6.4	2.7
Oven Baked, Weighed Frozen, McCain*	1 Piece/40g	60	2.4	150	1.6	21.3	6	2.1
Potatoes, From Restaurant, Average	*1 Portion/150g*	*489*	*32.5*	*326*	*2.6*	*32.1*	*21.6*	*2.7*
Uncooked, Average	*1 Piece/45g*	*78*	*3.7*	*173*	*2*	*22.5*	*8.3*	*1.9*
HAZELNUTS								
Blanched, Average	*1 Serving/25g*	*164*	*15.9*	*656*	*15.4*	*5.8*	*63.5*	*6.5*
Chopped, Average	*1 Serving/10g*	*67*	*6.4*	*666*	*16.8*	*5.6*	*64*	*6.6*
Roasted, Graze*	1 Pack/26g	173	16.9	665	14	6.1	65	0
Whole, Average	*10 Whole/10g*	*66*	*6.4*	*655*	*15.4*	*5.8*	*63.5*	*6.5*
HEART								
Lambs, Average	*1 Heart/75g*	*92*	*4.5*	*122*	*16*	*1*	*6*	*0*
Ox, Raw	*1oz/28g*	*23*	*0.8*	*82*	*14.4*	*0*	*2.8*	*0*
Ox, Stewed	*1oz/28g*	*44*	*1.4*	*157*	*27.8*	*0*	*5.1*	*0*
HERMESETAS								
Powdered, Hermes*	1 Tsp/0.8g	3	0	387	1	96.8	0	0
The Classic Sweetener, Hermes*	1 Tablet/0.5g	0	0	294	14.2	59.3	0	0
HERRING								
Canned in Tomato Sauce, Average	*1oz/28g*	*57*	*4.3*	*204*	*11.9*	*4.1*	*15.5*	*0.1*
Dried, Salted, Average	*1oz/28g*	*47*	*2.1*	*168*	*25.3*	*0*	*7.4*	*0*
Fillets, Raw, Average	*1 Herring/100g*	*139*	*9.4*	*139*	*13.8*	*0*	*9.4*	*0*
Fillets, Smoked, Peppered, Sainsbury's*	½ Pack/80g	163	8.7	204	22.8	3.5	10.9	0
Grilled, Average	*1oz/28g*	*51*	*3.1*	*181*	*20.1*	*0*	*11.2*	*0*
in Dill Marinade, Drained, Elsinore*	1 Jar/140g	336	15.4	240	9.8	27	11	0
Pickled in Mustard Sauce, Abba*	1 Serving/58g	150	10.9	260	7	16	19	0
Pickled, Average	*1oz/28g*	*42*	*2.9*	*149*	*8.1*	*5.5*	*10.3*	*0*
Whole, Raw, Average	*1 Serving/100g*	*95*	*6.6*	*95*	*8.9*	*0*	*6.6*	*0*
HOKI								
Grilled	*1oz/28g*	*34*	*0.8*	*121*	*24.1*	*0*	*2.7*	*0*
Raw	*1oz/28g*	*24*	*0.5*	*85*	*16.9*	*0*	*1.9*	*0*
HONEY								
Acacia Blossom, Sainsbury's*	1 Serving/24g	81	0	339	0.1	84.7	0.1	0.3
Acacia, Tesco*	1 Tsp/4g	12	0	307	0.4	76.4	0	0
Clear, with a Hint of Cinnamon, Rowse*	1 Tbsp/15g	49	0.1	329	0.5	81.5	0.5	0.5
Clover, New Zealand, M&S*	1 Tsp/5g	16	0	328	0.1	81.5	0.2	0.5
Greek, Waitrose*	1 Tsp/6g	18	0	307	0.4	76.4	0	0
Manuka, New Zealand, M&S*	1 Tsp/5g	17	0	348	0.1	86.9	0.1	0.3
Pure, Clear, Average	*1 Tbsp/20g*	*63*	*0*	*315*	*0.5*	*78.5*	*0*	*0*
Pure, Set, Average	*1 Tbsp/20g*	*62*	*0*	*312*	*0.4*	*77.6*	*0*	*0*
Raw, British Wildflower, Hilltop*	1 Tsp/5g	17	0	333	0.2	83.1	0.2	0
Scottish Heather, Waitrose*	1 Serving/20g	61	0	307	0.4	76.4	0	0
Spanish Orange Blossom, Sainsbury's*	1 Tbsp/15g	51	0	339	0.1	84.7	0	0.3
Wild Flower, M&S*	1 Tbsp/15g	49	0	328	0.1	81.5	0.2	0.5
HONEYCOMB								
Natural, Epicure*	1 Serving/100g	290	4.6	290	0.4	74.4	4.6	0
HOOCH*								
Vodka, Calculated Estimate, Hooch*	1 Bottle/330ml	145	0	44	0.3	5.1	0	0
HORLICKS								
Malted Drink, Chocolate, Extra Light, Dry Weight, Horlicks*	1 Serving/32g	95	2.5	296	9.2	47	7.8	17.3

H

	Measure INFO/WEIGHT	per Measure KCAL	FAT	Nutrition Values per 100g / 100ml KCAL	PROT	CARB	FAT	FIBRE
HORLICKS								
Malted Drink, Extra Light, Instant, Dry Weight, Horlicks*	1 Serving/11g	35	0.7	319	8.4	57.4	6.2	10.5
Malted Drink, Light, Dry Weight, Horlicks*	1 Serving/32g	116	1.2	364	14.8	72.2	3.8	1.9
Malted Drink, Light, Made Up, Horlicks*	1 Mug/200ml	116	1.2	58	2.4	11.6	0.6	0.3
Powder, Made Up with Semi-Skimmed Milk	*1 Mug/227ml*	*184*	*4.3*	*81*	*4.3*	*12.9*	*1.9*	*0*
Powder, Made Up with Whole Milk	*1 Mug/227ml*	*225*	*8.9*	*99*	*4.2*	*12.7*	*3.9*	*0*
HORSERADISH								
Creamed, Sainsbury's*	1 Tsp/10ml	25	1.4	253	2.8	26.9	14.3	2.3
Prepared, Average	*1 Tsp/5g*	*1*	*0*	*28*	*2*	*5*	*0.1*	*2.8*
HOT CHOCOLATE								
Belgian Choc Butterscotch, Made Up, Options*	1 Sachet/11g	39	0.9	353	2.7	52	8.1	8.5
Belgian Choc, Options*	1 Sachet/11g	40	0.8	365	8.9	59	7.3	0
Cadbury*	1 Serving/12g	44	0.7	370	6.3	73.3	5.9	0
Caramel, Whittards of Chelsea*	1 Serving/20g	71	1.5	355	7.5	64.5	7.5	13
Choc Mint, Highlights, Made Up, Cadbury*	1 Serving/200ml	40	1.4	20	1	2.5	0.7	0.3
Choca Mocha Drink, Options, Ovaltine*	1 Sachet/11g	39	1.3	359	14.1	50.1	11.4	7
Chocolate Au Lait, Options, Ovaltine*	1 Sachet/10g	36	1	355	11.8	54.5	10	7.3
Cocoa, Lidl*	1 Serving/20g	77	1.2	386	6.1	74.1	6.2	0
Dairy Fudge, Highlights, Dry Weight, Cadbury*	1 Serving/11g	38	1.2	347	16	41	11	9.7
Dairy Fudge, Highlights, Made Up, Cadbury*	1 Serving/200ml	40	1	20	1	2.7	0.5	0.2
Dark, Bournville, Highlights, Made Up, Cadbury*	1 Serving/200ml	35	0.9	18	1.2	2	0.4	0
Dreamy Caramel, Options, Ovaltine*	1 Sachet/11g	39	0.9	354	12.3	48.5	7.8	0
Drink, Organic, Green & Black's*	1 Tsp/5g	20	0.4	395	8.6	67	7.5	12
Fairtrade, Whittards of Chelsea*	4 Tsp/20g	68	0.8	342	7.8	69	3.9	10.9
From Coffee Shop, Waitrose*	1 Serving/298ml	217	5.9	73	3.6	10.9	2	0
Galaxy, Mars*	1 Sachet/25g	97	1.9	386	4.8	71.9	7.7	4.7
Highlights, Instant, Made Up, Cadbury*	1 Cup/200ml	40	1.4	20	1	2.5	0.7	0.3
Instant Break, Cadbury*	1 Sachet/28g	119	3.9	425	10.9	64.2	14	0
Instant, Highlights, Cadbury*	1 Sachet/22g	80	2.8	364	17.3	44.6	12.7	0
Instant, Tesco*	1 Serving/30g	120	2.5	401	7.1	71.6	8.4	5.4
Low Calorie, Dry Weight, As Sold, Average	*1 Sachet/11g*	*41*	*1.2*	*374*	*14.6*	*50*	*10.7*	*11.1*
Luxury, Skinny, Whittards of Chelsea*	1 Serving/28g	92	0.8	328	12.9	67.1	2.8	13.5
Made Up, Tassimo, Suchard*	1 Serving/280ml	88	2.4	31	0.3	5.5	0.9	0.2
Maltesers, Malt Drink, Instant, Made Up, Mars*	1 Serving/220ml	104	3	47	0.9	7.7	1.4	0
Mint Madness, Belgian, Options, Ovaltine*	1 Sachet/11g	38	0.8	348	12.3	49.2	6.9	20
Mint, Highlights, Cadbury*	1 Serving/200ml	40	1.4	20	1	2.5	0.7	0
Outrageous Orange, Options, Ovaltine*	1 Serving/11g	38	0.8	348	12.3	49.3	6.9	20
San Cristobal, Cafe Direct*	1 Serving/40g	158	3.4	396	8.9	65	8.4	0
Tempting Toffee, Options, Ovaltine*	1 Sachet/11g	43	1	391	13.6	66.4	9.1	0
Velvet, Cadbury*	1 Serving/28g	136	6.9	487	8.6	57.8	24.6	2
Wicked White, Options, Ovaltine*	1 Sachet/11g	44	1.1	398	10.5	64.6	10	3.7
Wispa, Hot Frothy, Cadbury*	1 Sachet/27g	107	1.4	395	11	74	5.3	2.9
HOT DOG								
Plain, From Restaurant, Average	*1 Sandwich/98g*	*242*	*14.5*	*247*	*10.6*	*18.4*	*14.8*	*0*
Sausage, American Style, Average	*1 Sausage/75g*	*180*	*14.3*	*241*	*11.6*	*6.2*	*19*	*0*
Sausage, Average	*1 Sausage/23g*	*40*	*3*	*175*	*10.8*	*4.3*	*12.8*	*0.3*
Vegetarian, Meat Free, Sainsbury's*	1 Sausage/30g	72	5.1	240	17.4	3.8	16.8	2
Vegetarian, Tesco*	1 Sausage/30g	66	4.7	222	17.1	1.6	15.8	2.2
HOT POT								
Beef, Classic, 800g, Asda*	1 Serving/400g	400	20.8	100	5.7	7.1	5.2	1.2
Beef, Healthy Options, Birds Eye*	1 Pack/350g	294	7	84	4.5	12	2	1.2
Beef, Minced, & Vegetable, COU, M&S*	1 Pack/400g	380	6.8	95	10.3	9	1.7	2.4
Beef, Minced, Bisto*	1 Pack/375g	363	13.5	97	4.1	11.3	3.6	1.4
Beef, Minced, Classic, Asda*	1 Pack/400g	424	18.4	106	6.8	8.7	4.6	1.1

H

	Measure INFO/WEIGHT	per Measure KCAL	FAT	Nutrition Values per 100g / 100ml KCAL	PROT	CARB	FAT	FIBRE
HOT POT								
Beef, Minced, Frozen, Tesco*	1 Pack/360g	377	10.1	105	5.2	11.7	2.8	1.6
Beef, Minced, HFC, Tesco*	1 Pack/362g	347	10	96	5.2	11.7	2.8	1.6
Beef, Minced, Iceland*	1 Pack/500g	500	20	100	2.8	12.1	4	1.8
Beef, Minced, Sainsbury's*	1 Pack/450g	464	22.1	103	5.3	9.5	4.9	2.2
Beef, Ross*	1 Pack/310g	255	11.2	82	2.2	9.4	3.6	1.5
Beef, Weight Watchers*	1 Pack/320g	231	7.7	72	3.6	8.4	2.4	1.6
Chicken & Mushroom, HL, Tesco*	1 Serving/450g	369	6.8	82	6.3	11.8	1.5	0.5
Chicken, Chunky, Weight Watchers*	1 Pack/320g	275	9	86	4.7	10.4	2.8	0.6
Chicken, Co-Op*	1 Pack/340g	289	10.2	85	6	9	3	0.7
Chicken, GFY, Asda*	1 Serving/400g	256	5.2	64	4.8	8.2	1.3	1.4
Chicken, Good Choice, Iceland*	1 Pack/400g	276	5.2	69	5	9.3	1.3	1
Chicken, LC, Tesco*	1 Pack/361g	250	4.6	70	5.1	9.1	1.3	1.5
Chicken, LC, Tesco*	1 Pack/363g	272	5.4	75	4.9	8.7	1.5	1.4
Chicken, Sainsbury's*	1 Pack/400g	340	11	85	5.2	9.8	2.8	1.3
Chicken, Weight Watchers*	1 Pack/320g	296	6.7	93	6.3	11.8	2.1	1.1
Corned Beef, 876, Oakhouse Foods Ltd*	1 Serving/340g	370	13.6	109	6	13.1	4	0.8
Lamb, & Vegetable, Asda*	1 Pot/500g	240	2	48	4	7	0.4	0
Lamb, Vegetable, Sliced, 035, Wiltshire Farm Foods*	1 Meal/179g	234	12.4	131	7	9.9	6.9	0
Lamb, British, Little Dish*	1 Pack/200g	206	7	103	5.1	11.8	3.5	2.1
Lamb, Classic, CBY, Asda*	1 Pack/399g	323	13.6	81	3.9	8.1	3.4	1.2
Lamb, Cumbrian, Look What We Found*	1 Pack/300g	276	5.4	92	8.9	10.1	1.8	3
Lamb, Diet Chef Ltd*	1 Pack/300g	276	5.4	92	8.9	10.1	1.8	3
Lamb, Keema, Microwaved, Mumbai Street Food, Iceland*	1 Meal/231g	296	15.5	128	5.6	9.6	6.7	3
Lamb, Minced, & Vegetable, COU, M&S*	1 Pack/400g	340	10.8	85	5.7	12.5	2.7	1.8
Lamb, Minced, Classic Kitchen, Tesco*	1 Pack/434g	389	10.8	90	5.2	11	2.5	1.3
Lamb, Minced, Morrison*	1 Pack/400g	376	11.6	94	4.1	11.7	2.9	2.2
Lamb, Minced, New Zealand, Sainsbury's*	1 Pack/450g	580	30.2	129	7.3	8.2	6.7	3.6
Lamb, Mini, Classics, Asda*	1 Pack/300g	223	10.5	74	5.3	5.4	3.5	3.3
Lamb, Organic, Great Stuff, Asda*	1 Pack/300g	327	10.2	109	8	11.6	3.4	1.1
Lamb, Shank, Extra Special, Asda*	1 Pack/450g	508	20.2	113	10.2	7.8	4.5	1.3
Lancashire, 305, Oakhouse Foods Ltd*	1 Serving/400g	344	14	86	5.6	7.4	3.5	1.1
Lancashire, Asda*	1 Pack/401g	269	5.2	67	3.8	10	1.3	0.9
Lancashire, M&S*	1 Pack/450g	441	13.5	98	8.4	8.8	3	1.3
Lancashire, Tesco*	½ Pack/225g	205	7	91	6	9.7	3.1	0.5
Lancashire, with Sliced Potatoes, Cooked, Aldi*	1 Pot/450g	460	17	108	7.3	9.3	4	2.7
Liver & Bacon, Tesco*	1 Pack/550g	693	31.4	126	6.4	12.3	5.7	1.5
Potato, Slim Save*	1 Pack/40g	147	2.2	368	36	26.6	5.5	11.3
Sausage, Aunt Bessie's*	¼ Pack/200g	212	9.2	106	3.6	12.6	4.6	1.9
Sausage, Smart Price, Asda*	1 Pack/300g	239	7	80	3.7	11	2.3	0.4
Sausage, with Baked Beans, Heinz*	1 Can/340g	354	10.9	104	4.6	14.3	3.2	2.4
Vegetable, Ready Meal, Average	**1 Serving/400g**	**261**	**7.4**	**65**	**1.9**	**10.7**	**1.9**	**1.9**
Vegetable, Weight Watchers*	1 Pack/335g	228	6.4	68	2.6	9.9	1.9	1.5
Vegetarian, Quorn*	1 Pack/400g	252	8	63	3.3	8	2	1.9
Vegetarian, Sausage & Vegetable, Linda McCartney*	1 Pot/400g	516	20.4	129	6.4	15.7	5.1	2.3
HOUMOUS								
Avocado, Fresh, San Amvrosia*	1 Serving/50g	172	16	344	5.4	8.5	32.1	2.5
Beetroot, Cannellini Bean, Mint, HL, Tesco*	¼ Tub/45g	82	5.1	183	5.9	11.2	11.3	6.5
Beetroot, Roasted, Mint, Sainsbury's*	¼ Pot/50g	130	10.2	261	5.8	11.5	20.3	4.9
Chilli, Smoked, Harissa, Moorish*	1 Pot/150g	432	34	288	7.2	11.9	22.7	3.5
Classic, Sainsburys*	¼ Pot/58g	161	12.8	278	6.7	10.6	22	5.3
Discover The Choice*	¼ Pot/43g	143	11.9	337	7.1	12	28	3.9
Jalapeno, Pepper, Hot Spicy, Tesco*	¼ Pot/46g	104	6.8	227	8.1	12.8	14.9	4.8
Jalapeno, Tesco*	½ Pot/100g	360	31.1	360	7.5	11.4	31.1	3.9

H

	Measure INFO/WEIGHT	per Measure KCAL	FAT	Nutrition Values per 100g / 100ml KCAL	PROT	CARB	FAT	FIBRE
HOUMOUS								
Lemon & Coriander, Sainsbury's*	¼ Tub/50g	146	12.6	291	7	9.1	25.1	6
Lemon Coriander, GFY, Asda*	1 Serving/50g	130	9.9	259	8.3	12	19.8	5.1
Lemon Coriander, M&S*	½ Pack/100g	296	24.5	296	6.5	9.1	24.5	6.3
Lemon Coriander, Tesco*	¼ Pot/46g	116	8.9	253	6.8	9.9	19.4	5.7
Moroccan, Chunky, Layered, M&S*	1 Serving/30g	66	4.7	219	5.7	9.2	15.7	9.1
Moroccan, Inspired, Finest, Tesco*	¼ Pot/43g	130	10.7	305	5.3	12	25.1	4.7
Moroccan, Sainsbury's*	¼ Pot/50g	114	8.3	229	6	11.1	16.6	5.5
Moroccan, with Coriander & Spices, Tesco*	¼ Pot/50g	131	9.9	262	9.4	11.6	19.8	5.2
Onion, Caramelised, Tesco*	¼ Pack/46g	118	8.9	256	5.2	12.4	19.4	5.8
Onion, Caramelised, The Deli, Aldi*	½ Pack/42g	94	5.9	224	7.4	15	14	4.1
Red Pepper, & Chilli, Chargrilled, 30% Less Fat, Asda*	1 Serving/50g	116	8.2	233	7.5	11.5	16.4	4.9
Red Pepper, Meadow Fresh, Lidl*	1 Serving/50g	158	12.9	307	7.1	11	25	5
Red Pepper, Reduced Fat, Tesco*	1 Serving/20g	44	2.9	220	7.7	11.9	14.4	5.7
Red Pepper, Roasted, Sainsbury's*	½ Pot/100g	317	27.2	317	6.2	9	27.2	5.7
Reduced Fat, Average	**1 Tbsp/30g**	**72**	**5**	**241**	**9.2**	**13.3**	**16.8**	**3.6**
Reduced Fat, with Crunchy Carrot Sticks, M&S*	1 Pack/130g	157	9.9	121	3.3	7.8	7.6	3.9
Smoked, Moorish*	1 Pack/150g	448	36.3	299	7.1	11.5	24.2	3.4
Sweet Chilli, Morrisons*	1 Serving/20g	58	4.1	290	7.1	17.5	20.3	4.3
Sweet Chilli, Sainsbury's*	¼ Pot/50g	151	11.8	302	5.8	14.1	23.6	4.8
Sweet Chilli, Tesco*	¼ Pot/46g	106	6.8	231	7.1	15	14.7	5.2
HULA HOOPS								
Beef Puft, Hula Hoops*	1 Pack/15g	72	3	478	9	64	20	4
Beef, 55% Less Saturated Fat, KP Snacks*	1 Pack/34g	172	9	505	3.7	61.8	26.4	2.2
Beef, Big Hoops, Hula Hoops*	1 Pack/50g	250	12	499	3.8	65	24	2.8
Cheese Onion 55% Less Saturated Fat, KP Snacks*	1 Bag/34g	175	9.7	515	3.6	61	28.5	1.9
Cheese, Puft, KP Snacks*	1 Pack/28g	132	5.6	471	8.8	61	20	4.1
Original, 55% Less Saturated Fat, KP Snacks*	1 Bag/34g	172	8.8	507	3.3	63	26	2.2
Ready Salted, Puft, KP Snacks*	1 Pack/15g	72	3.2	482	8.3	64	21	4
Salt Vinegar, 50% Less Saturated Fat, KP Snacks*	1 Pack/25g	128	7	510	3.1	60.9	28.2	1.8
Salt Vinegar, Puft, KP Snacks*	1 Pack/15g	72	3	478	8.1	63	20	3.9

H

ICE CREAM

	Measure INFO/WEIGHT	per Measure KCAL	FAT	Nutrition Values per 100g / 100ml KCAL	PROT	CARB	FAT	FIBRE
Praline, Carte d'Or*	1 Serving/100g	225	11	225	4	27	11	0
After Dinner, Mint, Dairy, Asda*	1 Serving/100g	182	8	182	3.4	24	8	0.4
Baked Alaska, Ben & Jerry's*	1 Serving/100g	260	15	260	4	29	15	0.1
Bananas Foster, Haagen-Dazs*	1 Serving/125ml	260	15	208	3.2	22.4	12	0
Banoffee Fudge, Sainsbury's*	1/8 Pot/67g	119	4	178	2.8	28.7	5.9	0.2
Banoffee, Haagen-Dazs*	1 Serving/120ml	274	15.6	228	4	23	13	0
Bar, Belgian Chocolate Vanilla, Giant, M&S*	1 Bar/120g	384	26.3	320	3.5	27.7	21.9	0.1
Belgian Chocolate, Haagen-Dazs*	1 Sm Tub/78g	249	16.2	318	4.6	28.4	20.7	0
Belgian Milk Chocolate, Tesco*	1 Lolly/75g	241	15.4	321	3	31.2	20.5	0
Berry Neighbourly, Ben & Jerry's*	1 Scoop/44g	123	7	279	3.5	29	16	0
Birthday Cake, High Protein, Halo Top*	1 Scoop/50g	30	1	59	4	12	2	2.5
Black Treacle, Northern Bloc*	1 Sm Tub/120ml	149	5.2	124	2.9	19.6	4.3	0
Blondie Brownie, Ben & Jerry's*	1 Scoop/43g	109	6	253	4.2	29	14	0
Bluberries, Cream, Haagen-Dazs*	1 Scoop/43g	105	6.9	245	4	20.7	16.1	0.5
Blueberries & Cream, Minicup, Haagen-Dazs*	1 Minicup/87g	212	14	244	4.1	20.3	16.1	0.5
Blueberry, Gelateria, Carte d'Or*	2 Scoops/56g	110	4.1	190	28	31	7	0
Bob Marleys One Love, Ben & Jerry's*	1 Scoop/45g	123	6.3	273	3.2	33	14	0
Bounty, Mini Bar, Mars*	1 Bar/25ml	72	4.8	288	4.5	24.8	19	1
Caffe Latte, The Best, Morrisons*	1/5 Tub/100ml	144	6.6	144	2.9	18	6.6	0.4
Candy Bar, Halo Top*	¼ Tub/118g	90	3.7	76	4.3	14	3.1	2.3
Cappuccino, Tesco*	1 Scoop/54g	121	4.5	224	2.3	34.8	8.3	0.2
Cappuccino, Thorntons*	1oz/28g	61	3.6	218	4.4	20.7	12.9	0
Caramel Biscuit & Cream, Minicup, Haagen-Dazs*	1 Minicup/87g	249	16.1	286	4.6	25.5	18.4	0.1
Caramel Chew Chew, Classic Mix, Minicup, Ben & Jerry's*	1 Minicup/100g	271	15	271	3.6	30	15	0
Caramel Craze, Organic, Tesco*	1 Serving/100g	253	15.3	253	3.3	25.5	15.3	0
Caramel Sensation, Baileys*	1 Ice Cream/73g	262	16.8	359	3.2	34	23	0
Caramel, Chew Chew, Ben & Jerry's*	1 Scoop/45g	122	6.8	270	3.5	28	15	0
Caramel, Cookie Fix, Moophoria, Ben & Jerry's*	2 Scoops/61g	128	4.3	210	3.5	33	7	0
Caramel, Pecan, Jude's*	1 Scoop/50g	90	5.2	180	3	18.6	10.3	0
Caramel, with Caramel Pieces, Carte d'Or*	1 Serving/100g	230	7.4	230	2.9	38	7.4	0
Caramella, Sundae, Tesco*	1 Sundae/80g	165	5.5	205	2.2	32.9	6.8	1.9
Caramella, Tesco*	1 Serving/51g	120	5.5	235	2.6	32	10.7	1.1
Cheeky Choc, Brownie, Skinny Cow*	1 Tub/500ml	590	5.5	118	3	23.9	1.1	4.1
Cheesecake Brownie, Ben & Jerry's*	1 Serving 100g	260	16	260	4	26	16	0
Cheesecake, Strawberry, Haagen-Dazs*	2 Scoops/86g	226	12.3	262	3.8	29.4	14.3	0.4
Choc Chip, Cookie Dough, Haagen-Dazs*	1oz/28g	74	4.7	266	3.8	24.9	16.9	0
Choc Choc Chip, Minicup, Haagen-Dazs*	1 Minicup/87g	245	15.9	281	4.5	24.3	18.2	0.9
Chocolate & Orange, Organic, Green & Black's*	1 Serving/100g	248	14.1	248	5	25.3	14.1	0.1
Chocolate Brownie with Walnuts, Haagen-Dazs*	1 Cup/101g	223	16.4	221	4.4	21	16.2	0
Chocolate Brownie, Salted Caramel, Kelly's Of Cornwall*	1 Serving/125ml	161	7.3	129	2.1	16.6	5.8	0.8
Chocolate Chip Cookie Dough, Halo Top*	1 Serving/118g	90	3.1	76	3.9	14	2.6	2.5
Chocolate Chip, Baskin Robbins*	1 Serving/75g	170	10	227	4	24	13.3	0
Chocolate Flavour, Average	*1 Serving/70g*	*149*	*7.9*	*212*	*4.1*	*23.7*	*11.3*	*0.6*
Chocolate Flavour, Soft Scoop, Sainsbury's*	1 Serving/70g	122	5.2	174	3.1	23.6	7.5	0.3
Chocolate Honeycomb, Co-Op*	¼ Pot/81g	186	10.5	230	4	26	13	0.3
Chocolate Ripple, PB, Waitrose*	1 Serving/125ml	205	3.1	164	4.8	30.5	2.5	4.1
Chocolate Salted Caramel, Minicup, Haagen-Dazs*	1 Minicup/87g	250	15.2	287	4.3	27.5	17.5	1.4
Chocolate, Caramel, Cookie Dough, Topped, Ben & Jerry's	1 Scoop/45g	137	7.6	305	3.9	33	17	0
Chocolate, Creamy, Breyer's Delights*	1 Serving/100ml	62	1.7	62	3.9	9.3	1.7	0
Chocolate, Dairy Free, Halo Top*	¼ Tub/119g	70	3.1	59	2.3	11	2.6	2.2
Chocolate, Finest, Tesco*	1 Scoop/70g	254	17.7	363	4.4	28.9	25.3	1.1
Chocolate, Fudge, Brownie, Ben & Jerry's*	1 Scoop/42g	102	5.4	245	4.2	29	13	0
Chocolate, Fudge, Brownie, Non-Dairy, Ben & Jerry's*	1 Scoop/40g	88	4.3	222	2.9	26	11	0

ICE CREAM

	Measure INFO/WEIGHT	per Measure KCAL	FAT	Nutrition Values per 100g / 100ml KCAL	PROT	CARB	FAT	FIBRE
Chocolate, Gelatelli, Lidl*	1 Portion/50g	126	6.8	251	3.8	27.3	13.6	2.1
Chocolate, Haagen-Dazs*	1 Serving/120ml	269	18	224	4	19	15	0
Chocolate, Heavenly, Non Dairy, Swedish Glace, Wall's*	1 Serving/100g	206	11	206	3.3	23	11	0
Chocolate, High Protein, Halo Top*	1 Scoop/50g	34	1.2	68	4.2	11	2.3	1.5
Chocolate, Inspiration, Gelateria, Carte d'Or*	1 Serving/100g	210	9	210	3.5	28	9	0
Chocolate, Organic, Green & Black's*	1 Serving/125g	310	17.6	248	5	25.3	14.1	1.1
Chocolate, Organic, M&S*	1oz/28g	71	4.5	255	5	24	16	1.5
Chocolate, Santo Domingo, 1, Waitrose*	1 Serving/66g	220	16.4	333	4.5	22.8	24.8	0.5
Chunky Monkey, Non-Dairy, Ben & Jerry's*	1 Scoop/42g	109	5.8	262	2.4	30	14	0
Cinnamon Oat Cluster, High Protein, Breyer's Delights*	1 Scoop/50g	64	1.6	127	7.5	18	3.1	0
Cinnamon Roll, Tub, Halo Top*	1 Serving/118g	90	3	76	4	15	2.5	2.5
Clotted Cream, Cornish, Kelly's Of Cornwall*	1 Serving/125g	282	18.6	226	2.9	20.1	14.9	0.1
Coconut, Alpro*	1 Serving/100g	167	8.2	167	0.2	16.1	8.2	12.5
Coconut, Carte d'Or*	1 Serving/100ml	125	7.1	125	1.8	14	7.1	0.5
Coconut, Toasted, Dairy Free, Halo Top*	1 Scoop/50g	34	1.8	68	2.2	14	3.5	4.2
Coffee Coffee Chip, Baskin Robbins*	1 Scoop/112g	264	15	236	3.8	25	13.4	0
Coffee Cupcake, High Protein, Breyer's Delights*	1 Scoop/50g	62	1.2	125	7.5	19	2.5	0
Coffee, Finest, Tesco*	¼ Pot/93g	236	14.9	254	4.9	22.5	16	0
Coffee, Haagen-Dazs*	1 Serving/120ml	271	18.4	226	4.1	17.9	15.3	0
Coffee, Waitrose*	¼ Tub/125ml	292	16.4	234	3.6	25.4	13.1	0
Cookie Dough, Ben & Jerry's*	1 Scoop/43g	115	6.4	270	4	30	15	0
Cookie Dough, Classic Mix, Minicup, Ben & Jerry's*	1 Minicup/100g	268	15	268	4	29	15	0
Cookie Dough, S'wich Up, Ben & Jerry's*	1 Scoop/41g	117	6.5	290	4.2	31	16	0
Cookie Dough, Tesco*	1 Serving/125g	301	14.2	241	3.3	31	11.4	0.6
Cookies Cream, Breyer's Delights*	1 Serving/100g	70	1.9	70	3.9	11	1.9	0
Cookies Cream, Haagen-Dazs*	1 Sm Tub/100ml	226	14.7	226	4	19.5	14.7	0
Cream Di Frutta, Noblissima, Lidl*	1 Scoop/50g	89	2.4	178	2.2	29.9	4.7	0
Crunchie, Blast, Cadbury*	1 Lolly/100ml	230	13.9	230	2.8	23.1	13.9	0.1
Dairy Cornish, Tesco*	1 Serving/49g	112	6	228	3.2	24.7	12.3	0.1
Dairy Milk, Orange, Cadbury*	1 Serving/120ml	259	13.9	216	3.5	26	11.6	0
Dairy, Flavoured	*1oz/28g*	*50*	*2.2*	*179*	*3.5*	*24.7*	*8*	*0*
Dark Chocolate, & Almonds, Minicup, Haagen-Dazs*	1 Minicup/87g	252	16.6	289	5	23.1	19	2.6
Dark Chocolate, Lolly, Minis, Multipack, G, Aldi*	1 Lolly/35g	131	8.8	373	3.8	31	25	2.3
Double Chocolate, Nestle*	1 Serving/78g	248	14.3	320	4.8	33.7	18.4	0
Dulce De Leche, Bar, Haagen-Dazs*	1 Bar/105g	370	24	352	3.8	32.3	22.9	0
Dulce De Leche, Minicup, Haagen-Dazs*	1 Minicup/87g	231	13.6	265	4.4	26.7	15.6	0.1
Eton Mess, Gelateria, Carte d'Or*	1 Serving/100g	181	5.8	181	2.2	30	5.8	0
Eton Mess, Kelly's Of Cornwall*	1 Serving/125ml	261	10.1	209	3.1	30.7	8.1	0.4
Exotic, Solero, Wall's*	1 Lolly/68g	98	2.1	144	1.7	27	3.1	0
Fig & Orange Blossom Honey, Waitrose*	1 Serving/100g	219	11.8	219	3.9	24.3	11.8	0.4
Fruit & Fresh Tropical, Carte d'Or*	1 Serving/83g	154	7.1	185	2.5	24.5	8.5	0
Galaxy, Mars*	1 Bar/60ml	203	13.4	339	4.7	29.7	22.4	0
Gelato, Vanilla	*1 Serving/100g*	*162*	*7.2*	*162*	*2.4*	*22.6*	*7.2*	*0.3*
Gingerbread, Specially Selected, Aldi*	1 Scoop/64g	169	8.3	264	4	33	13	0.6
Gingerbread, with Toffee Sauce, Sticky, Kelly's Of Cornwall*	1 Scoop/50g	62	3	123	1.8	15.3	6	0.1
Gold Digger Dynamite, Chokablok*	¼ Tub/125ml	288	14	230	3.2	28.2	11.2	0.9
Greek Yoghurt & Honey, Carte d'Or*	1 Serving/55g	114	4.8	207	2.7	29	8.8	0
Half Baked, Ben & Jerry's*	1 Scoop/41g	107	5.3	262	4.1	32	13	0
Hazelnut Chocolate, Alpro*	1 Serving/100g	177	9.4	177	0.8	17.2	9.4	8.6
Home Sweet Honeycomb, Ben & Jerry's*	1 Scoop/43g	114	6.4	266	3.8	30	15	0
Honeycomb Caramel, Dairy, Sainsbury's*	2 Scoops/76g	180	8	236	3.2	32	10.5	0.6
Honeycomb Harvest, Mackies*	1 Serving/100g	209	10	209	4	25	10	0
Hunky Punky Chocolate, Dairy Free, Booja-Booja*	1 Tub/500ml	685	35	137	3.3	17	7	0

ICE CREAM

	Measure INFO/WEIGHT	per Measure KCAL	FAT	Nutrition Values per 100g / 100ml KCAL	PROT	CARB	FAT	FIBRE
Jam Roly Poly Custard, Aunt Bessie's*	1 Scoop/50g	92	4.1	185	4	23	8.3	0.1
Karamel Sutra, Ben & Jerry's*	1 Scoop/43g	112	6	260	4	27	14	0
Knickerbocker Glory	**1oz/28g**	**31**	**1.4**	**112**	**1.5**	**16.4**	**5**	**0.2**
Kulfi Ice, Almond Pistachio, Tubzee*	1 Stick/62g	102	4.3	165	3.6	21.8	6.9	0.5
Kulfi Ice, Original, Tubzee*	1 Scoop/50g	82	3.4	165	3.6	21.8	6.9	0.5
Lavazza, Carte d'Or*	1 Serving/55g	120	5.4	218	3.5	29	9.9	0
Lemon Cream, Dairy, Sainsbury's*	1 Serving/100g	199	9.3	199	3	25.9	9.3	0.1
Lemon Curd Swirl, Duchy Originals*	¼ Pot/101g	247	14.2	245	3.7	25.8	14.1	0
Lemon Meringue Bar, Heston from Waitrose, Waitrose*	1 Serving/60g	108	2.8	181	1.8	32	4.7	1.5
Lemon Meringue Pie, Aunt Bessie's*	1 Serving/50g	101	4.6	202	3.6	26	9.1	0.1
Lemon Tart, Dessert, Carte d'Or*	1 Dessert/130g	212	9.6	163	1.6	22	7.4	0
Lemon, Haagen-Dazs*	1 Serving/120ml	144	0.2	120	0.3	29.3	0.2	0
Light Chocolate Ices, Co-Op*	1 Ice/62g	121	8.1	195	2	18	13	0.5
Log, Mint Chocolate, Sainsbury's*	1 Serving/51g	100	5.1	197	3	23.8	10	0.2
Luscious Mint Choc Chip, Morrisons*	1 Serving/50g	99	5.2	198	2.9	23.1	10.5	0.7
Lychee Cream & Ginger, Haagen-Dazs*	1 Serving/120ml	258	12.7	215	3.6	26.1	10.6	0
Macadamia Nut, Baskin Robbins*	1 Serving/113g	270	18	239	4.4	22.1	15.9	0.9
Magnum, Chocolate, Hazelnut Praline, Tub, Wall's*	2 Scoops/100g	233	16	233	3	19	16	0
Magnum, Classic, Tub, Wall's*	1 Scoop/50g	108	7	217	2.4	21	14	0
Magnum, White, Tub, Wall's*	1 Scoop/50g	109	6.5	218	2.5	23	13	0
Maltesers, Mars*	1 Scoop/50g	64	3	128	1.4	17	6	0
Mango & Raspberry, Minicup, Haagen-Dazs*	1 Minicup/87g	211	11.5	243	3.3	27.2	13.3	0.6
Mango, 98% Fat Free, Bulla*	1 Serving/70g	94	1.1	134	4.2	25.4	1.6	0
Maple & Walnut, American, Sainsbury's*	1/8 Pot/68g	121	4.9	179	3.1	25.6	7.2	0.2
Marshmallow, Tesco*	1 Scoop/53g	117	4.6	222	2.5	32.9	8.8	0.7
Milk Chocolate, & Chopped Almonds, Minis, Lolly, Aldi*	1 Lolly/38g	144	9.5	380	4.5	34	25	1.1
Milk Chocolate, Minis, Lolly, Multipack, G, Aldi*	1 Lolly/34g	120	7.5	353	3.4	35	22	0.5
Mince Pie, Farmhouse Dairy, TTD, Sainsbury's*	¼ Pot/100g	272	14.9	272	4.5	29.3	14.9	1.3
Mince Pie, Finest, Tesco*	¼ Pack/188g	476	22.1	254	3.9	33	11.8	1.1
Mini Mix, Chocolate Coated, Gelatelli, Lidl*	1 Lolly/36g	123	7.8	342	3.9	32	21.8	1.2
Mini Mix, Sorbet Coated, Gelatelli, Lidl*	1 Lolly/40g	64	2.4	160	1.7	24.7	5.9	0.6
Mini Sticks, Milk Chocolate, Weight Watchers*	1 Mini Stick/45ml	96	5	213	2.7	25.8	11.1	0.7
Mint Chocolate Flavour, Average	**1 Serving/70g**	**129**	**6.3**	**184**	**3**	**22.6**	**9**	**1.2**
Mint Chocolate, Sainsbury's*	1 Serving/71g	137	6.7	192	3.4	23.5	9.4	0.4
Mint Chip, Breyer*	1 Serving/100ml	68	2.1	68	4	10	2.1	0
Mint Choc Chip Soft Scoop, Asda*	1 Serving/46g	86	4.1	189	2.9	24	9	0.3
Mint Chocolate Chip, Baskin Robbins*	1 Scoop/113g	270	16	239	4.4	24.8	14.2	0.9
Mint Chocolate, with Dark Chocolate Pieces, Carte D'or*	2 Scoops/50g	109	5.5	218	2.8	28	11	0
Mint Crunch, Dairy Milk, Cadbury*	1 Serving/60ml	162	13.3	270	3	29	22.2	0
Mint Ripple, Good Choice, Iceland*	1 Scoop/50g	58	1	117	3	21.7	2.1	0.1
Mint, Majestic Luxury, Iceland*	1 Serving/80g	269	14.6	337	3.8	39.3	18.3	1.3
Mint, Viennetta, Wall's*	1 Scoop/50g	125	8	250	2.5	25	16	0
Minter Wonderland, Ben & Jerry's*	1 Scoop/44g	117	7.5	266	4	24	17	0
Mocha Coffee Indulgence, Sainsbury's*	¼ Pot/82g	178	10.6	217	3.2	22.1	12.9	0.1
Monster Mint, Sainsbury's*	1/8 Pot/67g	121	4.6	180	3	26.3	6.9	0.3
My Carte D'or, Chocolate, Carte d'Or*	1 Tub/200ml	220	11	110	1.8	12.5	5.5	0.4
Neapolitan, Average	**1 Serving/70g**	**111**	**4.6**	**158**	**3.1**	**21.9**	**6.5**	**0.6**
Neapolitan, Brick, Tesco*	1 Serving/50g	82	3.4	163	3.3	21.9	6.9	0.4
Neapolitan, Soft Scoop, Sainsbury's*	1 Serving/75g	124	5.2	165	2.8	22.8	6.9	0.2
Neopolitian, Soft Scoop, Tesco*	1 Serving/43g	70	3	163	3.3	21.9	6.9	0.4
Non-Dairy, Reduced Calorie	**1oz/28g**	**33**	**1.7**	**119**	**3.4**	**13.7**	**6**	**0**
Oatmeal, High Protein, Halo Top*	1 Scoop/50ml	30	1	59	4	13	1.9	2.5
Organic, Madagascan Vanilla, Yeo Valley*	1 Serving/40ml	45	2.5	112	2.4	11.4	6.3	0.1

ICE CREAM

Measure INFO/WEIGHT		per Measure		Nutrition Values per 100g / 100ml				
		KCAL	FAT	KCAL	PROT	CARB	FAT	FIBRE
Panna Cotta, & Raspberry Swirl, Haagen-Dazs*	1 Serving/120ml	250	14.9	208	3.2	21	12.4	0
Peanut Butter Crunch, Haagen-Dazs*	2 Scoops/100g	343	24.4	343	8.4	21.7	24.4	1.7
Peanut Butter Cup, Ben & Jerry's*	1 Scoop/43g	138	9	320	7	25	21	0
Peanut Butter Cup, Dairy Free, Halo Top*	1 Scoop/50g	34	1.6	68	2.5	13	3.3	3.9
Peanut Butter, Cookies, Non-Dairy, Ben & Jerry's*	1 Scoop/41g	113	6.5	280	4.3	29	16	0
Peanut Chip, Vegan, Northern Bloc*	1 Sm Tub/120ml	163	5.6	136	3	20.2	4.7	0
Phish Food, Ben & Jerry's*	1 Scoop/43g	116	5.2	270	3.5	36	12	0
Pistachio, Haagen-Dazs*	1 Serving/120ml	276	18.8	230	4.4	17.7	15.7	0
Pistachio, Joe Deluccis Gelato*	1 Scoop/70g	148	6.6	211	2.4	28	9.4	0
Pistachio, Seriously Nutty, Waitrose*	1 fl oz/30ml	48	3.2	161	3.2	12.6	10.8	0.3
Praline, Green & Black's*	1 Sm Pot/100g	191	10.8	191	3.5	20	10.8	0.9
Pralines Cream, Haagen-Dazs*	1 Sm Tub/78g	213	12.9	272	3.9	27.2	16.5	0
Protein, Banoffee, WheyHey*	1 Pot/150ml	149	4.4	99	13.4	7.8	2.9	0
Protein, Chocolate, WheyHey*	1 Pot/150ml	154	4.3	103	14	8	2.9	0
Protein, Chocolate, WheyHey*	1 Scoop/50g	40	1.8	81	7.3	7.6	3.6	0.8
Protein, Salted Caramel, WheyHey*	1 Scoop/50g	38	1.7	76	7.1	7.2	3.4	0.1
Protein, Vanilla, WheyHey*	1 Pot/150ml	149	4.4	99	13.4	7.8	2.9	0
Raspberries, Clotted Cream, Waitrose*	1 Tub/500ml	790	39.5	158	2.9	18.9	7.9	0.1
Raspberry Ripple Brick, Tesco*	1 Serving/48g	71	2.9	148	2.6	20.8	6	0.2
Raspberry Ripple, Average	*1 Serving/70g*	*93*	*3.3*	*134*	*1.9*	*20.8*	*4.7*	*0.1*
Raspberry Ripple, Soft Scoop, Asda*	1 Scoop/46g	78	3.2	170	2.5	24	7	0.3
Raspberry Ripple, Soft Scoop, Tesco*	1 Scoop/25g	39	1.5	157	2.5	23	6.1	0.2
Raspberry, Delightful, Non Dairy, Swedish Glace, Wall's*	1 Serving/100g	211	9.4	211	2.6	29	9.4	0
Raspberry, Easy Serve, Co-Op*	1oz/28g	43	1.7	152	2.5	22.3	5.9	0
Really Creamy Chocolate, Asda*	1 Serving/100g	227	11	227	4.1	28	11	0.4
Really Creamy Toffee, Asda*	1 Serving/120ml	146	6	122	1.8	17.5	5	0.1
Red Berries, Solero, Wall's*	1 Lolly/75g	111	2	148	1.4	29	2.7	0
Red Velvet, Halo Top*	1 Scoop/50g	38	1.2	76	4.2	14	2.5	2.5
Rhubarb Crumble, Aunt Bessie's*	1 Serving/50g	96	4.4	192	3.8	25	8.7	0.2
Rocky Road, M&S*	1 Tub/500g	1475	88.5	295	4.2	29.5	17.7	1.2
Rocky Road, Sainsbury's*	1/8 Pot/67g	137	4.9	205	3.8	30.9	7.3	1
Rum & Raisin, Haagen-Dazs*	1 Serving/120ml	264	17.6	220	3.4	18.6	14.7	0
Rum Raisin, TTD, Sainsbury's*	¼ Pot/100g	220	10.4	220	3.8	27.7	10.4	1
Run Raisin, with West Indies Rum, Carte d'Or*	1 Serving/100g	201	7.5	201	2.6	25	7.5	0
Salted Caramel Cake, High Protein, Breyers Delights*	1 Scoop/50ml	34	0.6	68	4	11	1.3	0
Salted Caramel, Almond, Alpro*	1 Scoop/50g	90	4.4	181	0.8	18.5	8.8	12.3
Salted Caramel, Brownie, Topped, Ben & Jerry's*	1 Scoop/45g	134	8	301	4.2	30	18	0
Salted Caramel, Minicup, Haagen-Dazs*	1 Minicup/87g	246	15	282	4.1	27.8	17.2	0
Salted Caramel, Tesco*	1 Lolly/68g	224	12.4	330	3.6	37.1	18.3	1.2
Salted Caramel, The Best, Morrisons*	1 Serving/100ml	188	11.5	188	2.8	17.9	11.5	0.5
Screwball, Asda*	1 Screwball/60g	122	6	203	3.3	25	10	1.5
Screwball, Farmfoods*	1 Lolly/72ml	127	4.4	177	3.3	27.1	6.1	0
Screwball, Tesco*	1 Screwball/61g	116	5.2	190	2.9	25.2	8.6	0.3
Sea Salt Caramel, Dairy Free, Halo Top*	1 Scoop/50g	34	1.2	68	2.2	14	2.5	4
Smarties Ice Cream Pot, Nestle*	1 Pot/69g	151	5.7	218	4.4	33.6	8.2	0
Smarties, Nestle*	1 Serving/50g	125	6	250	3.6	32.3	11.9	0.2
Sofa So Good , Ben & Jerry's*	1 Scoop/43g	110	5.5	259	4	31	13	0
Spagnola, Carte d'Or*	1 Serving/100g	187	5.7	187	2	32	5.7	0
Speculoos? Specu-Love, Ben & Jerry's*	1 Scoop/42g	129	8.3	310	3.8	28	20	0
Spice All Things N'ice, Ben & Jerry's*	1 Scoop/50g	116	9	233	3.9	27	18	0
Stem Ginger with Belgian Chocolate, Waitrose*	1 Lolly/110g	255	14.4	232	2.9	25.5	13.1	1.7
Sticky Toffee, Cream O' Galloway*	1 Serving/30g	80	4.4	266	4.7	28.7	14.7	0
Strawberries & Cream, Minicup, Haagen-Dazs*	1 Minicup/87g	211	13.5	243	3.9	21.8	15.5	0.3

ICE CREAM

INFO/WEIGHT	KCAL	FAT	KCAL	PROT	CARB	FAT	FIBRE
Strawberries Cream, Haagen-Dazs*	1 Scoop/50g	122	7.8	244	3.9	22.2	15.5	0.3
Strawberry & Cream, Mivvi, Nestle*	1 Serving/60g	118	4.6	196	2.6	29.4	7.6	0.2
Strawberry Cheesecake, Ben & Jerry's*	1 Serving 100g	240	14	240	3	27	14	0
Strawberry Cheesecake, Co-Op*	1/6 Pot/86g	163	6	190	3	29	7	0.2
Strawberry, Yuzu, Vegan, Northern Bloc*	1 Sm Tub/120ml	103	0	86	0	21.5	0	0
Strawberry, Carte d'Or*	1 Scoop/50g	46	1.4	91	1.4	15	2.9	0
Strawberry, Iced Dessert, Free From, Sainsbury's*	1 Serving/67g	106	6.3	159	1.7	16.4	9.5	0.5
Strawberry, Soft Scoop, Tesco*	1 Serving/46g	78	3.4	170	2.8	23.1	7.4	0.1
Summer Berries & Cream, Minicup, Haagen-Dazs*	1 Minicup/88g	225	14.1	255	3	24.4	16	0.8
Taste of Carrot Cake, Iced Dessert, Perfect World*	1 Tub/120ml	170	12	142	3.1	14	10	2.6
Taste Sensation, Mascarpone Forest Fruits, Aldi*	1 Pot/73g	159	7.4	217	1.8	29.6	10.1	0.6
Tiramisu, Haagen-Dazs*	1 Serving/120ml	303	19.6	253	3.8	22.7	16.3	0
Toffee & Biscuit, Weight Watchers*	1 Pot/100ml	93	2.7	93	1.5	14.9	2.7	0.1
Toffee Honeycomb Sundaes, Weight Watchers*	1 Pot/98g	119	1.8	122	1.7	18.1	1.8	5.9
Toffee Vanilla, Sainsbury's*	1 Serving/71g	146	6.8	205	3.1	26.7	9.5	0.1
Toffee Fudge, Soft Scoop, Asda*	1 Serving/50g	92	3.5	185	2.6	28	7	0
Toffee Vanilla, HE, Tesco*	1 Serving/73g	106	1.8	145	2.5	28.1	2.5	0.5
Triple Chocolate, Brownie, Skinny Cow*	1 Ice Cream/65g	93	1.7	144	3.5	24.1	2.6	5.3
Triple Chocolate, Carte d'Or*	1 Serving/58g	122	5.7	210	3.7	27	9.8	0
Triple Chocolate, Dairy, Morrisons*	1 Serving/100g	233	10.8	233	3.8	30	10.8	0.4
Vanilla & Cinnamon, Finest, Tesco*	1 Serving/50g	114	7.4	229	3.9	20.2	14.7	0.4
Vanilla & Cinnamon, Spar*	1 Serving/120g	247	10.3	206	3.8	28	8.6	0
Vanilla Caramel, Tesco*	1 Scoop/53g	117	4.4	222	2.4	34.5	8.3	0.1
Vanilla Bean, Light, Deluxe, Lidl*	1 Serving/64g	110	2.5	172	4.7	26.6	3.9	0
Vanilla Bean, Purbeck*	1 Serving/100g	198	11.5	198	4.8	18.7	11.5	0
Vanilla Caramel Brownie, Haagen-Dazs*	1 Serving/150g	410	24.8	273	4.5	26.8	16.5	0
Vanilla Caramel Brownie, Minicup, Haagen-Dazs*	1 Minicup/83g	228	13.7	275	4.4	26.9	16.5	0.4
Vanilla Chocolate, Taste Sensation, Frosty's, Aldi*	1 Pot/73g	164	7	224	2.1	32.4	9.6	0.7
Vanilla Flavour, Soft Scoop, Sainsbury's*	1 Serving/71g	96	3.9	136	2.9	18.8	5.5	0.2
Vanilla Florentine, Specially Selected, Aldi*	1 Scoop/62g	148	7.4	238	4.4	28	12	0.7
Vanilla with Strawberry Swirl, Mini Tub, Weight Watchers*	1 Mini Tub/57g	81	2.2	142	2.5	23.4	3.9	0.2
Vanilla, Chocolate Sauce, Organic, Green & Black's*	1 Serving/71g	170	9.8	240	4.3	24.6	13.9	0.6
Vanilla, Chocolate, Cone, Ms Mollys*	1 Cone/61g	169	7.1	278	3.2	39.7	11.6	0.7
Vanilla, Chocolate, Viennetta, Wall's*	1 Serving/100ml	125	7	250	2.5	27	14	0
Vanilla, Alpro*	1 Serving/100g	166	8	166	2.3	16.4	8	9.8
Vanilla, Ben & Jerry's*	1 Mini Tub/112g	258	16.8	230	4	20	15	0.1
Vanilla, Dairy Milk, Cadbury*	1 Serving/120g	259	13.9	216	3.5	26	11.6	0.1
Vanilla, Dairy, Average	*1 Scoop/40g*	*80*	*4.4*	*201*	*3.5*	*23.6*	*11*	*0.7*
Vanilla, Dairy, Finest, Tesco*	1 Serving/92g	227	16	247	4.5	18	17.4	0.3
Vanilla, Dairy, Organic, Yeo Valley*	1 Serving/100g	206	11.2	206	4.9	21.3	11.2	0
Vanilla, Haagen-Dazs*	1oz/28g	70	4.8	250	4.5	19.7	17.1	0
Vanilla, Light, Soft Scoop, Wall's*	1 Serving/100g	139	5.9	139	3	17	5.9	0
Vanilla, Low Fat, Average	*1 Scoop/50g*	*59*	*1.7*	*118*	*2.3*	*19.4*	*3.4*	*0.6*
Vanilla, Low Fat, Weight Watchers*	1 Scoop/125ml	75	2.1	60	1.1	9.7	1.7	0.1
Vanilla, Mackies*	1 Serving/100g	193	11	193	4	18	11	0
Vanilla, Madagascan, Carte d'Or*	1 Serving/100g	197	7.4	197	2.6	30	7.4	0
Vanilla, Madagascan, Light, 4.5% Fat, Carte d'Or*	1 Serving/100g	140	4.5	140	2.1	21	4.5	4
Vanilla, Made with Madagascan Vanilla, Sainsbury's*	1 Serving/56g	101	4	181	3	25.6	7.2	0.6
Vanilla, Ms Mollys*	1 Scoop/40g	58	1.9	146	2.5	23.1	4.7	0.6
Vanilla, Non-Dairy, Average	*1 Serving/60g*	*107*	*5.2*	*178*	*3.2*	*23.1*	*8.7*	*0*
Vanilla, Really Creamy, Asda*	1 Serving/50g	98	5	196	3.5	23	10	0.1
Vanilla, Smart Price, Asda*	1 Scoop/40g	55	2.4	137	2.8	19	6	0.2
Vanilla, Smooth, Soy, Non Dairy, Swedish Glace, Wall's*	1 Scoop/50g	46	1.6	91	0.5	15	3.1	0

ICE CREAM

INFO/WEIGHT	Measure	per Measure KCAL	FAT	Nutrition Values per 100g / 100ml KCAL	PROT	CARB	FAT	FIBRE
Vanilla, Soft Scoop, Tesco*	1 Serving/45g	69	2.3	153	2.5	23.6	5.2	0.7
Vanilla, Soft Scoop, Wall's*	1 Serving/100g	187	9.1	187	3	23	9.1	0
Vanilla, Toffee Crunch, Ben & Jerry's*	1 Tub/407g	1099	65.1	270	4	29	16	0.5
Vanilla, Vanilla Collection, Minicup, Haagen-Dazs*	1 Minicup/87g	217	14.7	249	4.3	19.9	16.9	0
Vanilla, Waitrose*	1 Serving/100ml	156	10.8	156	2.6	12	10.8	0
Venezuelan Chocolate, Truly Irresistible, Co-Op*	1 Serving/100g	329	21	329	4.5	30	21	0.5
White Chocolate, Minis, Lolly, Multipack, G, Aldi*	1 Lolly/35g	128	8.4	366	3.2	34	24	0.5
with Cherry Sauce, Tesco*	1 Scoop/56g	114	4.1	204	2.1	32.4	7.3	0.2

ICE CREAM BAR

INFO/WEIGHT	Measure	per Measure KCAL	FAT	Nutrition Values per 100g / 100ml KCAL	PROT	CARB	FAT	FIBRE
Bailey's, Haagen-Dazs*	1oz/28g	86	5.9	307	4.1	24.8	21.2	0
Bounty, 100 Ml Bar, Mars*	1 Bar/100ml	278	18.5	278	3.4	24.7	18.5	0.7
Chocolate Covered	***1 Bar/40g***	***128***	***9.3***	***320***	***5***	***24***	***23.3***	***0***
Crunchie, Cadbury*	1 Bar/60ml	165	9.7	275	3	29.5	16.2	0.5
Dairy Milk, Caramel, Cadbury*	1 Bar/60ml	175	10.3	290	3.6	30.2	17.1	0
Dairy Milk, Fruit Nut, Cadbury*	1 Bar/90ml	243	15.3	270	3.5	26.1	17	0
Dairy Milk, Lolly, Cadbury*	1 Lolly/100g	235	15	235	3	25.1	15	0
Dream, Cadbury*	1 Serving/118g	260	14	220	3.6	26	11.9	0
Galaxy, Mars*	1 Bar/54g	184	12.2	341	3.8	30.7	22.5	0.6
Lion, Nestle*	1 Bar/45g	166	9.9	370	4.2	39.1	21.9	1
Maltesers, Mars*	1 Bar/45ml	113	7	252	2.9	25	15.6	0.7
Snickers, Mars*	1 Bar/53ml	179	10.4	337	6.5	33.2	19.6	0
Twix, Mars*	1 Serving/43ml	128	7.3	301	4	32	17.1	1.2
Yorkie, Nestle*	1 Bar	144	8.7	359	4.8	36.5	21.6	0

ICE CREAM CONE

INFO/WEIGHT	Measure	per Measure KCAL	FAT	Nutrition Values per 100g / 100ml KCAL	PROT	CARB	FAT	FIBRE
Average	***1 Cone/75g***	***140***	***6.4***	***186***	***3.5***	***25.5***	***8.5***	***0***
Choc Chip with Hazelnut, Flirt, Cornetto, Wall's*	1 Cone/70g	223	11.2	320	4	40	16	0
Chocolate & Nut, Co-Op*	1 Cone/110g	307	17	279	3.9	31	15.5	0.6
Chocolate & Vanilla, Good Choice, Iceland*	1 Cone/110ml	161	7.2	146	2.7	22.9	6.5	0.8
Chocolate & Vanilla, M&S*	1oz/28g	83	4.8	295	4.2	31.8	17	0.7
Chocolate Fudge, Gooey, Extreme, Nestle*	1 Cone/73g	218	10.4	299	3.8	37.4	14.3	2.5
Chocolate, Caramel, Crunch, Cornetto, Wall's*	1 Cornetto/75g	247	15	329	3.6	34	20	0
Chocolate, M&S*	1oz/28g	94	6.4	335	4	28	23	2.3
Chocolate, Mini, Cornetto, Wall's*	1 Cone/36g	110	5.9	300	3.5	34	16	2
Chocolate, Vanilla & Hazelnut, Sainsbury's*	1 Cone/62g	190	10.5	306	4.5	33.9	16.9	0.6
Cookies Cream, Tesco*	1 Cone/71g	197	7.9	277	3.9	39.8	11.1	1.4
Cornet, Wafer Cone, Askeys*	1 Cone/4g	13	0.1	376	10.7	77.6	2.5	0
Cornetto, GFY, Asda*	1 Cone/67g	162	6	241	3	37	9	0.1
Cornetto, Wall's*	1 Cone/75g	195	9.7	260	3.7	34.5	12.9	0
Cup Cornet, Wafer Cone, Askeys*	1 Cone/4g	13	0.1	376	10.7	77.6	2.5	0
Dairy Milk Buttons, Cadbury*	1 Cone/100ml	204	10.4	204	0	24.6	10.4	0.6
Extreme Raspberry, Cornetto, Nestle*	1 Cone/76g	177	6.2	233	2.4	36.4	8.2	1.5
Flake 99, Cadbury*	1 Cone/125ml	238	12	190	2.6	23.1	9.6	0.5
Mint Choc Chip, Iceland*	1 Cone/72g	210	9.4	292	3.3	40.4	13	1
Mint, Cornetto, Wall's*	1 Cornetto/60g	169	8.4	282	3.4	37	14	0
Peanut Butter, Giannis, Aldi*	1 Cone/72g	230	11.5	320	4.7	39	16	1.6
Peanut Butter, Love, Cornetto, Wall's*	1 Cornetto/75g	245	15	326	3.3	33	20	0
Salted Butter Caramel, Gelatelli*	1 Cone/76g	216	8.1	284	3.6	43.4	10.6	0
Salted Caramel, White Chocolate, Extreme, Nestle*	1 Cone/73g	209	9.3	286	3.3	39.3	12.7	0.8
Strawberry & Vanilla, Iceland*	1 Serving/70g	182	7.6	260	3.3	37.5	10.8	0.7
Strawberry & Vanilla, Tesco*	1 Cone/69g	181	7	262	3.3	39	10.1	0.8
Strawberry, Cornetto, Wall's*	1 Cornetto/75g	198	8.2	264	2.1	40	11	0
Toffee Vanilla, Giannis, Aldi*	1 Cone/71g	195	7.1	275	4.5	42	10	0.6
Toffee, Vanilla, Free From, Tesco*	1 Cone/65g	185	8.9	285	2.1	38	13.7	0.6

	Measure INFO/WEIGHT	per Measure KCAL	FAT	Nutrition Values per 100g / 100ml KCAL	PROT	CARB	FAT	FIBRE
ICE CREAM CONE								
Vanilla, & Strawberry Sauce, Dairy Free, Swedish Glace*	1 Cone/105g	207	8.2	197	1.3	30	7.8	0
Vanilla, Chocolate, Classico, Cornetto, Wall's*	1 Cornetto/75g	233	12.7	311	3.3	36	17	0
ICE CREAM ROLL								
Arctic, Average	*1 Serving/70g*	*140*	*4.6*	*200*	*4.1*	*33.3*	*6.6*	*0*
ICE CREAM SANDWICH								
'Wich, Ben & Jerry's*	1 Pack/117g	398	19.9	340	4	44	17	1
Neapolitan, Gelatelli, Lidl*	1 Sandwich/106g	233	9.5	220	4.9	29	9	1.9
ICE CREAM STICK								
Belgian Milk Chocolate Ices , Waitrose*	1 Bar/62g	208	12.7	338	4	33.5	20.6	1.6
Chocolate, Almond, Tesco*	1 Stick/77g	268	18	348	4.5	29.2	23.4	1.2
Chocolate, Feast, Wall's*	1 Lolly/70g	245	16.1	350	3.6	31	23	0
Chocolate, Milk, Mini, Tesco*	1 Lolly/35g	119	7.7	341	3.1	31.9	22.2	0.9
Chocolate, Mini Milk, Wall's*	1 Lolly/23g	32	0.7	138	4.4	22	3.2	0
Chocolate, White, Tesco*	1 Lolly/75g	255	17.5	341	3.3	29.4	23.4	0
Mint Double Chocolate, Skinny Cow*	1 Stick/110ml	94	1.8	85	2.7	15.1	1.6	2.4
Peanut Butter, Haagen-Dazs*	1 Ice Cream/70g	290	22.1	414	8.4	23.1	31.5	2.3
Speculoos, Caramel Biscuti, Cream, Haagen-Dazs*	1 Bar/70g	258	18.4	369	4.9	28.1	26.3	0.1
Stem Ginger, 1, Waitrose*	1 Ice Cream/79g	287	17.2	364	4.1	37.5	21.8	0.6
Strawberry, Refreshing, Non Dairy, Swedish Glace, Wall's*	1 Lolly/37g	117	7.8	317	2.3	29	21	0
Vanilla, Mini Milk, Wall's*	1 Lolly/23g	30	0.7	130	3.9	22	3.1	0
ICE LOLLY								
Assorted, Iceland*	1 Lolly/51g	33	0	65	0	16.2	0	0
Baby, Tesco*	1 Lolly/32g	26	0	80	0.1	20	0	0.1
Berry Burst, Sainsbury's*	1 Serving/90ml	93	1.6	103	1.1	20.8	1.8	0.7
Blackcurrant Split, Iceland*	1 Lolly/75g	61	2.4	81	1.1	12	3.2	0.1
Blackcurrant, Dairy Split, Sainsbury's*	1 Lolly/73ml	88	2.6	121	1.8	20.4	3.6	0.1
Blackcurrant, Ribena*	1 Lolly/35ml	25	0	68	0	16.4	0	0
Bubblegum, Calippo, Wall's*	1 Calippo/106g	90	0.5	85	0.5	21	0.5	0
Bubblegum, Tesco*	1 Lolly/59g	60	1.1	102	1.8	19.2	1.9	0.6
Cherry Tango, Liquid Ice, Britvic*	1 Lolly/65ml	84	0.1	129	0.1	31	0.1	0.2
Choc & Almond, Mini, Tesco*	1 Lolly/31g	103	7.4	331	4.4	24.8	23.8	0.9
Choc Lime Split, Morrisons*	1 Lolly/73ml	120	6.1	164	1.6	20.4	8.4	0.1
Chocolate Wonderpops, Sainsbury's*	1 Lolly/43g	118	8.3	276	2.6	21.8	19.4	0.7
Chocolate, Plain, Mini, Tesco*	1 Lolly/31g	94	6.6	304	3.1	24.8	21.4	1.2
Chocolate, with Chocolate Coating, Core, Tesco*	1 Lolly/47g	157	10.6	335	3.1	29.2	22.6	1.5
Cider Refresher, Treats*	1 Lolly/70ml	54	0	77	0	19.2	0	0
Coconut, Creamy, Finest, Tesco*	1 Lolly/77g	77	1.6	100	0.4	19.6	2.1	0.6
Cola Lickers, Farmfoods*	1 Lolly/56ml	38	0	68	0	17	0	0
Exotic Fruit, Ice Cream, Gelatelli, Lidl*	1 Lolly/110g	148	2.8	135	1.8	25.6	2.5	0
Exotic Fruit, Mini, HL, Tesco*	1 Lolly/31g	41	0.6	131	1	26.4	2	1
Fab, Nestle*	1 Lolly/58g	82	2.9	142	0.6	23.1	5.1	0.3
Fab, Orange, Nestle*	1 Lolly/58g	81	2.7	140	0.6	24	4.7	0
Fab, Strawberry, Mini, Nestle*	1 Lolly/35ml	47	1.6	133	0.5	22.5	4.6	0.3
Frozen Yoghurt, Mango, Greek Style, Claudi & Fin*	1 Mini Lolly/26g	29	1.3	112	2.7	12.9	5.2	0.5
Fruit Flavour, Assorted, Basics, Sainsbury's*	1 Lolly/50g	33	0	66	0	16.5	0	0
Fruit Fusion, Mini, Farmfoods*	1 Lolly/45ml	36	0	79	0.2	19.2	0.1	0.2
Fruit Ices, Made with Orange Juice, Del Monte*	1 Lolly/75ml	69	0.1	92	1.2	21.5	0.1	0.2
Fruit Luxury, Mini, Co-Op*	1 Lolly/45g	58	2.7	130	2	18	6	0.2
Fruit Pastilles, Rowntree's*	1 Lolly/65ml	61	0	94	0.2	23.2	0	0
Fruit Split, Waitrose*	1 Lolly/73g	91	2.6	124	2.5	21.7	3.6	0.4
Fruit Splits, Treats*	1 Lolly/75ml	77	3.1	103	1.4	17.6	4.1	0
Fruits of the Forest, Ice Cream, Gelatelli, Lidl*	1 Lolly/110g	145	2.8	132	1.9	24.5	2.5	0
Fruity 'n' Freezy, Asda*	1 Lolly/30ml	24	0	80	0.1	20	0	0

ICE LOLLY

INFO/WEIGHT	Measure		Nutrition Values per 100g / 100ml				
	KCAL	FAT	KCAL	PROT	CARB	FAT	FIBRE
ICE LOLLY							
Fruity, Helter Skelter, Tesco* — 1 Lolly/70g	51	0.1	74	0.2	18.1	0.1	0
Ice Burst, Aldi* — 1 Lolly/60g	67	1.1	112	0.5	24	1.8	0.5
Ice Lolly, Twister, Choc, Wall's* — 1 Mini Lolly/27g	40	1.6	150	3.5	22	6	0.9
Icicles, All Flavours, Freezepops, Calypso* — 1 Lolly/50ml	1	0	1	0	0.3	0	0
Kiwi Burst, Pineapple Sorbet in Kiwi Ice, Sainsbury's* — 1 Serving/90ml	76	0.1	84	0.1	20.7	0.1	0.4
Lemon & Lime, Mini Bar, M&S* — 1 Lolly/50g	48	0	95	0.1	23.6	0.1	0.2
Lemon & Lime, Rocket Split, De Roma* — 1 Lolly/60ml	65	2.6	108	1	16	4.3	0.2
Lemon Blackcurrant, Twister, Wall's* — 1 Lolly/71g	68	0.4	96	0.7	21	0.6	0
Lemon Lime, Mini, Calippo, Wall's* — 1 Mini/78g	70	0.4	90	0.5	21	0.5	0
Lemon Lime, Mini, Lemon Core, Twister, Wall's* — 1 Mini/39g	42	0.5	107	0.6	22	1.2	0
Lemon Lime, Mini, Strawberry Core, Twister, Wall's* — 1 Mini/39g	41	0.5	105	0.6	22	1.2	0
Lemon Lime, Twister, Wall's* — 1 Lolly/71g	76	0.9	107	0.5	22	1.2	0
Lemon Sorbet, Mercadona* — 1 Lolly/63g	38	0.2	61	0.5	32.4	0.3	8
Lemonade & Cola, Morrisons* — 1 Lolly/55ml	36	0	65	0	16.2	0	0
Lemonade Flavour, R White* — 1 Lolly/75ml	56	1.1	75	0.5	15.1	1.5	0.1
Lemonade Sparkle, Wall's* — 1 Lolly/55g	40	0	73	0	18.2	0	0
Mango Passion Fruit Bursts, Sainsbury's* — 1 Lolly/89ml	75	0.1	84	0.2	20.4	0.1	0
Mango Passion Fruit Smoothie, Waitrose* — 1 Lolly/73g	60	0.3	82	0.7	18.9	0.4	0.7
Milk, Blue Parrot Cafe, Sainsbury's* — 1 Lolly/30ml	34	1	113	2.7	18	3.3	0.3
Mint Chocolate, Tesco* — 1 Lolly/47g	160	10.9	342	2.7	30	23.2	1.1
Mixed Berry, Helter Skelter, Tesco* — 1 Lolly/75g	77	0.1	104	0.1	25.5	0.1	0.1
Mixed Fruit, Vimto* — 1 Lolly/45ml	39	0.2	87	0.5	20.9	0.5	0.2
Morrisons* — 1 Lolly/100g	30	0	30	0	7.4	0	0
No Added Sugar, Tesco* — 1 Lolly/32g	26	0	80	0.1	20	0	0.1
Nobbly Bobbly, Nestle* — 1 Lolly/70ml	219	11.6	312	2.9	38.1	16.5	0.6
Orange Lemon Splits, Farmfoods* — 1 Lolly/56ml	69	2.4	124	1.6	19.8	4.3	0.2
Orange 'n' Cream, Tropicana* — 1 Lolly/65g	83	2.9	129	1.4	20.5	4.5	0.3
Orange Juice, Co-Op* — 1 Lolly/73g	51	0.1	70	0.4	17	0.1	0.1
Orange Juice, Freshly Squeezed, Finest, Tesco* — 1 Lolly/80ml	89	0	111	0.7	27	0	0
Orange Juice, Freshly Squeezed, Waitrose* — 1 Lolly/73g	88	0.1	120	0.6	29.7	0.1	0
Orange, Average — **1 Lolly/72g**	**66**	**0**	**92**	**0.4**	**22.4**	**0**	**0.1**
Orange, Calippo, Wall's* — 1 Calippo/105g	100	0.5	95	0.5	23	0.5	0
Orange, Lidl* — 1 Lolly/50g	50	0	100	0.5	24.4	0	0
Orange, Mini, Calippo, Wall's* — 1 Mini/79g	75	0.4	95	0.5	23	0.5	0
Pineapple Coconut Colada, Waitrose* — 1 Lolly/73ml	79	1.5	108	1	21	2.1	0.6
Pineapple, Dairy Split, Sainsbury's* — 1 Lolly/72ml	84	2.6	116	1.8	19	3.6	0.1
Pineapple, Fruit Split, Free From, Tesco* — 1 Split/55g	72	2.7	132	0.6	21.1	4.9	0.5
Pineapple, Real Fruit Juice, Sainsbury's* — 1 Lolly/73ml	55	0.1	76	0.1	19	0.1	0.1
Pop Up, CBY, Asda* — 1 Lolly/80ml	65	0	81	0	20.1	0	0.3
Raspberry & Apple, Sainsbury's* — 1 Lolly/57ml	39	0.1	68	0.1	17.1	0.1	0.1
Raspberry, Real Fruit Juice, Sainsbury's* — 1 Lolly/72g	62	0.1	86	0.3	21	0.1	0.1
Raspberry, Smoothie, Iced, Del Monte* — 1 Lolly/90ml	84	0	94	0.3	22.8	0	0.8
Real Fruit Juice, Rocket, Blue Parrot Cafe, Sainsbury's* — 1 Lolly/58ml	45	0	77	0.2	19.1	0	0.1
Real Fruit, Dairy Split, Sainsbury's* — 1 Lolly/73ml	100	3.1	137	2.1	22.8	4.2	0.1
Refresher, Fruit Flavour, Bassett's* — 1 Lolly/45g	56	0.7	125	1.6	26	1.6	0.3
Rocket, Co-Op* — 1 Lolly/60g	42	0	70	0	17	0	0
Rocket, Essential, Waitrose* — 1 Lolly/58ml	42	0.1	72	0.4	16.8	0.2	0.7
Rocket, Sainsbury's* — 1 Lolly/60g	50	0.3	83	0.5	19.9	0.5	0.5
Rocket, Tesco* — 1 Lolly/60g	39	0.1	66	0.4	15.2	0.2	0.6
Rolo, Nestle* — 1 Lolly/75ml	243	14.1	324	3.8	36.5	18.8	0
Salted Caramel, Tesco* — 1 Lolly/70g	227	12.5	324	3.6	36.7	17.9	1.1
Scooby Doo, Freezepops, Calypso* — 1 Lolly/45ml	13	0	28	0	7	0	0
Scottish Raspberry, The Best, Morrisons* — 1 Lolly/73ml	63	0.1	86	0.5	20.3	0.2	0.6

	Measure INFO/WEIGHT	per Measure KCAL	FAT	Nutrition Values per 100g / 100ml KCAL	PROT	CARB	FAT	FIBRE
ICE LOLLY								
Seriously Fruity, Mango Sorbet, Waitrose*	1 Lolly/100ml	79	0.3	79	0.8	18.4	0.3	0.5
Skinny Dippers Minis, Caramel Chocolate, Skinny Cow*	1 Lolly/38ml	62	1.9	162	3.4	24.3	5	3.3
Spotty Dotty, Sainsbury's*	1 Lolly/47g	111	6.5	236	1.8	25.5	13.8	1.3
Sprinkle Tops, Sainsbury's*	1 Lolly/40g	51	1.2	126	0.2	24.8	2.9	0.1
Strawberries & Cream, Cadbury*	1 Lolly/100ml	225	11.7	225	2.9	27	11.7	0
Strawberries 'n' Cream, Tropicana*	1 Lolly/50g	58	0.6	117	1.6	25	1.2	0
Strawberry & Banana, Smoothies, Sainsbury's*	1 Lolly/60g	100	3.2	166	1.5	28	5.3	0.2
Strawberry & Vanilla, 99% Fat Free, So-Lo, Iceland*	1 Lolly/92g	98	0.4	107	2.3	23.5	0.4	2.2
Strawberry Lemon, Shots, Calippo, Wall's*	1 Pack/81g	25	1	31	0.5	4.8	1.3	0
Strawberry Split, Average	***1 Lolly/72g***	***78***	***2.3***	***108***	***1.5***	***18.5***	***3.2***	***0.2***
Strawberry Split, Co-Op*	1 Lolly/71ml	75	2.1	105	1	17	3	0.1
Strawberry, Chocolate, with Sugar Balls, Tesco*	1 Lolly/47g	137	6.9	293	2.2	37.9	14.7	0.5
Strawberry, Blackcurrant Vanilla, Mini, Twister, Wall's*	1 Lolly/50ml	38	0.3	77	0.7	16	0.7	0
Strawberry, Dairy Split, Sainsbury's*	1 Lolly/73ml	86	2.6	118	1.7	19.8	3.6	0.1
Strawberry, Fruit Split, Free From, Tesco*	1 Split/55g	73	2.7	133	0.6	21.1	5	0.5
Strawberry, Fruit Split, Iceland*	1 Lolly/73g	77	2.4	105	0.9	17.8	3.3	0.5
Strawberry, Orange & Pineapple, Rocket, Iceland*	1 Lolly/47g	38	0	81	0	20.2	0	0.1
Tip Top, Calypso*	1 Lolly/20ml	6	0	30	0.1	7.1	0.1	0
Traffic Light, Co-Op*	1 Lolly/52g	55	0.4	105	0.4	25	0.8	0
Tropical Fruit Sorbet, Waitrose*	1 Lolly/110g	90	2.2	82	1.5	14.5	2	0.2
Tropical Fruit, Starburst, Mars*	1 Lolly/93ml	94	0.1	101	0.3	24.8	0.1	0
Tropical, Mmmm, Tesco*	1 Lolly/73g	109	3.1	150	1.2	26.6	4.3	0.4
Vimto, Ice Pop, Vimto*	1 Pop/50ml	4	0	7	0	1.7	0	0
Watermelon, Rowntree's*	1 Lolly/73ml	61	0.3	83	0.1	19	0.4	0.3
Whirlz, Giannis, Aldi*	1 Lolly/50g	49	0.9	98	0	17.4	1.8	0
Wonka Super Sour Tastic, Nestle*	1 Lolly/60ml	84	2.2	140	0	26.1	3.6	0
Zoom, Nestle*	1 Lolly/58ml	54	0.4	93	0.9	20.6	0.7	0
INDIAN MEAL								
Banquet for One, COU, M&S*	1 Pack/500g	400	6	80	6.7	10.2	1.2	3.1
for One, Asda*	1 Pack/550g	834	25.3	152	6.7	20.9	4.6	1.4
for One, Vegetarian, Asda*	1 Pack/499g	789	44.9	158	3.2	16	9	1.4
for Two, Hot, Takeaway, Tesco*	1 Pack/825g	1215	60.6	147	6.6	13.6	7.4	1.9
for Two, Menu, Tesco*	1 Serving/537g	811	34.4	151	6.3	17	6.4	0.8
Takeaway for One, Heated, HL, Tesco*	1 Pack/400g	410	6.4	103	7.2	14	1.6	2.1
IRN BRU								
Diet, Sugar Free, Barr's*	1 Can/330ml	2	0	1	0.5	0	0	0
Original, Barr's*	1 Bottle/500ml	214	0	43	0	10.5	0	0
Xtra, Barr's*	1 Serving/250ml	2	0	1	0.5	0	0	0

I

INFO/WEIGHT	Measure INFO/WEIGHT	per Measure KCAL	per Measure FAT	KCAL	PROT	CARB	FAT	FIBRE
JACKFRUIT								
Pulled, BBQ, Sweet Smoky, Sainsbury's*	½ Pack/175g	126	0.9	72	1.6	13.2	0.5	4.9
Raw, Average, Flesh Only	*1 Portion/165g*	*155*	*0.5*	*94*	*1.5*	*24.4*	*0.3*	*1.6*
JALFREZI								
Chicken, & Rice, Serves 1, Tesco*	1 Serving/475g	589	38	124	7.4	5.7	8	1.6
Chicken, Coriander Rice, TTD, Sainsbury's*	1 Pack/473g	501	15.1	106	6.2	13.2	3.2	3.1
Chicken, Pilau Rice, Sainsbury's*	1 Pack/417g	596	17.5	143	7	17.9	4.2	2.9
Chicken, Asda*	1 Pack/340g	415	20.4	122	10	7	6	1.6
Chicken, Canned, Tesco*	½ Can/200g	190	6.8	95	10.8	4.1	3.4	1.4
Chicken, Diet Chef Ltd*	1 Pack/300g	285	5.7	95	10.5	9	1.9	2.2
Chicken, Finest, Tesco*	1 Pack/350g	402	16.4	115	10.4	6.9	4.7	1.2
Chicken, Hot & Spicy, Sainsbury's*	½ Pack/200g	228	11.4	114	12.8	2.9	5.7	1
Chicken, Indian Takeaway, Tesco*	½ Pack/194g	162	7.8	84	7.1	3.9	4	1.8
Chicken, with Basmati Rice, Weight Watchers*	1 Pack/330g	238	1.6	72	5	11.8	0.5	0.5
Chicken, with Lemon Pilau Rice, Finest, Tesco*	1 Pack/493g	665	21.7	135	6.9	16.4	4.4	1.8
Chicken, with Pilau Rice, Charlie Bigham's*	½ Pack/422g	586	27.4	139	6.5	14.3	6.5	0
Chicken, with Pilau Rice, Indian Cuisine, Aldi*	1 Pack/450g	673	21.3	158	8.7	18	5	3.3
Chicken, with Pilau Rice, Taste of India, Tesco*	1 Pack/421g	445	10.1	106	7.3	12.2	2.4	3
Chicken, with Pilau Rice, Tesco*	1 Pack/460g	506	17.5	110	5.3	13.6	3.8	0.9
Chicken, with Rice, Ready Meal	*1 Serving/450g*	*557*	*18.9*	*124*	*6.9*	*14.5*	*4.2*	*1.5*
Chicken, with Rice, Ready Meal, Healthy Range	*1 Serving/400g*	*363*	*5.7*	*91*	*7.1*	*12.3*	*1.4*	*1.4*
Vegetable, Eastern Indian, Sainsbury's*	1 Pack/400g	208	13.6	52	3.4	2	3.4	1.7
Vegetable, Indian, Sainsbury's*	½ Pack/200g	156	9	78	2	5.3	4.5	4.2
Vegetable, Waitrose*	1 Pack/400g	256	16	64	2.2	4.7	4	3.7
JAM								
Apricot, Average	*1 Tbsp/15g*	*37*	*0*	*248*	*0.2*	*61.6*	*0*	*1.5*
Apricot, Reduced Sugar, Average	*1 Serving/20g*	*37*	*0.1*	*186*	*0.4*	*46*	*0.3*	*0.4*
Black Cherry, Average	*1 Tsp/5g*	*12*	*0*	*247*	*0.4*	*61.2*	*0.3*	*0.4*
Blackberry, Extra Special, Asda*	1 Tbsp/15g	29	0.1	190	0.9	45	0.7	0
Blackcurrant, Average	*1 Tbsp/15g*	*38*	*0*	*250*	*0.2*	*62.3*	*0*	*1*
Blackcurrant, Reduced Sugar, Average	*1 Tsp/6g*	*10*	*0*	*178*	*0.4*	*44.4*	*0.2*	*1*
Blueberry, Best, Hartley's*	1 Tsp/20g	49	0	244	0.3	60.6	0.1	0
Damson, Extra Fruit, Best, Hartley's*	1 Tsp/5g	12	0	244	0.2	60.8	0	0
Fig	*1 Tsp/15g*	*36*	*0*	*242*	*0.5*	*60*	*0*	*0*
Golden Peach, Rhapsodie De Fruit, St Dalfour*	1 Tsp/10g	23	0	227	0.5	56	0.1	1.3
Kiwi Gooseberry, 66% Fruit, Asda*	1 Serving/30g	56	0.2	187	0.5	45	0.5	0
Mixed Fruit, Average	*1 Tbsp/15g*	*38*	*0*	*252*	*0.3*	*63.5*	*0*	*0.5*
Peach, Pure, Summerland Sweets*	1 Tsp/5g	25	0	500	0	130	0	0
Plum, Damson, Soft Set, British, M&S*	1 Tsp/5g	13	0	264	0.4	63.7	0.5	1.3
Plum, Tesco*	1 Serving/50g	130	0	261	0.2	64.4	0	0.6
Raspberry, Average	*1 Tbsp/15g*	*36*	*0*	*239*	*0.6*	*58.6*	*0.1*	*0.9*
Raspberry, Reduced Sugar, Average	*1 Tsp/6g*	*10*	*0*	*160*	*0.5*	*39.3*	*0.2*	*0.6*
Raspberry, Seedless, Average	*1 Tsp/10g*	*26*	*0*	*257*	*0.4*	*63.6*	*0*	*0.3*
Rhubarb Ginger, Baxters*	1 Tsp/15g	40	0	264	0.4	65	0.1	0.8
Strawberry & Redcurrant, Reduced Sugar, Streamline*	1 Tbsp/15g	29	0	192	0.4	46.8	0.3	0
Strawberry, Average	*1 Tsp/10g*	*24*	*0*	*243*	*0.3*	*60.2*	*0.1*	*0.7*
Strawberry, Reduced Sugar, Average	*1 Tbsp/15g*	*28*	*0*	*187*	*0.4*	*45.8*	*0.3*	*0.2*
Summer Berry, Soft Set, British, M&S*	1 Tsp/5g	13	0	255	0.7	61.1	0.1	3.2
Wild Blackberry Jelly, Baxters*	1 Tsp/15g	32	0	210	0	53	0	1.2
JAMBALAYA								
American Style, Tesco*	1 Serving/275g	432	19.2	157	7.7	16	7	0.5
Cajun Chicken, Cooked, BGTY, Sainsbury's*	1 Pack/400g	381	7.2	100	6.2	12.7	1.9	3.3
Chicken Prawn, World Cafe, Waitrose*	1 Pack/350g	413	12.2	118	5.3	15.3	3.5	2.3
Chicken, HL, Tesco*	1 Pack/385g	319	5.2	83	7.7	9	1.3	2.1

J

	Measure INFO/WEIGHT	per Measure KCAL	FAT	Nutrition Values per 100g / 100ml KCAL	PROT	CARB	FAT	FIBRE
JAMBALAYA								
Ready Meal, Average	*1 Pack/450g*	*569*	*18.2*	*126*	*6.4*	*15.7*	*4*	*1.3*
JELLY								
Apple & Watermelon, Low Calorie, Hartley's*	1 Serving/175g	5	0	3	0	0.3	0	0.3
Apple, No Added Sugar, Hartley's*	1 Pot/115g	7	0.3	6	0	1.1	0.3	0
Blackberry, Unprepared, Morrisons*	1 Serving/20g	52	0	261	0.3	65	0	0
Blackcurrant Tahitian Vanilla, M&S*	¼ Pack/143g	77	0.4	54	0.3	12.1	0.3	0.6
Blackcurrant, Made Up, Rowntree's*	¼ Jelly/140ml	100	0.1	71	1.4	16.4	0.1	0
Blackcurrant, Made Up, Sainsbury's*	¼ Jelly/150g	98	0	65	1.2	15.1	0	0
Blackcurrant, Sugar Free, Unprepared, Rowntree's*	1 Pack/24g	73	0	305	50	25	0	25
Blackcurrant, Tesco*	1 Serving/100g	84	0.1	84	0.2	20.5	0.1	0.4
Bramble, Tesco*	1 Serving/100g	257	0.1	257	0.3	63.7	0.1	1.3
Cherry Flavoured, Waitrose*	1 Pot/175g	87	0.5	50	0.3	11.3	0.3	0.2
Cloudy Lemonade, Pot, Hartley's*	1 Pot/183g	11	0.9	6	0.5	0.9	0.5	0
Crystals, Orange, Sugar Free, Bird's*	1 Sachet/12g	39	0.1	335	62.5	6.4	0.9	0
Crystals, Strawberry, Made Up, Tesco*	1 Serving/145g	9	0	6	1.3	0.3	0	0
Exotic Fruit, M&S*	1 Pot/175g	140	0.4	80	0.1	18.9	0.2	0.9
Fresh Fruit, M&S*	1 Pot/175g	131	0.2	75	0.2	18.4	0.1	0.3
Fruitini, Del Monte*	1 Serving/120g	78	0.1	65	0.3	15.3	0.1	0.5
Lime Flavour, Cubes, Hartley's*	1 Cube/12g	36	0	296	5.1	68.9	0	0
Lime, Made Up, Rowntree's*	¼ Jelly/140ml	100	0.1	71	1.4	16.4	0.1	0
Lime, Unprepared, Co-Op*	1 Pack/135g	397	0.1	294	5.5	68.1	0	1
Made Up with Water, Average	*1oz/28g*	*17*	*0*	*61*	*1.2*	*15.1*	*0*	*0*
Mandarin & Pineapple, Sainsbury's*	1 Pot/125g	95	0.1	76	0.2	18.9	0.1	1.2
Mixed Berry, WT5, Sainsbury's*	1 Serving/160g	112	0.3	70	0.7	16.3	0.2	1.5
Orange, Sugar Free, Crystals, Dry Weight, Hartley's*	1 Pack/26g	66	0	254	57.4	6.1	0	0
Orange, Sugar Free, Made Up, Hartley's*	1 Serving/140ml	9	0	6	1.3	0.3	0	0
Orange, Sugar Free, Rowntree's*	1 Serving/140ml	8	0	6	1.4	0.1	0	0
Orange, Sugar Free, Unprepared, Asda*	1 Serving/12g	36	0	303	63.6	12	0.1	0.2
Orange, Unprepared, Rowntree's*	1 Square/11g	33	0	296	4.4	69.6	0	0
Orange, with Mandarin Pieces, Tesco*	1 Pot/120g	92	0.1	77	0.1	18.7	0.1	0.5
Peach Melba, Eat Well, M&S*	1 Pot/175g	114	0.4	65	0.2	15.9	0.2	0.2
Raspberry Elderflower, Seriously Fruity, Waitrose*	1/6 Pack/103g	71	0.3	69	2.3	13.9	0.3	0.5
Raspberry Flavour, Sugar Free, Made Up, Rowntree's*	1 Serving/140ml	9	0	6	1.4	0.1	0	0
Raspberry Flavour, Tesco*	1 Serving/34g	22	0	64	1	15	0	0.1
Raspberry Glitter, Made Up, Hartley's*	1 Serving/150g	94	0	63	0	15.4	0	0
Raspberry, Crystals, Vegetarian, Just Wholefoods*	1 Pack/85g	293	0	345	0.5	85.7	0	0
Raspberry, Individual Pot, Waitrose*	1 Pot/175g	92	1.2	53	0.3	10.7	0.7	1.1
Raspberry, Unprepared, Rowntree's*	1 Serving/135g	405	0.5	300	5.6	67.3	0.4	0
Redcurrant, Average	*1oz/28g*	*70*	*0*	*250*	*0.2*	*64.4*	*0*	*0*
Strawberry & Raspberry, Sainsbury's*	½ Pot/280g	230	0	82	0.2	20.2	0	1.2
Strawberry Flavour, Sugar Free, Made Up, Rowntree's*	1 Serving/140ml	10	0	7	1.5	0.1	0	0
Strawberry, Glitter, Made Up, Hartley's*	1 Serving/150g	94	0	63	0	15.4	0	0
Strawberry, Sugar Free, Crystals, Dry Weight, Hartley's*	1 Sachet/26g	73	0	280	56.8	13.1	0	0
Strawberry, Unprepared, Co-Op*	1 Pack/135g	402	0.1	298	5.5	69.1	0	0
Sugar Free, Dry, Tesco*	1 Pack/13g	36	0	285	55.4	15.6	0	0.2
JELLY BABIES								
Bassett's*	1 Sweet/6g	20	0	335	3.5	79.7	0	0
M&S*	1 Pack/125g	418	0	334	5.2	78	0	0
Mini, Rowntree's*	1 Sm Bag/35g	128	0	366	4.6	86.9	0	0
Waitrose*	1 Sweet/6g	20	0	342	4.6	79.6	0.5	0.5
JELLY BEANS								
Asda*	1 Bag/100g	364	0.4	364	0.1	90	0.4	0.2
Average	*1 Serving/100g*	*365*	*0.1*	*365*	*0.1*	*91.2*	*0.1*	*0.1*

J

	Measure INFO/WEIGHT	per Measure KCAL	per Measure FAT	Nutrition Values per 100g / 100ml KCAL	PROT	CARB	FAT	FIBRE
JELLY BEANS								
Jelly Belly*	35 Beans/40g	140	0	350	0	90	0	0
Rowntree's*	1 Pack/35g	128	0	367	0	91.8	0	0
JERKY								
Beef, BBQ Flavour, Kings*	1 Bag/40g	116	1.9	291	36.3	26.3	4.9	1.3
Beef, Honey BBQ, Wild West*	1 Pack/70g	216	2.2	308	29.6	39.6	3.2	1.1
Chicken, Chipotle Chilli, Eat Well, M&S*	1 Serving/25g	69	0.5	277	43.3	21	2.1	0.6
Salmon, Hot Spicy, Ready To Eat, Sainsbury's*	1 Pack/55g	263	17.5	479	27.8	20.1	31.9	0.5
JUICE								
Apple & Cranberry, Average	*1 Glass/250ml*	*114*	*0*	*46*	*0.1*	*10.2*	*0*	*0*
Apple & Elderflower, Copella*	1 Glass/250ml	108	0.2	43	0.4	10.2	0.1	0
Apple & Mango, Average	*1 Glass/200ml*	*108*	*0.1*	*54*	*0.3*	*12.6*	*0*	*0.1*
Apple & Orange, Fresh Up*	1 Serving/250ml	105	0	42	0	10.3	0	0
Apple & Raspberry, Average	*1 Serving/200ml*	*89*	*0.1*	*44*	*0.4*	*10.2*	*0*	*0.2*
Apple Cherry, Sainsbury's*	1 Serving/200ml	96	0	48	0.3	10.8	0	0.8
Apple Mango, 100% Pressed, Tesco*	1 Glass/150ml	72	0	48	0.4	10.7	0	0.9
Apple Mango, Pressed, Waitrose*	1 Glass/100ml	54	0	54	0.3	12.6	0	0
Apple Raspberry, Tropicana*	1 Glass/150ml	72	0	48	0.2	10.5	0	0.9
Apple Rhubarb, Caxton Vale*	1 Glass/250ml	115	1	46	0.2	9.7	0.4	0
Apple Rhubarb, Pressed, Cawston Press*	1 Serving/200ml	92	0.8	46	0.2	9.7	0.4	0
Apple, Cloudy, Pressed, Copella*	1 Glass/100ml	46	0	46	0.2	10.7	0	0.7
Apple, Concentrate, Average	*1 Tbsp/15ml*	*45*	*0*	*302*	*0*	*73.6*	*0.2*	*0*
Apple, Peach Pear, Innocent*	1 Serving/100ml	45	0.1	45	0.4	10	0.1	1.4
Apple, Pink Lady, Pressed, Eat Well, M&S*	1 Bottle/300ml	153	0.6	51	0.4	11.7	0.2	0.3
Apple, Pressed, 100%, Never From Concentrate, Tesco*	1 Glass/180ml	88	0	49	0.3	11.2	0	0.5
Apple, Pure, Average	*1 Glass/250ml*	*116*	*0.1*	*47*	*0.1*	*11.2*	*0*	*0*
Apple, Pure, Organic, Average	*1 Serving/200ml*	*92*	*0.1*	*46*	*0*	*11.2*	*0*	*0*
Apple, Pure, Value, Tesco*	1 Glass/200ml	94	0.2	47	0.1	11.1	0.1	0.1
Beetroot, Apple, Rhubarb, Morrisons*	1 Glass/150ml	68	0.2	45	0.7	9.9	0.1	0.7
Beetroot, Natural, So Organic, Sainsbury's*	1 Pack/250g	105	1.2	42	0.9	8.2	0.5	1.9
Breakfast, Ruby, Tropicana*	1 Glass/200ml	90	0	45	0.8	9.7	0	0.7
Carrot, Average	*1 Glass/200ml*	*48*	*0.2*	*24*	*0.5*	*5.7*	*0.1*	*0*
Carrot, Orange, Apple, Cold Pressed, B Fresh *	1 Bottle/250ml	65	0	26	0	6.2	0	0
Chia Watermelon Pomegranate, WOW, Planet Organic*	1 Bottle/250ml	122	3.8	49	2.3	5.6	1.5	2.2
Clementine, 100% Pure Squeezed, Tesco*	1 Serving/150ml	71	0	48	0.4	10.7	0	0.2
Clementine, Morrisons*	1 Serving/100ml	48	0.1	48	0.5	10.9	0.1	0.1
Cranberry, Average	*1 Bottle/250ml*	*139*	*0.2*	*56*	*0.1*	*13.4*	*0.1*	*0.3*
Cranberry, No Added Sugar, Average	*1 Glass/200ml*	*11*	*0.1*	*6*	*0.1*	*0.8*	*0*	*0*
Cranberry, No Added Sugar, M&S*	1 Serving/150ml	9	0.2	6	0.1	0.9	0.1	0.1
Exotic Fruit, Pure, Del Monte*	1 Glass/200ml	96	0	48	0.3	11.3	0	0
Exotic Fruit, Waitrose*	1 Glass/175ml	88	0	50	0.4	11.6	0	0
Exotic, No Added Sugar, Morrisons*	1 Glass/150ml	24	0	16	0	3.6	0	0
Froot Refresh, Orange & Passion Fruit, Minute Maid*	1 Bottle/330ml	79	0	24	0	6	0	0
Fruit, Tropical in Sparkling Spring Water, Light, Rio*	1 Can/330ml	17	0	5	0.1	1.1	0	0
Fruit, Tropical, Pure Premium, Tropicana*	1 Glass/200ml	98	0	49	0.5	11	0	0.8
Ginger, Boost, Shot, On the Go, Sainsbury's*	1 Shot/100ml	41	0.5	41	0.5	9.9	0.5	0.5
Grape, Purple, Welch's*	1 Serving/200ml	136	0	68	0.1	16.5	0	0
Grape, Red, Average	*1 Serving/100ml*	*62*	*0*	*62*	*0.2*	*15.2*	*0*	*0*
Grape, White, Average	*1 Can/160ml*	*95*	*0.1*	*60*	*0.2*	*14.3*	*0.1*	*0.1*
Grapefruit, Pink, Average	*1 Glass/200ml*	*81*	*0.1*	*40*	*0.6*	*9*	*0*	*0.2*
Grapefruit, Pure, Average	*1 Glass/200ml*	*77*	*0.2*	*38*	*0.5*	*8.5*	*0.1*	*0.1*
Lemon, Fresh, Average	*1 Lemon/36ml*	*2*	*0*	*7*	*0.3*	*1.6*	*0*	*0.1*
Lemon, from Concentrate	*1 Tsp/5ml*	*1*	*0*	*28*	*0.4*	*6.5*	*0*	*0*
Lemon, The Pantry, Aldi*	1 Tbsp/15ml	3	0.1	20	0.5	1.2	0.5	0.5

JUICE

	Measure INFO/WEIGHT	per Measure KCAL	FAT	KCAL	PROT	CARB	FAT	FIBRE
Lime, Fresh, Average	*1 Tsp/5ml*	*0*	*0*	*9*	*0.4*	*1.6*	*0.1*	*0.1*
Mandarin Orange, Tropicana*	1 Serving/200ml	94	0	47	0.6	10	0	0.8
Mango Veggie, Naked Juice Co*	1 Serving/240ml	150	1	62	1.2	15.8	0.4	2.1
Mango, Peach, Papaya, Pure, Premium, Tropicana*	1 Glass/200ml	88	0	44	0.5	9.8	0	0.1
Mango, Pure, Canned	*1 Glass/250ml*	*98*	*0.5*	*39*	*0.1*	*9.8*	*0.2*	*0*
Multivitamin, Fruit, Vitafit, Lidl*	1 Carton/250ml	135	0.2	54	0.3	12.5	0.1	0.5
Orange & Kiwi Fruit, Tropicana*	1 Serving/175ml	90	0	51	0.5	12	0	0
Orange & Pineapple, Average	*1 Glass/120ml*	*56*	*0.6*	*46*	*0.4*	*10.5*	*0.5*	*0.5*
Orange & Raspberry, Average	*1fl oz/30ml*	*15*	*0*	*50*	*0.6*	*11.4*	*0.1*	*0.2*
Orange Banana, Pure, Average	*1 Glass/150ml*	*79*	*0.1*	*53*	*0.7*	*12.1*	*0.1*	*0.2*
Orange Grapefruit, Average	*1 Glass/200ml*	*84*	*0.2*	*42*	*0.8*	*9.2*	*0.1*	*0.4*
Orange Lime, Tropicana*	1 Serving/250ml	115	0	46	1.1	9.4	0	0.6
Orange Mango, Average	*1 Bottle/375ml*	*176*	*0.4*	*47*	*0.5*	*10.7*	*0.1*	*0.2*
Orange Passionfruit, Tropicana*	1 Serving/200ml	94	0	47	0.8	10	0	0.7
Orange Raspberry, Tropicana*	1 Bottle/330ml	139	0	42	0.4	9	0	0.8
Orange 100% from Concentrate, Farmfoods*	1 Serving/200ml	84	0.2	42	0.6	9.1	0.1	0.1
Orange with Bits, Freshly Squeezed, TTD, Sainsbury's*	1 Serving/249g	132	0	53	0.7	11.4	0	0.2
Orange with Bits, Innocent*	1 Glass/250ml	120	0	48	0.8	10.9	0	0.3
Orange with Bits, Not From Concentrate, Tesco*	1 Glass/250ml	110	0	44	0.4	10.6	0	0
Orange, Apple & Mango, Calypso*	1 Carton/200ml	92	0.4	46	0	11	0.2	0.1
Orange, Carrot Passionfruit, Morrisons*	1 Glass/250ml	88	0.2	35	0.6	7.5	0.1	0.9
Orange, Freshly Squeezed, Average	*1 Serving/200ml*	*66*	*0*	*33*	*0.6*	*8.1*	*0*	*1*
Orange, Freshly Squeezed, with Bits, 1, Waitrose*	¼ Bottle/250ml	108	0.2	43	0.7	9.5	0.1	0.5
Orange, Mango Passionfruit, Pure Squeezed, Waitrose*	1 Serving/250ml	130	0.8	52	0.6	10.9	0.3	0.3
Orange, Pure from Concentrate, Carton, Value, Tesco*	1 Serving/250ml	115	0	46	0.5	10.4	0	0
Orange, Pure Premium, Smooth, No Bits, Tropicana*	1 Glass/200ml	96	0	48	0.8	10	0	0.4
Orange, Pure with Bits, Average	*1 Glass/200ml*	*90*	*0.1*	*45*	*0.6*	*10.2*	*0.1*	*0.1*
Orange, Pure, Smooth, Average	*1 Glass/200ml*	*88*	*0.1*	*44*	*0.7*	*9.8*	*0*	*0.2*
Orange, Pure, Smooth, From Concentrate, Sainsbury's*	1 Serving/200ml	84	0.2	42	0.5	9.1	0.1	0.1
Orange, Pure, Tesco*	1 Glass/200ml	94	0	47	0.5	10.5	0	0
Orange, Red, Average	*1 Glass/250ml*	*115*	*0.1*	*46*	*0.4*	*10.7*	*0*	*0.2*
Orange, Smooth, Freshly Squeezed, TTD, Sainsbury's*	1 Serving/249g	132	0	53	0.7	11.4	0	0.2
Orange, Smooth, Innocent*	1 Serving/200ml	76	0	38	0.7	8.2	0	0
Orange, Smooth, Pure, From Concentrate, Iceland*	1 Serving/200ml	94	0.2	47	0.5	10.4	0.1	0
Orange, Sparkling, 55, Britvic*	1 Bottle/275ml	135	0.3	49	0.3	11.3	0.1	0.1
Orange, Vitafit*	1 Glass/200ml	78	0.2	39	0.7	8.3	0.1	0.7
Passion Fruit, Average	*1 Glass/200ml*	*94*	*0.2*	*47*	*0.8*	*10.7*	*0.1*	*0*
Pear, Blackcurrant, Pressed, Eat Well, M&S*	1 Bottle/300ml	165	0.6	55	0.6	12.4	0.2	0.7
Pineapple, Average	*1 Glass/200ml*	*100*	*0.1*	*50*	*0.3*	*11.7*	*0.1*	*0.2*
Pineapple, Rugani*	1 Bottle/330ml	549	3.6	166	1.6	32	1.1	0.5
Pomegranate, Grape Apple, Tropicana*	1 Bottle/330ml	211	0	64	0.2	15.5	0	0.6
Pomegranate, Pomegreat*	1 Glass/200ml	88	0	44	0.1	11.1	0	0
Pomegranate, Pure, Organic, Biona*	1 Portion/100g	74	0.6	74	0.7	16.7	0.6	0.4
Prune, Average	*1 Serving/200ml*	*123*	*0.1*	*61*	*0.6*	*15.3*	*0.1*	*1.8*
Sweet Carrot & Orange, Shapers, Boots*	1 Serving/250ml	100	0.4	40	0.9	8.8	0.2	0.4
Tomato from Concentrate, Sainsbury's*	1 Glass/250ml	40	0.2	16	0.7	2.7	0.1	0.7
Tomato, Average	*1 Glass/200ml*	*40*	*0.1*	*20*	*0.8*	*4*	*0*	*0.4*
Tomato, Tangy, Princes*	1 Serving/200ml	34	0	17	0.8	3.1	0	0.6
Tomato, Vitafit, Lidl*	1 Serving/250ml	47	0.5	19	0.8	2.9	0.2	0.7
Tropical made from Concentrate, Sainsbury's*	1 Glass/250ml	120	0.2	48	0.5	10.7	0.1	0.1
Tropical, Pure, Sainsbury's*	1 Glass/200ml	104	0.2	52	0.5	12	0.1	0.1
Turmeric Booster, Cold Pressed, Moju*	1 Shot/60ml	22	0.1	36	0.8	7.5	0.1	0
V Fusion, Passion Fruit, Mango Carrot, V8*	1 Serving/150ml	72	0	48	0.3	11.8	0	0.4

J

	Measure INFO/WEIGHT	per Measure KCAL	FAT	Nutrition Values per 100g / 100ml KCAL	PROT	CARB	FAT	FIBRE
JUICE								
V Fusion, Raspberry Beetroot, V8*	1 Serving/150ml	68	0	45	0.3	10.8	0	0.3
Vegetable, Organic, Evernat*	1 Glass/200ml	36	0.2	18	0.9	3.5	0.1	0.2
Vegetable, Organic, James White*	1 Sm Glass/100g	22	0.2	22	0.6	4.4	0.2	0
Vegetable, Original, V8*	1 Glass/150ml	26	0.2	17	0.9	2.8	0.1	0.9
Watermelon, Mello Drinks*	1 Bottle/250ml	100	0.2	40	1	8.5	0.1	0.7
White Apple Ginger, James White*	1 Glass/250ml	122	0	49	0.1	11.8	0	0
White Grape, Raspberry Blackcurrant, Asda*	1 Serving/200ml	120	0.2	60	0.4	13.8	0.1	0.1
JUICE DRINK								
Aloe Vera, OKF*	1 Bottle/500ml	175	0	35	0	9	0	0
Apple & Blueberry, The Feel Good Drinks Co*	1 Serving/375ml	163	0.4	44	0.1	10.6	0.1	0
Apple & Elderflower, Tesco*	1 Serving/200ml	76	0	38	0	9.4	0	0
Apple & Raspberry, Sainsbury's*	1 Serving/200ml	112	0.2	56	0.1	13.8	0.1	0.1
Apple & Strawberry, Sainsbury's*	1 Serving/250ml	13	0.1	5	0	1	0	0
Apple Mango, CBY, Asda*	1 Carton/250ml	115	0	46	0	11	0	0
Apple Pomegranate, Sparkling Water, Sainsbury's*	1 Serving/200ml	4	0	2	0	0.3	0	0
Apple Raspberry, Light, Just Drink, Don Simon*	1 Glass/250ml	50	0	20	0.1	6.1	0	0.3
Apple Raspberry, Tesco*	1 Serving/300ml	138	0	46	0.1	11.2	0	0
Apple Lemonade, Cawston Press*	1 Glass/200g	106	0.2	53	0.2	11.9	0.1	0
Apple, Cranberry, & Blueberry, Waitrose*	1 Serving/150ml	75	0	50	0.1	11.9	0	0.1
Apple, No Added Sugar, Asda*	1 Glass/200ml	10	0	5	0	1	0	0
Apple, No Added Sugar, LC, Tesco*	1 Glass/250ml	12	0	5	0	0.9	0	0
Apple, Plum Pear, Pure Pressed, CBY, Asda*	1 Glass/200ml	92	0	46	0.4	10.5	0	0.2
Berry & Elderberry, Fusion, Oasis*	1 Bottle/375ml	11	0	3	0	0.4	0	0
Bitter Lemon, Sugar Free, Essential, Waitrose*	1 Serving/250ml	5	0	2	0	0	0	0
Blackcurrant Apple, Oasis*	1 Serving/500ml	90	0	18	0	4.1	0	0
Blackcurrant, 45% High, No Added Sugar, Asda*	1 Serving/250ml	50	1.2	20	0.5	4.5	0.5	0
Blackcurrant, Extra Light, Ribena*	1 Serving/200ml	8	0	4	0	0.5	0	0
Blackcurrant, Pouch, Sun Shots, Aldi*	1 Pouch/200ml	10	0.5	5	0.2	1.1	0.2	0.2
Blood Orange, Sparkling, Aranciata Rossa, San Pellegrino*	1 Can/330ml	73	0	22	0.1	4.9	0	0
Blueberry, BGTY, Sainsbury's*	1 Serving/250ml	15	0	6	0.1	1	0	0
Cherry Cinnamon Presse, CBY, Asda*	1 Can/250ml	95	1.3	37	0.5	9.2	0.5	0.5
Cherry, No Added Sugar, Sainsbury's*	1 Carton/250ml	25	0.1	10	0.2	1.9	0	0
Cranberry & Blackberry, Ocean Spray*	1 Glass/250ml	120	0.2	48	0.1	11.3	0.1	0.2
Cranberry & Blackcurrant, Ocean Spray*	1 Bottle/500ml	265	0	53	0.2	12.7	0	0
Cranberry & Orange, HE, Tesco*	1 Glass/200ml	10	0	5	0	0.8	0	0
Cranberry & Raspberry, BGTY, Sainsbury's*	1 Glass/250ml	10	0.2	4	0.1	0.7	0.1	0.1
Cranberry & Raspberry, Sainsbury's*	1 Serving/250ml	105	0	42	0.1	9.9	0	0
Cranberry & Raspberry, Tesco*	1 Serving/200ml	96	0	48	0	11.6	0	0
Cranberry Mango, Light, Ocean Spray*	1 Glass/250ml	22	0	9	0	2	0	0.1
Cranberry Pomegranate, Ocean Spray*	1 Glass/250ml	120	0	48	0	11.5	0	0
Cranberry Raspberry, No Add Sugar, LC, Tesco*	1 Serving/250ml	12	0	5	0	0.8	0	0
Cranberry Raspberry, Ocean Spray*	1 Glass/200ml	96	0	48	0	11.6	0	0
Cranberry Raspberry, with Spring Water, Zeo*	1 Serving/275ml	33	0	12	0	2.6	0	0
Cranberry Blend, Ocean Spray*	1 Glass/250ml	148	0	59	0.1	13.9	0	0
Cranberry, Asda*	1 Serving/200ml	40	0	20	0	4.5	0	0
Cranberry, Classic, Ocean Spray*	1 Bottle/500ml	245	0.5	49	0.1	11.7	0.1	0.1
Cranberry, Grape & Apple, Ocean Spray*	1 Glass/200ml	108	0	54	0.1	12.9	0	0
Cranberry, Light, Classic, Ocean Spray*	1 Glass/200ml	16	0	8	0	1.4	0	0
Cranberry, McEnnedy, Lidl*	1 Glass/200ml	98	0	49	0	11.7	0	0
Cranberry, Morrisons*	1 Glass/200ml	92	0	46	0	11.6	0	0
Cranberry, No Added Sugar, BGTY, Sainsbury's*	1 Glass/200ml	4	0	2	0	0.3	0	0
Cranberry, No Added Sugar, HL, Tesco*	1 Glass/200ml	8	0	4	0	1.1	0	0
Cranberry, Organic, Sainsbury's*	1 Serving/200ml	100	0	50	0	11.9	0	0

J

	Measure INFO/WEIGHT	per Measure KCAL	FAT	Nutrition Values per 100g / 100ml KCAL	PROT	CARB	FAT	FIBRE
JUICE DRINK								
Cranberry, Original, Concentrated, Ocean Spray*	1 Serving/15ml	27	0	183	0.2	44.1	0	0
Cranberry, Solevita*	1 Serving/200ml	98	0	49	0.5	11.7	0	0
Cranberry, Tesco*	1 Serving/250ml	50	0	20	0	4.4	0	0.1
Cranberry, Waitrose*	1 Serving/250ml	145	0	58	0.1	13.9	0	0.1
Exotic, Tesco*	1 Serving/250ml	128	0	51	0.1	12.3	0	0
Forest Fruits, Asda*	1 Serving/200ml	88	0	44	0.3	10.9	0	0.3
Fruit Cocktail, Sainsbury's*	1 Glass/200ml	90	0	45	0.2	10.6	0	0.1
Fruit Shoot, My-5, Apple Pear, Robinson's*	1 Bottle/200ml	78	0.2	39	0.2	8.9	0.1	0
Grape Elderflower, White, Sparkling, Shloer*	1 Glass/200ml	74	0	37	0	9.2	0	0
Grape, Apple & Raspberry, Co-Op*	1 Serving/150ml	75	0	50	0.4	12	0	0.1
Grape, Apple Raspberry, Asda*	1 Glass/200ml	82	1	41	0.5	9.8	0.5	0.5
Grape, Red, Sparkling, Shloer*	1 Glass/200ml	84	0	42	0	10.4	0	0
Grape, White, Sparkling, Light, Shloer*	1 Glass/125ml	28	0	22	0.7	5.3	0	0
Grape, White, Sparkling, Shloer*	1 Serving/120ml	59	0	49	0	11.6	0	0
Guava Exotic, Rubicon*	1 Carton/288ml	150	0.3	52	0.2	12.9	0.1	0
J20, Apple Mango, Britvic*	1 Bottle/275ml	83	0	30	0.1	6.8	0	0.2
J20, Apple Raspberry, Britvic*	1 Bottle/275ml	88	0	32	0.1	7.3	0	0.3
J20, Orange Passion Fruit, Britvic*	1 Bottle/275ml	88	0	32	0.3	7.2	0	0.2
J2O, Apple Blueberry, Britvic*	1 Bottle/275g	124	0	45	0.1	11	0	0.2
J2O, Apple Watermelon, Sparkling, Spritz, Britvic*	1 Serving/250ml	58	0	23	0	5.4	0	0
J2O, Glitterberry, Britvic*	1 Bottle/275ml	77	0	28	0	6.4	0	0
Lemon & Lime, Light, Oasis*	1 Bottle/250ml	6	0	3	0	0.2	0	0
Lemon, Cloudy, Lightly Carbonated, Zeo*	1 Serving/275ml	28	0	10	0.1	2.3	0	0
Lemon, Lime, Apple, Sparkling, Bubbles, Innocent*	1 Can/333ml	90	0	27	0	6.8	0	0
Lemon, The Feel Good Drinks Co*	1 Bottle/171ml	78	0.2	46	0.1	10.8	0.1	0
Lemonade, Asda*	1 Glass/200ml	88	0	44	0.1	11	0	0
Lychee, Sparkling, Rubicon*	1 Can/330g	182	0	55	0	13.6	0	0
Mango Passionfruit, Shot, Big Shotz*	1 Shot/120ml	67	0.5	56	0	12.1	0.4	3.4
Mango Madness, Snapple*	1 Bottle/227ml	104	0	46	0	12	0	0
Mango, Earl Grey Tea, Rio Doro, Aldi*	1 Bottle/ 330ml	3	0.3	1	0.1	0.3	0.1	0.1
Mango, from Mango Puree, Natura*	1 Bottle/500ml	290	0.5	58	0.2	13.9	0.1	0.5
Mango, Rubicon*	1 Serving/100ml	54	0.1	54	0.1	13.1	0.1	0
Mango, Sparkling, Rubicon*	1 Can/330ml	172	0	52	0	12.8	0	0
Mixed Berry Crush, Sparkling, CBY, Asda*	1 Glass/250ml	8	0	3	0	0.5	0	0
Mulled Lemonade, Sainsbury's*	1 Serving/150ml	67	0.8	44	0.5	10.8	0.5	0.5
Netar Multifruit, Light, Linessa, Lidl*	1 Glass /200ml	54	0.1	27	0.3	5.8	0.1	0
Orange Lime, Refresh'd, Robinson's*	1 Bottle/500ml	55	0	11	0	2.2	0	0
Orange Lime, Sparkling, Innocent*	1 Can/330ml	93	0	28	0.6	6.5	0	0
Orange Mango, Spring Water, Sparkling, Rubicon*	1 Bottle/500ml	15	0	3	0	0.5	0	0
Orange, Caprisun*	1 Pouch/200ml	89	0	45	0	10.8	0	0
Orange, Carrot & Lemon, Pago*	1 Serving/200g	90	0.2	45	0.2	10.5	0.1	0
Orange, Diluted, Mi Wadi*	1 Serving/250ml	26	0	10	0	2.3	0	0
Orange, Fruitish, Spar*	1 Carton/330ml	13	0.3	4	0.1	0.8	0.1	0
Orange, HE, Tesco*	1 Glass/200ml	56	0.2	28	0.3	6.1	0.1	0
Orange, Juice Burst, Purity Soft Drinks Co*	1 Bottle/500ml	220	0	44	1	10.2	0	0
Orange, Mango Lime, Fruit Crush, Shapers, Boots*	1 Bottle/330ml	150	0.6	45	0.4	10.6	0.2	0.4
Orange, Mango, Passionfruit, Morrisons*	1 Serving/200ml	6	0	3	0	0.2	0	0
Orange, Morrisons*	1 Serving/250ml	12	0.2	5	0.1	0.9	0.1	0.1
Orange, Sainsbury's*	1 Serving/250ml	18	0.2	7	0.1	1.4	0.1	0.1
Orange, Sun Shots, Sun Quench, Aldi*	1 Pouch/200ml	10	1	5	0.5	1.1	0.5	0.5
Orange, Value, Tesco*	1 Glass/250ml	32	0	13	0	3.3	0	0
Orange, Zero, Vive, Aldi*	1 Serving/200g	2	1	1	0.5	0.5	0.5	0.5

J

	Measure INFO/WEIGHT	per Measure		Nutrition Values per 100g / 100ml				
		KCAL	FAT	KCAL	PROT	CARB	FAT	FIBRE

JUICE DRINK

	Measure INFO/WEIGHT	KCAL	FAT	KCAL	PROT	CARB	FAT	FIBRE
Oranges Lemons, Juicy Water*	1 Bottle/420ml	134	0	32	0	8.1	0	0
Passion Fruit, Exotic, Rubicon*	1 Serving/200ml	110	0	55	0.1	13.6	0	0
Peach & Passionfruit Fruit, Sunmagic*	1 Serving/330ml	172	0	52	0.3	13	0	0.1
Peach Apricot, Sparkling, J2O Spritz, Britvic*	1 Serving/250ml	52	0	21	0	4.9	0	0
Peach Grapefruit, Lightly Carbonated, Zeo*	1 Serving/275ml	30	0	11	0	2.3	0	0
Peach Hibiscus, with Black Tea Extracts, Fuzetea*	1 Bottle/400ml	76	0	19	0	4.3	0	0
Peach, Passion Fruit, Extra Light, Oasis*	1 Bottle/500ml	18	0	4	0	0.6	0	0
Pear Raspberry, Sparkling, J2O Spritz, Britvic*	1 Serving/250ml	55	0	22	0	5.2	0	0
Pear, Partially Made with Concentrate, Tesco*	1 Glass/200ml	110	0	55	0	12.4	0	0.2
Pineapple & Grapefruit, Shapers, Boots*	1 Bottle/500ml	10	0.5	2	0.1	0.2	0.1	0
Pink Cranberry Lemonade, Diet, Sparkling, M&S*	1 Bottle/500ml	15	0.5	3	0.1	0.5	0.1	0.1
Pink Grapefruit, Juice Burst, Purity Soft Drinks Co*	1 Bottle/500ml	210	0	42	0.4	10	0	0
Pink Guava, Yuzu, Presse, Sparkling, M&S*	1 Serving/200ml	84	0.2	42	0.1	9.1	0.1	0.4
Pomegranate & Raspberry, Still, Shapers, Boots*	1 Bottle/500ml	45	0	9	0	2	0	0
Pomegranate, Rubicon*	1 Can/330ml	108	0	54	0	13.5	0	0
Purple Grape Mango, Welch's*	1 Glass/200ml	54	0	27	0	6.1	0	0.2
Raspberry & Pear, Tesco*	1 Serving/250ml	118	0	47	0	11.3	0	0
Raspberry, Ribena*	1 Bottle/500ml	215	0	43	0	10.4	0	0
Sicilian Lemon Garden Mint, Presse, Finest, Tesco*	1 Serving/250ml	50	0	20	0	5	0	0
Spirit, Lemon & Grapefruit, Tropicana*	1 Bottle/400ml	184	0	46	0.3	10.4	0	0.6
Strawberry, Mint, British, Agua Fresca, M&S*	1 Bottle/300ml	60	0.6	20	0.5	4	0.2	0.2
Summer Fruits, Fresh, Tesco*	1 Glass/250ml	112	0.2	45	0.1	10.8	0.1	0.3
Summer Fruits, Oasis*	1 Bottle/500ml	90	0	18	0	4.2	0	0
Tropical Fruit, Tesco*	1 Glass/250ml	118	0	47	0	11.4	0	0
Tropical Fruit, Waitrose*	1 Glass/250ml	118	0	47	0.2	11.2	0	0
Tropical, Be Light, Aldi*	1 Glass/250ml	62	0.2	25	0.2	5.4	0.1	0.2
Tropical, Naturis*	1 Carton/250ml	60	0.2	24	0.2	5.3	0.1	0.5
Tropical, No Added Sugar, Tesco*	1 Carton/250ml	12	0	5	0	1.1	0	0
White Cranberry & Lychee, Ocean Spray*	1 Glass/200ml	86	0	43	0	11.5	0	0
White Grape & Peach, Sainsbury's*	1 Glass/250ml	95	0.2	38	0.2	9	0.1	0.1
White Grape, Raspberry Cranberry, Sparkling, Shloer*	1 Serving/250ml	117	0	47	0	11	0	0

J

Food	Measure INFO/WEIGHT	per Measure KCAL	per Measure FAT	Nutrition Values per 100g / 100ml KCAL	PROT	CARB	FAT	FIBRE
KALE								
Black, Cavolo Nero, Aldi*	1 Serving/80g	23	0.9	29	2.4	1	1.1	2.8
Cavolo Nero, Boiled, Growers Selection, Asda*	½ Pack/150g	45	1.7	30	2.4	1	1.1	2.8
Curly, Boiled in Salted Water, Average	*1 Serving/60g*	*14*	*0.7*	*24*	*2.4*	*1*	*1.1*	*2.8*
Curly, Raw, Average	*1 Serving/90g*	*25*	*1.2*	*28*	*2.9*	*1.2*	*1.4*	*2.6*
Kalettes, Sprouts, Sweet Nutty Versatile, Waitrose*	1 Serving/80g	41	1.1	51	3.5	4.1	1.4	4.1
Leaf, Frozen, Tesco*	1 Serving/80g	19	0.9	24	2.4	1	1.1	0
Sprouts, Kalettes, Staples*	½ Bag/100g	53	1.5	53	3	5.2	1.5	3.5
KANGAROO								
Raw, Average	*1 Serving/200g*	*196*	*2*	*98*	*22*	*1*	*1*	*0*
KARELA								
Frozen, Shana*	1 Serving/80g	14	0.1	18	1.4	1.3	0.1	0
KATSU								
Chicken, Pot, Tesco*	1 Pack/132g	187	4.1	141	7.1	20.4	3.1	1.7
Coconut, Everdine*	1 Serving/450g	585	28.4	130	9.1	7.2	6.3	4.4
Curry, City Kitchen, Tesco*	1 Pack/385g	465	13.2	121	6	16.3	3.4	1.3
Sweet Potato, with Rice, Love Your Veg!, Sainsbury's*	1 Pack/393g	688	22	175	2.9	27.2	5.6	2.3
KEBAB								
Beef ,& Pepper, Kofta, Waitrose*	1 Kebab/138g	223	13.9	162	14.8	2.9	10.1	0.6
Beef, Kofta, Uncooked, Tesco*	1 Kebab/73g	163	12.5	225	14	3.2	17.3	1.2
Chicken, & Pineapple, Caribbean Style, Iceland*	1 Kebab/44g	41	0.6	93	11.6	8.7	1.4	1.4
Chicken, Chorizo, Waitrose*	1 Kebab/70g	135	8.2	195	20.4	1.3	11.8	1.1
Chicken, Breast, Moroccan Style, Sainsburys*	4 Kebabs/133g	170	2.5	128	26.8	0.9	1.9	0.5
Chicken, Mini Fillets, M&S*	1 Serving/150g	210	8.7	140	20.2	2	5.8	0.3
Chicken, Shish in Pitta Bread with Salad	*1 Kebab/250g*	*388*	*10.2*	*155*	*13.5*	*17.2*	*4.1*	*1*
Chicken, Shish, Meat Only, Average	*1 Kebab/250g*	*312*	*5.2*	*125*	*25.7*	*0.9*	*2.1*	*0.1*
Chicken, Spanish Style, Good to Go, Waitrose*	1 Pack/80g	148	4.6	185	18.3	13.8	5.7	2.6
Chicken, Sticky, Tesco*	1 Skewer/16g	31	1.4	198	23.7	5.7	8.8	0.5
Chicken, Thigh, Sticky Barbecue, M&S*	1 Pack/100g	189	6.8	189	26.3	5.7	6.8	0.1
Chicken, Tikka, Oakhurst, Aldi*	1 Kebab/59g	52	0.7	88	14	5.1	1.2	0.5
Doner, Frozen, Easy Chef*	1 Kebab/170g	493	44.2	290	14.9	1.5	26	1.7
Doner, Heat 'Em Up, Tesco*	1 Kebab/159g	346	10.6	218	8.4	30	6.7	2
Doner, in Pitta, with Salad, Average	*1 Serving/400g*	*1020*	*64.8*	*255*	*14.2*	*14*	*16.2*	*0.8*
Donner, Meat, Babek*	1 Portion/100g	300	28	300	14.7	8.1	28	0
Lamb, & Chicken, Kofta, Tesco*	2 Koftas/38g	97	5.3	255	14.6	16.8	13.9	2
Lamb, & Chicken, Kofta, with Mixed Grains, Finest, Tesco*	1 Pack/400g	549	22.4	137	8	12	5.6	3.1
Lamb, & Chicken, Seekh, Indian Kitchen, Heated, Tesco*	½ Pack/64g	145	7.9	226	15.4	11.8	12.3	3.4
Lamb, Kofta, Citrus Tikka, Sainsbury's*	1 Kebab/84g	199	11.6	235	18.1	9.8	13.7	2.6
Lamb, Kofta, Indian Style, Waitrose*	1 Kebab/125g	266	19.8	213	12.3	5.5	15.8	1.6
Lamb, Minted, Ashfield Farm, Aldi*	1 Kebab/54g	137	9.2	254	18.5	5.7	17	0
Lamb, Minted, Shish, As prepared, Waitrose*	1 Kebab/57g	123	7.3	217	17.2	7.9	12.9	0.1
Lamb, Shami with a Mint Raita Dip, M&S*	½ Pack/90g	189	12.1	210	12.8	9.7	13.4	3.5
Lamb, Shish, Sainsbury's*	1 Kebab/85g	178	11.3	210	19.7	2.8	13.3	0.7
Lamb, Spiced Harissa, Waitrose*	1 Kebab/69g	162	9.9	235	19.1	6.9	14.3	1.3
Lamb, with Mint, Tesco*	1 Serving/80g	192	13.4	240	16	5.5	16.7	0.4
Pork, BBQ, Sainsbury's*	1 Serving/90g	65	2.2	72	11	1.4	2.4	0.9
Shish with Onions & Peppers	*1oz/28g*	*59*	*4.5*	*212*	*12.9*	*3.9*	*16.2*	*1.2*
KEDGEREE								
Average	*1oz/28g*	*48*	*2.4*	*171*	*15.9*	*7.8*	*8.7*	*0.1*
COU, M&S*	1 Pack/370g	388	8.1	105	7.6	13.7	2.2	2.1
Smoked Haddock, Big Dish, M&S*	1 Pack/450g	585	22.5	130	8.5	13	5	1.9
KETCHUP								
Barbeque, Asda*	1 Tbsp/15g	20	0	136	0.9	33	0	0
BBQ, Heinz*	1 Serving/10g	14	0	137	1.3	31.3	0.3	0.3

K

	Measure INFO/WEIGHT	per Measure KCAL	FAT	Nutrition Values per 100g / 100ml KCAL	PROT	CARB	FAT	FIBRE
KETCHUP								
Chilli, Smoked, Gran Luchito*	1 Tsp/5g	18	0	358	1.8	18.4	0.9	0
Red Green Tomatoes, Hellmann's*	1 Tbsp/15g	13	0.1	86	1.7	19	0.6	0
Sweetened with Honey, Hellmann's*	1 Tbsp/15g	11	0.1	76	1.7	16	0.5	0
Tomato, Average	*1 Tsp/5g*	*6*	*0*	*120*	*1.5*	*28.1*	*0.2*	*0.8*
Tomato, Reduced Sugar, Average	*1 Tbsp/10g*	*9*	*0.1*	*87*	*2*	*16.9*	*1.2*	*0.9*
KIDNEY								
Lamb, Fried, Average	*1oz/28g*	*53*	*2.9*	*188*	*23.7*	*0*	*10.3*	*0*
Lamb, Raw, Average	*1oz/28g*	*25*	*0.7*	*91*	*17*	*0*	*2.6*	*0*
Ox, Raw	*1oz/28g*	*22*	*0.5*	*77*	*15.1*	*0*	*1.8*	*0*
Ox, Stewed	*1oz/28g*	*39*	*1.2*	*138*	*24.5*	*0*	*4.4*	*0*
Pig, Fried	*1oz/28g*	*57*	*2.7*	*202*	*29.2*	*0*	*9.5*	*0*
Pig, Raw	*1oz/28g*	*22*	*0.7*	*77*	*14*	*0*	*2.4*	*0*
Pig, Stewed	*1oz/28g*	*43*	*1.7*	*153*	*24.4*	*0*	*6.1*	*0*
Veal, Raw, Average	*1 Serving/100g*	*99*	*3.1*	*99*	*15.8*	*0.8*	*3.1*	*0*
KIEV								
Chicken, COU, M&S*	1 Kiev/150g	188	2.7	125	15.8	10.8	1.8	0.5
Chicken, Creamy Peppercorn, Tesco*	1 Kiev/132g	290	17.3	220	13.1	12.1	13.1	0.6
Chicken, Garlic & Parsley Butter, Breaded, Waitrose*	1 Kiev/156g	375	21.3	241	17.5	11.1	13.7	1.4
Chicken, Garlic Herb Sauce, Inspirations, Birds Eye*	1 Breast/125g	305	16.5	244	12.2	18.8	13.2	0.7
Chicken, Garlic Herb, Frozen, Birds Eye*	1 Piece/91g	240	11.9	264	15.3	20.6	13.1	1
Chicken, Garlic Herb, Sainsbury's*	1 Kiev/121g	350	26.2	289	13.8	9.6	21.6	0.7
Chicken, Garlic Parsley, BGTY, Sainsbury's*	1 Kiev/125g	267	15.5	213	14.7	10.6	12.4	0.5
Chicken, Garlic Butter, HL, Tesco*	1 Kiev/106g	318	22.3	300	13.6	14	21	0.7
Chicken, Garlic, Ashfield Farm, Aldi*	1 Kiev/131g	363	25.9	277	9.5	13.8	19.8	2.9
Chicken, Garlic, Whole Breast, Asda*	1 Pack/290g	638	38	220	15.2	10.4	13.1	0
Chicken, Garlic, Wild, & Cornish Butter, Gastropub, M&S*	1 Kiev/225g	493	32.2	219	17.3	5	14.3	0.6
Chicken, Ham, Cheese, Tesco*	1 Serving/143g	307	18.6	215	14.4	9.3	13	1.3
Chicken, with Cheese & Ham Sauce, Birds Eye*	1 Breast/124g	294	14.9	237	13	19	12	0.7
Mushroom Spinach, Good Life*	1 Kiev/125g	290	14	232	6.4	24.5	11.2	3.7
Vegetable, Veggie, M&S*	1 Kiev/155g	267	15.5	172	3.4	15.9	10	2.6
Vegetarian, Chicken Style, Cheesy, Garlic, Tesco*	1 Kiev/113g	249	13.4	221	13.1	13.3	11.8	4.3
Vegetarian, Mini, Quorn*	1 Kiev/20g	41	2.2	207	14	13	11	6.5
KIMCHI								
Unpasteurised , Kim Kong*	1 Serving/15g	6	0.1	37	2.3	4.4	0.7	2.1
KIPPER								
Baked, Average	*1oz/28g*	*57*	*3.2*	*205*	*25.5*	*0*	*11.4*	*0*
Fillets in Sunflower Oil, John West*	1 Can/140g	321	23.8	229	19	0	17	0
Fillets, Raw, Average	*1 Serving/200g*	*384*	*29.1*	*192*	*14.5*	*0*	*14.6*	*0*
Fillets, Scottish, with Butter, Youngs*	1 Pack/170g	350	25.9	226	18.9	0.1	16.7	0
Fillets, Smoked with Butter, Scottish, Boil in Bag, Tesco*	1 Serving/100g	225	17.2	225	17	0	17.2	0
Grilled, Average	*1oz/28g*	*71*	*5.4*	*255*	*20.1*	*0*	*19.4*	*0*
Smoked, Average	*1 Serving/150g*	*322*	*23*	*214*	*18.9*	*0*	*15.4*	*0*
Whole, with Bone, Grilled, Average	*1 Serving/100g*	*161*	*12.2*	*161*	*12.7*	*0*	*12.2*	*0*
KIT KAT								
2 Finger, Dark, Nestle*	2 Fingers/21g	107	5.4	510	5.4	62.2	25.5	5.4
2 Finger, Nestle*	2 Fingers/21g	104	5.1	502	6.7	62.7	24.4	2.1
4 Finger, Nestle*	4 Fingers/42g	208	10.2	502	6.7	62.7	24.5	2.1
Caramac, 4 Finger, Nestle*	4 Fingers/49g	259	14.1	532	5.9	61.9	29	0.6
Chunky, Caramel, Nestle*	1 Bar/48g	259	15.3	539	5.2	58.6	31.8	0
Chunky, Double Caramel, Nestle*	½ Bar/21g	109	5.8	520	6.5	61	27.6	1
Chunky, Nestle*	1 Bar/40g	206	10.2	516	5.4	65.1	25.6	1.7
Chunky, Orange, Nestle*	1 Bar/48g	247	12.5	515	5.8	62	26.1	0
Chunky, Peanut, Nestle*	1 Bar/42g	226	13.2	537	8.4	54.9	31.5	0

K

	Measure INFO/WEIGHT	per Measure KCAL	FAT	Nutrition Values per 100g / 100ml KCAL	PROT	CARB	FAT	FIBRE
KIT KAT								
Chunky, Snack Size, Nestle*	1 Bar/26g	133	7.1	513	6.6	60.4	27.2	1.1
Cookies & Cream, 2 Finger, Nestle*	1 Bar/21g	106	5.3	507	7.6	60.9	25.4	1.4
Cookies Cream, Snap Share, Nestle*	1 Row/16g	81	4.2	522	7.2	61.5	26.9	1.5
Dark, Mint, 2 Finger, Nestle*	1 Bar/21g	105	5.3	502	5.4	60.6	25.3	5.3
Editions, Mango Passionfruit, Nestle*	1 Bar/45g	225	10.5	499	4.7	69	23.4	0
Editions, Seville Orange, Nestle*	1 Bar/45g	223	10.4	496	4.6	69.3	23	0.8
Kubes, Nestle*	1 Pack/50g	258	13.8	515	5.9	60.9	27.5	1
Lemon Drizzle, Nestle*	1 Bar/21g	105	5.1	505	6.8	63.2	24.5	2.1
Low Carb, 2 Finger, Nestle*	2 Fingers/21g	92	6.6	438	9.2	28.3	31.3	1.3
Low Carb, 4 Finger, Nestle*	1 Finger/11g	46	3.3	438	9.2	28.3	31.3	1.3
Mini, Nestle*	1 Bar/15g	75	3.9	502	7.5	59.4	26	0
Mint, 4 Finger, Nestle*	4 Fingers/48g	244	12.7	508	6	61.5	26.4	1.1
Orange, 2 Finger, Nestle*	2 Fingers/21g	107	5.6	507	5.5	61.7	26.5	0
Peanut Butter, Bites, Nestle*	4 Pieces/23g	121	6.5	525	10.8	55.3	28.3	2.1
Senses, Nestle*	1 Bar/31g	165	9.5	531	7.5	56.3	30.7	0
White, Chunky, Nestle*	1 Bar/40g	206	10.6	516	8.1	60.8	26.4	0.5
KIWI BERRY								
Tesco*	1 Serving/80g	70	0.5	87	1.2	17.6	0.6	3.2
KIWI FRUIT								
Fresh, Raw, Flesh Seeds, Average	*1 Kiwi/60g*	*29*	*0.3*	*49*	*1.1*	*10.6*	*0.5*	*1.9*
Weighed with Skin, Average	*1 Kiwi/60g*	*25*	*0.3*	*42*	*0.9*	*9.1*	*0.4*	*1.6*
KOHLRABI								
Boiled in Salted Water	*1oz/28g*	*5*	*0.1*	*18*	*1.2*	*3.1*	*0.2*	*1.9*
Raw	*1oz/28g*	*5*	*0*	*16*	*1.1*	*2.6*	*0.1*	*1.5*
KORMA								
Chicken, & Basmati Rice, Tesco*	1 Pot/350g	588	32.6	168	4.3	16.9	9.3	2.3
Chicken, & Pilau Rice, Morrisons*	1 Pack/450g	889	48.2	198	9.4	15.9	10.7	1.4
Chicken, & Rice, 95% Fat Free, Birds Eye*	1 Pack/370g	444	7	120	6.2	19.6	1.9	1.1
Chicken, & Rice, Everyday, Value, Tesco*	1 Pack/400g	625	28.9	160	7.3	13.8	7.4	2.6
Chicken, & White Rice, BGTY, Frozen, Sainsbury's*	1 Pack/375g	341	3.8	91	5.6	14.9	1	0.5
Chicken, Pilau Rice, Charlie Bigham's*	½ Pack/405g	688	38.4	170	7.3	14.7	9.5	0
Chicken, Rice, Free From, Tesco*	1 Pack/369g	565	18.8	153	8.3	17.8	5.1	1.5
Chicken, Rice, Indian Meal for Two, Sainsbury's*	1 Pack/500g	785	40.5	157	6.8	14.3	8.1	3.1
Chicken, CBY, Asda*	1 Pack/316g	518	34.8	164	11	4.2	11	1.8
Chicken, Indian Meal for 2, Finest, Tesco*	½ Pack/200g	348	24	174	10.3	6.2	12	2.5
Chicken, Indian Takeaway for One, Sainsbury's*	1 Serving/300g	498	30.9	166	13	5.3	10.3	1.6
Chicken, Indian Takeaway, Iceland*	1 Pack/400g	656	44	164	11.8	4.5	11	1.4
Chicken, Indian, Takeaway, Tesco*	½ Pack/179g	280	18.8	156	9.7	5.2	10.5	1.1
Chicken, Indian, Waitrose*	½ Pack/175g	280	17.5	160	12.4	4.7	10	1.2
Chicken, M&S*	½ Pack/200g	316	19.2	158	13.1	4.4	9.6	1
Chicken, Morrisons*	1 Pack/350g	707	46.6	202	13.6	7	13.3	0.7
Chicken, with Peshwari Coriander Rice, Finest, Tesco*	1 Pack/550g	908	48.4	165	7.5	13.9	8.8	0.9
Chicken, with Pilau Rice, Co-Op*	1 Pack/450g	783	44.6	174	7.4	13	9.9	1.8
Chicken, with Pilau Rice, PB, Waitrose*	1 Pack/400g	452	6.8	113	8.9	15.4	1.7	1.3
Chicken, with Pilau Rice, Taste of India, Frozen, Tesco*	1 Pack/374g	478	16.7	128	6.6	14.9	4.5	0.7
Chicken, with Pilau Rice, Taste of India, Tesco*	1 Pack/426g	609	28.1	143	8.1	11.5	6.6	2.8
Chicken, with Rice, Ready Meal	*1 Pack/400g*	*740*	*34.7*	*185*	*8.4*	*18.1*	*8.7*	*1.7*
Chicken, with Rice, Ready Meal, Healthy Range	*1 Serving/400g*	*450*	*8.2*	*112*	*7.3*	*16.1*	*2.1*	*1.2*
Vegetable, Ready to Cook, Fresh, Sainsbury's*	½ Pack/255g	263	17.3	103	2.8	7.7	6.8	2.1
Vegetable, Roasted, Balanced for You, M&S*	1 Pack/355g	433	10.6	122	9.4	12.2	3	4.3
Vegetable, Takeaway or Restaurant	*1 Serving/300g*	*336*	*13.5*	*112*	*3.4*	*15.4*	*4.5*	*2.6*
KRISPROLLS								
Cracked Wheat, Original, Pagen*	1 Krisproll/13g	48	0.9	380	12	67	7	9

K

	Measure INFO/WEIGHT	per Measure KCAL	per Measure FAT	Nutrition Values per 100g / 100ml KCAL	PROT	CARB	FAT	FIBRE
KRISPROLLS								
Golden, Swedish Toasts, Pagen*	1 Krisproll/12g	48	1	400	11	69	8.5	5
Organic, Bio, Pagen*	1 Krisproll/12g	46	0.8	380	12	67	7	8
Swedish Toasts, Wholegrain, Pagen*	1 Toast/13g	51	0.8	390	11	67	6.5	8.5
KULFI								
Average	*1oz/28g*	*119*	*11.2*	*424*	*5.4*	*11.8*	*39.9*	*0.6*
KUMQUATS								
Raw	*1 Kumquat/20g*	*9*	*0.1*	*43*	*0.9*	*9.3*	*0.5*	*3.8*
KUNG PO								
Chicken, Sainsbury's*	½ Pack/175g	131	4.4	75	9.2	4	2.5	1
Chicken, Waitrose*	1 Pack/350g	318	3.9	91	8.2	12.1	1.1	1.2

K

LAGER

	INFO/WEIGHT	KCAL	FAT	KCAL	PROT	CARB	FAT	FIBRE
Alcohol Free, Becks*	1 Serving/275ml	55	0	20	0.7	5	0	0
Alcohol Free, Heineken*	1 Can/330ml	69	0	21	0	4.8	0	0
Amstel, Heineken*	1 Pint/568ml	227	0	40	0.5	3	0	0
Average	*½ Pint/284ml*	*117*	*0*	*41*	*0.3*	*3.1*	*0*	*0*
Basics, Sainsbury's*	1 Can/440g	71	0	16	0	1	0	0
Becks*	1 Can/275ml	113	0	41	0	3	0	0
Blanc, Kronenbourg*	½ pt/284ml	119	0	42	0	3.3	0	0
Boston, Samuel Adams*	1 Bottle/355ml	160	0	45	0	0	0	0
Bottled, Brahma*	1 Bottle/330ml	125	0	38	0	0	0	0
Budweiser, 66, Anheuser-Busch*	1 Bottle/330ml	102	0	31	0	0	0	0
C2, Carling*	½ Pint/284ml	80	0	28	0	3.5	0	0
Can, Carlsberg*	1 Can/440ml	141	0	32	0	2	0	0
Draught, Carling*	1 Pint/568ml	189	0	33	0	1.4	0	0
Export, Carlsberg*	1 Can/440ml	185	0	42	0.4	2.8	0	0.4
Export, Foster's*	1 Pint/568ml	210	0	37	0	2.2	0	0
Foster's*	1 Pint/568ml	193	0	34	0	3.1	0	0
German, Low Alcohol, Sainsbury's*	1 Bottle/330ml	92	0.3	28	0.4	5.9	0.1	0.1
Gold, Foster's, Heineken*	1 Can/440ml	145	0	33	0.3	1.2	0	0
Grolsch*	1 Sm Can/330ml	145	0	44	0	2.2	0	0
Heineken v 5, Heineken*	1 Pint/568ml	256	0	45	0.5	3	0	0
Heineken*, 5%, Heineken*	1 Bottle/250ml	110	0	44	0.4	3.4	0	0
Innis Gunn*	1 Bottle/330ml	132	0	40	0.3	3.5	0	0
Kaliber, Guinness*	1 Can/440ml	110	0	25	0.2	6	0	0
Kîlsch, Fr¼h*	1 Glass/200ml	112	0	56	0.5	4	0	0
Light, Coors*	1 Pint/568ml	170	0	30	0.3	1.5	0	0
Light, Corona*	1 Bottle/330ml	105	0	32	1.5	0	0	0
Lite, Carlsberg*	1 Bottle/330ml	89	0	27	0.1	0.5	0	0
Low Alcohol	*1 Can/440ml*	*44*	*0*	*10*	*0.2*	*1.5*	*0*	*0*
Organic, Tesco*	1 Bottle/500ml	215	0	43	0.2	3.5	0	0
Pils, Holsten*	1 Can/440ml	167	0	38	0.3	2.4	0	0
Pilsner, Efes*	1 Can/500ml	226	0	45	0	7.6	0	0
Pilsner, Premium, Bavaria*	1 Bottle/330ml	142	0	43	0.4	3.5	0	0
Polish, Tyskie*	1 Can/549ml	236	0	43	0	0	0	0
Premier, Kronenbourg*	½ Pint/284ml	136	0	48	0	0	0	0
Premium	*1 Can/440ml*	*260*	*0*	*59*	*0.3*	*2.4*	*0*	*0*
Premium, French, Biere Speciale, Tesco*	1 Serving/250ml	105	0	42	0.3	3.3	0	0
Premium, Light, Amstel*	1 Can/355ml	95	0	27	0	1.4	0	0
Premium, San Miguel*	1 Bottle/330ml	148	0	45	0.3	3.7	0	0
Premium, Tesco*	1 Can/440ml	145	0	33	0.3	4	0	0
Shandy, Traditional Style, Asda*	1 Serving/200ml	44	0	22	0	4.6	0	0
Skinny Brands*	1 Bottle/330ml	89	0.3	27	0	0.9	0.1	0
Stella Artois*	1 Can/550ml	220	0	40	0.4	3.1	0	0
Tuborg Green, Carlsberg*	1 Serving/200ml	78	0	39	0.5	2.5	0	0
Vier, Becks*	1 Bottle/275ml	110	0	40	0	3	0	0

LAKSA

	INFO/WEIGHT	KCAL	FAT	KCAL	PROT	CARB	FAT	FIBRE
Chicken Coconut Noodle, Cooked, Tesco*	1 Pack/351g	321	10.6	91	7.1	8.4	3	1.2
Chicken Prawn, Asian, Waitrose*	1 Pack/380g	505	19.8	133	4.6	15.7	5.2	2.3
Chicken, King Prawn, Chargrilled, Taste Singapore, M&S*	1 Pack/400g	436	21.2	109	6.2	8.7	5.3	0.9
Chicken, COU, M&S*	1 Pack/450g	360	9.9	80	7.5	7	2.2	1.1
Thai Noodle, with Chicken, M&S*	1 Pack/400g	460	21.6	115	7	9.8	5.4	1.1

LAMB

	INFO/WEIGHT	KCAL	FAT	KCAL	PROT	CARB	FAT	FIBRE
Breast, Lean, Roasted, Average	*1 Serving/100g*	*273*	*18.5*	*273*	*26.7*	*0*	*18.5*	*0*
Chops, Average	*1 Chop/82g*	*190*	*13.4*	*231*	*20.6*	*0.4*	*16.4*	*0*

L

INFO/WEIGHT	Measure	per Measure KCAL	FAT	Nutrition Values per 100g / 100ml KCAL	PROT	CARB	FAT	FIBRE

LAMB

	Measure INFO/WEIGHT	KCAL	FAT	KCAL	PROT	CARB	FAT	FIBRE
Chops, Minted, Average	1 Chop/100g	260	15.1	260	25.9	5.1	15.1	0.3
Cutlets, Neck, Raw, Lean Fat, Weighed with Bone	1 Pack 210g	359	31.7	171	8.8	0	15.1	0
Diced, From Supermarket, Healthy Range, Average	½ Pack/200g	277	8.9	138	24.6	0.1	4.5	0
Grill Steak, Average	1oz/28g	70	4.7	250	20.2	4.4	16.9	0.4
Grill Steak, Prime, Average	1 Steak/63g	197	16.1	312	18.5	2	25.5	0.1
Leg, Joint, Raw, Average	1 Joint/510g	858	45.5	168	20.9	1.4	8.9	0.2
Leg, Roasted, Lean & Fat, Average	1oz/28g	66	3.8	237	28.6	0	13.6	0
Leg, Roasted, Lean, Average	1oz/28g	58	2.7	206	29.9	0	9.6	0
Loin, Chop, Grilled, Lean Fat, Weighed with Bone	1 Serving/100g	193	14	193	16.8	0	14	0
Loin, Chops, Raw, Lean Fat, Weighed with Bone	1 Serving/100g	216	17.9	216	13.7	0	17.9	0
Mince, Average	1oz/28g	58	4.2	207	17.6	0.5	14.8	0
Mince, Extra Lean, Sainsbury's*	1 Serving/225g	324	11.9	144	24.1	0	5.3	0.1
Neck Fillet, Lean, Raw	1 Serving/100g	232	17.6	232	18.4	0	17.6	0
Rack, Raw, Lean & Fat	1oz/28g	79	6.7	283	17.3	0	23.8	0
Rack, Raw, Lean Only, Weighed with Bone	1oz/28g	21	1.1	73	8.6	0	4	0
Rack, Roasted, Lean	1oz/28g	63	3.6	225	27.1	0	13	0
Rack, Roasted, Lean & Fat	1oz/28g	102	8.4	363	23	0	30.1	0
Shank, Just Cook, Sainsbury's*	1 Shank/225g	394	18.7	175	22.9	1.8	8.3	0
Shanks, Slow Cook, Wine & Rosemary Gravy, Sainsbury's*	½ Pack/265g	374	15.1	141	19.8	2.6	5.7	0.5
Shoulder, Cooked, Lean & Fat	1oz/28g	84	6.3	301	24.4	0	22.5	0
Shoulder, Fillet, Average	1oz/28g	66	5.1	235	17.6	0	18.3	0
Shoulder, Raw, Average	1oz/28g	70	5.7	248	16.8	0	20.2	0
Shoulder, Roasted, Whole, Lean	1oz/28g	61	3.4	218	27.2	0	12.1	0
Sliced, in Rich Mint Gravy, Iceland*	½ Pack/150g	164	6.9	109	11.9	4.5	4.6	0.6
Steak, Leg, Raw, Average	1 Steak/150g	169	5.5	112	20	0	3.6	0
Steak, Minted, Average	1 Steak/125g	212	9	170	22.7	3.4	7.2	0.9
Steak, Raw, Average	1 Steak/140g	190	7.6	136	21.7	0.2	5.4	0
Stewing, Raw, Lean & Fat	1oz/28g	57	3.5	203	22.5	0	12.6	0
Stewing, Stewed, Lean	1oz/28g	67	4.1	240	26.6	0	14.8	0
Stewing, Stewed, Lean & Fat	1oz/28g	78	5.6	279	24.4	0	20.1	0
Trimmed Fat, Raw, Average	1 Serving/100g	518	51.6	518	13.3	0	51.6	0

LAMB IN

	Measure INFO/WEIGHT	KCAL	FAT	KCAL	PROT	CARB	FAT	FIBRE
Garlic Rosemary Gravy, Shank, Asda*	1 Shank/280g	451	23.2	161	19.8	1.7	8.3	0.5
Rich Minted Gravy, Shank, Morrisons*	1 Pack/400g	612	26.4	153	18.8	5.2	6.6	0

LAMB MOROCCAN

	Measure INFO/WEIGHT	KCAL	FAT	KCAL	PROT	CARB	FAT	FIBRE
with Cous Cous, PB, Waitrose*	1 Pack/400g	390	5.2	98	7.7	13.6	1.3	2.2

LAMB WITH

	Measure INFO/WEIGHT	KCAL	FAT	KCAL	PROT	CARB	FAT	FIBRE
Mint Butter, Leg Steaks, Waitrose*	1 Serving/155g	270	16.3	174	19.6	0.4	10.5	0
Mint Gravy, Leg Chops, Tesco*	1 Serving/175g	214	9.8	122	15	3.2	5.6	1.7

LANGOUSTINE

	Measure INFO/WEIGHT	KCAL	FAT	KCAL	PROT	CARB	FAT	FIBRE
Fishmongers, Frozen, Tesco*	½ Pack/229g	262	5.3	114	23	0.1	2.3	0.5

LARD

	Measure INFO/WEIGHT	KCAL	FAT	KCAL	PROT	CARB	FAT	FIBRE
Average	1oz/28g	249	27.7	891	0	0	99	0

LASAGNE

	Measure INFO/WEIGHT	KCAL	FAT	KCAL	PROT	CARB	FAT	FIBRE
Al Forno, Heated, Finest, Tesco*	1 Pack/400g	608	29.2	158	9.8	11.8	7.6	1.5
Al Forno, TTD, Sainsbury's*	1 Pack/400g	550	24.4	142	8.9	11.7	6.3	1.5
Asda*	1 Pack/398g	502	23.9	126	7.3	10.6	6	1.1
Beef, & Chunky Vegetable, HL, Tesco*	1 Pack/360g	356	8.9	99	6.5	12	2.5	1.2
Beef, Italian Veg, Musclefood*	1 Serving/380g	471	16	124	10.5	9.4	4.2	3
Beef, al Forno, Cooked, 1, Waitrose*	1 Pack/400g	663	34.7	170	9.5	12.2	8.9	1.7
Beef, BGTY, Sainsbury's*	1 Pack/390g	380	11.1	103	6.8	10.8	3	2.8
Beef, Calorie Controlled, As Prepared, Love Life, Waitrose*	1 Pack/400g	341	7.1	91	6.7	10.6	1.9	2.4
Beef, Cooked, Italian, Sainsbury's*	1 Serving/375g	555	32.2	148	7.8	6.8	8.6	6.7

L

	Measure INFO/WEIGHT	per Measure KCAL	FAT	Nutrition Values per 100g / 100ml KCAL	PROT	CARB	FAT	FIBRE
LASAGNE								
Beef, COU, M&S*	1 Pack/365g	394	9.1	108	6.6	13.9	2.5	1.7
Beef, Frozen, Eat Smart, Morrisons*	1 Pack/315g	343	10.4	109	5.9	13.1	3.3	1.4
Beef, Frozen, Tesco*	1 Pack/450g	608	25.2	135	7.5	12.6	5.6	0.8
Beef, GF, M&S*	1 Pack/400g	668	30.8	167	7.2	16.6	7.7	1.2
Beef, HFC, Tesco*	1 Pack/400g	552	26.8	138	5.8	13	6.7	1.5
Beef, Italian, Classic, Tesco*	1 Pack/600g	948	51	158	7.5	12.7	8.5	0.5
Beef, Meal to Share, 1kg, M&S*	1/3 Pack/333g	509	28	153	7.9	10.4	8.4	2
Beef, Meal to Share, 800g, M&S*	½ Pack/400g	644	33.2	161	8	12.7	8.3	1.6
Beef, Ready Meal, Average	*1 Serving/400g*	*553*	*24*	*138*	*8.2*	*12.7*	*6*	*1.4*
Beef, Ready Meals, Waitrose*	1 Pack/400g	444	20.5	111	5.8	10.4	5.1	0.8
Beef, Serves 2, TTD, Sainsbury's*	½ Pack/400g	626	31.9	159	8.4	12.1	8.1	1.7
Bolognese, Lidl*	1 Serving/200g	336	18	168	8	13.7	9	0
Charlie Bigham's*	½ Pack/369g	601	33.9	163	6.8	10.5	9.2	0
Extra Special, Asda*	½ Pack/291g	416	20.4	143	7	13	7	0.3
Family, Big Value Pack, Iceland*	¼ Pack/237g	322	14	136	5	15.9	5.9	1.4
Mushroom, & Spinach, Waitrose*	1 Pack/400g	373	14	93	3.1	12.3	3.5	1.3
Noci, Allplants*	½ Pack/380g	440	20.1	116	3.5	11	5.3	2.2
Primana, Aldi*	1 Serving/250g	422	22.5	169	8	14	9	0
Ricotta, & Vegetable, Creamy, HL, Tesco*	1 Pack/384g	407	10.8	106	5.5	14.6	2.8	3.6
Sheets, Dry, Average	*1 Sheet/20g*	*70*	*0.3*	*349*	*11.9*	*72.1*	*1.5*	*2.9*
Spinach, & Ricotta, Finest, Tesco*	1 Pack/350g	584	37.1	167	6.1	11.7	10.6	1.2
Vegetable, Free From, Sainsbury's*	1 Pack/376g	414	10.2	110	2.2	18.3	2.7	2.2
Vegetable, Healthy Range, Average	*1 Serving/400g*	*318*	*8.2*	*80*	*3.5*	*11.8*	*2.1*	*1.5*
Vegetable, Mediterranean, COU, M&S*	1 Pack/360g	306	9.7	85	3.4	11.5	2.7	1.4
Vegetable, Ready Meal, Average	*1 Serving/400g*	*408*	*17.6*	*102*	*4.1*	*12.4*	*4.4*	*1*
Vegetable, Roasted, M&S*	1 Pack/400g	408	14.4	102	3.6	13.2	3.6	1.4
Vegetarian, Butternut Squash, Ovenbaked, Asda*	1 Pack/400g	376	13.1	92	2.4	13	3.2	0.6
Vegetarian, Meat Free, Quorn*	½ Pack/250g	251	8.8	109	4.5	13.1	3.8	2.5
Vegetarian, Vegetable, Meat Free, Tesco*	1 Pack/349g	305	5.9	87	3.6	13.4	1.7	2
LAVERBREAD								
Average	*1oz/28g*	*15*	*1*	*52*	*3.2*	*1.6*	*3.7*	*0*
LEEKS								
Boiled, Average	*1oz/28g*	*6*	*0.2*	*21*	*1.2*	*2.6*	*0.7*	*1.7*
Creamed, Frozen, Waitrose*	1 Serving/225g	115	5.4	51	1.8	5.5	2.4	0
Raw, Unprepared, Average	*1 Leek/166g*	*37*	*0.8*	*22*	*1.6*	*2.9*	*0.5*	*2.2*
LEMON								
Fresh, Raw, Average	*1 Slice/5g*	*1*	*0*	*18*	*0.9*	*2.9*	*0.3*	*2.1*
Peel, Raw, Average	*1 Tbsp/6g*	*3*	*0*	*47*	*1.5*	*16*	*0.3*	*10.6*
Zest, Average	*1 Tsp/2g*	*2*	*0*	*100*	*0*	*25*	*0*	*0*
LEMON CURD								
Average	*1 Tbsp/15g*	*44*	*0.7*	*294*	*0.7*	*62.9*	*4.7*	*0.1*
Luxury, Average	*1 Tsp/7g*	*23*	*0.6*	*326*	*2.8*	*59.7*	*8.4*	*0.1*
LEMON GRASS								
Easy, Asda*	1 Tsp/10g	5	0.1	52	0.4	7.4	1.2	5.2
Stalks, Tesco*	1 Stalk/13g	12	0.1	99	1.8	25.3	0.5	0
LEMON SOLE								
Fillets, Raw, Average	*1 Serving/220g*	*177*	*2.8*	*81*	*17*	*0.2*	*1.3*	*0.3*
Goujons, Average	*1 Serving/150g*	*359*	*18.3*	*239*	*13.9*	*18.5*	*12.2*	*1*
Grilled, Average	*1oz/28g*	*27*	*0.5*	*97*	*20.2*	*0*	*1.7*	*0*
in Breadcrumbs, Average	*1 Fillet/142g*	*322*	*17.4*	*228*	*13.7*	*15.7*	*12.3*	*1*
in White Wine Herb Butter, Fillets, M&S*	1 Pack/220g	385	27.7	175	15.1	0.1	12.6	0
Steamed, Average	*1oz/28g*	*25*	*0.3*	*91*	*20.6*	*0*	*0.9*	*0*

L

INFO/WEIGHT	Measure	per Measure		Nutrition Values per 100g / 100ml				
		KCAL	FAT	KCAL	PROT	CARB	FAT	FIBRE

LEMONADE

	Measure	KCAL	FAT	KCAL	PROT	CARB	FAT	FIBRE
7 Up, Zero, Britvic*	1 Can/330ml	6	0	2	0.1	0.1	0	0
7-Up, Light, Britvic*	1 Can/330ml	4	0	1	0.1	0.2	0	0
Average	*1 Glass/250ml*	*52*	*0.2*	*21*	*0.1*	*5*	*0.1*	*0.1*
Cloudy, Diet, Sparkling, M&S*	1 Serving/250ml	8	0.2	3	0.1	0.1	0.1	0.1
Cloudy, Sparkling, Shapers, Boots*	1 Bottle/500ml	15	0.5	3	0.1	0.3	0.1	0.2
Cloudy, Waitrose*	1 Glass/250ml	125	0	50	0	12.2	0	0
Diet, Average	*1 Glass/250ml*	*4*	*0.1*	*2*	*0.1*	*0.2*	*0*	*0*
Diet, Premium, Tesco*	1 Glass/250ml	8	0	3	0.1	0.4	0	0
Diet, Toppers, Aldi*	1 Glass/100ml	1	0	1	0	0	0	0
Diet, Traditional Style, Tesco*	1 Glass/200ml	6	0	3	0	0.8	0	0
Low Calorie, Smart Price, Asda*	1 Glass/250ml	1	0	0	0	0.1	0	0
Pink, Still, Pure Premium, Tropicana*	1 Serving/200ml	90	0	45	0.2	10	0	0.7
Pink, Zero Calories, Lucozade*	1 Bottle/380ml	8	0	2	0.1	0.1	0	0
Pure Premium, Still, Tropicana*	1 Glass/200ml	86	2	43	0.2	9.5	1	0.7
R White*	1 Glass/250ml	65	0	26	0.1	6.2	0	0
Sainsbury's*	1 Glass/250ml	52	0.2	21	0.1	4.9	0.1	0.1
Schweppes*	1 Glass/250ml	45	0	18	0	4.2	0	0
Sicilian, Sainsbury's*	1 Glass/200ml	98	0.2	49	0.1	11.5	0.1	0.1
Sicilian, The Best, Morrisons*	1 Serving/150ml	52	0.2	34	0.1	7.9	0.1	0.5
Slimline, Schweppes*	1 Glass/300ml	6	0	2	0	0	0	0
Sparkling with Spanish Lemon Juice, Waitrose*	1 Glass/250ml	85	0	34	0	8.3	0	0
Sparkling, Co-Op*	1 Can/330ml	25	0	8	0	1.5	0	0
Sparkling, Morrisons*	1 Glass/250ml	63	0	25	0	6.1	0	0
Sparkling, Sicilian, The Best, Morrisons*	1 Serving/250ml	120	0.2	48	0.4	11.1	0.1	0.4
Still, Freshly Squeezed, M&S*	½ Bottle/250ml	100	0.5	40	0.1	9	0.2	0.5
Still, Raspberry, M&S*	1 Glass/250ml	112	0	45	0.2	10.3	0	0.1
Sugar Free, Everyday Value, Tesco*	1 Glass/250ml	1	0	0	0	0	0	0
Tesco*	1 Glass/200ml	30	0	15	0	3.6	0	0
Traditional Style, Tesco*	1 Glass/200ml	100	0	50	0	12.3	0	0
TTD, Sainsbury's*	1 Serving/248g	159	0	64	0.1	14.8	0	0.2
Victorian, Fentiman's*	1 Bottle/275ml	130	0	47	0	11.3	0	0

LEMSIP

	Measure	KCAL	FAT	KCAL	PROT	CARB	FAT	FIBRE
Beechams*	1 Sachet/3g	11	0	387	0	100	0	0

LENTILS

	Measure	KCAL	FAT	KCAL	PROT	CARB	FAT	FIBRE
Black Beluga, Ready to Eat, Merchant Gourmet*	1 Serving/63g	92	0.8	147	10.9	20.5	1.2	5.2
Good Grains, Aldi*	1 Pack/250g	242	5.2	97	6.6	10	2.1	5
Green & Brown, Dried, Boiled in Salted Water, Average	*1 Tbsp/30g*	*32*	*0.2*	*105*	*8.8*	*16.9*	*0.7*	*3.8*
Green or Brown in Water, Tinned, Average	*½ Can/132g*	*131*	*0.8*	*99*	*8.1*	*15.4*	*0.6*	*3.8*
Green or Brown, Dried, Average	*1 Serving/50g*	*150*	*0.8*	*301*	*22.8*	*49.8*	*1.5*	*9.6*
Puy, Green, Dry, Average	*1 Serving/100g*	*306*	*1.4*	*306*	*24.7*	*49.5*	*1.4*	*10.3*
Red, Boiled in Unsalted Water, Average	*1oz/28g*	*28*	*0.1*	*102*	*7.6*	*17.5*	*0.4*	*2.6*
Red, Split, Wholefoods, Tesco*	1 Serving/80g	81	0.3	102	7.6	16	0.4	1.9

LETTUCE

	Measure	KCAL	FAT	KCAL	PROT	CARB	FAT	FIBRE
Average, Raw	*½ Cup/28g*	*4*	*0.1*	*13*	*1*	*1.7*	*0.3*	*1.1*
Curly Leaf, Sainsbury's*	1 Serving/80g	11	0.4	14	0.8	1.7	0.5	0
Lamb's, Average	*1 Serving/80g*	*12*	*0.2*	*14*	*1.4*	*1.6*	*0.2*	*1*
Little Gem, Average	*1 Lettuce/90g*	*14*	*0.4*	*15*	*0.8*	*1.8*	*0.5*	*0.7*
Radicchio, Red, Raw, Average	*1 Head/220g*	*29*	*0.2*	*13*	*1.4*	*1.6*	*0.1*	*3*
Red Gem, Tesco*	½ Lettuce/45g	7	0.2	15	0.8	1.7	0.5	0.9
Romaine, Average	*1 Serving/80g*	*12*	*0.4*	*15*	*0.9*	*1.7*	*0.5*	*0.7*
Romaine, Hearts, Average	*1 Serving/80g*	*12*	*0.4*	*16*	*0.9*	*1.7*	*0.6*	*1*
Romaine, Sweet, Average	*1 Serving/80g*	*12*	*0.4*	*16*	*0.9*	*1.6*	*0.6*	*0.8*
Round, Average	*1 Serving/80g*	*10*	*0.2*	*13*	*1.4*	*2.2*	*0.2*	*1.1*

L

	Measure INFO/WEIGHT	per Measure KCAL	FAT	Nutrition Values per 100g / 100ml KCAL	PROT	CARB	FAT	FIBRE
LETTUCE								
Sweet Gem, TTD, Sainsbury's*	1 Serving/100g	15	0.5	15	0.8	1.7	0.5	0.9
LILT								
Fruit Crush, Coca-Cola*	1 Can/330ml	66	0	20	0	4.6	0	0
Fruit Crush, Zero, Coca-Cola*	1 Can/330ml	12	0	4	0	0.3	0	0
Z, Coca-Cola*	1 Can/330ml	10	0	3	0	0.4	0	0
LIME								
Peel, Raw	*1 Tbsp/6g*	*3*	*0*	*47*	*1.5*	*16*	*0.3*	*10.6*
Raw, Flesh Only, Average	*1 Lime/71g*	*18*	*0.1*	*25*	*0.6*	*8.8*	*0.2*	*2.4*
Raw, Weighed with Peel & Seeds, Average	*1 Lime/85g*	*21*	*0.1*	*25*	*0.6*	*8.9*	*0.2*	*2.4*
Zest, Average	*1 Tsp/2g*	*2*	*0*	*100*	*0*	*25*	*0*	*0*
LINGUINE								
Cooked	*1 Serving/100g*	*133*	*0.7*	*133*	*5.1*	*26.3*	*0.7*	*1.1*
Crab, Rocket Chilli, Italian, Heated, Finest, Tesco*	1 Serving/352g	410	12.7	117	5.7	14.8	3.6	1
Dry, Average	*1 Serving/100g*	*352*	*2.2*	*352*	*13.1*	*70*	*2.2*	*2.8*
Fresh, Dry, Average	*1 Pack/250g*	*681*	*6.5*	*272*	*12.3*	*51.7*	*2.6*	*4*
King Prawn, COU, M&S*	1 Meal/360g	400	9	111	5.9	16.4	2.5	0.8
Prawn, in a White Wine Sauce, Microwaved, HL, Tesco*	1 Pack/340g	326	7.5	96	4.5	14.2	2.2	0.8
Smoked Salmon, Sainsbury's*	1 Serving/400g	586	28.8	146	6.2	14.2	7.2	1.2
with Scallops, Pancetta Peas, Spirit of Summer, M&S*	1 Pack/380g	521	14.8	137	7	17.6	3.9	1.8
LINSEEDS								
Average	*1 Tsp/5g*	*23*	*1.7*	*464*	*21.7*	*18.5*	*33.5*	*26.3*
LION BAR								
Mini, Nestle*	1 Bar/16g	80	3.6	486	4.6	67.7	21.7	0
Nestle*	1 Bar/52g	248	11.2	478	6.5	64.6	21.6	0
Peanut, Nestle*	1 Bar/40g	195	10	488	8.1	57.1	25	2.3
LIQUEURS								
Amaretto, Average	*1 Pub Shot/25ml*	*97*	*0*	*388*	*0*	*60*	*0*	*0*
Aperol, Cocktail Mixer, Aperol*	1 Serving/150ml	142	0	95	0	6.7	0	0
Chambord*	1 Serving/35ml	79	0	225	0	29.3	0	0
Cointreau, Specialite De France	*1 Serving/37ml*	*80*	*0*	*215*	*0*	*8.5*	*0*	*0*
Cream, Average	*1 Shot/25ml*	*81*	*4*	*325*	*0*	*22.8*	*16.1*	*0*
Grand Marnier*	1 Pub Shot/35ml	94	0	268	0	22.9	0	0
High Strength, Average	*1 Shot/25ml*	*78*	*0*	*314*	*0*	*24.4*	*0*	*0*
Kirsch, Average	*1 Shot/25ml*	*67*	*0*	*267*	*0*	*20*	*0*	*0*
LIQUORICE								
Allsorts, Average	*1 Sm Bag/56g*	*195*	*2.9*	*349*	*3.7*	*76.7*	*5.2*	*2*
Allsorts, Bassett's*	1 Pack/225g	855	11	380	5.6	77.8	4.9	1.6
Catherine Wheels, Barratt*	1 Wheel/22g	65	0.1	290	3.8	67.2	0.3	0.7
Catherine Wheels, Sainsbury's*	1 Wheel/17g	49	0.1	286	3.8	67.2	0.3	0.7
Log, Raspberry, Choc, RJ's Licorice Ltd*	1 Log/45g	178	4.5	395	3.9	74	10	0.9
Panda*	1 Bar/32g	109	0.2	340	3.8	78	0.5	0
Shapes, Average	*1oz/28g*	*78*	*0.4*	*278*	*5.5*	*65*	*1.4*	*1.9*
Soft Eating, Australia, Darrell Lea*	1 Piece/20g	68	0.4	338	2.8	76.1	1.9	0
Torpedos, Panda*	1 Serving/25g	92	0	366	1.9	88	0.2	1.4
LIVER								
Calves, Fried	*1oz/28g*	*49*	*2.7*	*176*	*22.3*	*0*	*9.6*	*0*
Calves, Raw	*1oz/28g*	*29*	*1*	*104*	*18.3*	*0*	*3.4*	*0*
Chicken, Cooked, Simmered, Average	*1 Serving/100g*	*167*	*6.5*	*167*	*24.5*	*0.9*	*6.5*	*0*
Chicken, Fried, Average	*1oz/28g*	*47*	*2.5*	*169*	*22.1*	*0*	*8.9*	*0*
Chicken, Raw, Average	*1oz/28g*	*26*	*0.6*	*92*	*17.7*	*0*	*2.3*	*0*
Lamb's, Braised, Average	*1 Serving/100g*	*220*	*8.8*	*220*	*30.6*	*2.5*	*8.8*	*0*
Lamb's, Fried, Average	*1oz/28g*	*66*	*3.6*	*237*	*30.1*	*0*	*12.9*	*0*
Lamb's, Raw, Average	*1 Serving/125g*	*171*	*7.8*	*137*	*20.3*	*0*	*6.2*	*0*

L

	Measure INFO/WEIGHT	per Measure KCAL	FAT	Nutrition Values per 100g / 100ml KCAL	PROT	CARB	FAT	FIBRE
LIVER								
Ox, Raw	*1oz/28g*	*43*	*2.2*	*155*	*21.1*	*0*	*7.8*	*0*
Ox, Stewed	1oz/28g	55	2.7	198	24.8	3.6	9.5	0
Pig's, Raw	*1oz/28g*	*32*	*0.9*	*113*	*21.3*	*0*	*3.1*	*0*
Pig's, Stewed	1 Serving/70g	132	5.7	189	25.6	3.6	8.1	0
Veal, Deluxe, Lidl*	1 Slice/150g	188	5.2	125	19.6	3.8	3.5	0
LIVER & BACON								
Onions, Cook*	1 Portion/280g	372	21.3	133	11.8	4.3	7.6	0.5
Meal for One, M&S*	1 Pack/452g	430	16.7	95	7	8	3.7	1.2
with Fresh Mashed Potato, Waitrose*	1 Pack/400g	416	17.2	104	7.3	9	4.3	1.3
with Mash, Mini Meals, Tesco*	1 Pack/234g	262	9.1	112	5.8	12.9	3.9	1.1
with Mash, Serves 1, Classic, Sainsbury's*	1 Pack/450g	448	18.7	103	6.4	8.6	4.3	2.5
LIVER SAUSAGE								
Average	*1 Slice/10g*	*22*	*1.5*	*216*	*15.3*	*4.4*	*15.2*	*0.2*
LLAMA								
Steak, Average	*1 Steak/150g*	*158*	*2*	*105*	*23*	*0.2*	*1.3*	*0*
LOBSTER								
Boiled, Average	*1oz/28g*	*29*	*0.4*	*103*	*22.1*	*0*	*1.6*	*0*
Dressed, Canned, John West*	1 Can/43g	45	2.1	105	13	2	5	0
Raw, Average	*1 Serving/100g*	*92*	*1.4*	*92*	*18.7*	*0.3*	*1.4*	*0*
Thermidor, M&S*	1 Serving/140g	287	19.2	205	10.7	9.7	13.7	0
LOGANBERRIES								
Raw	*1oz/28g*	*5*	*0*	*17*	*1.1*	*3.4*	*0*	*2.5*
LOLLIPOPS								
Assorted, Co-Op*	1 Lolly/10g	40	0	400	0	97	0	0
Chupa Chups*	1 Lolly/12g	47	0	388	0	95	0.3	0
Cremosa, Sugar Free, Chupa Chups*	1 Lolly/10g	28	0.5	275	0.2	92.5	5.4	0
Drumsticks, Swizzels*	1 Lolly/12g	50	0.7	413	0.4	87.9	6.1	0
Refreshers, Bassett's*	1 Lolly/6g	25	0	417	0	108.3	0	0
LOQUATS								
Raw	*1oz/28g*	*5*	*0*	*18*	*0.4*	*4*	*0.1*	*0*
LOZENGES								
Blackcurrant Flavour, Fishermans Friend, Lofthouses*	1 Lozenge/1g	3	0	251	0.1	97.2	1.3	0
Original Extra Strong, Fishermans Friend, Lofthouses*	1 Lozenge/1g	4	0	382	0.3	94.9	0	0.5
Original, Victory V*	1 Lozenge/3g	9	0	350	0	91	0	0
LUCOZADE								
Caribbean Crush, Energy, Lucozade*	1 Bottle/380ml	217	0	57	0	13.9	0	0
Energy, Original, GlaxoSmithKline UK Limited*	1 Bottle/380ml	266	0	70	0	17.2	0	0
Orange Energy Drink, GlaxoSmithKline UK Limited*	1 Bottle/500ml	350	0	70	0	17.2	0	0
Orange, Sport Lite, GlaxoSmithKline UK Limited*	1 Serving/500g	50	0	10	0	2	0	0
Raspberry Sport Body Fuel, GlaxoSmithKline UK Limited*	1 Bottle/500ml	140	0	28	0	6.4	0	0
Summer Berries, Sport, Lite, GlaxoSmithKline UK Limited*	1 Serving/200ml	20	0	10	0	2	0	0
Tropical, GlaxoSmithKline UK Limited*	1 Bottle/380ml	266	0	70	0	17.2	0	0
Zero Calories, Lucozade*	1 Serving/250ml	10	0	4	0.1	0.5	0	0
LUNCHEON MEAT								
Pork, Average	*1oz/28g*	*81*	*6.8*	*288*	*13.3*	*4*	*24.3*	*0*
LYCHEES								
Fresh, Raw, Flesh Only	*1oz/28g*	*16*	*0*	*58*	*0.9*	*14.3*	*0.1*	*0.7*
in Juice, Amoy*	1oz/28g	13	0	46	0.4	10.9	0	0
in Syrup, Average	*1oz/28g*	*19*	*0*	*69*	*0.4*	*17.7*	*0*	*0.4*
Raw, Weighed with Skin & Stone	*1oz/28g*	*6*	*0*	*22*	*0.3*	*5.5*	*0.1*	*0.2*

L

	Measure INFO/WEIGHT	per Measure KCAL	FAT	Nutrition Values per 100g / 100ml KCAL	PROT	CARB	FAT	FIBRE
M&M'S								
Crispy, Mars*	1 Serving/36g	179	8.8	498	4.1	63.9	24.4	2.7
Mars*	1 Pack/45g	218	9.7	485	5	68	21.5	0
Mini, Mars*	1 Sm Pack/36g	176	8.4	489	6.3	63.6	23.2	0
Peanut Butter, Mars*	1 Pack/46g	240	14	520	8.7	56.3	30.3	2.2
Peanut, Mars*	1 Pack/45g	228	11.4	506	9.4	60.1	25.4	2.7
MACADAMIA NUTS								
Plain, Average	*1 Pack/100g*	*750*	*77.6*	*750*	*7.9*	*4.8*	*77.6*	*5.3*
Roasted, Salted, Average	*6 Nuts/10g*	*75*	*7.8*	*748*	*7.9*	*4.8*	*77.6*	*5.3*
MACARONI								
Dry, Average	*1oz/28g*	*99*	*0.5*	*354*	*11.9*	*73.5*	*1.7*	*2.6*
MACARONI CHEESE								
Jack Fruit, Love Your Veg!, Sainsbury's*	1 Pack/384g	537	22.2	140	5.3	15.1	5.8	2.8
Leeks, with Smoked Cheddar Crumb, Veggie, M&S*	1 Pack/400g	748	39.6	187	7	16.9	9.9	1.3
Bites, Mac N Cheese, Crispy, M&S*	½ Pack/100g	255	13.8	255	7.9	23.9	13.8	1.6
Canned	*1oz/28g*	*39*	*1.8*	*138*	*4.5*	*16.4*	*6.5*	*0.4*
Cheddar, Vintage, Rich Creamy, TTD, Sainsbury's*	1 Pack/375g	703	33.5	197	8.2	18.8	9.4	2.1
Chilled, HFC, Tesco*	1 Pack/400g	540	14.3	135	5.6	18	4.1	1.9
Creamy, Weight Watchers*	1 Pack/360g	344	9.7	96	4.4	12.9	2.7	1
Italian, Tesco*	1 Pack/450g	764	25.8	169	7.3	21.6	5.7	1.1
Meal for One, M&S*	1 Pack/400g	684	30.8	171	7.7	17.3	7.7	0.6
Ready Meal, Average	*1 Serving/400g*	*580*	*25.5*	*145*	*6*	*15.8*	*6.4*	*1*
Rice, GF, Amy's Kitchen*	1 Meal/255g	400	16.1	157	6.3	18	6.3	0.4
Triple, Finest, Tesco*	1 Pack/400g	645	22.2	174	7.3	22	6	1.4
Waitrose*	1 Pack/350g	466	32.9	133	6.8	5.2	9.4	0
with Pancetta, Crispy, Charlie Bigham's*	1 Pack/340g	740	44.8	205	9.3	13.7	12.4	0
MACAROONS								
Coconut, Tesco*	1 Macaroon/33g	143	6.3	432	4.5	58	19	5.5
French, Average	*1 Serving/60g*	*225*	*11*	*375*	*6.7*	*46.7*	*18.3*	*3.3*
MACKEREL								
Atlantic, Raw, Average	*1 Fillet/75g*	*154*	*10.4*	*205*	*18.6*	*0*	*13.9*	*0*
Fillets, in a Hot Chilli Dressing, Princes*	1 Pack/125g	370	33.8	296	13.3	0	27	0
Fillets, in Brine, Average	*1 Can/88g*	*206*	*15.3*	*234*	*19.4*	*0*	*17.4*	*0*
Fillets, in Curry Sauce, John West*	1 Can/125g	275	20.8	220	14.2	3.5	16.6	0.2
Fillets, in Hot Smoked Peppered, Asda*	1 Fillet/100g	341	28	341	19	3.3	28	0.6
Fillets, in Mustard Sauce, Average	*1 Can/125g*	*274*	*19.4*	*219*	*14.1*	*5.4*	*15.5*	*0*
Fillets, in Olive Oil, Average	*1 Serving/50g*	*149*	*12.2*	*298*	*18.5*	*1*	*24.4*	*0*
Fillets, in Spicy Tomato Sauce, Average	*1oz/28g*	*56*	*3.9*	*199*	*14.3*	*3.8*	*14*	*0*
Fillets, in Sunflower Oil, Average	*1 Can/94g*	*262*	*20.6*	*279*	*20.2*	*0.2*	*21.9*	*0.2*
Fillets, in Teriyaki Sauce, Boneless & Skinless, Tesco*	1 Can/125g	320	20.3	255	12.6	13.4	16.2	2
Fillets, in Tomato Sauce, Average	*1 Can/125g*	*251*	*18.3*	*200*	*14.3*	*2.7*	*14.7*	*0*
Fillets, Lemon Parsley, Smoked, Fishmonger, Aldi*	1 Pack/200g	700	60	350	19.6	0.9	30	0
Fillets, Mexican, Canned, Princes*	1 Can/125g	241	13.8	193	11.4	11.8	11	0.5
Fillets, Smoked, Average	*1 Fillet/75g*	*251*	*21.1*	*334*	*19.7*	*0.5*	*28.2*	*0.3*
Fried in Blended Oil	*1oz/28g*	*76*	*5.5*	*272*	*24*	*0*	*19.5*	*0*
Grilled	*1oz/28g*	*67*	*4.8*	*239*	*20.8*	*0*	*17.3*	*0*
King, Raw	*1 Fillet/198g*	*208*	*4*	*105*	*20.3*	*0*	*2*	*0*
Raw with Skin, Weighed with Bone, Average	*1oz/28g*	*64*	*4.7*	*227*	*18.9*	*0*	*16.8*	*0*
Smoked, Peppered, Average	*1oz/28g*	*87*	*7*	*310*	*20.4*	*0.3*	*25.2*	*0.2*
Whole, Raw, Average	*1 Serving/100g*	*156*	*11.4*	*156*	*13.3*	*0*	*11.4*	*0*
MADRAS								
Beef, Indian, Takeaway, CBY, Asda*	½ Pack/200g	246	14.2	123	8.9	4.7	7.1	2.5
Beef, Tesco*	1 Pack/460g	616	37.7	134	10.6	4.5	8.2	1.2
Beef, with Pilau Rice, Finest, Tesco*	1 Pack/418g	643	19.7	154	8.3	18.5	4.7	2.1

	Measure INFO/WEIGHT	per Measure KCAL	FAT	Nutrition Values per 100g / 100ml KCAL	PROT	CARB	FAT	FIBRE
MADRAS								
Chicken, M&S*	1 Pack/400g	492	25.2	123	12.7	2.7	6.3	2.2
Chicken, Sainsbury's*	1 Pack/400g	532	29.6	133	11	4.5	7.4	1.9
Chicken, Taste of India, Tesco*	½ Pack/215g	275	14.2	128	10.2	5.7	6.6	2.7
Chicken, Waitrose*	1 Pack/400g	672	42	168	14.6	3.7	10.5	1.8
Chicken, with Pilau Rice, Tesco*	1 Pack/372g	492	21.9	132	6.4	12.8	5.9	1.2
MAGNUM								
Almond, Mini, Wall's*	1 Mini/55g	155	9.4	281	3.9	27	17	0
Almond, Vegan, Wall's*	1 Magnum/90g	248	16.2	276	2.2	26	18	0
Almond, Wall's*	1 Magnum/73g	243	14.6	332	4.8	32	20	0
Bites, After Dinner Classic, Wall's*	1 Bite/29g	102	6.9	353	4	30	24	0
Caramel, Double, Mini, Wall's*	1 Mini/50g	174	10	348	3.2	37	20	0
Caramel, Double, Wall's*	1 Magnum/73g	246	14.6	338	3.2	36	20	0
Chocolate, Double, Mini, Wall's*	1 Mini/50g	182	11.5	365	4	33	23	0
Chocolate, Double, Wall's*	1 Magnum/69g	248	15.9	359	4.1	33	23	0
Classic, Mini, Wall's*	1 Mini/50g	168	11	336	3.7	31	22	0
Classic, Vegan, Wall's*	1 Magnum/90g	234	14.3	261	1.3	27	16	0
Classic, Wall's*	1 Magnum/79g	244	15	309	3.6	29	19	1.2
Dark, Mini, Wall's*	1 Mini/50g	165	11	329	3.8	29	22	0
Double Coconut, Wall's*	1 Magnum/88g	239	14.1	272	3.2	27	16	0
Espresso, Black, Mini, Wall's*	1 Mini/50g	159	10.5	317	3.7	29	21	0
Espresso, Black, Wall's*	1 Magnum/82g	237	15.6	289	3.4	27	19	0
Honeycomb, Wall's*	1 Magnum/78g	240	13.2	308	3.6	35	17	0
Mint, Mini, Wall's*	1 Mini/50g	165	10.5	330	4.2	30	21	0
Mint, Wall's*	1 Magnum/78g	244	14	313	3.1	33	18	0
Peanut Butter, Double, Mini, Wall's*	1 Mini/50g	173	11	346	4.3	32	22	0
Peanut Butter, Double, Wall's*	1 Magnum/73g	245	15.3	336	4.2	32	21	0
Pistachio, Wall's*	1 Magnum/75g	250	15.8	333	4.2	30	21	0
Raspberry, Pink, Mini, Wall's*	1 Mini/50g	166	11.5	332	2.9	31	23	0
Raspberry, Pink, Wall's*	1 Magnum/73g	239	15.3	328	2.9	30	21	0
Strawberry, White, Wall's*	1 Magnum/88g	250	13.2	284	3	34	15	0
White, Mini, Wall's*	1 Mini/55g	137	8.3	248	2.8	26	15	0
White, Wall's*	1 Magnum/79g	239	14.2	303	3.5	33	18	0
MAKHANI								
Chicken, Sainsbury's*	½ Pack/199g	313	21.3	157	12.2	2.9	10.7	2.5
Chicken, Tikka, Pilau Rice, BGTY, Sainsbury's*	1 Pack/400g	448	4	112	8.3	17.5	1	1.9
Chicken, Tikka, Waitrose*	1 Pack/400g	560	30.4	140	14	3.8	7.6	2.1
Prawn, King, Curry, M&S*	1 Pack/400g	732	51.6	183	8	8.1	12.9	1
Prawn, King, Finest, Tesco*	1 Pack/350g	514	38.8	147	6	6	11.1	1.3
MALTESERS								
MaltEaster, Chocolate Bunny, Mars*	1 Bunny/29g	156	9	539	6.9	57.6	31	1.2
Mars*	1 Reg Bag/37g	187	9.3	505	8	61.8	25	0.9
Mini Bunnies, Mars*	1 Bunny/12g	64	3.6	534	8	53.5	30.2	0
White Chocolate, Mars*	1 Pack/37g	186	9.4	504	7.9	61	25.4	0
MANDARIN ORANGES								
in Juice, Average	*1oz/28g*	*11*	*0*	*39*	*0.7*	*9*	*0*	*0.5*
in Light Syrup, Average	*1 Can/298g*	*201*	*0.1*	*68*	*0.6*	*16*	*0*	*0.1*
Weighed with Peel, Average	*1 Sm/50g*	*14*	*0*	*27*	*0.7*	*6.2*	*0.1*	*0.9*
MANGE TOUT								
& Sugar Snap Peas, Tesco*	1 Pack/150g	102	0.6	68	7	9.2	0.4	3.8
Boiled in Salted Water	*1oz/28g*	*7*	*0*	*26*	*3.2*	*3.3*	*0.1*	*2.2*
Raw, Average	*1 Serving/80g*	*25*	*0.2*	*31*	*3.5*	*4*	*0.2*	*1.1*
Stir-Fried in Blended Oil	*1oz/28g*	*20*	*1.3*	*71*	*3.8*	*3.5*	*4.8*	*2.4*

	Measure INFO/WEIGHT	per Measure KCAL	FAT	Nutrition Values per 100g / 100ml KCAL	PROT	CARB	FAT	FIBRE
MANGO								
Dried, Average	**1 Serving/50g**	**174**	**0.5**	**347**	**1.4**	**83.1**	**1**	**4.9**
in Syrup, Average	**1oz/28g**	**22**	**0**	**80**	**0.3**	**20.5**	**0**	**0.9**
Ripe, Raw, Weighed with Skin Stone, Average	**1 Mango/225g**	**60**	**0.2**	**27**	**0.3**	**6.5**	**0.1**	**1.2**
Ripe, Raw, without Peel Stone, Flesh Only, Average	**1 Mango/207g**	**118**	**0.4**	**57**	**0.7**	**14.1**	**0.2**	**2.6**
MANGOSTEEN								
Raw, Fresh, Average*	1 Serving/80g	50	0.5	63	0.6	15.6	0.6	5.1
MARINADE								
Barbeque, Sticky, Sainsbury's*	¼ Jar/77g	112	2.8	145	0.8	26.7	3.6	1
BBQ, Sticky, Newman's Own*	1/3 Jar/83ml	139	0.7	167	0.9	39	0.8	2.5
Cajun Spice, The English Provender Co.*	1 Serving/50g	94	6.7	187	1.3	15.3	13.4	1.6
Coat 'n Cook, Medium, Nando's*	1 Sachet/120g	94	5.4	78	1.1	9.6	4.5	2.8
Hickory Dickory Smokey, Ainsley Harriott*	1 Pot/300ml	360	0.3	120	0.6	28.1	0.1	0
Hoisin, Sharwoods*	¼ Jar/72g	123	0.9	171	1.5	37.6	1.3	1.4
Hot & Spicy Barbecue, M&S*	1 Serving/18g	23	0.1	130	1	31.1	0.3	0.8
Sticky Barbecue, Tesco*	¼ Jar/70g	80	0.1	115	0.7	26.7	0.2	0.6
Tandoori, Spice, Patak's*	1 Tbsp/15g	15	0.4	99	3.5	10.1	2.7	5.9
Tequila Chilli Lime, M&S*	1 Serving/75ml	116	1.2	155	0.6	34	1.6	0.5
Texan, Hickory Style, BBQ, Quick, Batts, Lidl*	1 Serving/16g	29	0.1	181	1.2	42.5	0.6	3.1
MARJORAM								
Dried	**1 Tsp/1g**	**2**	**0**	**271**	**12.7**	**42.5**	**7**	**0**
MARLIN								
Steaks, Chargrilled, Sainsbury's*	1 Steak/240g	367	14.6	153	23.6	0.8	6.1	0.6
MARMALADE								
3 Fruit, Thick Cut, Waitrose*	1 Tsp/15g	39	0	262	0.4	64.8	0.1	0.7
Blood Orange, TTD, Sainsbury's*	1 Tbsp/15g	40	0	264	0.3	65.7	0	0.8
Lemon & Lime, Average	**1 Tbsp/20g**	**53**	**0**	**267**	**0.2**	**66.4**	**0.1**	**0.4**
Lemon with Shred, Average	**1 Serving/20g**	**50**	**0**	**248**	**0.2**	**61.6**	**0**	**0.6**
Lime with Shred, Average	**1 Tbsp/15g**	**39**	**0**	**261**	**0.2**	**65**	**0.1**	**0.4**
Onion, Organic, Duchy Originals*	1 Serving/40g	103	1	257	1	57.8	2.4	2.6
Orange & Ginger, Average	**1 Tbsp/15g**	**40**	**0**	**264**	**0.2**	**65.7**	**0.1**	**0.3**
Orange & Tangerine, Tiptree, Wilkin & Sons*	1 Tsp/15g	40	0	268	0	67	0	0
Orange with Shred, Average	**1 Tsp/5g**	**13**	**0**	**263**	**0.2**	**65.2**	**0**	**0.3**
Orange, Fine Shred, Bonne Maman*	1 Tsp/5g	12	0	238	0.3	59	0.1	0.6
Orange, Reduced Sugar, Average	**1 Tbsp/15g**	**26**	**0**	**170**	**0.4**	**42**	**0.1**	**0.6**
Orange, Reduced Sugar, Thin Cut, Streamline*	1 Serving/10g	18	0	178	0.5	43	0.3	0
Orange, Seville, with Stem Ginger, Coarse Cut, M&S*	1 Tsp/5g	13	0	261	0.1	64.5	0.1	0.6
Orange, Shredless, Average	**1 Tsp/10g**	**26**	**0**	**261**	**0.2**	**65**	**0**	**0.1**
MARMITE*								
Yeast Extract, Marmite*	1 Tsp/9g	22	0	250	39	24	0.1	3.5
MARROW								
Boiled, Average	**1oz/28g**	**3**	**0.1**	**9**	**0.4**	**1.6**	**0.2**	**0.6**
Raw	**1oz/28g**	**2**	**0**	**6**	**0.3**	**1.2**	**0.1**	**0.3**
MARS								
Bar, 5 Little Ones, Mars*	1 Piece/8g	38	1.5	477	4.5	73.6	18.3	0
Bar, Duo, Mars*	1 Bar/42g	191	7.6	450	4.4	67.5	18	1.2
Bar, Funsize, Mars*	1 Bar/18g	80	3	446	3.5	70.1	16.8	1.1
Bar, Mars*	1 Std Bar/51g	229	8.7	449	4	69	17	1
Bar, Medium, 58g, Mars*	1 Bar/58g	263	10.5	453	4.6	67.9	18.1	0
Bar, Minis, Mars*	1 Bar/18g	80	11.6	444	3.3	0	64.4	1.1
Bar, Protein, Mars*	1 Bar/57g	200	4.6	351	33	39	8.1	0
Choc Brownie, Bar, Mars*	1 Bar/51g	231	9.4	452	4.6	66	18.3	0
Triple Choc, Bar, Limited Edition, Mars*	1 Bar/52g	233	9	448	4.5	67.7	17.3	2

M

MARSHMALLOWS

INFO/WEIGHT	Measure KCAL	FAT	per 100g KCAL	PROT	CARB	FAT	FIBRE
Average	*1 Mallow/5g*	*16*	*0*	*327*	*3.9*	*83.1*	*0*	*0*
Chocolate Mallows, Cadbury*	1 Mallow/13g	56	2.2	435	4.7	64.7	17.4	0.8
Dark Chocolate Covered, Mister Choc, Lidl*	1 Mallow/25g	95	2.5	380	4	68	10	0
Fat Free, Tesco*	1 Mallow/7g	24	0	339	3.4	80.8	0.2	0.5
Haribo*	1 Mallow/5g	16	0	330	3	80	0	0
No Added Sugar, Sainsbury's*	1 Mallow/2g	5	0	206	3.3	77	0.1	0
Pascall*	1 Mallow/5g	15	0	335	2.6	80	0	0
Pink White, Co-Op*	1 Mallow/7g	24	0	340	3	82	0	0
Princess*	1 Mallow/5g	16	0	314	3.4	80	0	0
Raspberry Cream, Sainsbury's*	1 Mallow/7g	23	0	330	4.1	78.5	0	0.5
Sainsbury's*	1 Mallow/7g	23	0	330	4.1	78.5	0	0.5
Snowballs, Lees*	1 Snowball/18g	79	3	432	3.4	65.2	16.6	3.9

MARZIPAN

INFO/WEIGHT	Measure KCAL	FAT	per 100g KCAL	PROT	CARB	FAT	FIBRE
Bar, Chocolate, Plain, Thorntons*	1 Bar/46g	206	8	448	5.2	69.1	17.4	2
Dark Chocolate, Thorntons*	1 Serving/46g	207	8	451	5.2	69.4	17.4	2.1
Plain, Average	*1oz/28g*	*115*	*4*	*412*	*5.8*	*67.5*	*14.2*	*1.7*

MASALA

INFO/WEIGHT	Measure KCAL	FAT	per 100g KCAL	PROT	CARB	FAT	FIBRE
Keema, Vegetable, Love Your Veg!, Sainsbury's*	1 Pack/382g	401	19.5	105	2.8	10.1	5.1	3.6
Mixed Vegetable, M&S*	½ Pack/200g	170	9	85	2.3	7.4	4.5	2.9
Paneer Butter, The City Kitchen*	½ Pack/347g	545	31.2	157	5.7	12.5	9	1.6
Prawn Mango, Waitrose*	½ Pack/175g	175	11.2	100	5.8	4.3	6.4	1.3
Vegetable, Indian, Sainsburys*	1 Pack/300g	273	17.7	91	2.2	5.5	5.9	3.7
Vegetable, Waitrose*	1 Serving/400g	288	19.2	72	2.2	4.9	4.8	2.5
Vegetable, with Cauliflower Rice, Goodlife*	1 Pack/400g	296	14	74	2.9	5.5	3.5	4.2

MAYONNAISE

INFO/WEIGHT	Measure KCAL	FAT	per 100g KCAL	PROT	CARB	FAT	FIBRE
Average	*1 Tsp/5g*	*35*	*3.8*	*690*	*0.9*	*1.6*	*75.5*	*0*
Branston, with a Twist of Pesto, Crosse & Blackwell*	1 Tbsp/30ml	124	11.6	412	1.2	14.1	38.6	0.2
Caramelised Onion, M&S*	1 Tsp/5ml	24	2.3	470	1.2	13.2	45.5	1.5
Extra Light, Average	*1 Tbsp/33g*	*34*	*2*	*102*	*0.7*	*10.5*	*6.2*	*0.8*
French, Light, Sainsbury's*	1 Serving/15ml	46	4.7	307	0.4	6.1	31.1	0.2
Garlic Herb, Reduced Calorie, Hellmann's*	1 Serving/25ml	58	4.8	233	0.7	13.1	19.3	0.4
Garlic, Hellmann's*	1 Tbsp/15g	40	4	267	0.7	6.7	27	0
Garlic, Retail, Average	*1 Tsp/11g*	*44*	*4.4*	*403*	*1.2*	*8.6*	*40.3*	*0*
Lemon, Waitrose*	1 Tsp/8ml	56	6.1	694	1.2	1.3	76	5.4
Reduced Calorie, Average	*1 Tsp/6g*	*18*	*1.7*	*301*	*0.7*	*8.9*	*29*	*0.1*
with a Spark of Chilli, Hellmann's*	1 Tbsp/15ml	41	4	276	0.8	7.5	27	0.3
with Dijon Mustard, Hellmann's*	1 Tbsp/15ml	32	3	210	2.9	5.1	19.7	0
with Mustard, Tesco*	1 Tbsp/15ml	68	6.4	450	1.6	13.3	43	1.6

MEAL REPLACEMENT

INFO/WEIGHT	Measure KCAL	FAT	per 100g KCAL	PROT	CARB	FAT	FIBRE
Banana Flavour Shake, Celebrity Slim*	1 Sachet/55g	214	2.4	389	34.5	51.5	4.4	0.6
Bars, Crispy Caramel Flavour, Slim & Save*	1 Bar/45g	169	5.3	377	26.7	37.5	11.8	6.9
Breakfast Shake, Banana, Be Fast*	1 Bottle/250ml	200	3.8	80	3.4	12	1.5	2.4
Breakfast Shake, Chocolate, Be Fast*	1 Bottle/250ml	200	3.8	80	3.3	12	1.5	2.5
Breakfast Shake, Strawberry, Be Fast*	1 Bottle/250ml	200	3.8	80	3.4	12	1.5	2.4
Breakfast Shake, Vanilla, Be Fast*	1 Bottle/250ml	190	3.8	76	3.6	10.9	1.5	2.6
Caramel Flavour Shake, Celebrity Slim*	1 Pack/55g	212	2.4	385	34.2	50.9	4.4	0.6
Chocolate Flavour Shake, Celebrity Slim*	1 Sachet/55g	211	2.5	383	34	49.1	4.6	2.2
Chocolate, Slender Shake, Boots*	1 Serving/30g	116	2.1	385	15	60	7	11
Chocolate, Weight Loss Shake, As Consumed, Yokobe*	1 Serving/300ml	302	7.2	101	9.6	9.4	2.4	1.4
Nutra Cookies, Chocolate Chip, Visalus Sciences*	1 Cookie/40g	170	7	425	22.5	45	17.5	10
Nutra Cookies, Peanut Butter, Visalus Sciences*	1 Cookie/40g	185	9	463	25	40	22.5	10
Scrambled Eggs, Slim Save*	1 Pack/40g	196	10.5	491	39.4	16.6	26.3	5
Shake Mix, Made with Water, Visalus Sciences*	1 Serving/31g	115	3	371	38.7	32.3	9.7	16.1

MEAL REPLACEMENT

	Measure INFO/WEIGHT	per Measure KCAL	FAT	KCAL	PROT	CARB	FAT	FIBRE
Shake, Chocolate, Advantage, Atkins*	1 Serving/34g	121	4.2	361	49	8.1	12.5	15.5
Shake, Chocolate, Ready to Drink, Advantage, Atkins*	1 Carton/330ml	172	9.2	52	6	0.6	2.8	1.2
Shake, Chocolate, Rich, Great Shape, Asda*	1 Bottle/330ml	198	6.3	60	5.2	4.8	1.9	1.5
Shake, Herbalife*	1 Serving/250ml	245	6.4	98	10	8.8	2.6	1
Shake, Latte, Smooth, Great Shape, Asda*	1 Bottle/330ml	208	6.9	63	5.5	4.8	2.1	1.6
Shake, Strawberry, Delight, Great Shape, Asda*	1 Serving/330ml	198	6.3	60	5.1	5.1	1.9	1.2
Shake, Vanilla, Ready to Drink, Advantage, Atkins*	1 Carton/330ml	175	8.9	53	6.2	0.6	2.7	0.9
Shake, Vanillla, Smooth, Great Shape, Asda*	1 Bottle/330ml	198	6.3	60	5.1	5.1	1.9	1.2
Strawberry Flavour Shake, Celebrity Slim*	1 Sachet/55g	214	2.4	389	34.4	51.6	4.4	0.6
Strawberry, High Protein, Energy Meal, Spiru-tein*	1 Serving/34g	99	0	291	41.2	32.4	0	2.9
Strawberry, Slender Shake, Boots*	1 Serving/30g	115	1.9	383	15	61	6.3	11
Strawberry, Weight Loss Shake, As Consumed, Yokobe*	1 Serving/300ml	302	7.2	101	9.4	9.6	2.4	1.2
Ultra Slim, Ready to Drink, Strawberry, Tesco*	1 Carton/330ml	231	3	70	4.2	10.5	0.9	1.5
Ultra Slim, Ready to Drink, Vanilla, Tesco*	1 Carton/330ml	224	3	68	4.2	10.5	0.9	1.5
Ultra-Slim, Ready to Drink, Chocolate, Tesco*	1 Carton/330ml	214	3.6	65	4	9.8	1.1	1.3
Vanilla Bean Sundae, Protein Shake, Skinnygirl*	1 Bottle/340ml	80	1.5	24	3.5	1.5	0.4	0.3
Vanilla Flavour Shake, Celebrity Slim*	1 Sachet/55g	215	2.4	391	34.2	52	4.4	0.6
Vanilla Flavoured, Shake, Mealpak, All About Weight*	1 Shake/32g	120	3.3	375	37.5	30.6	10.3	8.1

MEAT LOAF

	Measure INFO/WEIGHT	per Measure KCAL	FAT	KCAL	PROT	CARB	FAT	FIBRE
Beef & Pork, Co-Op*	¼ Loaf/114g	314	25.1	275	13	7	22	1
Iceland*	1 Serving/150g	332	23.6	221	10.8	9.3	15.7	0.9
Turkey & Bacon, Tesco*	1 Serving/225g	400	22.3	178	14.7	7.4	9.9	1.1

MEATBALLS

	Measure INFO/WEIGHT	per Measure KCAL	FAT	KCAL	PROT	CARB	FAT	FIBRE
Al Forno, Charlie Bigham's*	½ Pack/324g	532	32.4	164	7	11.5	10	1.1
Beef, Aberdeen Angus, 12 Pack, Waitrose*	1 Meatball/36g	93	7.1	259	18	2.3	19.8	0.1
Beef, As Sold, Tesco*	1 Meatball/28g	78	6.2	277	16.6	2.3	22.3	0.9
Beef, Ashfield Farm, Aldi*	1 Meatball/20g	45	2.7	232	23	3.9	14	0.5
Beef, in Onion Ale Gravy, Classic Kitchen, Tesco*	½ Pack/224g	331	17.6	148	10.5	8.5	7.9	0.5
Beef, in Tomato Sauce, with Parmigiano, Sainsbury's*	½ Pack/217g	467	33	215	13.8	5.5	15.2	0.5
Beef, Italian Style, As Consumed, Morrisons*	3 Meatballs/104g	235	14.7	226	19.7	4.5	14.1	0.9
Beef, Korean, Spicy, Sainsbury's*	3 Meatballs/68g	153	9.7	225	20.7	3	14.2	1.4
Beef, Mini, Oven Cooked, Finest, Tesco*	5 Meatballs/72g	149	8.2	207	21.8	4	11.4	0.8
Beef, Sainsbury's*	1 Meatball/24g	59	4	251	19.6	4.8	16.9	0.5
Beef, Skinny, Mini, 24, M&S*	½ Pack/120g	132	2.9	110	17.9	4.3	2.4	0.5
Beef, TTD, Sainsbury's*	1 Meatball/35g	73	5.2	208	16.7	1.5	15	0.1
Beef, with Italian Herbs, Finest, Tesco*	4 Meatballs/83g	184	11.2	222	23.6	1.6	13.5	0.1
Chicken, in Tomato Sauce, Average	*1 Can/392g*	*580*	*32.9*	*148*	*7.7*	*10.4*	*8.4*	*0*
in Gravy, Campbell's*	½ Can/205g	164	5.3	80	5.6	8.6	2.6	0
Lamb, Asda*	1 Pack/340g	928	71.4	273	16	5.1	21	0.6
Pork, & Beef, Swedish Style, Tesco*	1 Meatball/14g	34	2.5	245	14.3	6.5	17.7	2
Pork, Herb, Finest, Tesco*	6 Balls/168g	356	26.7	212	16	1	15.9	0.7
Pork, Duchy Originals, Waitrose*	5 Meatballs/68g	184	12.6	270	21.7	4	18.6	0
Pork, Italian, Al Forno, Sainsbury's*	1 Pack/450g	644	23.8	143	6.1	17.6	5.3	1.4
Pork, Mini, Richmond*	5 Meatballs/50g	128	8	255	14	13	16	14
Spanish, with Patatas Bravas, TTD, Sainsbury's*	1 Pack/391g	543	30.1	139	9.6	6.7	7.7	2.6
Swedish, Average	*¼ Pack/88g*	*198*	*13.8*	*224*	*14*	*7.4*	*15.7*	*1.3*
Turkey, Marinara, Frozen, Microwaved, Slimzone, Asda*	1 Pack/500g	448	4.1	99	7.1	14	0.9	2.6
Veal, with Parmesan, Mini, British, Waitrose*	½ Pack/110g	235	13.2	214	22.9	2.8	12	1.4
Vegetarian, Super Greens Balls, as Sold, Heck*	1 Ball/28g	43	0.5	153	6.5	30.3	1.8	5.4
Vegetarian, Swedish, Frozen, Quorn*	¼ Pack/75g	98	3.5	130	13.2	7.4	4.6	3
with Veggies, Tomato Sauce, Ella's Kitchen*	1 Meatball/26g	21	0.5	82	7.2	8.5	2.1	1.5

MEDLAR

	Measure INFO/WEIGHT	per Measure KCAL	FAT	KCAL	PROT	CARB	FAT	FIBRE
Raw, Flesh Only	*1 Fruit/28g*	*11*	*0.1*	*40*	*0.5*	*10.6*	*0.4*	*10*

M

MELBA TOAST

MELBA TOAST	Measure INFO/WEIGHT	per Measure KCAL	FAT	Nutrition Values per 100g / 100ml KCAL	PROT	CARB	FAT	FIBRE
Asda*	1 Slice/3g	13	0.2	395	12	76	4.8	4.6
Average	*1 Serving/3g*	*13*	*0.2*	*396*	*12*	*76*	*4.9*	*4.6*
Dutch, LC, Tesco*	1 Pack/20g	75	0.5	375	13.1	75	2.4	4.6
NUME, Morrisons*	6 Slices/20g	77	0.5	384	11.8	76.9	2.4	3.9
Original, Van Der Meulen*	1 Slice/3g	12	0.1	399	12.8	80.5	2.9	3.9
Thinly Sliced Toasted Wheat Bread, Sainsbury's*	1 Slice/3g	12	0.1	374	13.1	75.1	2.4	4.6
MELON								
Cantaloupe, Flesh Only, Average	*½ Melon/255g*	*87*	*0.5*	*34*	*0.8*	*8.2*	*0.2*	*0.9*
Cantaloupe, Weighed with Rind, Average	*1 Wedge/100g*	*18*	*0.2*	*18*	*0.4*	*4.2*	*0.2*	*0.4*
Galia	*1 Serving/240g*	*60*	*0.1*	*25*	*0.8*	*5.8*	*0*	*0.2*
Honeydew, Raw, Flesh Only, Average	*1oz/28g*	*8*	*0*	*30*	*0.7*	*7*	*0.1*	*0.5*
Medley, Pre Packed, Average	*1 Pack/240g*	*66*	*0.3*	*27*	*0.6*	*6*	*0.1*	*0.5*
MERINGUE								
Average	*1 Meringue/8g*	*30*	*0*	*379*	*5.3*	*95.4*	*0*	*0*
Bombe, Raspberry & Vanilla, M&S*	1 Bombe/100g	155	1.8	155	3.4	33.3	1.8	2.6
Coffee Fresh Cream, Asda*	1 Meringue/28g	109	4.7	396	3.8	57	17	0.3
Cream, Fresh, Sainsbury's*	1 Meringue/35g	142	5.1	407	3.5	65.4	14.6	0.5
Cream, M&S*	1 Meringue/34g	145	7.6	425	4.1	52.6	22.2	1.4
Mini, M&S*	1 Meringue/4g	15	0	395	6.1	91.6	0	0.2
Nests, Average	*1 Nest/16g*	*63*	*0*	*397*	*4.8*	*93.3*	*0.1*	*0.1*
Nests, Bakery, Sainsbury's*	1 Nest/12g	47	0.1	395	4.6	93.9	0.5	0.5
Nests, M&S*	1 Nest/12g	47	0	390	6.1	91.6	0	0
Nests, Mini, Tesco*	1 Nest/5g	19	0	386	4.8	91.2	0.2	0
Nests, Waitrose*	1 Nest/16g	62	0	386	4.8	91.2	0.2	0
Toffee Cream, Tesco*	1 Meringue/30g	114	5	380	4.2	52.9	16.5	0
MIDGET GEMS								
M&S*	1 Bag/113g	367	0.1	325	6.3	75.1	0.1	0
Smart Price, Asda*	1 Pack/178g	586	0.2	329	6	76	0.1	0
MILK								
Almond, & Rice, Almond Dream*	1 Glass/95ml	36	1.2	38	0.6	5.2	1.3	0.4
Almond, Dark Chocolate, Alpro*	1 Serving/200ml	94	2.6	47	0.8	7.6	1.3	0.8
Almond, Original, Alpro*	1 Serving/200ml	48	2.2	24	0.5	3	1.1	0.2
Almond, Original, Fresh, Alpro*	1 Serving/200ml	48	22	24	0.5	3	11	0.2
Almond, Original, Roasted, Alpro*	100ml	22	1.1	22	0.4	2.4	1.1	0.4
Almond, Unsweetened, Breeze, Blue Diamond*	1 Serving/250ml	32	2.8	13	0.5	0.2	1.1	0.3
Almond, Unsweetened, Roasted, Alpro*	1 Serving/200ml	26	2.2	13	0.4	0	1.1	0.4
Almond, Unsweetened, Roasted, Fresh, Alpro*	1 Serving/200ml	26	2.2	13	0.4	0	1.1	0.4
Almond, Unsweetened, Unroasted, Alpro*	1 Serving/200ml	26	2.6	13	0.5	0	1.3	0.2
Alternative, Original, Good Hemp*	1 Glass/250ml	90	6	36	1.3	2.2	2.4	0.2
Camel, 100% Raw, Fresh, Desert Farms*	100ml	53	3.5	53	3.4	3.4	3.5	0
Coconut, Almond, Fresh, Alpro*	1 Serving/200ml	48	2.6	24	0.3	2.6	1.3	0
Coconut, Average	*1 Can/400ml*	*698*	*69.7*	*174*	*1.4*	*2.9*	*17.4*	*2.9*
Coconut, Canned, Pride*	½ Can/200ml	284	30	142	1	1.6	15	0
Coconut, Canned, Tesco*	¼ Can/100ml	151	15	151	0.9	3.2	15	0
Coconut, Chocolate, Alpro*	1 Serving/200ml	82	2.2	41	0.4	7	1.1	0
Coconut, Frozen, Tesco*	¼ Pack/63g	115	8.6	183	8.5	6.3	13.6	0.7
Coconut, Half Fat, Waitrose*	½ Can/135ml	92	8.1	68	0.7	2.7	6	0
Coconut, KTC*	1 Can/400ml	516	73.2	129	1.3	1.8	18.3	0
Coconut, Light, Tesco*	1 Can/400ml	244	24	61	0.4	1.3	6	0
Coconut, Lighter, Sainsbury's*	¼ Can/100ml	75	6.5	75	0.9	2.9	6.5	0.5
Coconut, Organic, Canned, Coconut Merchant*	¼ Can/100g	161	17	161	1.6	2.6	17	0.5
Coconut, Organic, Tesco*	1/8 Can/49g	85	8.3	175	1.8	2.7	17	1.3
Coconut, Original, Fresh, Alpro*	1 Serving/200ml	40	1.8	20	0.1	2.7	0.9	0

MILK

Measure INFO/WEIGHT		per Measure KCAL	FAT	Nutrition Values per 100g / 100ml KCAL	PROT	CARB	FAT	FIBRE
Coconut, Pure, Kefir Cultures, Drink, Rhythm Health*	1 Bottle/126g	43	2.5	34	0.8	2.8	2	1.7
Coconut, Reduced Fat, Amoy*	1 Tin/400ml	440	44	110	1	2	11	1
Coconut, Reduced Fat, Average	*1 Serving/100g*	*104*	*10*	*104*	*1*	*2.4*	*10*	*0.4*
Coconut, Reduced Fat, Canned, Essential, Waitrose*	1 Can/400ml	244	24	61	0	1.8	6	0
Coconut, Rich Creamy, Canned, Kingfisher*	¼ Can/100ml	210	20	210	2.2	5.2	20	0
Condensed, Caramel, Carnation, Nestle*	1 Serving/50g	148	3	296	5.5	55.1	6	0
Condensed, Semi Skimmed, Sweetened	*1oz/28g*	*75*	*0.1*	*267*	*10*	*60*	*0.2*	*0*
Condensed, Skimmed, Unsweetened, Average	*1oz/28g*	*30*	*1.1*	*108*	*7.5*	*10.5*	*4*	*0*
Condensed, Squeezy, Carnation, Nestle*	1 Serving/50g	162	4	325	7.3	56	8	0
Condensed, Whole, Sweetened, Average	*1oz/28g*	*93*	*2.8*	*333*	*8.5*	*55.5*	*10.1*	*0*
Dried, Skimmed, Average	*1oz/28g*	*99*	*0.3*	*355*	*35.4*	*52.3*	*0.9*	*0*
Dried, Whole, Average	*1oz/28g*	*137*	*7.4*	*490*	*26.3*	*39.4*	*26.3*	*0*
Evaporated, Average	*1 Serving/85g*	*136*	*7.6*	*160*	*8.2*	*11.6*	*9*	*0*
Evaporated, Reduced Fat, Average	*1oz/28g*	*33*	*1.5*	*118*	*7.4*	*10.5*	*5.2*	*0*
Goat's, Semi Skimmed, St Helen's Farm*	1 Serving/200ml	88	3.2	44	3	4.3	1.6	0
Goat's, Skimmed, St Helen's Farm*	1 Serving/200ml	60	0.2	30	3	4.3	0.1	0
Goat's, Whole, St Helen's Farm*	1 Serving/200ml	122	7.2	61	2.8	4.3	3.6	0
Goats, Pasteurised	*1 fl oz/30ml*	*18*	*1*	*60*	*3.1*	*4.4*	*3.5*	*0*
Gold Top, Original, Graham's*	1 Tbsp/15ml	12	0.8	80	3.7	4.7	5	0
Kefir, Bibi's Homemade*	1 Glass/210g	128	7.4	61	3.3	4.3	3.5	0
Lattfil, Light, Sourmilk, Arla*	1 Serving/200ml	80	1	40	3.5	3.9	0.5	0
Oat, Original, Alpro*	1 Serving/200ml	88	3	44	0.3	6.8	1.5	1.4
Powder, Instant, Skimmed, Basics, Sainsbury's*	1 Serving/60g	209	0.4	349	35.6	50.4	0.6	0
Rice, Organic, Provamel*	1 Serving/250ml	122	3.8	49	0.1	9.5	1.5	0
Rice, Original, Alpro*	1 Glass/200ml	94	2	47	0.1	9.5	1	0
Rice, Original, Rice Dream*	1 Serving/150ml	70	1.5	47	0.1	9.4	1	0.1
Semi Skimmed, Average	*1fl oz/30ml*	*15*	*0.5*	*49*	*3.4*	*5*	*1.7*	*0*
Semi Skimmed, Long Life, Average	*1fl oz/30ml*	*15*	*0.5*	*49*	*3.4*	*5*	*1.7*	*0*
Semi Skimmed, Low Lactose, Lactofree, Arla*	1 Glass/125ml	50	1.9	40	3.6	3	1.5	0
Skimmed, Average	*1 Pint/568ml*	*194*	*0.5*	*34*	*3.3*	*5*	*0.1*	*0*
Skimmed, Lactofree, Arla*	1 Serving/200ml	66	0.8	33	3.8	3.6	0.4	0
Skimmed, Uht, Average	*1fl oz/30ml*	*10*	*0*	*34*	*3.4*	*5*	*0.1*	*0*
Soya, Banana Flavour, Provamel*	1 Serving/250ml	195	5.5	78	3.8	10.4	2.2	0.6
Soya, Choco Flavour, Provamel*	1 Serving/250ml	208	6	83	3.8	11.1	2.4	1.1
Soya, Chocolate, Alpro*	1 Serving/200ml	154	4.2	77	3.3	10.7	2.1	1
Soya, Chocolate, So Good Beverages*	1 Serving/250ml	160	2.5	64	3.6	10.8	1	0
Soya, Chocolate, UHT, Alpro*	1 Serving/200ml	122	3.6	61	3.1	7.8	1.8	0.9
Soya, Fat Free, Original, So Good Beverages*	1 Serving/250ml	100	0.2	40	3.6	6.4	0.1	0
Soya, Flavoured, Average	*1 Glass/250ml*	*100*	*4.2*	*40*	*2.8*	*3.6*	*1.7*	*0*
Soya, Growing Up Drink, Low in Sugars, Alpro*	1 Serving/200ml	128	4.4	64	2.5	8.3	2.2	0.4
Soya, Light, Alpro*	1 Serving/200ml	54	2.4	27	2.1	1.6	1.2	0.9
Soya, Light, Fresh, Alpro*	1 Serving/200ml	44	2.4	22	2	0.1	1.2	1.2
Soya, Mild, Simply, Alpro*	1 Serving/200ml	70	3.6	35	3	1.5	1.8	0.5
Soya, No Added Sugar, Unsweetened, Average	*1 Serving/250ml*	*85*	*4.8*	*34*	*3.3*	*0.9*	*1.9*	*0.4*
Soya, Omega Original, So Good Beverages*	1 Serving/250ml	98	3.8	39	2	4.4	1.5	0
Soya, Original, Alpro*	1 Serving/200ml	88	3.8	44	3.3	3	1.9	0.6
Soya, Original, Fresh, Alpro*	1 Serving/200ml	78	3.6	39	3	2.5	1.8	0.5
Soya, Original, Fresh, Organic, Alpro*	1 Serving/200ml	76	3.4	38	3	2.4	1.7	0.5
Soya, Plain, Organic, Kirkland*	1 Glass/250ml	118	5.5	47	4	3.7	2.2	0.5
Soya, Strawberry Flavour, Provamel*	1 Serving/250ml	160	5.2	64	3.6	7.7	2.1	1.2
Soya, Strawberry, Alpro*	1 Serving/200ml	124	3.6	62	3.3	7.6	1.8	0.5
Soya, Sweetened, Actileaf, Aldi*	1 Serving/200ml	98	5.2	49	3.5	2.6	2.6	0.5
Soya, Sweetened, Average	*1 Glass/200ml*	*94*	*4.2*	*47*	*3.4*	*3.7*	*2.1*	*0.4*

MILK

INFO/WEIGHT	Measure	per Measure KCAL	FAT	Nutrition Values per 100g / 100ml KCAL	PROT	CARB	FAT	FIBRE
MILK								
Soya, Sweetened, Calcium Enriched, Average	*1 Glass/200ml*	*91*	*3.9*	*46*	*3.4*	*3.7*	*2*	*0.3*
Soya, UHT, Non Dairy, Alternative to Milk, Waitrose*	1 Serving/250ml	102	4.8	41	3.3	2.7	1.9	0.2
Soya, Unsweetened, Actileaf, Aldi*	1 Serving/200ml	68	4.2	34	3.4	0.5	2.1	0.5
Soya, Unsweetened, Organic, Waitrose*	1 Serving/60ml	19	1.1	31	3.3	0.2	1.9	0
Soya, Unsweetened, Uht, Everyday Value, Tesco*	1 Serving/250ml	72	4	29	2.9	0.4	1.6	0.5
Soya, Unsweetened, Uht, Organic, Tesco*	1 Serving/150ml	50	2.8	33	3.4	0.4	1.9	0.6
Soya, Vanilla Flavour, Organic, Provamel*	1 Serving/250ml	150	5.5	60	3.8	6.2	2.2	0.6
Soya, Vanilla, Alpro*	1 Serving/200ml	108	3.4	54	3	6.5	1.7	0.5
Soya, Vanilla, Fat Free, So Good Beverages*	1 Serving/250ml	140	0.2	56	3.6	10.4	0.1	0
Soya, Vanilla, Organic, Heinz*	1 Serving/200ml	106	3.2	53	2.6	6.9	1.6	0.2
Soya, Vanilla, So Good Beverages*	1 Serving/250ml	180	5	72	3.6	10.4	2	0
Soya, Vitasoy*	1 Serving/250ml	130	3.8	52	3	5.5	1.5	2
Soya, Wholebean, Unsweetened, Alpro*	1 Serving/200ml	66	3.6	33	3.3	0	1.8	0.6
Soya, Wholebean, Unsweetened, Fresh, Alpro*	1 Serving/200ml	66	3.6	33	3.3	0	1.8	0.6
Soya, Wholebean, Unsweetened, Organic, Alpro*	1 Serving/200ml	66	3.6	33	3.3	0	1.8	0.6
Strawberry Flavoured, Essential, Waitrose*	1 Glass/200ml	136	3.4	68	3.3	9.5	1.7	0.5
Super Milk Low Fat 1%, Avonmore*	1 Litre/1000ml	420	10	42	3.4	5	1	0
Whole, Average	*1 Serving/200ml*	*134*	*7.8*	*67*	*3.3*	*4.7*	*3.9*	*0*
Whole, Lactose Free, Lactofree, Arla*	1 Serving/200ml	114	7	57	3.4	2.8	3.5	0
Whole, Uht, Tesco*	1 Serving/100ml	65	3.6	65	3.4	4.7	3.6	0
MILK DRINK								
Banana Flavour, Sterilised, Low Fat, Gulp*	1 Bottle/500ml	425	9	85	5.2	11.9	1.8	0
Chocolate Coconut, Free From, Tesco*	1 Serving/250ml	125	5.4	49	0.4	6.8	2.1	0.7
Chocolate Flavoured, Goodness for Kids, Tesco*	1 Bottlel/330ml	248	5.9	75	3.8	10.3	1.8	0.7
Chocolate Sterilised Skimmed, Happy Shopper*	1 Bottle/500ml	295	1.5	59	3.6	10.4	0.3	0
Chocolate, Break Time, Arla*	1 Bottle/500ml	290	1.5	58	3.6	10.2	0.3	0
Chocolate, Brekkie, Up Go, Life Health Foods*	1 Carton/330ml	218	3.3	66	3.8	9.1	1	2.4
Chocolate, Spar*	1 Serving/500ml	290	1.5	58	3.6	10.2	0.3	0
Chocolatte, Cafe Met*	1 Bottle/290ml	174	4.1	60	3.7	9.1	1.4	0.3
Oat, Oat Dream*	1 Serving/200ml	56	1.4	28	0.4	4.8	0.7	0
Original, Mars*	1 Serving/330g	284	6.9	86	3.1	13.7	2.1	0
Refuel, Mars*	1 Bottle/388ml	299	5.8	77	3.1	13.5	1.5	0
Semi Skimmed, Cholesterol Lowering, Pro Activ, Flora*	1 Serving/250ml	125	4.5	50	3.6	4.8	1.8	0
Strawberry Flavoured, Goodness for Kids, Tesco*	1 Bottle/330ml	248	5.6	75	4	9.9	1.7	0.4
Strawberry, Flavoured, Asda*	1 Bottle/330ml	211	3.6	64	3.6	10	1.1	0.5
MILK SHAKE								
Banana Flavour, Frijj*	1 Bottle/500ml	325	4.5	65	3.7	10.5	0.9	0
Banana Flavour, Shapers, Boots*	1 Bottle/250ml	201	1.9	80	5.6	12.8	0.8	1.9
Banana Flavour, Spar*	1 Bottle/500ml	250	0.5	50	3.3	9.1	0.1	0
Banana, Diet Chef Ltd*	1 Drink/330ml	225	3	68	4.2	10.5	0.9	1.5
Banana, Shudda, Aldi*	½ Bottle/236g	163	2.1	69	3.4	12	0.9	0.5
Banana, Yazoo, Campina*	1 Bottle/200ml	120	2.4	60	3.1	9.6	1.2	0
Chocolate Flavour, BGTY, Sainsbury's*	1 Bottle/500ml	290	2.5	58	5.3	8	0.5	0.9
Chocolate Flavour, Diet Chef Ltd*	1 Drink/330ml	210	2.3	64	4.1	8.5	0.7	1.9
Chocolate Flavoured, Fresh, Thick, Frijj*	1 Bottle/500ml	350	5	70	3.5	11.7	1	0
Chocolate, Asda*	1 Serving/250ml	198	9.2	79	4.4	7	3.7	0.4
Chocolate, Belgian, M&S*	1 Bottle/300ml	360	14.4	120	4.2	14.6	4.8	0.7
Chocolate, Extreme, Frijj*	1 Bottle/500g	425	10.5	85	3.9	12.7	2.1	0
Chocolate, Protein, Ufit*	1 Bottle/310ml	170	3.1	55	7.1	3.6	1	1.2
Honeycomb Choc Swirl Flavour, The Incredible, Frijj*	1 Bottle/500ml	450	12.5	90	4	13	2.5	0.2
Mount Caramel, Frijj*	1 Bottle/500ml	360	4.5	72	3.4	12.7	0.9	0
Powder, Made Up with Semi-Skimmed Milk	*1 Serving/250ml*	*172*	*4*	*69*	*3.2*	*11.3*	*1.6*	*0*
Powder, Made Up with Whole Milk	*1 Serving/250ml*	*218*	*9.2*	*87*	*3.1*	*11.1*	*3.7*	*0*

MILK SHAKE	Measure INFO/WEIGHT	per Measure KCAL	FAT	Nutrition Values per 100g / 100ml KCAL	PROT	CARB	FAT	FIBRE
Raspberry Strawberry, Protein 20g, Arla*	1 Serving/225ml	171	3.6	76	9	6.5	1.6	0
Strawberry Raspberry, Syrup, Robinson's*	1 Serving/50ml	20	0.7	39	2.9	4	1.4	0
Strawberry Flavour, Thick, Low Fat, Frijj*	1 Bottle/250ml	155	2	62	3.4	10.1	0.8	0
Strawberry, British, M&S*	1 Bottle/300ml	270	10.2	90	4	10.8	3.4	0.1
Strawberry, Diet Chef Ltd*	1 Drink/330g	225	3	68	4.2	10.5	0.9	1.5
Strawberry, High Protein, For Goodness Shakes*	1 Bottle/475ml	206	0.5	43	5.3	5.3	0.1	0.1
Strawberry, Protein, Euro Shopper*	1 Bottle/330ml	148	1.6	45	6.2	5.1	0.5	0.5
Strawberry, Yazoo, Campina*	1 Bottle/475ml	300	6	60	3.1	9.5	1.2	0
Thick, Milky Way, Mars*	1 Bottle/440ml	282	4.8	64	3.4	10	1.1	0.7
Vanilla, Diet Chef Ltd*	1 Pack/330ml	225	3	68	4.2	10.5	0.9	1.5
White Chocolate, Vanilla, M&S*	1 Bottle/300ml	315	12.9	105	3.8	12.4	4.3	0.6
MILKY BAR								
Buttons, Nestle*	1 Std Pack/30g	164	9.5	547	7.3	58.4	31.7	0
Chunky, Nestle*	¼ Bar/38g	207	12	547	7.3	58.4	31.7	0
Crunchies, Nestle*	1 Pack/30g	168	10.4	560	7	54.9	34.7	0
Funsize (17g), Mars*	1 Bar/17g	75	2.7	449	3.8	71.8	16.3	0.6
Milk Crunchy, Nestle*	1 Bar/21g	117	7.2	557	8.5	53.5	34.3	0.1
Mini Eggs, Nestle*	1 Pack/100g	501	22	501	5.4	70.1	22	0.5
Munchies, Nestle*	1 Serving/70g	392	24.3	560	7	54.9	34.7	0.1
Nestle*	1 Sm Bar/13g	68	4	547	7.3	58.4	31.7	0
MILKY WAY								
Fun Size, Mars*	1 Bar/17g	75	2.7	447	3.8	71.6	16.2	0
Funsize (15.5g), Mars*	1 Bar/16g	69	2.5	446	3.9	71.6	16.3	0.6
Mars*	1 Bar/22g	96	3.3	446	3.9	72.4	15.5	0.6
MINCEMEAT								
Average	*1oz/28g*	*77*	*1.2*	*274*	*0.6*	*62.1*	*4.3*	*1.3*
Sainsbury's*	1 Tbsp/20g	58	0.6	291	1.2	62.3	3.1	1.4
Traditional, Robertson*	1 Tbsp/24g	68	0.6	285	0.8	63.5	2.7	2.5
MINSTRELS								
Galaxy, Mars*	1 Serving/39g	196	8.6	498	5.2	69.1	21.9	0
MINT								
Dried, Average	*1 Tsp/5g*	*14*	*0.2*	*279*	*24.8*	*34.6*	*4.6*	*0*
Fresh, Average	*2 Tbsp/3.2g*	*1*	*0*	*43*	*3.8*	*5.3*	*0.7*	*0*
Spearmint, Fresh, Average	*2 Leaves/0.1g*	*0*	*0*	*44*	*3.3*	*8*	*0.7*	*7*
MINTS								
After Dinner, Dark, Elizabeth Shaw*	1 Sweet/9g	42	2.1	469	2.8	62.5	23.1	0
After Dinner, Sainsbury's*	1 Mint/7g	32	1.5	456	4.1	62.1	21.2	4.1
Butter Mintoes, M&S*	1 Sweet/9g	35	0.6	391	0	84	6.8	0
Butter Mintoes, Tesco*	1 Sweet/7g	24	0.5	349	0	71.3	7.1	0
Clear, Co-Op*	1 Sweet/6g	24	0	395	0	98	0	0
Cream, Luxury, Thorntons*	1 Sweet/13g	62	3.1	477	4.2	62.3	23.8	2.3
Creams, Bassett's*	1 Sweet/11g	40	0	365	0	91.8	0	0
Curiously Strong, M&S*	1 Sweet/1g	4	0	390	0.4	97.5	0	0
Doublemint, Sugarfree, Wrigleys*	1 Mint/3g	7	0	234	0	97.4	0	0
Everton, Co-Op*	1 Sweet/6g	25	0.2	410	0.6	92	4	0
Extra Strong, Peppermint, Trebor*	1 Mint/2g	10	0	395	0.3	98.5	0	0
Extra Strong, Spearmint, Trebor*	1 Pack/44g	174	0	395	0.4	98.7	0	0
Extra, Peppermint Coolburst, Wrigleys*	1 Pack/22g	53	0.2	240	0	98	1	0
Extra, Spearmint, Sugar Free, Wrigleys*	1 Sweet/1g	3	0	244	0	98.5	0.8	0
Extra, Wrigleys*	1 Sweet/1g	3	0	240	0	64	1	0
Glacier, Fox's*	1 Sweet/5g	19	0	386	0	96.4	0	0
Humbugs, Co-Op*	1 Sweet/8g	34	0.6	425	0.6	89.9	7	0
Humbugs, Grumpy Old Gits, Spencer Fleetwood Ltd*	1 Sweet/25g	92	0.4	366	0.2	87.5	1.5	0

M

MINTS

	Measure INFO/WEIGHT	per Measure KCAL	FAT	Nutrition Values per 100g / 100ml KCAL	PROT	CARB	FAT	FIBRE
Humbugs, M&S*	1 Sweet/9g	37	0.4	407	0.6	91.1	4.4	0
Humbugs, Thorntons*	1 Sweet/9g	31	0.4	340	1	87.8	4.4	0
Imperials, Co-Op*	1 Sweet/3g	12	0	395	0.3	98	0.2	0
Imperials, M&S*	1 Sweet/3g	12	0	391	0	97.8	0	0
Imperials, Sainsbury's*	1 Sweet/3g	10	0	374	0	92.1	0	0
Imperials, Tesco*	1 Sweet/3g	12	0	397	0.6	98.7	0	0
Mento, Sugar Free, Mentos*	1 Sweet/2g	5	0.1	260	1	87	5.5	0
Mighties, Sugar Free, Trebor*	1 Sweet/1g	1	0	235	0.4	97	0.2	0
Mint Assortment, M&S*	1 Sweet/7g	26	0.5	375	0.4	78.2	6.9	0
Mint Favourites, Bassett's*	1 Sweet/6g	22	0.4	367	0.9	77.4	5.9	0
Peppermints, Strong, Altoids*	1 Sweet/1g	3	0	385	0.5	96	0	0
Soft, Trebor*	1 Pack/48g	182	0	380	0	94.9	0	0
Softmints, Peppermint, Trebor*	1 Pack/48g	170	0	355	0	88.9	0	0
Softmints, Spearmint, Trebor*	1 Pack/45g	170	0	375	0	94.3	0	0
Thins, Chocolate, Waitrose*	1 Thin/5g	27	1.3	509	4.2	69.6	23.8	0.2
MIRIN								
Rice Wine, Sweetened, Average	*1 Tbsp/15ml*	*35*	*0*	*231*	*0.2*	*41.6*	*0*	*0*
MISO								
Average	*1oz/28g*	*57*	*1.7*	*203*	*13.3*	*23.5*	*6.2*	*0*
Paste, Red, AKA, Unpasteurised, Organic, Miso Tasty*	1 Tbsp/15g	31	0.8	208	10	25.3	5.6	4.1
MIXED HERBS								
Average	*1 Tsp/5g*	*13*	*0.4*	*260*	*13*	*37.5*	*8.5*	*6.7*
MOLASSES								
Average	*1 Tsp/5g*	*13*	*0*	*266*	*0*	*68.8*	*0.1*	*0*
MONKEY NUTS								
without Shell, Average	*1oz/28g*	*158*	*13.4*	*565*	*25.6*	*8.2*	*48*	*6.3*
MONKFISH								
Grilled	*1oz/28g*	*27*	*0.2*	*96*	*22.7*	*0*	*0.6*	*0*
Raw	*1oz/28g*	*18*	*0.1*	*66*	*15.7*	*0*	*0.4*	*0*
MONSTER MUNCH								
Pickled Onion, Walkers*	1 Std Bag/22g	108	5.5	490	6	60	25	1.7
Roast Beef, Walkers*	1 Std Bag/22g	108	5.5	490	7	59	25	1.7
Spicy, Walkers*	1 Std Bag/25g	125	7.2	500	5	55	29	1.3
MOUSSAKA								
Beef, BGTY, Sainsbury's*	1 Pack/400g	300	10.4	75	6.1	6.8	2.6	1.2
Charlie Bigham's*	½ Pack/328g	425	27.8	130	6.1	6.9	8.5	0
Lamb, Finest, Tesco*	½ Pack/334g	513	36.5	154	6.4	6.6	10.9	1.5
Lamb, Gastropub, M&S*	½ Pack/375g	735	51.4	196	7.9	9.7	13.7	1.1
Lamb, Serves 2, TTD, Sainsbury's*	½ Pack/400g	546	33.7	141	7.2	8	8.7	1.2
Vegetable, COU, M&S*	1 Pack/400g	280	10.8	70	2.7	9.1	2.7	2.4
Vegetarian, Quorn*	1 Pack/400g	364	16.4	91	3.6	9.8	4.1	1.2
MOUSSE								
Aero Chocolate, Nestle*	1 Pot/58g	101	3	174	4.8	27.3	5.1	1.1
Aero Twist Cappuccino & Chocolate, Nestle*	1 Pot/75g	135	8.1	180	4.2	16.8	10.8	0.2
Apricot, Lite, Onken*	1 Pot/150g	156	2.2	104	4.6	18	1.5	0.3
Banoffee, COU, M&S*	1 Pot/70g	102	1.5	145	2.9	28.8	2.1	1.5
Black Cherry, Lite, Onken*	1 Pot/150g	156	2.2	104	4.6	17.9	1.5	0.2
Blackcurrant, Onken*	1 Pot/150g	210	10.2	140	5.2	14.6	6.8	0
Cappuccino, Essential, Waitrose*	1 Pot/100g	279	16.7	279	4.2	27.7	16.7	0.5
Caramel, Meringue, Cadbury*	1 Pot/65g	181	6.7	277	4.6	42.4	10.3	1
Chocolate	*1 Pot/60g*	*83*	*3.2*	*139*	*4*	*19.9*	*5.4*	*0*
Chocolate, & Hazelnut, Creamy, Dr Oetker*	1 Pot/115g	158	6.9	137	3.3	17.6	6	0.6
Chocolate, & Hazelnut, Onken*	1 Pot/125g	171	7.5	137	3.3	17.8	6	0

MOUSSE

	Measure INFO/WEIGHT	per Measure KCAL	FAT	Nutrition Values per 100g / 100ml KCAL	PROT	CARB	FAT	FIBRE
Chocolate, & Mint, COU, M&S*	1 Pot/70g	84	1.8	120	6.2	18.7	2.5	1
Chocolate, & Orange, COU, M&S*	1 Pot/70g	77	1.8	110	5.9	16	2.6	0.9
Chocolate, & Vanilla, Belgian, Weight Watchers*	1 Pot/80g	106	2.2	132	4.4	22.2	2.8	0.9
Chocolate, Asda*	1 Pot/61g	134	6.1	219	3.7	26	10	1
Chocolate, Basics, Sainsbury's*	1 Pot/63g	94	3.8	150	5.1	18.9	6	0
Chocolate, Belgian, Finest, Tesco*	1 Pot/120g	360	22.7	300	5.1	26.6	18.9	1.1
Chocolate, BGTY, Sainsbury's*	1 Pot/63g	83	1.8	133	4.9	21.8	2.9	0.5
Chocolate, Cadbury*	1 Pot/55g	107	4.5	195	6.1	24.6	8.2	0
Chocolate, Finest, Tesco*	1 Pot/82g	321	26.4	391	3.7	21.7	32.2	0
Chocolate, GFY, Asda*	1 Pot/60g	70	1.7	117	4.8	17.9	2.9	3.5
Chocolate, Iceland*	1 Pot/62g	113	4.3	183	4	26.3	6.9	0
Chocolate, Italian Style, Tesco*	1 Pot/90g	243	11.9	270	5	32.8	13.2	2.4
Chocolate, Light, Cadbury*	1 Pot/55g	60	1.9	110	4.6	14.2	3.4	0
Chocolate, Low Fat, Danette, Danone*	1 Pot/60g	73	1.1	121	5.1	20.8	1.9	1.5
Chocolate, Milk, M&S*	1 Pot/90g	180	7.8	200	5.3	24.8	8.7	1.5
Chocolate, Mint, Cadbury*	1 Pot/45g	90	3.6	200	6	25.6	8.1	0
Chocolate, Minty, Bubbly, Dessert, Aero, Nestle*	1 Pot/58g	108	5.9	186	4.6	18.9	10.2	0.3
Chocolate, Orange, Low Fat, Cadbury*	1 Pot/100g	110	3	110	5.6	15.1	3	0
Chocolate, Pere & Fils*	1 Pot/80g	282	20.3	352	8.5	20.5	25.4	0
Chocolate, Plain, Low Fat, Nestle*	1 Pot/120g	71	0.9	59	2.4	10.4	0.8	0
Chocolate, Sainsbury's*	1 Pot/63g	119	5.3	190	4.7	23.8	8.5	1
Chocolate, Shapers, Boots*	1 Pot/70g	97	1.9	138	5.3	23	2.7	1.7
Chocolate, Tesco*	1 Pot/60g	120	5	200	3.6	27.6	8.4	0.9
Chocolate, Value, Tesco*	1 Pot/63g	101	3.3	161	4.9	23.3	5.2	1.3
Chocolate, White, Bubbly, Dessert, Aero, Nestle*	1 Pot/58g	99	4.4	170	4.3	21	7.5	0.2
Chocolate, with Mini Chunks of, Dairy Milk, Cadbury*	1 Pot/100g	215	9.9	215	6.1	25.7	9.9	0
Chocolate, with Vanilla Layer, Cadbury*	1 Pot/100g	162	6.1	162	4.8	21.9	6.1	0
Cocoa, Vegan, Sugar Free, As Prepared, Eco Free From*	1 Serving/80g	74	1.8	92	2.7	13.4	2.3	3.5
Lemon, Classic, Onken*	1 Pot/150g	210	9.4	140	5.1	15.8	6.3	0
Lemon, COU, M&S*	1 Pot/70g	91	1.8	130	3.1	23.7	2.5	0.6
Lemon, Dessert, Sainsbury's*	1 Pot/63g	114	5.9	182	3.6	20.7	9.4	0.6
Lemon, Fruit Juice, Shape, Danone*	1 Pot/100g	116	2.8	116	3.5	18.6	2.8	0
Lemon, Low Fat, Morrisons*	1 Pot/63g	99	5.8	158	3.7	15.4	9.3	0.3
Lemon, Ski, Nestle*	1 Tub/60g	76	2.8	127	3.7	17.6	4.7	0
Lemon, Tesco*	1 Pot/60g	67	1.6	111	3.4	18.2	2.7	0
Lemon, with Meringue Style Sauce, Ski, Nestle*	1 Pot/60g	81	2.8	137	3.1	19.8	4.8	0
Orange, Mango & Lime, Onken*	1 Pot/150g	207	9.4	138	5.1	15.3	6.3	0.1
Peach, Onken*	1 Pot/150g	204	9.4	136	5.1	15.1	6.3	0.2
Raspberry, Lite, Onken*	1 Pot/150g	156	2.2	104	4.6	17.3	1.5	0.1
Raspberry, Ripple, Ms Mollys*	1 Tub/50g	80	3.4	161	3.3	21.5	6.7	0.7
Raspberry, Ripple, Value, Tesco*	1 Pot/47g	70	2.9	149	2.1	21.3	6.1	0.1
Raspberry, Ripple, Value, Tesco*	1 Mousse/47g	77	3.1	163	2.9	23	6.6	0.3
Rhubarb, COU, M&S*	1 Pot/70g	88	1.5	125	2.9	25.7	2.1	4.2
Rolo, Nestle*	1 Pot/50g	80	3	158	4.7	21.6	5.9	0
Strawberry, & Vanilla, Weight Watchers*	1 Pot/80g	87	1.9	109	3.8	18.1	2.4	0.4
Strawberry, Asda*	1 Pot/64g	107	5.8	167	3.5	18	9	0.2
Strawberry, Layered, Co-Op*	1 Pot/100g	120	3	120	3	19	3	0.2
Strawberry, Light, Muller*	1 Pot/150g	147	0.6	98	4.3	19.4	0.4	0
Strawberry, Low Fat, Waitrose*	1 Pot/95g	112	2.7	118	3.2	20	2.8	0.6
Strawberry, Sainsbury's*	1 Pot/63g	106	5.9	168	3.4	17.5	9.4	0.1
Strawberry, Shape, Danone*	1 Pot/100g	44	1.8	44	3	4	1.8	0
Strawberry, Ski, Nestle*	1 Tub/60g	77	3.1	128	3.8	16.6	5.2	0
Strawberry, Tesco*	1 Pot/60g	97	4.6	162	2.7	20.2	7.7	0.5

	Measure INFO/WEIGHT	per Measure		Nutrition Values per 100g / 100ml				
		KCAL	FAT	KCAL	PROT	CARB	FAT	FIBRE
MOUSSE								
Strawberry, with Strawberry Sauce, Ski, Nestle*	1 Pot/60g	79	3.1	131	3.1	18.1	5.2	0
Summer Fruits, Light, Muller*	1 Pot/149g	143	0.6	96	4.3	18.7	0.4	0
Toffee, M&S*	1 Pot/90g	180	7.2	200	4.5	27.6	8	0.6
Vanilla, Finesse, Aero, Rowntree's*	1 Pot/57g	127	8.3	223	3.7	18.8	14.6	0
White Chocolate Raspberry, Gu*	1 Pot/83g	225	14.6	271	1.9	28.4	17.6	4.1
White Chocolate, Finest, Tesco*	1 Pot/92g	436	34.5	474	3.9	30.2	37.5	0
MUFFIN								
All Butter, M&S*	1 Muffin/65g	175	4.7	270	10.3	40.8	7.3	2.1
Banana Pecan, Organic, Honeyrose Bakery*	1 Muffin/110g	300	12.6	273	4.1	38.3	11.5	4.3
Blueberry, American Style, Aldi*	1 Muffin/85g	344	17.3	405	4.3	51.2	20.3	0
Blueberry, American Style, Sainsbury's*	1 Muffin/72g	256	13.1	355	5.1	42.7	18.2	1.9
Blueberry, Asda*	1 Muffin/77g	273	13.1	353	5	45	17	1.3
Blueberry, Bakery, Tesco*	1 Muffin/82g	307	13.1	374	4.3	52.2	16	1.9
Blueberry, Big, Asda*	1 Muffin/105g	342	11.2	326	7.5	49.8	10.7	2.3
Blueberry, GF, Genius*	1 Muffin/95g	352	16.2	370	3.6	51	17.1	1.6
Blueberry, M&S*	1 Muffin/75g	255	12.6	340	4.9	41.9	16.8	1.3
Blueberry, McVitie's*	1 Muffin/80g	328	18.6	405	4.7	47.9	23	1.3
Blueberry, Mini, Tesco*	1 Muffin/28g	104	5.4	370	5.6	43.5	19.3	1.2
Blueberry, PB, Waitrose*	1 Muffin/100g	225	2.2	225	4.6	46.5	2.2	1.8
Blueberry, Waitrose*	1 Muffin/65g	239	9.2	367	4.7	55.2	14.2	1.7
Caramel, Cadbury*	1 Muffin/116g	535	30.3	461	5.9	50.8	26.1	0
Caramel, Salted, Filled, Tesco*	1 Muffin/82g	320	15.5	390	4.7	49.5	18.9	1.6
Caramel, Salted, TTD, Sainsbury's*	1 Muffin/113g	447	22	396	4.8	49.6	19.5	1.5
Cheese, Courgette, Ella's Kitchen*	1 Muffin/25g	59	3	237	8.3	25.4	12	1.2
Chocolate Chip, BGTY, Sainsbury's*	1 Muffin/75g	282	12.3	376	5.2	51.8	16.4	1.6
Chocolate Chip, Double, Co-Op*	1 Muffin/60g	246	12.6	410	6	49	21	3
Chocolate Chip, Double, Mini, Asda*	1 Muffin/19g	76	3.7	400	7.4	48.5	19.6	2.7
Chocolate Chip, Double, Tesco*	1 Muffin/100g	360	17.9	360	6.1	44.9	17.9	5.4
Chocolate Chip, Mini, Asda*	1 Muffin/22g	77	2.9	349	7	51	13	2.1
Chocolate Chip, Mini, BGTY, Sainsbury's*	1 Muffin/30g	130	6.7	434	5.5	52.1	22.5	0.8
Chocolate Chip, Mini, Essential, Waitrose*	1 Muffin/27g	108	5.1	399	5.9	49.8	19	2.5
Chocolate Chip, Mini, Tesco*	1 Muffin/25g	108	5.6	436	5	52.5	22.5	1.6
Chocolate Chip, Plain, Tesco*	1 Muffin/72g	270	12.7	375	5	48.1	17.6	1.4
Chocolate, Double, Mini, M&S*	1 Muffin/32g	133	6.9	416	5.4	49.8	21.7	1.1
Cinnamon, & Sultana, Baked by Us, Morrisons*	1 Muffin/68g	166	1	244	8.3	48.2	1.4	2.9
English	1 Muffin/57g	120	1	211	7	43.9	1.8	1.8
English, Egg, Cheese, & Sausage, From Restaurant	*1 Muffin/165g*	*487*	*30.9*	*295*	*13.1*	*18.8*	*18.7*	*0*
English, Gluten, Wheat Milk Free, Free From, Livwell*	1 Muffin/50g	160	4.9	320	4.6	52.8	9.8	3.2
English, Kingsmill*	1 Muffin/75g	167	1.4	222	9.7	40.4	1.8	2.6
English, Mild Red Cheddar Cheese, Extra Special, Asda*	1 Muffin/70g	201	4.7	288	11	45	6.7	2.7
English, Tesco*	1 Muffin/72g	158	1.1	219	8.4	41.7	1.5	2.7
Lemon & Poppy Seed, Entenmann's*	1 Muffin/105g	417	20.3	397	5.6	52.8	19.3	2.5
Lemon Poppy Seed, Waitrose*	1 Muffin/121g	460	23.1	380	4.3	46.8	19.1	1.8
Lemon Curd, Patisserie, TTD, Sainsbury's*	1 Muffin/108g	418	20.9	386	5.4	47.1	19.3	1.4
Mini, Tesco*	1 Muffin/28g	120	6.3	428	6.4	50	22.6	1.2
Muesli, Breakfast, Love Life, Waitrose*	1 Muffin/68g	216	6.2	318	9.1	50	9.1	3.4
Orange, Apricot Almond, Organic, Honeyrose Bakery*	1 Muffin/110g	312	11.4	284	3.5	44.2	10.4	1.9
Oven Bottom, Aldi*	1 Muffin/68g	173	1	255	10	50.4	1.5	2.2
Oven Bottom, Asda*	1 Muffin/65g	175	1.8	269	9	51	2.7	2.1
Oven Bottom, Warburton's*	1 Muffin/63g	173	2.7	274	10.4	49.4	4.3	2.3
Plain, Co-Op*	1 Muffin/60g	135	1.1	225	11.2	41.3	1.9	2.4
Plain, Prepared From Recipe, Average	*1 Muffin/57g*	*169*	*6.5*	*296*	*6.9*	*41.4*	*11.4*	*2.7*
Raspberry, Cream, Sainsbury's*	1 Muffin/90g	314	19.8	349	3.9	33.8	22	1.3

	Measure INFO/WEIGHT	per Measure		Nutrition Values per 100g / 100ml				
		KCAL	FAT	KCAL	PROT	CARB	FAT	FIBRE
MUFFIN								
Raspberry, PB, Waitrose*	1 Muffin/101g	220	2.1	219	4.7	45.4	2.1	3.7
Sausage, Breakfast, All Day, Rustlers*	1 Pack/155g	386	13.8	249	11.8	29	8.9	0
Toasting, Warburton's*	1 Muffin/64g	138	1	216	8.9	41.4	1.6	2.9
Vanilla, & Choc Chip, GFY, Asda*	1 Muffin/59g	152	1.3	260	7	53	2.2	1.6
White Chocolate, & Strawberry Filled, Tesco*	1 Muffin/103g	415	20.3	405	5.2	51.3	19.8	1.3
White Chocolate, Chunk Lemon, Mini, M&S*	1 Muffin/28g	130	6.7	464	6.4	55.4	23.9	2.1
White, M&S*	1 Muffin/60g	135	1.1	225	11.2	43.7	1.9	2.9
White, Soft, Hovis*	1 Muffin/60g	145	1.7	241	8.9	44	2.8	2.4
White, Tesco*	1 Muffin/72g	173	2.3	240	11.3	41.6	3.2	2.8
Wholemeal, Tesco*	1 Muffin/65g	130	1.3	200	12.6	32.9	2	5.7
MULBERRIES								
Raw	*1oz/28g*	*10*	*0*	*36*	*1.3*	*8.1*	*0*	*0*
MULLET								
Grey, Grilled	*1oz/28g*	*42*	*1.5*	*150*	*25.7*	*0*	*5.2*	*0*
Grey, Raw	*1oz/28g*	*16*	*0.6*	*58*	*9.9*	*0*	*2*	*0*
Red, Grilled	*1oz/28g*	*34*	*1.2*	*121*	*20.4*	*0*	*4.4*	*0*
Red, Raw, Weighed Whole, Flesh Only	*1 Portion/100g*	*25*	*0.9*	*25*	*4.3*	*0*	*0.9*	*0*
MUNCHIES								
Original, Tube, Nestle*	1 Pack/55g	266	12.3	487	5.4	64.6	22.5	1.4
MUSHROOMS								
Breaded, Average	*3 Mushroom/51g*	*77*	*2.9*	*152*	*4.3*	*20.8*	*5.7*	*0.6*
Breaded, Crispy, in Panko Crumb, M&S*	½ Pack/100g	214	11.7	214	4.9	21.1	11.7	2.3
Breaded, Garlic, Average	*3 Mushroom/50g*	*92*	*4.9*	*183*	*5.2*	*18.7*	*9.7*	*1.7*
Button, Raw, Average	*1 Serving/50g*	*7*	*0.2*	*15*	*2.3*	*0.5*	*0.4*	*1.2*
Chestnut, Average	*1 Med/5g*	*1*	*0*	*13*	*1.8*	*0.4*	*0.5*	*0.6*
Chinese, Dried, Raw	*1oz/28g*	*80*	*0.5*	*284*	*10*	*59.9*	*1.8*	*0*
Closed Cup, Average	*1 Handful/30g*	*4*	*0.2*	*14*	*1.8*	*0.4*	*0.5*	*1.1*
Common, Boiled in Salted Water, Average	*1oz/28g*	*3*	*0.1*	*11*	*1.8*	*0.4*	*0.3*	*1.1*
Common, Fried, Average	*1oz/28g*	*44*	*4.5*	*157*	*2.4*	*0.3*	*16.2*	*1.5*
Common, Raw, Average	*1 Serving/80g*	*18*	*0.3*	*22*	*3.1*	*3.3*	*0.3*	*1*
Creamed, Average	*1oz/28g*	*23*	*1.5*	*82*	*1.3*	*6.8*	*5.5*	*0.5*
Dried	*1oz/28g*	*45*	*1.7*	*159*	*21.8*	*4.8*	*6*	*13.3*
Enoki, Average	*1 Serving/80g*	*34*	*0*	*42*	*3*	*7*	*0*	*3*
Flat, Large, Average	*1 Mushroom/52g*	*10*	*0.3*	*20*	*3.3*	*0.5*	*0.5*	*0.7*
Garlic, Average	*½ Pack/150g*	*159*	*14*	*106*	*2.1*	*3.7*	*9.3*	*1.7*
Garlic, Breaded, Frozen, Tesco*	1 Serving/54g	96	3	179	5.3	25.5	5.6	3
Oyster, Average	*1 Serving/80g*	*10*	*0.2*	*13*	*1.4*	*1.4*	*0.2*	*1.1*
Porcini, Wild, Dried, Merchant Gourmet*	1 Pack/50g	154	1.1	307	29.6	34.1	2.2	16.5
Portobello, Raw, Average	*1 Mushroom/50g*	*7*	*0.2*	*14*	*1.8*	*0.4*	*0.5*	*1.1*
Shiitake, Cooked	*1oz/28g*	*15*	*0.1*	*55*	*1.6*	*12.3*	*0.2*	*0*
Shiitake, Dried, Raw	*1oz/28g*	*83*	*0.3*	*296*	*9.6*	*63.9*	*1*	*0*
Sliced, Average	*1oz/28g*	*3*	*0.1*	*12*	*1.8*	*0.4*	*0.3*	*1.1*
Straw, Canned, Drained	*1oz/28g*	*4*	*0.1*	*15*	*2.1*	*1.2*	*0.2*	*0*
Stuffed, Cheesy, Asda*	1 Serving/290g	322	17.4	111	4.3	10	6	0
Stuffed, Garlic, Cream Cheese, Herb, Breadcrumbs, Aldi*	½ Pack/125g	184	10.1	147	6.4	11	8.1	2.2
Stuffed, with Leek Wensleydale, Loved by Us, Co-Op*	1 Mushroom/100g	85	3.6	85	4.3	7.8	3.6	2.1
MUSSELS								
Boiled, Flesh Only, Average	*1 Mussel/2g*	*2*	*0.1*	*104*	*16.7*	*3.5*	*2.7*	*0*
Boiled, Weighed in Shell, Average	*1 Mussel/7g*	*2*	*0.1*	*28*	*4.5*	*0.9*	*0.7*	*0*
Pickled, Drained, Average	*1oz/28g*	*32*	*0.6*	*112*	*20*	*1.5*	*2.2*	*0*
Raw, Weighed in Shell, Average	*1oz/28g*	*7*	*0.2*	*23*	*3.4*	*1*	*0.7*	*0*
MUSSELS IN								
Garlic Butter Sauce, Average	*½ Pack/225g*	*179*	*11.5*	*80*	*6.4*	*2*	*5.1*	*0.2*

	Measure INFO/WEIGHT	per Measure KCAL	per Measure FAT	Nutrition Values per 100g / 100ml KCAL	PROT	CARB	FAT	FIBRE
MUSSELS IN								
Oil, Smoked, Canned, Drained, John West*	1 Can/60g	117	7.3	196	19.9	1.6	12.2	0
Seasoned White Wine Sauce, Bantry Bay*	1 Serving/450g	270	9	60	6.3	4.1	2	0.1
White Wine Garlic Sauce , Scottish, Tesco*	1 Pouch/155g	130	6.2	84	9.8	1.9	4	0.6
White Wine Sauce, Sainsbury's*	½ Pack/250g	215	10.2	86	6.4	5.6	4.1	0.7
MUSTARD								
American, Average	*1 Tsp/5g*	*5*	*0.2*	*102*	*4.4*	*10.5*	*5*	*2.5*
Cajun, Colman's*	1 Tsp/6g	11	0.4	187	7	23	6.5	2.7
Coarse Grain, Average	*1 Tsp/5g*	*7*	*0.4*	*141*	*7.7*	*8.4*	*8.3*	*5.9*
Dijon, Average	*1 Tsp/5g*	*8*	*0.6*	*163*	*7.4*	*7.7*	*11.3*	*1.1*
English, Average	*1 Tsp/5g*	*9*	*0.4*	*173*	*6.8*	*19.2*	*7.6*	*1.2*
French, Average	*1 Tsp/5g*	*5*	*0.3*	*106*	*5.4*	*8.1*	*5.6*	*1.8*
German Style, Sainsbury's*	1 Serving/10g	9	0.6	92	5.5	2.8	6.5	0
Honey, Colman's*	1 Tsp/6g	12	0.5	208	7.4	24	8.2	0
Posh Dog, M&S*	1 Tsp/5g	4	0.3	83	5.1	1.5	5.4	4
Powder, Average	*1 Tsp/3g*	*15*	*0.9*	*452*	*28.9*	*20.7*	*28.7*	*0*
Smooth, Average	*1 Tsp/8g*	*11*	*0.7*	*139*	*7.1*	*9.7*	*8.2*	*0*
Whole Grain, Average	*1 Tsp/8g*	*11*	*0.8*	*140*	*8.2*	*4.2*	*10.2*	*4.9*
Yellow, Prepared	1 Tbsp/15ml	11	0.6	73	4	6	4	0
MUSTARD CRESS								
Raw	*1oz/28g*	*4*	*0.2*	*13*	*1.6*	*0.4*	*0.6*	*1.1*

	Measure INFO/WEIGHT	per Measure KCAL	FAT	Nutrition Values per 100g / 100ml KCAL	PROT	CARB	FAT	FIBRE
NACHOS								
American Chilli Beef, Asda*	1 Serving/200g	208	10	104	10	4.7	5	0.8
Cheesy with Salsa Soured Cream, Sainsbury's*	½ Pack/170g	449	26.9	264	8.8	21.5	15.8	1.4
Chilli, Sainsbury's*	½ Pack/250g	695	32.2	278	10.9	29.5	12.9	1.3
Kit, Old El Paso*	½ Pack/260g	598	26	230	4	31	10	0
with Cheese, From Restaurant, Average	**1 Nacho/16g**	**49**	**2.7**	**306**	**8**	**32.2**	**16.8**	**0**
NASI GORENG								
Indonesian, Asda*	1 Pack/360g	778	22.7	216	7.4	32.3	6.3	1.3
Vitasia, Lidl*	1 Bowl/250g	438	11	175	7.3	25.8	4.4	1.1
NECTARINES								
Fresh, Raw, Weighed with Stone, Average	**1 Med/140g**	**50**	**0.1**	**36**	**1.2**	**8**	**0.1**	**1.1**
NESQUIK								
Chocolate Flavour, Powder, Dry Weight, Nesquik, Nestle*	1 Serving/15g	56	0.5	372	3	82.9	3.1	6.5
Strawberry Flavour, Powder, Dry Weight, Nesquik, Nestle*	1 Serving/15g	59	0	393	0	98.1	0	0
NIK NAKS								
Cream 'n' Cheesy, KP Snacks*	1 Bag/34g	196	13	575	5.2	52.7	38.1	0.2
Nice 'n' Spicy, KP Snacks*	1 Bag/30g	171	11.5	571	4.6	51.6	38.4	1.6
Rib 'n' Saucy, Golden Wonder*	1 Sm Bag/25g	143	9.4	571	4.5	53.7	37.6	0.5
Scampi 'n' Lemon, KP Snacks*	1 Bag/25g	143	9.4	573	4.9	53.1	37.5	0.1
NOODLES								
Chicken, & Mushroom, Mugfull, Batchelors*	1 Portion245g	198	1.2	81	2.5	16	0.5	0.7
Bacon , Dry Supernoodles, Weight, Batchelors*	1 Pack/100g	526	23.6	526	9.4	69.2	23.6	1.6
Beef, Barbecue, Instant, Asda*	1 Pack/333g	420	16	126	2.6	18	4.8	0
Beef, BBQ, Instant, Cooked, Aldi*	1 Serving/324g	515	19.4	159	3.7	21.9	6	1.1
Beef, BBQ, Made Up, Supernoodles, Batchelors*	1 Serving/100g	156	6.7	156	3.2	20.9	6.7	1.1
Beef, BBQ, to Go, 98% Fat Free, Supernoodles, Batchelors	1 Pack/380g	308	0.6	81	2.4	17.6	0.2	0.6
Beef, Chilli, Finest, Tesco*	1 Pack/450g	486	8.6	108	7.7	15.2	1.9	0.9
Beef, Chilli, Ramen, M&S*	1 Pack/484g	532	17.4	110	8.1	11.9	3.6	0.8
Beef, Instant, Prepared, Heinz*	1 Pack/384g	257	0.4	67	2.1	14.4	0.1	0.6
Beef, Oriental, GFY, Asda*	1 Pack/400g	372	6.8	93	7.4	12.1	1.7	1.7
Beef, Shanghai, COU, M&S*	1 Pack/400g	380	6.4	95	6.8	13.1	1.6	1.5
Beef, Szechuan, Dry, Blue Dragon*	½ Pack/100g	350	1.2	350	10.5	72.3	1.2	0
Beef, Teriyaki, Taste of Japan, Tesco*	½ Pack/221g	253	9.1	114	6.9	12	4.1	0.9
Chicken & Herb, Dry Weight, Supernoodles, Batchelors*	½ Pack/43g	161	0.8	379	12.2	78.4	1.9	2.4
Chicken, & Coconut & Lime, Fuller Longer, M&S*	1 Pack/390g	448	17.6	115	8.7	10	4.5	1.6
Chicken, & Ham, Dry Weight, Supernoodles, Batchelors*	1 Pack/100g	472	20.2	472	9.4	63.2	20.2	1.5
Chicken, & Herb, Made Up, Supernoodles, Batchelors*	1 Pack/170g	322	1.6	189	6.1	39.2	0.9	1.2
Chicken, & Mushroom, Speedy, Newgate, Lidl*	1 Pot/302g	438	14.8	145	3.6	21	4.9	1.1
Chicken, & Noodle, Sweet Chilli, Tesco*	1 Pot/240g	323	4.3	134	6.4	22.5	1.8	1.3
Chicken, & Red Thai, Easy Steam, Tesco*	1 Serving/400g	556	28.4	139	10.3	8.6	7.1	1.1
Chicken, & Sweetcorn, Snack Pot, Morrisons*	1 Pot/247g	249	1.5	101	4.1	19.8	0.6	1.6
Chicken, Chilli, GFY, Asda*	1 Pack/415g	461	3.3	111	6	20	0.8	1
Chicken, Chinese Style, GFY, Asda*	1 Pack/393g	295	6.7	75	6	9	1.7	0.6
Chicken, Chinese, As Consumed, Fresh Ideas, Morrisons*	1 Pot/375g	394	10.9	105	6.3	12.2	2.9	2.7
Chicken, Chinese, Asda*	1 Pot/302g	305	4.2	101	6	16	1.4	0.8
Chicken, Curry Flavour, Instant, Sainsbury's*	1 Pack/85g	167	6.2	196	4.6	27.9	7.3	0.8
Chicken, Firecracker, Made Up, Naked, Symingtons*	1 Pot/338g	301	2	89	2.7	17.5	0.6	1.3
Chicken, Flavour, 3 Minute, Dry, Blue Dragon*	1 Pack/85g	403	18.2	475	9.3	61.2	21.4	0
Chicken, Flavour, Dry, Princes*	1 Pack/85g	395	16	465	10	63.8	18.8	0
Chicken, Flavour, Instant, Cooked, Smart Price, Asda*	1 Serving/246g	293	11.1	111	2.8	14.9	4.2	1
Chicken, Flavour, Instant, Made Up, Tesco*	½ Pack/168g	285	10.6	170	4.1	23.7	6.3	1.5
Chicken, Flavour, Instant, Sainsbury's*	½ Pack/335g	549	21.4	164	4.4	22.3	6.4	1.3
Chicken, Instant, Basics, Sainsbury's*	½ Pack/132g	209	7	158	4	23.5	5.3	0.6
Chicken, Instant, Cooked, Aldi*	½ Pack/150g	248	10.6	165	3.3	21	7.1	1.3

NOODLES

	Measure INFO/WEIGHT	KCAL	FAT	KCAL	PROT	CARB	FAT	FIBRE
Chicken, Instant, Made Up, Everyday Value, Tesco*	1 Pack/265g	437	15.6	165	3.8	19.4	5.9	3.2
Chicken, Laksa, Made Up, Kabuto*	1 Pot/450g	342	6.3	76	2.6	13.2	1.4	0.6
Chicken, Made Up, Supernoodles, Batchelors*	1 Serving/150g	264	11.8	176	3.1	23	7.9	0.4
Chicken, Oriental Style, Instant, Cooked, Koka*	1 Pack/485g	393	16.5	81	1.9	10.4	3.4	0.5
Chicken, Pad Thai, Tesco*	1 Pack/378g	558	20.8	148	9.1	14.8	5.5	1.2
Chicken, Spicy, King Prawn, Bowl, Tesco*	1 Pack/355g	353	2.2	100	7.1	15.2	0.6	2.3
Chicken, Sweet Chilli, Cooked, My Goodness, Sainsbury's*	1 Pack/380g	321	5.5	87	5.9	11.6	1.5	2
Chicken, Teriyaki, Pot, Tesco*	1 Pot/300g	315	4.8	105	5.8	15.9	1.6	1.8
Chicken, Yellow Thai, Taste Thailand, Banquet Box, M&S*	½ Pack/125g	182	9.6	146	8.7	9.5	7.7	2
Chilli Infused, Blue Dragon*	1 Serving/150g	286	1	191	6.1	33.6	0.7	0.3
Chinese, & Veggies, Cashew Cream Sauce, Amy's Kitchen*	1 Pack/271g	490	21.9	181	6	21	8.1	2
Chow Mein, Classic, As Prepared, Fusian, Maggi*	½ Pack/190g	273	11.8	144	3.3	18	6.2	1.7
Chow Mein, Instant, Made Up, Morrisons*	½ Pack/168g	210	7.9	125	3	17.1	4.7	1.2
Chow Mein, Made Up, Supernoodles, Batchelors*	½ Pack/150g	262	11.8	175	3	23	7.9	0.4
Chow Mein, Sainsbury's*	1 Pack/125g	136	2.2	109	3.9	19.2	1.8	0.8
Chow Mein, Snack in a Pot, LC, Tesco*	1 Pot/235g	235	1.2	100	3.7	19.4	0.5	1.8
Crispy, Dry, Blue Dragon*	1 Box/125g	438	0.6	350	2.4	84	0.5	0
Curry, Chicken, Thai Green, Made Up, Kabuto Noodles*	1 Pot/408g	298	4.9	73	1.6	13.9	1.2	0.5
Curry, Instant, Dry, Asda*	1 Serving/65g	415	11	638	20	101.5	16.9	0.9
Curry, Instant, Dry, Heinz*	1 Serving/85g	261	0.3	307	9.5	66.4	0.4	2.7
Curry, Instant, Sainsbury's*	1 Pack/335g	412	15.4	123	2.6	17.8	4.6	0.1
Curry, Instant, Vitasia, Lidl*	1 Pack/108g	124	5.3	115	2.5	15.3	4.9	0
Curry, Mild, Dry Weight, Supernoodles, Batchelors*	½ Pack/50g	260	11.7	520	9.4	67.8	23.4	1.4
Curry, Mild, Made Up, Supernoodles, Batchelors*	1 Serving/100g	157	6.7	157	3.2	20.9	6.7	1
Curry, Singapore, Made Up, Naked Noodle Snack Pot*	1 Pot/329g	270	2	82	2.9	15.7	0.6	0.9
Curry, Spicy, Dry, Princes*	1 Pack/85g	395	16	465	9.6	64.1	18.8	0
Curry, Spicy, Speedy, Newgate, Lidl*	1 Pot/312g	443	13.7	142	3.6	21	4.4	2.1
Duck, Hoisin, Shredded, Tesco*	1 Pack/388g	384	10.1	99	5.6	12.3	2.6	2
Egg, & Bean Sprouts, Cooked, Tesco*	1 Pack/250g	238	5.2	95	4.4	14.6	2.1	1.5
Egg, Asda*	¼ Pack/176g	319	1.1	181	5.4	38	0.6	0.8
Egg, Boiled	**1oz/28g**	**17**	**0.1**	**62**	**2.2**	**13**	**0.5**	**0.6**
Egg, Chilli Ginger, Asian Fusion, Waitrose*	½ Pack/137g	188	3.3	137	4.4	24	2.4	0.8
Egg, Dry, Average	**1 Block/63g**	**218**	**1.2**	**348**	**12.1**	**70.1**	**1.9**	**2.6**
Egg, Fine Thread, Dry, M&S*	1 Serving/63g	220	0.6	350	14.3	71.6	0.9	5.1
Egg, Fine, Blue Dragon*	1 Serving/100g	356	1.7	356	13.8	70	1.7	3.4
Egg, Fine, Dry Weight, Sharwood's*	1 Block/63g	216	1.3	346	12	70	2.1	2.5
Egg, Fine, Fresh, M&S*	1 Pack/275g	330	6.1	120	4.4	20.7	2.2	1.5
Egg, Fine, Waitrose*	¼ Pack/63g	221	1.6	353	15	67.3	2.6	3.8
Egg, Free Range, Asda*	1 Serving/125g	209	4.9	167	5.1	27	3.9	1.8
Egg, Free Range, Fresh, Sainsbury's*	½ Pack/205g	340	7	166	5	28	3.4	1.8
Egg, Free Range, Morrisons*	1 Pack/300g	372	8.7	124	4.9	19.7	2.9	1.3
Egg, Fresh, Tesco*	½ Pack/205g	287	3.9	140	4.9	25.3	1.9	2
Egg, M&S*	½ Pack/110g	165	1.9	150	4.9	28.3	1.7	2.8
Egg, Medium, Asda*	1 Serving/83g	125	0.7	150	4.8	31	0.8	1.3
Egg, Medium, Dry Nests, Cooks' Ingredients, Waitrose*	1 Nest/54g	189	0.9	350	13.2	70.4	1.7	2.4
Egg, Medium, Dry, Blue Dragon*	1 Serving/50g	158	1.2	317	10.1	62.3	2.4	3.1
Egg, Medium, Dry, Sharwood's*	1 Serving/63g	229	1.4	367	13.2	71.2	2.3	4.1
Egg, Medium, Sainsbury's*	1 Serving/63g	236	1.2	375	12.5	76.4	1.9	1.3
Egg, Raw, Medium, Waitrose*	¼ Pack/63g	221	1.6	353	15	67.3	2.6	3.8
Egg, Singapore Curry, Made Up, Aldi*	1 Pot/338g	341	1.9	88	2.7	18	0.5	1
Egg, Thick, Dry Weight, Sharwood's*	1 Serving/63g	214	1.1	342	10.8	71	1.7	2.5
Egg, Tossed in Sesame Oil, Asda*	½ Pack/150g	174	10.5	116	2.3	11	7	0.6
Fine, Chicken Breast, Sweet Chilli Sauce, Tesco*	1 Pack/329g	462	11.9	140	8.5	17.7	3.6	1.6

NOODLES

Measure INFO/WEIGHT	per Measure KCAL	FAT	Nutrition Values per 100g / 100ml KCAL	PROT	CARB	FAT	FIBRE
Fried, Average							
Fried, Average — 1oz/28g	*43*	*3.2*	*153*	*1.9*	*11.3*	*11.5*	*0.5*
Garlic, Chilli Ginger, Tesco* — 1 Serving/350g	508	11.2	145	4.8	24.1	3.2	2.6
Glass, Dry Weight — 1 Serving/100g	*351*	*0.1*	*351*	*0.1*	*86.1*	*0.1*	*0.5*
Madras, Mighty Spicy, Made Up, Mug Shot, Symingtons* — 1 Pot/320g	278	1	87	2.5	18.1	0.3	0.8
Medium, Soft, Ready to Wok, Asia Specialities, Aldi* — 1 Serving/150g	232	0.9	155	6.6	30	0.6	1.6
Medium, Traditional, Straight to Wok, Amoy* — 1 Serving/150g	243	2.2	162	4.3	34.3	1.5	1.3
Miso, Mushroom, Kit, Itsu* — 1 Serving/237g	298	4.7	126	6	21	2	0
Nest, Medium, Cooked, Waitrose* — 1 Nest/63g	88	0.3	139	5	28.6	0.5	0.6
Oriental, Snack Pot, Made Up, HL, Tesco* — 1 Serving/238g	221	0.7	93	3.1	19.4	0.3	0.6
Plain, Boiled — 1oz/28g	*17*	*0.1*	*62*	*2.4*	*13*	*0.4*	*0.7*
Plain, Dry — 1oz/28g	*109*	*1.7*	*388*	*11.7*	*76.1*	*6.2*	*2.9*
Pork, Chinese, CBY, Asda* — 1 Pack/400g	380	6.4	95	6.7	12.6	1.6	1.8
Pork, Spicy BBQ, Snack Pot, Tesco* — 1 Pack/280g	351	7.3	125	4.8	19.7	2.6	2
Prawn, Chilli, King, Finest, Tesco* — 1 Pack/400g	340	8	85	4	11.9	2	0.9
Prawn, Hot & Sour, King, Bowl, My Goodness, Sainsbury's* — 1 Pack/360g	324	3.2	90	4.7	15.1	0.9	1.1
Prawn, King, Singapore, Free From, Tesco* — 1 Pack/338g	352	11.8	104	3.8	13.8	3.5	1.2
Prawn, Tiger, Stir Fry, Tesco* — 1 Pack/400g	596	14.8	149	6	23	3.7	2.7
Ramen, Chicken, Miso, The City Kitchen* — 1 Pack/368g	303	8.1	82	6.5	8.3	2.2	1.6
Ramen, Morrisons* — 1/3 Pack/83g	289	0.7	348	11.1	72.7	0.8	2.8
Ramen, Sesame, Kit, Itsu* — 1 Serving/239g	323	6.7	135	7.1	19	2.8	2.8
Ribbon, Pad Thai, Ready to Wok, Sharwood's* — 1 Serving/150g	206	1.7	137	5	26.3	1.1	1
Ribbon, Soft, Sharwood's* — 1 Portion/150g	225	1.8	150	5.7	25.7	1.2	6.6
Rice, Cooked — 1 Cup/176g	*192*	*0.4*	*109*	*0.9*	*24.9*	*0.2*	*1*
Rice, Cooked, Sharwood's* — 1 Serving/200g	239	0.6	120	2	27.2	0.3	0.8
Rice, Dry, Amoy* — 1oz/28g	101	0.3	361	6.5	86.6	1	0
Rice, Dry, Blue Dragon* — 1 Serving/30g	113	0	376	7	84	0	0
Rice, Fresh, Sainsbury's* — ½ Pack/150g	202	3.3	135	2.2	25.9	2.2	1.4
Rice, in Curry Sauce, Instant, Made Up, Free From, Tesco* — 1 Pot/374g	292	0.7	78	1.6	17	0.2	1
Rice, Medium, Blue Dragon* — 1 Serving/63g	235	0	376	7	84	0	0
Rice, Oriental, Thai, Stir Fry, Dry Weight, Sharwood's* — 1 Serving/63g	226	0.6	361	6.5	86.8	1	2.4
Rice, Stir Fry, Tesco* — ½ Pack/190g	304	10.8	160	2	24.8	5.7	1
Rice, Thick, Thai, Dry, M&S* — 1 Serving/100g	355	0.7	355	6.5	80.6	0.7	1.4
Rice, Vermicelli, Mama* — 1 Serving/45g	166	0.4	370	7	81	1	0
Rice, with Spring Onions, Fresh Tastes, Asda* — ½ Pack/188g	248	4.1	132	2.2	25.9	2.2	1.4
Singapore, BGTY, Sainsbury's* — 1 Pack/369g	317	10	86	7.2	8.2	2.7	2.1
Singapore, Sainsbury's* — 1 Pack/450g	540	18	120	6.4	13.3	4	2.7
Singapore, Style, Asda* — 1 Pack/400g	688	32	172	7	18	8	1
Singapore, Style, Sainsbury's* — ½ Pack/150g	320	10.8	214	3.2	33.2	7.2	1.3
Singapore, with Chicken, Pork, Egg, Prawns, M&S* — 1 Pack/400g	560	25.6	140	5.7	14.1	6.4	1.4
Soba, with Yakisoba Sauce, Instant, Made Up, Nissin* — 1 Pot/180g	394	17.6	219	5.3	26.1	9.8	0
Soybean, GF, Organic, Yutaka* — 1 Serving/50g	167	3.3	334	44	15	6.6	20
Special, Chinese Takeaway, Iceland* — 1 Pack/340g	422	10.9	124	6.5	17.2	3.2	0.6
Spicy, Sainsbury's* — 1 Serving/180g	182	8.3	101	10.4	4.5	4.6	0.9
Stir Fry, Tesco* — 1 Serving/150g	202	3.6	135	5.3	23	2.4	1.5
Straight to Wok, Medium, Amoy* — 1 Pack/150g	240	2.2	160	5.8	31.7	1.5	0
Straight to Wok, Rice, Amoy* — 1 Pack/150g	174	0.2	116	1.6	27.4	0.1	0
Straight to Wok, Singapore, Amoy* — 1 Serving/150g	206	3.3	137	6.4	21.6	2.2	2.8
Straight to Wok, Thread, Fine, Amoy* — 1 Pack/150g	237	3.9	158	5	28.7	2.6	0
Straight to Wok, Udon, Amoy* — 1 Pack/150g	212	2	141	4.4	28.8	1.3	0
Sweet Sour, Asian, Veggie Bowl, Birds Eye* — 1 Meal/380g	323	6.8	85	3.5	12.8	1.8	1.7
Sweet Chilli, Thai, Dry Weight, Supernoodles, Batchelors* — 1 Pack/85g	292	1	343	10.6	72.5	1.2	3
Sweet Chilli, Thai, Made Up, Aldi* — 1 Pot/338g	301	1.7	89	2.9	18	0.5	1
Teriyaki, Japanese, Made Up, Naked Noodle, Symingtons* — 1 Pot/327g	268	2	82	2.9	15.8	0.6	0.7

N

	Measure INFO/WEIGHT	per Measure KCAL	per Measure FAT	Nutrition Values per 100g / 100ml KCAL	PROT	CARB	FAT	FIBRE
NOODLES								
Thai, Spicy, Instant, Heinz*	1 Pack/385g	262	0.4	68	2.1	14.6	0.1	0.6
Thai, Spicy, Stir Fry, HL, Tesco*	½ Pack/250g	220	5.5	88	4.1	12.9	2.2	1.7
Thai, Style, Sainsbury's*	1 Pack/340g	381	7.8	112	3.3	19.4	2.3	0.7
Thai, Style, Snack, Cupshotz, Aldi*	1 Pack/55g	215	2.8	391	11.4	71.4	5.1	6.9
Thai, Waitrose*	1 Pack/300g	357	6.3	119	6.8	18.4	2.1	1.7
Tom Yum, Vegetable, Made Up, Kabuto Noodles*	1 Pot/405g	263	0.8	65	1.3	14.6	0.2	0.5
Udon, Curry, Kit, Itsu*	1 Serving/238g	319	5.2	134	5.9	21	2.2	3
Udon, Japanese & Dashi Soup Stock, Yutaka*	1 Pack/230g	290	1.2	126	3	26.8	0.5	0
Udon, Japanese, Sainsbury's*	1 Serving/150g	210	2.7	140	3.9	27.1	1.8	1.2
Udon, Style, Thick, Ready to Wok, Sharwood's*	1 Pack/150g	233	0.6	155	5.4	32.5	0.4	2.1
Udon, Wheat, Organic, Explore Asian*	1 Serving/56g	202	1.2	361	14.3	71.4	2.1	1.8
Udon, with Chicken, Indian Inspired, Pot, Itsu*	1 Pot/492g	295	3.4	60	2.1	10.3	0.7	1.8
Udon, Yasai Yaki, Allplants*	½ Pack/380g	494	24.3	130	4.4	12	6.4	2.1
Vegetable, Savoury, COU, M&S*	1 Pack/450g	270	2.7	60	2.9	11.5	0.6	1.2
Wholewheat, Cooked Weight, Sharwoods*	1 Portion/161g	215	1.5	134	5	24.8	0.9	2.7
Wholewheat, Dry, Sharwoods*	1 Portion/63g	224	1.4	356	13	66.2	2.3	9.2
NOUGAT								
Average	*1 Sm Bar/28g*	*108*	*2.4*	*384*	*4.4*	*77.3*	*8.5*	*0.9*
Raspberry Orange Hazelnut, Thorntons*	1 Sweet/9g	39	1.8	433	4.8	60	20	2.2
Soft, Bar, Bassett's*	1 Bar/25g	94	1	375	4	82	4	0
NUT ROAST								
Average	*1 Serving/200g*	*704*	*51.4*	*352*	*13.3*	*18.3*	*25.7*	*4.2*
Courgette & Spiced Tomato, Cauldron Foods*	1 Serving/100g	208	12.3	208	11.7	12.5	12.3	4.9
Lentil, Average	*1oz/28g*	*62*	*3.4*	*222*	*10.6*	*18.8*	*12.1*	*3.8*
Vegan, GF, Clive's*	1 Serving/140g	216	13.7	154	5.1	20.8	9.8	0
NUTMEG								
Ground, Average	*1 Tsp/3g*	*16*	*1.1*	*525*	*5.8*	*45.3*	*36.3*	*0*
NUTS								
Assortment, Eat Well, M&S*	1 Pack/70g	441	41.2	630	16.7	8.5	58.9	5.3
Cashews Peanuts, Honey Roasted, Average	*1 Serving/50g*	*290*	*21.4*	*579*	*21.6*	*26.6*	*42.9*	*4.2*
Chopped, Mixed, M&S*	1 Serving/30g	185	15.2	616	27.1	9.6	50.8	6
Medley, On the Go, Sainsbury's*	1 Pack/20g	127	11.2	636	19.8	9.2	56.1	7.5
Mixed	*1 Pack/40g*	*243*	*21.6*	*607*	*22.9*	*7.9*	*54.1*	*6*
Mixed, Almonds, Brazil, Hazel Walnuts, M&S*	1 Serving/25g	168	16	670	16	4.8	64	5.4
Mixed, Delicious, Boots*	1 Pack/50g	332	29	663	16	16	58	8.1
Mixed, Natural, Asda*	1 Snack/30g	197	18.8	656	18	4.3	62.7	7.4
Mixed, Natural, Luxury, Tesco*	1oz/28g	179	16.2	639	22.6	6.9	57.9	5.6
Mixed, Roasted, Salted, On the Go, Sainsbury's*	1 Serving/30g	186	15.6	620	23.1	10.5	52	8.9
Mixed, Roasted, Salted, Waitrose*	1 Pack/200g	1252	116.8	626	13.7	11.3	58.4	4.4
Mixed, Unsalted, Sainsbury's*	1 Serving/50g	311	28.8	622	18.5	7.2	57.7	8.7
Pine, Tesco*	1 Pack/100g	699	68.6	699	16.5	4	68.6	1.9
NUTS & RAISINS								
Mixed, Average	*1 Serving/30g*	*144*	*10.2*	*481*	*14.1*	*31.5*	*34.1*	*4.5*
Peanuts, Mixed, Average	*1 Pack/40g*	*174*	*10.4*	*435*	*15.3*	*37.5*	*26*	*4.4*
Yoghurt Coated, Waitrose*	1 Serving/50g	264	18.4	527	10.9	38.2	36.7	3

	Measure INFO/WEIGHT	per Measure KCAL	FAT	Nutrition Values per 100g / 100ml KCAL	PROT	CARB	FAT	FIBRE
OAT CAKES								
Cheese, GF, Nairn's*	1 Oatcake/9g	45	2.3	498	14.8	44.4	25.7	7.3
Cheese, Nairn's*	1 Cake/8g	39	2.3	471	13.2	43.3	27.2	6.8
Fine Milled, Nairn's*	1 Cake/8g	35	1.7	449	10.5	52.6	21.8	8.6
Herb Pumpkin Seed, Nairn's*	1 Cake/10g	43	2.1	426	12.2	46.8	21.1	13
Highland, Walkers*	1 Cake/12g	54	2.5	451	10.3	56	20.6	6.7
Oatmeal, Rough, Nairn's*	1 Cake/11g	45	1.8	431	10.2	58.6	17.3	8
Oatmeal, Rough, Organic, Nairn's*	1 Cake/10g	43	1.7	418	10.2	57.7	16.3	7.5
Orkney, Thick, Stockan's*	1 Oatcake/27g	122	5.2	487	8.7	66.7	20.6	6.3
Orkney, Thin, Stockan's*	1 Oatcake/100g	453	23	453	11.1	50.3	23	6
Retail, Average	*1 Cake/13g*	*57*	*2.4*	*441*	*10*	*63*	*18.3*	*2*
Rough Scottish, Sainsbury's*	1 Cake/11g	51	2.1	462	12.3	59.9	19.3	6.5
Rough with Olive Oil, Paterson's*	1 Cake/13g	55	2.1	440	11.7	54.7	17	0
Rough, Sainsbury's*	1 Oatcake/10g	47	2	454	9.8	55.4	19.2	10
Rough, Scottish, Tesco*	1 Cake/10g	45	1.9	435	11.4	55.3	18.4	8
Scottish, Asda*	1 Oatcake/13g	58	2.3	461	11	59	18	9.8
Scottish, Rough, Waitrose*	1 Cake/13g	55	2.3	438	10.4	57.4	18.5	8
Scottish, Tower Gate, Lidl*	1 Oatcake/13g	60	2.5	465	10	60	19	6.8
Traditional, M&S*	1 Cake/11g	49	2	445	11	59.3	18.3	6.6
OAT DRINK								
Barista Edition, Oatly*	100ml	59	3	59	1	6.6	3	0.8
Healthy, Enriched, Oatly*	1 Serving/250ml	112	3.8	45	1	6.5	1.5	0.8
Oat Milk, Organic, Healthy, Oatly*	1 Serving/250ml	100	1.2	40	1	6.7	0.5	0.8
OCTOPUS								
Chunks in Olive Oil, Palacio De Oriente*	1 Tin/111g	148	4	133	21.6	4.5	3.6	0
Raw	*1oz/28g*	*18*	*0.3*	*66*	*14.1*	*0*	*1*	*0*
OIL								
Avocado, Olivado*	1 Tsp/5ml	40	4.4	802	0	0	88	0
Black Truffle, Grapeseed, Cuisine Perel*	1 Tsp/5ml	43	5	857	0	7.1	100	0
Chilli, Average	*1 Tsp/5ml*	*41*	*4.6*	*824*	*0*	*0*	*91.5*	*0*
Chinese Stir Fry, Asda*	1 Tbsp/15ml	123	13.7	823	0	0	91.4	0
Coconut, Average	*1 Tsp/5ml*	*45*	*5*	*899*	*0*	*0*	*99.9*	*0*
Coconut, Cold Pressed, Virgin, Waitrose*	1 Tbsp/15g	135	15	900	0	0	100	0
Cod Liver, Average	*1 Capsule/1g*	*9*	*1*	*900*	*0*	*0*	*100*	*0*
Corn, Average	*1 Tsp/5ml*	*43*	*4.8*	*864*	*0*	*0*	*96*	*0*
Evening Primrose, Average	*1 Serving/1g*	*9*	*1*	*900*	*0*	*0*	*100*	*0*
Fish, Average	*1 Serving/1g*	*9*	*1*	*900*	*0*	*0*	*100*	*0*
Flax Seed, Average	*1 Tbsp/15ml*	*124*	*13.9*	*829*	*0*	*0*	*92.6*	*0*
Garlic, Infuse, Fry Light*	1 Spray/0.2ml	1	0.1	507	0	0.4	52.9	0
Grapeseed, Average	*1 Tsp/5ml*	*43*	*4.8*	*866*	*0*	*0*	*96.2*	*0*
Groundnut, Average	*1 Tsp/5ml*	*41*	*4.6*	*824*	*0*	*0*	*91.8*	*0*
Hazelnut, Average	*1 Tsp/5ml*	*45*	*5*	*899*	*0*	*0*	*99.9*	*0*
Linseed, Organic, Biona*	1 Serving/10ml	84	9.3	837	0	0	93	0
Mustard, Average	*1 Serving/100g*	*884*	*100*	*884*	*0*	*0*	*100*	*0*
Olive, Average	*1 Tsp/5ml*	*43*	*4.7*	*855*	*0*	*0*	*94.9*	*0*
Olive, Basil Infused, Tesco*	1 Serving/20ml	180	20	900	0	0	100	0
Olive, Evo Filtered, Italian, Parioli, Cucina*	1 Serving/100ml	825	91.6	825	0	0	91.6	0
Olive, Extra Virgin, Average	*1 Tsp/5ml*	*42*	*4.7*	*848*	*0*	*0*	*94.5*	*0*
Olive, Extra Virgin, Only 1 Cal, Spray, Fry Light*	1 Spray/0.2ml	1	0.1	498	0	0	55.2	0
Olive, Extra Virgin, Spray, Sainsbury's*	10 Sprays	10	1.1	823	0	0	91.4	0
Olive, Garlic, Average	*1 Tbsp/15ml*	*127*	*14.1*	*848*	*0*	*0*	*94.3*	*0*
Olive, Mild, Average	*1 Tbsp/15ml*	*129*	*14.4*	*862*	*0*	*0*	*95.7*	*0*
Olive, Spray, Average	*10 Sprays/2ml*	*10*	*1.1*	*508*	*0*	*0*	*54.6*	*0*
Olive, Spray, Fry Light*	5 Sprays/1ml	5	0.5	520	0	0	54.2	0

	Measure INFO/WEIGHT	per Measure KCAL	FAT	Nutrition Values per 100g / 100ml KCAL	PROT	CARB	FAT	FIBRE
OIL								
Palm, Average	*1 Tsp/5ml*	*45*	*5*	*899*	*0*	*0*	*99.9*	*0*
Peanut, Average	*1 Tsp/5ml*	*45*	*5*	*899*	*0*	*0*	*99.9*	*0*
Rapeseed, Average	*1 Tbsp/15ml*	*130*	*14.4*	*864*	*0*	*0*	*96*	*0*
Rice Bran, Average	*1 Tbsp/14g*	*120*	*13.6*	*884*	*0*	*0*	*100*	*0*
Safflower, Average	*1 Tsp/5ml*	*45*	*5*	*899*	*0*	*0*	*99.9*	*0*
Sesame, Average	*1 Tsp/5ml*	*45*	*5*	*892*	*0.1*	*0*	*99.9*	*0*
Soya, Average	*1 Tsp/5ml*	*45*	*5*	*899*	*0*	*0*	*99.9*	*0*
Sunflower, Average	*1 Tsp/5ml*	*43*	*4.8*	*869*	*0*	*0*	*96.6*	*0*
Sunflower, Spray, Fry Light*	1 Spray/0.2ml	1	0.1	519	0	0.2	53.9	0
Ultimate Blend, Udo's Choice*	1 Capsule/1ml	9	1	900	1.3	0	96.8	0
Vegetable, Average	*1 Tbsp/15ml*	*129*	*14.3*	*858*	*0*	*0*	*95.3*	*0*
Walnut, Average	*1 Tsp/5ml*	*45*	*5*	*899*	*0*	*0*	*99.9*	*0*
OKRA								
Boiled in Unsalted Water, Average	*1 Serving/80g*	*22*	*0.7*	*28*	*2.5*	*2.7*	*0.9*	*3.6*
Raw, Average	*1 Serving/80g*	*18*	*0.6*	*23*	*2.1*	*2.2*	*0.7*	*3*
Stir-Fried in Corn Oil, Average	*1 Serving/80g*	*215*	*20.9*	*269*	*4.3*	*4.4*	*26.1*	*6.3*
OLIVES								
Black Green with Greek Feta Cheese, Tesco*	1 Pot/100g	200	20.1	200	3.4	0.3	20.1	4.6
Black, Pitted, Average	*½ Jar/82g*	*135*	*13.3*	*164*	*1*	*3.5*	*16.2*	*3.1*
Black, Pitted, Hojiblanca, in Brine, Specially Selected, M&S*	1 Serving/25g	32	3.3	127	0.5	0	13.2	3
Green Harissa, Graze*	1 Punnet/44g	110	11.6	255	0.8	2	27	3
Green, Garlic Stuffed, Asda*	1 Olive/3g	6	0.6	174	1.8	3.5	17	0
Green, Lightly Flavoured with Lemon & Garlic, Attis*	1 Serving/50g	82	8.2	164	1.7	2.2	16.5	0
Green, Manzanilla, Stuffed with Jalapeno, Fragata *	½ Can/100g	169	18	169	0.8	0	18	0
Green, Pitted, Average	*1 Olive/3g*	*4*	*0.4*	*130*	*1.1*	*0.9*	*13.3*	*2.5*
Green, Stuffed with Almonds, Pitted, Waitrose*	1 Serving/50g	90	8.4	180	3.8	3.2	16.9	2.5
Halkidiki, Stuffed with Garlic, Tesco*	¼ Pack/40g	66	6.7	164	1.3	0.3	16.8	3
Kalamata, Pitted, Greek, Drained, Sainsbury's*	1 Serving/15g	31	3.2	205	1.6	0.5	21.4	3.2
Marinated, Mixed, M&S*	1 Serving/20g	33	3	165	1.6	6.5	14.9	3
Marinated, Selection, M&S*	4 Olives/20g	44	4.4	225	1.4	3.9	22.6	2.1
Mixed, Greek Feta, Sainsburys*	1 Serving/50g	114	10.8	227	5.8	1.3	21.6	2
Mixed, Chilli Garlic, Asda*	1 Serving/30g	43	4.7	144	0.9	0	15.6	6.1
Nocellara, Green, Unearthed*	1 Serving/30g	62	6.4	206	1.1	0.4	21.5	0
Spanish, Extra Virgin Olive Oil, Hint of Lemon, M&S*	1 Serving/25g	51	5.4	205	1	0.1	21.4	3.8
Stuffed, Pimiento, Finest, Tesco*	3 Olives/16g	23	2.1	142	1.1	3.8	13	2.7
with Chipotle Manchego, Unearthed*	1 Pack/184g	482	44.7	262	8.1	4	24.3	0
OMELETTE								
Cheese & Mushroom, Apetito*	1 Serving/320g	486	25	152	6.2	14.4	7.8	1.9
Cheese, 2 Egg, Average	*1 Omelette/180g*	*479*	*40.7*	*266*	*15.9*	*0*	*22.6*	*0*
Cheese, Asda*	1 Omelette/119g	268	22.6	225	12	1.5	19	0
Cheese, HFC, Tesco*	1 Omelette/95g	214	16.4	226	13.2	4.1	17.3	0.6
Ham & Mushroom, Farmfoods*	1 Omelette/120g	200	16.7	167	8.7	1.8	13.9	0.1
Mushroom & Cheese, Tesco*	1 Omelette/120g	248	21.5	207	9.8	1.6	17.9	0.2
Plain, 2 Egg	*1 Omelette/120g*	*229*	*19.7*	*191*	*10.9*	*0*	*16.4*	*0*
Spanish	*1oz/28g*	*34*	*2.3*	*120*	*5.7*	*6.2*	*8.3*	*1.4*
Spanish, Potato, Rapido, Unearthed*	1 Pack/300g	492	32.7	164	5.2	10.5	10.9	2.2
ONION POWDER								
Average	*1 Tsp/2g*	*7*	*0*	*341*	*10.4*	*79.1*	*1*	*15.2*
ONION RINGS								
Battered, Free From, Tesco*	3 Rings/63g	190	9.5	303	3.1	37.3	15.2	2.1
Battered, Mini, Frozen, Tesco*	4 Rings/34g	87	3.9	259	4.2	32.8	11.6	3.3
Battered, Oven Baked, Tesco*	1 Serving/50g	110	5	219	3.9	28.4	10	3.5
Battered, Sainsbury's*	1 Ring/12g	26	1.2	219	3.9	28.4	10	3.5

	Measure INFO/WEIGHT	per Measure KCAL	per Measure FAT	Nutrition Values per 100g / 100ml KCAL	PROT	CARB	FAT	FIBRE
ONION RINGS								
Beer Battered, Frozen, Tesco*	3 Rings/75g	213	10	284	4.6	36	13.3	0.8
Breaded & Fried, From Restaurant	**1 Ring/12g**	**40**	**2.2**	**332**	**4.5**	**37.7**	**18.7**	**0**
Breaded, Asda*	1 Serving/67g	180	7.4	267	4.3	36	11	3.3
Breaded, Iceland*	1 Ring/11g	33	1.7	293	4.4	34.2	15.4	2.7
Oven Crisp Batter, Tesco*	1 Ring/17g	44	1.9	259	4.1	34.4	11.2	2.1
Whole, Battered, Frozen, Aunt Bessies*	5 Rings/90g	195	10.8	217	2.5	24	12	1.8
ONIONS								
Baked	**1oz/28g**	**29**	**0.2**	**103**	**3.5**	**22.3**	**0.6**	**3.9**
Boiled in Unsalted Water	**1oz/28g**	**5**	**0**	**17**	**0.6**	**3.7**	**0.1**	**0.7**
Dried, Raw, Average	**1oz/28g**	**88**	**0.5**	**313**	**10.2**	**68.6**	**1.7**	**12.1**
Flakes, Dried, Average	**1 Tbsp/15g**	**52**	**0.1**	**349**	**9**	**83.3**	**0.5**	**9.2**
Fried, Average	**1oz/28g**	**46**	**3.1**	**164**	**2.3**	**14.1**	**11.2**	**3.1**
Pickled, Average	**1 Onion/15g**	**3**	**0**	**19**	**0.7**	**4.1**	**0.1**	**0.6**
Pickled, Red, Sliced, in Vinegar, M&S*	¼ Jar/38g	28	0	75	0.7	17.3	0.1	1.2
Raw, Average	**1 Med/180g**	**69**	**0.4**	**38**	**1.2**	**7.9**	**0.2**	**1.3**
Red, Raw, Average	**1 Med/180g**	**66**	**0.4**	**37**	**1.2**	**7.9**	**0.2**	**1.5**
Spring, Raw, Average	**1 Med/15g**	**4**	**0.1**	**24**	**1.9**	**2.9**	**0.5**	**1.4**
ORANGE CURD								
Baxters*	1 Tbsp/15g	51	1.1	343	2	67	7.4	0.1
Florida, Finest, Tesco*	1 Tbsp/15g	52	1.3	348	2.9	63.8	9	0.2
Jaffa, Luxury, Waitrose*	1 Tbsp/15g	54	1.5	357	3	63.5	10.1	0.1
Sainsbury's*	2 Tsps/12g	34	0.5	282	1.1	59.2	4.4	0.4
ORANGES								
Blood, Average	**1 Orange/140g**	**82**	**0**	**58**	**0.8**	**13.3**	**0**	**2.5**
Fresh, Weighed with Peel, Average	**1 Med/220g**	**97**	**0.5**	**44**	**0.9**	**10.8**	**0.2**	**3.2**
Fresh, without Peel, Average	**1 Med/154g**	**97**	**0.5**	**63**	**1.3**	**15.5**	**0.3**	**4.5**
Peel Only, Raw, Average	**1 Tbsp/6g**	**6**	**0**	**97**	**1.5**	**25**	**0.2**	**10.6**
Ruby Red, Tesco*	1 Med/130g	51	0.1	39	1.1	8.5	0.1	1.7
Segments, in Juice, Canned, Morrisons*	1 Portion/80g	36	0.1	45	0.4	10.3	0.1	0.5
Zest, Average	**1 Tsp/2g**	**2**	**0**	**100**	**0**	**25**	**0**	**0**
OREGANO								
Dried	**1 Tsp/1g**	**3**	**0.1**	**306**	**11**	**49.5**	**10.3**	**0**
Fresh	**1 Tsp/1.3g**	**1**	**0**	**66**	**2.2**	**9.7**	**2**	**0**
OSTRICH								
Steak, Fillet, Klein Karoo*	1 Fillet/125g	141	2.6	113	23.1	1	2.1	1
Steaks, in Marrakesh Marinade, South African, Deluxe*	1 Steak/150g	158	1.4	105	20	4.1	0.9	0
OVALTINE*								
Chocolate, Light, Ovaltine*	1 Serving/20g	76	1.2	380	8.5	70.5	6	4.5
Chocolate, Light, Sachet, Ovaltine*	1 Sachet/25g	96	1.5	384	7.4	73	5.9	4.7
Hi Malt, Light, Instant Drink, Ovaltine*	1 Sachet/20g	72	1.2	358	9.1	67.1	5.9	2.8
Powder, Made Up with Semi-Skimmed Milk, Ovaltine*	1 Mug/227ml	179	3.9	79	3.9	13	1.7	0
Powder, Made Up with Whole Milk, Ovaltine*	1 Mug/227ml	220	8.6	97	3.8	12.9	3.8	0
OXTAIL								
Raw	**1oz/28g**	**18**	**1.1**	**65**	**7.6**	**0**	**3.8**	**0**
Stewed, Bone Removed	**1oz/28g**	**68**	**3.8**	**243**	**30.5**	**0**	**13.4**	**0**
OYSTERS								
Raw, Shelled, Shucked	**1 Oyster/14g**	**9**	**0.2**	**65**	**10.8**	**2.7**	**1.3**	**0**

	Measure INFO/WEIGHT	per Measure KCAL	FAT	Nutrition Values per 100g / 100ml KCAL	PROT	CARB	FAT	FIBRE
PAELLA								
Bistro, Waitrose*	1 Serving/300g	534	19.8	178	7.4	22.2	6.6	0.7
Chicken, & Chorizo, & Prawn, City Kitchen, Tesco*	1 Pack/400g	540	20	135	4.7	17	5	1.4
Chicken, & Chorizo, Asda*	1 Pack/390g	484	8.6	124	10	16	2.2	2.6
Chicken, & Prawn, King, Balanced for You, M&S*	1 Pack/390g	425	8.6	109	8.3	13.4	2.2	1.2
Chicken, & Prawn, Meal in a Bag, Cooked, Iceland*	½ Bag/373g	500	18.3	134	4.4	17.1	4.9	1.7
Chicken, Chorizo, Rice Pot, Tesco*	1 Pack/330g	469	10.6	142	5.5	22	3.2	1.4
Chicken, Prawn, King, Mix, Simply Bistro, Aldi*	½ Bag/309g	303	4	98	5.3	16	1.3	1.6
Chicken, Chorizo King Prawn, Finest, Tesco*	1 Pack/450g	590	14	131	6.2	18.9	3.1	1.1
Cooked, Quorn*	1 Pack/376g	361	8.3	96	4.1	13.6	2.2	2.9
Pepper, & Courgette, Smoky Piquillo, Tesco*	1 Pack/393g	322	4.3	82	2.1	14.8	1.1	2
Roja, Bowl, Allplants*	½ Pack/380g	410	9.5	108	3.9	16	2.5	3
Seafood, Finest, Tesco*	1 Pack/400g	756	23.6	189	6.8	27.2	5.9	1
Vegetarian, Quorn*	1 Pack/400g	384	8.8	96	4.1	13.6	2.2	2.9
PAIN AU CHOCOLAT								
All Butter, Tesco*	1 Pain/58g	235	11.6	406	8.3	46.8	20	3
Average	**1 Pastry/60g**	**253**	**13.7**	**422**	**8**	**45.8**	**22.8**	**3.1**
M&S*	1 Pastry/60g	210	11.5	350	5.9	38	19.2	1.6
Mini, Asda*	1 Pastry/23g	96	5.5	420	8	43	24	3.3
Sainsbury's*	1 Pastry/58g	241	13.8	415	7.9	42.5	23.7	3.3
Waitrose*	1 Pastry/52g	226	12.7	435	8.3	44.2	24.4	2.9
PAIN AU RAISIN								
Bakery, Tesco*	1 Pastry/107g	351	14.7	328	6.9	43.3	13.7	1.8
Takeaway, Average	**1 Pastry/100g**	**313**	**13.2**	**313**	**5.2**	**43**	**13.2**	**1.3**
Twist, Extra Special, Asda*	1 Pastry/110g	421	20.9	383	7	46	19	2.5
PAK CHOI								
Raw, Average	**1 Leaf/14g**	**2**	**0**	**11**	**1.3**	**1.9**	**0.2**	**0.9**
PAKORA								
Bhaji, Onion, Fried in Vegetable Oil	**1oz/28g**	**76**	**4.1**	**271**	**9.8**	**26.2**	**14.7**	**5.5**
Bhajia, Potato Carrot & Pea, Fried in Vegetable Oil	**1oz/28g**	**100**	**6.3**	**357**	**10.9**	**28.8**	**22.6**	**6.1**
Bhajia, Vegetable, Retail	**1oz/28g**	**66**	**4.1**	**235**	**6.4**	**21.4**	**14.7**	**3.6**
Chicken, Indian, Sainsbury's*	½ Pack/45g	95	3.3	211	27.7	7.8	7.4	1
Chicken, Taste of India, Tesco*	1 Pack/150g	345	10.8	230	26.6	13.8	7.2	1.8
Chicken, Tikka, Asda*	1 Pack/350g	696	38.5	199	16	9	11	1.1
Vegetable, Indian Starter Selection, M&S*	1 Pakora/20g	43	0.6	214	1.2	4.1	3.2	0.9
PANCAKE								
Asda*	1 Pancake/23g	59	1.6	254	4.8	43	7	4
Big, Crafty, Genesis*	1 Pancake/70g	149	3.6	213	5.6	38.4	5.2	4.1
Blueberry, Tesco*	1 Pancake/75g	195	3.1	260	4.8	49.5	4.1	2
Buttermilk, Large, Tesco*	1 Pancake/65g	176	3.9	270	6.7	46.8	6	1.2
Chocolate, M&S*	1 Pancake/80g	125	4.9	156	3.1	22.1	6.1	0.2
Lemon, M&S*	1 Pancake/38g	90	2.8	235	4.5	38.5	7.2	2.8
Maple Raisin, M&S*	1 Pancake/35g	102	2.4	290	5.6	50.4	6.9	2.2
Mini, Scotch, Tesco*	1 Pancake/16g	44	0.9	277	6.7	50	5.6	1.4
Plain, Prepared From Recipe, Average	**1 Pancake/38g**	**86**	**3.7**	**227**	**6.4**	**28.3**	**9.7**	**0**
Raisin & Lemon, Asda*	1 Serving/30g	92	2.4	304	6	52	8	1.4
Raisin & Lemon, Sainsbury's*	1 Pancake/35g	95	1.5	272	6.3	51.8	4.4	2.2
Ready Made, Average	**1 Sm/30g**	**77**	**1.9**	**258**	**6.1**	**44.2**	**6.4**	**1.7**
Savoury, Made with Skimmed Milk, Average	**6"Pancake/77g**	**192**	**11.3**	**249**	**6.4**	**24.1**	**14.7**	**0.8**
Savoury, Made with Whole Milk, Average	**6"Pancake/77g**	**210**	**13.5**	**273**	**6.3**	**24**	**17.5**	**0.8**
Scotch	**1 Pancake/50g**	**146**	**5.8**	**292**	**5.8**	**43.6**	**11.7**	**1.4**
Scotch, Hovis*	1 Pancake/30g	88	2.5	295	5.5	48.1	8.4	2.3
Scotch, M&S*	1 Pancake/34g	95	1.4	280	6.5	54.5	4	1.6
Scotch, Sainsbury's*	1 Pancake/30g	78	1.3	260	5.9	48.8	4.4	1

	Measure INFO/WEIGHT	per Measure		Nutrition Values per 100g / 100ml				
		KCAL	FAT	KCAL	PROT	CARB	FAT	FIBRE
PANCAKE								
Scotch, Tesco*	1 Pancake/30g	81	2	271	5.5	46.7	6.5	1.8
Sweet, Tesco*	1 Pancake/60g	157	6.7	263	5	33.9	11.2	3.5
Syrup, Tesco*	1 Pancake/30g	80	2.5	265	4.7	42.1	8.2	1.5
Vegetable Roll	**1 Roll/85g**	**185**	**10.6**	**218**	**6.6**	**21**	**12.5**	**0**
with Syrup, American Style, Large, Tesco*	1 Pancake/38g	102	1.3	268	5.1	54.2	3.4	0.9
PANCETTA								
Average	**½ Pack/65g**	**212**	**18.7**	**326**	**17**	**0.1**	**28.7**	**0**
Oak Beech Smoked, Dry Cure, Finest, Tesco*	1 Rasher/8g	24	1.9	294	18	1.1	24.1	0.6
PANINI								
Cheese, Tesco*	1 Panini/100g	249	9.1	249	10.5	31.3	9.1	3.1
Chicken, Pesto, Rustlers*	1 Panini/143g	415	19.6	290	13.3	27.8	13.7	0
Chicken, Arrabiata, Ginsters*	1 Panini/200g	489	16.8	245	12.8	29.4	8.4	2.4
Chicken, Chargrilled, Mozzarella, & Pesto, Udo's Choice*	1 Panini/170g	389	14.6	229	16.4	21.6	8.6	2
Ham, & Cheese, Ginsters*	1 Panini/200g	567	25.6	283	13.3	28.7	12.8	1.6
Mozzarella, & Tomato, M&S*	1 Serving/176g	484	28.5	275	11.3	21.3	16.2	2.1
Tuna, & Sweetcorn, Tesco*	1 Serving/250g	559	16.4	224	12	29.3	6.6	1.4
PANNA COTTA								
BGTY, Sainsbury's*	1 Pot/150g	150	2.8	100	2.4	18.2	1.9	1.4
Caramel, Sainsbury's*	1 Serving/120g	319	15.1	266	4	31.8	12.6	0.7
Raspberry, COU, M&S*	1 Pot/140g	146	3.5	104	2.6	17.5	2.5	0.6
Sainsbury's*	1 Pot/100g	304	15.7	304	3	41.5	15.7	4
Strawberry, COU, M&S*	1 Pot/145g	145	3.8	100	2.6	15.7	2.6	0.8
PAPAYA								
Dried, Pieces, Nature's Harvest*	1 Serving/50g	178	0	355	0.2	85.4	0	2.6
Raw, Flesh Only, Average	**1 Serving/140g**	**37**	**0.1**	**26**	**0.4**	**6.6**	**0.1**	**1.2**
PAPPARDELLE								
Beef Chianta, Finest, Tesco*	1 Pack/362g	513	14.4	142	10.9	14.9	4	1.6
Egg, Dry, Average	**1 Serving/100g**	**364**	**3.7**	**364**	**14.1**	**68.5**	**3.7**	**2.1**
Egg, Fresh, Waitrose*	¼ Pack/125g	350	3.4	280	12.9	51	2.7	1.9
Mushroom, in a Rich Sauce, Meal for One, M&S*	1 Pack/375g	578	30.7	154	4.8	14.6	8.2	1.3
with Salmon, COU, M&S*	1 Pack/358g	340	6.8	95	6.3	13	1.9	0.8
PAPRIKA								
Average	**1 Tsp/2g**	**6**	**0.3**	**289**	**14.8**	**34.9**	**13**	**0**
PARATHA								
Average	**1 Paratha/80g**	**258**	**11.4**	**322**	**8**	**43.2**	**14.3**	**4**
Roti, Plain, Crown Farms*	1 Slice/80g	250	10	312	5	46.2	12.5	1.2
PARCELS								
Chicken, Bacon, Sainsbury's*	½ Pack/170g	406	28.6	239	21.9	0.1	16.8	0
Filo, Feta Spinach, Sainsbury's*	1 Parcel/27g	83	5.6	307	5.8	23.8	20.7	1.8
Salmon, Puff Pastry, Cream Cheese Sauce & Dill, Tesco*	1 Parcel/124g	334	19.4	269	10.7	20.5	15.6	1.8
PARSLEY								
Dried	**1 Tsp/1g**	**2**	**0.1**	**181**	**15.8**	**14.5**	**7**	**26.9**
Fresh, Average	**1 Tbsp/3.8g**	**1**	**0**	**27**	**2.4**	**2.2**	**1**	**4**
Root, Raw, Average	**1 Avg Root/33g**	**18**	**0.2**	**55**	**2.3**	**12.3**	**0.6**	**4.3**
PARSNIP								
Boiled, Average	**1 Serving/80g**	**53**	**1**	**66**	**1.6**	**12.9**	**1.2**	**4.7**
Honey Glazed, Roast, Baked, Aunt Bessie's*	1 Serving/100g	158	12	158	1.1	8.6	12	5.1
Honey Glazed, Roasting, Cooked, Betty Smith's*	1 Serving/80g	177	11.9	221	1.4	18.7	14.9	3.4
Honey Roasted, Tesco*	½ Pack/142g	159	5	112	1.2	16.8	3.5	4.2
Raw, Unprepared, Average	**1 Serving/100g**	**62**	**1**	**62**	**1.7**	**11.6**	**1**	**4.3**
PARTRIDGE								
Meat Only, Roasted	**1 Partridge/260g**	**551**	**18.7**	**212**	**36.7**	**0**	**7.2**	**0**

	Measure INFO/WEIGHT	per Measure KCAL	FAT	Nutrition Values per 100g / 100ml KCAL	PROT	CARB	FAT	FIBRE
PASSATA								
Classic, Italian with Onion Garlic, Sainsbury's*	¼ Carton/125g	29	0.6	23	1.3	3.6	0.5	1.2
Mutti Di Pomodoro , Mutti*	1/5 Jar/140g	50	0.4	36	1.6	5.1	0.3	0
Napolina*	1 Bottle/690g	172	0.7	25	1.4	4.5	0.1	0
Smart Price, Asda*	1 Serving/100g	30	0.1	30	1.1	5.6	0.1	0.9
Tomato, Freshona, Lidl*	1 Carton/500g	170	2.5	34	1.5	4.6	0.5	1.3
PASSION FRUIT								
Raw, Fresh, Average	*1 Fruit/30g*	*11*	*0.1*	*36*	*2.6*	*5.8*	*0.4*	*3.3*
Weighed with Skin, Average	*1 Fruit/30g*	*7*	*0.1*	*22*	*1.6*	*3.5*	*0.2*	*2*
PASTA								
Basil, & Parmesan, Parcels, Fresh, Sainsbury's*	1 Serving/162g	357	13.5	220	10	26.4	8.3	3.3
Cappelletti, Prosciutto, Italian, Sainsbury's*	½ Pack/200g	362	9.4	181	9.6	23.9	4.7	2.2
Cheese, Leek, & Ham, Pasta n Sauce, Batchelors*	½ Pack/184g	235	3.9	128	5	21.9	2.1	0.7
Cheese, Macaroni, Dry, Pasta n Sauce, Batchelors*	1 Pack/108g	402	5.1	372	17.2	65.2	4.7	2.7
Chicken, & Chorizo, Average	*1 Pack/400g*	*174*	*5.7*	*174*	*10.1*	*20.3*	*5.7*	*1.5*
Chicken, & Chorizo, Quadrotti, TTD, Sainsbury's*	1 Pack/320g	616	25.3	192	9.6	19.5	7.9	2.4
Chicken, Mushroom, Free From, Tesco*	1 Pack/373g	393	5.6	105	4.4	18.1	1.5	0.9
Chicken, Chilli, Spicy, Tesco*	1 Pack/275g	387	4.4	141	6.2	24.4	1.6	2.1
Chicken, Peri Peri, No Mayonnaise, Tesco*	1 Pack/300g	363	5.1	121	4.3	21.4	1.7	1.4
Chicken, Piri Piri, On the Go, Sainsbury's*	1 Pack/350g	514	10.8	147	7.7	21.2	3.1	1.9
Chicken, Roast, As Consumed, Mug Shot, Symingtons*	1 Serving/258g	201	2.6	78	2.8	14.2	1	0.5
Chicken, Tomato, Basil, On the Go, Sainsbury's*	1 Pack/350g	581	22.4	166	6.7	19.7	6.4	1.5
Chicken, Tomato, Basil, Tesco*	1 Pack/300g	471	11.1	157	6.7	23.3	3.7	1.6
Feta, & Slow Roasted Tomatoes, M&S*	1 Pack/190g	332	13.3	175	6	22.3	7	2.5
Green Pea, GF, As Prepared, Love Life, Waitrose*	1 Serving/175g	276	1.6	158	10.5	24.1	0.9	5.5
Mac Cheese, Pot, Tesco*	1 Pack/315g	482	13.6	153	5.6	22.1	4.3	1.6
Margherite, Basil, & Pinenut, TTD, Sainsbury's*	½ Pack/125g	259	10.9	207	7.8	23.5	8.7	1.5
Meat, Cappelletti, Sainsbury's*	1 Pack/420g	816	23.9	195	10	25.8	5.7	2.3
Orzo, Dry, Average	*1 Serving/100g*	*348*	*1.5*	*348*	*12.4*	*71.9*	*1.5*	*3*
Pesto, with Semi Dried Tomatoes, Tesco*	1 Pack/225g	432	18.2	192	5.6	23.4	8.1	1.7
Pumpkin, & Pine Nut, Stuffed, Fiorelli, Fresh, Waitrose*	½ Pack/125g	225	7.5	180	8	22.3	6	2.3
Pumpkin, & Sage, Quadrotti, Fresh, TTD, Sainsbury's*	½ Pack/125g	271	7.4	217	7.9	32.4	5.9	1.2
Seafood, Retail	*1 Serving/100g*	*110*	*4.8*	*110*	*8.9*	*7.6*	*4.8*	*0.4*
Tomato 'n' Herb, Mug Shot, Symingtons*	1 Serving/253g	223	2	88	3	16.6	0.8	1
Tuna, Sweetcorn, Tesco*	½ Pot/150g	253	11.6	169	6.5	17.9	7.7	0.9
Vegetable, Mediterranean, Cooked, BGTY, Sainsbury's*	1 Pack/400g	347	5.5	89	2.8	15.2	1.4	1.9
Veggie, Venetian Style, Hello Fresh*	1 Serving/567g	771	29	136	5.5	17.8	5.1	0
Wholewheat, Cooked, Tesco*	1 Serving/200g	284	1.8	142	5.7	27.9	0.9	4.5
PASTA BAKE								
Bacon Leek, Average	*1 Serving/400g*	*633*	*32.3*	*158*	*6.7*	*14.8*	*8.1*	*1.3*
Beef, Bolognese, Meal to Share, M&S*	½ Pack/400g	700	30.8	175	9.3	16.6	7.7	1.2
Bolognese, Nisa Heritage*	1 Pack/400g	524	24	131	7	11	6	1.6
Cheese, & Tomato, Italiano, Tesco*	1 Bake/300g	354	12.6	118	3.9	16.1	4.2	1
Chicken, & Bacon, Asda*	¼ Pack/374g	610	26.2	163	9	16	7	4.1
Chicken, & Bacon, Asda*	1 Pack/400g	592	25.2	148	8.6	14.2	6.3	3
Chicken, & Bacon, Average	*1 Serving/400g*	*627*	*28.7*	*157*	*9*	*13.7*	*7.2*	*1.6*
Chicken, & Broccoli, Morrisons*	1 Pack/400g	452	16	113	6.1	13.3	4	0.6
Chicken, Bacon, Taste of Italy, Tesco*	1 Pack/429g	606	19	141	10	15	4.4	0.7
Chicken, Bacon Mushroom, Average	*1 Serving/400g*	*632*	*29.2*	*158*	*7.8*	*15.1*	*7.3*	*2.3*
Chicken, Pesto, & Mozzarella, Meal to Share, M&S*	½ Pack/400g	632	24.4	158	8.3	16.7	6.1	1.3
Creamy, Tomato, Dolmio*	1 Serving/125g	141	9	113	2.3	8.4	7.2	0
Meat Feast, Average	*1 Serving/400g*	*601*	*21.4*	*150*	*5.8*	*19.2*	*5.4*	*1.4*
Meatball, Aberdeen Angus, Waitrose*	½ Pack/350g	501	28	143	5.2	12.5	8	0.9
Pepperoni, Taste of Italy, Tesco*	1 Pack/450g	651	23.3	145	5.9	18	5.2	1.1

	Measure INFO/WEIGHT	per Measure KCAL	FAT	Nutrition Values per 100g / 100ml KCAL	PROT	CARB	FAT	FIBRE
PASTA BAKE								
Sausage, Average	*1 Serving/400g*	*591*	*24*	*148*	*5.5*	*17.7*	*6*	*1.9*
Tomato, & Bacon, Creamy, Italian, Asda*	1 Serving/125g	131	11.2	105	2	3.9	9	0.6
Tomato, & Mozzarella, Average	*1 Serving/400g*	*500*	*12.4*	*125*	*5.3*	*17.3*	*3.1*	*1.5*
Tomato, & Pepperoni, Spicy, Asda*	1 Pack/440g	431	26.4	98	1.1	10	6	1.2
Tomato, Mozzarella, Taste of Italy, Tesco*	1 Pack/450g	535	13.7	119	5	17	3	1.8
Tuna, & Sweetcorn, Average	*1 Pack/400g*	*423*	*22.4*	*106*	*5*	*8.6*	*5.6*	*1.9*
Tuna, Co-Op*	1 Serving/340g	306	6.8	90	7	12	2	1
Tuna, Counted, As Consumed, Eat Smart, Morrisons*	1 Pack/348g	310	5.9	89	5.2	12.4	1.7	1.5
Vegetable, M&S*	1 Pack/350g	396	13.3	113	4.4	14.5	3.8	1.4
PASTA QUILLS								
Dry, Average	*1 Serving/75g*	*256*	*0.9*	*342*	*12*	*72.3*	*1.2*	*2*
GF, Salute*	1 Serving/75g	269	1.4	359	7.5	78	1.9	0
PASTA SALAD								
Basil Pesto Dressing, & Mixed Leaf, Tesco*	1 Pack/220g	528	37.6	240	4.7	16.9	17.1	0.7
Cheese, Tomato, On the Go, Sainsbury's*	1 Pot/300g	519	18.6	173	5.8	22.6	6.2	1.5
Cheese, Average	*1 Serving/370g*	*782*	*56.8*	*211*	*5.5*	*12.8*	*15.4*	*1.2*
Cheese, Layered, Asda*	1 Pack/440g	647	40.9	147	4.5	11.4	9.3	0
Chicken, & Bacon Caesar, Tesco*	1 Pack/265g	418	18.3	158	11.5	12.1	6.9	0.7
Chicken, & Bacon, Tesco*	½ Pack/233g	487	28.6	209	6.6	17.6	12.3	0.9
Chicken, Bacon, Sainsbury's*	1 Serving/83g	157	9.2	189	6.2	15.7	11.1	0.6
Chicken, Bacon, Sweetcorn, M&S*	1 Pack/380g	680	33.1	179	8.2	16.1	8.7	1.7
Chicken, Chilli, Boots*	1 Serving/189g	331	13.2	175	7.7	18	7	1.2
Chicken, Honey & Mustard, M&S*	1 Serving/190g	304	4.8	160	8.7	26.7	2.5	1.5
Chicken, Honey & Mustard, Sainsbury's*	1 Pack/350g	649	34	185	7	16.6	9.7	1.8
Chicken, Spicy, On the Go, Sainsbury's*	1 Pot/300g	455	10.8	152	6.4	22.7	3.6	1.5
Chicken, Tomato, Basil, 205g Pot, M&S*	1 Pack/205g	340	14.6	166	8	16.7	7.1	1.4
Chicken, Tomato, Basil, 380g Pot, M&S*	1 Pot/380g	559	21.7	147	7.9	15.3	5.7	1.6
Chicken, Tomato, Basil, Tesco*	1 Pack/260g	235	3.9	90	7.7	10.8	1.5	1.1
Chicken, Chargrilled, & Red Pepper, Tesco*	1 Pack/270g	554	24	205	9.8	20.3	8.9	3.1
Feta, Slow Roasted Tomato, M&S*	1 Tub/190g	344	13.3	181	6.5	22.3	7	2.5
Goats Cheese, & Mixed Pepper, Sainsbury's*	1 Pack/200g	366	18.8	183	6.4	18.2	9.4	1.5
Italian Style, Sainsbury's*	1/3 Pot/84g	129	5.3	153	3.5	20.5	6.3	1.4
Italian Style, Snack, Asda*	1 Pack/150g	141	6	94	3.4	11	4	4.1
Italian, Tesco*	¼ Pack/138g	186	4.7	135	4	21.6	3.4	1.3
Mozzarella, & Sun Dried Tomato, Waitrose*	1 Serving/150g	312	18.3	208	5.8	18.8	12.2	1.3
Mozzarella, Basil, Tomato, On the Go, Sainsbury's*	1 Pack/260g	437	16.1	168	6.6	20.4	6.2	1.9
Orzo, Roast Tomato, Pepper, TTD, Sainsbury's*	½ Pot/150g	234	8.4	156	3.6	22.1	5.6	1.7
Pesto, Creamy, Pot, Diet Chef*	1 Pot/248g	236	3.7	95	3.6	16.2	1.5	1
Pesto, Mini, 293, Oakhouse Foods Ltd*	1 Serving/225g	758	37.1	337	12.4	33.8	16.5	2.1
Pesto, Spicy Chilli, Sainsbury's*	¼ Pot/63g	170	12.3	272	3.8	20.1	19.6	1.6
Prawn Cocktail, Layered, Shapers, Boots*	1 Pot/210g	181	5.2	86	3.6	13	2.5	1.3
Prawn, Growers Selection, Asda*	1 Pack/380g	365	9.1	96	5.1	13	2.4	1.2
Spinach Pine Nut, Sainsbury's*	½ Pot/100g	226	11.6	226	6.4	23	11.6	2.2
Tomato, & Basil, Sainsbury's*	1 Serving/83g	121	3.4	145	3.7	22.7	4.1	1.6
Tuna, & Sweetcorn, HE, Tesco*	1 Pot/200g	230	5.4	115	5.7	17	2.7	1.3
Tuna, Sweetcorn, GF, Tesco*	1 Pack/275g	405	19.3	147	5.1	15.7	7	0.6
Tuna, Sweetcorn, On the Go, Sainsbury's*	1 Pack/300g	492	17.1	164	5.9	21.6	5.7	1.4
Vegetable, Chargrilled, & Tomato, Shapers, Boots*	1 Pack/175g	187	5.4	107	2.8	17	3.1	1.5
Vegetable, Chargrilled, Sainsbury's*	1 Serving/178g	192	4.8	108	2.7	15.9	2.7	4.7
PASTA SAUCE								
Amatriciana, Italiano, Tesco*	½ Pot/175g	124	6.6	71	4.1	5.3	3.8	0.9
Amatriciana, M&S*	1 Jar/340g	425	32.3	125	3.4	6.3	9.5	2.9
Arrabiata, Barilla*	1 Serving/100g	47	3	47	1.5	3.5	3	0

P

PASTA SAUCE

	Measure INFO/WEIGHT	per Measure KCAL	FAT	Nutrition Values per 100g / 100ml KCAL	PROT	CARB	FAT	FIBRE
Arrabiata, Fresh, Co-Op*	½ Pot/150g	82	4.5	55	1	5	3	1
Arrabiata, Fresh, M Kitchen, Morrisons*	½ Pot/175g	89	4.2	51	1.4	5	2.4	1.8
Arrabiata, GFY, Asda*	1 Serving/350g	133	3.9	38	1.1	6	1.1	0
Arrabiata, M&S*	1 Jar/320g	240	17	75	1.2	6.2	5.3	0.8
Aubergine, & Mascarpone, Roasted, Stir Through, M&S*	½ Jar/95g	111	8.9	117	1	6.3	9.4	1.7
Bacon, Smoky, Loyd Grossman*	½ Jar/175g	142	8.4	81	3	6.1	4.8	0.8
Bolognese, Extra Onion & Garlic, Dolmio*	1 Serving/125g	51	0.8	41	1.4	6.6	0.6	1
Bolognese, Free From, Tesco*	¼ Jar/125g	63	0.9	51	1.9	8.4	0.7	1.5
Bolognese, Garlic Onion, Intense, Dolmio*	1 Jar/500g	210	1	42	1.7	7.4	0.2	1.8
Bolognese, Mushroom, Chunky, Dolmio*	½ Jar/375g	165	0.8	44	1.7	7.9	0.2	2
Bolognese, Organic, Seeds of Change*	1 Jar/500g	290	6	58	1.3	10.4	1.2	0.8
Bolognese, Original, Light, Low Fat, Dolmio*	1 Serving/125g	41	0.1	33	1.2	6	0.1	1.3
Bolognese, Original, Sainsbury's*	¼ Jar/136g	90	2.9	66	1.9	9.9	2.1	1.3
Bolognese, Smooth, Hidden Vegetables, Dolmio*	1 Portion/125g	60	1	48	1.4	7.7	0.8	1.9
Bolognese, Tesco*	1 Serving/100g	41	0.7	41	1.4	6.6	0.7	1.3
Bolognese, Tomato, Beef & Red Wine, Fresh, Waitrose*	1 Pot/350g	301	17.2	86	5.4	5.3	4.9	2
Bolognese, with Beef, Tesco*	½ Can/213g	179	10	84	4.9	5.5	4.7	0
Cacciatore, Fresh, Sainsbury's*	½ Pot/150g	152	8.8	101	5.4	8.1	5.9	1.5
Carbonara, Asda*	½ Pot/175g	359	29.8	205	7	6	17	0.1
Carbonara, Co-Op*	½ Pot/150g	270	25.5	180	3	4	17	0.1
Carbonara, Creamy, Dolmio Express, Dolmio*	1 Pack/150g	166	13.2	111	3.3	4.7	8.8	0.1
Carbonara, Creamy, Stir in Sauce, Dolmio*	1 Serving/75g	98	8	130	3.3	5.2	10.6	0.2
Carbonara, Italian, Fresh, Sainsbury's*	½ Pot/176g	209	16.3	119	5.4	3.4	9.3	0.9
Cheese, Four, Sainsbury's*	1 Serving/150g	296	25.5	197	6.6	4.5	17	0.8
Cheese, Fresh, PB, Waitrose*	½ Pot/175g	144	5.1	82	6.1	7.9	2.9	0.5
Cheese, Three, Co-Op*	1 Pack/300g	405	27	135	6	6	9	0.1
Cherry Tomato, Parmesan, Seeds of Change*	1 Serving/175g	103	5.1	59	1.5	5.9	2.9	1.3
Lasagne, Tomato, Red, Ragu, Knorr*	1 Jar/500g	215	0	43	1.1	9.7	0	1.1
Lasagne, White, Ragu, Knorr*	1 Jar/475g	755	72.2	159	0.5	5.1	15.2	0.3
Mediterranean, Fresh, Waitrose*	1 Pot/350g	214	13.6	61	1.4	5	3.9	2.4
Mushroom, & Cream, M&S*	1oz/28g	45	4	160	1.5	6.6	14.3	0.6
Mushroom, Creamy, Dolmio*	1 Pack/150g	166	15	111	1.3	3.7	10	0
Mushroom, Creamy, Express, Dolmio*	1 Serving/150g	160	14.4	107	1.4	3.8	9.6	0
Mushroom, Italian, Sainsbury's*	1 Serving/85g	56	1.8	66	2	9.8	2.1	1.7
Mushroom, Sainsbury's*	1 Serving/100g	66	2.1	66	2	9.8	2.1	1.7
Mushroom, Tesco*	1/6 Jar/120g	48	0.6	40	1.2	6.9	0.5	1.5
Napoletana, Fresh, Sainsbury's*	1oz/28g	25	1.6	91	1.9	7.9	5.8	1.1
Napoletana, Morrisons*	1 Serving/175g	82	2.6	47	2.6	6.7	1.5	0
Napoletana, Sainsbury's*	½ Pot/150g	126	8.4	84	1.9	6.6	5.6	0.9
Olive, & Tomato, Sacla*	½ Jar/95g	182	17.8	192	1.5	2.9	18.7	2.8
Pomodoro, Cirio*	1 Serving/200g	116	4.6	58	1.4	8.4	2.3	0
Puttanesca, Loyd Grossman*	½ Jar/175g	117	6	67	1.4	5.5	3.4	0.7
Red Pepper, & Tomato, Roasted, Finest, Tesco*	1 Serving/145g	117	7.8	81	1.2	6.8	5.4	2.2
Red Pepper, Sweet, Loyd Grossman*	1 Jar/350g	304	19.6	87	1.7	7.3	5.6	1.2
Tomato, & Basil, Dolmio*	1 Serving/170g	95	3.6	56	1.4	7.9	2.1	0
Tomato, & Basil, Loyd Grossman*	½ Jar/175g	107	6	61	1.5	5.8	3.4	0.8
Tomato, & Basil, Morrisons*	½ Jar/140g	76	0.7	54	1.7	10.1	0.5	1.3
Tomato, & Basil, Sun Dried, Organic, Seeds of Change*	½ Jar/100g	155	13.1	155	1.6	7.7	13.1	0
Tomato, & Basil, Sun Ripened, Dolmio*	1 Serving/150g	117	6.9	78	1.3	7.9	4.6	0
Tomato, & Basil, Sun Ripened, Express, Dolmio*	1 Pouch/170g	88	2.7	52	1.5	7.9	1.6	0
Tomato, & Chilli, Pour Over, M&S*	1 Jar/330g	231	12.5	70	1.3	7.6	3.8	1.8
Tomato, & Chilli, Whole Cherry Tomatoes, Classic, Sacla*	½ Jar/175g	238	19.2	136	2	7.2	11	3.1
Tomato, & Garlic, CBY, Asda*	½ Jar/160g	74	0.8	46	1.6	7.9	0.5	1.7

PASTA SAUCE

	Measure INFO/WEIGHT	per Measure KCAL	FAT	per 100g KCAL	PROT	CARB	FAT	FIBRE
Tomato, & Garlic, Roasted, CBY, Asda*	1 Pot/350g	122	2.1	35	1.5	5	0.6	1.7
Tomato, & Garlic, Roasted, Loyd Grossman*	½ Jar/175g	133	5.6	76	2	9	3.2	1.4
Tomato, & Mascarpone, Finest, Tesco*	1 Serving/175g	135	8.8	77	2.7	5.4	5	0.8
Tomato, & Mascarpone, Fresh, Sainsbury's*	1 Serving/150g	177	15.4	118	2.2	4.2	10.3	1.1
Tomato, & Mascarpone, Italiano, Tesco*	½ Pot/175g	168	12.2	96	2.8	5.5	7	0.7
Tomato, & Mascarpone, Sainsbury's*	½ Pot/150g	137	9.9	91	2.1	5.9	6.6	1.2
Tomato, & Mascarpone, Tesco*	¼ Jar/125g	101	5.2	81	1.4	8.8	4.2	1
Tomato, & Mascarpone, Waitrose*	½ Pot/175g	184	14.7	105	1.9	5.5	8.4	1.1
Tomato, & Mushroom, Wild, Loyd Grossman*	½ Jar/175g	107	6	61	1.4	5.8	3.4	0.6
Tomato, & Onions, Original, Morrisons*	1 Serving/125g	51	1.4	41	1.4	6.3	1.1	1.2
Tomato, & Parmesan, Seeds of Change*	1 Serving/150g	100	4.4	67	2.5	7.8	2.9	1.1
Tomato, & Ricotta, Italian, Sainsbury's*	1 Pack/390g	238	11.7	61	2.5	6.1	3	1.2
Tomato, & Tuna, Loyd Grossman*	½ Jar/175g	154	7.7	88	4.4	7.5	4.4	0.8
Tomato, Herb, HFC, Tesco*	¼ Jar/110g	36	0.8	33	0.8	5.5	0.7	0.8
Tomato, Bacon, & Mushroom, Asda*	½ Pot/50g	33	1.8	66	2.5	6	3.6	0
Tomato, Courgette, Basil, Veggie Goodness, Dolmio*	½ Pack/170g	70	1.2	41	1.7	6.2	0.7	1.4
Tomato, Onion, Garlic, Baresa, Lidl*	1 Jar/500g	240	2.5	48	2.1	7.8	0.5	1.8
Tomato, Sun Dried, Stir In, Light, Dolmio*	1 Serving/75g	62	3.5	83	1.7	9.8	4.7	0
Tomato, with Basil Pesto, Rich, Express, Dolmio*	1 Pack/170g	146	10	86	2	6.2	5.9	0
Vegetable, Chunky, Tesco*	1 Jar/500g	235	5	47	1.8	6.8	1	1.8
Vegetable, Mediterranean, Organic, Seeds of Change*	1 Jar/350g	210	10.2	60	1.2	6.6	2.9	1.4
Vegetable, Mediterranean, Tesco*	1 Serving/166g	95	2.8	57	1.4	9	1.7	1.2
Vegetable, Roasted, Sainsbury's*	½ Pot/151g	103	5.9	68	1.6	6.7	3.9	0.4

PASTA SHAPES

	Measure INFO/WEIGHT	per Measure KCAL	FAT	per 100g KCAL	PROT	CARB	FAT	FIBRE
Alphabetti, in Tomato Sauce, Heinz*	1 Can/200g	118	1	59	1.8	11.7	0.5	1.5
Bob The Builder in Tomato Sauce, Heinz*	1 Can/205g	111	0.6	54	1.7	11.3	0.3	1.5
Cooked, Tesco*	1 Serving/260g	356	2.1	137	5.1	26.3	0.8	1.1
DC Heroes, in Tomato Sauce, Snap Pots, Heinz*	1 Pot/190g	122	0.6	64	1.8	13.2	0.3	0.6
Disney Princess in Tomato Sauce, Heinz*	1 Can/200g	114	0.6	57	1.8	11.9	0.3	1.5
Dried, Tesco*	1 Serving/100g	345	2	345	13.2	68.5	2	2.9
Durum Wheat, Dry, Basics, Sainsbury's*	1 Serving/75g	260	1.5	346	12	70	2	4
Spiderman with Mini Sausages in Tomato Sauce, Heinz*	1 Can/200g	178	6.2	89	3.6	11.6	3.1	0.5

PASTA SHELLS

	Measure INFO/WEIGHT	per Measure KCAL	FAT	per 100g KCAL	PROT	CARB	FAT	FIBRE
Dry, Average	**1 Serving/75g**	**265**	**1.5**	**353**	**11.1**	**71.8**	**2**	**2**
Egg, Fresh, Average	**1 Serving/125g**	**344**	**3.6**	**275**	**11.5**	**49.8**	**2.8**	**3.4**
Wholewheat, Healthy Living, Co-Op*	1 Serving/75g	232	0.8	310	11	64	1	12

PASTA TWISTS

	Measure INFO/WEIGHT	per Measure KCAL	FAT	per 100g KCAL	PROT	CARB	FAT	FIBRE
Dry, Average	**1oz/28g**	**99**	**0.4**	**354**	**12.2**	**71.8**	**1.5**	**2.2**
Wheat GF, Glutafin*	1 Serving/75g	262	1.5	350	8	75	2	0.1

PASTE

	Measure INFO/WEIGHT	per Measure KCAL	FAT	per 100g KCAL	PROT	CARB	FAT	FIBRE
Beef, Asda*	1 Serving/37g	72	5.2	194	17	0.1	14	0
Beef, Princes*	1 Serving/18g	42	3.1	231	15.2	3.4	17.4	0
Beef, Sainsbury's*	1 Jar/75g	142	9.9	189	16	1.5	13.2	1.4
Chicken, & Ham, Princes*	1 Jar/100g	233	18.6	233	13.6	2.8	18.6	0
Chicken, & Ham, Tesco*	1 Serving/19g	44	3.7	231	12.5	1.4	19.5	0
Chicken, & Mushroom, Princes*	1 Serving/50g	94	5.5	187	17.1	5	11	0
Chicken, & Stuffing, Asda*	½ Jar/35g	71	4.9	203	16	3.3	14	0
Chicken, & Stuffing, Princes*	1 Jar/100g	229	17	229	15.7	3.3	17	0
Chicken, Asda*	1 Thin Spread/7g	13	0.9	184	16	0.8	13	0
Chicken, Tesco*	1 Serving/12g	30	2.4	248	14.8	2.3	20	0.1
Chilli, Sainsbury's*	1 Tsp/6g	5	0.4	82	1	2.9	5.8	7.3
Crab, Sainsbury's*	1 Spread/5g	6	0.2	115	16.5	1.7	4.7	0.5
Curry, Katsu, Mild, M&S*	¼ Jar/48g	88	4.2	186	4.8	19.6	8.8	4.7

P

	Measure INFO/WEIGHT	per Measure KCAL	FAT	Nutrition Values per 100g / 100ml KCAL	PROT	CARB	FAT	FIBRE
PASTE								
Curry, Korma, Mild, M&S*	¼ Jar/50g	112	8.2	224	2.5	13.9	16.3	5.7
Curry, Thai, Red, Shots, M&S*	1 Pot/45g	61	4	135	1.2	10.6	9	3.3
Red Pepper, Mild, 1001 Delights, Lidl*	1 Tsp/6g	4	0	70	3	10.5	0.8	0
Salmon, & Shrimp, Tesco*	1 Jar/75g	83	2.6	111	15.1	5	3.4	0.1
Salmon, Value, Tesco*	1 Serving/10g	16	1	165	14	4.6	10.1	0.8
Sardine, & Tomato, Asda*	1 Thin Spread/9g	11	0.5	123	14	3.3	6	0
Sardine, & Tomato, Princes*	1 Jar/75g	130	8.1	173	13.9	3.4	10.8	3.2
Sardine, & Tomato, Sainsbury's*	1 Mini Pot/35g	60	3.8	170	16.9	1.2	10.8	1.3
Stroganoff, Recipe Paste, M&S*	¼ Jar/45g	72	5.2	161	2.2	10	11.5	4.3
Tamarind, M&S*	¼ Jar/30g	38	0	125	0.9	30.1	0.1	0.5
Tikka, M&S*	¼ Jar/50g	110	7.8	219	2.8	13.8	15.5	6.4
Tuna, & Mayonnaise, Tesco*	1 Serving/15g	32	2.3	215	15.8	0.7	15.6	2.2
PASTILLES								
Fruit, 30% Less Sugar, Rowntree's*	1 Sweet/3g	9	0	325	6.5	68.8	0.1	9.5
Fruit, Average	*1 Tube/33g*	*108*	*0*	*327*	*2.8*	*84.2*	*0*	*0*
Fruit, Rowntree's*	1 Tube/53g	186	0	351	4.4	83.7	0	0
Fruit, Sainsbury's*	4 Sweets/23g	79	0.1	344	4.1	80.6	0.5	0.6
PASTRAMI								
Beef, Average	*1 Serving/40g*	*51*	*1.4*	*128*	*23.1*	*1.1*	*3.6*	*0.2*
Turkey, Average	*½ Pack/35g*	*38*	*0.5*	*107*	*21.8*	*1.7*	*1.5*	*0.5*
PASTRY								
Apricot, Custard, Lattice, Bakery, Tesco*	1 Pastry/95g	311	12.9	328	4.8	46.1	13.6	1
Beef, Red Wine, Lattice, Mini, Tesco*	1 Lattice/28g	95	5.3	340	10.7	30.3	18.9	2.7
Beef, Chilli, Mexican, Slice, Ginsters*	1 Slice/170g	491	32.3	289	8.5	20.2	19	0
Beef, Slow Cooked, Christmas Cracker, Tesco*	¼ Cracker/184g	553	32.1	300	13	21.6	17.4	2.3
Block, GF, Ready to Roll, Sillyyak *	1 Block/325g	1170	73.1	360	0.7	40.1	22.5	2.7
Brie, Cranberry, Plaits, Tesco*	1 Plait/91g	316	15.9	347	8.3	38	17.4	2.5
Cannoli, Shells, Hand Rolled, Large, Alessi*	1 Shell/21g	90	4.5	429	4.8	47.6	21.4	0
Case, From Supermarket, Average	*1 Case/230g*	*1081*	*58.9*	*470*	*5.8*	*55.9*	*25.6*	*1.2*
Chicken, Mushroom, Lattice, Tesco*	1 Lattice/110g	222	6	202	8.4	28.8	5.5	2.1
Choux, Cooked, Average	*1oz/28g*	*91*	*5.5*	*325*	*8.5*	*29.8*	*19.8*	*1.2*
Choux, Raw, Average	*1oz/28g*	*59*	*3.6*	*211*	*5.5*	*19.4*	*12.9*	*0.8*
Cinnamon Swirls, Bake it Fresh, Jus-Rol*	1 Swirl/45g	162	7.1	360	6.2	47.7	15.7	1.6
Cinnamon Swirls, Danish Selection, Tesco*	1 Swirl/35g	151	8.8	432	6.4	43.5	25.2	1.2
Coronets, Chocolate, Cherry, Danish Selection, Tesco*	1 Coronet/36g	128	7.1	357	5.5	38.1	19.7	2.7
Feta, Herb, Spinach, Tesco*	2 Pastries/65g	168	8.3	258	7.4	27.2	12.8	2.3
Filo, Average	*1 Sheet/45g*	*137*	*1.2*	*304*	*9*	*61.4*	*2.7*	*0.9*
Flaky, Cooked, Average	*1oz/28g*	*157*	*11.4*	*560*	*5.6*	*45.9*	*40.6*	*1.8*
Flaky, Raw, Average	*1oz/28g*	*119*	*8.6*	*424*	*4.2*	*34.8*	*30.7*	*1.4*
Ginger Bread Latte, Plait, Bakery, Tesco*	1 Plait/87g	370	21.5	425	5.4	44.3	24.7	1.9
Horn, Filled with Cream, Jam, Sainsbury's*	1 Horn/49g	196	10.9	401	4.1	45.4	22.3	1
Pain Au Chocolat, Bake it Fresh, Jus-Rol*	1 Pain/46g	170	8.7	369	7.4	41	19	2.2
Pork, Pulled, Topped with Cheese Parsley, Tesco*	1 Pasty/23g	60	1.9	265	10.3	35.4	8.5	3
Puff, Frozen, Average	*1 Serving/47g*	*188*	*12*	*400*	*5*	*29.2*	*25.6*	*0*
Puff, Light, Frozen, Ready Roll Sheets, Jus-Rol*	1/6 Sheet/53g	176	8.7	332	6.4	38.3	16.5	2.3
Puff, Light, Sheet, Jus-Rol*	1 Serving/50g	166	8.2	332	6.4	38.3	16.5	2.3
Salted Caramel, Mini, Danish Selection, Tesco*	1 Plait/31g	136	8.1	440	5.4	44.6	26.1	2.3
Shortcrust, Cooked, Average	*1oz/28g*	*146*	*9*	*521*	*6.6*	*54.2*	*32.3*	*2.2*
Shortcrust, Raw, Average	*1oz/28g*	*127*	*8.1*	*453*	*5.6*	*44*	*29.1*	*1.3*
Spring Roll Wrapper, TYJ Food Manufacturing*	1 Lge Sheet/18g	54	0	300	0	73	0	0
Steak, Onion, Lattice, Pastry, Tesco*	1 Serving/167g	374	17.9	223	12	18.9	10.7	1.7
Vanilla Slice, Frozen, Tesco*	1 Slice/38g	136	6	359	4.7	48.9	15.8	1.5
Vol-Au-Vents, Jus-Rol*	1 Pastry/17g	67	4.3	392	5	36	25.1	1.1

	Measure INFO/WEIGHT	per Measure KCAL	FAT	Nutrition Values per 100g / 100ml KCAL	PROT	CARB	FAT	FIBRE
PASTRY								
Wholemeal, Cooked, Average	*1oz/28g*	*140*	*9.2*	*499*	*8.9*	*44.6*	*32.9*	*6.3*
PASTY								
Cauliflower, Curried, Wicked Kitchen, Tesco*	1 Pasty/150g	361	19.5	241	4.1	26.2	13	1.1
Cheese, & Onion, Average	*1 Pasty/150g*	*435*	*27.6*	*290*	*7.3*	*24.5*	*18.4*	*1.4*
Cheese, & Onion, Tesco*	1 Pasty/150g	416	26.4	277	5.9	23.7	17.6	2.2
Cornish, Average	*1 Pasty/160g*	*450*	*27.7*	*281*	*7*	*24.2*	*17.3*	*1.6*
Cornish, Mini, Sainsbury's*	1 Pasty/70g	280	20.1	400	7.3	28.1	28.7	1.5
Cornish, Multi Pack, Ginsters*	1 Pasty/130g	358	24.3	275	6	20.6	18.7	2.6
Cornish, Original, Ginsters*	1 Pasty/227g	549	32.2	242	5.3	23.2	14.2	3.1
Cornish, Tesco*	1 Pasty/150g	466	32.7	311	6.8	21.9	21.8	1.6
Cornish, Traditional Style, Geo Adams*	1 Pasty/165g	488	30.4	296	7.1	25.4	18.4	1.3
Vegetable	*1oz/28g*	*77*	*4.2*	*274*	*4.1*	*33.3*	*14.9*	*1.9*
Vegetarian, Cornish Style, Quorn*	1 Pasty/150g	320	15	213	6.9	22.5	10	3
PATE								
Ardennes, BGTY, Sainsbury's*	1 Serving/30g	59	4.5	197	12.3	3.2	15	0.5
Ardennes, Reduced Fat, Waitrose*	¼ Pack/42g	94	7.1	224	15.4	2.6	16.9	0.5
Ardennes, Tesco*	1 Tbsp/15g	53	5	354	13.3	0.5	33.2	1.2
Ardennes, with Bacon, Tesco*	½ Pack/85g	241	20.6	284	11.4	5.1	24.2	1.1
Avocado, Cashew, Findlater's Fine Foods*	1 Serving/25g	95	9	380	4	8	36	0
Brussels, & Garlic, Tesco*	1 Serving/40g	145	13.5	363	8.7	6	33.8	0
Brussels, 25% Less Fat, Morrisons*	¼ Pack/43g	106	8.8	249	14.2	0.7	20.6	0
Brussels, Co-Op*	1 Serving/15g	51	4.6	340	11	4	31	2
Brussels, M&S*	1 Thin Spread/7g	23	2.1	323	9.9	1.9	30.5	0.5
Brussels, Sainsbury's*	1 Pack/170g	663	64.9	390	10.6	1.1	38.2	0.1
Brussels, Smooth, Reduced Fat, Tesco*	1 Serving/40g	98	7.5	245	12	6.4	18.7	0.5
Brussels, Smooth, Reduced, Tesco*	1 Serving /40g	82	6.4	205	10.7	4.5	16	0.6
Brussels, Smooth, Spreadable, Sainsbury's*	1 Serving/30g	97	8.7	323	10.7	4.7	29	0
Butternut Squash, Red Pepper, Roasted, Waitrose*	1 Pack/160g	259	16.8	162	2.6	12.9	10.5	2.5
Chicken, Liver, M&S*	1oz/28g	79	6.7	281	14	1.9	24.1	0.1
Chicken, Liver, Organic, Waitrose*	½ Tub/88g	204	16.1	233	12.6	1.8	18.4	1.4
Chicken, Liver, Parfait, Specially Selected, Aldi*	1 Portion/85g	278	26.4	327	11	2.1	31	0.6
Chicken, Liver, Parfait, Waitrose*	1 Pack/100g	258	22.9	258	7.5	4.8	22.9	1.1
Chicken, Liver, with Madeira, Sainsbury's*	1 Serving/30g	84	7.3	279	13.1	1.9	24.3	0
Crab, M&S*	1oz/28g	63	4.8	225	12.1	5.9	17.3	0
Crab, Waitrose*	1 Pot/113g	218	16.7	193	12.4	2.5	14.8	0.9
De Campagne, Sainsbury's*	1 Serving/55g	129	10	235	16.3	1.4	18.2	0
Duck, & Orange, Smooth, Tesco*	1 Serving/50g	188	17.7	377	10.5	4	35.4	0.5
Duck, Liver, Grand Marnier & Orange Jelly, M&S*	½ Pot/75g	218	18.5	291	8.7	8.2	24.7	0.6
Farmhouse, with Mushrooms & Garlic, Tesco*	1 Serving/90g	256	22.8	285	13.8	0.6	25.3	1.3
Farmhouse, with Mushrooms, Sainsbury's*	1 Serving/30g	76	6.8	252	11.3	1.2	22.5	0.5
Layered, Duck, Pork, Sainsbury's*	1 Serving/30g	94	8	313	11.3	6.8	26.7	0.5
Mackerel, Smoked	*1oz/28g*	*103*	*9.6*	*368*	*13.4*	*1.3*	*34.4*	*0*
Mackerel, Smoked, Sainsbury's*	½ Pot/57g	176	14.7	308	15	3.7	25.8	0
Mackerel, Smoked, Scottish, M&S*	½ Pot/58g	158	13.3	275	15.9	0.6	23.2	0.1
Mackerel, Tesco*	1 Serving/29g	102	9.5	353	14.3	0.5	32.6	0
Mushroom, Sainsbury's*	½ Pot/58g	85	6.7	147	3.9	5.8	11.6	0
Salmon, Smoked, Tesco*	1 Pack/115g	282	22	245	15	3	19.1	1
Tomato, Lentil, & Basil, Cauldron Foods*	1 Pot/115g	161	7.8	140	6.8	14	6.8	3.2
Trout, Smoked, Waitrose*	1 Serving/34g	59	3.7	176	18.3	0.6	11.1	0
Tuna, M&S*	1oz/28g	106	9.5	380	17	0.8	33.8	0.7
Tuna, Tesco*	1 Pack/115g	332	26.7	289	19.8	0.3	23.2	0.2
Tuna, with Butter & Lemon Juice, Sainsbury's*	½ Pot/58g	145	11.5	251	15.5	2.2	19.9	0.6
Turkey, Pork, Duck, Liver, Deluxe, Lidl*	1 Pack/125g	366	30.6	293	13.1	4.5	24.5	1

INFO/WEIGHT	Measure	per Measure KCAL	FAT	Nutrition Values per 100g / 100ml KCAL	PROT	CARB	FAT	FIBRE

PATE

	Measure INFO/WEIGHT	per Measure KCAL	FAT	KCAL	PROT	CARB	FAT	FIBRE
Vegetable	**1oz/28g**	**48**	**3.8**	**173**	**7.5**	**5.9**	**13.4**	**0**
Walnut, Basil, Organic, GranoVita*	1 Serving/20g	48	4.4	241	8.3	11.5	22	3.6
Yeast, Garlic & Herb, Tartex*	1 Serving/30g	69	5.4	230	7	10	18	0
Yeast, Wild Mushroom, GranoVita*	1oz/28g	60	4.8	213	10	5	17	0

PATTY

Beef, Jamaican, Port Royal*	1 Patty/140g	350	17.4	250	6.1	28.1	12.4	1.3
Beef, Jerk, Jamaican, Patty, Island Delight*	1 Patty/50g	155	8.6	310	7.6	31.9	17.3	0
Chicken, Jamaican, Port Royal*	1 Patty/140g	346	16.2	247	6.9	28	11.6	1.3
Fish, Salt, Jamaican, Port Royal*	1 Patty/130g	300	13.4	231	6.8	27.8	10.3	0
Jerk, Jamaican, Crust Pattie, Island Delight*	1 Patty/140g	420	23.8	300	6.5	30	17	1
Lamb, Curried, Island Delight*	1 Patty/140g	451	28	322	6.4	28	20	1.4
Lamb, Jamaican, Port Royal*	1 Patty/130g	352	17.4	271	7.2	30.5	13.4	0
Pattie, Chilli, Island Delight*	1 Patty/140g	424	26.6	303	7.3	26	19	1.5
Vegetable, Jamaican, Patty, Island Delight*	1 Patty/140g	423	22.4	302	5.2	35	16	0
Vegetarian, Jamaican, Port Royal*	1 Patty/130g	315	13.8	242	12.5	24.1	10.6	0

PAVLOVA

Maltesers, Mars*	1 Serving/50g	205	8.1	410	3.6	61.7	16.2	0
Raspberry, Individual, M&S*	1 Pavlova/65g	133	1.6	205	4	41.8	2.4	0.2
Raspberry, M&S*	1 Serving/84g	193	8.1	230	2.3	33.3	9.6	0.3
Raspberry, Tesco*	1 Serving/65g	191	8.4	294	2.7	41.8	12.9	1.1
Sticky Toffee, Sainsbury's*	1/6 Pavlova/60g	249	9.8	415	3.7	63.1	16.4	0.9

PAW-PAW

Raw, Fresh	**1oz/28g**	**10**	**0**	**36**	**0.5**	**8.8**	**0.1**	**2.2**
Raw, Weighed with Skin & Pips	**1oz/28g**	**6**	**0**	**20**	**0.3**	**5**	**0.1**	**1.3**

PEACH

Dried, Average	**1 Pack/250g**	**472**	**1.6**	**189**	**2.6**	**45**	**0.6**	**6.9**
in Fruit Juice, Average	**1oz/28g**	**13**	**0**	**47**	**0.5**	**11.2**	**0**	**0.7**
in Light Syrup, Canned, As Sold	**1 Serving/100g**	**66**	**0**	**66**	**0.4**	**15.9**	**0**	**1**
in Strawberry Jelly, Hartleys*	1 Pot/120g	86	0	72	0.2	14.5	0	0
in Syrup, Average	**1oz/28g**	**19**	**0**	**67**	**0.4**	**16.3**	**0.1**	**0.4**
Pieces in Strawberry Jelly, Fruitini, Del Monte*	1 Can/140g	91	0.1	65	0.3	15.3	0.1	0
Raw, Stoned, Average	**1oz/28g**	**9**	**0**	**33**	**1**	**7.6**	**0.1**	**1.5**
Raw, Weighed with Stone, Average	**1 Peach/125g**	**39**	**0.1**	**31**	**1**	**7.2**	**0.1**	**1.3**
Slices in Fruit Juice, Average	**1 Serving/100g**	**49**	**0**	**49**	**0.6**	**11.6**	**0**	**0.5**

PEANUT BUTTER

30% Less Fat, Tesco*	1 Tbsp/15g	86	5.7	570	18.4	37.1	37.9	3.6
Crunchy , Hi-pro*	1 Serving/15g	93	7.4	618	33.9	5.6	49.1	7.3
Crunchy, Natural, No Added Sugar or Salt, Average	**1 Tsp/5g**	**30**	**2.4**	**606**	**27.6**	**12.2**	**48.4**	**7**
Crunchy, So Organic, Sainsbury's*	1 Serving/15g	93	7.6	619	29.4	5.8	51	9.9
Crunchy, Tesco*	1 Tbsp/15g	95	8	634	24.2	9.6	53.4	9.2
Smooth, Average	**1 Serving/20g**	**125**	**10.7**	**623**	**22.6**	**13.1**	**53.7**	**5.4**
Smooth, No Added Sugar, Organic, Whole Earth*	1 Serving/20g	126	10.2	628	25.6	13.7	51.2	4.9
Smooth, No Added Sugar, Sunpat*	1 Serving/30g	183	14.6	610	24.4	14.7	48.8	7.2
Smooth, Simply, M&S*	1 Tbsp/15g	93	7.6	623	24	14.8	50.6	6.4
Smooth, Unsalted, Biona Organic*	1 Thin Spread/7g	42	3.4	594	25.8	16.1	49.2	8.5
Whole Nut, Crunchy, Average	**1 Tsp/10g**	**61**	**5.3**	**606**	**24.9**	**7.7**	**53.1**	**6**
with Cocoa, Nature's Energy, Meridian Foods*	1 Tbsp/15g	93	7.5	617	24	15.8	50.2	6

PEANUTS

Chilli, Average	**½ Pack/50g**	**303**	**25.3**	**605**	**28.2**	**9.3**	**50.6**	**6.8**
Chilli, Smoked, Mexican, Coated, Sensations, Walkers*	1 Serving/30g	171	11.8	569	14.2	38.4	39.3	2.8
Dry Roasted, Average	**1 Serving/20g**	**117**	**9.8**	**587**	**25.7**	**11.5**	**48.8**	**6.5**
Honey Roasted, Average	**1oz/28g**	**169**	**13.2**	**605**	**26.8**	**23.6**	**47**	**5.5**
Plain, Average	**10 Whole/10g**	**59**	**5**	**592**	**24.7**	**11**	**50**	**6.3**

	INFO/WEIGHT	KCAL	FAT	KCAL	PROT	CARB	FAT	FIBRE
PEANUTS								
Roast, Salted, Average	**10 Whole/12g**	**74**	**6.3**	**614**	**27.8**	**7.9**	**52.4**	**4.9**
Salted, Average	**10 Whole/6g**	**37**	**3.1**	**609**	**27**	**8.3**	**52**	**5.4**
Sweet Chilli, Nobby's*	1 Bag/40g	214	13.6	535	15	42	34	3
Sweet Chilli, Thai, Coated, Sensations, Walkers*	1 Serving/30g	172	11.9	574	14.2	38.7	39.8	2.7
PEARL BARLEY								
Boiled	**1oz/28g**	**34**	**0.1**	**123**	**2.3**	**28.2**	**0.4**	**3.8**
Cooked, Average	**1 Serving/150g**	**184**	**0.7**	**123**	**2.3**	**28.2**	**0.4**	**3.8**
Raw, Average	**1oz/28g**	**99**	**0.3**	**352**	**9.9**	**77.7**	**1.2**	**15.6**
PEARS								
Abate Fetel, Average	**1 Med/133g**	**48**	**0.1**	**36**	**0.4**	**8.3**	**0.1**	**2.2**
Asian, Nashi, Raw, Average	**1 Lge/209g**	**80**	**0.4**	**38**	**0.5**	**9.7**	**0.2**	**3.3**
Blush, Tesco*	1 Pear/133g	62	0.1	47	0.3	10	0.1	2.2
Comice, Raw, Weighed with Core	**1 Med/170g**	**56**	**0**	**33**	**0.3**	**8.5**	**0**	**2**
Conference, Average	**1 Lge/209g**	**88**	**0.2**	**42**	**0.3**	**10.1**	**0.1**	**2**
Dessert, Green, Sainsbury's*	1 Sm/135g	53	0.1	39	0.3	9.2	0.1	2
Dried, Average	**1 Pear Half/16g**	**33**	**0.1**	**204**	**1.9**	**48.4**	**0.5**	**9.7**
in Fruit Juice, Average	**1 Serving/225g**	**102**	**0.1**	**45**	**0.3**	**10.9**	**0**	**1.2**
in Syrup, Average	**1oz/28g**	**16**	**0**	**58**	**0.2**	**14.4**	**0.1**	**1.4**
Prickly, Raw, Fresh	**1oz/28g**	**8**	**0.1**	**30**	**0.4**	**7**	**0.2**	**0**
Raw, Weighed with Core, Average	**1 Med/166g**	**58**	**0.2**	**35**	**0.3**	**8.4**	**0.1**	**1.3**
Red, Tesco*	1 Med/180g	65	0.2	36	0.4	8.3	0.1	2.2
William, Raw, Average	**1 Med/170g**	**58**	**0.2**	**34**	**0.4**	**8.3**	**0.1**	**2.2**
PEAS								
Dried, Boiled in Unsalted Water, Average	**1oz/28g**	**31**	**0.2**	**109**	**6.9**	**19.9**	**0.8**	**5.5**
Dried, Raw, Average	**1oz/28g**	**85**	**0.7**	**303**	**21.6**	**52**	**2.4**	**13**
Edible Podded, Raw	**1 Cup/63g**	**25**	**0.1**	**39**	**2.6**	**7.1**	**0.2**	**2.4**
Frozen, Average	**1 Serving/85g**	**62**	**0.8**	**73**	**6**	**9.7**	**1**	**4.5**
Frozen, Boiled, Average	**1 Serving/75g**	**51**	**0.7**	**68**	**6**	**9.4**	**0.9**	**5.1**
Garden, Canned with Sugar Salt, Average	**1 Serving/90g**	**59**	**0.6**	**66**	**5.3**	**9.3**	**0.7**	**5.1**
Garden, Canned, No Sugar Or Salt, Average	**1 Can/80g**	**36**	**0.3**	**45**	**4.4**	**6**	**0.4**	**2.8**
Garden, Frozen, Average	**1 Serving/90g**	**66**	**1**	**74**	**6.3**	**9.8**	**1.1**	**3.3**
Garden, Minted, Average	**1 Serving/80g**	**59**	**0.9**	**74**	**6.3**	**9.7**	**1.1**	**5.9**
Marrowfat, Average	**1 Sm Can/160g**	**134**	**0.9**	**84**	**6.1**	**13.7**	**0.6**	**3.7**
Mushy, Average	**1 Can/200g**	**173**	**1**	**86**	**6.2**	**14.4**	**0.5**	**2.2**
Processed, Canned, Average	**1 Sm Can/220g**	**162**	**1.6**	**74**	**5.6**	**11.3**	**0.7**	**3.4**
Roasted, Paprika, Chilli, Brave*	1 Pack/35g	132	3.8	378	19	41	11	20
Roasted, Sea Salt, Vinegar, Brave*	1 Pack/35g	134	3.8	383	19	41	11	19
Roasted, Sea Salt, Classic, Brave*	1 Pack/35g	134	3.8	382	20	41	11	20
Roasted, Sour Cream, Chive, Brave*	1 Pack/35g	132	3.8	377	20	41	11	20
Snow	**1 Serving/80g**	**24**	**0.2**	**29**	**3.3**	**3.9**	**0.2**	**2.1**
Sugar Snap, Average	**1 Serving/80g**	**27**	**0.2**	**33**	**3.2**	**4.8**	**0.2**	**1.4**
Wasabi, Average	**1 Serving/28g**	**114**	**3.8**	**406**	**15.2**	**54**	**13.7**	**8.6**
Wasabi, Ranch, Snapea Crisp, Harvest Snaps, Calbee*	1 Serving/28g	120	5	429	17.9	57.1	17.9	14.3
PEASE PUDDING								
Canned, Re-Heated, Drained	**1oz/28g**	**26**	**0.2**	**93**	**6.8**	**16.1**	**0.6**	**1.8**
PECAN NUTS								
Average	**3 Nuts/6g**	**42**	**4.2**	**692**	**10**	**5.6**	**70.1**	**4.7**
PENNE								
Arrabiata, BGTY, Sainsbury's*	1 Pack/450g	414	7.2	92	2.9	16.5	1.6	1.9
Brown Rice, GF, Pasta, Waitrose*	¼ Pack/125g	250	2.1	200	4.1	41	1.7	1.9
Chickpea, Peaz*	1 Portion/75g	264	4.4	352	26	43	5.8	11
Cooked, Average	**1 Serving/185g**	**244**	**1.3**	**132**	**4.7**	**26.7**	**0.7**	**1.1**
Dry, Average	**1 Serving/100g**	**352**	**1.9**	**352**	**12.4**	**71.3**	**1.9**	**2.7**

	Measure INFO/WEIGHT	per Measure KCAL	per Measure FAT	Nutrition Values per 100g / 100ml KCAL	PROT	CARB	FAT	FIBRE
PENNE								
Egg, Fresh, Average	*1 Serving/125g*	*352*	*4*	*282*	*11.1*	*52.2*	*3.2*	*2*
Free From, Tesco*	1 Serving/100g	340	2	340	8	72.5	2	2.5
Fresh, Dry, Average	*1 Serving/125g*	*222*	*2.4*	*178*	*7.3*	*32.2*	*1.9*	*1.6*
Organic, Dry, Average	*1 Serving/100g*	*352*	*1.8*	*352*	*12.4*	*71.6*	*1.8*	*1.9*
Red Pepper, Roasted, GFY, Asda*	1 Pack/400g	212	2.4	53	1.9	10	0.6	0.8
Rigate, Dry Weight, Average	*1 Serving/90g*	*318*	*1.6*	*353*	*12.3*	*72.1*	*1.8*	*1.8*
Sausage, Tuscan, Spicy Tomato , Meal for One, M&S*	1 Pack/400g	640	36.8	160	4.7	13.9	9.2	1.6
Vegetable, Roasted, Waitrose*	1 Pack/400g	424	15.6	106	2.8	15	3.9	0.8
Wholewheat, Asda*	1 Serving/100g	333	2.1	333	12.1	66.3	2.1	6.9
Wholewheat, Authentic, Italiano, Tesco*	1 Portion/75g	244	1.9	325	12.5	62.5	2.5	9
PEPERAMI*								
Hot, Peperami*	1 Stick/23g	112	9.9	497	22	3.2	44	1.2
Lunchbox Minis, 30% Less Fat, Peperami*	1 Stick/10g	40	3.1	400	26	5.5	31	3
Original, Peperami*	1 Stick/25g	126	11	504	24	2.5	44	0.1
PEPPER								
Black, Freshly Ground, Average	*1 Tsp/2g*	*5*	*0.1*	*255*	*11*	*64.8*	*3.3*	*26.5*
Cayenne, Ground	*1 Tsp/2g*	*6*	*0.3*	*318*	*12*	*31.7*	*17.3*	*0*
Pimento, Puree, Carrefour*	1 Tsp/5g	2	0	38	1.5	3.6	1	4.3
White	*½ Tsp/1g*	*3*	*0*	*296*	*10.4*	*68.6*	*2.1*	*26.2*
PEPPERCORNS								
Black, Schwartz*	1 Tsp/2g	11	0.4	529	13	68.7	22.5	27
Green, Average	*1 Tsp/10g*	*4*	*0.1*	*44*	*1.6*	*5.3*	*0.8*	*4.7*
PEPPERS								
Chargrilled, Spirit of Summer, M&S*	1 Pack/105g	45	1.5	43	1	5.6	1.4	2
Chargrilled, Sunflower Oil, Antipasto, Drained, Sainsbury's*	1 Serving/70g	82	5.4	118	1.7	9.5	7.7	1.8
Chilli, Dried, Flakes, Average	*1 Tsp/3g*	*13*	*0.4*	*425*	*16*	*56*	*15*	*44*
Chilli, Green, Raw, Unprepared, Average	*1 Med/13g*	*4*	*0*	*29*	*1.5*	*6.9*	*0.1*	*1.1*
Chilli, Red, Raw, Unprepared, Average	*1 Med/45g*	*13*	*0.1*	*29*	*1.5*	*6.9*	*0.1*	*1.1*
Chilli, Red, Very Lazy, The English Provender Co.*	1 Serving/15g	17	0.6	114	4.2	15.3	4	0.5
Green, Boiled in Salted Water	*1oz/28g*	*5*	*0.1*	*18*	*1*	*2.6*	*0.5*	*1.8*
Green, Raw, Unprepared, Average	*1 Med/160g*	*20*	*0.4*	*13*	*0.7*	*2.2*	*0.3*	*1.3*
Jalapeno, Raw	*1 Pepper/14g*	*4*	*0.1*	*28*	*1.2*	*5.4*	*0.4*	*2.6*
Mixed Bag, From Supermarket, Average	*1oz/28g*	*7*	*0.1*	*25*	*1*	*4.4*	*0.4*	*1.7*
Orange, Sweet, Raw, Average	*1oz/28g*	*8*	*0.1*	*30*	*1.8*	*5*	*0.3*	*1.5*
Red, Boiled in Salted Water	*1oz/28g*	*10*	*0.1*	*34*	*1.1*	*7*	*0.4*	*1.7*
Red, Raw, Unprepared, Average	*½ Med/80g*	*21*	*0.3*	*27*	*0.8*	*5.3*	*0.3*	*1.3*
Red, Sweet Pointed, Organic, Tesco*	1 Serving/100g	33	0.4	33	1	6.4	0.4	1.6
Roasted, in Oil, M&S*	1 Serving/50g	56	4.5	112	0.8	6.2	9	1.5
Stuffed, Cream Cheese, Sweet, Aldi*	1 Serving/60g	92	7.2	154	3.7	6.9	12	2.1
Stuffed, Red, Filled, Halves, Vegetarian, M&S*	1 Pack/295g	239	9.7	81	2.4	9.7	3.3	1.6
Stuffed, with Rice Based Filling, Average	*1oz/28g*	*24*	*0.7*	*85*	*1.5*	*15.4*	*2.4*	*1.3*
Stuffed, with Vegetables, Cheese Topping, Average	*1oz/28g*	*31*	*1.9*	*111*	*3.4*	*9.8*	*6.7*	*1.5*
Sweet, Pointed, Tesco*	1 Pepper/90g	24	0.2	27	0.8	4.3	0.2	2.2
Yellow, Raw, Unprepared, Average	*1 Med/160g*	*35*	*0.3*	*22*	*1*	*4.4*	*0.2*	*1.4*
PERCH								
Raw, Atlantic	*1oz/28g*	*26*	*0.5*	*94*	*18.6*	*0*	*1.6*	*0*
PERNOD*								
19% Volume, Pernod*	1 Pub Shot/35ml	46	0	130	0	0	0	0
Ricard Pastis, Pernod Ricard*	1 Pub Shot/25ml	64	0	257	0	36.7	0	0
PESTO								
Chilli, Fiery, Sacla*	1 Tbsp/15g	50	4.8	334	2.8	7.2	32	2.8
Green, Alla Genovese, Finest, Tesco*	1 Serving/65g	188	25.7	290	5.7	1.5	39.6	2.8
Green, Alla Genovese, Sacla*	1 Serving/30g	116	12.1	388	5.2	0.8	40.4	5.7

	Measure INFO/WEIGHT	per Measure KCAL	FAT	Nutrition Values per 100g / 100ml KCAL	PROT	CARB	FAT	FIBRE
PESTO								
Green, Average	*1 Tbsp/20g*	*103*	*9.5*	*517*	*20.4*	*2*	*47.5*	*0*
Green, Classic, Sacla*	1 Serving/40g	185	18.6	462	5.2	7.6	46.5	0
Green, Organic, Sacla*	1 Tbsp/15g	68	6.8	451	4.3	6.4	45	1.8
Green, Reduced Fat, Tesco*	¼ Jar /49g	96	9.5	195	2.6	0.7	19.4	3.4
Green, Sainsbury's*	1 Tsp/5g	17	1.8	347	4.8	1.9	35.1	2
Green, Tesco*	1 Tbsp/15g	50	4.8	331	4.7	4.4	31.9	3.7
Olive, Black, Sacla*	1oz/28g	115	11.8	409	2.9	4.3	42.2	0
Red, Morrisons*	1 Tbsp/15g	47	4.4	311	5.7	6.6	29	5.9
Red, Rosso, Bertolli*	1 Jar/185g	703	64.8	380	6.8	9.5	35	2
Wild Rocket, Sacla*	1 Serving/30g	128	13	425	5.2	3.2	43.5	4.5
PETIT POIS								
Baby Carrots, Canned, Drained, Average	*½ Can/122g*	*58*	*0.8*	*47*	*2.9*	*7*	*0.7*	*3.2*
Canned, Drained, Average	*1 Sm Can/200g*	*125*	*1*	*63*	*4.8*	*8.9*	*0.5*	*2.6*
Fresh, Frozen, Average	*1 Serving/80g*	*51*	*0.8*	*63*	*5.4*	*7.1*	*1*	*4.8*
PHEASANT								
Meat Only, Roasted	*1oz/28g*	*62*	*3.4*	*220*	*27.9*	*0*	*12*	*0*
Meat Only, Roasted, Weighed with Bone	*1oz/28g*	*32*	*1.7*	*114*	*14.5*	*0*	*6.2*	*0*
Stuffed, Easy Carve, Finest, Tesco*	1 Serving/200g	540	37.4	270	23.2	2.2	18.7	0.9
PHYSALIS								
Goldenberries, Dried, Neal's Yard*	1 Serving/20g	60	1.6	302	6	42.8	8	17.4
Raw, without Husk, Average	*5 Fruits/30g*	*16*	*0.2*	*53*	*1.9*	*11.2*	*0.7*	*0.4*
PICCALILLI								
Haywards*	1 Serving/28g	18	0.2	66	0.6	12	0.7	0.7
Heinz*	1 Serving/10g	10	0.1	99	1	20.5	0.6	0.6
Morrisons*	1 Serving/50g	38	0.4	75	1.6	15	0.7	0.6
Sweet Mild, Haywards*	2 Tbsp/40g	41	0.3	102	0.5	21	0.8	1
PICKLE								
Branston, Original, Crosse & Blackwell*	1 Serving/12g	19	0.1	157	0.5	34	0.7	1.8
Branston, Red Onion Cranberry, Crosse & Blackwell*	1 Tbsp/14g	13	0.1	92	0.6	21.4	0.4	0.8
Branston, Red Pepper Tomato, Crosse & Blackwell*	1 Tbsp/14g	12	0	84	1.2	17.7	0.3	1.1
Branston, Sm Chunk, Squeezy, Crosse & Blackwell*	1 Serving/15g	19	0	127	0.9	29.8	0.2	1.1
Branston, Smooth, Squeezy, Crosse & Blackwell*	1 Serving/15g	19	0	127	0.9	29.8	0.2	1.1
Brinjal, Patak's*	1 Tsp/16g	61	4	381	2.1	34.5	24.8	0
Chilli, Patak's*	1 Tsp/16g	52	5.4	325	4.3	1.3	33.7	0
Cornichons, Freshona, Lidl*	1 Serving/50g	18	0.2	35	1.2	5.5	0.3	0
Cornichons, with Mustard Seeds, in Vinegar, Drained, M&S*	¼ Jar/39g	17	0.2	44	1.5	8.1	0.4	1.1
Cucumber, Dill, Krakus*	1 Portion/80g	19	0	24	0	5.4	0	1.2
Garlic, Patak's*	1 Tsp/16g	42	3	261	3.6	20	18.5	1.6
Hot Chilli Jam, What A Pickle*	1 Tsp/8g	14	0	178	0.6	44	0.1	1.2
Lime, Hot, Patak's*	1 Tsp/16g	31	3	194	2.2	4	18.7	0.4
Lime, Oily	*1 Serving/39g*	*70*	*6.1*	*178*	*1.9*	*8.3*	*15.5*	*0*
Lime, Sharwood's*	1 Tbsp/20g	28	2	142	1.7	11.5	9.9	1.3
Mild Mustard, Heinz*	1 Tbsp/10g	13	0.1	129	2.2	25.7	1.3	0.9
Mixed, Drained	*1 Serving/100g*	*14*	*0.2*	*14*	*1*	*1.9*	*0.2*	*1*
Mixed, Drained, Haywards*	½ Jar/120g	22	0.4	18	1.4	2.4	0.3	0
Mixed, Patak's*	1 Serving/30g	78	7.7	259	2.3	4.7	25.7	0.8
Red Cabbage, Asda*	1 Serving/50g	16	0	32	1.6	6	0.1	0
Sandwich, Tesco*	1 Tbsp/30g	38	0	126	0.7	29.5	0.1	1.9
Sweet	*1 Tsp/10g*	*14*	*0*	*141*	*0.6*	*36*	*0.1*	*1.2*
Sweet, Batts, Lidl*	1 Serving/15g	17	0.1	114	0.8	26	0.5	1.1
Sweet, Bramwells*	1 Tbsp/15g	20	0.1	130	0.7	30	0.5	1.7
Sweet, Country, Morrisons*	1 Tbsp/15g	20	0	130	0.9	31.1	0.2	0
Sweet, Original, Tesco*	1 Tbsp/15g	20	0	135	0.5	31.5	0.1	2.1

P

INFO/WEIGHT	Measure	per Measure KCAL	FAT	Nutrition Values per 100g / 100ml KCAL	PROT	CARB	FAT	FIBRE

PICKLE

	Measure INFO/WEIGHT	per Measure KCAL	FAT	KCAL	PROT	CARB	FAT	FIBRE
Sweet, Savers, Morrisons*	1 Tbsp/15g	18	0	121	0.9	27.2	0.3	1.6
Tangy, Sandwich, Heinz*	1 Tsp/10g	13	0	134	0.7	31.4	0.2	0.9
PICNIC								
Cadbury*	1 Bar/48g	230	10.9	475	7.3	60.9	22.6	2.1
PIE								
Admiral's, Ross*	1 Pie/340g	357	15.6	105	4.8	10.9	4.6	0.7
Aloo Gobi, GF, Clive's*	1 Pie/235g	486	29.3	207	3	19.2	12.5	0
Apple, & Blackberry, Co-Op*	1 Serving/138g	338	15.2	245	3	33	11	2
Apple, & Blackberry, Lattice Topped, BGTY, Sainsbury's*	¼ Pie/100g	256	7.5	256	2.8	44.4	7.5	3.1
Apple, & Blackberry, Shortcrust, M&S*	1 Serving/142g	469	17.8	330	4.3	50.2	12.5	1.1
Apple, Bramley, Aunt Bessie's*	¼ Pie/138g	386	15.1	281	2.4	42	11	1.1
Apple, Bramley, Bakery, Tesco*	1/6 Pie/87g	234	9.7	269	3	38.4	11.1	1.5
Apple, Bramley, Free From, Tesco*	1 Serving/67g	173	7.6	260	0.6	37.5	11.4	2.6
Apple, Bramley, Individual, Mr Kipling*	1 Pie/60g	210	7.9	351	3.4	54	13.2	1.4
Apple, Bramley, Individual, Sainsbury's*	1 Pie/54g	165	5	307	3.6	52.2	9.3	1.3
Apple, Bramley, Individual, Tesco*	1 Pie/60g	221	7.6	362	4	57.5	12.5	1.9
Apple, Bramley, Large, Tesco*	1/8 Pie/87g	311	13	358	3.9	51.9	15	1.9
Apple, Commercially Prepared	*1 Slice/125g*	*296*	*13.8*	*237*	*1.9*	*34*	*11*	*1.6*
Apple, Pastry Top & Bottom	*1oz/28g*	*74*	*3.7*	*266*	*2.9*	*35.8*	*13.3*	*1.7*
Apple, Prepared From Recipe, Average	*1oz/28g*	*74*	*3.5*	*265*	*2.4*	*37.1*	*12.5*	*0*
Apple, with Custard	*1 Serving/217g*	*353*	*18.8*	*163*	*2.4*	*25.2*	*8.7*	*1.1*
Banoffee, Mini, Waitrose*	1 Pie/26g	115	5.8	444	3.3	57	22.5	1.2
Beef, & Onion, Minced, Tesco*	1 Pie/150g	454	28.5	303	5.7	27.4	19	1.7
Beef, & Onion, Pukka Pies Ltd*	1 Serving/231g	529	32.6	229	7.6	17.9	14.1	3
Beef, Bourguignon, Deluxe, Lidl*	1 Pie/190g	591	37.6	311	9.6	22.7	19.8	1.8
Beef, Minced, Aberdeen Angus, Shortcrust, M&S*	1 Pie/171g	435	26.6	255	9.3	19.3	15.6	3
Cheese, & Onion, Hollands*	1 Pie/200g	516	24.4	258	6.3	30.9	12.2	0
Cheese, & Onion, Oven Baked, Average	*1 Serving/200g*	*654*	*40*	*327*	*8.2*	*30.4*	*20*	*1.2*
Cheese, & Potato	*1oz/28g*	*39*	*2.3*	*139*	*4.8*	*12.6*	*8.1*	*0.7*
Cherry, Bakery, Tesco*	1/6 Pie/87g	240	9.7	276	2.6	40.5	11.2	1.3
Chicken, & Asparagus, Tesco*	1 Serving/170g	468	28.7	275	8.3	22.4	16.9	0.8
Chicken, & Bacon, Puff Pastry, Deep Fill, Sainsbury's*	1/3 Pie/200g	532	34	266	9.1	19.1	17	1.3
Chicken, & Gravy, Just, Fray Bentos*	½ Pie/215g	267	7.3	124	5.6	17.2	3.4	0.6
Chicken, & Gravy, Roast, Deep Fill, Tesco*	¼ Pie/157g	358	16	228	9.7	23.7	10.2	1.5
Chicken, & Gravy, Shortcrust Pastry, Serves 3, Sainsbury's*	1 Serving/184g	552	33.3	300	10.8	22.7	18.1	1.7
Chicken, & Gravy, Shortcrust Pastry, Tesco*	1 Pie/250g	618	34.5	247	6.8	23.9	13.8	1
Chicken, & Ham, & Leek, Pot, Higgidy*	1 Pie/250g	670	39.8	268	11.1	21.4	15.9	1.2
Chicken, & Ham, Deep Filled, Sainsbury's*	1 Pie/210g	594	37.2	283	8	23	17.7	1
Chicken, & Leek, & Bacon, Aldi*	1 Pie/210g	601	37.6	286	10.9	19.7	17.9	1
Chicken, & Leek, & Bacon, Deluxe, Lidl*	1/3 Pie/171g	511	30.8	299	11	22	18	2.7
Chicken, & Leek, & Ham, Morrisons*	1 Serving/113g	305	16.6	270	8.8	25.7	14.7	1.1
Chicken, & Leek, LC, Tesco*	1 Pie/350g	298	5.6	85	6.6	10.3	1.6	1.3
Chicken, & Leek, M&S*	1oz/28g	70	4.2	250	10.1	18.8	15.1	1.1
Chicken, & Mushroom, Average	*1 Serving/200g*	*540*	*31.7*	*270*	*8*	*23.8*	*15.9*	*1*
Chicken, & Mushroom, Pukka Pies Ltd*	1 Pie/226g	475	29.2	210	7.6	15.7	12.9	3.5
Chicken, & Wiltshire Ham, Finest, Tesco*	1 Pie/250g	688	37.2	275	11.6	22.7	14.9	1.1
Chicken, Bacon, Puff Pastry Lid, Tesco*	1 Pie/131g	300	15.7	229	7.6	22	12	1.4
Chicken, Mushroom, Serves 1, BGTY, Sainsbury's*	1 Pack/400g	359	9.2	94	7.1	10.5	2.4	1.1
Chicken, Vegetable, Frozen, Tesco*	1 Pie/129g	282	14.4	219	7.2	21.6	11.2	1.4
Chicken, Deep Filled, Puff Pastry, Sainsbury's*	1 Pie/210g	538	31.9	256	10	19.9	15.2	3.1
Chicken, Individual, Ready Made, Average	*1 Pie/155g*	*392*	*22.3*	*253*	*9.5*	*20.9*	*14.4*	*1.6*
Chicken, Shortcrust, Oven Baked, Birds Eye*	1 Pie/155g	417	23.1	271	8.4	25	15	1.2
Chilli, Three Bean, GF, Twinpack, Clive's*	1 Pie/185g	326	21.3	176	3.2	19.8	11.5	0

PIE

	Measure INFO/WEIGHT	per Measure KCAL	FAT	Nutrition Values per 100g / 100ml KCAL	PROT	CARB	FAT	FIBRE
Cod, & Haddock, Smoked, COU, M&S*	1 Pack/400g	320	9.6	80	6.1	9	2.4	1.2
Cottage, 1, Waitrose*	1 Pack/400g	580	30.4	145	8.2	10.3	7.6	1.6
Cottage, Aberdeen Angus, Large, Chilled, Finest, Tesco*	½ Pack/400g	420	17.2	105	7.1	8.7	4.3	1.8
Cottage, Aldi*	1 Pack/440g	484	27.3	110	4.1	9.5	6.2	0.2
Cottage, Beef, Delicious, Annabel Karmel*	1 Pack/200g	206	9.6	103	4.7	9.8	4.8	1.1
Cottage, Classic British, Sainsbury's*	1 Pack/450g	414	14.8	92	5.8	9.3	3.3	1
Cottage, COU, M&S*	1 Pack/400g	340	8	85	6	11	2	1.5
Cottage, Diet Chef Ltd*	1 Pack/270g	235	9.7	87	3.7	9.8	3.6	1.7
Cottage, Finest, Tesco*	1 Pack/400g	447	15.7	114	6.8	12.2	4	0.9
Cottage, Frozen, Weight Watchers*	1 Pack/320g	252	6.4	79	5.2	9.5	2	1
Cottage, HFC, Tesco*	1 Pack/388g	283	5	73	2.6	12.3	1.3	1.1
Cottage, Lentil Vegetable, Linda McCartney*	1 Pot/398g	374	10.3	94	2.8	13.5	2.6	2.5
Cottage, Lentil, with Sweet Potato Mash, Sainsbury's*	1 Pack/382g	283	6.1	74	2.6	10.4	1.6	4
Cottage, Little Dish*	1 Pack/200g	188	7.2	94	3.9	10.5	3.6	1.9
Cottage, Meal for One, M&S*	1 Pack/445g	356	16	80	5.4	6.2	3.6	1.7
Cottage, Morrisons*	1 Pack/450g	450	18.4	100	5.2	10.7	4.1	1.2
Cottage, Retail, Average	*1 Pack/400g*	*399*	*15.7*	*100*	*5.5*	*10.5*	*3.9*	*1.3*
Cottage, Serves 1, Basics, Sainsbury's*	1 Pack/286g	269	8.3	94	3.9	12.3	2.9	1.5
Cottage, with Cheddar Mash, TTD, Sainsbury's*	1 Pack/400g	525	27.2	131	8.6	7.9	6.8	1.8
Cumberland, Asda*	1 Pack/400g	504	22.4	126	6.3	12.7	5.6	1.5
Fish	*1 Serving/250g*	*262*	*7.5*	*105*	*8*	*12.3*	*3*	*0.7*
Fish, Admirals, Frozen, Oven Baked, Youngs*	1 Pie/291g	338	12.8	116	4.9	13.7	4.4	1
Fish, Charlie Bigham's*	½ Pack/328g	499	29.9	152	8.4	9.6	9.1	0
Fish, Classic Kitchen, Tesco*	½ Pack/386g	457	19.8	119	8.7	8.8	5.1	1.3
Fish, Crunchy Topped, Menu, Waitrose*	1 Pack/400g	444	19.2	111	7.5	8.4	4.8	1.8
Fish, Extra Special, Asda*	1 Pack/400g	540	30.8	135	9.8	6.5	7.7	1.1
Fish, HL, Tesco*	1 Pack/384g	311	7.7	81	3.9	11.4	2	0.9
Fish, Little Dish*	1 Pack/200g	206	8.8	103	4.5	10.5	4.4	1.5
Fish, Main for One, Gastropub, M&S*	1 Pie/420g	483	20.6	115	8	9.3	4.9	0.8
Fish, Mariner's, Frozen, Oven Baked, Youngs*	1 Pack/340g	444	20.3	140	5.1	15.1	6.4	1
Fish, Meal for One, Oven Baked, Gastro, Youngs*	1 Pie/317g	412	20.3	130	8.5	9.2	6.4	1
Fish, Serves 1, BGTY, Sainsbury's*	1 Pie/450g	369	8.6	90	6.7	10.2	2.1	1.6
Fisherman's, Youngs*	1 Pack/340g	377	13.6	111	5.6	12.8	4	0.8
Fruit, Pastry Top & Bottom	*1oz/28g*	*73*	*3.7*	*260*	*3*	*34*	*13.3*	*1.8*
Fruit, Selection, Mr Kipling*	1 Pie/66g	232	9	350	3.5	53.5	13.6	1.3
Homity, GF, Clive's*	1 Pie/235g	390	22.6	166	4.2	14.4	9.6	0
Lemon Meringue	*1 Portion/120g*	*383*	*17.3*	*319*	*4.5*	*45.9*	*14.4*	*0.7*
Lemon Meringue, Sainsbury's*	¼ Pie/110g	351	9.9	319	2.3	57.3	9	0.5
Lemon Meringue, Tesco*	1 Serving/79g	223	6.2	283	3.4	49.1	7.8	1.3
Lentil, & Olive, Greek, Clive's*	1 Pie/235g	477	25.4	203	4.5	20	10.8	0
Macaroni Cheese, Countryside*	1 Serving/144g	282	10.1	196	4.9	28.3	7	1.2
Meat, & Potato, Hollands*	1 Pie/175g	410	19.2	234	6.1	27.5	11	0
Meat, & Potato, Tesco*	1 Serving/150g	414	26.8	276	5.1	23.6	17.9	1.6
Mince, All Butter Pastry, Extra Special, Asda*	1 Pie/70g	278	11.1	400	3.6	59	16	3.2
Mince, All Butter, 1, Waitrose*	1 Pie/61g	238	8.9	391	3.3	60	14.6	3.3
Mince, All Butter, Average	*1 Pie/65g*	*251*	*8.9*	*386*	*4*	*60.2*	*13.8*	*2.4*
Mince, All Butter, Mini, 1, Waitrose*	1 Pie/28g	111	3.8	392	3.1	63.6	13.4	2.5
Mince, All Butter, Mini, Average	*1 Pie/20g*	*78*	*2.8*	*389*	*4.3*	*61.6*	*13.8*	*2.8*
Mince, All Butter, Mini, The Best, Morrisons*	1 Pie/32g	127	4.7	402	4	62	14.9	2
Mince, All Butter, Puff Pastry, Average	*1 Pie/60g*	*228*	*10.5*	*381*	*4.3*	*51.1*	*17.4*	*2.2*
Mince, All Butter, Puff Pastry, Extra Special, Asda*	1 Pie/51g	195	10.1	386	3.8	47	20	1.3
Mince, Butter Enriched, Puff Pastry, Bakery, Sainsbury's*	1 Pie/65g	246	9.7	379	4.7	55.4	14.9	2.2
Mince, Christmas, Classic, Asda*	1 Pie/57g	229	9.1	401	3.5	59	16	3.5

INFO/WEIGHT	Measure	per Measure		Nutrition Values per 100g / 100ml				
		KCAL	FAT	KCAL	PROT	CARB	FAT	FIBRE
PIE								
Mince, Christmas, Finest, Tesco*	1 Pie/64g	255	9.4	395	4.6	60.3	14.5	1.4
Mince, Christmas, Sainsbury's*	1 Pie/37g	147	6	397	4.5	58	16.3	2.6
Mince, Deep Fill, Holly Lane, Aldi*	1 Pie/65g	265	10.4	407	3.9	61	16	3.3
Mince, Deep Filled, All Butter Pastry, Finest, Tesco*	1 Pie/65g	259	10.8	401	5	56.2	16.7	2.7
Mince, Deep Filled, All Butter, The Best, Morrisons*	1 Pie/67g	263	10.3	395	3.8	59.4	15.4	1.9
Mince, Deep, Morrisons*	1 Pie/65g	243	9.1	371	3.7	57.8	13.9	1.5
Mince, Dusted, Mini, Finest, Tesco*	1 Pie/20g	76	2.4	379	7.3	62.9	12.2	5
Mince, Free From, Sainsbury's*	1 Pie/58g	226	7.5	393	2.3	64	13	2.5
Mince, Iced Top, Asda*	1 Pie/55g	220	7.7	399	2.8	63	14	4.7
Mince, Individual, Average	**1 Pie/65g**	**260**	**11**	**400**	**4.2**	**56.3**	**17**	**1.6**
Mince, Individual, Mr Kipling*	1 Pie/66g	253	9.2	381	3.7	59.5	13.8	1.3
Mince, Luxury, Deep Filled, M&S*	1 Pie/65g	234	9	360	4.3	55	13.8	3.8
Mince, Luxury, Extra Special, Asda*	1 Pie/64g	247	8.9	387	4.2	60	14	2.3
Mince, Luxury, Iceland*	1 Pie/60g	230	8.3	383	4.1	59.3	13.8	2.6
Mince, Mini, M&S*	1 Pie/28g	105	4	380	4.3	57.8	14.6	4
Mince, Puff Pastry, Co-Op*	1 Pie/72g	245	11.9	340	5	43.1	16.5	2.6
Mince, Shortcrust, Essential, Waitrose*	1 Pie/53g	226	9.5	423	4	60.1	17.7	3.4
Mince, Tesco*	1 Pie/54g	211	7.5	389	3.8	61.2	13.8	2.6
Mushroom, Camembert, Puff Pastry Topped, Tesco*	1 Pie/162g	434	26.2	268	5.6	24	16.2	2.1
Mushroom, Leek, GF, Clive's*	1 Pie/235g	456	26.8	194	3.2	18.3	11.4	0
Mushroom, Onion, with Parsley Mash, Veggie, M&S*	1 Pack/400g	288	8.4	72	1.7	10.6	2.1	1.9
Mushroom, Feta, Spinach, Little, Higgidy*	1 Pie/160g	385	24.4	241	6.8	20.1	15.3	1.3
Mushroom, Tomato, & Red Wine, Kevin, Pieminister*	1 Pie/270g	562	25.7	208	4.4	25	9.5	0
Mushroom, Wild Shroom, Pieminister*	1 Pie/270g	513	26.2	190	5.2	19.5	9.7	2.7
Plum, Cinnamon, Tesco*	1 Pie/66g	239	8.2	360	3.9	56.6	12.3	3.7
Pork, & Egg, M&S*	¼ Pie/110g	411	31	374	10.9	18.4	28.2	1.5
Pork, BBQ, Mini, Tesco*	1 Pie/50g	198	13.2	396	10.7	28.2	26.3	1.9
Pork, Cheese & Pickle, Mini, Tesco*	1 Pie/49g	191	12.8	389	9.2	29.3	26.1	1.2
Pork, Individual	**1 Pie/75g**	**272**	**19.3**	**363**	**10.8**	**23.7**	**25.7**	**0.9**
Pork, Melton Mowbray, Chef Select, Lidl*	1 Pie/50g	204	14.4	407	10.3	25.9	28.9	1.2
Pork, Melton Mowbray, Cured, Mini, M&S*	1 Pie/50g	192	12.2	385	9.8	32.6	24.4	1
Pork, Melton Mowbray, Individual, Sainsbury's*	½ Pie/70g	234	15.1	334	11.1	22.8	21.6	1.8
Pork, Melton Mowbray, Lattice, Sainsbury's*	1 Serving/100g	342	23.6	342	10.8	21.7	23.6	1.2
Pork, Melton Mowbray, Mini, Co-Op*	1 Pie/49g	189	13.2	385	11	24	27	2
Pork, Melton Mowbray, Mini, M&S*	1 Pie/50g	185	12.1	370	11.6	26.1	24.2	1.6
Pork, Melton Mowbray, Mini, Morrisons*	1 Pie/50g	197	12.5	393	10.9	31.3	24.9	0.9
Pork, Melton Mowbray, Mini, Tesco*	1 Pie/50g	192	12.8	383	10.6	26.9	25.6	1.5
Pork, Melton Mowbray, Mini, TTD, Sainsbury's*	1 Pie/50g	204	14.2	407	10.6	26.5	28.4	1.7
Pork, Mini, Retail, Average	**1 Mini/50g**	**198**	**13.7**	**396**	**10.8**	**26.4**	**27.4**	**2.4**
Pork, Mini, Tesco*	1 Pie/45g	162	10.7	359	10.2	25.9	23.8	1
Pork, Sliced	**1 Slice/100g**	**380**	**29.9**	**380**	**10.2**	**18.7**	**29.9**	**0**
Rhubarb, Shortcrust Pastry, Bakery, Tesco*	1 Slice/87g	219	9.3	251	3.1	34.8	10.7	1.7
Scotch, Co-Op*	1 Pie/132g	408	24.9	309	7.3	27.3	18.9	1.5
Shepherd's, Average	**1oz/28g**	**31**	**1.7**	**112**	**6**	**9.3**	**5.9**	**0.7**
Shepherd's, British Classic, Meal For One, Aldi*	1 Pie/450g	614	35.5	142	5.4	11	8.2	1
Shepherd's, Chilled, Finest, Tesco*	½ Pack/400g	414	14	103	6.3	11.1	3.5	1.2
Shepherd's, Vegetarian, Average	**1 Serving/400g**	**371**	**14.6**	**93**	**4**	**10.4**	**3.6**	**2.5**
Steak, & Ale with Chips & Gravy	**1 Serving/400g**	**825**	**42.2**	**206**	**7.2**	**20.5**	**10.6**	**0.5**
Steak, & Ale, Average	**1 Pie/200g**	**507**	**28.7**	**253**	**9.8**	**21.1**	**14.4**	**1.3**
Steak, & Ale, Pub Style, Co-Op*	1 Pie/250g	538	30	215	9	17	12	2
Steak, & Ale, Sainsbury's*	1 Serving/190g	445	23.4	234	8.3	22.6	12.3	0.9
Steak, & Kidney with Puff Pastry, 425g, Fray Bentos*	1 Pie/425g	622	16.6	131	5.6	17.4	3.5	0.6
Steak, & Kidney, Individual	**1 Pie/200g**	**646**	**42.4**	**323**	**9.1**	**25.6**	**21.2**	**0.9**

	Measure INFO/WEIGHT	per Measure KCAL	FAT	Nutrition Values per 100g / 100ml KCAL	PROT	CARB	FAT	FIBRE
PIE								
Steak, & Kidney, Puff Pastry, Sainsbury's*	1 Pie/150g	423	23.6	282	8.2	26.9	15.7	0.9
Steak, & Kidney, Pukka Pies Ltd*	1 Pie/239g	537	28.2	225	9.7	17.7	11.8	4.5
Steak, Ale, Charlie Bigham's*	1 Pie/300g	742	39.7	247	13.2	17	13.2	0
Steak, Ale, Puff Pastry, Serves 3, Sainsbury's*	1 Serving/183g	464	24.9	253	9.5	22.7	13.6	0.9
Steak, Aberdeen Angus, Top Crust, Waitrose*	½ Pie/280g	476	24.1	170	10	13.4	8.6	4.1
Steak, All, Pukka Pies Ltd*	1 Pie/233g	495	24.5	212	11.1	17.7	10.5	2.5
Steak, Mini, Asda*	1 Serving/67g	117	5.3	176	9	17	8	0.9
Steak, Puff Pastry Lid, Frozen, Tesco*	1 Pie/131g	304	14.9	232	8.5	23.1	11.4	1.5
Steak, Puff Pastry, Serves 3, Sainsbury's*	1 Serving/183g	512	30	280	9.8	22.6	16.4	1.3
Steak, Scotch, Bell's Bakery*	1 Serving/150g	378	20.2	252	13.6	18.6	13.5	0.7
Steak, Short Crust, Sainsbury's*	½ Pie/117g	314	24.1	267	10.9	22.2	20.5	1.7
Steak, Tesco*	1 Pie/150g	408	21.4	272	9.5	25.5	14.3	1.8
Vegetable	*1oz/28g*	*42*	*2.1*	*151*	*3*	*18.9*	*7.6*	*1.5*
Vegetable, & Cheese, Asda*	1 Pie/141g	330	16.2	234	5.8	26.9	11.5	1
Vegetable, & Feta, Moroccan, Little, Higgidy*	1 Pie/180g	418	22.5	232	5.1	24.7	12.5	0.6
Vegetable, Retail, Average	*1 Serving/200g*	*348*	*19*	*174*	*3.7*	*18.6*	*9.5*	*1.1*
Vegetarian, Chicken Style, Mushroom, Quorn*	1 Pie/235g	588	33.2	250	5.5	23.7	14.1	3
Vegetarian, Deep Country, Linda McCartney*	1 Pie/166g	413	23.6	249	5.2	24.9	14.2	2.6
Vegetarian, Mince Potato, Quorn*	1 Pie/200g	388	16	194	6.5	22.5	8	3
Vegetarian, Mushroom Ale, Linda McCartney*	1 Pie/200g	439	23.5	219	4.1	25	11.7	1.2
Vegetarian, Shepherd's, Linda McCartney*	1 Pack/340g	286	7.5	84	3.7	12.3	2.2	2.3
Vegetarian, Steak, Meat Free, Quorn*	1 Pie/235g	439	18.8	187	5.6	22	8	2
PIE FILLING								
Apple, Sainsbury's*	1 Serving/75g	67	0.1	89	0.1	22.1	0.1	1
Cherry	*1oz/28g*	*23*	*0*	*82*	*0.4*	*21.5*	*0*	*0.4*
Fruit	*1oz/28g*	*22*	*0*	*77*	*0.4*	*20.1*	*0*	*1*
Pistachio, Mix, Avidhipro*	1 Pack/25g	91	0.6	364	74.8	9.6	2.4	2
Summer Fruits, Fruit, Tesco*	1 Can/385g	377	0	98	0.4	24.1	0	0.9
PIGEON								
Meat Only, Roasted, Average	*1 Pigeon/115g*	*215*	*9.1*	*187*	*29*	*0*	*7.9*	*0*
Meat Only, Roasted, Weighed with Bone, Average	*1oz/28g*	*12*	*0.5*	*41*	*6.4*	*0*	*1.7*	*0*
PIKELETS								
Free From, Tesco*	1 Pikelet/30g	58	1.3	194	2.8	36.2	4.3	1.4
Sainsbury's*	1 Pikelet/24g	55	0.3	230	7.6	45.1	1.4	3.3
Tesco*	1 Pikelet/27g	52	0.3	193	6.6	38.1	1	2.4
PILAF								
Bulgur Wheat, Sainsbury's*	1 Pack/381g	347	11.1	91	3.9	12.3	2.9	6.3
Vegetables, with Coconut Lentil, City Kitchen, Tesco*	1 Pack/385g	474	20.8	123	2.6	14.9	5.4	2.3
with Tomato, Average	*1oz/28g*	*40*	*0.9*	*144*	*2.5*	*28*	*3.3*	*0.4*
PILCHARDS								
Fillets in Tomato Sauce, Average	*1 Can/120g*	*158*	*7.8*	*132*	*16.2*	*2.2*	*6.5*	*0.1*
Fillets in Virgin Olive Oil, Glenryck*	1 Serving/92g	223	14.4	242	23.3	2	15.7	0
in Brine, Average	*½ Can/77g*	*114*	*5.6*	*148*	*20.8*	*0*	*7.3*	*0*
PIMMS*								
Lemonade, Premixed, Canned, Pimms*	1 Can/250ml	160	0	64	0	8.4	0	0
25% Volume, Pimms*	1 Serving/50ml	80	0	160	0	5	0	0
PINE NUTS								
Average	*1 Tbsp/8g*	*56*	*5.5*	*695*	*15.7*	*3.9*	*68.6*	*1.9*
PINEAPPLE								
Chunks, Average	*1 Serving/100g*	*66*	*0.1*	*66*	*0.5*	*15.5*	*0.1*	*0.3*
in Juice, Canned, Average	*1 Can/106g*	*57*	*0*	*53*	*0.3*	*12.9*	*0*	*0.6*
Raw, Flesh Only, Average	*1 Med Slice/80g*	*40*	*0.1*	*50*	*0.5*	*13.1*	*0.1*	*1.4*

P

	Measure INFO/WEIGHT	per Measure KCAL	FAT	Nutrition Values per 100g / 100ml KCAL	PROT	CARB	FAT	FIBRE
PISTACHIO NUTS								
Raw, Average, without Shells	*1 Serving/20g*	*111*	*8.9*	*557*	*20.6*	*28*	*44.4*	*10.3*
Roasted Salted, without Shells, Average	*1 Serving/25g*	*152*	*13.6*	*608*	*19.6*	*9.9*	*54.5*	*6.1*
Salted, Roasted, Weighed with Shell	*1 Serving/100g*	*331*	*30.5*	*331*	*9.8*	*4.5*	*30.5*	*3.4*
Salted, Roasted, without Shells	*1 Serving/100g*	*601*	*55.4*	*601*	*17.9*	*8.2*	*55.4*	*6.1*
PIZZA								
American Hot, Thin Crispy, Stonebaked, Aldi*	½ Pizza/149g	357	16.4	240	9.7	25	11	2.8
American, Supermarket, Pizza Express*	½ Pizza/130g	352	14.5	271	11.3	30.5	11.2	1.5
Aubergine, Spinach, & Tomato, Pizzeria, Waitrose*	½ Pizza/193g	403	7.7	209	7.8	35.4	4	3.6
Bacon, & Mushroom, Pizzeria, Sainsbury's*	1 Pizza/355g	880	24.8	248	11.7	34.5	7	3.7
Bacon, & Mushroom, Thin & Crispy, Sainsbury's*	½ Pizza/150g	396	15.9	264	12.9	29.2	10.6	1.7
BBQ, Cola, Sticky Sweet, Stuffed Crust, Chicago Town*	¼ Pizza/155g	426	13.7	274	11	37	8.8	0
Beef, Chilli, Classic Crust, Tex Mex, Tesco*	½ Pizza/260g	655	26.5	252	10.9	27.9	10.2	2.5
Cheese & Tomato, Average	*1 Serving/300g*	*711*	*35.4*	*237*	*9.1*	*25.2*	*11.8*	*1.4*
Cheese & Tomato, Baguette, Tesco*	1 Baguette/125g	275	8.5	220	11	28	6.8	2.8
Cheese & Tomato, Deep Pan, Goodfella's*	¼ Pizza/102g	259	10.8	253	11.5	29.6	10.5	3.7
Cheese & Tomato, Everyday Value, Tesco*	1 Pizza/150g	423	9.2	282	9.6	46	6.1	2.2
Cheese & Tomato, French Bread, Findus*	1 Serving/143g	322	11.6	225	9.4	29	8.1	0
Cheese & Tomato, Frozen, Sainsbury's*	1 Serving/122g	300	10.7	246	13.7	28	8.8	3
Cheese & Tomato, Meltingly Good, M&S*	½ Pizza/227g	613	22.5	270	10.8	33.5	9.9	2
Cheese & Tomato, Mini, Bruschetta, Iceland*	1 Pizza/34g	63	2.3	188	8	23	7	2.8
Cheese & Tomato, Mini, M&S*	1 Pizza/95g	233	5.5	245	10	38.7	5.8	1.6
Cheese & Tomato, Range, Italiano, Tesco*	1 Pizza/380g	969	35	255	11.4	31.7	9.2	3.3
Cheese & Tomato, Retail, Frozen	*1oz/28g*	*70*	*3*	*250*	*7.5*	*32.9*	*10.7*	*1.4*
Cheese & Tomato, Sainsbury's*	1 Pizza/247g	706	24.5	286	13.7	35.4	9.9	2.4
Cheese & Tomato, Slice, Ross*	1 Slice/77g	148	6.6	192	6.5	22.2	8.6	2
Cheese & Tomato, Slices, CBY, Asda*	1 Slice/14g	62	2.5	453	8.2	63.2	18.1	2.3
Cheese & Tomato, Stonebaked, Organic, Co-Op*	1 Pizza/330g	676	23.1	205	9	26	7	4
Cheese & Tomato, Stonebaked, Thin & Crispy, Tesco*	½ Pizza/161g	388	13.8	241	11.6	29.4	8.6	2.1
Cheese & Tomato, Thin & Crispy, Asda*	1 Pizza/366g	827	36.6	226	11	23	10	2
Cheese & Tomato, Thin & Crispy, Sainsbury's*	1 Serving/135g	344	10	255	14.9	32.2	7.4	5
Cheese & Tomato, Thin & Crispy, Waitrose*	1 Pizza/280g	658	28.3	235	12.3	23.6	10.1	2.3
Cheese & Tomato, Thin, HFC, Tesco*	½ Pizza/144g	361	9.6	250	10.9	35.5	6.7	2.3
Cheese Tomato, Mini, HFC*	1 Mini Pizza/241g	709	27.7	294	11.1	35.1	11.5	3
Cheese Tomato, Mini, HFC, Tesco*	1 Mini Pizza/82g	241	9.5	294	11.1	35.1	11.5	3
Cheese Feast, Deep Crust, Carlos, Aldi*	1 Pizza/155g	432	14.9	279	9.7	37.3	9.6	2.1
Cheese Feast, Deep Pan, Asda*	½ Pizza/210g	422	18.9	201	13	17	9	2.3
Cheese Feast, Stuffed Crust, Garlic Herb Dip, Sainsbury's*	¼ Pizza/148g	387	13.9	261	12.1	31	9.4	1.8
Cheese Feast, Stuffed Crust, Take Away, Carlos, Aldi*	½ Pizza/238g	650	27	273	11.8	29.4	11.3	2.7
Cheese Feast, Thin Crust, Chilled, Tesco*	½ Pizza/175g	467	22.4	267	14.7	23.4	12.8	2.5
Cheese, & Garlic, Tesco*	½ Pizza/102g	304	11.7	298	9.2	38.1	11.5	2.4
Cheese, Four, Deep Dish, Chicago Town*	1 Pizza/148g	433	17.8	292	12	33	12	0
Cheese, Four, Finest, Tesco*	½ Pizza/230g	575	21.2	250	12.1	29.8	9.2	1.3
Cheese, Four, Stonebaked, Thin, Carlos, Aldi*	½ Pizza/176g	498	17.4	283	13	34	9.9	2.8
Cheese, Four, Stuffed Crust, Takeaway, Chicago Town*	¼ Pizza/158g	433	17	275	10.8	33	10.8	1.9
Cheese, Four, Thin & Crispy, Iceland*	½ Pizza/148g	354	12.6	239	10.7	29.1	8.5	1.6
Cheese, Loaded, Stuffed Crust, Takeaway, Chicago Town*	¼ Pizza/150g	436	17.9	292	12	33	12	0
Cheese, Reg Crust, From Restaurant, Average	*1 Pizza/905g*	*2018*	*46.2*	*223*	*12.2*	*32.5*	*5.1*	*0*
Cheese, Simply, Goodfella's*	¼ Pizza/82g	226	11	276	16.3	22.5	13.4	1.9
Cheese, Stuffed Crust, Sainsbury's*	1 Pizza/525g	1428	52.5	272	14	31.5	10	2
Cheese, Stuffed Crust, Takeaway, Tesco*	½ Pizza/203g	521	17.7	256	11.5	31.8	8.7	2.5
Cheese, Thick Crust, From Restaurant, Average	*1 Pizza/976g*	*2655*	*107.3*	*272*	*12*	*31.3*	*11*	*1.8*
Cheese, Thin Crust, From Restaurant, Average	*1 Pizza/627g*	*1906*	*98.3*	*304*	*14.2*	*26.5*	*15.7*	*2*
Cheese, Three, & Tomato, Stonebaked, Co-Op*	1 Pizza/415g	888	33.6	214	10	25.2	8.1	1.5

PIZZA

	Measure INFO/WEIGHT	KCAL	FAT	KCAL	PROT	CARB	FAT	FIBRE
Cheese, Triple, Deep Dish, Chicago Town*	1 Serving/170g	418	18.2	246	9.9	27.6	10.7	0
Chicken, & Bacon, Loaded, Tesco*	1 Serving/258g	622	25.3	241	12.8	25.4	9.8	1.9
Chicken, & Bacon, Pizzeria, Italian, Sainsbury's*	½ Pizza/170g	508	24.1	300	13.6	29.4	14.2	2.7
Chicken, & Chorizo, 12", TTD, Sainsbury's*	½ Pizza/290g	702	20.9	242	12.2	32.1	7.2	2.6
Chicken, & Chorizo, Sourdough, Carlos, Aldi*	½ Pizza/165g	406	14.2	246	12	29	8.6	4.7
Chicken, & Pesto, Californian Style, Asda*	½ Pizza/235g	533	16.4	227	10	31	7	2
Chicken, & Sweetcorn, Stonebaked, Tesco*	1 Serving/177g	354	9.6	200	11.9	26	5.4	2
Chicken, & Vegetable, Leggera, Pizza Express*	1 Pizza/191g	396	12.8	207	9.9	25.6	6.7	2.5
Chicken, & Vegetable, Stone Baked, GFY, Asda*	½ Pizza/161g	349	3.7	217	13	36	2.3	1.7
Chicken, Bacon, Large, Takeaway, Chicago Town*	¼ Pizza/123g	355	14.7	289	13	32	12	0
Chicken, Arrabiata, with Nduja, TTD, Sainsbury's*	½ Pizza/163g	408	14.4	250	12.5	28.9	8.8	2.8
Chicken, BBQ, M&S*	½ Pizza/210g	430	11.8	205	11.6	27.5	5.6	1.8
Chicken, BBQ, Stonebaked, Tesco*	½ Pizza/158g	285	9.5	180	10.5	20.9	6	3.9
Chicken, BBQ, Texan, Thin & Crispy, Co-Op*	½ Pizza/190g	418	14.1	220	11	27	7.4	2.1
Chicken, BBQ, Thin & Crispy, Sainsbury's*	½ Pizza/167g	399	12.4	238	11.4	30.4	7.4	2.2
Chicken, Cajun Style, Stonebaked, Tesco*	1 Pizza/561g	1318	55	235	11.9	24.8	9.8	1.4
Chicken, Cajun, Sainsbury's*	½ Pizza/146g	285	2.6	195	12.9	31.8	1.8	2.6
Chicken, Chargrilled, Iceland*	1 Pizza/381g	804	25.5	211	12.3	25.4	6.7	2
Chicken, Chargrilled, Thin & Crispy, Asda*	1 Pizza/373g	780	18.6	209	9	32	5	1.6
Chicken, Club, Deep Dish, Chicago Town*	1 Pizza/155g	404	14.9	261	11	32	9.6	0
Chicken, Fajita, 10 Inch, CBY, Asda*	½ Pizza/151g	319	9.8	211	10.7	26.3	6.5	2.4
Chicken, Fajita, Thin & Crispy, Iceland*	1 Pizza/361g	729	21.3	202	9.6	26.5	5.9	1.8
Chicken, Garlic, Thin & Crispy, Stonebake, Sainsbury's*	½ Pizza/160g	386	17.3	241	10.7	25.2	10.8	3.5
Chicken, Hot & Spicy, Deep Pan, Morrisons*	½ Pizza/233g	521	13	224	10.5	32.9	5.6	1
Chicken, Hot & Spicy, Deep Pan, Tesco*	½ Pizza/222g	423	7.3	191	10.5	30	3.3	2.1
Chicken, Provencal, Goodfella's*	½ Pizza/143g	388	18	272	13.7	25.9	12.6	2.1
Chicken, Romano, Goodfella's*	½ Pizza/189g	447	17.6	236	11	26	9.3	0
Chicken, Smoky BBQ, Stonebaked, M&S*	½ Pizza/230g	513	15.2	223	11.3	28.5	6.6	2.1
Chicken, Sweet Chilli, BGTY, Sainsbury's*	½ Pizza/138g	276	2.3	200	13	33.2	1.7	2.1
Chicken, Tandoori, Thin Crust, Halal, Gino's*	1 Pizza/300g	663	27.3	221	10.3	24.8	9.1	0
Chicken, Tikka, Protein Base, Musclefood*	1 Pizza/200g	380	16	190	16.5	11.8	8	2.4
Chocolate, Dessert, Chicago Town*	¼ Pizza/35g	128	5.6	369	7.1	49	16	0
Diavolo, Takeaway, Goodfella's*	¼ Pizza/129g	388	19.3	301	11	29	15	0
Falafel, Vegan, Stonebaked, Goodfellas *	½ Pizza/182g	397	12.7	218	6.4	30	7	0
Four Seasons, Stonebaked, Truly Irresistible, Co-Op*	½ Pizza/245g	502	16.2	205	9.5	26.6	6.6	2.6
Funghi, Ristorante, Dr Oetker*	1 Pizza/365g	847	43.4	232	7.6	22.5	11.9	1.8
Goats Cheese, Protein Base, Musclefood*	1 Pizza/200g	386	13.2	193	17.9	17.1	6.6	3.3
Ham, & Cheese, Ultra Thin, Sodebo*	1 Pizza/200g	400	8.6	200	11.3	29.1	4.3	0
Ham, & Mushroom & Tomato, BGTY, Sainsbury's*	½ Pizza/150g	309	6.1	206	11.8	30.4	4.1	1.2
Ham, & Mushroom Slices, Farmfoods*	1 Slice/89g	170	2.3	191	8	34	2.6	0.9
Ham, & Mushroom, Average	*1 Serving/250g*	*533*	*16*	*213*	*10.5*	*28.4*	*6.4*	*2.1*
Ham, & Mushroom, Finest, Tesco*	½ Pizza/240g	576	26.4	240	9.5	25.9	11	2.2
Ham, & Mushroom, Smoked, Thin & Crispy, Co-Op*	1 Pizza/400g	792	18	198	9	30.3	4.5	1.7
Ham, & Mushroom, Thin & Crispy, Asda*	1 Pizza/360g	760	25.2	211	11	26	7	2.4
Ham, & Mushroom, Thin & Crispy, Tesco*	½ Pizza/185g	380	11.1	205	11.2	25.6	6	2.3
Ham, & Pineapple, Average	*1 Serving/250g*	*555*	*16.8*	*222*	*11*	*29.2*	*6.7*	*2.1*
Ham, & Pineapple, Stone Bake, M&S*	1 Pizza/345g	690	19.7	200	10.1	28.3	5.7	1.6
Ham, & Pineapple, Stonebaked, Tesco*	1 Pizza/161g	293	9.2	182	9.2	23.5	5.7	3.5
Ham, & Pineapple, Tesco*	1/6 Pizza/56g	134	4.6	240	10.4	30.9	8.3	2.1
Ham, & Pineapple, Thin & Crispy Italian, Morrisons*	1 Pizza/375g	746	22.9	199	10.2	24.9	6.1	0
Ham, & Pineapple, Thin & Crispy, Iceland*	1 Serving/110g	301	13.1	274	9.9	31.9	11.9	3
Ham, & Pineapple, Thin & Crispy, Sainsbury's*	½ Pizza/165g	371	13.8	226	11.6	24.9	8.4	2
Ham, & Pineapple, Thin Crust, Tesco*	½ Pizza/175g	385	10	220	12.3	29.6	5.7	2.5

P

PIZZA

	Measure INFO/WEIGHT	per Measure KCAL	FAT	Nutrition Values per 100g / 100ml KCAL	PROT	CARB	FAT	FIBRE
Ham, Pepperoni & Milano, M&S*	1 Pizza/290g	696	28.4	240	14	23.3	9.8	1.1
Hawaii, Ristorante, Dr Oetker*	¼ Pizza/91g	206	7.7	226	8.8	28	8.5	0
Hawaiian, Stonebaked, Cucina, Aldi*	½ Pizza/165g	326	5.6	198	9.5	32	3.4	1.6
Hawaiian, Thin Crust, Tesco*	½ Pizza/192g	365	9.4	190	10.3	25.6	4.9	1.8
Italian Style, Oumph!*	½ Pizza/200g	362	11.8	181	6.6	24	5.9	2.1
La Reine, Supermarket, Pizza Express*	½ Pizza/153g	322	9.3	211	10.2	27.7	6.1	2.3
Margherita, 12", Finest, Tesco*	½ Pizza/255g	433	9.2	170	8.1	26.4	3.6	2.7
Margherita, Average	*1 Slice/108g*	*239*	*8.6*	*239*	*11*	*30.5*	*8.6*	*1.2*
Margherita, Cheese Tomato, San Marco*	½ Pizza/200g	454	14.4	227	10.7	29.8	7.2	1.2
Margherita, Classic, Kirstys*	1 Pizza/290g	658	24.9	227	10.3	26.5	8.6	1.4
Margherita, Classico, Italiano, Tesco*	½ Pizza/191g	414	11.8	217	11.2	29.1	6.2	2.5
Margherita, Free From, Tesco*	½ Pizza/144g	375	11.5	261	2.6	42.1	8	5.2
Margherita, GF, Goodfella's*	¼ Pizza/74g	203	8.2	273	11	32	11	0
Margherita, Lactose Free,, Schar*	1 Pizza/300g	690	27.6	230	7.5	27	9.2	3.8
Margherita, Large, Supermarket, Pizza Express*	½ Pizza/228g	511	17.1	224	10.6	28.6	7.5	2.5
Margherita, Pizzeria, Italian, Sainsbury's*	½ Pizza/169g	426	17.4	253	12.2	27.9	10.3	2.5
Margherita, Speciale, Supermarket, Pizza Express*	½ Pizza/169g	438	17.2	259	11.6	28.5	10.2	3.2
Margherita, Stone Baked, Goodfella's*	1 Slice/36g	95	4.1	263	10.9	31.9	11.4	7.6
Margherita, Stonebaked, 10", Sainsbury's*	½ Pizza/139g	359	11.3	258	12.4	32.2	8.1	3.5
Margherita, Supermarket, Pizza Express*	½ Pizza/127g	312	10.8	245	10	31.5	8.5	1.4
Margherita, The Best, Morrisons*	½ Pizza/216g	569	20.8	263	9.8	32.7	9.6	3.5
Margherita, Thin & Crispy, Iceland*	½ Pizza/170g	391	14.4	230	12.7	25.9	8.5	2.8
Margherita, Thin Crust, Takeaway, Goodfella's*	½ Pizza/206g	594	26.7	289	13	29	13	0
Margherita, Thin Crust, Tesco*	1 Serving/170g	354	13.4	208	10.1	24.1	7.9	3.6
Meat Feast, Deep & Loaded, Sainsbury's*	½ Pizza/298g	818	30	275	13.2	32.7	10.1	2.6
Meat Feast, Italian, Thin & Crispy, Waitrose*	1 Pizza/182g	477	22.9	262	10.7	26.5	12.6	1.8
Meat Feast, Large, Tesco*	1 Pizza/735g	1904	69.1	259	10.9	32.6	9.4	2
Meat Feast, Mega, Asda*	½ Pizza/428g	1044	33.8	244	9.5	33.6	7.9	3.2
Meat Feast, Thin & Crispy, Asda*	½ Pizza/183g	410	14.6	224	11	27	8	1.4
Meat Feast, Thin Crust, Stonebakes, Goodfella's*	½ Pizza/171g	450	17.1	263	12	28	10	0
Meat Feast, Thin Crust, Tesco*	½ Pizza/178g	430	20.2	242	13.6	21.3	11.4	2.3
Meat Mayhem, Goodfella's*	1 Pizza/437g	1100	41.9	252	10.6	30.9	9.6	2.5
Meatball, Marinari, Deep Loaded, M&S*	¼ Pizza/389g	930	45.1	239	10.2	22.5	11.6	1.7
Meats, Italian, Finest, Tesco*	½ Pizza/217g	449	8.5	207	13.6	29.4	3.9	1.3
Mediterranean, Thin Crispy, Stonebaked, Tesco*	½ Pizza/179g	350	10.7	195	7.1	27.3	6	2.1
Mega Meaty, Deep Dish, Chicago Town*	1 Pizza/157g	442	18.9	281	11	31	12	0
Mini, Party, Tesco*	1 Pizza/11g	26	1.1	248	11.4	28.6	10.5	1.9
Mozzarella, & Sunblush Tomato, 12", TTD, Sainsbury's*	½ Pizza/251g	638	17.8	254	12.4	35	7.1	2.6
Mozzarella, Ristorante, Dr Oetker*	½ Pizza/184g	472	23.9	257	10	25	13	0
Mushroom, & Ricotta, Leggera, Pizza Express*	1 Pizza/170g	371	11.1	218	8.9	29.4	6.5	2.9
Mushroom, Garlic, Classico, Tesco*	½ Pizza/208g	415	13.9	200	10	24.9	6.7	2.6
Mushroom, Garlic, Tesco*	1 Pizza/425g	829	34	195	9.3	21.6	8	5.3
Mushroom, Garlic, Thin Crust, Tesco*	½ Pizza/163g	340	14.6	209	11	21.1	9	3.6
Napoletana, Sainsbury's*	½ Pizza/186g	424	14.3	228	9.7	29.9	7.7	3.1
Napoli, Tesco*	½ Pizza/184g	431	11.6	235	11.9	32.6	6.3	1.4
Onion, Caramelised, & Feta, & Rosemary, Bistro, Waitrose*	½ Pizza/230g	607	32	264	8.6	26.1	13.9	2.4
Pepperoni, & Cheese, Asda*	½ Pizza/150g	386	13.5	257	10	34	9	2.7
Pepperoni, & Jalapeno Chill, Asda*	1 Pizza/277g	742	22.2	268	10	39	8	1.8
Pepperoni, Aldi*	1 Serving/55g	123	4.3	224	8.7	29.5	7.9	1.4
Pepperoni, Asda*	½ Pizza/150g	386	13.5	257	10	34	9	2.7
Pepperoni, Average	*1 Serving/250g*	*671*	*28.4*	*269*	*11.8*	*29.6*	*11.4*	*2.1*
Pepperoni, Baguette, Ovenbaked, Asda*	1 Baguette/123g	243	7.3	197	9.7	25	5.9	2.4
Pepperoni, Deep & Crispy, Iceland*	1 Serving/175g	490	21	280	11.9	31.1	12	1.8

PIZZA

INFO/WEIGHT	Measure	per Measure KCAL	per Measure FAT	Nutrition Values per 100g / 100ml KCAL	PROT	CARB	FAT	FIBRE
Pepperoni, Deli, The Pizza Kitchen, Chicago Town*	½ Pizza/174g	544	26.2	312	13	29	15	0
Pepperoni, Double, Thin & Crispy, Loved by Us, Co-Op*	½ Pizza/173g	389	18.9	225	10.5	27.3	10.9	3.4
Pepperoni, Hot & Spicy, Stuffed Crust, Asda*	1 Pizza/245g	666	30	272	13.9	26.5	12.2	2.4
Pepperoni, Mini, Tesco*	1 Serving/22g	71	3.7	323	11.8	30.5	16.8	2.7
Pepperoni, Mushroom, & Ham, GF, Goodfellas*	½ Pizza/175g	450	17.5	257	10	30	10	0
Pepperoni, Passion, Thin Crust, Takeaway, Goodfella's*	½ Pizza/212g	637	31.8	300	13	28	15	0
Pepperoni, Picante, Bella Italia*	1 Pizza/425g	1016	48.9	239	12.7	20.7	11.5	1.6
Pepperoni, Reg Crust, From Restaurant, Average	**1 Pizza/959g**	**2445**	**94**	**255**	**14.3**	**28**	**9.8**	**0**
Pepperoni, Salame, Ristorante, Dr Oetker*	½ Pizza/165g	465	23.2	281	10	28	14	0
Pepperoni, Stone Baked, Carlos*	1 Pizza/330g	832	39.6	252	13	23	12	0
Pepperoni, Stonebaked Ciabatta, Goodfella's*	½ Pizza/181g	503	26.1	278	11.9	27.4	14.4	2.4
Pepperoni, Stonebaked, 10", Sainsbury's*	½ Pizza/143g	373	15.1	260	12.2	27.7	10.5	2.7
Pepperoni, Stonebaked, 12", Sainsbury's*	¼ Pizza/103g	301	13.3	292	13.2	29.2	12.9	3.1
Pepperoni, Stonebaked, Chef Select, Lidl*	¼ Pizza/85g	209	7.4	246	11.1	29.5	8.7	2.4
Pepperoni, Takeaway, Fully Loaded, Goodfella's*	½ Pizza/251g	800	47.6	319	11	25	19	0
Pepperoni, Thin & Crispy, Sainsbury's*	½ Pizza/139g	393	18.3	282	12.5	27.6	13.1	1.8
Pepperoni, Thin Crispy, Cucina, Aldi*	½ Pizza/170g	503	23.8	296	12	29	14	2.4
Pepperoni, Thin Crispy, Essential, Waitrose*	½ Pizza/133g	380	18	286	12.3	28.8	13.5	1
Pepperoni, Thin Crispy, HFC, Tesco*	½ Pizza/148g	383	13.2	258	10.6	32.8	8.9	2.4
Pollo, ad Astra, Supermarket, Pizza Express*	½ Pizza/144g	315	8.7	218	11.3	28.9	6	1.8
Pollo, Primavera, Wood Fired, Ultra Thin, M&S*	1 Pizza/185g	414	15.9	224	10.4	25.3	8.6	1.9
Pollo, Ristorante, As Sold, Dr Oetker*	½ Pizza/183g	408	16.5	223	8.8	25.7	9	1.8
Pork, 'n' Pineapple, Punchy, Freshly Prepared, Tesco*	½ Pizza/186g	510	18	274	12.4	32.9	9.7	2.7
Pork, Pulled, BBQ, Fully Loaded, Takeaway, Sainsbury's*	½ Pizza/262g	691	26.7	264	10.5	31.4	10.2	2.2
Prosciutto, Italian Style, Co-Op*	½ Pizza/183g	421	12.8	230	13	29	7	3
Prosciutto, Ristorante, Dr Oetker*	1 Pizza/330g	752	32.3	228	10.3	24.6	9.8	0
Quattro Formaggi, Ristorante, Dr Oetker*	½ Pizza/170g	457	23.8	269	10.8	24.1	14	1.6
Salame, Ristorante, Dr Oetker*	½ Pizza/160g	455	24.5	285	10.4	26.3	15.3	0
Salami, & Ham, Pizzeria, Waitrose*	½ Pizza/205g	443	13.7	216	10.1	28.7	6.7	1.8
Salami, & Pepperoni, Waitrose*	½ Pizza/190g	578	30.8	304	13.4	23.9	16.2	2.1
Salami, Napoli Diavolo, Pizza, Wood Fired, M&S*	½ Pizza/244g	549	24.9	225	10.8	21.7	10.2	1.7
Salami, Romano, Goodfella's*	½ Pizza/177g	481	21.3	271	13	27	12	0
Salami, Ultra Thin Italian, Tesco*	1 Serving/263g	692	25.5	263	12	31.9	9.7	1
Selection, Slices, M&S*	1 Serving/52g	120	4.1	230	9.4	30.3	7.8	1.9
Sloppy Giuseppe, Supermarket, Pizza Express*	½ Pizza/151g	333	10.9	220	10	28.1	7.2	1.6
Spinach, & Bacon & Mushroom, GFY, Asda*	1 Serving/270g	618	12.2	229	13	34	4.5	2.6
Spinach, & Ricotta, Classic Italian, Stonebaked, Tesco*	½ Pizza/190g	460	16.3	240	10.3	29	8.5	1.2
Spinach, & Ricotta, Extra Special, Asda*	1 Pizza/400g	940	28	235	9	34	7	1.9
Spinach, & Ricotta, Italian, Chilled, Sainsbury's*	1 Pizza/361g	859	34.7	238	9.3	28.7	9.6	2.3
Spinach, & Ricotta, Thin Crust, Italian, Tesco*	½ Pizza/190g	365	16.7	192	9.6	18.7	8.8	1.9
Spinach, Ricotta, Stonebaked, M&S*	½ Pizza/253g	543	17.4	215	8	29.2	6.9	2.1
Supreme, Deep Dish, Individual, Chicago Town*	1 Pizza/170g	456	20.4	268	9.2	30.8	12	1
The Whole Hog, Deep Loaded, M&S*	½ Pizza/345g	823	33.4	239	12.3	24.9	9.7	1.5
Vegetable, & Peppers, Fire Roasted, Waitrose*	½ Pizza/235g	442	16.7	188	9.8	21.3	7.1	2.7
Vegetable, & Pesto, Chargrilled, Specially Selected, Aldi*	½ Pizza/305g	756	29	248	9.2	30	9.5	2.9
Vegetable, Average	**1 Serving/250g**	**475**	**13.1**	**190**	**8.2**	**27.5**	**5.2**	**2.4**
Vegetable, Balsamic Roast, & Mozzarella, Sainsbury's*	½ Pizza/200g	444	15.6	222	8.5	29.4	7.8	2.4
Vegetable, Chargrilled, Frozen, BGTY, Sainsbury's*	1 Pizza/290g	548	13.3	189	10.2	26.7	4.6	3
Vegetable, Deep Pan, Co-Op*	1 Pizza/425g	829	29.8	195	8	25	7	2
Vegetable, Frozen, HL, Tesco*	1 Pizza/400g	604	10.8	151	8.1	23.5	2.7	4.4
Vegetable, GFY, Asda*	¼ Pizza/94g	141	2.7	150	7	24	2.9	3.7
Vegetable, Mediterranean, Pizzeria, Sainsbury's*	1 Serving/211g	397	13.5	188	8	24.7	6.4	3.2
Vegetable, Mediterranean, Stonebaked, Carlos, Aldi*	½ Pizza/173g	323	8.7	187	7.5	26.6	5	2.9

P

	Measure INFO/WEIGHT	per Measure KCAL	FAT	Nutrition Values per 100g / 100ml KCAL	PROT	CARB	FAT	FIBRE
PIZZA								
Vegetable, Mediterranean, Stonebaked, Sainsbury's*	½ Pizza/260g	622	16.4	239	9.8	35.7	6.3	3.1
Vegetable, Romano, Goodfella's*	½ Pizza/195g	419	15	215	9	26	7.7	0
Veggie Supreme, Takeaway, Tesco*	1 Slice/106g	280	11.8	264	10.4	29.9	11.1	1.4
Veggie, Very, Stonebaked, M&S*	½ Pizza/274g	537	15.9	196	7.9	27	5.8	2.1
Vegi Supreme, Stuffed Crust, Medium	*1 Slice/87g*	*209*	*7*	*240*	*12*	*29.3*	*8*	*2.2*
PIZZA BASE								
Deep Pan, Italian, Sainsbury's*	1 Base/220g	684	11	311	7	59.5	5	1.4
Deep Pan, Napolina*	1 Base/260g	757	7.8	291	7.9	58	3	0.2
Everyday Value, Tesco*	½ Base/125g	401	2.8	320	9.6	65.2	2.2	0.7
Garlic Bread, Sainsbury's*	¼ Base/59g	109	4.2	186	5.1	25.4	7.1	1.8
Gluten, Wheat Dairy Free, Free From, Livwell*	1 Base/100g	237	2.6	237	5.2	48.3	2.6	4.7
Italian, Classic, Sainsbury's*	1 Base/150g	452	7.2	301	7.6	57	4.8	1.5
Light & Crispy, Napolina*	1 Base/150g	436	4.5	291	7.9	58	3	0.2
M&S*	1 Base/150g	418	8.1	279	9.2	47.5	5.4	1.9
Mini, Napolina*	1 Base/75g	218	2.2	291	7.9	58	3	0.2
Stone Baked, GF, BFree*	½ Pizza/90g	231	2.6	257	3.5	49.2	2.9	10
Thin Crispy, Sainsbury's*	1 Base/150g	504	7.8	336	9.9	62.3	5.2	4.3
Wholemeal, Dough, Frozen, The Northern Dough Co*	1 Base/110g	226	1.8	205	9.7	38.9	1.6	0
with Tomato Sauce, Crosta Mollica*	½ Pizza/135g	282	4.9	209	6	40.7	3.6	3
PIZZA BASE MIX								
Morrisons*	1 Serving/77g	313	3.8	407	12.7	77.9	5	3.6
Sainsbury's*	1 Pack/145g	486	5.5	335	12.8	62.3	3.8	2.9
PLAICE								
Fillets in Breadcrumbs, Average	*1 Serving/150g*	*331*	*17.9*	*221*	*12.8*	*15.5*	*11.9*	*0.8*
Fillets, Lightly Dusted, Average	*1 Fillet/113g*	*188*	*9.2*	*166*	*12.9*	*10.4*	*8.2*	*0.6*
Fillets, Raw, Average	*1oz/28g*	*24*	*0.4*	*87*	*18.2*	*0*	*1.5*	*0*
Goujons, Baked	*1oz/28g*	*85*	*5.1*	*304*	*8.8*	*27.7*	*18.3*	*0*
Goujons, Fried in Blended Oil	*1oz/28g*	*119*	*9*	*426*	*8.5*	*27*	*32.3*	*0*
Grilled	*1oz/28g*	*27*	*0.5*	*96*	*20.1*	*0*	*1.7*	*0*
in Batter, Fried in Blended Oil	*1oz/28g*	*72*	*4.7*	*257*	*15.2*	*12*	*16.8*	*0.5*
Steamed	*1oz/28g*	*26*	*0.5*	*93*	*18.9*	*0*	*1.9*	*0*
PLANTAIN								
Boiled in Unsalted Water	*1oz/28g*	*31*	*0.1*	*112*	*0.8*	*28.5*	*0.2*	*1.2*
Raw, Average	*1 Med/179g*	*218*	*0.7*	*122*	*1.3*	*31.9*	*0.4*	*2.3*
Ripe, Fried in Vegetable Oil	*1oz/28g*	*75*	*2.6*	*267*	*1.5*	*47.5*	*9.2*	*2.3*
PLUMS								
Average, Stewed without Sugar	*1oz/28g*	*8*	*0*	*30*	*0.5*	*7.3*	*0.1*	*1.3*
Fresh, Raw, Weighed without Stone, Average	*1 Plum/66g*	*24*	*0.1*	*36*	*0.6*	*8.6*	*0.1*	*1.9*
Weighed with Stone, Average	*1 Plum/90g*	*31*	*0.1*	*34*	*0.5*	*8.1*	*0.1*	*1.8*
Yellow, Waitrose*	1 Plum/50g	20	0	39	0.6	8.8	0.1	1.5
POLENTA								
Dry, Merchant Gourmet*	1 Serving/65g	232	0.9	357	7.4	78.8	1.4	1.3
Organic, Dry, Kallo*	1 Serving/150g	543	2.7	362	8.5	78	1.8	0
POLLOCK								
Fillets, Breaded, Cooked, Tesco*	1 Fillet/125g	315	12.2	250	15	24.4	9.7	2
Fillets, British, Sainsbury's*	1 Pack/218g	157	1.3	72	16.6	0	0.6	0
Fillets, in Batter, Frozen, Chip Shop, Youngs*	1 Fillet/106g	241	14.1	228	11.6	15	13.3	1.1
POLO								
Fruits, Nestle*	1 Tube/37g	142	0	383	0	96	0	0
Mints, Clear Ice, Nestle*	1 Sweet/4g	16	0	390	0	97.5	0	0
Mints, Original, Nestle*	1 Sweet/2g	8	0	402	0	98.2	1	0
Spearmint, Nestle*	1 Tube/35g	141	0.4	402	0	98.2	1.1	0

P

	Measure INFO/WEIGHT	KCAL	FAT	Nutrition Values per 100g / 100ml				
				KCAL	PROT	CARB	FAT	FIBRE
POMEGRANATE								
Raw, Fresh, Flesh Only, Average	*1 Sm Fruit/86g*	*59*	*0.3*	*68*	*1*	*17.2*	*0.3*	*0.6*
Raw, Weighed with Rind Skin, Average	*1 Sm Fruit/154g*	*59*	*0.3*	*38*	*0.5*	*9.6*	*0.2*	*0*
POMELO								
Fresh, Raw, Weighed with Skin Seeds	*100 Grams/100g*	*11*	*0.1*	*11*	*0.2*	*2.5*	*0.1*	*0*
Raw, Flesh Only, Average	*1 Fruit/340g*	*129*	*0.1*	*38*	*0.8*	*9.6*	*0*	*1*
POP TARTS								
Bustin' Berry, Kellogg's*	1 Tart/50g	200	6	400	4	69	12	2
Chocolate Chip Cookie Dough, Kellogg's*	1 Pastry/50g	190	5	380	4	70	10	2
Chocolate Chip, Kellogg's*	1 Pastry/52g	210	6	404	5.8	69.2	11.5	1.9
Chocolate, Kellogg's*	1 Pastry/50g	198	8.5	396	5	136	17	2
Cinnamon Roll, Kellogg's*	1 Pastry/50g	210	7	420	4	68	14	2
Cookies 'n' Creme, Kellogg's*	1 Pastry/50g	190	5	380	4	70	10	2
Frosted Blueberry, Kellogg's*	1 Pastry/52g	200	5	385	3.8	73.1	9.6	1.9
Frosted Blueberry, Mini Crisps, Kellogg's*	1 Pouch/23g	100	2.5	435	4.4	78.3	10.9	0
Frosted Brown Sugar Cinnamon, Kellogg's*	1 Tart/50g	210	7	420	6	68	14	2
Frosted Cherry, Kellogg's*	1 Pastry/52g	200	5	385	3.8	73.1	9.6	2.3
Frosted Chocolate Fudge, Kellogg's*	1 Pastry/52g	200	5	385	5.8	71.2	9.6	1.9
Frosted Cinnamon with Wholegrain, Low Fat, Kellogg's*	1 Pastry/50g	180	3	360	4	74	6	6
Frosted Hot Fudge Sundae, Kellogg's*	1 Pastry/48g	190	4.5	396	4.2	70.8	9.4	2.1
Frosted Raspberry, Kellogg's*	1 Pastry/52g	200	5	385	3.8	73.1	9.6	1.9
Frosted S'mores, Kellogg's*	1 Pastry/52g	200	5	385	5.8	69.2	9.6	1.9
Frosted Strawberry, Oatmeal Delights, Kellogg's*	1 Pastry/50g	200	5	400	4	72	10	6
Pumpkin Pie, Frosted, Kellogg's*	1 Pastry/50g	200	5	400	4	70	10	2
Strawberry Sensation, Kellogg's*	1 Tart/50g	198	5.5	395	4	70	11	2
Wild! Fruit Fusion, Frosted, Kellogg's*	1 Pastry/50g	200	5	400	4	72	10	2
Wild! Grape, Kellogg's*	1 Tart/50g	200	5	400	4	72	10	2
POPCORN								
94% Fat Free, Orville Redenbacher's*	1 Bag/76g	220	0	289	13.2	65.8	0	0
Air Popped, Plain, Average	*1 Sm Bag/17g*	*66*	*0.8*	*387*	*12.9*	*77.9*	*4.5*	*14.5*
Butter Toffee, Belgian Milk Chocolate Coated, M&S*	1 Pack/100g	505	25	505	6.5	60.4	25	4.1
Butter Toffee, Snack-A-Jacks, Quaker*	1 Bag/35g	149	3.2	425	3.5	86	9	4.5
Butter Toffee, Tesco*	1 Pack/175g	709	13.5	405	2.2	81.7	7.7	4.3
Butter, Microwave, 94% Fat Free, Act II*	½ Bag/41g	130	2.5	317	9.8	68.3	6.1	12.2
Butter, Microwave, Act II*	1 Bag/90g	425	16.2	472	9	69	18	9
Butter, Microwave, Butterkist*	1 Bag/70g	305	12.7	436	8.5	55.2	18.1	9.6
Butter, Microwave, Popz*	1 Serving/100g	480	27.5	480	7.5	51.1	27.5	9.2
Caramel, Crunch, Sugar Free, with Sweeteners, Free'ist*	1 Portion/26g	94	1.5	362	3.1	73.8	5.8	0
Caramel, Salted, Bloom's*	1 Bag/28g	135	6.6	483	4.9	60.3	23.4	5.8
Caramel, Salted, Butterkist*	1 Serving/20g	83	1.9	417	3.4	77.7	9.5	3.5
Caramel, Salted, Skinny, Metcalfe's Food Co*	¼ Bag/19g	85	3.6	455	8.9	57	19	10.3
Chocolate, & Pecan, M&S*	1 Pack/27g	130	5.2	480	3.3	72.9	19.3	3.6
Chocolate, & Toffee, Snack-A-Jacks, Quaker*	1 Bag/35g	126	3.4	359	2.2	65	9.8	3
Irish Cream, Epic Snacks*	1 Serving/30g	122	2.1	407	2.4	82	7.1	3.7
Maize, Unpopped, Love Life, Waitrose*	1 Serving/33g	200	14.1	605	6.2	48.7	42.8	12.7
Maple, Shapers, Boots*	1 Bag/20g	94	3.6	469	12	59	18	10
Organic Amaranth*	1 Serving/10g	36	0.9	365	14.6	26.8	8.8	0
Paprika, Smoked, Sainsbury's*	1 Bag/11g	53	2.9	480	8.7	46.6	26.1	12.1
Peanut, & Almond, Smooth, Propercorn*	1 Serving/25g	120	5.9	481	11.9	49.4	23.5	12.2
Plain, Oil Popped, Average	*1 Bag/74g*	*439*	*31.7*	*593*	*6.2*	*48.7*	*42.8*	*0*
Popping Corn, Average	*1 Serving/30g*	*112*	*1.3*	*375*	*10.9*	*73.1*	*4.3*	*12.7*
Salt & Vinegar, Sea Salt, Sainsbury's*	1 Bag/11g	52	2.7	474	4.8	53.6	24.6	9.7
Salt Vinegar, Sainsbury's*	1 Bag/11g	52	2.7	474	4.8	53.6	24.6	9.7
Salt Vinegar, Snack-A-Jacks, Quaker*	1 Sm Pack/13g	47	1.3	360	12	55	9.9	14

POPCORN

INFO/WEIGHT	Measure	per Measure		Nutrition Values per 100g / 100ml				
		KCAL	FAT	KCAL	PROT	CARB	FAT	FIBRE
Salted, Blockbuster*	1 Bowl/25g	99	2.9	397	10.6	62.2	11.7	8.6
Salted, Crunch Corn, Propercorn*	1 Serving/30g	140	7.9	468	5	52.1	26.4	12.2
Salted, Diet Chef Ltd*	1 Pack/23g	107	3.8	465	10.5	68.6	16.6	14
Salted, Light, Microwave, Act II*	1 Pack/85g	336	6.5	395	10.6	71	7.6	15.8
Salted, Lightly, Popping Corn, Graze*	1 Punnet/28g	127	7	454	8	44	25	13
Salted, Lightly, Sea Salt, Wholegrain, Sunbites, Walkers*	1 Pack/20g	84	2.6	419	8.6	59.3	12.9	15.7
Salted, Lightly, Sea, Propercorn*	1 Bag/20g	85	3	424	9.3	54	15.1	17.6
Salted, Lightly, Snack-A-Jack, Quaker*	1 Bag/13g	48	1.3	370	12.1	58	9.9	14.6
Salted, Lime & Sea Salt, Captain Theodore's, Ten Acre*	1 Pack/28g	139	7	497	5.3	63.8	25	6.1
Salted, M&S*	1 Pack/25g	132	7.8	530	9.4	50.4	31.1	6.4
Salted, Manhatten Peanuts Limited*	1 Bag/30g	135	4.3	450	10	70	14.3	13.7
Salted, Microwave, Popz*	1 Serving/20g	101	6	504	7	51.5	30	9.2
Salted, Microwave, Sunsnacks*	1 Pack/100g	498	22.9	498	10.7	51.3	22.9	10.8
Salted, Sea Salt, Skinny, Topcorn, Metcalfe's Food Co*	1 Pack/23g	108	5.6	471	6.6	63.7	24.4	15.2
Salted, Simply, Protein, Natural Nutrients*	1 Bag/30g	145	6.4	483	14.7	48.7	21.3	0
Salted, Sold At Cinema, Playtime Popcorn*	1 Sm/74g	384	24.9	519	8.3	45.9	33.6	0
Sesame, & Salt, Bloom's*	1 Pack/40g	200	11.5	501	4.8	48.6	28.8	14
Sour Cream & Onion, Creamy, Ranch Kern Pops, Graze*	1 Punnet/25g	139	7.3	554	5	56	29	12
Sour Cream Black Pepper, Propercorn*	1 Bag/20g	88	3.7	440	10.8	50.1	18.3	15.9
Super, Perri*	1 Pack/30g	139	7	464	8.4	55.5	23.2	8.5
Sweet & Salty, Microwave, Butterkist*	1 Pack/70g	298	14.1	425	8.2	48.5	20.2	8.4
Sweet & Salty, Propercorn*	1 Bag/30g	129	4.7	431	6.5	64.4	15.8	9.9
Sweet Salty, Bloom's*	1 Portion/28g	138	7	492	4	58.6	25	8.5
Sweet Salty, M&S*	1 Bag/15g	73	3.7	488	7.7	55.4	24.4	7.8
Sweet Salty, Shapers, Boots*	1 Bag/20g	89	3.2	443	5.8	65	16	10
Sweet Salty, Skinny Pop*	1 Pack/23g	98	3.4	424	7.2	66.7	14.8	8.9
Sweet Maple, Diet Chef Ltd*	1 Pack/23g	111	3.6	483	9.7	75.2	15.7	13
Sweet, Best-In*	1 Serving/34g	161	5.8	473	7.3	72.6	17	0
Sweet, Butterkist, Butterkist*	1 Pack/120g	612	29.8	510	2.8	68.5	24.8	5.6
Sweet, Cinema Style, Basics, Sainsbury's*	1 Handful/20g	90	4.4	450	5.9	57.5	21.8	11.1
Sweet, Cinema Style, Butterkist*	1 Bag/85g	447	22	526	5.2	65.2	25.9	5.8
Sweet, Coconut Vanilla, Propercorn*	1 Bag/25g	122	5.5	486	6	61.6	22.1	7.7
Sweet, Deli, Passions, Aldi*	1 Bag/27g	121	4.2	448	7	74.8	15.6	10.7
Sweet, Microwave, Butterkist*	1 Pack/70g	316	15.4	452	7	53	22	7.2
Sweet, Microwave, Cinema, Popz*	1 Bag/85g	420	21.7	494	6	60	25.5	8.2
Sweet, Slightly, Popping Corn, Graze*	1 Punnet/26g	116	5.4	447	7.5	53	21	9.3
Sweet, Vanilla & Sugar, Microwave, Act II*	1 Pack75g	369	18.1	492	7.9	60.8	24.1	10.4
Toffee, Butterkist*	1 Sm Bag/50g	212	4.7	424	3.1	80.1	9.4	3.2
Toffee, Chicago Joes*	1 Serving/10g	31	0.5	314	3.1	84.6	4.8	0
Toffee, Milk Chocolate Coated, Sainsbury's*	¼ Bag/25g	130	6.6	520	6.5	64.1	26.4	1.3
Toffee, Sainsbury's*	1 Serving/50g	208	6.4	415	1.8	73.8	12.7	3.3
Toffee, Snack Pack, Butterkist*	1 Bag/25g	106	2.4	424	3.1	80.1	9.4	3.2
Tomato, Sun Dried, Chilli, Propercorn*	1 Bag/20g	88	3.7	439	8.7	50.9	18.6	16.6
Twist of Black Pepper, Graze*	1 Punnet/28g	127	7	452	8	44	25	13
Vanilla, Cinema Sweet Microwave, Act II*	½ Pack/50g	234	8	468	9	71	16	12
Vanilla, Sweet, Protein, Natural Nutrients*	1 Pack/30g	156	7.9	522	15.7	49.5	26.5	9.7
Wasabi, Skinny, Topcorn, Metcalfe's Food Co*	1 Bag/25g	121	6.6	484	8.4	54.1	26.2	9.7
Wholegrain, Sweet Salty, Sunbites, Walkers*	1 Pack/30g	127	3.1	424	6.3	67.5	10.4	12.8
Yoghurt Coated, Butterkist*	1 Pack/20g	96	3.6	479	3.2	74.6	18.2	2.1

POPPADOMS

INFO/WEIGHT	Measure	per Measure		Nutrition Values per 100g / 100ml				
Cracked Black Pepper, Ready to Eat, Sharwood's*	1 Poppadom/9g	41	2.4	461	16.7	37.2	27.3	7.3
Fried in Vegetable Oil, Takeaway, Average	**1 Poppadom/13g**	**65**	**5**	**501**	**11.5**	**28.3**	**38.8**	**5.8**
Garlic Coriander, Ready To Eat, Pappadums, Patak's*	1 Poppadom/10g	45	2.3	453	18.5	37.1	23.4	9.9

POPPADOMS

INFO/WEIGHT	Measure	per Measure		Nutrition Values per 100g / 100ml				
		KCAL	FAT	KCAL	PROT	CARB	FAT	FIBRE
Garlic Coriander, Ready to Eat, Sharwood's*	1 Poppadom/9g	39	1.9	438	18.4	43	21.4	6.5
Indian, Asda*	1 Pack/45g	232	15.7	516	14.5	36.2	34.8	7.8
Mango Chutney Flavour, Mini, M&S*	1 Poppadom/25g	130	8.3	518	13.1	39.9	33	4.5
Mini, Sainsbury's*	½ Pack/50g	249	16.2	498	14.9	36.9	32.3	7.6
Plain, Asda*	1 Poppadom/9g	44	2.5	484	18	40	28	0
Plain, Bilash, Aldi*	1 Poppadom/8g	36	1.8	448	20	38	22	9.7
Plain, Cook to Eat, Sharwood's*	1 Poppadom/12g	32	0.1	273	21.9	45.7	1	10.1
Plain, Indian to Go, Sainsbury's*	1 Poppadom/8g	34	1.5	405	18.4	43.4	17.5	9
Plain, Mini, Cook to Eat, Sharwood's*	1 Poppadom/4g	11	0	273	21.9	45.7	0.3	10.1
Plain, Ready to Eat, Average	2 Poppadom/16g	68	2.8	427	19.8	46.6	17.3	6.6
Plain, Ready to Eat, Sharwood's*	1 Poppadom/8g	37	1.8	461	19.4	46.3	22	5.6
Plain, Tesco*	1 Serving/9g	41	2	439	17.8	44.4	21.1	4.6
Plain, Waitrose*	1 Serving/9g	37	1.7	408	21	39.3	18.6	9.1
Spicy, Cook to Eat, Sharwood's*	1 Poppadom/12g	30	0.1	257	20.2	43	0.5	13
Spicy, COU, M&S*	1 Pack/26g	84	0.6	325	23.5	51.9	2.4	8.1
Tesco*	1 Poppadom/9g	39	1.9	440	17.8	44.4	21.1	4.6

POPPETS*

INFO/WEIGHT	Measure	per Measure		Nutrition Values per 100g / 100ml				
Chocolate Raisins, Poppets*	1 Pack/35g	140	4.7	401	4.9	65.4	13.3	0
Mint Cream, Poppets*	1oz/28g	119	3.6	424	2	75	13	0
Peanut, Poppets*	1 Box/100g	544	37	544	16.4	37	37	0
Strawberry Milkshake, Payne's*	1 Box/40g	180	5.3	450	2	79.1	13.2	3.3
Toffee, Milk Chocolate, Poppets*	1 Box/100g	491	23	491	5.3	68	23	0

PORK

INFO/WEIGHT	Measure	per Measure		Nutrition Values per 100g / 100ml				
Belly, Fresh, Raw, Weighed with Skin, Average	1 Serving/100g	518	53	518	9.3	0	53	0
Belly, Roasted, Lean Fat	1oz/28g	82	6	293	25.1	0	21.4	0
Bites, Smoky BBQ, Fridge Raiders, Mattessons*	1 Pack/80g	196	13.6	245	17	5.7	17	0
Chilli, Thai, with Rice, The City Kitchen*	1 Pack/337g	706	36	210	8.9	18.8	10.7	1.3
Chitterlings, Raw, Average	1 Serving/100g	182	16.6	182	7.6	0	16.6	0
Chop, Lean Fat, Boneless, Raw, Average	1oz/28g	67	3.8	240	29.2	0	13.7	0
Chopped, Canned, Pek*	1 Can/240g	497	37.2	207	16.9	0.1	15.5	0
Diced, Lean, Average	1oz/28g	31	0.5	109	22	0	1.8	0
Escalope, Average	1 Escalope/75g	108	1.7	144	31	0	2.2	0
Escalope, Lean, Healthy Range, Average	1 Escalope/75g	80	1.5	106	22	0	2	0
Ham, Hock, Raw, Weighed with Bone, Fat & Skin	100g	124	5	124	18.4	0	5	0
Joint with Crackling, Ready to Roast, Average	1 Joint/567g	1283	80.1	226	24.2	0.8	14.1	0
Joint, Ready to Roast, Average	½ Joint/254g	375	18	148	19.2	2.3	7.1	0.2
Leg, Joint, Healthy Range, Average	1 Serving/200g	206	4.4	103	20	0.6	2.2	0
Loin, Applewood Smoked, Asda*	1 Slice/15g	18	0.5	122	21.8	0.5	3.6	0
Loin, Chops, Boneless, Grilled, Average	1oz/28g	83	4.1	298	27	0	14.6	0
Loin, Chops, Grilled, Lean	1oz/28g	52	1.8	184	31.6	0	6.4	0
Loin, Chops, Raw, Lean Fat, Weighed with Bone	1 Chop/130g	248	19.9	191	13.2	0	15.3	0
Loin, Joint, Mini, with Sage Onion Stuffing, Waitrose*	½ Pack/200g	510	34.8	255	21.6	3	17.4	0.1
Loin, Joint, Roast, Lean	1oz/28g	51	1.9	182	30.1	0	6.8	0
Loin, Joint, Roasted, Lean & Fat	1oz/28g	71	4.3	253	26.3	0	15.3	0
Loin, Roasted, Slices, M&S*	½ Pack/50g	72	2.6	144	22.9	1.3	5.2	0.5
Loin, Steak, Fried, Lean	1oz/28g	53	2	191	31.5	0	7.2	0
Loin, Steak, Fried, Lean & Fat	1oz/28g	77	5.2	276	27.5	0	18.4	0
Loin, Steak, Lean, Raw, Average	1 Serving/175g	345	19.6	197	22.7	0	11.2	0.4
Loin, Steaks, Mediterranean, Grilled, Ashfield Farm, Aldi*	1 Steak/100g	288	17	288	30	3.4	17	0.5
Loin, Stuffed, Roast, M&S*	1 Slice/12g	22	0.9	180	24.4	2.4	7.9	0
Loin, with Rind, Uncooked, Average	1 Serving/100g	246	18.8	246	19.3	0	18.8	0
Medallions, Average	1 Medallion/125g	140	2.6	112	22.6	0	2	0
Mince, Lean, Healthy Range, Average	1 Pack/400g	504	20.2	126	19.8	0.4	5	0.3

P

PORK

INFO/WEIGHT	Measure	per Measure KCAL	FAT	Nutrition Values per 100g / 100ml KCAL	PROT	CARB	FAT	FIBRE
Mince, Raw	*1oz/28g*	*46*	*2.7*	*164*	*19.2*	*0*	*9.7*	*0*
Mince, Stewed	*1oz/28g*	*53*	*2.9*	*191*	*24.4*	*0*	*10.4*	*0*
Pulled, with BBQ Beans, Musclefood*	1 Serving/395g	486	20.5	123	14.5	3	5.2	3.2
Pulled, with BBQ Sauce, Boneless, British, Tesco*	1 Serving/150g	256	11.2	171	17.3	8.5	7.5	0
Pulled, with BBQ Sauce, Shoulder, British, Sainsbury's*	1 Serving/120g	290	18.1	242	24.6	1.6	15.1	0.5
Raw, Lean, Average	*1oz/28g*	*42*	*1.2*	*151*	*28.6*	*0*	*4.1*	*0*
Roast, Lean Only, Average	*1oz/28g*	*34*	*0.9*	*121*	*22.7*	*0.3*	*3.3*	*0*
Roast, Slices, Average	*1 Slice/30g*	*40*	*1.4*	*134*	*22.7*	*0.4*	*4.5*	*0*
Shoulder, Boneless, Average	*1 Piece/430g*	*127*	*3.4*	*127*	*22.5*	*0*	*3.4*	*0*
Shoulder, Slices, Cured	*1oz/28g*	*29*	*1*	*103*	*16.9*	*0.9*	*3.6*	*0*
Shoulder, Steak, Boneless, Frozen, Grilled, Tesco*	1 Steak/125g	156	4.9	125	0	0	3.9	0
Shoulder, Whole, Lean Fat, Raw, Average	*100g*	*236*	*18*	*236*	*17.2*	*0*	*18*	*0*
Shoulder, Whole, Lean Only, Roasted	*1 Serving/150g*	*345*	*20.3*	*230*	*25.3*	*0*	*13.5*	*0*
Steak, Lean & Fat, Average	*1oz/28g*	*61*	*3.8*	*219*	*23.8*	*0*	*13.7*	*0.1*
Steak, Lean, Stewed	*1oz/28g*	*49*	*1.3*	*176*	*33.6*	*0*	*4.6*	*0*
Steak, Loin, BBQ Chinese, Tesco*	1 Steak/81g	219	14.4	270	21.9	5.3	17.7	1.1
Steak, Loin, Thick Cut, Finest, Tesco*	1 Steak/200g	450	32.3	224	19.9	0	16.1	0
Stir Fry Strips, Lean, Healthy Range, Average	*¼ Pack/113g*	*118*	*2.3*	*104*	*21.3*	*0*	*2*	*0*
Tenderloin, Lean, Boneless, Raw, Average	*1 Serving/100g*	*109*	*2.2*	*109*	*21*	*0*	*2.2*	*0*

PORK DINNER

	Measure	KCAL	FAT	KCAL	PROT	CARB	FAT	FIBRE
Roast, 103, Oakhouse Foods Ltd*	1 Dinner/400g	376	14.8	94	6.7	8.3	3.7	1.4
Roast, Birds Eye*	1 Pack/340g	410	12	121	7.6	14.7	3.5	1.6

PORK IN

	Measure	KCAL	FAT	KCAL	PROT	CARB	FAT	FIBRE
Gravy, & Baby Potatoes, Carrots, & Savoy Cabbage, M&S*	1 Pack395g	288	9.9	73	6.2	5.7	2.5	1.6
Mustard & Cream, Chops	*1oz/28g*	*73*	*6*	*261*	*14.5*	*2.4*	*21.6*	*0.3*

PORK SCRATCHINGS

	Measure	KCAL	FAT	KCAL	PROT	CARB	FAT	FIBRE
Crunch, Mr Porky*	1 Pack/25g	129	6.9	515	65.7	0.6	27.7	0
KP Snacks*	1 Pack/20g	125	9.6	624	47.3	0.5	48.1	0.5
Pn, Proteinium*	1 Bag/30g	156	7.9	520	69.7	0.1	26.2	0

PORT

	Measure	KCAL	FAT	KCAL	PROT	CARB	FAT	FIBRE
Average	*1 Serving/50ml*	*78*	*0*	*157*	*0.1*	*12*	*0*	*0*
White, Average	*1 Glass/125ml*	*182*	*0*	*146*	*0.1*	*11*	*0*	*0*

POT NOODLE*

	Measure	KCAL	FAT	KCAL	PROT	CARB	FAT	FIBRE
Beef Tomato, King, Made Up, Pot Noodle*	1 Pot/420g	543	19.8	129	3.3	18.5	4.7	1.1
Beef Tomato, Made Up, Pot Noodle*	1 Pot/320g	426	14.7	133	3.4	19.4	4.6	1.3
Beef Tomato, Mini, Made Up, Pot Noodle*	1 Pot/190g	254	9.5	134	3.5	18.7	5	1.7
Bombay Bad Boy, King, Made Up , Pot Noodle*	1 Pot/420g	542	19.7	129	3.3	18.5	4.7	1.1
Bombay Bad Boy, Made Up, Pot Noodle*	1 Pot/320g	415	15.3	130	3.3	18.4	4.8	1.1
Chicken Mushroom, King, Made Up, Pot Noodle*	1 Pack/420g	545	19.3	130	3.3	18.8	4.6	1
Chicken Mushroom, Made Up, Pot Noodle*	1 Pot/305g	430	18	141	3	19	5.9	1
Chicken, Roast, in a Mug, Made Up, Pot Noodle*	1 Mug/227g	141	1.8	62	2.1	11.5	0.8	0.4
Chilli Beef, Made Up, Pot Noodle*	1 Pot/305g	384	14.6	126	3	17.7	4.8	0.8
Chow Mein Chinese, Made Up, Pot Noodle*	1 Pot/320g	416	14.7	130	3.2	19	4.6	1.3
Curry, Balti, Made Up, Pot Noodle*	1 Pot/301g	268	1.5	89	3.1	17.8	0.5	0.5
Curry, Chicken, Hot, Made Up, Pot Noodle*	1 Pot/300g	384	14.1	128	2.8	18.7	4.7	1.1
Curry, Original, King, Made Up, Pot Noodle*	1 Pot/420g	507	18.1	121	2.6	17.9	4.3	1
Curry, Original, Made Up, Pot Noodle*	1 Pot/320g	431	15	135	3.1	20	4.7	1.2
Curry, Spicy, Made Up, Pot Noodle*	1 Pot/300g	393	14.4	131	2.9	19.1	4.8	1.1
Jamaican Jerk, Made Up, Pot Noodle*	1 Pot/310g	430	15.4	140	3	21	5	1.5
Piri Piri Chicken, Made Up, Pot Noodle*	1 Pot/307g	430	15.4	140	3	20	5	0
Sweet Sour, Oriental, Posh, Made Up, Pot Noodle*	1 Pot/300g	375	13.8	125	1.7	19.2	4.6	0.5

POTATO BOMBAY

	Measure	KCAL	FAT	KCAL	PROT	CARB	FAT	FIBRE
Average	*½ Pack/150g*	*176*	*10.2*	*117*	*2*	*13.7*	*6.8*	*1.2*

	Measure INFO/WEIGHT	per Measure KCAL	FAT	Nutrition Values per 100g / 100ml KCAL	PROT	CARB	FAT	FIBRE
POTATO BOMBAY								
Indian, Cooked, Sainsbury's*	½ Pack/150g	132	7.4	95	1.6	7.8	5.3	4.9
Indian, Waitrose*	½ Pack/150g	125	5.4	83	1.6	9.7	3.6	3
Tesco*	1 Pack/300g	240	12.6	80	1.3	9.3	4.2	2.1
POTATO CAKES								
Average	*1 Cake/70g*	*127*	*1.2*	*180*	*3.8*	*37.5*	*1.7*	*2.4*
Fried, Average	*1oz/28g*	*66*	*2.5*	*237*	*4.9*	*35*	*9*	*0.8*
POTATO SALAD								
& Egg, with Mayonnaise, Tesco*	½ Tub/150g	115	8.5	77	2.9	3.1	5.7	1.2
Yoghurt, Meadow Fresh, Lidl*	1 Portion/50g	72	4	144	1.8	15.4	8	1.8
Asda*	¼ Pot/57g	67	4	117	0.9	12.5	7	1.1
Baby, Finest, Tesco*	¼ Pack/69g	143	11.8	206	1.4	11.3	17	0.7
Charlotte, Yoghurt Dressed, Waitrose*	1 Serving/90g	191	15.5	212	1.6	11.7	17.2	1.8
Creamy, Asda*	½ Tub/150g	226	16	151	1.1	11.3	10.7	2.5
Creamy, Waitrose*	1 Serving/100g	163	11.9	163	1.3	12.7	11.9	1.1
From Restaurant, Average	*1/3 Cup/95g*	*108*	*5.7*	*114*	*1.5*	*13.5*	*6*	*0*
HL, Tesco*	1 Tub/250g	288	12	115	1.7	15.4	4.8	1.2
M&S*	1oz/28g	55	4.8	195	1.2	8.5	17.3	1.3
New, Free Range Egg, Side, Sainsbury's*	1 Pack/290g	174	12.2	60	2.5	3.1	4.2	1.4
New, Co-Op*	1 Serving/50g	98	8	195	1	10	16	2
Reduced Calorie, Pre Packed	*1oz/28g*	*27*	*1.1*	*97*	*1.3*	*14.8*	*4.1*	*0.8*
Tesco*	1 Serving/50g	90	7.1	179	1	11.1	14.2	1.3
with Mayonnaise, Retail	*1oz/28g*	*80*	*7.4*	*287*	*1.5*	*11.4*	*26.5*	*0.8*
with Onions Chives, Co-Op*	1 Serving/50g	80	6	160	1	12	12	1
POTATO SKINS								
American Style, Loaded, Asda*	1 Serving/78g	294	18	375	15	27	23	2.4
¼ Cut, Deep Fried, McCain*	1oz/28g	52	1.7	186	3	30.1	6	0
Cheese & Bacon, Loaded, Asda*	½ Pack/125g	275	15	220	13	15	12	3.3
Cheese Bacon, Loaded, Tesco*	1 Skin/59g	133	7.5	226	9.3	17.3	12.7	2.4
Cheese Chive, Sainsbury's*	2 Skins/150g	286	17.8	191	7.7	13.3	11.9	2.8
Cheese Ham, Iceland*	2 Skins/108g	155	4.9	143	6.3	19.3	4.5	2
Cheese Onion, Loaded, Tesco*	1 Skin/60g	114	6.5	190	5.8	17.6	10.8	1.4
with Sour Cream	*1 Serving/275g*	*541*	*34.6*	*197*	*7.2*	*13.8*	*12.6*	*2.2*
POTATO WAFFLES								
Frozen, Cooked	*1oz/28g*	*56*	*2.3*	*200*	*3.2*	*30.3*	*8.2*	*2.3*
Uncooked, Average	*1 Waffle/62g*	*113*	*5.1*	*182*	*2.4*	*24.4*	*8.3*	*1.8*
POTATO WEDGES								
Aldi*	1 Serving/100g	150	6.8	150	2.1	20.2	6.8	0
Crispy, M&S*	1 Serving/200g	340	14.2	170	1.3	25.3	7.1	1.7
Frozen, Average	*1 Serving/120g*	*145*	*4.1*	*121*	*2*	*20.5*	*3.4*	*2.2*
Garlic & Herb, COU, M&S*	1 Pack/300g	300	7.8	100	2.3	16.4	2.6	3.2
Harvest Basket, Lidl*	1 Serving/100g	147	5.7	147	2.2	20.5	5.7	0
Smoky Paprika, Ridged, Frozen, Mccain *	1 Serving/100g	156	6.2	156	2.4	21.1	6.2	2.8
Spicy, Asda*	1 Serving/100g	145	5.7	145	1.8	21.8	5.7	2.1
with Cheese, Bacon, Tesco*	½ Pack/188g	305	12.8	162	5.6	18.5	6.8	2.3
POTATOES								
Alphabites, Captain Birds Eye, Birds Eye*	9 Bites/56g	75	3	134	2	19.5	5.3	1.4
Anya, Raw, TTD, Sainsbury's*	1 Serving/100g	75	0.3	75	1.5	17.8	0.3	1.1
Baby, Herby, Microwave, Nature's Pick, Aldi*	½ Pack/193g	171	3.5	89	2.2	15	1.8	2.2
Baby, Herby, Microwaved, Growers Selection, Asda*	1 Pack/360g	198	4.7	55	2	7.4	1.3	2.8
Baby, New with Butter, Mint Parsley, Organic, Asda*	1 Pack/360g	414	10.4	115	1.7	20.4	2.9	2.5
Baby, New, Ocado*	¼ Bag/188g	141	0.6	75	1.7	16.1	0.3	1.3
Baby, Pearl, As Sold, Waitrose*	½ Pack/100g	79	0.3	79	1.7	16.1	0.3	2.4
Baby, with Butter & Herbs, Sainsbury's*	¼ Pack/148g	103	0.9	70	1.9	14.2	0.6	2

P

POTATOES

	Measure INFO/WEIGHT	per Measure KCAL	FAT	Nutrition Values per 100g / 100ml KCAL	PROT	CARB	FAT	FIBRE
Baby, with Herbs & Butter, Morrisons*	1 Serving/100g	94	2.3	94	1.9	14.6	2.3	1.9
Baked, & Cheese, Waitrose*	½ Pack/220g	281	8.6	128	3.7	18.1	3.9	2.6
Baked, Chilli Con Carne, COU, M&S*	1 Pack/300g	270	6.3	90	6	11.1	2.1	1.2
Baked, Flesh Skin, Average	*1 Med/200g*	*218*	*0.2*	*109*	*2.3*	*25.2*	*0.1*	*2.4*
Baked, Flesh Only, Weighed with Skin, Average	*1oz/28g*	*20*	*0*	*72*	*1.5*	*16.6*	*0.1*	*1.2*
Baked, Frozen, Lidl*	1 Potato/200g	184	0.8	92	2.3	18	0.4	3.4
Baked, Ham & Cheddar Cheese, Asda*	1 Pack/300g	435	11.1	145	7	21	3.7	1.6
Baked, in Microwave, Flesh & Skin, Average	*1oz/28g*	*29*	*0*	*105*	*2.4*	*24.1*	*0.1*	*2.3*
Baked, in Microwave, Flesh Only, Average	*1oz/28g*	*28*	*0*	*100*	*2.1*	*23.3*	*0.1*	*1.6*
Baked, in Microwave, Skin Only, Average	*1oz/28g*	*37*	*0*	*132*	*4.4*	*29.6*	*0.1*	*5.5*
Baked, Jacket, Naked, Bannisters*	1 Potato/151g	119	0.8	79	1.8	15.8	0.5	2.1
Baked, Mature Cheddar Cheese, M&S*	½ Pack/206g	225	6.6	109	3.6	16.9	3.2	1
Baked, Skin Only, Average	*1oz/28g*	*55*	*0*	*198*	*4.3*	*46.1*	*0.1*	*7.9*
Baked, Stuffed, Mini, Tesco*	1 Serving/108g	130	6.3	120	2.3	14.6	5.8	2.3
Baked, Tuna & Sweetcorn, Average	*1 Serving/300g*	*273*	*6.8*	*91*	*5*	*12.6*	*2.2*	*0.9*
Baked, Tuna & Sweetcorn, BGTY, Sainsbury's*	1 Pack/350g	360	9.4	103	6.5	13.2	2.7	1.3
Baked, Tuna & Sweetcorn, Morrisons*	1 Serving/300g	243	2.1	81	5.1	13.5	0.7	0
Baked, with Cheese & Bacon, Finest, Tesco*	1 Potato/245g	360	19.6	147	6	12.6	8	2.5
Baked, with Cheese & Butter, Tesco*	1 Potato/214g	212	4.2	99	3	16.4	2	1.9
Baking, Raw, Average	*1 Med/250g*	*198*	*0.2*	*79*	*2.1*	*18*	*0.1*	*1.6*
Boiled with Skin	*1 Potato/125g*	*98*	*0.1*	*78*	*2.9*	*17.2*	*0.1*	*3.3*
Boiled, Average	*1 Serving/120g*	*86*	*0.1*	*72*	*1.8*	*17*	*0.1*	*1.2*
Boulangere, M&S*	½ Pack/225g	180	2	80	2.8	15.9	0.9	0.9
Charlotte, Average	*1 Serving/184g*	*139*	*0.5*	*76*	*1.6*	*17.4*	*0.2*	*3.3*
Chorizo, Roast, Tesco*	¼ Pack/125g	189	9	151	4.8	16.4	7.2	1
Crispy Slices, M&S*	1 Pack/450g	922	53.1	205	2.5	21.5	11.8	1.4
Crispy, Pops, HFC, Tesco*	¼ Pack/111g	215	8.2	194	2.8	27.8	7.4	2.2
Crunchies, Oven, Ross*	1 Serving/100g	240	11.7	240	3.6	30	11.7	2.4
Dauphinoise, Average	*1 Serving/200g*	*335*	*23.9*	*168*	*2.2*	*12.8*	*12*	*1.5*
Dauphinoise, Cook*	1 Pack /225g	320	18.7	142	5.3	11	8.3	1.8
Dauphinoise, Creamy, Oven Baked, Extra Special, Asda*	½ Pack/167g	162	8.9	97	2.7	9	5.3	1.2
Dauphinoise, Finest, Tesco*	½ Pack/186g	299	18.6	161	2.9	13.9	10	1.5
Dauphinoise, Rich Creamy, TTD, Sainsbury's*	½ Pack/200g	189	10	104	3.2	9.5	5.5	2.2
Desiree, Average	*1 Serving/200g*	*152*	*0.4*	*76*	*2.2*	*16.4*	*0.2*	*0.6*
Fritters, Crispy, Oven Baked, Birds Eye*	1 Fritter/20g	29	1.6	145	2	16.3	8	1.2
Hasselback, Average	*1 Serving/175g*	*182*	*1.6*	*104*	*1.9*	*22*	*0.9*	*2.9*
Hassleback, Dine in Side, Eat Well, M&S*	½ Pack/175g	195	6	110	2.1	18.3	3.4	1.9
Jacket, Ready Baked, Frozen, McCain*	1 Potato/213g	202	1.1	95	1.7	20.9	0.5	1.4
Jersey Royal, Canned, Average	*1 Can/186g*	*116*	*0.2*	*62*	*1.4*	*14*	*0.1*	*1.2*
Jersey Royal, New, Raw, Average	*1oz/28g*	*21*	*0.1*	*75*	*1.6*	*17.2*	*0.2*	*1.5*
Lattices, Tesco*	¼ Pack/103g	221	8.4	215	3	29.8	8.2	5.2
Maris Piper, Mashed, Eat Fresh, Tesco*	½ Pack/213g	191	4	90	1.9	14.7	1.9	1.6
Maris Piper, Raw, Average	*1 Serving/200g*	*151*	*0.4*	*75*	*2*	*16.5*	*0.2*	*1.4*
Mashed, Buttery, Seasoned, Classic Cuisine, Aldi*	½ Pack/225g	207	8.6	92	1.6	12	3.8	1.3
Mashed, Cheddar, TTD, Sainsbury's*	½ Pack/226g	323	19.7	143	3.8	11.5	8.7	1.9
Mashed, Dry, Tesco*	1 Serving/70g	225	0.1	321	7.7	72	0.2	7.1
Mashed, Fresh, Tesco*	1 Pack/500g	395	8	79	2.3	13.1	1.6	1.9
Mashed, From Restaurant, Average	*1/3 Cup/80g*	*66*	*1*	*83*	*2.3*	*16.1*	*1.2*	*0*
Mashed, From Supermarket, Average	*½ Pack/200g*	*197*	*8.1*	*98*	*1.8*	*13.3*	*4.1*	*1.5*
Mashed, From Supermarket, Healthy Range, Average	*1 Serving/200g*	*160*	*3.1*	*80*	*1.8*	*14.6*	*1.6*	*1.3*
Mashed, From Supermarket, Premium, Average	*1 Serving/225g*	*305*	*17.8*	*136*	*1.7*	*14.4*	*7.9*	*1.1*
Mashed, Home Prepared with Whole Milk	*1 Cup/210g*	*162*	*1.2*	*77*	*1.9*	*17.6*	*0.6*	*2*
Mashed, Jersey Butter & Black Pepper, TTD, Sainsbury's*	½ Pack/225g	243	13.7	108	1.4	11.2	6.1	1.5

	Measure INFO/WEIGHT	per Measure KCAL	FAT	Nutrition Values per 100g / 100ml KCAL	PROT	CARB	FAT	FIBRE
POTATOES								
Mashed, Made Up with Water, Average	*1 Serving/180g*	*118*	*0.3*	*66*	*1.7*	*14.5*	*0.2*	*1.3*
Mashed, Mash Direct*	½ Pack/200g	190	3.8	95	1.7	17.7	1.9	1.3
Mashed, Original, Dry Weight, Smash*	1 Serving/30g	101	0.3	343	8.3	71.8	1	6.7
Mashed, with Cream Butter, Ultimate, M&S*	½ Pack/225g	268	13.7	119	2.5	12.8	6.1	1.2
New, Average	*1 Serving/100g*	*75*	*0.3*	*75*	*1.5*	*17.8*	*0.3*	*1.1*
New, Baby, Average	*1 Serving/180g*	*135*	*0.5*	*75*	*1.7*	*17*	*0.3*	*1.6*
New, Baby, Canned, Average	*1 Can/120g*	*69*	*0.2*	*58*	*1.4*	*12.9*	*0.2*	*1.4*
New, Canned, in Water, Drained, Hob Heated, Asda*	1 Serving/108g	69	0.5	64	1.1	14	0.5	1.5
New, Easy Steam with Herbs Butter, Tesco*	1 Serving/125g	94	3.5	75	1.8	9.6	2.8	1.7
New, Garlic, Herb & Parsley Butter, Co-Op*	1 Serving/100g	115	5	115	1	15	5	2
New, with Herbs & Butter, Asda*	½ Pack/170g	146	2.9	86	1.7	16	1.7	1.5
Pan Fried, Aldi*	1 Serving/250g	182	2	73	2.7	13.7	0.8	0
Raw, Peeled, Flesh Only	*1 Serving/100g*	*75*	*0.2*	*75*	*2*	*17.3*	*0.2*	*1.4*
Red, Flesh Only, Average	*1 Serving/300g*	*218*	*0.4*	*72*	*2*	*16.4*	*0.2*	*1.2*
Roast, Basted in Beef Dripping, Waitrose*	1 Serving/165g	213	8.9	129	2.2	18	5.4	1.9
Roast, Dry, No Oil, No fat	*1 Serving/100g*	*79*	*0.1*	*79*	*2.7*	*18*	*0.1*	*1.6*
Roast, Extra Crispy, Oven Baked, Aunt Bessie's*	1 Serving/100g	223	11.8	223	2.9	26.1	11.8	3.6
Roast, Frozen, As Consumed, Harvest Basket, Lidl*	1 Serving/165g	190	4	115	2.4	20	2.4	2
Roast, Frozen, Average	*1 Potato/70g*	*105*	*3.5*	*149*	*2.6*	*23.5*	*5*	*1.4*
Roast, Frozen, Healthy Range, Average	*1 Potato/70g*	*70*	*1.7*	*100*	*2.6*	*18.2*	*2.4*	*2.1*
Roast, Garlic Rosemary, Miniature, Tesco*	¼ Pack/125g	85	0.9	68	1.8	12.5	0.7	2.3
Roast, in Lard, Average	*1oz/28g*	*42*	*1.3*	*149*	*2.9*	*25.9*	*4.5*	*1.8*
Roast, in Oil, Average	*1oz/28g*	*42*	*1.3*	*149*	*2.9*	*25.9*	*4.5*	*1.8*
Roast, New, Rosemary, Ainsley Harriott*	1 Serving/150g	133	4	89	2	16	2.7	1.3
Roast, Roasties, Mini, Midweek, as Sold, Aunt Bessie's*	1 Serving/100g	129	2.7	129	2.1	23	2.7	2
Roast, Scrumptiously Crispy & Fluffy, Frozen, McCain*	1 Serving/200g	446	28.6	223	1.8	20.7	14.3	2
Roast, with Goose Fat, TTD, Sainsbury's*	½ Pack/185g	216	4.4	117	2.7	21.1	2.4	3
Roasting, Average	*1 Serving/150g*	*202*	*5.2*	*135*	*2.5*	*23.4*	*3.5*	*1.6*
Saute, Oven Baked, McCain*	1oz/28g	56	1.1	199	4.4	36.9	3.8	0
Saute, with Onion & Bacon, Country Supper, Waitrose*	¼ Pack/100g	112	4.3	112	1.9	16.4	4.3	1.3
Scallops, Battered, Deep Fried, Average	*1 Scallop/67g*	*216*	*14.5*	*323*	*5.4*	*27.3*	*21.6*	*0*
Slices, in Rich Crispy Batter, Crispy, Chilled, Sainsbury's*	¼ Pack/100g	223	10.8	223	2.6	27.3	10.8	2.8
Smiles, Weighed Baked, McCain*	1 Serving/100g	237	10.1	237	3.4	33.4	10.1	3.1
Smiles, Weighed Frozen, McCain*	1 Serving/100g	191	8	191	2.6	27	8	2.7
Vivaldi, Baked with Skin, TTD, Sainsbury's*	1 Potato/180g	248	0.4	138	3.8	28.8	0.2	2.7
White, Raw, Flesh Skin	*1 Lge/369g*	*284*	*0.3*	*77*	*2*	*17.5*	*0.1*	*2.2*
White, Raw, Weighed with Skin, Flesh Only, Average	*1 Med/213g*	*153*	*0.3*	*72*	*1.9*	*16.1*	*0.2*	*1.2*
POUSSIN								
Meat & Skin, Raw, Average	*1oz/28g*	*57*	*3.9*	*202*	*19.1*	*0*	*13.9*	*0*
Spatchcock, British, Waitrose*	½ Poussin/225g	364	20.2	162	19	1.2	9	0
POWERADE								
Berry & Tropical Fruit, Coca-Cola*	1 Bottle/500ml	90	0	18	0	4.1	0	0
Isotonic, Sports Drink, Coca-Cola*	1 Bottle/500ml	120	0	24	0	5.6	0	0
Zero, Coca-Cola*	1 Bottle/500ml	5	0	1	0	0	0	0
PRAWN COCKTAIL								
BGTY, Sainsbury's*	½ Pot/85g	119	7.9	140	9.1	4.7	9.3	0.5
Delicious, Boots*	1 Pack/250g	285	6.5	114	5.5	17	2.6	1.2
in Marie Rose Sauce, Rich Creamy, Waitrose*	½ Pot/100g	338	32.2	338	9.1	2.7	32.2	0.5
LC, Tesco*	1 Pot/140g	210	16	150	7.5	4.3	11.4	1.3
Reduced Fat, M&S*	1 Pack/200g	296	20	148	9.9	4.5	10	0.5
PRAWN CRACKERS								
Asda*	1 Serving/25g	134	8.8	535	2	53	35	0
M&S*	1 Bag/50g	262	15.6	525	2.8	57.4	31.3	0.8

	Measure INFO/WEIGHT	per Measure KCAL	FAT	Nutrition Values per 100g / 100ml KCAL	PROT	CARB	FAT	FIBRE
PRAWN CRACKERS								
Meal for Two, Meal Box, Tesco*	½ Pack/23g	127	8	554	2	57.3	35	1.1
Ready to Eat, Sharwood's*	1 Bag/60g	316	18.5	527	0.5	62	30.8	1.2
Sainsbury's*	1 Cracker/3g	16	1	537	2.4	60.4	31.7	0.8
PRAWN TOAST								
from Chinese Selection, Ken Hom, Tesco*	1 Toast/14g	50	3.8	364	11	17.1	27.4	2.6
Mini, Oriental Selection, Party, Iceland*	1 Toast/15g	52	3.6	345	10.5	22	23.9	2.1
Oriental Selection, Sainsbury's*	1 Toast/31g	119	9.1	385	10.1	18.8	29.5	2.1
Sesame Prawn, Toasted Triangles, M&S*	1 Pack/220g	616	39.6	280	12.4	17.3	18	2
Sesame, Oriental Snack Selection, Sainsbury's*	1 Toast/12g	40	2.7	335	9.3	23	22.9	5.1
PRAWNS								
Batter Crisp, Lyons*	1 Pack/160g	350	20.3	219	8	18.2	12.7	1.1
Boiled	**1 Prawn/3g**	**3**	**0**	**99**	**22.6**	**0**	**0.9**	**0**
Cooked & Peeled, Average	**1oz/28g**	**21**	**0.2**	**77**	**17.6**	**0.2**	**0.6**	**0**
Hot & Spicy, Average	**1 Serving/170g**	**461**	**26.9**	**271**	**9.4**	**22.8**	**15.8**	**2.2**
Icelandic, Raw, Average	**1oz/28g**	**30**	**0.4**	**106**	**22.7**	**0**	**1.6**	**0**
King, & Scallops, Lemon & Pink Peppercorn Butter, Youngs	½ Pack/81g	155	10.5	191	17.9	0.6	12.9	0.8
King, Breaded	**1 Prawn/13g**	**33**	**1.8**	**260**	**15.1**	**17.8**	**14**	**1.2**
King, Garlic Marinated, Specially Selected, Aldi*	½ Pack/95g	114	2.8	120	21	1.6	3	0.5
King, Raw, Average	**1 Bag/200g**	**145**	**1.9**	**72**	**15.8**	**0.2**	**1**	**0.1**
King, Tandoori, Average	**1 Prawn/59g**	**33**	**0.6**	**55**	**5.7**	**5.9**	**1.1**	**0.7**
King, with Lemon, Garlic, Parsley, Waitrose*	½ Pack/75g	70	2	93	16.9	0.4	2.6	0.1
North Atlantic, Peeled, Cooked, Average	**1oz/28g**	**22**	**0.3**	**80**	**17.5**	**0**	**1.1**	**0**
North Atlantic, Raw, Average	**1oz/28g**	**17**	**0.1**	**62**	**14.4**	**0**	**0.4**	**0**
Tiger, Cooked & Peeled, Average	**1 Pack/180g**	**151**	**2**	**84**	**18.4**	**0.1**	**1.1**	**0**
Tiger, Jumbo, Average	**1 Serving/50g**	**39**	**0.2**	**78**	**18.2**	**0.3**	**0.5**	**0**
Tiger, Raw, Average	**1 Prawn/30g**	**19**	**0.2**	**64**	**14.2**	**0**	**0.7**	**0**
PRAWNS CHILLI								
& Coriander, Cooked & Peeled, Tesco*	1 Pack/160g	144	3.4	90	16.7	0.2	2.1	0.5
Crispy, with Sweet Chilli Dipping Sauce, M&S*	1 Pack/240g	490	20.2	204	8.2	23.6	8.4	0.6
King, Chilli Coriander, Marinated, Just Add, M&S*	1 Pack/80g	82	2.1	102	19	0.1	2.6	0
King, with a Sweet Chilli Sauce, Succulent, Birds Eye*	1 Serving/140g	251	17.2	179	10.5	6.5	12.3	0.1
Skewers, Sweet Chilli, King, BBQ Favourites, Asda*	1 Skewer/48g	48	0.5	100	16.6	5.4	1.1	1
PRAWNS IN								
Creamy Garlic Sauce, Youngs*	1 Serving/158g	261	22.9	165	8.5	0.3	14.5	0
PRAWNS WITH								
Chilli, Coriander Lime, King, Waitrose*	1 Pack/140g	143	3.2	102	19.9	0.5	2.3	0.6
Ginger & Spring Onion, Sainsbury's*	1 Pack/300g	198	9.3	66	4.7	4.7	3.1	0.3
King, with a Creamy Cocktail Sauce, M&S*	1 Pack/120g	278	23.3	232	12.6	1.3	19.4	1.1
King, with Garlic Butter, M&S*	1 Serving/100g	165	9	165	12.5	9.1	9	0.5
PRESERVE								
Ginger Shred, Robertsons*	1 Tsp/15g	40	0	267	0.1	66	0	0
Ginger, Asda*	1 Serving/15g	39	0.1	261	0.5	63	0.5	1.7
Ginger, Stem, Extra Fruity, Waitrose*	1 Tbsp/15g	39	0.1	258	2.5	60.4	0.6	0.3
Greengage, Extra Fruity, Waitrose*	1 Serving/15g	36	0.1	243	0.2	59.2	0.4	0.8
Rhubarb Ginger, Mackays Ltd*	1 Serving/10g	27	0	269	0.3	66.7	0	0
PRETZELS								
American Style, Salted, Sainsbury's*	1 Serving/50g	202	2.2	403	10.8	79.7	4.5	1.8
Cheddar Cheese, Penn State Pretzels*	1 Sm Bag/30g	124	2.8	412	10	71.6	9.3	3.8
Jumbo, Tesco*	1 Serving/50g	194	3.4	388	9.7	71.9	6.8	5.4
Mini, M&S*	1 Pack/45g	194	6	430	10.4	66.6	13.4	4.9
Plain, Bakery, Tesco*	1 Pretzel/108g	316	5.8	293	9.5	50.3	5.4	2.7
Salted, Average	**1 Serving/30g**	**114**	**0.8**	**380**	**10.3**	**79.8**	**2.6**	**3**
Salted, Mini, M&S*	1 Pack/25g	96	0.5	382	10.9	78	2.1	3.9

	Measure INFO/WEIGHT	per Measure KCAL	FAT	Nutrition Values per 100g / 100ml KCAL	PROT	CARB	FAT	FIBRE
PRETZELS								
Salted, Sainsbury's*	1 Serving/30g	118	1.3	393	10.3	76.7	4.2	3.6
Snacks, Fabulous Bakin' Boys*	1 Pack/24g	96	1.2	401	9	79.5	4.9	2.5
Soft, Cheddar Red Onion, Knot, New York Bakery Co*	1 Pretzel/59g	168	2.5	284	11.8	46.7	4.3	5.3
Soft, Cinnamon Sugar, Auntie Anne's*	1 Pretzel/112g	380	1	339	7.1	75	0.9	1.8
Soft, Salted, Original, Auntie Anne's*	1 Pretzel/112g	310	1	277	7.1	58	0.9	1.8
Sour Cream & Onion, M&S*	1 Serving/30g	136	4.4	455	11	70.9	14.5	0.7
Sour Cream Chive, Penn State Pretzels*	1 Serving/25g	111	3.2	443	8.9	71.8	12.9	2
Turkey, Emmental, Avocado, Finest, Tesco*	1 Pretzel/192g	487	21.9	254	13.1	23.9	11.4	1.6
Wheat, GF, Trufree*	1 Bag/60g	282	12	470	0.5	72	20	0.7
PRINGLES*								
Barbecue, Pringles*	1 Serving/50g	266	18	533	4.9	48	36	5.1
BBQ Spare Rib, Rice Infusions, Pringles*	1 Pack/23g	108	5.3	469	5.1	60	23	2.6
Burger, Take Aways, Pringles*	1 Serving/25g	129	8	516	4.2	52	32	2.5
Cheese & Onion, Pringles*	1 Serving/25g	132	8.5	528	4.1	50	34	3.4
Chip n Ketchup, Pringles*	1 Serving/25g	129	8	516	3.9	52	32	2.5
Hot & Spicy, Pringles*	1 Serving/25g	132	8.5	530	4.6	49	34	3.7
Light, Aromas, Greek Cheese Avocado Oil, Pringles*	1 Serving/25g	122	6.2	488	4.6	57	25	3.6
Light, Original, Pringles*	1 Serving/25g	121	6.2	484	4.3	59	25	3.6
Light, Sour Cream & Onion, Pringles*	1 Serving/25g	122	6.2	487	4.7	57	25	3.6
Margarita Pizza, Classic Takeaways, Pringles*	1 Serving/25g	134	8	538	3.9	53	32	2.6
Minis, Original, Pringles*	1 Pack/23g	118	6.9	514	5.1	55	30	3.7
Minis, Salt & Vinegar, Pringles*	1 Pack/23g	115	6.4	502	4.5	55	28	3.6
Minis, Sour Cream & Onion, Pringles*	1 Pack/23g	118	6.7	511	5.2	56	29	3.5
Original, Pringles*	1 Serving/25g	130	8.5	522	3.8	51	34	2.6
Paprika, Pringles*	1 Serving/25g	132	8.5	529	4.9	49	34	6.5
Prawn Cocktail, Pringles*	1 Serving/25g	130	8	518	4.1	53	32	2.5
Salt Vinegar, Pringles*	1 Serving/25g	128	8	512	3.9	52	32	2.4
Sour Cream Onion, Pringles*	1 Serving/30g	153	9.6	509	3.9	52	32	2.6
Texas BBQ Sauce, Pringles*	1 Serving/25g	132	8.5	527	4.2	50	34	3.5
PROFITEROLES								
12 Chocolate, Waitrose*	3 Profiteroles/65g	284	21.4	437	6	28.7	33	0.4
Asda*	1 Serving/64g	218	17.2	343	5	20	27	0
Black Forest, Tesco*	1 Profiterole/19g	71	4.3	374	4.9	37.4	22.6	0.7
Chocolate Covered, Tesco*	1 Serving/72g	295	21.2	410	5.7	29.3	29.5	2
Chocolate, 8 Pack, Co-Op*	¼ Pack/112g	330	17.9	295	6	31	16	2
Chocolate, Sainsbury's*	1/6 Pot/95g	192	8.5	202	5.4	25.1	8.9	0.8
Chocolate, Stack, Sainsbury's*	¼ Pack/76g	311	19.5	409	5.3	39.3	25.6	2
Chocolate, Tesco*	4 Profiteroles/59g	202	16.1	343	5.2	18.5	27.4	1
Choux & Chocolate Sauce, Tesco*	1 Serving/77g	295	22	386	5.1	26.9	28.7	0.5
Classic French, Sainsbury's*	1 Serving/90g	284	15.5	316	6.6	33.7	17.2	0.1
Dairy Cream, Co-Op*	¼ Pack/70g	242	17.5	345	6	24	25	0.5
Filled with Cream, Stack, Fresh, M&S*	1 Serving/75g	303	22.8	404	5.6	26.3	30.4	1.5
in a Pot, Waitrose*	1 Pot/80g	207	11.3	259	6.3	25.6	14.1	2.9
Salted Caramel, Baileys*	1 Profiterole/18g	69	4.5	384	4	35.5	25	0.5
Savoury with Cheese Chive, CBY, Asda*	¼ Pack/15g	95	7.7	634	9.1	32.1	51.3	3.5
Waitrose*	4 Profiteroles/75g	269	17.9	359	4.8	31.1	23.9	0.7
PRUNES								
Dried, Average	*1 Prune/7g*	*11*	*0*	*158*	*2.5*	*36.4*	*0.4*	*5.8*
in Apple Juice, Average	*1 Serving/90g*	*76*	*0.1*	*84*	*0.8*	*19.8*	*0.1*	*1.4*
in Fruit Juice, Average	*1oz/28g*	*24*	*0*	*86*	*0.9*	*20.9*	*0.2*	*2.9*
in Syrup, Average	*1oz/28g*	*25*	*0*	*89*	*0.9*	*21.5*	*0.2*	*2.6*
Stewed with Sugar	*1oz/28g*	*29*	*0.1*	*103*	*1.3*	*25.5*	*0.2*	*3.1*
Stewed without Sugar	*1oz/28g*	*23*	*0.1*	*81*	*1.4*	*19.5*	*0.3*	*3.3*

P

INFO/WEIGHT	Measure	per Measure KCAL	per Measure FAT	Nutrition Values per 100g / 100ml KCAL	PROT	CARB	FAT	FIBRE

PUDDING

	Measure INFO/WEIGHT	KCAL	FAT	KCAL	PROT	CARB	FAT	FIBRE
Apple, & Sultana, Steamed, BGTY, Sainsbury's*	1 Pudding/110g	294	3.2	267	2.9	57.4	2.9	0.8
Beef, & Onion, Minced, Hollands*	1 Pudding/165g	353	19	214	6.5	20.6	11.5	0
Black Forest, Brilliant, Graze*	1 Punnet/37g	97	3.3	262	4	40	9	2
Bread, Retail Average	*1 Slice/120g*	*301*	*8*	*251*	*8.4*	*41.8*	*6.7*	*0.5*
Chocolate, Fudge, Pot, Pots & Co*	1 Pot/125g	495	30	396	3.8	40	24	2.4
Chocolate, Ganache, Mini Pot, Gu*	1 Pot/45g	199	16.6	442	3.3	26.4	36.8	2.3
Chocolate, M&S*	¼ Pudding/76g	265	12	350	4.1	48	15.8	2.1
Chocolate, Melt in The Middle, Frozen, Waitrose*	1 Pudding/90g	310	14.4	344	6.7	41.4	16	3.5
Chocolate, Melt in The Middle, Mini, Tesco*	1 Pudding/20g	85	5.9	427	7.5	30.2	29.5	5.5
Chocolate, Melting Middle, Hot, Puds, Gu*	1 Pud/100g	409	26.9	409	6	36	26.9	2.7
Chocolate, Melting Middle, M&S*	1 Pudding/155g	510	27.8	330	5.8	36.2	18	3.1
Chocolate, Sponge with Rich Caramel Sauce, Cadbury*	1 Pudding/110g	352	16.6	320	4	41.1	15.1	1.2
Eve's, Average	*1oz/28g*	*67*	*3.7*	*241*	*3.5*	*28.9*	*13.1*	*1.4*
Gingerbread, Butterscotch, Melt, Finest, Tesco*	½ Pudding/113g	440	14.6	390	4.9	62.6	12.9	1.7
Golden Syrup, Steamed, Aunty's*	1 Pudding/100g	293	4.1	293	3.3	57.3	4.1	0.8
Jam, Roly Poly, Sainsbury's*	¼ Pack/81g	291	11.5	359	4.4	53.3	14.2	0.5
Queen of Puddings	*1oz/28g*	*60*	*2.2*	*213*	*4.8*	*33.1*	*7.8*	*0.2*
Roly Poly, Jam, Aunt Bessie's*	1 Serving/75g	278	9	370	3.6	62	12	1.4
Souffle, Hot Chocolate, Gu*	1 Pot/65g	298	23.5	458	6	24.1	36.2	2.5
Sponge, with Golden Syrup, Individual, Mr Kipling*	1 Pudding/95g	395	16.7	366	3.1	53.1	15.5	0.6
Sponge, with Raspberry Jam, Individual, Mr Kipling*	1 Pudding/108g	392	16.8	363	3.1	52.4	15.6	0.7
Sticky Toffee, Co-Op*	¼ Pudding/100g	355	20	355	3	40	20	0.7
Sticky Toffee, Deluxe, Lidl*	½ Pudding/225g	806	36	358	2.5	50	16	2.1
Sticky Toffee, Extra Special, Asda*	¼ Pudding/100g	378	18	378	1.9	52	18	1.8
Sticky Toffee, Indulgent, Specially Selected, Aldi*	¼ Pudding/112g	387	14.6	344	2.6	54	13	1.5
Sticky Toffee, Steamed, Aunty's*	1 Pudding/110g	331	5.3	301	2.6	58.4	4.8	1.2
Sticky Toffee, Tesco*	1 Serving/110g	287	14.7	261	3.3	31.8	13.4	0.7
Strawberry, Jelly Pud, with Devon Custard, Ambrosia*	1 Pot/150g	129	1.2	86	0.7	19.4	0.8	0
Suet, Average	*1oz/28g*	*94*	*5.1*	*335*	*4.4*	*40.5*	*18.3*	*0.9*
Summer Fruits, Eat Well, M&S*	1 Pudding/135g	128	0.7	95	1.7	20.8	0.5	3
Summer, BGTY, Sainsbury's*	1 Pot/110g	223	5.1	203	3.2	40.9	4.6	2.4
Summer, Waitrose*	1 Pot/120g	125	0.5	104	2	23.1	0.4	1.4
Syrup, M&S*	1 Serving/105g	370	10.5	352	3.9	61.7	10	0.8
Torte, Cheeky Little Chocolate, Gu*	1 Pud/50g	211	14.6	422	5.7	31.6	29.1	1.8
Truffle, Chocolate with Raspberry Compote, Gu*	1 Pot/80g	250	14.6	312	2.8	28.8	18.2	1.8

PUMPKIN

Boiled in Salted Water	*1oz/28g*	*4*	*0.1*	*13*	*0.6*	*2.1*	*0.3*	*1.1*
Potimarron, Raw, Average	*1 Serving/80g*	*21*	*0.1*	*26*	*1*	*6.5*	*0.1*	*1.9*
Puree, Baking Buddy*	1 Serving/53g	22	0	42	1.7	6.7	0	2.5

	Measure INFO/WEIGHT	per Measure KCAL	FAT	KCAL	PROT	CARB	FAT	FIBRE
QUAVERS								
Cheese, Walkers*	1 Bag/20g	107	6	534	2.7	62.5	30.1	1.1
Prawn Cocktail, Walkers*	1 Bag/16g	88	5.1	537	2.1	62	31	1.2
Salt Vinegar, Walkers*	1 Bag/16g	86	4.9	527	1.9	62	30	1.2
QUESADILLA								
Chicken, from Restaurant, Average	*1 Serving/300g*	*867*	*46.7*	*289*	*15.6*	*22.2*	*15.6*	*1.7*
Meal Kit, Toasted Cheese, Old El Paso*	1 Quesadilla/63g	135	2.1	215	6.6	38.4	3.4	2.2
QUICHE								
Asparagus, & Mushroom, Tesco*	½ Quiche/200g	474	32.8	237	5.1	17.2	16.4	1.2
Asparagus, & Vegetable, Herby Summer, Higgidy*	1 Quiche/400g	848	50	212	5.9	18.9	12.5	2.7
Bacon, & Cheese, Sainsbury's*	¼ Quiche/100g	237	15	237	7	18.6	15	0.7
Bacon, & Leek, From Our Deli, As Consumed, Morrisons*	1 Quiche/160g	435	28	272	7.8	20	17.5	1.6
Bacon, Leek & Mushroom, M&S*	¼ Quiche/100g	245	16.4	245	6.9	17.2	16.4	1.3
Bacon, Smoked Mature Cheddar, Higgidy*	1 Quiche/400g	1096	74	274	8.4	18.6	18.5	1.5
Broccoli, Tesco*	1 Serving/100g	249	17.2	249	6	17.6	17.2	1.4
Broccoli, Tomato and Cheese, Classic, Sainsbury's*	1 Serving/100g	223	14.5	223	5.3	17.1	14.5	1.6
Cheese, & Bacon, Crustless, Tesco*	¼ Quiche/85g	196	13.4	230	9.8	11.8	15.7	1.5
Cheese, & Broccoli, Morrisons*	1/3 Quiche/134g	338	22.4	253	7.1	18.4	16.8	1.7
Cheese, & Egg	*1oz/28g*	*88*	*6.2*	*314*	*12.5*	*17.3*	*22.2*	*0.6*
Cheese, & Leek, & Chive, Sainsbury's*	1/3 Quiche/125g	292	20.2	234	7.1	14.9	16.2	1.3
Cheese, & Onion, Asda*	½ Quiche/200g	578	39.6	289	9	18.6	19.8	1.5
Cheese, & Onion, Caramelised Onion, Finest, Tesco*	¼ Quiche/100g	300	18.6	300	9.4	22.4	18.6	1.7
Cheese, & Onion, Co-Op*	¼ Quiche/88g	262	19.2	300	10	17	22	1
Cheese, & Onion, Crustless, Deli, Morrisons*	1 Quiche/388g	1005	68.3	259	9.7	14.9	17.6	1
Cheese, & Onion, Crustless, Weight Watchers*	1 Quiche/160g	267	12.3	167	11.3	11.1	7.7	4.3
Cheese, & Onion, Finest, Tesco*	1 Serving/130g	346	24.3	266	9.1	15.3	18.7	2.5
Cheese, & Onion, HL, Tesco*	¼ Quiche/100g	180	7.8	180	9.4	17.6	7.8	1.8
Cheese, & Onion, Individual, Sainsbury's*	1 Quiche/170g	434	26	255	7.3	21.7	15.3	1.2
Cheese, & Onion, M&S*	1 Slice/100g	250	17.2	250	8.2	16.1	17.2	1.5
Cheese, & Onion, Mature Cheddar, Crustless, Higgidy*	¼ Quiche/95g	254	16.9	267	7.4	18.7	17.8	1
Cheese, & Onion, Reduced Fat, Eat Smart, Morrisons*	1 Quiche/400g	824	36.8	206	7.7	16.9	9.2	0.7
Cheese, & Onion, Retail, Average	*¼ Quiche/100g*	*262*	*17.8*	*262*	*8.4*	*17.1*	*17.8*	*1.3*
Cheese, & Onion, Value, Tesco*	½ Quiche/200g	526	36.4	263	8.6	16.1	18.2	0.7
Cheese, & Onion, Weight Watchers*	1 Quiche/165g	325	15.3	197	7	21.2	9.3	1.6
Cheese, & Tomato, Asda*	¼ Quiche/105g	274	17.8	261	8	19	17	0.9
Cheese, & Tomato, Crustless, Iceland*	¼ Quiche/203g	483	34.7	238	7.5	12.8	17.1	1.9
Cheese, & Tomato, Retail, Average	*¼ Quiche/100g*	*268*	*17.1*	*268*	*8*	*20.2*	*17.1*	*1.1*
Cheese, Onion, Crustless, Tesco*	¼ Quiche/85g	211	14.4	249	10.8	12.8	16.9	1.2
Lorraine, 400g, Morrisons*	¼ Quiche/100g	323	23.7	323	9	17.9	23.7	0.9
Lorraine, Asda*	¼ Quiche/100g	246	16.2	246	6.6	18.5	16.2	4.2
Lorraine, BGTY, Sainsbury's*	1 Serving/128g	273	14	213	10.9	17.7	10.9	0.7
Lorraine, Castle Grove, Lidl*	½ Pie/200g	578	40	289	11	16	20	0.5
Lorraine, Classics, M&S*	¼ Quiche/100g	251	16.4	251	10.3	15	16.4	0.9
Lorraine, Co-Op*	¼ Quiche/100g	275	20.6	275	8.1	14.9	20.6	2.6
Lorraine, Crustless, Asda*	1 Quiche/160g	259	12.6	162	9.3	13.5	7.9	1.1
Lorraine, Crustless, LC, Tesco*	1 Pack/160g	280	13.4	175	12.6	11.8	8.4	2.5
Lorraine, Crustless, You Count, Love Life, Waitrose*	1 Quiche/160g	295	15.4	185	8.9	15.2	9.6	0.9
Lorraine, Extra Special, Asda*	¼ Quiche/100g	270	18	270	8	19	18	2.3
Lorraine, Finest, Tesco*	1 Serving/100g	330	25.1	330	8.4	17.5	25.1	1.5
Lorraine, Individual, Tesco*	1 Quiche/160g	424	27.1	265	10.6	16.9	16.9	1.5
Lorraine, Quiche Selection, M&S*	1 Slice/56g	160	11.5	285	12.8	12.3	20.6	2.1
Lorraine, Retail, Average	*¼ Quiche/100g*	*280*	*19.5*	*280*	*9*	*16.8*	*19.5*	*2*
Lorraine, Smoked Bacon & Cheese, M&S*	¼ Quiche/100g	270	18.4	270	9.7	16.4	18.4	1.6
Lorraine, Tesco*	½ Quiche/88g	249	16.6	285	9.3	18.2	19	1.9

Q

	Measure INFO/WEIGHT	per Measure KCAL	FAT	Nutrition Values per 100g / 100ml KCAL	PROT	CARB	FAT	FIBRE
QUICHE								
Lorraine, TTD, Sainsbury's*	¼ Quiche/100g	286	18.9	286	10.2	18.4	18.9	1.2
Mushroom	*1oz/28g*	*80*	*5.5*	*284*	*10*	*18.3*	*19.5*	*0.9*
Mushroom, Medley, Waitrose*	¼ Quiche/100g	222	15.2	222	6.4	15	15.2	2.9
Salmon, & Broccoli, Tesco*	1 Serving/133g	311	20.1	234	7.9	16.6	15.1	0.9
Salmon, & Spinach, Sainsbury's*	1/3 Quiche/125g	318	21.9	254	8.2	15.9	17.5	1
Salmon, & Spinach, Smoked, Little, Higgidy*	1 Quiche/155g	448	31.5	289	8.6	17.5	20.3	0.9
Spinach, & Red Pepper, Goats Cheese, Waitrose*	1 Serving/100g	218	14.3	218	6.5	15.8	14.3	2.6
Spinach, & Ricotta, Tesco*	¼ Quiche/100g	237	14.9	237	5.8	19.9	14.9	1
Spinach, & Roast Red Pepper, Little, Higgidy*	1 Quiche/155g	397	27.3	256	9.1	15.2	17.6	1.2
Spinach, Edamame, Kale, Crustless, Tesco*	1 Quiche/160g	350	22.2	219	8.7	13.9	13.8	2.2
Spinach, Feta, Roasted Red Pepper, Higgidy*	½ Quiche/200g	526	35.8	263	8.8	17.4	17.9	1.8
Vegetable, Sundried Tomato, Tesco*	¼ Quiche/100g	211	12.9	211	6.7	16.4	12.9	1.3
Vegetable, Mediterranean Style, Classic, Sainsbury's*	1 Quiche/400g	868	50.4	217	6.2	19.8	12.6	2.2
QUINCE								
Average	*1 Avg fruit/209g*	*37*	*0.1*	*18*	*0.2*	*4.3*	*0.1*	*1.3*
QUINOA								
Black Rice Edamame Soya Beans, Eat Well, M&S*	1 Pack/240g	283	9.4	118	4.1	13.9	3.9	5.6
Cooked, Love Life, Waitrose*	1 Serving/180g	216	3.5	120	9.9	4.4	1.9	2.8
Dry Weight, Average	*1 Serving/70g*	*258*	*4.2*	*368*	*14.1*	*64.2*	*6.1*	*7*
Red	*1 Serving/100g*	*358*	*6*	*358*	*12.9*	*62.2*	*6*	*9.7*
Red White, with Bulgur Wheat, Tesco*	½ Pack/125g	233	4.9	186	6.7	28.9	3.9	4.6
Tomato, Spiced, Tesco*	½ Pack/150g	186	7.2	124	3.6	14.8	4.8	3.5

Q

	Measure INFO/WEIGHT	per Measure KCAL	per Measure FAT	Nutrition Values per 100g / 100ml KCAL	PROT	CARB	FAT	FIBRE
RABBIT								
Meat Only, Raw	1oz/28g	38	1.5	137	21.9	0	5.5	0
Meat Only, Raw, Weighed with Bone	1 Serving/200g	164	6.6	82	13.1	0	3.3	0
Meat Only, Stewed	1oz/28g	32	0.9	114	21.2	0	3.2	0
Meat Only, Stewed, Weighed with Bone	1oz/28g	11	0.3	41	7.6	0	1.1	0
RADISH								
Black, Raw, Average	1 Lge/9g	1	0	16	1	3	0	2
Red, Unprepared, Average	1 Radish/8g	1	0	11	0.6	1.7	0.2	0.8
White, Mooli, Raw	1oz/28g	4	0	13	0.7	2.5	0.1	0
RAISINS								
Sultanas, Jumbo, M&S*	1 Serving/80g	212	0.4	265	2.4	62.4	0.5	2.6
Sultanas, The Fruit Factory*	1 Box/14g	43	0.1	305	3	72.3	0.5	4
Lime Infused, Tangy, Nak'd*	1 Pack/25g	68	0	272	2.1	69.3	0	0
Milk Chocolate, Belgian, M&S*	½ Pack/63g	274	9.6	438	4.6	68.9	15.3	2.9
Seedless, Average	1 Serving/75g	215	0.4	287	2.2	68.5	0.5	3.2
Yoghurt Coated, Fruit Bowl*	1 Pack/25g	114	4.8	455	2	67	19	3
RAITA								
Cucumber & Mint, Patak's*	1oz/28g	18	0.5	64	3.4	8.4	1.8	0
Dip, Indian, Asda*	1 Pot/70g	120	11.5	172	2.6	3.6	16.4	0.5
Plain, Average	1oz/28g	16	0.6	57	4.2	5.8	2.2	0
RASPBERRIES								
Dried, Graze*	1 Pack/30g	85	0.8	284	3.2	62	2.6	0
Freeze Dried, Simply*	1 Serving/10g	37	0	370	10	80	0	20
Fresh, Raw, Average	1 Serving/80g	20	0.2	25	1.3	4.7	0.3	6.5
Frozen, Average	1 Serving/100g	27	0.3	27	1.3	4.7	0.3	5.2
in Juice, Canned, Morrisons*	½ Can/150g	81	0.3	54	0.4	12	0.2	1.4
in Syrup, Canned	1oz/28g	25	0	88	0.6	22.5	0.1	1.5
RATATOUILLE								
Average	1oz/28g	23	2	82	1.3	3.8	7	1.8
Chicken, Finest, Tesco*	1 Pack/550g	407	11.6	74	7.8	5.9	2.1	0
RAVIOLI								
Asparagus, & Cheese, Waitrose*	1 Serving/100g	242	7.2	242	12.6	31.7	7.2	2.4
Asparagus, Waitrose*	1 Serving/150g	303	9	202	10.5	26.4	6	2
Beef	1 Serving/300g	501	13.7	167	6.4	25	4.6	1.4
Beef, & Red Wine, Italiano, Tesco*	½ Pack/200g	424	13	212	7.3	30	6.5	2.3
Beef, in Tomato Sauce, Heinz*	½ Can/200g	147	3.2	74	2.5	12	1.6	0.8
Beef, in Tomato Sauce, Minced, Rich, Corale, Aldi*	½ Can/200g	172	2	86	2.8	16.4	1	0.5
Butternut Squash, Marjoram , M&S*	½ Pack/125g	336	15.5	269	8.9	29.2	12.4	2.5
Cheese, Four, in Tomato Sauce, COU, M&S*	1 Pack/345g	352	7.6	102	7.5	12.3	2.2	1.5
Cheese, Four, Meal for One, M&S*	1 Pack/375g	668	36.8	178	6.2	15.6	9.8	1.1
Chicken, & Bacon, Cucina, Aldi*	1 Pack/250g	455	14	182	6.9	24.7	5.6	2.7
Goat's Cheese, & Pesto, Asda*	½ Pack/150g	204	5.4	136	6	20	3.6	0
in Tomato Sauce, Canned, Sainsbury's*	½ Can/200g	166	2	83	3.1	15.5	1	0.5
Mushroom, Portobello, Waitrose*	½ Pack/125g	201	5.1	161	7.5	22.3	4.1	2.6
Pancetta, & Mozzarella, Finest, Tesco*	1 Serving/125g	344	13.2	275	12.2	32.8	10.6	1.8
Salmon, & Dill, Smoked, Sainsbury's*	1 Serving/125g	256	8.9	205	8.7	26.5	7.1	0.7
Spinach, & Ricotta, Waitrose*	1 Serving/125g	309	9	247	10.5	35	7.2	1.9
Vegetable, Roasted, Asda*	½ Pack/150g	218	0.8	145	6	29	0.5	0
Vegetable, Tesco*	½ Can/200g	164	1.4	82	2.6	16.3	0.7	0.7
RAVIOLINI								
Pumpkin, Sage, GF, Ugo*	½ Pack/125g	214	3.4	171	2.3	29.8	2.7	9.3
REDCURRANTS								
Raw, Average	1oz/28g	6	0	20	1.1	4.3	0	3.3
Raw, Stalks Removed	1 Serving/100g	21	0	21	1.1	4.4	0	0

R

	Measure INFO/WEIGHT	per Measure KCAL	FAT	Nutrition Values per 100g / 100ml KCAL	PROT	CARB	FAT	FIBRE
REEF*								
Orange & Passionfruit, Reef*	1 Bottle/275ml	179	0	65	0	9.5	0	0
RELISH								
Barbeque, Sainsbury's*	1 Serving/50g	50	1	100	1	19.3	2.1	1.1
Branston, Sweet Onion, Crosse & Blackwell*	1 Serving/10g	15	0	153	1	36.3	0.4	0.7
Burger, Caramelised Red Onion, Branston*	1 Squeeze/15g	23	0.2	151	0.8	32	1.4	1.4
Caramelised Red Onion, Tesco*	1 Serving/10g	28	0	280	0.6	69.1	0.1	0.7
Corn, Spicy, Stonewall Kitchen*	1 Tbsp/15g	18	0	117	0	26.7	0	0
Onion, M&S*	1oz/28g	46	0.8	165	1	32.1	3	1.1
Onion, Sainsbury's*	1 Serving/15g	23	0.1	151	0.9	36	0.4	0.7
Sweetcorn, American Style, Maryland, Tesco*	1 Serving/15g	15	0	101	1.1	23.9	0.1	0.9
Sweetcorn, Bick's*	1 Tbsp/22g	23	0	103	1.3	24.3	0.2	0
Tomato Spicy, Bick's*	1 Serving/28g	28	0.1	99	1.3	23.2	0.2	0
Tomato, Sweet, Heinz*	1 Serving/25g	34	0	136	0.9	32.6	0.2	0.9
REVELS								
Mars*	1 Pack/35g	169	7.4	483	5.2	67.6	21	0
RHUBARB								
In Juice, Canned, Drained, Average	*1 Serving/100g*	*46*	*0*	*46*	*0.5*	*10.8*	*0*	*0.8*
Raw, Average	*1 Stalk/51g*	*4*	*0.1*	*7*	*0.9*	*0.8*	*0.1*	*1.4*
Stewed with Sugar, Average	*1oz/28g*	*32*	*0*	*116*	*0.4*	*31.2*	*0*	*2*
RIBENA*								
Apple Juice Drink, Ribena*	1 Carton/287ml	132	0	46	0	11.1	0	0
Blackcurrant Juice Drink, Ready Made, Ribena*	1 Carton/200ml	82	0	41	0	10.6	0	0
Blackcurrant, Diluted with Water, Ribena*	1 Serving/100ml	46	0	46	0	11.4	0	0
Blackcurrant, No Added Sugar, Diluted, Ribena*	1 Serving/250ml	11	0	4	0	0.6	0	0
Blackcurrant, Original, Undiluted, Ribena*	1 Serving/50ml	108	0	216	0	53	0	0
Blackcurrant, Really Light, No Added Sugar, Ribena*	1 Carton/250ml	8	0	3	0	0.8	0	0
Light, Ribena*	1 Carton/288ml	26	0	9	0.1	2.1	0	0
Orange, Juice Drink, Ribena*	1 Serving/288ml	98	0	34	0.1	8.1	0	0
Pineapple Passion Fruit, Juice Drink, Ribena*	½ Bottle/250ml	103	0	41	0	9.9	0	0
Plus, Apple Peach, Immunity Support, Ribena*	1 Carton/200ml	2	0	1	0	0.2	0	0
Really Light, Undiluted, Ribena*	1 Serving/25ml	20	0	80	0	2.5	0	0
Strawberry Juice Drink, Ribena*	1 Carton/288ml	12	0	4	0	0.5	0	0
RIBS								
Peking, Taste of China, Tesco*	½ Pack/104g	222	12.4	214	16.4	10.1	12	0
Pork, Barbecue, Meat Only, Cooked, Average	*1 Serving/130g*	*360*	*23.4*	*275*	*21.4*	*7.2*	*17.9*	*0.3*
Pork, Chinese Style, Average	*1 Serving/300g*	*736*	*44.7*	*245*	*17.9*	*10*	*14.9*	*0.7*
Pork, Chops, Raw, Lean Fat, Weighed with Bone	*1 Chop/130g*	*241*	*16.1*	*186*	*18.5*	*0*	*12.4*	*0*
Pork, Full Rack, Sainsbury's*	1 Serving/225g	567	38.7	252	18	6.5	17.2	0.9
Pork, Smokey BBQ, Slow Cooked, Sainsbury's*	½ Pack/165g	455	25.6	276	24.8	8.7	15.5	1
Rack, Pork, Smoky BBQ, Tex Mex, Tesco*	½ Pack/158g	337	21.1	213	17.6	5.6	13.3	0.2
Spare, Barbecue, Chinese Style, Farmfoods*	1 Pack/400g	464	25.2	116	9.3	5.6	6.3	0.1
Spare, Cantonese, Mini, Sainsbury's*	1 Rib/38g	97	5	259	17.2	17.3	13.4	1
Spare, Chinese Style, Summer Eating, Asda*	1 Serving/116g	334	18.6	288	32	4.1	16	0.8
Spare, Sweet, Sticky, Mini, M&S*	½ Pack/75g	215	12.9	286	22.7	9.8	17.2	0.8
RICE								
Arborio, Dry, Average	*1 Serving/80g*	*279*	*0.6*	*348*	*7.1*	*78.3*	*0.8*	*0.8*
Basmati, & Wild, Cooked, Sainsbury's*	½ Pack/125g	150	0.8	120	3.1	25.7	0.6	1.3
Basmati, & Wild, Dry Weight, Tilda*	1 Serving/70g	244	0.3	349	9.4	77	0.5	1
Basmati, Boil in the Bag, Dry, Average	*1 Serving/50g*	*176*	*0.4*	*352*	*8.4*	*77.8*	*0.8*	*0.4*
Basmati, Brown, Dry, Average	*1 Serving/50g*	*177*	*1.5*	*353*	*9.5*	*71.8*	*3*	*2.2*
Basmati, Cooked, Average	*1 Serving/140g*	*189*	*1*	*135*	*3.1*	*29*	*0.7*	*0.4*
Basmati, Dry Weight, Average	*1 Serving/60g*	*212*	*0.6*	*353*	*8.1*	*77.9*	*1*	*0.6*
Basmati, Indian, Dry, Average	*1 Serving/75g*	*260*	*0.7*	*346*	*8.4*	*76.1*	*0.9*	*0.1*

R

RICE

INFO/WEIGHT	Measure	per Measure KCAL	FAT	Nutrition Values per 100g / 100ml KCAL	PROT	CARB	FAT	FIBRE
Basmati, Microwave, Cooked, Average	**1 Serving/125g**	**182**	**2.3**	**146**	**2.7**	**30**	**1.8**	**0**
Basmati, Original, Pure, GF, Dry, Tilda*	1 Serving/60g	211	0.5	351	7.8	77.7	0.8	1
Basmati, White, Dry, Average	**1 Serving/75g**	**262**	**0.4**	**349**	**8.1**	**77.1**	**0.6**	**2.2**
Basmati, Wholegrain & Wild, Pouch, Tilda*	½ Pack/125g	160	2.6	128	3	23.4	2.1	1.7
Basmati, Wholegrain, Cooked, Tilda*	1 Portion/180g	203	1.6	113	3.3	23	0.9	3.2
Basmati, with Mushroom, Dine In, Veetee*	1 Pack/280g	372	6.4	133	3.3	24.4	2.3	1.2
Black Bean, Jerk Coconut, Pulses Rice, Tilda*	1 Pack/140g	178	5.5	127	4	16.5	3.9	4.9
Brown, Cooked, Average	**1 Serving/140g**	**173**	**1.5**	**123**	**2.6**	**26.6**	**1.1**	**0.9**
Brown, Dry, Average	**1 Serving/75g**	**266**	**2.3**	**355**	**7.5**	**76.2**	**3**	**1.4**
Brown, Long Grain, Dry, Average	**1 Serving/50g**	**182**	**1.4**	**364**	**7.6**	**76.8**	**2.8**	**2**
Brown, Short Grain, Dry, Average	**1 Serving/50g**	**176**	**1.4**	**351**	**6.8**	**77.6**	**2.8**	**1**
Brown, Whole Grain, Cooked, Average	**1 Serving/170g**	**223**	**1.9**	**132**	**2.6**	**27.8**	**1.1**	**1.2**
Brown, Whole Grain, Dry, Average	**1 Serving/40g**	**138**	**1.2**	**344**	**7.4**	**71.6**	**2.9**	**3**
Cauliflower, Parsley, Lets Cook, Aldi*	1 Pack/250g	85	0	34	2.9	2.1	0	2.7
Cauliflower, Frozen, Tesco*	1 Sachet/125g	30	0.2	24	1.8	2.1	0.2	3.2
Cauliflower, Mediterranean, Cauli Rice*	½ Pack100g	46	1.1	46	4	5.8	1.1	2.5
Cauliflower, Microwaved, Good & Balanced, Asda*	½ Pack/200g	68	1.8	34	2.9	2.1	0.9	2.7
Cauliflower, Original, Cauli Rice*	1 Serving/100g	34	0.9	34	3.6	3	0.9	1.8
Chicken, Sweetcorn, Microwave, Sainsbury's*	½ Pack/125g	204	2.6	163	3.9	31.2	2.1	1.9
Chicken, Fried, Chinese Takeaway, Iceland*	1 Pack/340g	510	15.6	150	6.5	20.7	4.6	0.6
Chicken, Savoury, Batchelors*	1 Pack/124g	455	1.9	367	8.9	79.4	1.5	2.6
Chickpea, Harissa Lemon, Pulses Rice, Tilda*	1 Pack/140g	139	4.3	99	3.8	11.6	3.1	4.9
Chilli, Garlic, One Pan, Meal Kit, Old El Paso*	¼ Pack/89g	185	1.1	208	4.7	43.1	1.2	2.8
Chinese Style, Express, Uncle Ben's*	1 Pack/250g	392	5.5	157	3.4	30.9	2.2	0.4
Coconut, Thai, Sainsbury's*	½ Pack/100g	178	9.1	178	2.6	21.3	9.1	1.9
Duck, Chicken, & Pork, Fried, Celebration, Sainsbury's*	1 Pack/450g	544	16.2	121	7.9	14.2	3.6	1.5
Egg Fried, Average	**1 Serving/300g**	**624**	**31.8**	**208**	**4.2**	**25.7**	**10.6**	**0.4**
Egg Fried, Chinese Takeaway, Tesco*	1 Serving/250g	462	15.8	185	3.8	27.2	6.3	2.1
Egg Fried, Express, Uncle Ben's*	½ Pack/125g	216	5.2	173	4	29.9	4.2	0.3
Egg Fried, M&S*	1 Pack/300g	543	12	181	4.4	31	4	1.6
Egg Fried, Micro, Tesco*	1 Pack/250g	312	9.2	125	4.6	18.3	3.7	6.4
Egg Fried, Wholegrain, Pouch, Uncle Ben's*	½ Pouch/125g	194	4.5	155	4.3	25	3.6	1.8
Egg, Fried, 2 Minute Meals, Sainsbury's*	1 Pack/250g	342	1.5	137	3.8	29.2	0.6	0.8
Ghee, Average	**1oz/28g**	**63**	**2.2**	**225**	**3.1**	**35.3**	**7.9**	**0**
Golden Savoury, Dry Weight, Batchelors*	1 Pack/120g	437	3.4	364	10.1	74.7	2.8	2.4
Jasmine, Curry Meal Box, Tesco*	½ Pack/194g	250	0.3	129	2.8	28.9	0.1	0.5
Jasmine, Taste of Thailand, Tesco*	1 Pack/242g	312	0.3	129	2.8	28.9	0.1	0.5
Long Grain, & Wild, Dry, Average	**1 Serving/75g**	**254**	**1.5**	**338**	**7.6**	**72.6**	**2**	**1.7**
Long Grain, Wild, Microwave, Uncle Ben's*	½ Pack/125g	188	1.6	150	3.2	30.9	1.3	0.9
Long Grain, American, Cooked, Average	**1 Serving/160g**	**229**	**2.8**	**143**	**3**	**28.8**	**1.8**	**0.2**
Long Grain, American, Dry, Average	**1 Serving/50g**	**175**	**0.5**	**350**	**7.2**	**77.8**	**1.1**	**0.6**
Long Grain, Dry, Average	**1 Serving/50g**	**169**	**0.5**	**337**	**7.4**	**75.5**	**1**	**1.7**
Long Grain, Microwavable, Cooked, Average	**1 Serving/150g**	**180**	**0.9**	**120**	**2.7**	**25.8**	**0.6**	**0.7**
Mexican Inspired, Micro, Tesco*	1 Bag/142g	184	2	130	3.2	25.5	1.4	1.1
Mexican, Style, Cooked, Express, Uncle Ben's*	1 Pack/250g	385	4.8	154	3.2	31.1	1.9	0.7
Mushroom, Pilau, Bombay Brasserie, Sainsbury's*	1 Pack/400g	672	17.2	168	3.7	28.6	4.3	0.7
Mushroom, Pilau, Indian, Sainsbury's*	1 Serving/100g	119	2.4	119	3	21.3	2.4	1.9
Mushroom, Roasted, Taste of India, Tesco*	½ Pack/135g	177	3.5	131	3.2	23	2.6	1.6
Paella, Spanish, Dry, Tesco*	1 Serving/75g	262	0.4	349	6.3	78.9	0.6	1.5
Pilaf, Royal, Microwaved, Mumbai Street Food, Iceland*	1 Meal/158g	463	12.8	293	5.3	48.6	8.1	2.3
Pilau, Cooked, Average	**1 Serving/200g**	**349**	**8.8**	**174**	**3.5**	**30.3**	**4.4**	**0.8**
Pilau, Dry, Average	**1oz/28g**	**101**	**0.7**	**362**	**8.4**	**78.2**	**2.4**	**3.4**
Pilau, Microwavable, Golden Sun, Lidl*	½ Pack/125g	199	3.5	159	3.7	29.3	2.8	1.1

	Measure INFO/WEIGHT	per Measure KCAL	FAT	Nutrition Values per 100g / 100ml KCAL	PROT	CARB	FAT	FIBRE
RICE								
Pilau, Takeaway, Tesco*	½ Pack/250g	357	5	143	3.2	27.7	2	0.8
Pilau, Taste of India, Tesco*	1 Pack/270g	429	9.2	159	2.8	28.8	3.4	1.1
Pudding, Dry Weight, Average	**1 Serving/100g**	**356**	**1.1**	**356**	**6.9**	**82**	**1.1**	**0.4**
Red, Dry, Ingredients, Tesco*	1 Serving/60g	209	1.8	349	8.2	69.8	3	5
Risotto, Dry, Average	**1 Serving/50g**	**174**	**0.6**	**348**	**7.8**	**76.2**	**1.3**	**2.4**
Saffron, Cooked, Average	**1 Serving/150g**	**208**	**4.7**	**139**	**2.6**	**25.3**	**3.2**	**0.5**
Special Fried, Chinese Takeaway, Iceland*	1 Pack/350g	630	17.5	180	5.5	28.2	5	1.2
Special Fried, Chinese, Tesco*	1 Serving/300g	618	33.3	206	6.5	19.9	11.1	0.8
Special Fried, M&S*	½ Pack/150g	300	12.3	200	6.7	24.2	8.2	1.2
Spinach, & Carrot, Pilau, Waitrose*	1 Pack/350g	466	8.4	133	3.1	24.8	2.4	1.2
Sweet & Spicy, Szechuan, Naked Rice, Symingtons*	1 Pot/259g	285	4.1	110	2.3	21.3	1.6	0.9
Thai, Black, Sainsbury's*	1 Serving/180g	205	2	114	3.7	20.4	1.1	3.8
Thai, Cooked, Average	**1 Serving/100g**	**136**	**1.8**	**136**	**2.5**	**27.4**	**1.8**	**0.3**
Thai, Dry, Average	**1 Serving/50g**	**174**	**0.2**	**348**	**7.1**	**78.9**	**0.4**	**0.9**
Thai, Fragrant, Dry, Average	**1 Serving/75g**	**272**	**0.5**	**363**	**7.2**	**82**	**0.7**	**0.3**
Thai, Glutinous, Sticky, White, Dry, Raw	**1 Serving/100g**	**370**	**0.6**	**370**	**6.8**	**81.7**	**0.6**	**2.8**
Vegetable, Golden, Freshly Frozen, Asda*	1 Sachet/200g	238	2.6	119	3.2	23.6	1.3	1.3
Vegetable, Mediterranean, SteamFresh, Birds Eye*	1 Bag/190g	218	4.9	115	2.4	20	2.6	1.2
Vegetable, Original, Birds Eye*	1oz/28g	29	0.2	105	4	20.8	0.6	1.1
Vegetable, Savoury, Mixed, Dry Weight, Tesco*	1 Pack/120g	450	3.2	375	7.8	79.1	2.7	2.9
Vegetable, Sunshine, Tilda*	1 Sachet/125g	130	2.9	104	1.9	18.3	2.3	1.4
White, Cooked, Average	**1 Serving/140g**	**182**	**1.1**	**130**	**2.6**	**28.7**	**0.8**	**0.2**
White, Cooked, Frozen, Average	**1 Serving/150g**	**168**	**0.8**	**112**	**2.9**	**23.8**	**0.6**	**1.2**
White, Flaked, Dry Weight, Average	**1oz/28g**	**97**	**0.3**	**346**	**6.6**	**77.5**	**1.2**	**0**
White, Fried	**1oz/28g**	**37**	**0.9**	**131**	**2.2**	**25**	**3.2**	**0.6**
White, Long Grain, Dry Weight, Average	**1 Serving/50g**	**181**	**1**	**362**	**7.1**	**79.1**	**1.9**	**0.4**
White, Microwave, Cooked, Average	**½ Pack/125g**	**185**	**2.4**	**148**	**3.3**	**29.4**	**1.9**	**1.4**
Whole Grain, Dry, Average	**1 Serving/50g**	**171**	**1.2**	**342**	**8.2**	**72**	**2.3**	**4**
Wholegrain, Quinoa, Tomato Basil, Uncle Ben's*	½ Pack/110g	176	2.5	160	4.3	29.2	2.3	2.5
Wholegrain, 3, Beans, Chilli, Uncle Ben's*	½ Pack/110g	176	2.5	160	4.6	28.9	2.3	3
Wholegrain, Microwave, Eat Well, M&S*	½ Pack/125g	181	1.5	145	2.5	31	1.2	2.2
Wild, Cooked, Average	**1 Cup/164g**	**166**	**0.6**	**101**	**4**	**21.3**	**0.3**	**1.8**
With Red Kidney Beans, Average	**1oz/28g**	**49**	**1**	**175**	**5.6**	**32.4**	**3.5**	**2.5**
RICE CAKES								
Asda*	1 Cake/8g	31	0.2	386	8.7	81.1	3	2.8
Caramel, Flavour, Kallo*	1 Cake/10g	38	0.5	383	6.2	78.9	4.8	3.9
Caramel, Free From, Tesco*	1 Rice Cake/11g	41	0.3	373	5.9	80.9	2.5	1.8
Caramel, Jumbo, Snack-A-Jacks, Quaker*	1 Cake/13g	51	0.3	390	5.5	87	2.1	1.4
Caramel, Jumbo, Tesco*	1 Cake/10g	34	0.3	340	7	74	3	5
Cheese, & Onion, Snack, Snack-A-Jacks, Quaker*	1 Bag/30g	120	2.2	400	6.7	77	7.5	1.5
Chocolate, Chip, Jumbo, Snack-A-Jacks, Quaker*	1 Cake/15g	62	1	410	6	81	7	1.7
Chocolate, Dark, Mint, Nature's Store*	1 Rice Cake/17g	82	3.9	485	6.3	61	23.1	5.1
Chocolate, Dark, Organic, Kallo*	1 Cake/12g	57	2.9	471	6.8	57.2	24.1	7.4
Chocolate, Milk, Minis, Kids, Kallo*	1 Pack/14g	69	3.3	496	6.6	62.6	23.8	0
Chocolate, Milk, Organic, Kallo*	1 Cake/11g	57	3.2	509	6.5	56.2	28.7	3.5
Chocolate, Milk, Slices, Morrisons*	1 Slice/11g	53	2.5	469	7.3	58.8	22	3.3
Idly, Average	**1 Idly/40g**	**59**	**0.4**	**149**	**4.1**	**30.8**	**1**	**1.3**
Multigrain, Ryvita*	3 Cakes/11g	43	0.5	384	9.1	76.2	4.7	5.3
Rye, Multigrain, High Fibre, Ryvita*	1 Cake/7g	23	0.2	352	9.4	66.3	2.5	13.3
Salt Vinegar, Tesco*	1 Cake/12g	47	0.7	392	6.3	78	5.7	1.8
Salt, & Vinegar, Balsamic, Sea, Kallo*	1 Cake/9g	32	0.2	361	6.5	78.1	2.5	3
Salt, & Vinegar, Jumbo, Snack-A-Jacks, Quaker*	1 Cake/10g	41	0.6	391	7.4	75.4	5.7	1.6
Salt, & Vinegar, Jumbo, Tesco*	1 Cake/9g	31	0.2	347	8.4	72.7	2.5	6

R

	Measure INFO/WEIGHT	per Measure KCAL	FAT	Nutrition Values per 100g / 100ml KCAL	PROT	CARB	FAT	FIBRE
RICE CAKES								
Salt, & Vinegar, Wholegrain, Tesco*	1 Cake/9g	28	0.2	314	8.4	61.9	2.6	6
Salted, Lightly, Thick Slice, Low Fat, Kallo*	1 Cake/8g	28	0.2	372	8	78.7	2.8	5.1
Salted, Sea, Harvest Morn, Aldi*	1 Cake/7g	27	0.2	379	8.7	78	2.2	5.1
Salted, Slightly, Organic, Thin Slice, Kallo*	1 Cake/5g	17	0.1	372	8	78.7	2.8	5.1
Salted, Slightly, Thick Slice, Organic, Kallo*	1 Cake/8g	28	0.2	372	8	78.7	2.8	5.1
Sesame, No Added Salt, Thick Sliced, Organic, Kallo*	1 Cake/10g	37	0.3	373	8	78	3.2	5.4
Sesame, Toasted, Ryvita*	1 Pack/11g	43	0.5	391	8.4	78.4	4.9	3.5
Thin Slice, No Added Salt, Organic, Kallo*	1 Cake/5g	19	0.1	372	8	78.7	2.8	5.1
Wholegrain, No Added Salt, BGTY, Sainsbury's*	1 Cake/8g	30	0.2	372	8	78.7	2.8	5.1
RICE CRACKERS								
Barbecue, Sakata*	½ Pack/50g	204	1.3	407	7.3	85.2	2.6	1.6
Cracked Pepper, Sakata*	½ Pack/50g	200	1.5	400	7.3	84.4	3	2
Japanese Style, Mix, Asda*	1 Serving/25g	96	0.2	385	6.8	88	0.6	0.5
Japanese, Mini, Sunrise*	1 Serving/50g	180	0	360	7	83	0	7
Japanese, Philon*	1 Serving/20g	77	0.1	383	0.4	85.8	0.6	8.3
Lightly Salted, The Snack Organisation*	1 Serving/25g	100	0.9	401	6.9	85	3.6	0.9
Pretzel Mix, Tesco*	1 Serving/25g	108	3	432	18	61	12	3.8
Sainsbury's*	1 Serving/20g	87	1.9	433	11.2	74.3	9.4	1
Seaweed, Woolworths Homebrand*	12 Crackers/25g	100	0.7	398	7.3	85	2.7	0
Sour Cream & Chive, Sakata*	1 Serving/25g	107	2	430	7.8	80.6	7.9	0
Sweet Chilli, The Snack Organisation, Hansells Foods*	1 Serving/25g	106	1.7	424	7.1	83	6.8	1
Thai, M&S*	1 Serving/55g	209	1.8	380	7	80.2	3.3	1.2
Thai, Wakama*	1 Cracker/2g	8	0.1	400	6.9	86.9	2.7	0.5
Thin, Blue Dragon*	3 Crackers/5g	20	0.2	395	6.1	84.4	3.7	0
RICE PUDDING								
Jam, Fat Free, Aunt Bessie's*	¼ Pack/131g	136	0.3	104	2.4	23	0.2	0.6
50% Less Fat, Asda*	½ Can/212g	180	1.7	85	3.3	16.2	0.8	0.2
Apple Strudel Flavour Sauce, Muller Rice, Muller*	1 Pot/190g	205	4.4	108	3.2	18.6	2.3	0.4
Apple, Ambrosia*	1 Pot/150g	125	2.3	104	2.7	18.8	1.9	0.5
Banana Toffee (Limited Edition), Muller Rice, Muller*	1 Pot/190g	207	4.2	109	3.1	19.3	2.2	0.4
Canned, Average	***1oz/28g***	***25***	***0.7***	***89***	***3.4***	***14***	***2.5***	***0.2***
Canned, Basics, Sainsbury's*	½ Can/213g	157	1.7	74	3.1	13.7	0.8	1.4
Creamed, Canned, Ambrosia*	1 Can/425g	382	8.1	90	3.1	15.2	1.9	0
Creamed, Pot, Ambrosia*	1 Pot/150g	156	3.8	104	3.3	17	2.5	0.1
Creamed, Value, Tesco*	1 Can/425g	348	3.4	82	3.2	15.5	0.8	0
Creamed, with British Milk, Canned, Simply, M&S*	½ Can/200g	230	9.8	115	3.2	13.9	4.9	1.2
Creamy, Tesco*	1 Pudding/190g	278	14.1	146	2.3	17.5	7.4	0.1
Low Fat, Devon, Creamed, Ambrosia*	½ Can/213g	193	2.8	91	3.2	16.5	1.3	0
Low Fat, Tesco*	1 Can/425g	404	5.5	95	3.2	16.9	1.3	0.1
Original, Muller Rice, Muller*	1 Pot/190g	196	4.9	103	3.6	16.3	2.6	0.3
Pot, Ambrosia*	1 Pot/125g	126	3.1	101	3.3	16.3	2.5	0
Raspberry, Mullerice, Muller*	1 Pot/190g	201	4.4	106	3.2	18.2	2.3	0.5
Strawberry, Muller*	1 Pot/180g	191	4	106	3	18.6	2.2	0
Toffee, Smooth, Muller Rice, Muller*	1 Pot/190g	201	4.4	106	3.3	18	2.3	0.3
Vanilla Custard, Mullerrice, Muller*	1 Pot/200g	230	5	115	3.4	19.8	2.5	0.3
RICE WINE								
Sake, Average	***1 Tbsp/15ml***	***20***	***0***	***134***	***0.5***	***5***	***0***	***0***
RIGATONI								
Dry, Average	***1 Serving/80g***	***272***	***1.2***	***340***	***11.4***	***68.4***	***1.5***	***2.7***
RISOTTO								
Beetroot, & Goats Cheese, Lovely Vegetables, M&S*	1 Pack/379g	530	17	140	4.4	20.7	4.5	3.6
Butternut Squash, Fresh Ideas, M Kitchen, Morrisons*	1 Pot/350g	371	11.9	106	1.8	16.8	3.4	0.7
Butternut Squash, Italian Style, Aldi*	½ Pack/252g	323	12.6	128	2.6	17	5	1.6

R

INFO/WEIGHT	Measure	per Measure KCAL	FAT	Nutrition Values per 100g / 100ml KCAL	PROT	CARB	FAT	FIBRE

RISOTTO

	Measure INFO/WEIGHT	per Measure KCAL	FAT	KCAL	PROT	CARB	FAT	FIBRE
Cheese, Onion, & Wine, Rice & Simple, Ainsley Harriott*	1 Pack/140g	253	7	181	3.1	31	5	1.6
Chicken	*1 Serving/380g*	*494*	*17.4*	*130*	*7.2*	*15.2*	*4.6*	*1.3*
Chicken, & Lemon, Weight Watchers*	1 Pack/320g	353	6.3	107	6.3	15.8	1.9	0.7
Chicken, Mushroom, Finest, Tesco*	1 Pack/387g	472	17	122	7.3	12.7	4.4	1
Chicken, Mushroom, Meal for One, M&S*	1 Pack/400g	468	13.2	117	8.1	13.3	3.3	0.8
Chicken, Mushroom, Sainsbury's*	1 Pack/383g	387	11.1	101	6.3	11.9	2.9	1.3
Chicken, Chargrilled, Ready Meal, M&S*	1 Pack/365g	493	25.2	135	6.4	11.6	6.9	0.7
Green Bean, Asparagus Pecorino, Finest, Tesco*	1 Pack/400g	460	15.6	115	4.4	15	3.9	1.5
Haddock, Smoked, Finest, Tesco*	1 Pack/362g	399	9.8	110	7	14.1	2.7	0.7
Mushroom, HL, Tesco*	1 Pack/366g	339	8.3	93	3.4	14	2.3	1.4
Prawn, COU, M&S*	1 Pack/350g	378	7.7	108	4.3	17.3	2.2	0.8
Prawn, Pea & Mint, King, M&S*	½ Pack/300g	405	18.6	135	3.8	15.9	6.2	0.9
Red Pepper, & Italian Cheese, Roasted, M&S*	1 Pack/400g	500	13.2	125	2.9	20.4	3.3	1
Seafood, Youngs*	1 Pack/350g	424	13	121	4.5	17.4	3.7	0.1
Vegetable, Average	*1oz/28g*	*41*	*1.8*	*147*	*4.2*	*19.2*	*6.5*	*2.2*
Vegetable, Brown Rice, Average	*1oz/28g*	*40*	*1.8*	*143*	*4.1*	*18.6*	*6.4*	*2.4*

ROCK SALMON

Raw, Flesh Only, Average	*1oz/28g*	*43*	*2.7*	*154*	*16.6*	*0*	*9.7*	*0*

ROCKET

Fresh, Raw, Average	*1 Serving/80g*	*12*	*0.4*	*16*	*0.8*	*1.7*	*0.5*	*1.2*

ROE

Cod, Average	*1 Can/100g*	*96*	*2.8*	*96*	*17.1*	*0.5*	*2.8*	*0*
Cod, Hard, Coated in Batter, Fried	*1oz/28g*	*53*	*3.3*	*189*	*12.4*	*8.9*	*11.8*	*0.2*
Cod, Hard, Fried in Blended Oil	*1oz/28g*	*57*	*3.3*	*202*	*20.9*	*3*	*11.9*	*0.1*
Herring, Soft, Fried in Blended Oil	*1oz/28g*	*74*	*4.4*	*265*	*26.3*	*4.7*	*15.8*	*0.2*
Herring, Soft, Raw	*1oz/28g*	*22*	*0.1*	*78*	*18.2*	*0.5*	*0.4*	*0*

ROGAN JOSH

Chicken Breast, Chunks, Hot, Sainsbury's*	½ Pack/114g	143	2	126	23.6	3.9	1.8	1
Chicken with Pilau Rice, Farmfoods*	1 Pack/325g	354	6.8	109	5.3	17.1	2.1	0.4
Lamb, Indian, Takeaway, CBY, Asda*	½ Pack/200g	218	12	109	8	5.1	6	1.4
Lamb, Sainsbury's*	1 Pack/400g	660	44.4	165	11.3	4.9	11.1	1.9
Lamb, Takeaway, Tesco*	½ Pack/192g	228	14	119	6.3	5.7	7.3	2.5
Prawn, COU, M&S*	1 Pack/400g	360	2.4	90	4.9	16.2	0.6	0.8

ROLL

Beef, Roast Onion Mayo, Soft White, M&S*	1 Pack/215g	522	17.6	243	11.5	30	8.2	1.5
Cheese, & Onion, Asda*	1 Serving/67g	199	12	298	7	27	18	2
Cheese, & Onion, Co-Op*	1 Roll/66g	195	11.9	295	7	26	18	2
Cheese, & Onion, Iceland*	1 Roll/67g	222	13.6	332	7.5	29.6	20.4	1.5
Cheese, & Onion, M&S*	1 Roll/25g	80	5.1	320	9.6	24.7	20.5	1.3
Cheese, & Onion, Tesco*	1 Roll/67g	203	12.1	305	7.3	28	18.1	1.9
Cheese, & Pickle, Sainsbury's*	1 Roll/136g	359	13.6	264	10.6	35.1	10	0
Cheese, Onion, Frozen, Tesco*	1 Roll/12g	45	2.9	375	7.2	31.8	23.8	2.8
Cheese, Onion, Sainsbury's*	1 Roll/66g	190	9.8	288	6.9	30.6	14.8	2.5
Cheese, Tomato & Onion, Sainsbury's*	1 Pack/100g	518	28.1	518	18.4	47.9	28.1	0
Cheese, Tomato, Pickle, Cheese Topped Roll, M&S*	1 Roll/177g	480	26.4	271	10	22.8	14.9	2.8
Chicken, & Mayonnaise, Roast, Big, Sainsbury's*	1 Pack/185g	479	27.4	259	9.6	21.8	14.8	0
Chicken, & Salad, HE, Tesco*	1 Serving/224g	289	5.8	129	10.3	16	2.6	1.1
Chicken, & Salad, Mini, Selection Pack, British, M&S*	1 Roll/61g	134	4.1	220	11.9	28.1	6.8	2.1
Chicken, & Salad, Roast, Improved, Shapers, Boots*	1 Pack/188g	302	3.6	161	11	25	1.9	1.6
Cornish, in Pastry, Pork Farms*	1 Roll/75g	226	15.1	301	6.6	24.5	20.1	0
Egg Mayo, & Cress, Fullfillers*	1 Roll/125g	266	11.8	213	10	25.7	9.4	0
Egg Mayonnaise, & Cress, Sub, Delicious, Boots*	1 Pack/205g	399	14.1	195	10	23	6.9	2.4
Egg, & Cress, HL, Tesco*	1 Pack/175g	322	6.8	184	9.6	27.7	3.9	1.2

R

	Measure INFO/WEIGHT	per Measure KCAL	FAT	Nutrition Values per 100g / 100ml KCAL	PROT	CARB	FAT	FIBRE
ROLL								
Ham, & Cheese, Leicester, Sub, Waitrose*	1 Pack/206ml	582	31.2	282	12.6	24	15.1	13
Ham, & Egg Mayo, Smoked, Soft White Seeded, M&S*	1 Pack/190g	371	9.5	195	12.7	23.4	5	3
Ham, & Salad, BGTY, Sainsbury's*	1 Roll/178g	292	3.4	164	10.8	25.9	1.9	0
Ham, & Salad, J D Gross, Lidl*	1 Roll/154g	293	9.2	190	7.7	29.1	6	1.9
Ham, & Tomato, Taste!*	1 Serving/112g	211	4.8	188	10.4	27	4.3	0
Ham, Darwins Deli*	1 Serving/125g	298	7.5	238	11	37.4	6	0
Ploughman's, Large, Ginsters*	1 Pack/140g	473	33.5	338	10.2	20.5	23.9	1.8
Pork, Stuffing, & Apple Sauce, Roast, Boots*	1 Roll/218g	602	26.2	276	10	32	12	1.8
Salmon, Oak Smoked, M&S*	1 Roll/55g	139	6.2	252	14.6	23.1	11.3	1.2
Sausage, Lincolnshire, COU, M&S*	1 Roll/175g	280	4.7	160	10	23.2	2.7	2.6
Soya, Organic, Vegan, Clive's*	1 Roll/110g	375	21.4	341	6.5	32.6	19.5	0
Tuna Mayo, & Cucumber, Taste!*	1 Serving/111g	274	12.5	247	9	27.3	11.3	0
Tuna Mayonnaise, with Cucumber, Yummies*	1 Serving/132g	340	18.6	257	10.4	22.5	14	0
Tuna, & Cucumber, Seasoned Mayo, Soft Sub Roll, M&S*	1 Pack/216g	435	16.4	201	9.4	22.5	7.6	2.3
Tuna, & Sweetcorn, with Mayonnaise, Shell*	1 Pack/180g	536	26.3	298	13.1	28.6	14.6	0
Tuna, Cheese Melt, Boots*	1 Roll/199g	612	35.8	308	13	23	18	1.2
Turkey, Salad, Northern Bites*	1 Roll/231g	323	8.3	140	8.6	19.6	3.6	3
ROLO								
Chocolate, Nestle*	2 Pieces/20g	102	5.3	509	4.1	62.6	26.6	1.3
Little, Nestle*	1 Pack/40g	196	9.4	491	4	65.5	23.5	0.5
Nestle*	1 Sweet/5g	24	1	478	4.4	68.2	20.4	1.1
ROOT BEER								
Average	*1 Can/330ml*	*135*	*0*	*41*	*0*	*10.6*	*0*	*0*
ROSE WATER								
The English Provender Co.*	1 Tsp/5g	0	0	2	0.1	0.6	0.1	0.1
ROSEMARY								
Dried	*1 Tsp/1g*	*3*	*0.2*	*331*	*4.9*	*46.4*	*15.2*	*0*
Fresh	*1 Tsp/0.7g*	*1*	*0*	*99*	*1.4*	*13.5*	*4.4*	*0*
ROSTI								
Cheese, Onion, Tesco*	1 Rosti/92g	202	10.9	220	5.1	21.6	11.9	3.2
Maris Piper Onion, M&S*	1 Rosti/35g	77	4.2	219	1.9	24.7	12	2.4
Potato Root Vegetable, COU, M&S*	1 Rosti/100g	85	2.7	85	1.6	13.3	2.7	1.5
Potato Cakes, Baby, M&S*	1 Rosti/23g	40	1.5	175	3.5	25.1	6.7	1.6
Potato, McCain*	1 Rosti/95g	161	8.6	169	2.2	19.6	9.1	0
Potato, Mini, Party Bites, Sainsbury's*	1 Serving/100g	218	11.5	218	2.5	26.2	11.5	3
Sweet Potato, Tesco*	½ Pack/91g	258	16	283	2.7	26.2	17.6	4.4
Vegetable, Waitrose*	1 Pack/400g	248	9.2	62	1.4	8.8	2.3	1.3
ROULADE								
Black Forest, Finest, Tesco*	1/8 Roulade/74g	206	6.5	280	3.2	46.4	8.8	1
Chocolate, Finest, Tesco*	1 Serving/80g	222	4.5	277	3.4	53.2	5.6	2.3
Chocolate, Sainsbury's*	1 Serving/72g	264	15.7	367	5.7	36.9	21.8	1.8
Passion Fruit, M&S*	1oz/28g	83	2.6	295	2.8	50	9.2	0.2
Raspberry, Finest, Tesco*	1/6 Roulade/75g	220	9.2	295	2.7	41.5	12.4	2.7
RUM								
37.5% Volume	*1 Pub Shot/35ml*	*72*	*0*	*207*	*0*	*0*	*0*	*0*
40% Volume	*1 Pub Shot/35ml*	*78*	*0*	*222*	*0*	*0*	*0*	*0*
Captain Morgans Cola, Premixed, Canned, Diageo*	1 Can/250ml	180	0	72	0	9.1	0	0
Malibu, 21% Volume, Pernod Ricard*	1 Pub shot/25ml	50	0	200	0	29	0	0
White	*1 Pub Shot/35ml*	*72*	*0*	*207*	*0*	*0*	*0*	*0*

R

INFO/WEIGHT	Measure	per Measure KCAL	FAT	Nutrition Values per 100g / 100ml KCAL	PROT	CARB	FAT	FIBRE

SAAG

	Measure INFO/WEIGHT	KCAL	FAT	KCAL	PROT	CARB	FAT	FIBRE
Aloo, M&S*	½ Pack/125g	121	7.1	97	1.6	8.7	5.7	2.1
Chicken, Microwaved, Slimming World, Iceland*	1 Pack/500g	395	8	79	11.5	3.9	1.6	1.6
Paneer, Sainsbury's*	1 Pack/300g	441	32.7	147	7.1	3.9	10.9	2.5
SAFFRON								
Average	*1 Tsp/1g*	*2*	*0*	*310*	*11.4*	*61.5*	*5.9*	*0*
SAGE								
Dried, Ground	*1 Tsp/1g*	*3*	*0.1*	*315*	*10.6*	*42.7*	*12.7*	*0*
Fresh	*1oz/28g*	*33*	*1.3*	*119*	*3.9*	*15.6*	*4.6*	*0*
SAGO								
Raw	*1oz/28g*	*99*	*0.1*	*355*	*0.2*	*94*	*0.2*	*0.5*
SALAD								
American, Style, Sweet & Crispy, Morrisons*	1 Serving/25g	7	0.1	28	1.2	4.2	0.3	2
Avocado, & Egg, Nourish Bowl, M&S*	1 Pack/285g	333	15.4	117	6.3	6.6	5.4	8.3
Avocado, & Feta, & Rice, Good to Go, Waitrose*	1 Pack/240g	350	13.4	146	3.4	18.4	5.6	4.1
Avocado, & Feta, Gourmet To Go, M&S*	1 Pack/320g	512	32	160	5.4	12.1	10	3.1
Baby Leaf, & Beetroot, Bistro, M&S*	1 Pack/165g	41	0	25	2	3.6	0	2
Baby Leaf, & Herb, Asda*	1 Serving/50g	7	0.1	14	2.3	0.7	0.2	2.4
Baby Leaf, Rocket, Florette*	1 Serving/25g	5	0.1	20	2.1	0.9	0.5	2
Baby Leaf, Aldi*	1 Serving/50g	11	0	22	3.5	1	0.1	1.5
Baby Leaf, Asda*	1 Serving/80g	10	0.2	12	2.1	0.2	0.3	1.7
Baby Leaf, Florette*	1 Serving/40g	5	0.1	12	2	0.4	0.3	1
Baby Leaf, Italian Style, M&S*	1 Serving/55g	11	0.3	20	1.3	2.3	0.5	1.3
Baby Leaf, Mild, Seasonal, Tesco*	½ Pack/42g	9	0.3	21	1.5	1.6	0.6	1.8
Baby Leaf, Seasonal, Morrisons*	½ Pack/50g	10	0.3	21	1.4	1.6	0.6	1.8
Baby Leaf, Sweet, Seasonal, M&S*	½ Bag/60g	9	0.2	15	2.4	0.6	0.4	1.8
Baby Leaf, with Watercress, Tesco*	1 Serving/30g	6	0.2	19	1.8	1.3	0.7	1.8
Bag, Tesco*	1 Serving/200g	38	0.8	19	0.9	3	0.4	1.4
Bean, 3, Sainsbury's*	1 Tub/270g	281	6.2	104	7.1	13.6	2.3	5.9
Bean, 3, with Mint Vinaigrette, Spirit of Summer, M&S*	1 Pack/250g	250	6	100	5.9	8.2	2.4	11.1
Bean, Four, Sainsbury's*	½ Pot/125g	121	3.2	107	6.6	11.5	2.8	4.8
Bean, Minty, Asda*	½ Pack/150g	154	4	103	6	9.8	2.7	7.9
Bean, Mixed, in Water, Drained, Essential, Waitrose*	1 Serving/80g	78	0.6	97	6.5	12.9	0.8	6.2
Bean, Three, with Mint Vinaigrette, M&S*	1 Pack/250g	250	6	100	5.9	8.2	2.4	11.1
Beetroot, & Feta, Veggie Pot, Eat Well, M&S*	1 Pot/140g	182	10.5	130	4.4	8.9	7.5	4.7
Beetroot, & Lettuce, Asda*	1 Serving/30g	5	0	16	1.4	2.7	0	2.5
Beetroot, Goats Cheese, Mixed Grain, Morrisons*	½ Pack/125g	165	4.5	132	5.5	16.4	3.6	5.8
Beetroot, Co-Op*	1 Pack/250g	100	0.8	40	0.9	8	0.3	2
Beetroot, Morrisons*	1 Tsp/10g	6	0.1	62	0.8	10.5	1.3	2.3
Beetroot, Roast with Quinoa Feta, Tesco*	1 Pack/250g	310	12.3	124	5.3	13.1	4.9	3.1
Beetroot, Squash, & Feta, Superbowl	*1 Bowl/266g*	*343*	*14.6*	*129*	*6.7*	*11.4*	*5.5*	*2.7*
Bistro, Asda*	1 Serving/180g	29	0	16	1.4	2.7	0	2.5
Broccoli, & Peanut, Finest, Tesco*	½ Pack/105g	196	9.2	187	6.9	18.4	8.8	3.3
Broccoli, Kale, & Quinoa, Tenderstem, Side, Waitrose*	1 Pack/165g	173	7.6	105	6.9	6.8	4.6	4.2
Bulgur Wheat, Lentil, & Edamame Shaker, Waitrose*	1 Pack/190g	217	10.6	114	4.7	11.1	5.6	4.4
Burrito, BBQ, Bowl, Allplants*	½ Pack/380g	543	12.2	143	4.2	21	3.2	5.3
Butternut Falafel, Rainbow Grains, Houmous, Asda*	1 Pack/235g	268	13.2	114	3.1	12	5.6	2.3
Caesar	*1 Serving/200g*	*352*	*27.8*	*176*	*4.8*	*8.1*	*13.9*	*0.7*
Caesar, Chicken, Fresh, Sainsbury's*	1 Serving/200g	278	20	139	6	6.2	10	1.2
Caesar, Chicken, Shapers, Boots*	1 Pack/200g	205	5.8	102	8.2	10	2.9	1
Caesar, Kit, Asda*	½ Pack/113g	154	9	136	5	11	8	1.4
Caesar, Kit, Tesco*	1 Pack/262g	404	31.7	154	3.4	7.3	12.1	1.2
Caesar, Kit, Waitrose*	1 Bag/250g	436	36.1	174	4.4	6.1	14.4	1.3
Caesar, Morrisons*	½ Pack/100g	136	10.1	136	4.7	6.1	10.1	1.2

S

SALAD

INFO/WEIGHT	Measure	per Measure		Nutrition Values per 100g / 100ml				
		KCAL	FAT	KCAL	PROT	CARB	FAT	FIBRE
Caesar, Roast Chicken, Bacon, High Protein, M&S*	1 Pack/220g	187	7	85	11.9	1.9	3.2	0.6
Caesar, with Dressing, Croutons & Parmesan, M&S*	1 Serving/115g	190	15.5	165	4.3	6.4	13.5	1.4
Caesar, with Parmigiano Reggiano, Tesco*	1 Bag/275g	552	49	201	4.1	5.8	17.8	1.3
Carrot, & Beetroot, with a Balsamic Dressing, Asda*	1 Pack/160g	101	6.6	63	0.9	5.6	4.1	1
Carrot, Pumpkin Seed, Bites, Eat Well, M&S*	1 Pack/220g	275	14.5	125	7.9	5.3	6.6	6.5
Celeriac, Delhaize*	¼ Jar/45g	80	7.4	177	3.3	3.1	16.5	1.5
Cheese, Layered, M&S*	½ Pack/230g	300	20.5	130	4.6	9.3	8.9	1.2
Cheese, Ploughman's, Asda*	1 Bowl/300g	246	10.8	82	3.6	8.9	3.6	1
Chick Pea, & Butter Bean, & Tomato, Chilli, Tesco*	1 Pack/130g	146	6	112	3.4	14.3	4.6	0.5
Chicken, & Coleslaw, Roast, Boots*	1 Serving/245g	392	34.3	160	4.5	3.9	14	1.3
Chicken, & Edamame, & Peanut Drizzle, Protein Pot, M&S*	1 Pot/130g	191	9.8	147	14.2	3.5	7.5	4.5
Chicken, & Noodle, Sweet Chilli, Shapers, Boots*	1 Pack/197g	266	5.1	135	12	16	2.6	0.9
Chicken, & Noodle, Sweet, Aldi*	1 Serving/295g	362	9.4	123	6.7	16	3.2	18
Chicken, Basil, with Peas, Broad Beans, M&S*	1 Pack/215g	228	11	106	5.3	1.5	5.1	0.8
Chicken, Chargrilled, Wholefood, M&S*	1 Pot/219g	230	4.2	105	10.1	11.6	1.9	4.8
Chickpea, Bean, Green White, Good Health, Waitrose*	1 Pack/180g	203	6.5	113	4.8	12.8	3.6	4.9
Classic, Asda*	1 Pack/185g	43	1.5	23	1	2.4	0.8	1.1
Cous Cous, & Pepper, Sweety Drop, Asda*	½ Pack/140g	162	0.7	116	4.2	22	0.5	2.8
Cous Cous, & Vegetable, Roasted, Waitrose*	1 Pack/220g	396	13.4	180	5.1	26.1	6.1	1.2
Crisp, Mixed, Morrisons*	1 Pack/230g	39	0.7	17	1	2.8	0.3	0
Crisp, Mixed, Tesco*	1 Pack/200g	40	0.6	20	1.1	3.2	0.3	2
Crispy, Co-Op*	1 Serving/80g	13	0.2	16	0.8	3	0.3	1
Crispy, Florette*	1 Portion/100g	22	0.3	22	1.5	3.4	0.3	3
Crunchy, & Crisp, Asda*	1 Pack/250g	55	1.5	22	0.8	3.3	0.6	1.4
Crunchy, Mini, Co-Op*	1 Pack/80g	16	0.4	20	1	2.5	0.5	1.7
Duck, & Herb, Crispy, M&S*	½ Pack/140g	378	25.6	270	20.7	3.7	18.3	1.4
Edamame, & Black Rice, Nourish Bowl, Eat Well, M&S*	1 Pack/295g	395	16.2	134	5.6	12.8	5.5	5.3
Edamame, & Petit Pois, Finest, Tesco*	½ Pack/100g	108	4.3	108	6	9.3	4.3	3.9
Edamame, Butter Bean, TTD, Sainsbury's*	½ Pot/93g	112	4.5	121	6.5	11	4.9	3.5
Edamame, Feta, High Protein, M&S*	1 Pack/215g	209	9	97	7.5	5.1	4.2	4.3
Edamame, Miso Cauliflower, Crush , Finest, Tesco*	½ Pack/95g	118	7.6	125	3.2	7	8	5.9
Edamame, Asda*	½ Pack/110g	90	3.3	82	5.9	4.8	3	5.9
Egg, & Ham, with Salad Cream Dressing, M&S*	1 Pack/240g	149	7.2	62	4.9	3.2	3	1.2
Egg, & Spinach, Baby, Waitrose*	1 Pack/215g	167	13.5	78	3.5	1.8	6.3	1
Egg, & Spinach, Protein Pot, Free Range, M&S*	1 Pot/105g	152	10.7	145	12.1	1.1	10.2	0.1
Egg, Avocado, & Quinoa, & Soy Sauce, Protein Pot, M&S*	1 Pot/140g	185	8.1	132	7.2	11.1	5.8	3.5
Egg, Surimi, Daunat*	1 Pack/250g	255	18.8	102	4.1	3.7	7.5	0
English Garden, Tesco*	1 Serving/180g	22	0.4	12	0.7	1.8	0.2	0.7
Falafel, Bulgur Wheat Houmous, Eat Well, M&S*	1 Pack/300g	375	15.3	125	4.1	13.2	5.1	4.8
Feta, & Sunblushed Tomato, M&S*	1 Serving/190g	361	21.1	190	5.5	17.2	11.1	2.1
Fine Cut, Asda*	1 Serving/100g	24	0.3	24	1.2	4.3	0.3	2.3
Greek	*1oz/28g*	*36*	*3.5*	*130*	*2.7*	*1.9*	*12.5*	*0.8*
Greek, Style, Bowl, M&S*	1 Bowl/223g	212	18.3	95	2.5	2.4	8.2	0.7
Greek, Style, Feta, Tip & Mix, M&S*	1 Pack/195g	214	18.3	110	4	2.5	9.4	1.6
Green Bean, Aldi*	½ Pack/80g	62	2.7	77	4.6	5	3.4	3.9
Green, Average	*1oz/28g*	*4*	*0.1*	*13*	*0.8*	*1.8*	*0.3*	*0.9*
Green, Complete, Sainsbury's*	1/3 Pack/55g	92	6.7	168	4.2	10.3	12.2	1.4
Green, Mixed, Average	*1 Serving/100g*	*12*	*0.3*	*12*	*0.7*	*1.8*	*0.3*	*1*
Green, Side, M&S*	1 Serving/200g	30	0.4	15	0.9	2.5	0.2	0
Ham, & Egg, Free Range, Good & Balanced, Asda*	1 Pack/265g	148	6.3	56	5.3	2.8	2.4	0.9
Ham, & Egg, with Salad Cream, Sainsbury's*	1 Pack/240g	216	14.1	90	4.8	4	5.9	1
Ham, Hock, Waitrose*	1 Pack/350g	245	9.5	70	6.6	4.8	2.7	2
House, Tesco*	½ Pack/60g	18	0.4	30	1.7	3.5	0.6	2.1

S

SALAD

INFO/WEIGHT	Measure	per Measure		Nutrition Values per 100g / 100ml				
		KCAL	FAT	KCAL	PROT	CARB	FAT	FIBRE
Italian, Tomatoes, Balsamic, & Italian Cheese, Sainsbury's*	½ Pack/80g	56	3.6	70	3.3	3.6	4.5	0.8
Large, Bowl, Sainsbury's*	1/6 Pack/52g	12	0.2	23	0.9	4.3	0.3	1.1
Lentil, Sprout, Toppers, Good4U*	1 Serving/30g	44	0.1	146	12	20	0.2	8.9
Lettuce, Lambs, Pea Shoot, Good Health, Waitrose*	1 Bag/100g	21	0.5	21	1.9	1.3	0.5	1.7
Mediterranean, Bowl, Sainsbury's*	½ Pack/71g	17	0.4	24	1.2	3.9	0.5	1.1
Mediterranean, Style, Asda*	½ Pack/135g	22	0	16	1	3	0	0
Mixed Grains, Chipotle, Tesco*	1 Pack/250g	348	4.5	139	5	22.4	1.8	6.5
Mixed Leaf, Essential, Waitrose*	1 Serving/30g	5	0.2	17	1	2	0.7	1.4
Mixed Leaf, Medley, Waitrose*	1 Serving/25g	4	0.1	15	0.8	1.7	0.5	1.4
Mixed Leaf, Spar*	1 Serving/20g	4	0	20	1.3	2.9	0.2	0.9
Mixed Leaf, Tesco*	1 Serving/20g	3	0.1	14	0.9	1.6	0.4	0.9
Mixed Leaf, Tomato & Olive, Tesco*	1 Serving/170g	150	13.3	88	1	3.4	7.8	2
Mixed Leaf, with Beetroot, Earthy, Waitrose*	1 Bag/140g	34	0.6	24	1.5	3.6	0.4	2.1
Mixed, Bowl, Waitrose*	¼ Pack/64g	9	0.3	14	0.8	1.6	0.5	1.4
Mixed, Crispy, Nightingale, Tesco*	½ Pack/60g	11	0.1	19	1.5	1.7	0.2	2.2
Mixed, Green Leaf, Lasting Leaf*	1 Serving/69g	12	0.3	17	0.8	1.8	0.4	1.5
Mixed, Medley, Bowl, Waitrose*	¼ Pack/60g	9	0.3	15	0.9	1.7	0.5	1
Mixed, Sweet & Crispy, Tesco*	1 Serving/200g	48	0.6	24	1	4.2	0.3	2
Mixed, Sweet Crunchy, Lasting Leaf*	1 Serving/62g	15	0.2	24	0.8	3.6	0.3	1.9
Moroccan, Mouthwatering, Jamie Oliver*	1 Portion/125g	211	6.5	169	5.5	21.7	5.2	6.6
New Potato, Tomato, & Egg with Salad Cream, M&S*	1 Pack/300g	165	7.2	55	2.9	5.4	2.4	1.3
New Potato, Tuna, & Egg, M&S*	1 Pack/340g	255	12.9	75	3.8	6.7	3.8	0.7
Nut, & Grain, Aldi*	½ Pack/100g	138	5.1	138	6	14	5.1	5.9
Pasta, Mediterranean Orzo, Love Life, Waitrose*	1 Pack/220g	299	10.8	136	3.9	19	4.9	3.2
Pea Shoot, & Baby Leaves, Steve's Leaves*	1 Pack/60g	14	0.4	24	2.7	2	0.6	2
Pea Shoot, Baby Cos & Batavia Lettuce, Bagged, M&S*	1 Bag/120g	24	0.6	20	2.6	0.8	0.5	2.3
Prawn, & Avocado, M&S*	1 Serving/240g	254	16.3	106	3	2	6.8	3.1
Prawn, Avocado, with Marie Rose Sauce, Waitrose*	1 Pack/240g	334	18.5	139	4.4	11.1	7.7	3.8
Prawn, Cocktail, Tesco*	1 Pack/300g	360	18	120	5.7	10.9	6	0.8
Prawn, Layer, Eat Well, M&S*	1 Pack/220g	205	8.2	93	4.1	10.5	3.7	0.6
Prawn, Layered, Co-Op*	1 Pack/300g	375	18	125	4	14	6	2
Prawn, Layered, M&S*	1 Pack/455g	410	17.7	90	4.5	8.9	3.9	1.2
Quinoa, & Avocado, Chipotle, Finest, Tesco*	½ Pack/113g	151	7	135	2.4	16.1	6.3	2
Quinoa, Supergreen, Eat Well, M&S*	1 Pack/180g	180	10.4	100	4.3	5	5.8	5.3
Quinoa, Tomato, Red Pepper, & Mango, Lidl*	1 Pot/210g	191	4.2	91	2.6	14.1	2	2.5
Rainbow, Morrisons*	½ Bowl/72g	20	0.1	27	1.4	3.7	0.2	2.5
Rocket, & Parmesan, Wild, Italian, Sainsbury's*	1 Serving/50g	88	7.4	177	7.5	3.4	14.8	0.5
Salmon, Moroccan Style, Light Lunch, John West*	1 Pack/220g	299	11.7	136	11.7	8.8	5.3	3.4
Side, Garden, with Cherry Tomatoes, Waitrose*	1 Pack/170g	25	0.7	15	0.8	2	0.4	1.3
Simple, Bowl, Tesco*	1 Bowl/135g	32	0.4	24	1.3	2.9	0.3	2.1
Slaw, Rainbow, Wicked Kitchen, Tesco*	½ Pack/75g	60	3.2	80	2	7.3	4.3	2.1
Spicy Mix, Fresh Naked *	1 Serving/45g	7	0.2	16	2.7	0.4	0.4	1.5
Sweet & Crispy, M&S*	1 Serving/140g	49	1.4	35	1.7	4.7	1	1.6
Sweet & Crispy, Side, Sainsbury's*	¼ Bag/93g	23	0.2	25	1.3	4.4	0.2	2.2
Sweet Crunchy, Bowl, Sainsbury's*	¼ Pack	42	0.6	49	1.6	8.2	0.7	2
Sweet Crunchy, Mixed, Prepared, Co-Op*	1 Serving/120g	42	0.4	35	1.1	5.9	0.3	1.8
Sweet Crunchy, Side, Eat Well, M&S*	1 Pack/145g	48	0.9	33	1.5	4.3	0.6	2.3
Sweet Leaf, Fully Prepared, Fresh, Sainsbury's*	¼ Pack/75g	12	0.1	16	0.8	3	0.1	2.1
Sweet Leaf, Nightingale Farms, Tesco*	½ Bag/130g	31	0.3	24	1	3.6	0.2	1.8
Sweet Potato, & Red Pepper, Deli, M&S*	1 Serving/250g	113	5.6	45	0.8	5.6	2.2	0.9
Tomato, & Onion	**1oz/28g**	**20**	**1.7**	**72**	**0.8**	**4**	**6.1**	**1**
Tomato, Cherry, Tesco*	1 Pack/210g	136	9.4	65	0.9	4.2	4.5	1.1
Tuna, Bowl, Fresh, Asda*	1 Serving/160g	184	11.2	115	8	5	7	0

	Measure INFO/WEIGHT	per Measure KCAL	FAT	Nutrition Values per 100g / 100ml KCAL	PROT	CARB	FAT	FIBRE
SALAD								
Tuna, French Style, Light Lunch, John West*	1 Pack/220g	218	6.2	99	7.5	9.8	2.8	2.5
Tuna, Italian Style, Light Lunch, John West*	1 Pack/220g	205	5.7	93	7.3	9.8	2.6	0.5
Tuna, Mediterranean Inspired, Tesco*	1 Pack/220g	200	2	91	8.5	10.5	0.9	3.4
Tuna, Mediterranean Style, Light Lunch, John West*	1 Pack/220g	211	4.2	96	8.5	10	1.9	2.4
Tuna, Mediterranean Style, Nixe, Lidl*	1 Pack/220g	254	5.5	116	10	12	2.5	2.8
Tuna, Mexican Style, Nixe, Lidl*	1 Tub/220g	293	11	133	11	9.4	5	3
Tuna, Nicoise, No Mayonnaise, Shapers, Boots*	1 Pack/276g	133	3.6	48	4	5	1.3	0.8
Tuna, Nicoise, Tesco*	1 Pack/240g	392	29	163	6.2	6.8	12.1	1.2
Vegetable, Mixed, without Dressing, From Restaurant	*1 ½ Cups/207g*	*33*	*0.1*	*16*	*1.2*	*3.2*	*0.1*	*2.1*
Waldorf, Average	*1 Serving/100g*	*193*	*17.7*	*193*	*1.4*	*7.5*	*17.7*	*1.3*
Watercress, Spinach Rocket, Prepared , Tesco*	½ Pack/40g	10	0.3	26	2.5	1.1	0.8	2
Watercress, Spinach Rocket, Waitrose*	1 Bag/145g	30	1.2	21	2.2	1.2	0.8	1.5
Wholefood, Super, Creamy Lemon & Mint Dressing, M&S*	1 Pack/290g	371	10.2	128	9.8	9.1	3.5	10.3
SALAD CREAM								
Average	*1 Tsp/5g*	*17*	*1.4*	*335*	*1.7*	*18.6*	*27.8*	*0.1*
Free From, Tesco*	1 Tbsp/15g	35	2.6	232	0.3	18.8	17.2	0.5
Reduced Calorie, Average	*1 Tsp/5g*	*6*	*0.4*	*130*	*1*	*12.9*	*7.9*	*0.2*
SALAMI								
Average	*1 Slice/5g*	*18*	*1.3*	*360*	*28.4*	*1.8*	*26.2*	*0*
Danish, Average	*1 Serving/17g*	*89*	*8.8*	*524*	*13.2*	*1.3*	*51.7*	*0*
German, Average	*1 Serving/60g*	*200*	*16.4*	*333*	*20.3*	*1.6*	*27.3*	*0.1*
German, Peppered, Average	*3 Slices/25g*	*86*	*6.8*	*342*	*22.2*	*2.5*	*27.1*	*0.2*
Healthy Range, Average	*4 Slices/25g*	*55*	*3.6*	*220*	*22.4*	*0.6*	*14.3*	*0*
Milano, Average	*1 Serving/70g*	*278*	*22.6*	*397*	*25.9*	*0.9*	*32.2*	*0*
Napoli, Average	*1 Slice/5g*	*17*	*1.3*	*342*	*27.1*	*0.8*	*25.5*	*0*
SALMON								
Cooked, Prepacked, Average	*1 Fillet/93g*	*180*	*11.1*	*194*	*21.8*	*0*	*11.9*	*0*
Fillets ,Soft Cheese, Pea & Mint, & Puff Pastry, Waitrose*	1 Serving/114g	233	14.2	204	18.3	4	12.5	1.1
Fillets, & Sweet Chilli Sauce, Simply Steam, Youngs*	1 Pack/258g	299	6.2	116	9.7	13.4	2.4	1
Fillets, Alaskan, Wild, Sockeye, 1, Waitrose*	1 Serving/101g	162	6.5	160	25.3	0.1	6.4	0.6
Fillets, Black Pepper, Kiln Roasted, Fishmonger, Aldi*	1 Fillet/93g	226	15.8	243	22	0.5	17	0.5
Fillets, Boneless, Scottish, Oven Cooked, Waitrose*	1 Serving/93g	166	8.8	178	23.4	0	9.4	0
Fillets, Hot Smoked, with Teriyaki, Good Health, Waitrose*	1 Fillet/71g	165	8.9	233	26.2	4	12.5	0
Fillets, in Teriyaki Marinade, Good Health, Waitrose*	1 Fillet/91g	176	9.2	193	23	2.1	10.1	0.9
Fillets, in Thai Marinade, Good Health, Waitrose*	1 Fillet/98g	185	10.3	188	22.1	1	10.5	0.6
Fillets, Lemon Dill Sauce, Pink, Inspirations, Birds Eye*	1 Fillet/225g	349	20.5	155	17.9	0.3	9.1	0.1
Fillets, Lemon Herb, Poached, Skinless, Scottish, Waitrose*	1 Fillet/79g	159	10.1	201	21.4	0.1	12.8	0.1
Fillets, Lightly Smoked, Scottish, Good Health, Waitrose*	1 Serving/95g	170	8.6	179	24.1	0	9.1	0
Fillets, Lightly Smoked, Scottish, Waitrose*	1 Serving/175g	382	26.6	218	18.7	1.3	15.2	0.6
Fillets, Orkney, Whole, Organic, Duchy Originals, Waitrose*	1 Serving/140g	224	11.1	160	22.2	0	7.9	0
Fillets, Poached , Sainsbury's*	1 Fillet/90g	218	15.4	242	20.9	0.9	17.1	0.5
Fillets, Prime, Scottish, As Prepared, 1, Waitrose*	1 Serving/107g	222	14	207	22.4	0	13.1	0
Fillets, Raw, Average	*1 Sm Fillet/120g*	*227*	*14*	*189*	*20.9*	*0.1*	*11.7*	*0.1*
Fillets, Skin On, Boneless, Individual, Sainsbury's*	1 Fillet/97g	259	19.4	267	21.5	0.4	20	0.4
Fillets, Skin On, TTD, Sainsbury's*	1 Fillet/126g	249	14.3	197	23.5	0.2	11.3	0
Fillets, Skinless, Scottish, Prime, As Sold, Waitrose*	1 Serving/100g	212	14.8	212	19.6	0.2	14.8	0
Fillets, Sweet Chilli, Hot Smoked, Ready to Eat, Tesco*	1 Fillet/90g	211	12.4	234	22.7	4.6	13.8	0.4
Fillets, Wild Alaskan, Keta, Sainsbury's*	1 Fillet/115g	178	6.4	155	25.9	0.2	5.6	0.3
Fillets, Wild, Sockeye, TTD, Sainsbury's*	1 Fillet/104g	198	10.2	191	25.5	0.5	9.8	0.5
Fillets, with Garlic & Rosemary, As Sold, Waitrose*	1 Serving/175g	405	28.9	231	19	1.7	16.5	0
Fillets, with Lemon Garlic Butter, Easy to Cook, Waitrose*	½ Pack/92g	196	11.9	214	21.4	2.6	13	0.6
Fillets, with Pesto, Scottish, Easy to Cook, Waitrose*	1 Serving/92g	199	12.1	216	23.5	0.5	13.1	0.7
Flakes, Honey Roast, Average	*1oz/28g*	*56*	*3*	*198*	*24*	*1.9*	*10.7*	*0.2*

S

	Measure INFO/WEIGHT	per Measure KCAL	per Measure FAT	Nutrition Values per 100g / 100ml KCAL	PROT	CARB	FAT	FIBRE
SALMON								
Flakes, Hot Smoked, with Honey, Tesco*	½ Pack/50g	104	5	208	22.8	6.3	10.1	0.5
Flakes, Sweet Chilli, M&S*	½ Pack/70g	143	4.6	204	24.5	11.7	6.6	0.6
Goujons, Average	*1 Pack/150g*	*321*	*16.4*	*214*	*16.4*	*12.4*	*11*	*1.1*
Gravadlax with Mustard Sauce, Waitrose*	1 Pack/200g	382	22.2	191	21.8	1	11.1	0.4
Gravadlax, Cured with Salt, Sugar Herbs	*1 Serving/100g*	*119*	*3.3*	*119*	*18.3*	*3.1*	*3.3*	*0.4*
Grilled	*1oz/28g*	*60*	*3.7*	*215*	*24.2*	*0*	*13.1*	*0*
Hot Smoked, Average	*1 Serving/62g*	*103*	*4.4*	*166*	*24*	*0.9*	*7.2*	*0.1*
in Watercress Sauce, with Potatoes, Tesco*	1 Pack/399g	342	12.5	86	8.9	5	3.1	0.9
Mild Oak Smoked, Average	*1 Slice/25g*	*46*	*2.5*	*182*	*22.6*	*0.1*	*10.2*	*0*
Mousse, Tesco*	1 Mousse/57g	100	7	177	13.5	2.9	12.4	0.2
Pink in Brine, Average	*1 Sm Can/105g*	*129*	*5.5*	*122*	*18.8*	*0*	*5.3*	*0*
Pink, Canned, Average	*1 Serving/125g*	*162*	*7.2*	*130*	*19.5*	*0.1*	*5.8*	*0.1*
Poached, Average	*1 Serving/90g*	*176*	*10.5*	*195*	*22.5*	*0.2*	*11.7*	*0.3*
Portions, Lemon Pepper, Fish of the Day, Iceland*	1 Portion/130g	281	18.3	216	22.2	0	14.1	0
Red in Brine, Average	*1oz/28g*	*42*	*2.2*	*149*	*19.7*	*0*	*7.8*	*0*
Red, Average	*½ Can/90g*	*141*	*7.4*	*156*	*20.4*	*0.1*	*8.2*	*0.1*
Skewers, Teriyaki, Sweet, M&S*	1 Skewer/48g	96	5.9	201	17.1	5.8	12.2	0
Smoked, Average	*1 Serving/70g*	*126*	*7*	*179*	*21.9*	*0.5*	*10*	*0.1*
Smoked, Juniper & Birch, TTD, Sainsbury's*	½ Pack/60g	132	8.4	220	23.3	0.3	14	0.1
Smoked, Trimmings, Average	*1 Serving/55g*	*101*	*5.7*	*184*	*22.8*	*0.2*	*10.3*	*0*
Steaks	*1 Serving/100g*	*180*	*11*	*180*	*20.2*	*0*	*11*	*0*
Steamed	*1oz/28g*	*55*	*3.6*	*197*	*20.1*	*0*	*13*	*0*
Teriyaki, Jasmine Rice, Charlie Bigham's*	½ Pack/400g	608	10.8	152	7.1	25.5	2.7	0
SALMON EN CROUTE								
Frozen, Tesco*	1 Serving/166g	365	18.4	220	10.1	19.1	11.1	1.1
Retail, Average	*1oz/28g*	*81*	*5.3*	*288*	*11.8*	*18*	*19.1*	*0*
SALMON IN								
Lime & Coriander, Fillets, Good Choice, Iceland*	½ Pack/150g	189	4.4	126	19.8	5.1	2.9	0.8
Tomato Mascarpone Sauce, Fillets, Asda*	½ Pack/181g	279	19.9	154	13	0.8	11	0.6
White Wine & Cream Sauce, Tesco*	1 Serving/170g	279	19.2	164	13.5	2	11.3	1.2
SALMON WITH								
Garlic Herb Butter, Tesco*	1 Fillet/112g	291	23.1	260	17.6	0	20.6	0
Giant Cous Cous Lentils, Creations, John West*	1 Pack/180g	297	15.5	165	7.6	13	8.6	2.5
Scottish Lochmuir with Soy Ginger, Fuller Longer, M&S*	1 Pack/360g	415	18	115	8	7.8	5	3.1
SALSA								
Chunky, Sainsbury's*	½ Pot/84g	43	1.4	51	1.1	7.8	1.7	1.2
Mango, Habanero, Hot, Tostitos*	1 Tbsp/15g	8	0.1	56	0.3	12.5	0.4	0.6
Mediterranean, with Roasted Aubergine, Sabra*	1 Serving/30g	58	4.9	192	2	9.2	16.3	1.7
Medium Hot, Discovery*	1 Serving/30g	17	0.1	56	1.4	11.7	0.4	0.8
Mild, Original, Old El Paso*	1 Sachet/144g	60	0.7	42	1.6	9	0.5	0
Original from Dinner Kit, Old El Paso*	1 Jar/226g	71	0.7	32	1.2	6	0.3	0
Pineapple, Chipotle, Stonewall Kitchen*	1 Tbsp/15g	10	0	67	0	16.7	0	0
Red, Medium, M&S*	¼ Jar/49g	34	1.5	69	1.4	8.3	3	1.8
Spicy Mango & Lime, Morrisons*	½ Pot/85g	62	0.3	73	1	15.9	0.4	1.3
Spicy Red Pepper, Fresh, Waitrose*	½ Pot/85g	27	0.8	32	1.9	4.1	0.9	1.6
Tomato, Chunky, Tesco*	1 Pot/170g	68	2.2	40	1.1	5.9	1.3	1.1
Tomato, Cool, Asda*	1 Pot/215g	84	1.1	39	1.4	6.4	0.5	1.5
Tomato, Onion, Coriander & Chilli, Fresh, Waitrose*	1 Tub/170g	110	5.3	65	1.3	8	3.1	1.2
Tomato, Sun Ripened, Tesco*	1 Serving/40g	46	1.7	115	5	14.2	4.2	4.6
Tomato, with Coriander Garlic, Sainsbury's*	1 Serving/50g	31	0.9	62	1	9.9	1.8	1.2
SALT								
Alternative, Reduced Sodium, Losalt*	½ Tsp/1g	0	0	0	0	0	0	0
Rock, Average	*¼ Tsp/1g*	*0*	*0*	*0*	*0*	*0*	*0*	*0*

S

	Measure INFO/WEIGHT	per Measure		Nutrition Values per 100g / 100ml				
		KCAL	FAT	KCAL	PROT	CARB	FAT	FIBRE
SALT								
Table, Average	*1 Tsp/5g*	*0*	*0*	*0*	*0*	*0*	*0*	*0*
SAMBUCA								
Average	*1 Pub Shot/35ml*	*122*	*0*	*348*	*0*	*37.2*	*0*	*0*
SAMOSAS								
Chicken, Tikka, Indian, Sainsbury's*	1 Samosa/55g	131	5.5	237	9.4	25	10	4.6
Indian Style Selection, Co-Op*	1 Samosa/21g	50	2.7	240	5	27	13	3
Meat, Takeaway, Average	*1 Samosa/110g*	*299*	*19*	*272*	*11.4*	*18.9*	*17.3*	*2.4*
Vegetable, Average	*1 Samosa/110g*	*258*	*12.8*	*235*	*4.8*	*26.9*	*11.6*	*2.5*
Vegetable, Indian Starter Selection, M&S*	1 Samosa/21g	53	2.5	254	5.3	29.3	12.1	3.3
Vegetable, Large, Individual, Sainsbury's*	1 Samosa/110g	254	16.5	231	3.3	20.7	15	2.1
Vegetable, Large, Tesco*	1 Samosa/98g	214	8.9	219	5.3	27.6	9.1	2.8
Vegetable, M&S*	1 Samosa/95g	227	13.2	239	4.1	22.6	13.9	3.5
Vegetable, Mini, Asda*	1 Samosa/23g	52	2	233	6	32	9	2.6
Vegetable, Mini, Indian Snack Selection, Sainsbury's*	1 Samosa/25g	70	4	280	4.7	29.8	15.8	3.2
Vegetable, Mini, Indian Snack Selection, Tesco*	1 Samosa/32g	76	4.2	238	4.7	25.5	13	3.3
Vegetable, On the Go, Sainsbury's*	1 Samosa/50g	124	5.8	248	4.8	29.2	11.5	4.6
Vegetable, Waitrose*	1 Samosa/58g	129	6.6	223	4.5	23.8	11.4	3.8
SANDWICH								
All Day Breakfast, Shapers, Boots*	1 Pack/207g	323	5.2	156	11	23	2.5	2.2
All Day Breakfast, Tesco Classic*	1 Pack/374g	636	29.9	170	8	14.5	8	3
Avo-Lafel, Urban Eat*	1 Pack/184g	453	18.6	246	7.4	29.5	10.1	4.2
Bacon, & Egg, Co-Op*	1 Pack/188g	536	32	285	13	20	17	2
Bacon, & Egg, Sainsbury's*	1 Pack/160g	384	17.8	240	13	22	11.1	1.8
Bacon, & Egg, Tesco*	1 Pack/213g	494	19.6	232	14.8	21.6	9.2	1.8
Bacon, Lettuce, & Tomato, Loved by Us, Co-Op*	1 Pack/195g	410	14.2	210	10.2	25.1	7.3	2.3
Bacon, Maple Cured, Lettuce, & Tomato, Sainsbury's*	1 Pack/191g	425	19.1	222	9.2	22.3	10	2.8
Bacon, On the Go, Sainsbury's*	1 Pack/163g	454	17.9	279	13.2	30.9	11	1.6
Beef, & Horseradish Mayonnaise, Roast, Rare, Waitrose*	1 Pack/197g	415	15.3	211	12.2	23.1	7.8	2
Beef, & Horseradish, & Tomato, Asda*	1 Pack/169g	255	4.4	151	10	22	2.6	2.7
Beef, & Horseradish, Sainsbury's*	1 Pack/187g	391	12.5	209	12.5	23.8	6.7	1.5
Beef, & Pate, M&S*	1 Pack/188g	310	7.3	165	11.2	21.6	3.9	2.4
Beef, & Salad, Roast, Daily Bread*	1 Pack/202g	319	8.3	158	9	21.4	4.1	0
Beef, Horseradish Mayo, Soft White Bread, M&S*	1 Pack/200g	398	12.2	199	13	22.4	6.1	1.4
Beef, Horseradish, Onion Bloomer, Booths*	1 Pack/199g	493	23.9	248	1.4	20	12	1.8
Beef, Horseradish, Tesco*	1 Pack/175g	364	9.6	208	13.2	25.7	5.5	1.6
Beef, Salt, with Gherkins & Mustard Mayo, Sainsbury's*	1 Pack/242g	486	18.2	201	9.3	24.1	7.5	3.1
BLT, Asda*	1 Pack/172g	325	11.9	189	9.9	21.8	6.9	4.6
BLT, Made Without Wheat, M&S*	1 Pack/206g	476	25.1	231	7.2	21.2	12.2	4
BLT, on Malted Brown Bread, Tesco*	1 Pack/185g	454	21.7	245	10.9	22.9	11.7	2.4
BLT, Waitrose*	1 Pack/184g	398	16.4	216	9.5	24.5	8.9	2.3
BLT, with Mayo, Malted Bread, Just Tasty, Aldi*	1 Pack/186g	437	17.9	235	14	22	9.6	2.4
Brie, & Cranberry, Morrisons*	1 Pack/178g	438	20.3	246	10.4	24.4	11.4	2.2
Brie, & Grape, Finest, Tesco*	1 Pack/209g	527	31.6	252	8.5	20.6	15.1	1.5
Brie, & Wild Cranberry, Delicious, Boots*	1 Pack/168g	413	18.5	246	9.1	27	11	3.3
Cheddar, & Ham, M&S*	1 Pack/165g	396	18.6	240	15.1	20	11.3	1.7
Cheddar, Tomato, Red, Tesco*	1 Pack/165g	474	23.8	287	9.2	29.2	14.4	1.9
Cheddar, Oldfields*	1 Pack/121g	384	17.3	317	12.8	33.2	14.3	1.5
Cheddar, Red Leicester, & Onion, Tesco*	1 Pack/182g	604	38.9	332	11	23.8	21.4	2.5
Cheese, & Coleslaw, M&S*	1 Pack/186g	498	32.4	268	10.2	17.6	17.4	3.2
Cheese, & Ham, & Pickle, Healthy Range, Average	*1 Pack/185g*	*299*	*5.1*	*162*	*13.6*	*20.6*	*2.8*	*2.5*
Cheese, & Ham, & Pickle, HL, Tesco*	1 Pack/201g	312	4.2	155	13.1	21	2.1	1.7
Cheese, & Ham, & Pickle, Tesco*	1 Pack/215g	497	24.7	231	11.7	20.3	11.5	1.8
Cheese, & Ham, Smoked, Co-Op*	1 Pack/167g	334	8.4	200	15	24	5	2

S

SANDWICH

	Measure INFO/WEIGHT	per Measure KCAL	FAT	Nutrition Values per 100g / 100ml KCAL	PROT	CARB	FAT	FIBRE
Cheese, & Marmite, No Mayonnaise, Boots*	1 Pack/156g	420	20	269	12.2	26.3	12.8	1.7
Cheese, & Onion, Eat Smart, Morrisons*	1 Pack/144g	340	10.9	236	13.1	27.8	7.6	2.1
Cheese, & Onion, Essential, Waitrose*	1 Pack/158g	432	21.5	273	11.5	25.2	13.6	2
Cheese, & Onion, Tesco*	1 Pack/172g	505	28.3	294	10.2	24.5	16.5	3.3
Cheese, & Pickle, Shapers, Boots*	1 Pack/165g	342	8.1	207	9.8	31	4.9	2.3
Cheese, & Pickle, Tesco*	1 Pack/140g	400	19.3	286	12.7	27.8	13.8	1.4
Cheese, & Pickle, Virgin Trains*	1 Pack/158g	444	19.6	281	11.5	31.1	12.4	0
Cheese, & Salad, & Reduced Fat Mayonnaise, Waitrose*	1 Pack/180g	301	9	167	9.8	20.8	5	3.1
Cheese, & Salad, COU, M&S*	1 Pack/188g	244	3	130	12.1	17	1.6	2.4
Cheese, & Spring Onion, Three, Shell*	1 Pack/168g	672	50.9	400	11.1	20.8	30.3	0
Cheese, & Tomato, Asda*	1 Pack/154g	388	19.7	252	11	23.2	12.8	3.7
Cheese, & Tomato, Co-Op*	1 Pack/155g	365	18.5	235	10.6	21.8	11.9	1.9
Cheese, & Tomato, Organic, M&S*	1 Pack/165g	559	35.3	339	11.8	24.8	21.4	1.9
Cheese, Apple Slaw, Wholemeal, Nutritious, Boots*	1 Pack/252g	400	14.3	159	8.1	17	5.7	3
Cheese, Onion, Soft Oatmeal Bread, M&S*	1 Pack/170g	497	30.1	292	10.3	21.9	17.7	2.1
Cheese, Cheddar, & Celery, Malted Brown Bread, M&S*	1 Pack/200g	506	26.4	253	9.6	23.4	13.2	1
Cheese, Cheddar, White Bread, On the Go, Sainsbury's*	1 Pack/131g	417	21.3	319	13.6	28.8	16.3	1.2
Cheese, Simply, Boots*	1 Pack/138g	375	13.9	272	13.8	30.4	10.1	2.2
Chicken Mayo, on Malted Bread, On the Go, Sainsbury's*	1 Pack/170g	369	11.4	217	12.6	25.3	6.7	2.6
Chicken Salad, BLT, Cheese Tomato, Triple, Tesco*	1 Pack/297g	714	31.5	240	12.1	23	10.6	2.2
Chicken, & Avocado, Roast, on Soft Malted Bread, M&S*	1 Pack/200g	412	14.2	206	11.2	23	7.1	2.7
Chicken, & Avocado, Roast, Tesco*	1 Pack/173g	360	13.3	208	12.1	21.4	7.7	2.4
Chicken, & Bacon, & Avocado, M&S*	1 Pack/242g	508	28.3	210	10.7	15.8	11.7	3.2
Chicken, & Bacon, COU, M&S*	1 Pack/179g	250	3.6	140	13.5	15.8	2	3.8
Chicken, & Bacon, Deep Filled, Co-Op*	1 Pack/166g	556	33.2	335	16	23	20	3
Chicken, & Bacon, Tesco*	1 Pack/195g	486	24.2	249	14.3	20	12.4	2.7
Chicken, & Bacon, with Mayo, Malted Grain, Ginsters*	1 Pack/183g	400	14.7	218	12.8	23.4	8	1
Chicken, & Mayo, Simply, Delicious, Boots*	1 Pack/148g	318	8.6	215	14	25	5.8	2.2
Chicken, & Salad, Aldi*	1 Pack/195g	338	4.5	173	11.5	23.8	2.3	2
Chicken, & Salad, Co-Op*	1 Pack/195g	448	21.4	230	10	24	11	2
Chicken, & Salad, Deep Fill, Ginsters*	1 Pack/203g	364	12.4	179	10.3	20.8	6.1	2.1
Chicken, & Salad, Healthy Living, Co-Op*	1 Pack/196g	265	3.5	135	10.4	19.1	1.8	3.9
Chicken, & Salad, M&S*	1 Pack/226g	350	9.3	155	10.6	18.8	4.1	3
Chicken, & Salad, Roast, Shapers, Boots*	1 Pack/183g	274	4.4	150	12	20	2.4	3.4
Chicken, & Salad, Roast, Waitrose*	1 Pack/217g	482	24.1	222	9.4	21.1	11.1	2
Chicken, & Salad, Sainsbury's*	1 Pack/241g	402	11.8	167	11.9	17.7	4.9	2.1
Chicken, & Stuffing, Co-Op*	1 Pack/208g	420	13	202	13.5	22.6	6.2	2.4
Chicken, & Stuffing, Pork Sage & Onion, Tesco*	1 Pack/136g	376	17	276	12.1	28.1	12.5	1.4
Chicken, & Stuffing, Roast, Boots*	1 Pack/235g	669	39.9	285	12	22	17	1.9
Chicken, & Stuffing, Waitrose*	1 Pack/183g	450	18.8	246	12.8	25.6	10.3	1.5
Chicken, & Sweetcorn, British, Eat Well, M&S*	1 Pack/194g	340	10.5	175	11.4	19.6	5.4	3.1
Chicken, & Sweetcorn, Malted Bread, Sainsbury's*	1 Pack/193g	370	9.8	192	12.3	22.9	5.1	2.6
Chicken, & Sweetcorn, Roast, Good to Go, Waitrose*	1 Pack/189g	321	6.2	170	12.1	21.3	3.3	3.3
Chicken, & Sweetcorn, Tesco*	1 Pack/174g	355	11	204	10.8	24.6	6.3	3
Chicken, Avocado, Limited Edition, Co-Op*	1 Pack/192g	362	11.9	188	10	21	6.2	2.9
Chicken, Salad, Roast, Soft Malted Brown Bread, M&S*	1 Pack/256g	440	13.6	172	12	17.6	5.3	2.7
Chicken, Stuffing, LC, Tesco*	1 Pack/172g	275	4.8	160	14.4	18.7	2.8	6.9
Chicken, Asian, Shapers, Boots*	1 Pack/190g	273	4.6	144	12	19	2.4	2.9
Chicken, Club, The, Tesco*	1 Pack/246g	613	29.8	249	12.9	21.1	12.1	2.1
Chicken, Coronation, M&S*	1 Pack/210g	420	20.4	200	11.2	20.2	9.7	3.1
Chicken, Coronation, on Onion Bread, M&S*	1 Pack/260g	458	16.9	176	10.6	17.7	6.5	2
Chicken, in White Bread, Tesco*	1 Pack/131g	279	4.6	213	10.8	34.1	3.5	1.1
Chicken, Jerk, Sunshine Slaw, Boots*	1 Pack/202g	349	7.7	173	10	23	3.8	2

S

SANDWICH

	Measure INFO/WEIGHT	per Measure KCAL	FAT	Nutrition Values per 100g / 100ml KCAL	PROT	CARB	FAT	FIBRE
Chicken, Just, No Mayonnaise, Tesco*	1 Pack/146g	298	6.3	204	14.6	25.8	4.3	1.6
Chicken, No Mayo, M&S*	1 Pack/142g	248	3.3	175	16.6	20.6	2.3	3.2
Chicken, Pesto, Shapers, Boots*	1 Pack/181g	311	4.2	172	12	26	2.3	1.7
Chicken, Roast, Chorizo, Finest, Tesco*	1 Pack/201g	431	14.1	214	12.6	24.1	7	1.9
Chicken, Tikka, & Mango Chutney, Tesco*	1 Pack/201g	352	4.8	175	11.6	25.4	2.4	2.6
Chicken, Tikka, COU, M&S*	1 Pack/185g	268	3.3	145	12.1	20.5	1.8	3.2
Chicken, Tikka, on Pepper Chilli Bread, Shapers, Boots*	1 Pack/172g	296	4.5	172	13	25	2.6	2.5
Chicken, Triple, On the Go, Sainsbury's*	1 Pack/296g	669	28.4	226	12	22	9.6	19
Chicken, with Pork, Sage & Onion Stuffing, Sainsbury's*	1 Pack/187g	423	18	226	12	22	9.6	1.9
Club, New York Style, Sainsbury's*	1 Pack/212g	608	33.5	287	13.3	22.8	15.8	2.7
Corned Beef, on White, Simply, Brambles*	1 Pack/126g	325	10.8	258	14.2	30.8	8.6	1.4
Corned Beef, Tomato Onion, Salad Garden*	1 Pack/137g	338	14.8	247	14.2	23	10.8	0
Crayfish, & Rocket, Finest, Tesco*	1 Pack/178g	365	10.5	205	9.8	27.5	5.9	2.1
Egg Mayo, & Salad, You Count, Love Life, Waitrose*	1 Pack/196g	314	10.2	160	8.8	18.5	5.2	2.2
Egg Mayo, Free Range, Asda*	1 Pack/178g	311	10.1	175	9.3	21.5	5.7	2.1
Egg Mayo, Free Range, on Oatmeal Bread, M&S*	1 Pack/180g	315	12.2	175	9.4	18.2	6.8	2.8
Egg Mayonnaise, & Cress, Co-Op*	1 Pack/159g	405	24	255	8.8	20.8	15.1	1.9
Egg Mayonnaise, & Cress, Go Simple, Asda*	1 Pack/169g	370	18.6	219	10	20	11	1.7
Egg Mayonnaise, & Cress, HL, Tesco*	1 Pack/149g	271	7.7	182	9	23.5	5.2	2.6
Egg Mayonnaise, Free Range, Soft Oatmeal Bread, M&S*	1 Pack/176g	345	12.3	196	9.9	21.9	7	3.1
Egg, & Avocado, & Chilli Chutney, M&S*	1 Pack/209g	368	15.1	176	7.7	18.3	7.2	3.5
Egg, & Bacon, Handmade, Tesco*	1 Pack/217g	489	20.4	225	13.4	20.8	9.4	2
Egg, & Cress, BGTY, Sainsbury's*	1 Pack/145g	268	7.5	185	9.1	25.4	5.2	2.7
Egg, & Cress, Co-Op*	1 Pack/159g	398	23.8	250	9	21	15	2
Egg, & Cress, COU, M&S*	1 Pack/192g	240	5.2	125	9.8	15.5	2.7	2.8
Egg, & Cress, Free Range, M&S*	1 Pack/192g	307	9	160	10.7	17.8	4.7	3
Egg, & Cress, Free Range, Sainsbury's*	1 Pack/183g	346	13	189	9.7	20.5	7.1	2.2
Egg, & Cress, No Mayo, LC, Tesco*	1 Pack/160g	280	7.2	175	9.4	23.7	4.5	3
Egg, & Ham, Deli Club, Tesco*	1 Pack/220g	433	15.4	197	11.4	20.5	7	2.7
Egg, & Salad, Co-Op*	1 Pack/190g	285	7.6	150	7	22	4	4
Egg, & Salad, on Softgrain Bread, HL, Tesco*	1 Pack/197g	290	4.7	147	7	23.6	2.4	1.7
Egg, & Tomato & Salad Cream, M&S*	1 Pack/214g	402	14.8	188	7.8	22.6	6.9	2
Egg, & Watercress, Bloomer, Freshly Prepared, M&S*	1 Pack/221g	465	26.1	210	10.2	15.3	11.8	3
Egg, & Watercress, GF Seeded Bread, Eat Well, M&S*	1 Pack/192g	382	16.9	199	8	20.6	8.8	2.9
Egg, Tomato, with Salad Cream, Delicious, Boots*	1 Pack/205g	410	16	200	7.8	23.4	7.8	2.6
Feta Cheese, & Salad, Tastte*	1 Pack/178g	367	13.4	206	10.6	24	7.5	0
Goat's Cheese, & Cranberry, Shapers, Boots*	1 Pack/150g	323	6.3	216	8.4	36	4.2	2.6
Ham, & Cheese, & Pickle, & Lettuce, No Mayo, Tesco*	1 Pack/207g	435	16.2	210	12.2	23	7.8	2.7
Ham, & Cheese, & Pickle, Average	**1 Pack/220g**	**524**	**25.1**	**238**	**12.2**	**21.6**	**11.4**	**2.5**
Ham, & Cheese, Honey Roast, Soft Oatmeal Bread, M&S*	1 Pack/188g	466	21.6	248	13.9	20.9	11.5	2.7
Ham, & Cheese, on a Croissant, Smoked, M&S*	1 Croissant/105g	341	22.7	325	13.4	22.2	21.6	3.9
Ham, & Edam, Smoked, Shapers, Boots*	1 Pack/183g	315	11.9	172	9.3	19	6.5	2.7
Ham, & Egg, Honey Roast, Tesco*	1 Pack/192g	355	9.8	185	12.8	20.6	5.1	2.5
Ham, & Mustard Mayo, Smoked, Oatmeal Bread, M&S*	1 Pack/150g	282	6.4	188	13.2	23.2	4.3	2
Ham, & Mustard, Ginsters*	1 Pack/140g	307	9.4	219	11.8	28	6.7	2.5
Ham, & Mustard, Loved by Us, Co-Op*	1 Pack/162g	310	7.9	191	13.2	22.4	4.9	1.8
Ham, & Mustard, Salad, BGTY, Sainsbury's*	1 Pack/183g	261	3.8	143	8.7	22.4	2.1	2.6
Ham, & Mustard, Tesco*	1 Pack/147g	437	27.9	297	10.6	20.8	19	1.2
Ham, & Mustard, Wiltshire, The Ultimate, M&S*	1 Pack/246g	344	11.8	140	9.8	15	4.8	1.4
Ham, & Salad, Bap, Co-Op*	1 Bap/164g	295	4.9	180	8	30	3	2
Ham, & Salad, On the Go, Sainsbury's*	1 Pack/174g	244	3	140	10.1	20	1.7	2
Ham, & Salad, Shapers, Boots*	1 Pack/195g	269	2.7	138	9.4	22	1.4	1.8
Ham, & Soft Cheese, Tesco*	1 Pack/164g	333	12.1	203	11.6	22.5	7.4	2.2

S

SANDWICH

INFO/WEIGHT	Measure	per Measure KCAL	FAT	Nutrition Values per 100g / 100ml KCAL	PROT	CARB	FAT	FIBRE
Ham, & Turkey with Salad, Co-Op*	1 Pack/188g	263	5.6	140	9	21	3	2
Ham, Cheese, Honey Roast, Seeded Bread, GF, M&S*	1 Pack/196g	499	26.6	255	11.9	19.6	13.6	3.1
Ham, Cheese, Morrisons*	1 Pack/183g	273	4.6	149	12.5	19.2	2.5	4.1
Ham, Coleslaw, Smoked, Soft Malted Brown Bread, M&S*	1 Pack/175g	388	16.3	222	9.2	24.2	9.3	2.5
Ham, Mustard Mayo, Smoked, Good to Go, Waitrose*	1 Pack/160g	309	8	193	12.9	23	5	2.2
Ham, Egg, Chips, Delicious, Boots*	1 Pack/206g	390	11.8	189	10	23	5.7	2.2
Ham, Honey Roast, Egg, Finest, Tesco*	1 Pack/271g	523	24.1	193	12.3	15	8.9	1.9
Ham, No Mayo, Just Ham, Tesco*	1 Pack/122g	250	4.9	205	11.6	30.4	4	2.1
Ham, No Mayo, On the Go, Sainsbury's*	1 Pack/131g	256	5.4	195	13.7	24.9	4.1	1.9
Houmous, & Carrot, Shapers, Boots*	1 Pack/204g	323	10.2	158	7.5	21	5	5.2
Houmous, Salad, Vegan, Chop Chop*	1 Pack/208g	300	6	144	5.2	21.5	2.9	3.8
New Yorker, TTD, On the Go, Sainsbury's*	1 Pack/248g	486	17.6	196	10.2	21.8	7.1	2.1
Pastrami, New York Deli, Finest, Tesco*	1 Pack/231g	500	22.7	216	11.9	18.7	9.8	2.9
Ploughman's, Cheese, Cheddar, Deep Fill, Asda*	1 Pack/229g	471	22.9	206	9	20	10	4.3
Ploughman's, Cheese, Deep Fill, Ginsters*	1 Pack/213g	491	24.2	231	8.4	23.8	11.4	2.2
Ploughman's, Red Leicester, On the Go, Sainsbury's*	1 Pack/219g	518	26.3	236	8.8	2	12	2.2
Ploughmans, Cheddar, Tesco*	1 Pack/186g	418	18.6	225	9	23.4	10	2.8
Pork, Roast, Stuffing, Apple, Roll, Finest, Tesco*	1 Pack/192g	397	8.4	207	8.9	31.9	4.4	1.9
Prawn Mayonnaise, Co-Op*	1 Pack/154g	285	6	185	9.7	27.3	3.9	3.2
Prawn Mayonnaise, Morrisons*	1 Pack/157g	234	3.9	149	9	22.7	2.5	3
Prawn Mayonnaise, Oatmeal Bread, Sainsbury's*	1 Pack/174g	357	15.3	205	10.3	20.1	8.8	2.3
Prawn Mayonnaise, Seeded Bread, GF, M&S*	1 Pack/203g	386	16.5	190	9	18.7	8.1	3
Prawn Mayonnaise, Shapers, Boots*	1 Pack/160g	293	7.5	183	9.4	25.6	4.7	2.5
Prawn Mayonnaise, Soft Malted Brown Bread, M&S*	1 Pack/197g	347	8.9	176	11.6	21.1	4.5	2.3
Prawn, & Salmon, Smoked, M&S*	1 Pack/445g	1135	63.6	255	11.7	19.3	14.3	1.4
Prawn, King, Sainsbury's*	1 Pack/204g	424	16.3	208	11.6	22.3	8	0
Prawn, Marie Rose, Waitrose*	1 Pack/164g	226	5.6	138	8.8	18	3.4	1.9
Rib, BBQ, Pork, Rustlers*	1 Pack/157g	355	14.1	226	10.2	25.3	9	0
Salami, & Cheese, Migrolino*	1 Pack/140g	486	26.6	347	14	29	19	2
Salmon, & Cream Cheese, Smoked, Morrisons*	1 Pack/160g	342	13.1	214	11	22	8.2	4
Salmon, & Cucumber, M&S*	1 Pack/168g	329	13.9	196	11	19.5	8.3	2.6
Salmon, & Cucumber, Red, Tesco*	1 Pack/144g	284	9.2	197	11.1	23.8	6.4	1.9
Salmon, & Soft Cheese, Smoked, Waitrose*	1 Pack/180g	416	18	231	11.5	22.6	10	2.2
Salmon, & Watercress, Poached, Lochmuir, M&S*	1 Pack/192g	355	11.7	185	10.3	22.3	6.1	1.6
Salmon, Cream Cheese, Smoked, Sainsbury*	1 Pack/168g	408	17.5	243	11.7	24.5	10.4	2.2
Salmon, Cucumber, Good to Go, Waitrose*	1 Pack/185g	316	9.2	171	12.1	18	5	2.8
Salmon, Smoked, Cream Cheese, Finest, Tesco*	1 Pack/200g	483	19.2	242	11.5	26.4	9.6	1.9
Sausage, Pigs Under Blankets, Delicious, Boots*	1 Pack/181g	453	16.7	250	11	29	9.2	2.5
Seafood, Medley, M&S*	1 Pack/227g	468	28.1	206	7.2	16.3	12.4	3.5
Steak	**1 Serving/204g**	**459**	**14.1**	**225**	**14.9**	**25.5**	**6.9**	**0**
Sub, Cold Cuts, From Restaurant	**1 Serving/228g**	**456**	**18.6**	**200**	**9.6**	**22.4**	**8.2**	**0**
Sub, Ham, & Tomato Salad, Shapers, Boots*	1 Pack/170g	286	3.9	168	9.2	28	2.3	1.4
Sub, Tuna, & Salad, From Restaurant, Average	**1 Serving/256g**	**584**	**28**	**228**	**11.6**	**21.6**	**10.9**	**0**
Tastes of Christmas, Selection, M&S*	1 Pack/205g	484	21.5	236	12.3	22	10.5	1.9
Tofu, Fiery, Slaw, Wicked Kitchen, Tesco*	1 Pack/236g	425	11.6	180	6.5	26.4	4.9	2.3
Tuna Mayo, Essential, Waitrose*	1 Pack/133g	283	7.4	213	13.3	25.9	5.6	2.9
Tuna Mayonnaise, & Cucumber, Finest, Tesco*	1 Pack/180g	394	17.1	219	10.2	22	9.5	2.3
Tuna Mayonnaise, & Cucumber, Simply, Boots*	1 Pack/200g	498	26	249	12	21	13	2.4
Tuna Mayonnaise, & Salad, Serious About Sandwiches*	1 Pack/192g	305	9	159	8.6	20.5	4.7	2.9
Tuna Mayonnaise, Menu, Boots*	1 Pack/182g	451	20	248	13	23	11	1.1
Tuna Mayonnaise, Sainsbury's*	1 Pack/150g	314	9.9	209	11.4	24.5	6.6	2.8
Tuna, & Cucumber, BGTY, Sainsbury's*	1 Pack/178g	268	3.2	151	11.3	22.3	1.8	3.1
Tuna, & Cucumber, COU, M&S*	1 Pack/204g	294	5.1	144	9.1	20.6	2.5	1.5

S

SANDWICH

INFO/WEIGHT	Measure		per Measure		Nutrition Values per 100g / 100ml				
			KCAL	FAT	KCAL	PROT	CARB	FAT	FIBRE
Tuna, & Cucumber, Healthy Living, Co-Op*	1 Pack/192g		250	3.5	130	10.9	17.9	1.8	3
Tuna, & Cucumber, NUME, Morrisons*	1 Pack/151g		255	3.5	169	12	23.7	2.3	2.5
Tuna, & Cucumber, On Oatmeal Bread, Ginsters*	1 Pack/175g		290	7.2	166	11.7	20.7	4.1	2.4
Tuna, & Cucumber, On the Go, Sainsbury's*	1 Pack/196g		284	5.5	145	9.6	19.4	2.8	2.1
Tuna, & Cucumber, You Count, Love Life, Waitrose*	1 Pack/195g		321	5.3	165	13	21.4	2.7	1.4
Tuna, & Sweetcorn, Loved by Us, Co-Op*	1 Pack/200g		380	9.2	190	11.7	24.1	4.6	2.4
Tuna, & Sweetcorn, Malted Bread, Asda*	1 Pack/202g		365	10.7	181	11	21	5.3	2.5
Tuna, Sweetcorn, BGTY, Sainsbury's*	1 Pack/187g		309	5.1	165	10.8	24.7	2.7	2.8
Tuna, Sweetcorn, Ginsters*	1 Pack/169g		348	11.4	205	9.6	26.4	6.7	2.4
Tuna, Sweetcorn, on Malt Bread, Tesco*	1 Pack/170g		425	20.4	250	11.4	22.5	12	3.3
Tuna, Crunch, HL, Tesco*	1 Pack/180g		261	4.3	145	11	19.9	2.4	0.5
Turkey, & Bacon, COU, M&S*	1 Pack/165g		256	4	155	12	21	2.4	1.7
Turkey, & Cranberry, COU, M&S*	1 Pack/180g		279	3.1	155	12.1	22.8	1.7	2.9
Turkey, & Pastrami, HL, Tesco*	1 Pack/185g		286	4.8	155	9.6	22.1	2.6	2.6
Turkey, & Salad, Fullfillers*	1 Pack/218g		320	7	147	10.3	18.6	3.2	0
Turkey, & Salad, Healthy Eating, Wild Bean Cafe*	1 Pack/230g		315	2.5	137	10	21.5	1.1	1.8
Turkey, & Trimmings, Christmas, Tesco*	1 Pack/209g		476	16.5	228	12.5	25.5	7.9	2.3
Turkey, & Trimmings, Light Choices, HL, Tesco*	1 Pack/154g		256	4.3	166	10.1	24.1	2.8	2.2

SANDWICH FILLER

Cheese & Spring Onion, M&S*	1 Serving/56g		199	18.8	355	8.5	5	33.6	0.2
Cheese Onion, Reduced Fat, Supermarket, Average	*1 Serving/100g*		*227*	*18.1*	*227*	*11.8*	*4.4*	*18.1*	*1.7*
Cheese Onion, Supermarket, Average	*1 Serving/100g*		*405*	*38.6*	*405*	*10.2*	*4.1*	*38.6*	*1.3*
Cheese Onion, Tesco*	1 Pack/250g		1060	106.5	424	10	0.2	42.6	1.5
Chicken & Bacon with Sweetcorn, Sainsbury's*	1 Serving/60g		123	9.4	205	12	4	15.7	0.9
Chicken & Bacon, Asda*	1 Serving/100g		341	29	341	17	3	29	0.5
Chicken Tikka, HE, Tesco*	1 Serving/100g		110	3.6	110	7.1	12.4	3.6	1
Chicken, Coronation, Deli, Meadow Fresh, Lidl*	1 Serving/30g		78	5.7	261	12	9.8	19	1.2
Chicken, Sweetcorn & Bacon, Tesco*	1 Serving/50g		167	14.8	334	12.3	4.3	29.7	1.6
Coronation Chicken, Sainsbury's*	¼ Tub/60g		183	14.8	305	12.1	8.9	24.6	1.2
Coronation Chicken, Tesco*	1 Tbsp/30g		88	7	293	11.4	9.2	23.2	0.7
Egg & Bacon, Fresh, Tesco*	1 Serving/45g		112	9	248	12.7	4.2	20.1	0.6
Egg Bacon, Free Range, Deli, Essential, Waitrose*	½ Pot/85g		267	23.6	314	12.7	3.3	27.8	0.5
Egg Mayonnaise, BGTY, Sainsbury's*	1 Serving/63g		71	4.1	113	10.2	3.4	6.5	0.1
Egg Mayonnaise, Chunky Free Range, Tesco*	1 Serving/50g		104	8.9	209	11.3	0.9	17.8	1.6
Egg Mayonnaise, Country Fresh, Aldi*	¼ Pack/50g		106	8.9	211	9.8	2.9	17.8	0
Egg Mayonnaise, Free Range, Co-Op*	1 Pack/200g		260	17.6	130	10.1	2.4	8.8	0.5
Egg Mayonnaise, Morrisons*	1 Serving/50g		71	5.3	142	10	1.7	10.6	0
Egg Mayonnaise, Tesco*	1 Serving/50g		100	7.8	199	10.9	3.5	15.6	0.5
Prawn Marie Rose, Sainsbury's*	1 Serving/60g		121	10.6	201	8.1	2.5	17.6	0.9
Prawn Mayonnaise, Deli, Asda*	1 Serving/50g		170	16.5	339	9	1.6	33	0.4
Seafood Cocktail, Sainsbury's*	1 Serving/55g		99	6.9	180	5.9	10.6	12.6	0.5
Smoked Salmon & Soft Cheese, M&S*	1 Pack/170g		450	40.6	265	11.1	4.9	23.9	0
Tuna & Sweetcorn, Reduced Fat, Supermarket	*1 Serving/100g*		*119*	*5.4*	*119*	*11.5*	*5.8*	*5.4*	*1.2*
Tuna & Sweetcorn, Supermarket	*1 Serving/100g*		*228*	*17.8*	*228*	*11.6*	*5.7*	*17.8*	*1.4*
Tuna Sweetcorn, Tesco*	1 Serving/54g		127	9.8	235	8.6	8.1	18.1	0.6
Tuna Mayonnaise Cucumber, Choice, Tesco*	1 Serving/200g		463	22.8	232	12.8	23.2	11.4	1.6
Tuna Mayonnaise, BGTY, Sainsbury's*	1 Serving/100g		114	3.4	114	17.6	3.5	3.4	0.1

SANDWICH SPREAD

Beef, Classic, Shippam's Foods*	1 Pot/75g		133	8.8	177	15.5	2.2	11.8	0
Chicken, Classic, Shippam's Foods*	1 Serving/35g		64	4.4	182	15.5	1.8	12.5	0
Heinz*	1 Tbsp/10ml		22	1.3	220	1	24	13	1
Light, Heinz*	1 Tbsp/10g		16	0.9	161	1.1	18.2	9.2	0.9

S

	Measure INFO/WEIGHT	per Measure KCAL	FAT	Nutrition Values per 100g / 100ml KCAL	PROT	CARB	FAT	FIBRE
SARDINES								
A La Antigua, Tinned, in Olive Oil, Ortiz, Brindisa*	1 Tin/140g	267	15.4	191	23	0	11	0
Grilled	*1oz/28g*	*55*	*2.9*	*195*	*25.3*	*0*	*10.4*	*0*
in Brine, Canned, Drained	*1oz/28g*	*38*	*2.1*	*136*	*17*	*0*	*7.6*	*0*
in Oil, Canned, Drained	*1oz/28g*	*51*	*3.2*	*180*	*19.1*	*0*	*11.6*	*0*
in Spring Water, Portuguese, Sainsbury's*	1 Can/90g	176	10.5	195	21.3	1.2	11.6	0.5
in Tomato Sauce, Canned	*1oz/28g*	*45*	*2.8*	*162*	*17*	*1.4*	*9.9*	*0*
Raw, Whole with Head	*1oz/28g*	*22*	*1.2*	*78*	*9.7*	*0*	*4.3*	*0*
SATAY								
Chicken with Peanut Sauce, Waitrose*	1 Pack/250g	492	27	197	18.9	6	10.8	0.5
Chicken, 12 Mini, Taste Original*	½ Pack/60g	102	3.9	170	23.3	4.4	6.5	0.7
Chicken, Indonesian, Mini, Sainsbury's*	1 Stick/10g	17	0.7	171	23	4	7	0.7
Chicken, Sticks, Asda*	1 Stick/20g	43	2.8	216	18	4.5	14	0
Chicken, with Peanut Dip, Sainsbury's*	1 Pack/90g	171	10	190	15.4	6.3	11.1	1.5
Spicy Chicken Noodles, Microwaved, Asda*	1 Portion/380g	361	10.3	95	6.4	10	2.7	1.4
SATSUMAS								
Fresh, Raw, Flesh Only, Average	*1 Sm/56g*	*21*	*0*	*37*	*0.9*	*8.6*	*0.1*	*1.3*
Weighed with Peel, Average	*1 Sm/60g*	*16*	*0*	*26*	*0.6*	*6.1*	*0.1*	*0.6*
SAUCE								
Aioli, with Extra Virgin Olive Oil, Spirit of Summer, M&S*	1 Tbsp/15g	102	11	683	1.5	3.5	73.5	0.9
Apple, Bramley, Colman's*	1 Tbsp/15ml	16	0	107	0.2	26.5	0	1.3
Apple, Bramley, Sainsbury's*	1 Tsp/15g	17	0	111	0.2	27.2	0.1	1.8
Apple, Everyday Value, Tesco*	1 Tbsp/15g	15	0	105	0.1	24.8	0.1	0.5
Arrabiata, Italian, Tesco*	½ Pot/175g	74	0.9	42	1.1	7.9	0.5	1
Bacon & Tomato, Smoked, Stir in, Dolmio*	½ Tub/75g	74	4.2	98	4.6	7.2	5.6	1.3
Balti, Cooking, Sharwood's*	¼ Jar/140g	120	8.3	86	1.2	7.1	5.9	1.4
Balti, Curry, Tesco*	1 Serving/200g	126	9.2	63	1.7	4.3	4.6	1.7
Balti, Loyd Grossman*	½ Jar/175g	180	11.7	103	1.3	8.4	6.7	1.7
Barbecue, Asda*	1 Tbsp/15g	19	0.1	126	0.9	30	0.5	0
Barbecue, Sticky, Marinade Sauce, M&S*	1 Tbsp/15g	27	0.1	179	0.9	42	0.6	1.2
Barbeque, Cook in, Homepride*	1 Can/500g	375	7.5	75	0.7	14.6	1.5	0.6
BBQ, Heinz*	1 Serving/20g	28	0.1	139	1.1	31.7	0.3	0.5
BBQ, Jerk, Reggae Reggae, Levi Roots*	1 Jar/310g	375	0.3	121	1.1	28.8	0.1	0.5
BBQ, Sticky, Spread & Bake, Heinz*	¼ Jar/78g	131	0.5	168	1	39.6	0.6	1.2
Bearnaise, Sainsbury's*	1 Tbsp/15g	59	6.2	393	0.6	5	41	0
Bechamel, M&S*	1 Jar/425g	480	34.8	113	2.1	7	8.2	1.6
Bhuna, Cooking, Sharwood's*	¼ Jar/105g	83	4.9	79	1.1	7.1	4.7	1.9
Biryani, Med Aromati, Oven Bake, Patak's*	½ Jar/175g	140	9.3	80	1.1	6.1	5.3	0
Black Bean, & Red Pepper, Sharwood's*	½ Jar/213g	132	3	62	1.9	10.5	1.4	1.2
Black Bean, Asda*	1 Serving/55g	55	0.8	100	2.9	19	1.4	0
Black Bean, Canton, Stir Fry, Blue Dragon*	½ Pack/60g	53	1.2	88	2.8	14.8	2	1.5
Black Bean, M&S*	½ Jar/140g	130	3.8	93	2.9	14.1	2.7	0.5
Black Bean, Stir Fry, Sharwood's*	1 Jar/195g	127	0.6	65	2.3	12.9	0.3	0
Bolognese, Dolmio*	1 Serving/100g	33	0.2	33	1.5	6.3	0.2	1.3
Bolognese, Loyd Grossman*	¼ Jar/106g	80	3.1	75	2	10.2	2.9	1.4
Bouillabaisse, M&S*	½ Pouch/100g	132	11.8	132	1.8	4.3	11.8	0.7
Bread, Christmas, Tesco*	1 Serving/60g	64	3.2	107	3.3	11.8	5.3	0.5
Bread, Made with Semi-Skimmed Milk	*1 Serving/45g*	*42*	*1.4*	*93*	*4.3*	*12.8*	*3.1*	*0.3*
Brown, Bottled	*1 Tsp/6g*	*6*	*0*	*99*	*1.1*	*25.2*	*0*	*0.7*
Brown, Bramwells, Aldi*	1 Tbsp/15g	17	0.1	115	0.5	27	0.5	1
Brown, Original, HP*	1 Tbsp/15g	18	0	122	0.9	28.3	0.1	0.4
Brown, Reduced Salt Sugar, HP*	1 Tbsp/15g	13	0	87	0.7	20	0.1	0.3
Brown, Tesco*	1 Tsp/10g	10	0	104	0.7	25.1	0.1	0.6
Brown, Value, Value, Tesco*	1 Serving/15g	13	0	86	0.7	18.8	0.1	0.3

S

SAUCE

INFO/WEIGHT	Measure	per Measure KCAL	FAT	Nutrition Values per 100g / 100ml KCAL	PROT	CARB	FAT	FIBRE
Burger, Heinz*	1 Tbsp/15g	56	5.3	372	0.9	12	35.5	0
Burger, Hellmann's*	1 Tbsp/15g	36	3.2	240	1.1	12	21	0
Butter Tarragon, Chicken Tonight, Knorr*	¼ Jar/125g	132	13	106	1	2.1	10.4	0.7
Carbonara, Frozen, Tesco*	1 Serving/90g	142	11.4	157	5.8	4.9	12.6	0.6
Carbonara, TTD, Sainsbury's*	½ pot/175g	347	31	198	5.2	4.5	17.7	0.5
Cheese, Cornish Cruncher, M&S*	½ Pouch/100g	159	12.9	159	4.8	5.7	12.9	0.5
Cheese, Four, for Pasta, Waitrose*	1 Pot/350g	546	41	156	6.7	5.8	11.7	0.1
Cheese, Fresh, Waitrose*	1 Pot/350g	458	34.3	131	5.1	5.7	9.8	0
Cheese, Made with Semi-Skimmed Milk	*1 Serving/60g*	*107*	*7.6*	*179*	*8.1*	*9.1*	*12.6*	*0.2*
Cheese, Made with Whole Milk	*1 Serving/60g*	*118*	*8.8*	*197*	*8*	*9*	*14.6*	*0.2*
Cheese, Sainsbury's*	1 Serving/125g	140	9.4	112	5	6.1	7.5	1.2
Chilli & Garlic, Blue Dragon*	1 Serving/30ml	26	0.1	85	1.1	19.7	0.2	0
Chilli & Garlic, Lea & Perrins*	1 Tsp/6g	4	0	60	1	14.9	0	0
Chilli Con Carne, Homepride*	½ Jar/250g	145	1.2	58	1.6	11.1	0.5	1.6
Chilli Con Carne, Hot, Uncle Ben's*	1 Jar/500g	295	3	59	2.3	10.9	0.6	1.7
Chilli, Barbeque, Encona*	1 Tbsp/15ml	19	0.1	129	1.3	30.7	0.1	0
Chilli, Hot, Blue Dragon*	1 Tbsp/15ml	14	0	96	0.5	23	0.2	0
Chilli, Hot, Mexican, Morrisons*	¼ Jar/125g	72	0.6	58	2.2	11.2	0.5	2
Chilli, Mild, Tesco*	1 Jar/550g	302	1.6	55	2.3	10	0.3	3.4
Chilli, Sweet, Thai, Dipping, Original, Blue Dragon*	1 Serving/30ml	69	0.2	230	0.6	55.1	0.7	1.6
Chilli, Tesco*	1 Tsp/5ml	4	0.2	90	1.3	14	3.2	1.1
Chilli, Tomato Based, Bottled, Average	*1 Tbsp/15g*	*16*	*0*	*104*	*2.5*	*19.8*	*0.3*	*5.9*
Chinese Stir Fry, Sainsbury's*	½ Sachet/75g	61	1.9	81	0.4	14.1	2.5	1
Chocolate, Dessert, M&S*	1 Dtsp/11g	35	1	330	2.1	59.3	9.4	1.9
Chow Mein, Stir Fry, Blue Dragon*	1 Sachet/120g	110	3.5	92	1.1	15.4	2.9	0.4
Chow Mein, Stir Fry, Straight to Wok, Amoy*	1 Pack/120g	172	7	143	0.9	21.9	5.8	0.5
Country French, Chicken Tonight, Knorr*	¼ Jar/125g	110	8.8	89	0.4	5.3	7.1	0.8
Cranberry Jelly, Morrisons*	1 Tsp/12g	23	0	189	0.2	47	0	0.1
Cranberry, Sainsbury's*	1 Tsp/15g	26	0.1	170	0.5	41.5	0.5	0.5
Cranberry, Tesco*	1 Tsp/15g	23	0	156	0.1	38.8	0	0.9
Cream, Gradds¥s, Ikea*	1 Serving/60ml	72	6.6	120	1	4	11	0
Curry, Asda*	1 Tbsp/15g	62	2.1	414	13	59	14	1.3
Curry, Basics, Sainsbury's*	¼ Jar/110g	70	2.8	64	0.7	9.7	2.5	0.9
Curry, Chinese Style, Tesco*	¼ Jar/125g	63	0.5	50	0.6	10.8	0.4	0.5
Curry, Chip Shop, Knorr*	1 Sachet/150g	146	6.9	97	1.7	12.4	4.6	0.7
Curry, Chip Shop, Prepared, CBY, Asda*	1 Serving/62ml	50	3	80	0.5	8.6	4.8	0.2
Curry, Cook in, Homepride*	½ Can/250g	170	6.2	68	0.8	10.5	2.5	0.7
Curry, Green Thai, Finest, Tesco*	1 Serving/350g	420	37.1	120	1.4	4.8	10.6	0.3
Curry, Medium, Uncle Ben's*	1 Jar/500g	330	10	66	0.9	10.9	2	0
Curry, Red Thai, Finest, Tesco*	1 Jar/350g	388	31.5	111	1.3	6.2	9	0.9
Curry, Thai Coconut, Uncle Ben's*	1 Serving/125g	128	6	102	1.4	13.2	4.8	0
Curry, Thai, Red, Mild, M&S*	½ Jar/135g	158	12	117	1.6	7.1	8.9	0.8
Damson, Fruity, Jelly, Tracklements*	1 Tsp/10g	28	0	281	0.2	70.2	0	0
Dhansak, Sharwood's*	1 Jar/445g	668	34.7	150	4.7	15.2	7.8	1.4
Dill Lemon, Delicate for Fish, Schwartz*	1 Pack/300g	387	34.2	129	1.1	5.6	11.4	0.5
Fajita, Asda*	¼ Jar/125g	79	5.4	63	1	5	4.3	1
Fruity, HP*	1 Tbsp/15g	20	0	135	0.9	31.5	0	0.3
Garlic Chive, Table Dip, Heinz*	1 Serving/10ml	32	3	323	1	12.1	29.9	0.2
Garlic, Creamy, Sainsbury's*	1 Tbsp/15g	44	4.3	296	0.5	7.6	29	1.5
Garlic, Heinz*	1 Tbsp/15g	60	5.4	398	2.2	15	36	0.3
Habanero, Hot Boy, Glorious!*	1 Pot/300g	342	26.4	114	1.6	6.8	8.8	1.3
Hoisin, & Garlic, Blue Dragon*	1 Serving/60g	80	1.6	133	1.2	26.1	2.6	0
Hoisin, & Plum, Stir Fry, HL, Tesco*	1 Serving/250g	148	3.2	59	2.1	9.7	1.3	1.3

S

SAUCE

INFO/WEIGHT	Measure KCAL	FAT	Nutrition Values per 100g / 100ml KCAL	PROT	CARB	FAT	FIBRE
Hoisin, & Spring Onion, Stir Fry, Sharwood's*	1 Jar/165g	196	1.5	119	1.3	26.5	0.9	0.8
Hoisin, Plum, Deliciously Versatile, M&S*	½ Bottle/75g	112	1.1	149	2.7	29.3	1.5	2.4
Hoisin, Sharwood's*	1 Tbsp/15g	32	0	211	2.7	49.5	0.3	0.1
Hoisin, Stir Fry, Amoy*	½ Pouch/60g	66	1.4	110	2.1	20.3	2.3	0.1
Hoisin, Stir Fry, Asda*	1 Pack/120g	103	0.7	86	0.6	18	0.6	3.1
Hollandaise, Finest, Tesco*	1 Serving/98g	473	44.5	485	1.4	17.2	45.6	0.3
Hollandaise, Fresh, Average	*1 Pack/150g*	*342*	*32.4*	*228*	*2.4*	*6.1*	*21.6*	*0*
Hollandaise, M&S*	½ Pouch/100g	327	34	327	1	4	34	0.5
Honey Mustard, Chicken Tonight, Knorr*	¼ Jar/125g	132	6.6	106	1	12.6	5.3	1.8
Horseradish, Colman's*	1 Tbsp/15ml	17	0.9	112	1.9	9.8	6.2	2.6
Horseradish, Creamed, M&S*	1 Tsp/5g	16	1.5	325	2.4	12.1	29.3	2.5
Horseradish, Creamed, Waitrose*	1 Tbsp/16g	30	1.6	185	2.4	19.6	9.9	2.3
Horseradish, Creamy, Sainsbury's*	1 Tsp/5g	11	0.6	223	2.8	28.9	11.8	1.6
Horseradish, Hot, Morrisons*	1 Serving/20g	31	1.5	157	2.2	19.1	7.7	1.7
Horseradish, Hot, Tesco*	1 Tsp/5g	12	0.8	233	1.8	17.4	16.9	2.1
Hot Pepper, Encona*	1 Tsp/5ml	3	0.1	52	0.5	10.5	1.2	0
Hot, Original, Cholula Hot Sauce*	1 Tsp/5ml	1	0	19	0.9	0.4	0.9	2.8
Hunters Chicken, Cooking, Tesco*	1/3 Jar/163g	155	0.3	95	1.2	20.6	0.2	0.8
Jalfrezi, Average	*1 Sm Jar/350g*	*326*	*23.7*	*93*	*1.3*	*6.7*	*6.8*	*1.6*
Jalfrezi, M&S*	½ Jar/170g	207	15.1	122	1.8	7.1	8.9	2.9
Korma, Coconut Cream, Mild, in Glass Jar, Patak's*	½ Jar/225g	326	25	145	1.2	9.4	11.1	0
Korma, Curry, Loyd Grossman*	½ Jar/175g	224	14.5	128	1.5	11.3	8.3	0.8
Korma, Curry, Uncle Ben's*	1 Jar/500g	630	42	126	1.4	11.1	8.4	0
Korma, Mild Curry, BFY, Morrisons*	¼ Jar/118g	150	7.2	127	1.3	16.8	6.1	1.5
Korma, Tesco*	¼ Jar/125g	192	14.6	154	2.4	9.9	11.7	1.3
Lemon & Ginger, Stir Fry, Finest, Tesco*	¼ Jar/85g	144	0.2	169	0.2	41.7	0.2	0.2
Madeira, Wild Mushroom, Atkins Potts*	½ Pack/175g	136	4.6	78	1	7.5	2.6	1.1
Madras, Aldi*	1 Serving/113g	68	2.3	60	1.5	9	2	0
Madras, Cooking, Sharwood's*	1 Tsp/2g	2	0.1	86	1.5	6.9	5.8	1.3
Madras, M&S*	½ Jar/170g	264	20.1	155	2	8.5	11.8	3.2
Makhani, Butter, M&S*	½ Jar/170g	291	22.6	171	1.9	10	13.3	1.9
Mint, Bramwells, Aldi*	1 Serving/30g	28	0.2	93	0.5	21	0.5	0
Mint, Reduced Sugar, Tesco*	1 Tbsp/15g	12	0.1	81	1.8	16.2	0.5	2.1
Mint, Sainsbury's*	1 Dtsp/10g	13	0	126	2.5	28.7	0.1	4
Mint, Smart Price, Asda*	1 Serving/15g	6	0.1	39	0.5	7.2	0.5	1.6
Mint, Value, Tesco*	1 Serving/10g	4	0	41	1.1	9	0.1	1.8
Mushroom, Creamy, Chicken Tonight, Knorr*	¼ Jar/125g	100	7.4	80	0.8	5.7	5.9	0.6
Oyster Spring Onion, Stir Fry, Blue Dragon*	1 Sachet/120g	134	0	112	1.5	26.3	0	0
Oyster, Blue Dragon*	1 Tsp/5ml	6	0	121	3.4	26.9	0	0
Parsley, Fresh, Microwaved, Sainsbury's*	1/3 Pot/100g	78	5.4	78	1.7	5.3	5.4	0.5
Parsley, Tesco*	½ Pack/89g	85	5.1	95	2.8	8.1	5.7	1.1
Pasta Bake, Tuna, Homepride*	½ Jar/250g	208	13	83	1.4	7.6	5.2	0.9
Peanut, Sainsbury's*	1 Sachet/70g	185	9.2	264	1.9	34.7	13.1	1.6
Pepper, As Prepared, Colman's*	1 Portion/75ml	89	4.7	119	4.7	11	6.3	0
Pepper, Creamy, Tesco*	1 Serving/85ml	128	11.4	151	1.2	6.4	13.4	0.5
Pepper, Southern, Curry, The Spice Tailor*	1 Serving/100g	167	13	167	2.4	8.4	13	3.8
Peppercorn, with a Dash of Brandy, M&S*	½ Pouch/100g	100	7.9	100	1.5	5.4	7.9	0.5
Peri Peri, Garlic, Nando's*	1 Serving/15g	9	0.5	59	0.5	6.6	3.4	0.8
Peri Peri, Medium, Nando's*	1 Serving/20g	14	0.7	69	0.5	8.4	3.7	0.8
Pesto, with Basil, Buitoni*	1 Serving/62g	290	27	467	11.3	8.1	43.5	0
Plum, Dipping, M&S*	1 Tbsp/15g	34	0	228	0.1	56.2	0.2	0.3
Plum, Sticky, Stir Fry, Blue Dragon*	1 Serving/60g	145	0.2	242	0.1	35.6	0.3	0
Prawn Cocktail, Frank Cooper*	1 Tbsp/15g	47	4	316	0.8	18.3	26.7	0.1

SAUCE

INFO/WEIGHT	Measure	per Measure		Nutrition Values per 100g / 100ml				
		KCAL	FAT	KCAL	PROT	CARB	FAT	FIBRE
Prawn Cocktail, Morrisons*	1 Portion/15ml	81	8.5	540	1.4	5.5	56.9	1.1
Raspberry, Dessert, M&S*	1 Serving/20g	24	0.1	120	0.5	28.7	0.3	2.6
Red Hot, Buffalo Wings, Bramwells, Aldi*	1 Tbsp/15g	8	0.4	53	1.5	4.6	2.6	2.5
Red Hot, Wings, Buffalo, Franks*	1 Tbsp/15g	4	0.2	30	0.8	2	1.5	2.5
Red Wine, Cooking, BGTY, Sainsbury's*	1 Serving/125g	52	0.6	42	0.5	8.8	0.5	0.8
Redcurrant, Colman's*	1 Tsp/12g	44	0	368	0.7	90	0	0
Rogan Josh, M&S*	½ Jar/170g	216	15.8	127	1.8	7.6	9.3	2.8
Rogan Josh, Medium, Sharwood's*	½ Jar/210g	151	7.6	72	1.4	8.6	3.6	0.5
Rogan Josh, Spice Simmer, Asda*	1/3 Jar/120g	101	5.6	84	1.3	8.3	4.7	1.5
Salted Caramel, Dipping, Waitrose*	1 Tsp/5g	21	1.2	425	2.4	46.4	24.5	4.4
Satay, Peanut, M&S*	1 Serving/15g	33	2.3	221	6.4	8.6	15.2	12.2
Satay, Peanut, Roast, Stir Fry, Straight to Wok, Amoy*	½ Pack/60g	106	6.4	176	4	16.3	10.6	1.3
Satay, Peanut, Roasted, Stir Fry Sensations, Amoy*	1 Pouch/160g	354	19.8	221	4.7	21.9	12.4	1
Satay, Tesco*	1 Jar/180g	265	14	147	4.7	10.9	7.8	7.1
Sausage Casserole, Cook in, Homepride*	½ Jar/250g	92	0.5	37	0.7	8	0.2	0.6
Seafood, Average	*1 Tsp/5g*	*20*	*1.9*	*410*	*1.4*	*15.4*	*38*	*0.2*
Seafood, Colman's*	1 Tbsp/15g	44	3.4	296	0.9	21.5	22.9	0.4
Seafood, Sainsbury's*	1 Tbsp/15g	53	4.5	356	1.2	20.1	30	0.5
Soy, & Garlic, Stir Fry, Fresh Tastes, Asda*	1 Pack/180g	175	6.7	97	1.7	14.1	3.7	0.5
Soy, & Plum, Stir Fry Additions, COOK!, M&S*	½ Sachet/60g	48	0.2	80	1.5	17.5	0.3	1.5
Soy, Garlic, Spiced, Deliciously Vesatile, M&S*	¼ Bottle/38g	156	14.8	415	2.3	10.3	39.5	4.6
Soy, Average	*1 Tsp/5ml*	*3*	*0*	*64*	*8.7*	*8.3*	*0*	*0*
Soy, Dark, Average	*1 Tsp/5g*	*4*	*0*	*84*	*4*	*16.7*	*0.1*	*0.2*
Soy, Light, Amoy*	1 Tsp/5ml	3	0	52	2.5	10.5	0	0
Soy, Reduced Salt, Amoy*	1 Tsp/5ml	3	0	56	4	10	0	0
Spanish Chicken, Batts, Lidl*	½ Jar/250g	122	4.8	49	1.3	5.9	1.9	1.4
Spanish Chicken, Chicken Tonight, Knorr*	¼ Jar/125g	68	2	55	1.6	7.3	1.6	2.3
Spare Rib, Lee Kum Kee*	2 Tbsp/38g	80	1	211	2.6	39.5	2.6	2.6
Sriracha, M&S*	1 Tsp/5g	6	0	125	1.4	25.4	1	4.2
Stroganoff, Cooking, Loyd Grossman*	½ Pack/165g	203	14.8	123	1.6	8.6	9	0.7
Stroganoff, Creamy, M&S*	1 Pouch/200g	190	15.2	95	0.6	4.6	7.6	1.8
Sweet & Sour, Chinese, Sainsbury's*	½ Jar/150g	222	0.2	148	0.2	36.6	0.1	0.1
Sweet & Sour, Cook In, Glass Jar, Homepride*	1 Jar/500g	335	0.5	67	0.3	16.2	0.1	0.5
Sweet & Sour, Cooking, Chinese, Sainsbury's*	¼ Jar/125g	155	0.1	124	0.6	30.1	0.1	0.7
Sweet & Sour, Spicy, Sharwood's*	1 Serving/138g	142	0.7	103	0.7	23.8	0.5	0.4
Sweet & Sour, Spicy, Uncle Ben's*	1 Jar/400g	364	0.4	91	0.6	22.1	0.1	0
Sweet & Sour, Stir Fry Additions, Tesco*	1 Sachet/50g	84	0.5	167	0.8	38.7	1	0.5
Sweet & Sour, Stir Fry, Asda*	1 Serving/63g	146	3.2	232	0.8	46	5	0
Sweet & Sour, Stir Fry, Sharwood's*	1 Jar 160g	168	0.8	105	0.6	24.5	0.5	0.8
Sweet & Sour, Stir Fry, Tesco*	½ Jar/222g	164	0.4	74	0.6	17	0.2	0.4
Sweet & Sour, Take-Away	*1oz/28g*	*44*	*1*	*157*	*0.2*	*32.8*	*3.4*	*0*
Sweet Sour, Cooking, HL, Tesco*	½ Jar/250g	98	1	39	0.2	8.3	0.4	0.6
Sweet Sour, Cooking, LC, Tesco*	1 Jar/510g	357	0.5	70	0.3	16.1	0.1	0.5
Sweet Sour, Extra Pineapple, Uncle Ben's*	1 Serving/165g	147	0.3	89	0.3	21.2	0.2	0.7
Sweet Sour, Light, Uncle Ben's*	¼ Jar/125g	71	0.1	57	0.4	12.6	0.1	0.9
Sweet Sour, M&S*	½ Jar/145g	144	1	99	1.1	22	0.7	0.5
Sweet Sour, No Added Sugar, Uncle Ben's*	1 Jar/440g	123	0.4	28	0.4	5.5	0.1	0.8
Sweet Sour, Stir Fry, Pouch, Average	*1 Pouch/120g*	*148*	*2.3*	*124*	*0.8*	*25.7*	*1.9*	*1*
Sweet Sour, Stir Fry, Sachet, Blue Dragon*	1 Sachet/120g	145	0.1	122	0.2	29.7	0.1	0.3
Sweet Chilli & Garlic, Stir Fry & Dipping, Tesco*	½ Jar/95ml	78	0	82	0.3	20.1	0	0.1
Sweet Chilli, Dipping, M&S*	1 Tbsp/15g	34	0.1	225	0.9	53.2	0.7	0.6
Sweet Chilli, Heinz*	1 Serving/25g	38	0.1	150	0.3	36.5	0.4	6.4
Sweet Chilli, Stir Fry, Additions, Tesco*	1 Serving/50g	106	3.8	211	0.3	35.2	7.6	0.6

S

SAUCE	Measure INFO/WEIGHT	per Measure KCAL	FAT	Nutrition Values per 100g / 100ml KCAL	PROT	CARB	FAT	FIBRE
Sweet Chilli, Thai, Blue Dragon*	1 Serving/15g	28	0.1	188	0.5	45.5	0.6	0
Sweet Curry, Eazy Squirt, Heinz*	1 Serving/10ml	12	0	124	0.7	29	0.3	0.5
Sweet Pepper, Stir in, Dolmio*	½ Pot/75g	77	4.6	103	1.4	9.6	6.2	1.6
Szechuan Style, Stir Fry, Fresh Ideas, Tesco*	1 Sachet/50g	114	4.8	228	1.9	33.4	9.7	0.1
Szechuan, Spicy Tomato, Stir Fry, Blue Dragon*	½ Sachet/60g	59	1.8	98	1.3	15.8	3	0.9
Szechuan, Tomato, Spicy, Stir Fry, Sharwoods*	½ Jar/98g	56	0.3	57	1.1	12	0.3	0.8
Tamari, Soya, Clearspring*	1oz/28g	55	0.1	196	14	34	0.2	0
Tamarind & Lime, Stir Fry, Sainsbury's*	1 Serving/75g	88	5.6	117	1.1	11.4	7.4	0.8
Tartare	*1oz/28g*	*84*	*6.9*	*299*	*1.3*	*17.9*	*24.6*	*0*
Tartare, Colman's*	1 Tbsp/15g	45	3.7	290	1.5	17	24	0.6
Tartare, Finest, Tesco*	1 Tbsp/15g	47	4.7	312	1.3	5.7	31.1	2.1
Tartare, Mild Creamy, Heinz*	1 Tbsp/15g	47	4.2	312	0.9	13.4	28.3	0.1
Tartare, Rich, Colman's*	1 Tsp/5ml	14	1.2	284	1.2	17	23	0.6
Tartare, Sainsbury's*	1 Tbsp/15ml	42	3.6	281	1.4	15.4	23.7	0.5
Tartare, Tesco*	1 Tbsp/15g	47	3.9	312	0.7	18.7	25.8	1.1
Teriyaki, Asda*	1 Serving/98g	99	0.1	101	2.1	23	0.1	0
Teriyaki, Deliciously Versatile, M&S*	1 Tbsp/15g	19	0.2	127	2.6	25.7	1.3	0
Teriyaki, Japanese Grill, Kikkoman*	1 Serving/15ml	24	0	158	4.5	30.8	0.1	0
Teriyaki, Lee Kum Kee*	1 Serving/15g	27	0	178	2.2	42.4	0	0.5
Teriyaki, Stir Fry, Blue Dragon*	1 Pack/120g	131	0.2	109	0.9	25.9	0.2	0
Teriyaki, Stir Fry, Fresh Ideas, Tesco*	1 Serving/25g	33	0.6	133	1.1	26.9	2.3	0
Tiger, TryMe*	1 Serving/5ml	10	0	200	0	40	0	0
Tikka Masala, Cooking, HL, Tesco*	¼ Jar/125g	78	3.1	62	0.4	9	2.5	0.7
Tikka Masala, GFY, Asda*	½ Jar/250g	190	8	76	2.9	9	3.2	0.5
Tikka Masala, M&S*	½ Jar/170g	309	26.9	182	1.8	7.2	15.8	2
Tikka Masala, Medium, Cooking, Sharwood's*	1/3 Jar/140g	150	9.7	107	1.3	9.7	6.9	0.5
Tikka Masala, Ready Made, Average	*1 Sm Jar/350g*	*422*	*28.8*	*121*	*2*	*9.6*	*8.2*	*1.2*
Toffee, GFY, Asda*	1 Serving/5g	15	0.1	306	2.2	68	2.8	0
Toffee, Luxury, Rowse*	1 Serving/20g	67	0.7	336	1.9	73.9	3.7	0.4
Tomato & Cheese, Pasta Bake, Dolmio*	¼ Jar/125g	70	1.5	56	2.1	9.1	1.2	1.2
Tomato & Herb, Creamy, Pasta Bake, Homepride*	1 Serving/125g	128	8.8	102	1.5	8.3	7	0.9
Tomato & Marscapone, Finest, Tesco*	1 Serving/350g	270	17.5	77	2.7	5.4	5	0.8
Tomato & Mushroom, Pasta, Cucina, Aldi*	¼ Jar/125g	59	0.6	47	2	8.2	0.5	1.4
Tomato Basil Sauce, Fresh, Tesco*	1 Pot/500g	245	9	49	1.5	6.8	1.8	0.9
Tomato Basil, for Meatballs, Dolmio*	¼ Jar/125g	48	0.2	38	1.5	6.9	0.2	1.3
Tomato Basil, Italian, Fresh, Asda*	½ Tub/175g	107	5.7	60	1.5	6.1	3.2	0.6
Tomato Basil, Italian, Sainsbury's*	½ Pot/175g	88	3	50	1.9	6.2	1.7	1
Tomato Garlic, for Meatballs, Dolmio*	1 Portion/125g	46	0.1	37	1.6	6.5	0.1	0
Tomato, Bacon, Pasta Bake, Aldi*	¼ Jar/123g	107	6.8	87	1.5	7.4	5.5	0.9
Tomato, Heinz*	1 Tbsp/17g	18	0	103	0.9	24.1	0.1	0.7
Tomato, Pizza Topping, Napolina*	1 Serving/70g	34	1.5	49	0.9	6.3	2.2	0.6
Tomato, Pomodorini, Finest, Tesco*	½ Pot/125g	79	3.9	63	1.2	5.8	3.1	3.7
Tomato, Smokehouse, M&S*	1 Tbsp/15g	28	0	185	2.3	42.5	0.2	1.9
Vindaloo, Hot, Patak's*	1 Jar/540g	518	34.6	96	1.5	6.4	6.4	0
Watercress, Stilton, Creamy for Fish, Schwartz*	1 Pack/300g	141	12.3	47	0.6	2	4.1	0.7
Watercress, Sainsbury's*	1 Serving/100g	87	6.4	87	2.8	4.2	6.4	0.5
White Wine, & Cream, Cook in, Classic, Homepride*	¼ Can/125g	101	5.1	81	1	8	4.1	0.4
White Wine, & Mushroom, BGTY, Sainsbury's*	¼ Jar/125g	81	2.5	65	2.8	9	2	0.3
White Wine, & Parsley, Pour Over, Loyd Grossman*	½ Sachet/85g	94	7.9	111	1	5.6	9.3	0.5
White, Savoury, Made with Semi-Skimmed Milk	*1oz/28g*	*36*	*2.2*	*128*	*4.2*	*11.1*	*7.8*	*0.2*
White, Savoury, Made with Whole Milk	*1oz/28g*	*42*	*2.9*	*150*	*4.1*	*10.9*	*10.3*	*0.2*
Worcestershire Sauce, Sainsbury's*	1 Tbsp/15ml	16	0	107	0.7	23.3	0.1	0.3
Worcestershire, Average	*1 Tsp/5g*	*3*	*0*	*65*	*1.4*	*15.5*	*0.1*	*0*

	Measure INFO/WEIGHT	per Measure KCAL	FAT	Nutrition Values per 100g / 100ml KCAL	PROT	CARB	FAT	FIBRE
SAUCE								
Worcestershire, Lea & Perrins*	1 Tsp/5ml	5	0	96	0.8	21	0.9	0
SAUCE MIX								
Beef Bourguignon, Colman's*	1 Pack/40g	136	0.8	340	7	72	2	3
Beef Stroganoff, Colman's*	1 Pack/40g	140	3.6	350	11.6	56.1	8.9	2.7
Bread, As Sold, M&S*	¼ Pack/18g	64	1.2	368	11.4	62.4	6.9	5.5
Bread, Made Up, Colman's*	1 Serving/75ml	70	1.5	95	5	14	2	0.6
Cheddar Cheese, Colman's*	1 Pack/40g	164	6	410	19	51	15	2
Cheddar Cheese, Dry Mix, Schwartz*	1 Pack/40g	144	3	361	18.4	55.1	7.4	2.3
Cheese Flavour, Dairy Free, Free & Easy*	4 Teasp/15g	4	0.1	26	0.6	4.9	0.4	0.3
Cheese, Made Up with Skimmed Milk	**1 Serving/60g**	**47**	**1.4**	**78**	**5.4**	**9.5**	**2.3**	**0**
Chicken Chasseur, Schwartz*	1 Pack/40g	126	1.8	316	9.6	59.1	4.6	6.8
Chilli Con Carne, Asda*	1 Sachet/50g	157	0.8	314	7	68	1.6	2.5
Chilli Con Carne, Recipe Mix, Bramwells, Aldi*	1 Pack/38g	130	1.1	341	6.2	70	2.8	5.3
Chilli Con Carne, Recipe Mix, Schwartz*	1 Pack/41g	133	1.5	324	8.2	60.8	3.6	0
Chip Shop Curry, Dry Weight, Bisto*	1 Dtsp/9g	38	1.6	427	3.4	63.5	17.7	1.3
Cream, for Meatballs, Ikea*	1 Pack/40g	179	9.4	448	9.6	49.2	23.6	0
Dauphinoise Potato Bake, Schwartz*	1 Pack/40g	161	10.5	402	6.8	34.7	26.3	15.8
Four Cheese, Colman's*	1 Pack/35g	127	3.9	362	17.1	48.4	11.1	1.8
Hollandaise, Colman's*	1 Pack/28g	104	3.1	372	6.4	61.6	11.1	1.8
Hollandaise, Made Up, Schwartz*	1 Serving/79g	58	2	73	3.9	8.7	2.5	0
Korma, Schwartz*	1 Pack/35g	124	4	354	8.4	47.6	11.4	13.5
Lemon Butter for Fish, Schwartz*	1 Pack/38g	136	3	357	6.1	65.3	8	5.8
Mixed Herbs for Chicken, So Juicy, Maggi*	1 Pack/34g	97	1	285	8.3	53.8	2.8	5.5
Paprika For Chicken, So Juicy, Maggi*	1 Pack/34g	91	1.4	267	8.8	45.5	4	7.1
Parsley Chive for Fish, Schwartz*	1 Pack/38g	150	4.3	394	9.4	61.8	11.4	3.5
Parsley, Creamy, Made Up, Schwartz*	1 Serving/79g	59	2	75	4.2	8.7	2.5	0.3
Parsley, Made Up, Bisto*	1 Serving/50ml	43	2.5	86	1	9.6	5	1
Pepper, Creamy, Schwartz*	1 Pack/25g	86	1.7	342	17.9	52	6.9	7
Peppercorn, Made Up with Water, CBY, Asda*	1 Serving/63ml	52	3.9	84	0.7	5.4	6.2	1.7
Peppercorn, Mild, Creamy, Schwartz*	1 Pack/25g	88	2.2	352	13.8	55	8.6	5
Savoury Mince, Schwartz*	1 Pack/35g	108	0.7	310	14.6	58.3	2	1.8
Shepherd's Pie, Schwartz*	1 Pack/38g	118	0.9	311	8.2	60.3	2.3	11.1
Shepherds Pie, Bramwells*	1 Pack/50g	168	3	336	8.6	62	6	6.9
Spaghetti Bolognese, Colman's*	1 Pack/40g	120	0.4	300	8.9	64.1	0.9	5.2
Spaghetti Bolognese, Schwartz*	1 Pack/40g	114	0.6	285	9.2	59	1.6	7
Spaghetti Carbonara, Schwartz*	1 Pack/32g	135	6.4	421	10.4	49.4	20.1	7.2
Stroganoff, Beef, Schwartz*	1 Pack/35g	125	3.6	358	15.6	50.8	10.3	4.4
Stroganoff, Mushroom, Schwartz*	1 Pack/35g	121	3.1	345	10.9	52.4	8.9	5.9
Thickening Granules, McDougalls*	1 Tbsp/10g	46	1.9	463	0	73.7	18.7	0
Tuna Napolitana, Schwartz*	1 Pack/30g	107	3.9	357	10.3	49.6	13.1	0.5
White, Dry Weight, Bisto*	1 Dtsp/9g	45	2.5	496	3.2	57.4	28.2	0.4
White, Instant, Made Up, Sainsbury's*	1 Serving/90ml	65	2.5	72	0.8	10.9	2.8	0.1
White, Made Up with Semi-Skimmed Milk	**1oz/28g**	**20**	**0.7**	**73**	**4**	**9.6**	**2.4**	**0**
White, Made Up with Skimmed Milk	**1oz/28g**	**17**	**0.3**	**59**	**4**	**9.6**	**0.9**	**0**
White, Savoury, Colman's*	1 Pack/25g	105	3.8	420	9	63	15	2
SAUERKRAUT								
Average	**1oz/28g**	**3**	**0**	**11**	**1.1**	**1.6**	**0**	**0.9**
SAUSAGE								
Asda*	1 Sausage/43g	81	3.9	189	20	7	9	2.9
Beef, Average	**1 Sausage/60g**	**151**	**11.1**	**252**	**14.5**	**7**	**18.5**	**0.6**
Beetroot, The Beet Goes On, Vegetarian, Heck*	2 Sausages/80g	138	6.9	173	5.5	10.8	8.6	15.1
Best Of British, Quorn*	1 Sausage/56g	115	5.8	206	15	10.4	10.4	5.4
Bierwurst, Average	**1 Slice/10g**	**25**	**2.1**	**252**	**14.4**	**1**	**21.2**	**0**

S

	Measure INFO/WEIGHT	per Measure KCAL	FAT	Nutrition Values per 100g / 100ml KCAL	PROT	CARB	FAT	FIBRE
SAUSAGE								
Billy Bear, Kids, Tesco*	1 Slice/20g	37	2.2	185	13.7	7.5	11.2	0.4
Bockwurst, Average	*1 Sausage/45g*	*114*	*10.4*	*253*	*10.8*	*0.8*	*23*	*0*
Bollywood Bangers, Indian Style, Vegetarian, Heck*	2 Sausages/76g	123	4.8	162	6.9	13.2	6.3	12.4
Braai Flavour, Fry's Special Vegetarian*	1 Sausage/63g	86	4.4	138	16.5	10	7	4
Bratwurst, Frozen, Lidl*	1 Sausage/80g	235	21.4	294	12.8	0.5	26.8	0
Bratwurst, Nuremberg, Dulano, Lidl*	1 Sausage/22g	77	7	349	14	1	32	0.5
Bratwurst, Tesco*	1 Sausage/90g	264	23.5	293	12.8	1.5	26.1	0.3
Chicken, Italia, Grilled, Heck*	1 Sausage/34g	49	0.9	145	28.5	2.4	2.6	0
Chicken, Manor Farm*	1 Sausage/65g	126	8.1	194	13.7	6.6	12.5	1.2
Chicken, Sundried Tomoato Basil, As Consumed, Mor*	1 Sausage/34g	43	1.3	127	12.4	9.6	3.9	2.2
Chipolata, Average	*1 Sausage/28g*	*81*	*6.5*	*291*	*12.1*	*8.7*	*23.1*	*0.7*
Chipolata, Chicken, Smoky Paprika, Grilled, Heck*	2 Chipolatas/68g	109	1.7	159	27.3	5.8	2.5	0
Chipolata, Lamb, & Rosemary, Tesco*	1 Sausage/32g	69	4.9	218	11.3	8.3	15.5	0
Chipolata, Pork, & Honey, Finest, Tesco*	2 Sausages/64g	170	12.3	265	14	8.7	19.2	0.7
Chipolata, Pork, Black Pepper & Nutmeg, Waitrose*	1 Sausage/22g	50	2.4	229	20	12.7	10.9	0.5
Chipolata, Premium, Average	*1 Serving/80g*	*187*	*13.8*	*234*	*14.8*	*4.7*	*17.3*	*1.2*
Chorizo, Average	*1 Serving/80g*	*250*	*19.4*	*313*	*21.1*	*2.6*	*24.2*	*0.2*
Chorizo, Lean, Average	*1 Sausage/67g*	*131*	*9.2*	*195*	*15.7*	*2.3*	*13.7*	*0.8*
Cocktail, Average	*1 Sausage/7g*	*23*	*1.9*	*323*	*12.1*	*8.6*	*26.7*	*0.9*
Cocktail, Vegetarian, Grilled, Linda McCartney*	1 Sausage/16g	26	0.9	161	18.8	5.8	5.6	6.3
Cocktail, Vegetarian, Tivall*	1 Portion/70g	156	9.8	223	18	5.5	14	1.5
Cumberland, Average	*1 Sausage/57g*	*167*	*13*	*293*	*13.8*	*8.6*	*22.8*	*0.8*
Cumberland, Cauldron Foods*	1 Sausage/46g	75	4	163	14	6.5	8.6	2
Cumberland, Healthy Range, Average	*1 Sausage/53g*	*75*	*2.1*	*142*	*17.4*	*9*	*4*	*0.9*
Cumberland, Meat Free, Quorn*	1 Sausage/47g	105	4.7	222	17.9	12.5	9.9	5.9
Cumberland, Naked, Finnebrogue*	3 Sausages/200g	532	44	266	15	0.5	22	1.5
Debrecziner, Spicy Smoked, Gebirgsjager*	1 Sausage/37g	118	10.4	320	16	1	28	0
Free From, Wheat & Gulten, Sainsbury's*	2 Sausages/104g	268	20	257	13.3	7.2	19.2	1
Garlic, Average	*1 Slice/11g*	*25*	*2*	*227*	*15.7*	*0.8*	*18.2*	*0*
German, Extrawurst, Selection, Sainsbury's*	1 Slice/3g	9	0.8	279	13.1	0.5	25	0.1
German, Schinkenwurst, Selection, Sainsbury's*	1 Slice/3g	8	0.7	251	13.1	0.3	21.9	0.1
Grilled, Linda McCartney*	1 Sausage/50g	80	2.7	160	17.9	7.5	5.4	5
Irish, Average	*1 Sausage/40g*	*119*	*8.3*	*298*	*10.7*	*17.2*	*20.7*	*0.7*
Italian, Tofurky*	1 Sausage/63g	167	8	270	29	12	13	8
Lamb, & Mint, M&S*	1oz/28g	63	4.6	225	13.3	6.6	16.3	1.7
Lincolnshire, Average	*1 Sausage/42g*	*122*	*9.1*	*291*	*14.6*	*9.2*	*21.8*	*0.6*
Lincolnshire, Cauldron Foods*	1 Sausage/46g	84	4.5	182	16.1	5.5	9.8	3.6
Lincolnshire, Frozen, Tesco*	1 Sausage/50g	78	2.5	155	15.5	10.8	5	3
Lincolnshire, Healthy Range, Average	*1 Sausage/50g*	*89*	*4.3*	*177*	*15.8*	*9*	*8.6*	*0.8*
Lincolnshire, Meat Free, Quorn*	1 Sausage/41g	60	2.7	146	13.5	7.2	6.6	5.2
Lorne, Average	*1 Sausage/25g*	*78*	*5.8*	*312*	*10.8*	*16*	*23.1*	*0.6*
Merguez	*1 Merguez/55g*	*165*	*14.3*	*300*	*16*	*0.6*	*26*	*0*
Outrageously Succulent, Grilled, Linda Mccartney's*	2 Sausage/88g	148	5.3	168	18.2	8.7	6	3
Patties, Quorn*	1 Pattie/42g	53	2	127	12.8	5.8	4.9	4.7
Pigs in Blankets, Cooked, Morrisons*	1 Roll/22g	52	2.9	235	22.9	5.2	13.3	1.5
Pigs In Blankets, Cooked, Sainsbury's*	1 Roll/15g	42	2.8	280	3.1	11.2	18.5	1
Polish Kabanos, Sainsbury's*	1 Sausage/25g	92	7.6	366	23	0.1	30.4	0.1
Pork & Beef, Average	*1 Sausage/45g*	*133*	*10.2*	*295*	*8.7*	*13.6*	*22.7*	*0.5*
Pork & Herb, Average	*1 Sausage/75g*	*231*	*19.5*	*308*	*13.2*	*5.4*	*26*	*0.4*
Pork & Herb, Healthy Range, Average	*1 Sausage/59g*	*75*	*1.4*	*126*	*16*	*10.8*	*2.4*	*1.1*
Pork & Tomato, Grilled, Average	*1 Sausage/47g*	*127*	*9.7*	*273*	*13.9*	*7.5*	*20.8*	*0.4*
Pork Apple, Average	*1 Sausage/57g*	*146*	*10.7*	*256*	*14.5*	*7.5*	*18.8*	*1.9*
Pork, & Caramelised Onion, Thick, Cooked, Morrisons*	1 Sausage/45g	125	8.3	279	20.1	7.1	18.6	0.9

S

SAUSAGE

	INFO/WEIGHT	KCAL	FAT	KCAL	PROT	CARB	FAT	FIBRE
Pork, & Leek, Thick, Signature, Morrisons*	1 Sausage/55g	127	8.6	231	20.5	1.5	15.6	1.4
Pork, Apple, Frozen, Tesco*	2 Sausages/80g	167	10.3	209	14.8	8.1	12.9	0.7
Pork, Bramley Apple, 80% Pork, M&S*	1 Sausage/134g	330	34.3	246	12.4	5.5	25.6	1
Pork, Average	*1 Sausage/45g*	*139*	*11.2*	*309*	*11.9*	*9.8*	*25*	*0.8*
Pork, Battered, Thick, Average	*1oz/28g*	*126*	*10.2*	*448*	*17.3*	*21.7*	*36.3*	*2*
Pork, Beetroot, & Bramley Apple, Mor*	2 Sausages/118g	205	11.7	174	10	10	9.9	2.4
Pork, Black Pudding, Apple, Aldi*	1 Sausage/59g	134	9.4	227	13	6.6	16	1.8
Pork, Extra Lean, Average	*1 Sausage/54g*	*84*	*3.7*	*155*	*17.3*	*6.1*	*6.8*	*0.8*
Pork, Frozen, Fried	*1oz/28g*	*88*	*6.9*	*316*	*13.8*	*10*	*24.8*	*0*
Pork, Frozen, Grilled	*1oz/28g*	*81*	*5.9*	*289*	*14.8*	*10.5*	*21.2*	*0*
Pork, Garlic & Herb, Average	*1 Sausage/76g*	*203*	*16.5*	*268*	*12*	*6*	*21.8*	*1.2*
Pork, Premium, Average	*1 Sausage/74g*	*191*	*13.6*	*258*	*14.9*	*8.3*	*18.4*	*1*
Pork, Reduced Fat, Chilled, Grilled	*1 Sausage/45g*	*104*	*6.2*	*230*	*16.2*	*10.8*	*13.8*	*1.5*
Pork, Reduced Fat, Healthy Range, Average	*1 Sausage/57g*	*86*	*3.4*	*151*	*15.6*	*9*	*6*	*0.9*
Pork, Skinless, Average	*1oz/28g*	*81*	*6.6*	*291*	*11.7*	*8.2*	*23.6*	*0.6*
Pork, Thick, Average	*1 Sausage/39g*	*115*	*8.7*	*296*	*13.3*	*10*	*22.4*	*1*
Pork, Thick, Reduced Fat, Healthy Range, Average	*1 Sausage/52g*	*90*	*3.8*	*172*	*14*	*12.3*	*7.4*	*0.8*
Pork, Thick, Reduced Salt Fat, Grilled, Richmond*	1 Sausage/38g	78	3.8	204	14	12	10	0
Pork. Cocktail, British, Finest, Tesco*	3 Sausages/37g	112	9.8	303	15.3	0.6	26.4	0.9
Premium, Chilled, Fried	*1oz/28g*	*77*	*5.8*	*275*	*15.8*	*6.7*	*20.7*	*0*
Premium, Chilled, Grilled	*1oz/28g*	*82*	*6.3*	*292*	*16.8*	*6.3*	*22.4*	*0*
Saveloy, Unbattered, Takeaway, Average	*1 Saveloy/65g*	*192*	*14.5*	*296*	*13.8*	*10.8*	*22.3*	*0.8*
Smoked Pork, Reduced Fat, Mattessons*	1 Serving/50g	120	10	240	16	0	20	0
Smoked, Average	*1 Sausage/174g*	*588*	*52.2*	*338*	*13*	*4*	*30*	*0*
Spinach, Leek & Cheese, Gourmet, Wicken Fen*	1 Sausage/46g	92	4.7	201	10.3	17	10.2	1.9
Toulouse, TTD, Sainsbury's*	2 Sausages/113g	314	24.3	278	19.8	0.9	21.5	1.1
Toulouse, with Bacon, Red Wine, Garlic, Waitrose*	2 Sausages/106g	275	19.4	260	20.8	2.4	18.3	1
Turkey & Chicken, Average	*1 Sausage/57g*	*126*	*8.2*	*222*	*14.4*	*8.2*	*14.6*	*1.8*
Turkey, Average	*1 Sausage/57g*	*90*	*4.6*	*157*	*15.7*	*6.3*	*8*	*0*
Vegetarian, Bangers, Quorn*	1 Sausage/50g	58	2.4	116	11.7	6.6	4.8	3
Vegetarian, Cocktail, Quorn*	1 Sausage/15g	31	1.7	206	12.4	11.6	11.3	4.3
Vegetarian, Quorn*	1 Sausage/40g	79	4.5	198	11.2	10.6	11.1	5.5
Venison Pork, Waitrose*	1 Sausage/64g	93	4	146	16.5	5.3	6.3	1.1
Wiejska, Polish, Sainsbury's*	1/8 Pack/50g	78	4.5	157	18.7	0.4	9	0.5
Wild Boar	*1 Sausage/85g*	*220*	*17*	*259*	*16.5*	*1.2*	*20*	*0*

SAUSAGE & MASH

2 British Pork Rich Onion Gravy, M&S*	1 Pack/400g	340	6.8	85	5.7	12.2	1.7	1.3
British Classic, Tesco*	1 Pack/450g	675	42.8	150	5.1	11.1	9.5	0.9
Classic Kitchen, Tesco*	1 Pack/450g	510	23.2	113	4	12	5.1	1.3
Frozen, HFC, Tesco*	1 Pack/380g	371	8.4	98	3.3	15.5	2.2	1.4
LC, Tesco*	1 Pack/400g	360	8.8	90	4.4	11.8	2.2	1.4
Lincolnshire, Root Vegetable Mash, Weight Watchers*	1 Pack/380g	294	8	77	5.3	8.6	2.1	1.4
with Ale Gravy, & Champ Potato, Pork, Gastropub, M&S*	1 Pack/400g	728	50.8	182	8.1	8.1	12.7	1.3
with Beans, Little Dish*	1 Pack/200g	204	7.4	102	4.7	11.4	3.7	2.1
with Onion Gravy, Bangers, British Classic, Sainsbury's*	1 Pack/450g	562	30.6	125	4.8	9.9	6.8	2.6

SAUSAGE MEAT

Pork, Average	*1oz/28g*	*96*	*8.2*	*344*	*9.9*	*10.2*	*29.4*	*0.6*

SAUSAGE ROLL

Bacon, Cheddar, Smoked, Vintage, Finest, Tesco*	1 Roll/47g	199	15.1	423	12.6	20.2	32.1	1.3
Buffet, HE, Tesco*	1 Roll/30g	83	3.8	278	9.6	31.2	12.8	1.5
Cocktail, Average	*1 Roll/15g*	*57*	*3.7*	*378*	*8.9*	*29.4*	*24.9*	*1.9*
Frozen, Greggs Iceland Exclusive*	1 Roll /103g	349	24.7	339	8	22	24	1.5
GF, Genius*	1 Roll/100g	281	17.5	281	8.2	21.8	17.5	1.7

S

INFO/WEIGHT	Measure	per Measure KCAL	FAT	Nutrition Values per 100g / 100ml KCAL	PROT	CARB	FAT	FIBRE

SAUSAGE ROLL

	Measure INFO/WEIGHT	per Measure KCAL	FAT	KCAL	PROT	CARB	FAT	FIBRE
Jumbo, Sainsbury's*	1 Roll/145g	456	26.3	314	9.5	27.2	18.1	2.3
Kingsize, Pork Farms*	½ Roll/50g	241	15.9	483	10.5	39.9	31.8	0
Lincolnshire, Snack, Chef Select, Lidl*	1 Roll/30g	110	7.4	368	8.9	27.2	24.6	1.2
Linda McCartney*	1 Roll/52g	145	7.1	278	13.1	26	13.7	1.6
Mini, 40 Pack, Tesco*	1 Roll/14g	48	2.9	349	8.3	30.3	21.1	2.4
Mini, Linda McCartney*	1 Roll/14g	41	2.2	293	11.3	23.7	15.8	5.2
Mini, Oven Baked, Greggs, Iceland*	1 Roll/25g	76	6	303	7.9	21	24	0
Mini, Tesco*	1 Roll/15g	53	3.7	356	9	23.9	24.9	1.5
Mini, Waitrose*	1 Roll/35g	124	9.2	353	13	16.1	26.3	1
Pork, Finest, Tesco*	1 Roll/47g	174	11.5	371	12.2	24.9	24.4	1.5
Pork, Morrisons*	1 Roll/70g	195	9	278	9.6	31.2	12.8	1.5
Pork, TTD, Sainsbury's*	1 Roll/65g	242	16.8	372	11.5	22.9	25.8	1.1
Puff Pastry	*1 Med/60g*	*230*	*16.6*	*383*	*9.9*	*25.4*	*27.6*	*1*
TTD, Sainsbury's*	1 Roll/27g	103	7	383	12.3	23.9	26.1	1.4
Vegetarian, Chilled, Quorn*	1 Roll/130g	293	12.1	225	12.3	21.2	9.3	3.8

SCALLOPS

Breaded, Thai Style with Plum Sauce, Finest, Tesco*	1 Serving/210g	401	14.7	191	11.5	20.6	7	0.8
Lemon Grass & Ginger, Tesco*	½ Pack/112g	90	1.1	80	15.2	2.5	1	0.6
Patagonian, Raw, Sainsbury's*	½ Pack/93g	112	2.5	120	22.5	1.2	2.7	0.5
Queen, Minted Pea, Oven Cooked, TTD, Sainsbury's*	½ Pack/92g	98	2.3	107	10.7	9.1	2.5	2.8
Raw, Bay or Sea with Roe, Average	*1 Scallop/15g*	*13*	*0.1*	*88*	*16.8*	*2.4*	*0.8*	*0*
Raw, Tesco*	½ Pack/72g	111	3.9	155	25.1	1.1	5.4	0.5
Steamed, Average	*1oz/28g*	*33*	*0.4*	*118*	*23.2*	*3.4*	*1.4*	*0*

SCAMPI

Chips, Chunky, Finest, Tesco*	1 Pack/280g	420	15.4	150	5.9	18.3	5.5	1.4
Chips, with Peas	*1 Serving/490g*	*822*	*43.6*	*168*	*10.1*	*11.3*	*8.9*	*1.2*
Bites, Everyday, Value, Tesco*	½ Pack/125g	262	10	210	9.4	23.4	8	1.2
Breaded, Baked, Average	*½ Pack/255g*	*565*	*27.4*	*222*	*10.7*	*20.5*	*10.7*	*1*
Breaded, Fried in Oil, Average	*1 Serving/100g*	*237*	*13.6*	*237*	*9.4*	*20.5*	*13.6*	*0*
Breaded, Oven Baked, Whitby Seafoods*	1 Pack/220g	447	15.4	203	9.3	24.5	7	0
Provencale	*1 Serving/100g*	*500*	*49*	*500*	*7*	*4*	*49*	*1*
Wholetail, Crispy, in Breadcrumbs, Ocean Trader, Lidl*	½ Pack/125g	270	10.8	216	11.9	22.2	8.6	1.1
Wholetail, Jumbo, Oven Baked, Gastro, Youngs*	1 Serving/103g	228	10.1	221	9.4	23	9.8	1.6

SCHNAPPS

Vodkat, Intercontinental Brands Ltd*	1 Serving/25ml	31	0	124	0	0.8	0	0

SCONE

All Butter, Cherry, Finest, Tesco*	1 Scone/70g	245	7.2	349	7.1	56	10.3	1.9
All Butter, Finest, Tesco*	1 Scone/70g	258	10.5	369	7.5	50.1	15	1.8
All Butter, Sultana, TTD, Sainsbury's*	1 Scone/70g	241	7	344	7.7	54	10	3.7
All Butter, Tesco*	1 Scone/60g	222	7.6	371	6.4	56.7	12.7	2
Cheddar, Cheese, Farmhouse, TTD, Sainsbury's*	1 Scone/70g	235	9.7	335	12	39.4	13.8	2.8
Cheese & Black Pepper, Mini, M&S*	1 Scone/18g	67	3.3	370	10.2	41.1	18.3	1.7
Cheese, Average	*1 Scone/40g*	*145*	*7.1*	*363*	*10.1*	*43.2*	*17.8*	*1.6*
Cherry, Double Butter, Genesis Crafty*	1 Scone/63g	198	4.8	314	6.8	54.5	7.6	1.4
Cherry, Genesis Crafty*	1 Scone/81g	226	5.8	279	4.9	50.5	7.1	0
Cherry, Haywood Padgett*	1 Scone/50g	178	4.6	357	6.1	61.6	9.1	2
Cherry, M&S*	1 Scone/60g	202	7.3	337	6.9	49.7	12.2	1.9
Clotted Cream, Cornish, TTD, Sainsbury's*	1 Scone/70g	269	12.7	384	8.4	46.6	18.2	2.1
Devon, M&S*	1 Scone/59g	225	9.6	380	7.1	50.8	16.2	1.5
Fresh Cream with Strawberry Jam, Tesco*	1 Scone/83g	290	15.6	352	4.7	40.7	18.9	1.1
Fruit, Aldi*	1 Scone/65g	239	5.8	367	6.3	64.4	9	1.6
Fruit, Average	*1 Scone/40g*	*126*	*3.9*	*316*	*7.3*	*52.9*	*9.8*	*0*
Fruit, Smart Price, Asda*	1 Scone/41g	139	4.1	338	7	55	10	3

S

	Measure INFO/WEIGHT	per Measure KCAL	FAT	Nutrition Values per 100g / 100ml KCAL	PROT	CARB	FAT	FIBRE
SCONE								
Fruit, Waitrose*	1 Scone/59g	190	4.8	325	6.3	56.5	8.2	2.2
Plain, All Butter, Sainsbury's*	1 Scone/58g	213	7.4	366	8.1	54.1	12.7	1.6
Plain, Average	*1 Scone/40g*	*145*	*5.8*	*362*	*7.2*	*53.8*	*14.6*	*1.9*
Plain, Butter Enriched, Tesco*	1 Scone/90g	317	8	352	7.7	59.8	8.9	1.2
Plain, Genesis Crafty*	1 Scone/74g	227	7.4	307	6.8	49.1	10	0
Potato, Average	*1 Scone/40g*	*118*	*5.7*	*296*	*5.1*	*39.1*	*14.3*	*1.6*
Potato, Mother's Pride*	1 Scone/37g	77	0.8	207	4.7	42	2.2	4.3
Red Berry, Mixed, Finest, Tesco*	1 Scone/110g	344	9.5	313	7.8	50.1	8.6	1.9
Strawberry, Fresh Cream, BGTY, Sainsbury's*	1 Scone/50g	154	5.6	309	5.1	47	11.2	1.1
Sultana, All Butter, Tesco*	1 Scone/60g	216	6.5	360	4.6	59.1	10.9	3.5
Sultana, Finest, Tesco*	1 Scone/70g	238	7.6	340	8.9	50.9	10.9	2.1
Sultana, H.W. Nevill's*	1 Scone/41g	136	3.1	334	6.8	58.6	7.5	2.3
Sultana, Haywood Padgett*	1 Scone/70g	254	6.2	363	6.8	63.8	8.8	1.6
Sultana, M&S*	1 Scone/66g	231	8.2	350	6.5	53	12.5	2
Sultana, Rowan Hill Bakery, Lidl*	1 Scone/60g	220	7.2	367	7.1	57	12	1.1
Sultana, Tesco*	1 Scone/90g	304	6.8	338	7.2	59.5	7.6	1.6
Sultana, Value, Tesco*	1 Scone/40g	134	4	335	6.5	53.8	10.1	2.7
Tattie, Scottish, Nick Nairn's*	1 Scone/21g	42	0.3	199	4	34.7	1.6	0.7
Wholemeal	*1 Scone/40g*	*130*	*5.8*	*326*	*8.7*	*43.1*	*14.4*	*5.2*
Wholemeal, Fruit	*1 Scone/40g*	*130*	*5.1*	*324*	*8.1*	*47.2*	*12.8*	*4.9*
SEA BASS								
Cooked, Dry Heat, Average	*1 Fillet/100g*	*124*	*2.6*	*124*	*23.6*	*0*	*2.6*	*0*
Fillets, Caramelised Ginger & Lime Butter, Sainsbury's*	1 Fillet/115g	258	18.1	224	19.9	0.5	15.7	0.5
Fillets, with Butter, Cooked, Tesco*	1 Fillet/86g	189	13	220	19.4	1	15.1	1.7
Raw, Fillet, Average	*1 Fillet/95g*	*108*	*3.4*	*113*	*20.3*	*0*	*3.5*	*0.1*
SEA BREAM								
Fillet, Cooked, Dry Heat, Average	*1 Serving/100g*	*124*	*3*	*124*	*24*	*0*	*3*	*0*
Fillets, Raw, Average	*1oz/28g*	*27*	*0.8*	*96*	*17.5*	*0*	*2.9*	*0*
SEAFOOD								
Cocktail, Average	*1oz/28g*	*24*	*0.4*	*87*	*15.6*	*2.9*	*1.5*	*0*
Selection, Fresh, Tesco*	1 Pack/234g	187	2.3	80	17.7	0.1	1	0
Selection, Sainsbury's*	½ Pack/125g	85	1.2	68	14.6	0.8	1	2.5
SEAFOOD STICKS								
Average	*1 Stick/15g*	*16*	*0*	*106*	*8*	*18.4*	*0.2*	*0.2*
SEASONING MIX								
All Purpose, Dunns River*	1 Tbsp/15g	37	1.5	248	8.3	26.7	9.9	9.3
Cajun, Perfect Shake, As Sold, Schwartz*	1 Tbsp/1g	2	0.1	249	9.9	27.2	7	19
Cajun, Tesco*	1 Tsp/5g	16	0.3	314	10.9	45.9	6.5	14
Chicken Provencal, Schwartz*	1 Pack/35g	104	0.7	296	9.3	55.3	2	9.9
Chicken, Blends, Bart*	1 Tbsp/15g	39	0.2	258	10.9	42.6	1.3	0
Chimichurri, Schwartz*	1 Pack/13g	37	0.4	283	10.7	46.8	3.2	0
Dukkah, Cooks' Ingredients, Waitrose*	1 Serving/5g	19	0.8	388	18.3	30.7	17	19.6
Dukkah, Cooks' Ingredients, Waitrose*	1 Serving/5g	19	0.8	388	18.3	30.7	17	19.6
Fajita, Fiery, Asda*	¼ Pack/9g	29	0.5	331	6.3	58	6	9.9
Fajita, Mild, M&S*	1 Pack/35g	112	2.2	319	10.2	44.7	6.2	21.9
Fajita, Original, Mild, Latin American Kitchen, Santa Maria*	¼ Sachet/7g	20	0.4	283	8.6	46	5	11
Garlic, For Chicken, So Juicy, Maggi*	1 Pack/30g	95	0.8	316	9.4	58.9	2.8	8.7
Garlic, Papyrus Sheets, SoTender, Maggi*	1 Sheet/6g	25	1.9	438	6.3	24.4	32.5	11.4
Italian Herb, Schwartz*	1 Tsp/1g	3	0	338	11	64.5	4	0
Italian Herbs, Papyrus Sheets, SoTender, Maggi*	1 Sheet/6g	26	2	440	7.3	22.1	34.1	7.7
Jamaican Jerk Chicken, Recipe, Schwartz*	1 Pack/27g	75	0.8	276	9.8	69.8	3	17.2
Jerk, Tesco*	1 Tsp/5g	15	0.2	304	5	53.8	3.3	19.5
Lamb Hot Pot, Colman's*	¼ Pack/10g	32	0.2	320	12	61	1.5	4

INFO/WEIGHT	Measure	per Measure KCAL	FAT	Nutrition Values per 100g / 100ml KCAL	PROT	CARB	FAT	FIBRE

SEASONING MIX

	Measure INFO/WEIGHT	per Measure KCAL	FAT	KCAL	PROT	CARB	FAT	FIBRE
Lemon Herb, for Chicken, Cook in Bag, Average	*1 Bag/34g*	*121*	*1.9*	*356*	*10.8*	*63.7*	*5.5*	*4.1*
Mediterranean Chicken, Season & Shake, Colman's*	1 Pack/33g	99	0.7	300	10.3	56.8	2.1	5.9
Mediterranean, for Chicken, Cook in Bag, Average	*1 Bag/33g*	*99*	*0.7*	*302*	*10.6*	*56.6*	*2*	*7*
Mexican Chicken, As Sold, So Juicy, Maggi*	1 Pack/40g	123	1.7	308	7.4	57.2	4.2	6
One Pan Rice Meal, for Chicken, Old El Paso*	¼ Pack/89g	203	4.3	228	4.4	40.9	4.8	1.7
Paprika, for Chicken, Cook in Bag, Average	*1 Bag/34g*	*96*	*1.3*	*283*	*12.3*	*45.8*	*4*	*8.1*
Paprika, Papyrus Sheets, SoTender, Maggi*	1 Sheet/6g	25	2	431	9.1	12.2	35.2	14.5
Potato Wedges, Garlic & Herb, Schwartz*	1 Pack/38g	106	1.9	278	11.4	47.1	4.9	11.7
Shepherd's Pie, Colman's*	1 Pack/50g	170	1	340	13	60	2	5
Smoked Paprika Chicken, As Sold, Schwartz*	1 Pack/28g	87	1.6	309	10.3	44.4	5.7	0
Spaghetti Bolognaise, Naturally Tasty, As Sold, Knorr*	1 Pack/43g	132	1.8	306	8.5	54	4.3	12
Taco, Old El Paso*	¼ Pack/9g	30	0.4	334	5.5	69	4	0

SEAWEED

	Measure INFO/WEIGHT	per Measure KCAL	FAT	KCAL	PROT	CARB	FAT	FIBRE
Chuka Wakame, Daiwa*	1 Serving/100g	70	3.3	70	1.3	8.8	3.3	1.4
Crispy, Average	*1oz/28g*	*182*	*17.3*	*651*	*7.5*	*15.6*	*61.9*	*7*
Mixed, Trimmed, Sea Vegetables, Waitrose*	1 Pack/80g	15	0.2	19	2.1	1	0.3	1.8
Nori, Dried, Raw	*1oz/28g*	*38*	*0.4*	*136*	*30.7*	*0*	*1.5*	*44.4*
Snack, Honey Sesame, Selwyn's*	1 Pack/4g	14	0.5	350	33	10.6	12.9	29.8
Spaghetti, Dry Weight, Tesco*	½ Pack/40g	89	0.2	223	10	29	0.5	31
Wakame, Dried, Raw	*1oz/28g*	*20*	*0.7*	*71*	*12.4*	*0*	*2.4*	*47.1*

SEED MIX

	Measure INFO/WEIGHT	per Measure KCAL	FAT	KCAL	PROT	CARB	FAT	FIBRE
Chia Flaxseed, Sprinkles, Tesco*	1 Serving/26g	135	9.2	518	24.2	15.9	35.3	20.2
Omega, Morrisons*	¼ Pack/25g	138	11.4	554	20.9	15	45.6	6.4
Omega, Munchy Seeds*	1 Bag/30g	184	14.9	613	28.4	13.1	49.7	2.2
Original, The Food Doctor*	1 Serving/30g	157	13.3	522	28.2	3.7	44.4	17.7
Roasted Sunflower Pumpkin, Salad Sprinkles, Tesco*	1 Serving/20g	112	8.5	561	30	9.4	42.6	10.2

SEEDS

	Measure INFO/WEIGHT	per Measure KCAL	FAT	KCAL	PROT	CARB	FAT	FIBRE
Chia, White, The Chia Co*	1 Tbsp/15g	67	4.7	447	20.7	4.7	31.3	37.3
Fiery, Graze*	1 Pack/34g	173	14.8	510	21.8	17.3	43.5	7.9
Flaxseed, Sunflower Pumpkin, Milled, Linwoods*	1 Scoop/10g	54	4.9	542	22.7	2.4	49.1	16.2
Hemp, Shelled, Linwoods*	2 Tbsps/30g	178	14.8	593	35.1	7.6	49.5	5.9
Mixed, Wholesome, Love Life, Waitrose*	1 Serving/30g	166	13.6	554	21.3	15.5	45.2	8
Mustard, Average	*1 Tsp/3.3g*	*15*	*0.9*	*469*	*34.9*	*34.9*	*28.8*	*14.7*
Nigella, Average	*1 Tsp/5g*	*20*	*1.7*	*392*	*21.3*	*1.9*	*33.3*	*8.4*
Poppy, Average	*1 Tbsp/9g*	*47*	*3.9*	*533*	*18*	*23.7*	*44.7*	*10*
Pumpkin, Sunflower, Toasted, Sainsbury's*	1 Serving/10g	64	5.6	643	28	1.9	56	9.8
Pumpkin, Alesto, Lidl*	1 Serving/25g	128	9	511	34.5	4.2	36.2	15.2
Pumpkin, Average	*1 Tbsp/10g*	*57*	*4.6*	*568*	*27.9*	*13*	*45.9*	*3.8*
Sesame, Average	*1 Tsp/2g*	*12*	*1.1*	*610*	*22.3*	*3.6*	*56.4*	*7.8*
Sesame, Tesco*	1 Tsp/4g	24	2.3	598	18.2	0.9	58	7.9
Sunflower, Average	*1 Tbsp/10g*	*59*	*4.9*	*585*	*23.4*	*15*	*48.7*	*5.7*

SEMOLINA

	Measure INFO/WEIGHT	per Measure KCAL	FAT	KCAL	PROT	CARB	FAT	FIBRE
Average	*1oz/28g*	*98*	*0.5*	*348*	*11*	*75.2*	*1.8*	*2.1*
Pudding, Creamed, Ambrosia*	1 Can/425g	344	7.2	81	3.3	13.1	1.7	0.2
Pudding, Creamed, Co-Op*	1 Can/425g	382	8.5	90	4	15	2	0

SHALLOTS

	Measure INFO/WEIGHT	per Measure KCAL	FAT	KCAL	PROT	CARB	FAT	FIBRE
Pickled in Hot Spicy Vinegar, Tesco*	1 Onion/18g	14	0	77	1	18	0.1	1.9
Raw, Average	*1 Serving/80g*	*16*	*0.2*	*20*	*1.5*	*3.3*	*0.2*	*1.4*

SHANDY

	Measure INFO/WEIGHT	per Measure KCAL	FAT	KCAL	PROT	CARB	FAT	FIBRE
Bitter, Original, Ben Shaws*	1 Can/330ml	89	0	27	0	6	0	0
Canned, Morrisons*	1 Can/330ml	36	0	11	0	1.8	0	0
Homemade, Average	*1 Pint/568ml*	*148*	*0*	*26*	*0.2*	*2.9*	*0*	*0*
Lemonade, Traditional Style, Tesco*	1 Can/330ml	63	0	19	0	4.7	0	0

	Measure INFO/WEIGHT	per Measure KCAL	FAT	Nutrition Values per 100g / 100ml KCAL	PROT	CARB	FAT	FIBRE
SHARK								
Raw	*1oz/28g*	*29*	*0.3*	*102*	*23*	*0*	*1.1*	*0*
SHARON FRUIT								
Average	*1oz/28g*	*19*	*0*	*68*	*0.7*	*17.3*	*0*	*1.5*
SHERRY								
Dry, Average	*1 Glass/120ml*	*139*	*0*	*116*	*0.2*	*1.4*	*0*	*0*
Medium	*1 Serving/50ml*	*58*	*0*	*116*	*0.1*	*5.9*	*0*	*0*
Sweet	*1 Serving/50ml*	*68*	*0*	*136*	*0.3*	*6.9*	*0*	*0*
SHORTBREAD								
All Butter, Deans*	1 Biscuit/15g	77	3.8	511	4.9	65.7	25.4	1.2
All Butter, Finger, Highland, TTD, Sainsbury's*	1 Biscuit/20g	103	5.5	515	4.6	61.8	27.4	1.2
All Butter, Fingers, Highland, Sainsbury's*	2 Biscuits/40g	208	11.5	521	4.8	59.4	28.8	2.7
All Butter, Fingers, Scottish, M&S*	1 Finger/18g	90	4.9	510	5.7	58.9	27.8	4.7
All Butter, Giant, Fingers, Higland, Sainsbury's*	1 Biscuit/35g	182	10.1	520	4.8	59.4	28.8	1.8
All Butter, Petticoat Tails, Co-Op*	1 Biscuit/13g	68	3.8	520	5	60	29	2
All Butter, Round, Luxury, M&S*	1 Biscuit/20g	105	5.8	525	6.2	60	29	2
All Butter, Selection, Waitrose*	1 Biscuit/18g	95	11	527	5.3	58.3	61.1	3
All Butter, Trufree*	1 Biscuit/11g	58	3.1	524	2	66	28	0.9
Average	*1oz/28g*	*139*	*7.3*	*498*	*5.9*	*63.9*	*26.1*	*1.9*
Belgian Chocolate Chunk, Asda*	1 Biscuit/20g	106	6.2	531	7	56	31	1.8
Butter Enriched, Bites, Bakery, Sainsbury's*	1 Bite/16g	84	4.7	527	6	58	29.8	1.4
Butter, with Real Lemons, Mini, Deluxe, Lidl*	3 Biscuits/24g	125	7	521	5.6	57.6	29.1	3.2
Caramel, Millionaires, Fox's*	1 Serving/16g	75	3.9	483	6.1	57.9	25.3	0.1
Choc Chip, Fair Trade, Co-Op*	1 Biscuit/19g	100	6	526	5.3	57.9	31.6	2.6
Chocolate Chip, Jacob's*	1 Biscuit/17g	87	4.7	513	5.2	61.2	27.5	1.8
Chocolate Chip, Tesco*	1 Serving/20g	105	6.1	525	7.5	55	30.6	3
Chocolate, Belgian, Chunky, TTD, Sainsbury's*	1 Piece/70g	353	19	505	5.5	58.8	27.2	1.4
Chocolate, Triple, Finest, Tesco*	1 Square/63g	325	18.5	516	5.8	56.3	29.4	1.5
Clotted Cream, Finest, Tesco*	1 Biscuit/20g	109	6.4	543	5.2	58	32.2	1.7
Clotted Cream, with Chocolate Pieces, Cornish, Furniss*	1 Biscuit/20g	107	5.7	534	5.8	61.6	28.4	0
Demerara, Rounds, TTD, Sainsbury's*	1 Biscuit/22g	113	5.9	508	5.1	62.2	26.5	1.8
Double Choc Chip, Petit Four, Scottish, Tesco*	1 Serving/50g	266	15	531	5.1	60.4	30	1.7
Fingers, Asda*	1 Finger/18g	93	5.1	519	5.8	60.3	28.3	18
Fingers, Scottish, Finest, Tesco*	1 Biscuit/21g	104	5	498	5.1	65.5	23.9	2
Mini Bites, Co-Op*	1 Biscuit/10g	53	3	530	7	59	30	2
Mini, Bites, Tesco*	1 Bite/12g	63	3.5	528	7.2	58.1	29.3	1.3
Pecan All Butter, Sainsbury's*	1 Biscuit/18g	99	6.5	548	5.3	49.9	36.3	2.5
Petticoat Tails, All Butter, Highland, Sainsbury's*	1 Biscuit/12g	65	3.6	521	6.3	58	28.8	2.2
Raspberry & Oatmeal, Deans*	1 Biscuit/20g	103	5.7	514	4.7	63.1	28.6	1.4
Rings, Handbaked, Border*	1 Biscuit/17g	86	4.9	520	6.2	61.2	29.5	0
Rose Petal, Chinese Tea, 1, Waitrose*	1 Biscuit/10g	53	2.9	527	5.8	59.6	29	2.1
Spotty Scottie Dogs, with Chocolate Chips, Sainsbury's*	1 Biscuit/12g	62	3.3	515	5.1	60.5	27.5	2.5
Wheat & GF, Free From Range, Tesco*	1 Shortbread/18g	93	4.9	521	5.4	61.7	27.6	1.9
SHORTCAKE								
Caramel, Baked in the Tray, Tesco*	1 Slice/49g	247	13.2	504	3.4	61.6	26.9	1.1
Caramel, Mini, Thorntons*	1 Piece/14g	69	4.1	491	5	50.6	29.5	0
SHRIMP								
Boiled, Average	*1 Serving/60g*	*70*	*1.4*	*117*	*23.8*	*0*	*2.4*	*0*
Frozen, Average	*1oz/28g*	*20*	*0.2*	*73*	*16.5*	*0*	*0.8*	*0*
in Brine, Canned, Drained, Average	*1oz/28g*	*17*	*0.2*	*61*	*13.5*	*0*	*0.8*	*0*
SKATE								
Grilled	*1oz/28g*	*22*	*0.1*	*79*	*18.9*	*0*	*0.5*	*0*
in Batter, Fried in Blended Oil	*1oz/28g*	*47*	*2.8*	*168*	*14.7*	*4.9*	*10.1*	*0.2*
Raw, Edible Portion	*1oz/28g*	*18*	*0.1*	*64*	*15.1*	*0*	*0.4*	*0*

S

	Measure INFO/WEIGHT	per Measure KCAL	FAT	Nutrition Values per 100g / 100ml KCAL	PROT	CARB	FAT	FIBRE
SKIPS								
Cheesy, KP Snacks*	1 Bag/17g	89	5	524	6.2	58.5	29.5	1
Prawn Cocktail, KP Snacks*	1 Bag/17g	92	5.4	544	4.9	58	32	0.7
SKITTLES								
Mars*	1 Pack/55g	223	2.4	406	0	90.6	4.4	0
Sweet Heat, Mars*	¼ Pack/49g	196	2.1	399	0	89.8	4.2	0
SLICES								
Bacon Cheese, Pastry, Tesco*	1 Slice/165g	480	32	291	7.4	21.7	19.4	1
Beef, Minced Steak & Onion, Tesco*	1 Slice/150g	424	27.2	283	8.7	21.3	18.1	1.6
Cheese Onion, Pastry, Tesco*	1 Slice/150g	502	37	335	8	20.1	24.7	1.4
Chicken & Mushroom, Tesco*	1 Slice/165g	457	28.9	277	9.2	20.6	17.5	0.9
Chicken Bacon, Wall's*	1 Slice/225g	576	33.5	256	10.5	19.9	14.9	0
Chicken Mushroom, Ginsters*	1 Slice/180g	439	26.8	244	8.3	19.1	14.9	1.8
Chicken Mushroom, Sainsbury's*	1 Slice/164g	427	26.5	259	7.3	21.3	16.1	1
Chicken Fajita, Puff Pastry, Sainsbury's*	1 Pack/180g	452	23	251	9.1	23.6	12.8	2.5
Custard, Pastry, Tesco*	1 Slice/94g	266	10.7	283	3.2	41.6	11.3	0.9
Fresh Cream, Tesco*	1 Slice/75g	311	21	414	3.5	37.4	27.9	1
Goats Cheese Spinach, Crisp Creamy, Waitrose*	1 Slice/100g	351	22.7	351	7.6	28.3	22.7	1.8
Ham Cheese, Ginsters*	1 Pack/180g	511	33.7	284	8.5	20.4	18.7	2.5
Minced Beef Onion, Crestwood, Aldi*	1 Slice/165g	543	40.1	329	6.3	19.7	24.3	3.1
Minced Steak & Onion, Sainsbury's*	1 Slice/165g	475	29.9	288	15.2	16	18.1	2.5
Raisin, Crispy, LC, Tesco*	1 Biscuit/15g	56	0.6	370	6	76.6	3.9	5.5
Spicy Chicken, Ginsters*	1 Slice/180g	448	27.4	249	6.7	21.4	15.2	1.9
Steak, Peppered, Ginsters*	1 Slice/180g	457	27	254	8.4	21.3	15	1.6
SLIM FAST*								
Bars, Chocolate Caramel Treat, Snack, Slim Fast*	1 Bar/26g	95	2.6	360	3.5	63	10	1.5
Bars, Chocolate Peanut, Meal, Slim Fast*	1 Bar/56g	210	7.2	380	24	50	13	5
Bars, Chocolate, Nutty, Nougat, Snack, Slim Fast*	1 Bar/25g	95	3	380	4	63	12	1.5
Bars, Heavenly Chocolate Delight, Snack, Slim Fast*	1 Bar/24g	95	3.2	390	5	58	13	7
Bars, Heavenly Chocolate, Crunch Snack, Slim Fast*	1 Bar/24g	95	3.2	390	5	58	13	7
Bars, Nutty Salted Caramel, Meal, Slim Fast*	1 Bar/60g	218	6.8	364	25.4	26.9	11.3	18.7
Bars, Summer Berry, Meal, Slim Fast*	1 Bar/60g	210	5	350	23.3	51.7	8.3	5.8
Chunky Chocolate, Shake, Ready to Drink, Slimfast*	1 Shake/325ml	204	5.2	63	4.6	6.6	1.6	1.5
Crackers, Cheddar Flavour Bites, Snack Bag, Slim Fast*	1 Pack/22g	92	2	417	9.6	72.8	9.2	2.5
Milk Shake, Blissful Banana, Powder, Dry, Slim Fast*	2 Scoops/37g	131	2.4	359	13.4	60.2	6.7	11
Milk Shake, Chunky Chocolate, Powder, Dry, Slim Fast*	2 Scoops/37g	132	2.7	363	13.9	59	7.5	10.9
Milk Shake, Simply Vanilla, Powder, Dry, Slim Fast*	2 Scoops/37g	131	2.4	360	13.4	60.9	6.5	11
Milk Shake, Summer Strawberry, Powder, Dry, Slim Fast*	2 Scoops/37g	139	2.4	380	13.5	60.1	6.6	11.1
Milk Shake,Caramel Temptation, Powder, Dry, Slim Fast*	1 Serving/37g	139	2.2	380	14	62	6	11
Noodles, Chicken Tikka Masala, Box, Slim Fast*	1 Box/250g	81	2.2	33	2.3	2.7	0.9	2.5
Noodles, Spicy Thai, Slim Fast*	1 Box/240g	70	3.1	29	0.9	2.4	1.3	2.4
Pretzels, Sour Cream Chive, Snack Bag, Slim Fast*	1 Pack/23g	99	2.2	432	9.7	74.9	9.5	4.1
Tortillas, Barbecue Flavour, Snack Bag, Slim Fast*	1 Bag/22g	96	2.6	435	6.5	73.9	11.8	3.6
SLUSH PUPPY								
Raspberry, Blue, Manchester Drinks Co.*	1 Serving/250ml	95	0	38	0.5	8.3	0	0
Sour Cherry, Manchester Drinks Co.*	1 Serving/250ml	95	0	38	0.5	8.4	0	0
SMARTIES								
Biscuits, Nestle*	1 Biscuit/5g	26	1.4	519	7.7	57.6	28.6	0
Mini Eggs, Nestle*	5 Eggs/17g	85	3.5	499	3.9	73.5	20.4	2.8
Mini, Treat Size, Smarties, Nestle*	1 Carton/14g	68	2.8	471	5	68.1	19.6	1
Nestle*	1 Tube/40g	188	7.1	469	3.9	72.5	17.7	2.4
Tree Decoration, Nestle*	1 Chocolate/18g	95	5.4	529	5.6	58.9	30.1	0.8
SMOOTHIE								
Apples Blackcurrants for Kids, Innocent*	1 Carton/180ml	104	0.2	58	0.3	14.1	0.1	0.1

S

SMOOTHIE	Measure INFO/WEIGHT	per Measure KCAL	FAT	Nutrition Values per 100g / 100ml KCAL	PROT	CARB	FAT	FIBRE
Banana Fruit with Yoghurt, Tesco*	1 Bottle/1000ml	610	7	61	2.1	11.3	0.7	0.4
Blackberries & Blueberries, Innocent*	1 Bottle/250ml	120	0.2	48	0.5	12	0.1	2.1
Cherries & Strawberries, Innocent*	1 Bottle/250ml	122	0.2	49	0.6	12.6	0.1	0
Coconut, Pineapple Banana, Coldpress*	1 Serving/150ml	96	1.2	64	0.7	12.7	0.8	0
Cucumber, Avocado, Lime, M&S*	1 Bottle/250ml	148	3.5	59	0.4	10.4	1.4	1.4
Fruit, Cereal, Forest Fruits, Morning Boost , Tropicana*	1 Serving/250ml	152	0	61	0.7	13	0	2.4
Kefir, Raspberry, Bio-tiful Dairy*	1 Bottle/250ml	162	6.8	65	3	7.2	2.7	0
Magnificent Mango, Innocent*	1 Bottle/250ml	136	0	54	0.4	12	0	1.4
Mango, Pineapple, Passion Fruit, Eat Well, M&S*	1 Bottle/250g	170	1.2	68	0.5	14.9	0.5	0.9
Mangoes Passion Fruits, Pure Fruit, Innocent*	1 Bottle/250ml	135	0	54	0.4	12	0	1.4
Mixed Berry, CBY, Asda*	1 Glass/250ml	143	0	57	0.6	12.6	0	1.6
Orange, Banana, Mango, Morning Boost, Tropicana*	1 Serving/250ml	125	0	50	0.1	9.2	0	2.3
Orange, Mango, Passionfruit, On the Go, Sainsbury's*	1 Serving/150g	84	0.8	56	0.5	12.8	0.5	0.7
Oranges, Mangoes Pineapples For Kids, Innocent*	1 Carton/180ml	94	0.2	52	0.7	11.7	0.1	0.9
Peaches Passionfruit, for Kids, Innocent*	1 Carton/180ml	95	0	53	0.6	14.7	0	0.9
Peaches, Bananas & Passionfruit, PJ Smoothies*	1 Bottle/250g	128	0.2	51	0.4	12.1	0.1	0
Pineapple, Banana Coconut, CBY, Asda*	1 Glass/250ml	178	2.8	71	0.7	13.6	1.1	1
Pineapples, Bananas Coconuts, Innocent*	1 Bottle/250ml	172	2.8	69	0.7	13.6	1.1	1
Pomegranates, Blueberries Acai, Special, Innocent*	1 Serving/250ml	170	0.5	68	0.6	15.6	0.2	0.8
Protein Superfood, Mango Banana, PhD Nutrition*	1 Serving/130g	175	7.7	135	15.4	4.2	5.9	1.4
Raspberry & Blueberry, Plus, Tesco*	1 Serving/100ml	59	0.3	59	2.6	11.6	0.3	0.5
Strawberries Bananas, Pure Fruit, Innocent*	1 Bottle/250ml	132	0.2	53	0.7	13.1	0.1	1.3
Strawberries, Blackberries, Raspberries, Kids, Innocent*	1 Carton/180ml	81	0.2	45	0.5	9.9	0.1	1.3
Strawberry & Banana, Tesco*	1 Bottle/250ml	112	0.5	45	0.6	10.1	0.2	0.8
Strawberry Banana, Prepacked, Average	*1 Serving/250ml*	*131*	*0.2*	*53*	*0.6*	*11.9*	*0.1*	*0.9*
Super Orange, Cold Pressed, Raw Fruit Veg, Savse*	1 Bottle/250ml	110	0.2	44	0.9	9.8	0.1	0.7
Super Red, Cold Pressed, Raw Fruit Veg, Savse*	1 Bottle/250ml	98	0.2	39	0.8	8.4	0.1	0.7
Superfruits, Pomegranates, Blueberries Acai, Innocent*	1 Serving/250ml	170	0.5	68	0.5	15.6	0.2	0.8
Tropical, High Protein, Naked Juice Co*	1 Bottle/450ml	292	0.9	65	4.4	11.4	0.2	0.5
Vanilla Bean, M&S*	1 Bottle/500ml	450	13	90	3.3	13.9	2.6	0
SMOOTHIE MIX								
Banana, Kale Mango, As Sold, Iceland*	1 Sachet/150g	90	0.4	60	1.1	12.2	0.3	2.3
Berry, Frozen, Love Life, Waitrose*	1 Serving/80g	31	0	39	1.1	7.2	0	2.9
Mango Pineapple, CBY, Asda*	1 Portion/80g	48	0.4	59	0.6	12	0.5	1.9
Strawberry Banana, Frozen, Love Life, Waitrose*	1 Serving/80g	37	0.3	46	0.7	8.2	0.4	3.4
Tropical, Frozen, Love Life, Waitrose*	1 Serving/80g	45	0.2	57	0.7	11.8	0.3	1.9
Yellow Frozen, Morrisons*	1 Portion/80g	41	0.2	51	0.5	10.9	0.2	1.9
SNACKS								
Box, Smokehouse BBQ, Crunch, Graze*	1 Pack/31g	137	4.6	441	9.9	60	15	7.3
Corn, Original, Mister Corn*	1 Serving/30g	145	6.3	482	7.6	63	21	5.5
Mild Green Curry, Baked Pea Sticks, Yushoi *	1 Serving/21g	87	3	415	19.1	45.7	14.2	14.3
Mix, Sweet Salty, Reese's*	½ Pack/28g	139	7.6	496	12.4	54.7	27.1	0
Pea, Malaysian Sweet Curry Flavour, Passions, Aldi*	1 Pack/21g	89	3.2	422	19	47	15	13
Pea, Thai Red Curry Flavour, Passions, Aldi*	1 Pack/21g	88	2.9	421	19	48	14	12
Slightly Salted, Baked Pea Sticks, Yushoi *	1 Serving/21g	88	0.6	419	19.2	9.9	2.9	13.4
Smoky Barbecue, Crunch, Retail, Graze*	1 Pack/31g	137	5	443	11	57	16	7.9
Smoky Salt Pepper, Baked Pea Sticks, Yushoi *	1 Serving/21g	86	2.7	409	19.3	46.5	13	14.3
Sour Cream Onion, Lentil Curls, Passions Deli, Aldi*	1 Pack/20g	91	3.4	454	11	63	17	3.6
Soy Balsamic Vinegar, Baked Pea Sticks, Yushoi *	1 Serving/21g	88	2.9	417	18.6	47.9	13.7	13.5
Sweet Chilli Lemon, Baked Pea Sticks, Yushoi *	1 Serving/21g	88	3	420	19.2	46.7	14.3	13.7
Teddy Faces, Snackrite, Aldi*	1 Bag/19g	96	5.1	505	3.4	61	27	2.7
Thai Sriracha Mix, Natural Selection*	1 Pack/26g	109	3.4	420	11	60	13	9.3
Veggie Caesar, Graze*	1 Punnet/24g	115	4.6	478	17	52	19	9.4

S

INFO/WEIGHT	Measure	per Measure KCAL	FAT	Nutrition Values per 100g / 100ml KCAL	PROT	CARB	FAT	FIBRE
SNAILS								
in Garlic Butter, Average	**6 Snails/50g**	**219**	**20.8**	**438**	**9.7**	**8**	**41.5**	**1**
Raw, Average	**1 Snail/5g**	**4**	**0.1**	**90**	**16.1**	**2**	**1.4**	**0**
SNAPPER								
Red, Fried in Blended Oil	**1oz/28g**	**35**	**0.9**	**126**	**24.5**	**0**	**3.1**	**0**
Red, Weighed with Bone, Raw	**1oz/28g**	**12**	**0.2**	**42**	**9.2**	**0**	**0.6**	**0**
SNICKERS								
Hazelnut, Snickers*	1 Bar/49g	240	11.7	489	8.1	59.5	23.9	0
Mars*	1 Single/48g	245	13.4	510	9.5	54.3	27.9	1.3
Protein, Mars*	1 Bar/51g	199	7.1	391	35.6	36.1	13.9	0
SOLE								
Fillet, Yellowfin, Lightly Dusted, Northern Catch, Aldi*	1 Fillet/114g	171	4.6	150	20	7.6	4	2.5
Yellow, Fillet, Lightly Dusted, As Consumed, Morrisons*	1 Fillet/124g	218	8.5	176	14	13.9	6.9	1
SOPOCKA								
Sliced, Cured, Pork Loin	**1 Serving/100g**	**101**	**2.9**	**101**	**17.8**	**0.8**	**2.9**	**0**
SORBET								
Blackcurrant, Yorvale Ltd*	1 Serving/100g	120	0.2	120	0	28.8	0.2	0
Exotic Fruit, Sainsbury's*	1 Serving/75g	90	1.5	120	1.2	24.1	2	0
Jamaican Me Crazy, Ben & Jerry's*	1 Serving/100g	130	0	130	0.2	32	0	0.4
Lemon	**1 Scoop/60g**	**79**	**0**	**131**	**0.9**	**34.2**	**0**	**0**
Lemon, Sainsbury's*	¼ Pot/89g	100	0	112	0	28.1	0	0.1
Lemon, Tesco*	1 Scoop/68g	81	0.2	120	0.1	28.8	0.3	0.5
Mandarin Orange, Yorvale Ltd*	1 Serving/100g	125	0.2	125	0.1	30.5	0.2	0
Mango, Tesco*	1 Scoop/50g	57	0.4	113	0.5	25.6	0.8	0.8
Mango, Waitrose*	1 Pot/100g	90	0	90	0.1	22.1	0	0.6
Orange, Del Monte*	1 Sorbet/500g	625	0.5	125	0.2	32.1	0.1	0
Passion Fruit, Yorvale Ltd*	1 Serving/100g	109	0.2	109	0.1	26.6	0.2	0
Pink Grapefruit, Bergamot, Northern Bloc*	1 Sm Tub/120ml	100	0.1	83	0	20.9	0.1	0
Raspberry & Blackberry, Fat Free, M&S*	1 Sorbet/125g	140	0	112	0.4	27.5	0	0.6
Raspberry, Haagen-Dazs*	½ Cup/105g	120	0	114	0	28.6	0	1.9
Raspberry, Tesco*	1 Scoop/70ml	79	0.4	114	0.2	26.8	0.5	0.5
SOUFFLE								
Cheese	**1oz/28g**	**71**	**5.4**	**253**	**11.4**	**9.3**	**19.2**	**0.3**
Cheese, Alizonne*	1 Serving/33g	129	3.4	392	60.5	14.5	10.2	0.2
Cheese, Mini, Waitrose*	1 Souffle/14g	32	2.4	232	16	2.9	17.4	2.4
Chocolate, Gu*	1 Pot/70g	307	24.9	439	6.3	24.4	35.6	2.9
Lemon, Finest, Tesco*	1 Pot/80g	270	20.5	338	2.9	24.1	25.6	0.2
Plain	**1oz/28g**	**56**	**4.1**	**201**	**7.6**	**10.4**	**14.7**	**0.3**
Raspberry & Amaretto, M&S*	1oz/28g	83	4.7	298	2.8	33.1	16.7	0.1
Ricotta & Spinach, M&S*	1 Serving/120g	186	13.3	155	8	6.2	11.1	2.1
Strawberry, M&S*	1 Serving/95g	171	10.1	180	1.6	19.5	10.6	0.9
SOUP								
Asparagus, Cream of, Canned, M&S*	½ Can/200g	108	7.2	54	0.9	4.3	3.6	0.2
Asparagus, New Covent Garden Food Co*	½ Carton/300g	132	7.2	44	1.5	4.1	2.4	0.9
Asparagus, Wellness, Natural Balance, Oriflame*	1 Serving/20g	76	1.3	380	35.4	44	6.3	2.7
Asparagus, with Croutons, Aldi*	1 Sachet/229ml	96	3.7	42	0.5	6.5	1.6	0.5
Bacon, & Bean, Smoked, Diet Chef Ltd*	1 Pack/300g	162	3.3	54	2.8	8.2	1.1	2.1
Bacon, & Bean, Three, Smoked, Chunky, Baxters*	1 Can/400g	232	4.8	58	2.9	8.8	1.2	1.8
Bacon, & Lentil, CBY, Asda*	½ Pot/300g	177	4.2	59	3.8	7.2	1.4	1.2
Bean, & Sweet Potato, Mexican, Super, Glorious!*	½ Pot/300g	137	0.6	46	2.3	6.9	0.2	3.4
Bean, & Vegetable, Three, HL, Tesco*	1 Portion/200g	90	0.6	45	2.1	7.5	0.3	1.9
Bean, & Vegetable, Three, LC, Tesco*	½ Can/200g	110	0.6	55	2.6	9.7	0.3	1.9
Bean, Veg, Stew, Mighty, Big Soup, Heinz*	1 Can/500g	355	4.5	71	3	11.8	0.9	3
Bean, Butter, & Chorizo, Meal, Sainsbury's*	1 Pot/400g	257	9.6	64	3.9	5.6	2.4	2.3

S

SOUP

INFO/WEIGHT	Measure	per Measure		Nutrition Values per 100g / 100ml				
		KCAL	FAT	KCAL	PROT	CARB	FAT	FIBRE
Bean, Chilli, Mexican, Tesco*	1 Carton/600g	270	6.6	45	2.2	6.4	1.1	1.9
Bean, Chilli, Three, Fresh, Tesco*	½ Pot/300g	128	0.3	42	3.3	6	0.1	2.2
Bean, Hearty, Italian Inspired, Love Life, Waitrose*	½ Pot/300g	151	6.6	50	1.5	5.2	2.2	1.8
Bean, Italian Style, Tesco*	1 Can/300g	153	3.6	51	2.8	7.3	1.2	1.1
Bean, Mexican, Fresh, Morrisons*	½ Pot/300g	171	3.9	57	2.1	8.3	1.3	1.9
Bean, Smoky Chipotle, with Quinoa, Meal, Sainsbury's*	1 Pot/400g	369	12.8	92	3.5	10.5	3.2	3.7
Bean, Tuscan, Canned, HL, Tesco*	½ Can/200ml	140	3.6	70	3.5	10.3	1.8	1.3
Bean, Tuscan, Chunky, Love Life, Waitrose*	½ Can/200g	101	1	50	2.6	7.6	0.5	2.3
Bean, Tuscan, Organic, Fresh, Sainsbury's*	1 Pack/400g	171	3.2	43	2.6	6.3	0.8	2
Bean, Tuscan, Slimming World, Iceland*	½ Pot/250g	100	0.5	40	2.6	5.1	0.2	3.7
Bean, Tuscan, Tesco*	1 Can/400g	272	3.2	68	3.6	10.3	0.8	2.6
Bean, Tuscan, with Roasted Garlic & Tomatoes, Heinz*	1 Can/400g	188	3.6	47	1.3	7.7	0.9	1.1
Beef, & Bean, Chilli, Mexican, Soups of the World, Heinz*	1 Can/515g	360	9.3	70	4.5	9	1.8	1.6
Beef, & Mushroom, Big Soup, Heinz*	1 Can/515g	216	2.6	42	2.3	7	0.5	0.7
Beef, & Tomato in a Cup, Sainsbury's*	1 Serving/210ml	61	1.1	29	0.6	5.6	0.5	0.2
Beef, & Tomato, Cup a Soup, Made Up, Batchelors*	1 Serving/252g	83	1.6	33	0.6	6.3	0.6	0.4
Beef, & Vegetable, Big Soup, Heinz*	1 Can/400g	212	4	53	3.5	7.5	1	0.9
Beef, Vegetables, Chunky, Newgate, Lidl*	1 Tin/400g	232	3.2	58	3.6	8.2	0.8	1.8
Beef, Broth, Big Soup, Heinz*	1 Can/400g	184	2.8	46	2.5	7	0.7	0.9
Beef, Broth, Classic, Heinz*	1 Can/400g	180	2	45	1.9	7.6	0.5	0.8
Beef, Broth, Rich, with Smoky Paprika, Heinz*	½ Can/200g	82	1	41	1.8	6.9	0.5	0.7
Beef, Chilli, Bean, Rice, M&S*	½ Pot/300g	159	2.4	53	2.7	7.8	0.8	1.9
Beef, Chilli, Chunky, Asda*	1 Can/400g	212	4	53	4.2	5.7	1	2.4
Beef, Chilli, Chunky, Greggs*	1 Serving/300g	216	5.1	72	4.1	9.7	1.7	0
Black Bean, Mexican, Extra Special, Asda*	½ Pot/263g	194	10.8	74	2.3	7	4.1	1.7
Broccoli, & Stilton, Canned, Sainsbury's*	½ Can/200g	84	4	42	1.5	4.2	2	0.6
Broccoli, & Stilton, Canned, Tesco*	1 Can/400g	240	14	60	1.7	5	3.5	0.4
Broccoli, & Stilton, Classics, Fresh, Tesco*	½ Pot/300g	156	10.8	52	2.4	1.8	3.6	1.5
Broccoli, & Stilton, Cup Soup, Ainsley Harriott*	1 Satchet/229ml	87	1.8	38	1	7	0.8	1.3
Broccoli, & Stilton, Fresh, Sainsbury's*	½ Pot/300ml	141	9.9	47	2.7	1.8	3.3	1.5
Broccoli, & Stilton, New Covent Garden Food Co*	1 Carton/600ml	240	14.4	40	2.2	1.9	2.4	1.1
Broccoli, & Stilton, Tesco*	1 Can/400g	192	10.4	48	1.9	4.2	2.6	1.2
Broccoli, & Zucinni, Cream Of, Canned, Italiamo*	½ Can/195ml	84	5.1	43	0.9	3.8	2.6	0.5
Broccoli, Pea Pesto, New Covent Garden Food Co*	½ Pack/350g	182	7.4	52	2.3	5.2	2.1	1.4
Broccoli, Salmon Watercress, Stay Full, Baxters*	1 Can/400g	244	8.8	61	3.3	5.8	2.2	2.4
Broccoli, Spinach & Pea, Super, M&S*	1 Serving/300g	102	3.9	34	2.1	2.7	1.3	1.6
Broccoli, with Kale, & Watercress, Naked Locals*	½ Pack/250ml	130	6.8	52	1.7	3.9	2.7	2.8
Butternut Squash, & Chilli, Sainsbury's*	½ Pot/300g	112	7.2	37	0.7	3.1	2.4	0.2
Butternut Squash, & Lentil, Curried, Seeds of Change*	1 Pack/400g	164	1.2	41	2.3	7.2	0.3	1.9
Butternut Squash, & Red Pepper, Canned, Sainsbury's*	½ Can/195g	99	4.3	51	1	6.6	2.2	3.6
Butternut Squash, & Red Pepper, Vegetarian, Baxters*	1 Can/415g	149	2.5	36	0.9	6.6	0.6	0.5
Butternut Squash, & Sage, New Covent Garden Food Co*	½ Carton/300g	153	6.9	51	0.9	6.6	2.3	0.7
Butternut Squash, & Tarragon, Waitrose*	½ Pot/300g	123	6.6	41	0.8	4.5	2.2	1
Butternut Squash, Chickpea, Spiced, Heinz*	½ Can/200g	69	1	35	1.1	6.3	0.5	1.2
Butternut Squash, Chilli, Musclefood*	1 Serving/400g	128	6	32	0.7	4.2	1.5	0.9
Butternut Squash, Creamy, New Covent Garden Food Co*	½ Carton/300g	153	7.5	51	0.8	6.4	2.5	0.9
Butternut Squash, Fresh, Waitrose*	½ Pot/300g	153	8.7	51	0.5	5.8	2.9	0.8
Butternut Squash, New England, Skinnylicious, Glorious!*	½ Pot/300g	87	2.1	29	0.5	4.5	0.7	1.4
Butternut Squash, Soupreme, Aldi*	½ Pot/300g	60	3.3	20	0.5	1.5	1.1	1.5
Butternut Squash, Tesco*	½ Pot/300g	82	4.3	27	0.4	2.5	1.4	1.5
Carrot ,& Coriander, Weight Watchers*	1 Pouch/300g	102	3.9	34	0.4	5.1	1.3	0.6
Carrot, & Butter Bean, Vegetarian, Baxters*	1 Can/415g	237	7.9	57	1.5	7.2	1.9	2.2

SOUP

INFO/WEIGHT	Measure	per Measure		Nutrition Values per 100g / 100ml				
		KCAL	FAT	KCAL	PROT	CARB	FAT	FIBRE
Carrot, & Coriander, Average	**1 Can/400g**	**167**	**8.6**	**42**	**0.6**	**4.8**	**2.2**	**1**
Carrot, & Coriander, Blended, Heinz*	½ Can/200g	104	5.4	52	0.7	6.2	2.7	0.6
Carrot, & Coriander, Canned, BGTY, Sainsbury's*	½ Can/200g	62	2	31	0.8	4.8	1	0.9
Carrot, & Coriander, Canned, M&S*	½ Can/210g	94	5	45	0.4	5.9	2.4	0.9
Carrot, & Coriander, Canned, Tesco*	1 Can/400g	220	11.6	55	0.7	5.7	2.9	0.8
Carrot, & Coriander, Classic Homestyle, M&S*	1 Can/425g	170	8.5	40	0.6	5.6	2	0.7
Carrot, & Coriander, Classic, Classic, Heinz*	1 Can/400g	164	6.4	41	0.4	5.8	1.6	0.9
Carrot, & Coriander, Fresh, New Covent Garden Food Co*	½ Carton/300g	129	6	43	0.5	5.2	2	1.1
Carrot, & Coriander, Fresh, Organic, Simply Organic*	1 Pot/600g	276	18	46	0.5	4.5	3	1.3
Carrot, & Coriander, Fresh, Tesco*	½ Pot /300g	99	4.8	33	0.6	2.9	1.6	2.2
Carrot, & Coriander, Less Than 5% Fat, Asda*	1 Serving/300g	96	0.9	32	1	6	0.3	0.8
Carrot, & Ginger, Fresh, Sainsbury's*	1 Pot/600g	150	5.4	25	0.4	3.9	0.9	1
Carrot, & Lentil, Weight Watchers*	1 Can/295g	87	0.3	29	1.3	5.5	0.1	0.7
Carrot, & Parsnip, Chantenay, Fresh, Extra Special, Asda*	½ Pot/300g	153	8.4	51	1.2	4.8	2.8	0.8
Carrot, Coconut, Thai, Fragrant, Soup of the Day, Heinz*	½ Carton/200g	104	5.6	52	0.9	5.5	2.8	1.8
Carrot, Coriander, Fresh, Asda*	½ Pot/300g	117	7.5	39	0.5	3.1	2.5	1.2
Carrot, Lentil, Farmers Market, Heinz*	1 Serving/200g	84	0.3	42	1.7	7.8	0.2	0.9
Carrot, Coriander Ginger, So Organic, Sainsbury's*	½ Can/197g	75	3.3	38	0.3	5.3	1.7	0.7
Carrot, Red Lentil Cumin, Organic, Waitrose*	1 Pack/350g	175	8.8	50	0.2	6.7	2.5	0.5
Carrot, Thai, Skinny, Aldi*	½ Pot/300g	90	4.8	30	0.5	3.3	1.6	0.6
Cauliflower, & Celeriac, Love Life, Waitrose*	1 Pot/350g	79	3.1	23	1.6	1.4	0.9	1.3
Cauliflower, Chickpea, & Turmeric, Indian, Glorious!*	½ Pot/300g	114	2.4	38	2	4.4	0.8	2.7
Cauliflower, Onion, Potato, Soup of the Day, Heinz*	½ Carton/200g	76	3.2	38	1.4	4.4	1.6	1
Celeriac, Velvety, Waitrose*	½ Pot/300g	151	11.5	50	0.8	2.8	3.8	0.9
Chicken Noodle, Canned, Sainsbury's*	½ Can/217g	78	0.7	36	1.7	7.4	0.3	0.7
Chicken Noodle, Classic, Heinz*	1 Can/400g	124	1.2	31	1.2	6	0.3	0.2
Chicken Noodle, Clear, Weight Watchers*	1 Can/295g	51	0.6	17	0.8	3.1	0.2	0.2
Chicken Noodle, Cup Soup, Dry, Heinz*	1 Sachet/20g	48	0.5	240	8	46	2.5	1.5
Chicken Noodle, Cup Soup, Made Up, Heinz*	1 Serving/218ml	48	0.4	22	0.7	4.3	0.2	0.1
Chicken Noodle, Dry, Nissin*	1 Pack/85g	364	14.1	428	9.5	62	16.6	3.3
Chicken Noodle, Fresh, CBY, Asda*	½ Pot/297g	98	1.2	33	2.5	4.3	0.4	0.9
Chicken Noodle, In a Cup, BGTY, Sainsbury's*	1 Sachet/219ml	59	1.1	27	1.7	4.9	0.5	0.5
Chicken Noodle, in a Cup, You Count, Love Life, Waitrose*	1 Cup/205ml	43	0.2	21	0.7	4.5	0.1	0.1
Chicken Noodle, Soup in a Cup, Made Up, Sainsbury's*	1 Serving/200ml	44	0.2	22	0.7	4.7	0.1	0.2
Chicken Noodle, Super Good, Baxters*	1 Can/400g	200	5.2	50	3.1	6.6	1.3	0.5
Chicken Noodle, Super, Dry, Knorr*	1 Pack/56g	182	2.7	325	14.3	56	4.9	1.8
Chicken Noodle, Teriyaki, Musclefood*	1 Serving/400g	140	6.8	35	4.6	0.2	1.7	0.1
Chicken Noodle, Thai Green, Yorkshire Provender*	½ Pot/300g	159	6	53	2.9	5.6	2	0
Chicken Noodle, with Sweetcorn, Canned, M&S*	1 Can/400g	184	3.2	46	2.8	6.8	0.8	0.4
Chicken, & Bean, Mexican Spiced, Eat Smart, Morrisons*	1 Can/400g	200	2	50	2.9	7.3	0.5	1.9
Chicken, & Black Eyed Pea, Gumbo, Hearty, Baxters*	1 Can/400g	184	2	46	2.6	6.7	0.5	1.5
Chicken, & Chorizo, New Covent Garden Food Co*	½ Pack/300g	132	4.5	44	1.9	5.3	1.5	0.9
Chicken, & Leek, Cup a Soup, Made Up, Batchelors*	1 Serving/259g	96	4.7	37	0.5	4.7	1.8	0.7
Chicken, & Multigrain, Finest, Tesco*	½ Pot/298g	125	3.6	42	3.2	3.9	1.2	1.3
Chicken, & Mushroom, Grain Soup , Sainsbury's*	1 Pot/600g	332	14.5	55	3.8	4.4	2.4	0.5
Chicken, & Mushroom, in a Cup, Sainsbury's*	1 Sachet/223ml	107	4.2	48	0.7	7.1	1.9	0.1
Chicken, & Orzo, Tuscan, Glorious!*	½ Pot/300g	120	1.2	40	2.8	6.2	0.4	0.7
Chicken, & Sweetcorn, Canned, HL, Tesco*	½ Can/200g	70	0.6	35	1.6	6.4	0.3	0.3
Chicken, & Sweetcorn, Cup Soup, Asda*	1 Sachet/200ml	109	3.9	54	0.7	8.5	2	0.3
Chicken, & Sweetcorn, Fresh, Average	**1 Serving/300g**	**146**	**3.1**	**48**	**2.4**	**7.3**	**1**	**0.6**
Chicken, & Sweetcorn, Light Choice, Tesco*	½ Can 200g	84	0.8	42	1.7	7.9	0.4	0.2
Chicken, & Vegetable Broth, Fresh, M Kitchen, Morrisons*	½ Pot/298g	131	4.5	44	2.8	4	1.5	1.6
Chicken, & Vegetable, Big Soup, Heinz*	½ Can/200g	110	2.4	55	3.3	7.2	1.2	0.8

SOUP

INFO/WEIGHT	Measure	per Measure		Nutrition Values per 100g / 100ml				
		KCAL	FAT	KCAL	PROT	CARB	FAT	FIBRE
Chicken, & Vegetable, Canned, Average	**1 Can/400g**	**192**	**8.5**	**48**	**2.5**	**4.6**	**2.1**	**0.8**
Chicken, & Vegetable, Chunky, Canned, Soupreme, Aldi*	1 Can/400g	184	2.4	46	3	6.4	0.6	1.3
Chicken, & Vegetable, Chunky, Meal Soup, Tesco*	1 Can/400g	184	7.2	46	2.5	4.6	1.8	1
Chicken, & Vegetable, Fresh, M&S*	½ Pot/300g	123	5.1	41	3.5	2.3	1.7	1.2
Chicken, & Vegetable, Fresh, Tesco*	½ Pack/300g	118	3.3	39	3.6	3.2	1.1	1.1
Chicken, & Vegetable, Healthy, Baxters*	1 Can/415g	170	2.1	41	1.9	6.3	0.5	1.8
Chicken, & Vegetable, Mighty, Asda*	1 Can/410g	176	5.3	43	2.5	6.8	1.3	0.7
Chicken, & Vegetable, Moroccan, Love Life, Waitrose*	½ Pot/300g	192	5.7	64	3.7	7.9	1.9	1.9
Chicken, & Vegetable, with Pasta, Select, Campbell's*	1 Can/480ml	220	1	46	2.9	7.9	0.2	0.8
Chicken, Barley, Broth, Heinz*	1 Can/400g	128	1.2	32	1.3	5.9	0.3	0.8
Chicken, Sweetcorn, Musclefood*	1 Serving/400g	176	5.2	44	4.5	3.8	1.3	0.3
Chicken, Vegetable, Chunky, Canned, Asda*	½ Can/200g	90	2	45	4.3	4.3	1	0.8
Chicken, Balti, Meal, Sainsbury's*	1 Pack/400g	242	7.1	61	3.9	6.3	1.8	1.8
Chicken, Broth, Favourites, Baxters*	1 Can/400g	140	1.2	35	1.7	5.9	0.3	1
Chicken, Chardonnay Wine Tarragon, Finest, Tesco*	½ Pot/300g	171	9.6	57	3.1	3.7	3.2	0.3
Chicken, Classic, New Covent Garden*	½ Pack/213g	151	9.6	71	2.9	4.8	4.5	0.5
Chicken, Courgette Orzo Pasta, Meal Soup, Glorious!*	½ Pot/300g	141	4.2	47	3.5	5.1	1.4	0.8
Chicken, Cream of, Canned, Tesco*	1 Can/400g	192	12	48	2.5	2.8	3	0.1
Chicken, Cream of, Reduced Salt, Heinz*	1 Can/400g	216	12	54	1.7	4.9	3	0.1
Chicken, Cream of, Soupreme, Aldi*	1 Can/400g	228	15.2	57	1.8	3.8	3.8	0.4
Chicken, Green Thai, Spiced, M&S*	½ Pot/300g	195	11.4	65	2	6.3	3.8	0.6
Chicken, Green Thai, Waitrose*	1 Pot/600g	462	30	77	4.4	3.5	5	1.6
Chicken, Hot Sour, New Covent Garden Food Co*	½ Carton/300g	69	0.6	23	1.2	3.5	0.2	1
Chicken, Hotpot, Chunky, Big Soup, Heinz*	½ Can/258g	126	3.1	49	2.3	7.4	1.2	0.8
Chicken, Jamaican Jerk, TTD, Sainsbury's*	½ Carton/300g	198	5.1	66	3.9	7.6	1.7	2.6
Chicken, Keralan, Sainsburys*	½ Carton/300g	252	15.3	84	3.5	5.5	5.1	1.1
Chicken, Miso, Noodle, Waitrose*	1 Pot/400g	268	8.8	67	5.9	5.9	2.2	0.9
Chicken, Mix, Telma*	1 Serving/7g	20	0.5	286	14.3	42.9	7.1	0
Chicken, Moroccan Inspired, Love Life, Waitrose*	½ Pot/300g	136	2.4	45	2.7	6.1	0.8	1.4
Chicken, Moroccan, Finest, Tesco*	½ Pot/300g	201	5.1	67	4.2	8.1	1.7	1.2
Chicken, Moroccan, Harira, Hearty, Baxters*	1 Can/400g	236	2.8	59	3.2	9.5	0.7	1.9
Chicken, Mulligatawny, Finest, Tesco*	½ Pot/300g	237	9.9	79	5	6.7	3.3	1
Chicken, Mushroom Rice, M&S*	1 Pack/350g	206	7.7	59	2.7	6.6	2.2	0.9
Chicken, Mushroom, Potato, Big Soup, Heinz*	½ Can/200g	132	4.6	66	3.4	8.1	2.3	0.4
Chicken, Potato Bacon, Big Soup, Heinz*	1 Can/515g	294	11.3	57	3	6.1	2.2	0.5
Chicken, Potato Leek, Weight Watchers*	1 Can/295g	97	2.4	33	1.1	5.1	0.8	0.3
Chicken, Spicy Thai, Nupo*	1 Serving/32g	114	2.4	356	38	39	7.6	9.3
Chicken, Thai Style, Canned, Soupreme, Aldi*	1 Can/400g	200	10.8	50	2.5	3.8	2.7	1.1
Chicken, Thai Style, Thick & Creamy, in a Mug, Tesco*	1 Sachet/28g	107	4	390	3.7	61.3	14.5	5.1
Chicken, Thai, Fresh, Finest, Tesco*	½ Tub/300g	176	9.9	59	3.2	3.4	3.3	1.3
Chicken, Tomato Red Pepper, Italian, Big Soup, Heinz*	½ Can/200g	78	1.8	39	1.6	6.2	0.9	0.7
Chicken, Tomato, & Grains, Tuscan, Glorious!*	½ Pack/300g	111	2.1	37	2	4.9	0.7	1.5
Chicken, Weight Watchers*	1 Can/295g	97	3	33	1.6	4.4	1	0
Chilli, Tomato, & Pasta, COU, M&S*	1 Serving/300g	150	5.7	50	1.3	7.2	1.9	0.9
Chorizo, & Butter Bean, Chunky, Sainsbury's*	½ Can/200g	150	5.6	75	3.4	7.8	2.8	2.7
Chowder, Corn, Spicy, New Covent Garden Food Co*	½ Carton/300g	132	5.4	44	1.6	4.3	1.8	2.2
Chowder, Ham Sweetcorn, Diet Chef Ltd*	1 Pack/300g	165	3.6	55	1.9	9.2	1.2	0.9
Chowder, Seafood, Waitrose*	1 Can/404g	226	11.3	56	2.2	5.6	2.8	0.6
Chowder, Smoked Haddock Salmon, Cully Sully*	1 Pack/400g	232	9.2	58	2.6	6.2	2.3	0.9
Chowder, Sweetcorn, Microwaved, Slimming World*	1 Pot/500g	160	2.5	32	1.1	5.3	0.5	0.7
Cock-A-Leekie, Favourites, Baxters*	1 Can/400g	116	2.4	29	1.1	4.7	0.6	0.3
Coconut, Lime, Chilli, Glorious!*	½ Tub/300g	168	2.4	56	3.4	6.7	0.8	4.1
Country Garden, Canned, Vegetarian, Baxters*	1 Can/400g	144	2	36	1	6.2	0.5	1

S

SOUP

INFO/WEIGHT	Measure	per Measure KCAL	FAT	Nutrition Values per 100g / 100ml KCAL	PROT	CARB	FAT	FIBRE
Courgette, & Parmesan, Fresh, Sainsbury's*	1 Pack/300ml	198	16.8	66	1.5	2.5	5.6	0.4
Cucumber, Gazpacho, Innocent*	1 Bowl/200ml	70	3.6	35	0.7	3	1.8	2.1
Daal, Lentil, Bangalore, Glorious!*	1 Pot/600g	294	8.4	49	2	6.1	1.4	2.2
Fish, Bouillabaise, Bistro, M&S*	1 Pack/820g	2665	18	325	10	4.3	2.2	1.3
Game, Royal, Favourites, Baxters*	1 Can/400g	152	0.8	38	1.8	6.9	0.2	0.3
Haddock, Smoked, Chowder, M&S*	½ Pot/300g	180	7.2	60	3.1	6.4	2.4	0.8
Ham Hock, & Vegetable, Broth, Crosse & Blackwell*	1 Can/400g	158	2	40	2.7	5.7	0.5	0.8
Ham Hock, Leek Potato, Chunky, Soup Pot, Tesco*	1 Pot/350g	174	6.3	50	2.5	5.5	1.8	1
Highlander's Broth, Favourites, Baxters*	1 Can/400g	192	5.6	48	1.7	6.3	1.4	0.9
Hot & Sour	*1 Serving/233g*	*90*	*2.8*	*39*	*2.6*	*4.3*	*1.2*	*0.5*
Kumara, Vegetable, Ready to Serve, Wattie's*	½ Can/265g	136	2.4	51	0.8	9.6	0.9	0.9
Lamb, & Vegetable, Big Soup, Heinz*	½ Can/200g	120	2.6	60	3	9.1	1.3	1.3
Lamb, Minted, Hot Pot, Big Soup, Heinz*	1 Can/500g	236	5.2	59	2.8	8.5	1.3	1
Leek, & Chicken, Knorr*	1 Serving/300ml	82	5.2	27	0.6	2.4	1.7	0.1
Leek, & Maris Piper Potato, Chilled, M&S*	1 Serving/300g	165	11.4	55	0.6	4.5	3.8	0.9
Leek, & Potato	*1oz/28g*	*15*	*0.7*	*52*	*1.5*	*6.2*	*2.6*	*0.8*
Leek, & Potato, Canned, Asda*	1 Can/400g	160	3.6	40	0.9	6.5	0.9	1
Leek, & Potato, Canned, Sainsbury's*	½ Can/200g	92	3.2	46	1	6.7	1.6	0.3
Leek, & Potato, Classics, Canned, Heinz*	1 Can/400g	184	7.2	46	0.8	6.7	1.8	0.6
Leek, & Potato, Cup a Soup, Batchelors*	1 Sachet/28g	121	4.9	432	5.2	63.2	17.6	1.8
Leek, & Potato, Favourites, Baxters*	1 Can/400g	192	7.2	48	1	6.6	1.8	0.9
Leek, & Potato, Fresh with Cream, Tesco*	½ Tub/300g	146	8.4	49	0.7	4.6	2.8	1.2
Leek, & Potato, Fresh, Sainsbury's*	½ Pot/300ml	141	7.2	47	1	5.3	2.4	0.4
Leek, & Potato, Fresh, Sainsbury's*	½ Pot/300g	114	3.6	38	0.7	6.1	1.2	1.3
Leek, & Potato, Fresh, Waitrose*	½ Pot/300g	108	5.1	36	0.7	4.6	1.7	0.9
Leek, & Potato, Soup in a Mug, HL, Tesco*	1 Serving/16g	54	0.9	336	4.3	67.1	5.6	7.4
Leek, Potato, Fresh, Soupreme, Aldi*	½ Pot/300g	192	11.1	64	0.8	6.4	3.7	0.8
Leek, Cream of, Favourites, Baxters*	1 Can/400g	228	16.8	57	1.1	3.8	4.2	0.7
Lentil, & Bacon, Canned, Sainsbury's*	½ Can/200g	102	1.4	51	4.1	6.6	0.7	1
Lentil, & Bacon, Canned, Tesco*	1 Serving/200g	96	1.4	48	3.2	7.2	0.7	0.5
Lentil, & Bacon, Chunky, Canned, M&S*	1 Can/400g	204	2.4	51	3.3	7.2	0.6	1.8
Lentil, & Bacon, Classic, Heinz*	1 Can/400g	232	5.6	58	2.7	8.4	1.4	0.9
Lentil, & Bacon, Favourites, Baxters*	1 Can/400g	208	2.8	52	3.4	7.3	0.7	0.8
Lentil, & Barley, Superbean, M&S*	1 Pack /600g	270	9	45	1.8	5.1	1.5	2.1
Lentil, & Chick Pea, Fresh, Organic, Tesco*	1 Serving/300ml	117	2.4	39	1.9	6.1	0.8	0.5
Lentil, & Ham, Red, Waitrose*	½ Pot/300g	147	3.3	49	3.9	5.8	1.1	2
Lentil, & Smoked Bacon, Fresh, Tesco*	1 Pack/600g	420	11.4	70	3.9	8.5	1.9	1.6
Lentil, & Tomato, New Covent Garden Food Co*	½ Pack/284g	162	3.1	57	3.6	8.1	1.1	0.7
Lentil, & Tomato, Spicy, Chunky, Fresh, Tesco*	½ Pot/300g	195	5.4	65	2.6	9.7	1.8	1.3
Lentil, & Vegetable Soup, Healthy, Baxters*	1 Can/415g	174	1.2	42	1.9	7.4	0.3	1.2
Lentil, & Vegetable, LC, Tesco*	1 Can/400g	188	0.8	47	2.5	8.8	0.2	1.1
Lentil, & Vegetable, Spicy, Chilled, M&S*	½ Serving/300g	150	2.4	50	2.7	8	0.8	1.1
Lentil, Bacon, Smoked, New Covent Garden Food Co*	1 Carton/350g	178	3.5	51	3.7	8.9	1	4.3
Lentil, Vegetable, Spiced, Protein Boosting, Bol*	1 Serving/500g	200	3	40	3.3	7.2	0.6	3.8
Lentil, Vegetable, Vegetarian, Baxters*	½ Can/200g	86	0.6	43	2.1	7.4	0.3	1.3
Lentil, Asda*	½ Can/202g	89	0.4	44	2.6	8	0.2	0.7
Lentil, Bacon Mixed Bean, Low Fat, Aldi*	1 Serving/400g	260	3.6	65	4.7	9.5	0.9	1.6
Lentil, Classic, Heinz*	1 Can/400g	180	0.8	45	2.4	8.5	0.2	0.8
Lentil, Dhal, Canned, Asda*	½ Can/200g	117	3	59	2.4	7.7	1.5	2.3
Lentil, Red, with Carrots, Potato & Onion, Asda*	1 Can/400g	192	0.8	48	1.4	10.2	0.2	1.2
Lentil, Scotty Brand*	1 Pot/550g	374	1.6	68	3.9	10.4	0.3	3.8
Lentil, Spiced, High Protein, Cup a Soup, Batchelors*	1 Pack/255g	97	1.5	38	1.9	6	0.6	0.5
Lentil, Spicy, M&S*	1 Serving/100g	50	1.1	50	2.6	6.3	1.1	2.1

SOUP

	Measure INFO/WEIGHT	per Measure KCAL	FAT	Nutrition Values per 100g / 100ml KCAL	PROT	CARB	FAT	FIBRE
Lobster, Bisque, Waitrose*	½ Carton/300g	201	13.8	67	0.9	5.5	4.6	0.6
Lobster, Bisque, with Brandy & Fresh Cream, Baxters*	½ Can/200g	150	8.6	75	3.3	4.2	4.3	0.2
Minestrone, Canned, Average	*1 Can/400g*	*252*	*12*	*63*	*1.8*	*7.6*	*3*	*0.9*
Minestrone, CBY, Asda*	½ Can/200g	70	1	35	0.4	6.4	0.5	1.6
Minestrone, Chunky, Fresh, Sainsbury's*	½ Pot/300g	93	0.6	31	1.4	6.1	0.2	2.3
Minestrone, Chunky, Love Life, Waitrose*	1 Can/400g	166	0.4	42	1.3	8.7	0.1	1.9
Minestrone, Classic, Heinz*	1 Can/400g	128	0.8	32	1	6.2	0.2	0.8
Minestrone, Diet Chef Ltd*	1 Pack/300g	123	1.8	41	1.4	7.5	0.6	1.2
Minestrone, Favourites, Baxters*	1 Can/400g	168	2.4	42	1.6	7	0.6	1.2
Minestrone, Fresh, Asda*	½ Pot/300g	138	2.1	46	1.8	8.2	0.7	1.2
Minestrone, Fresh, Average	*1 Carton/600g*	*244*	*4.9*	*41*	*1.7*	*6.8*	*0.8*	*1.2*
Minestrone, Fresh, Co-Op*	1 Pot/600g	260	8.4	43	1	6.2	1.4	1.3
Minestrone, Fresh, Morrisons*	1 Pot/506ml	182	2	36	1.9	6.4	0.4	0.2
Minestrone, Fresh, Tesco*	½ Carton/300g	132	3	44	1.8	6.3	1	1.4
Minestrone, Fresh, Waitrose*	1 Pack/600g	240	8.4	40	1.1	5.8	1.4	0.8
Minestrone, Loved by Us, Co-Op*	½ Pot/300g	135	4.2	45	1	6.2	1.4	1.3
Minestrone, Pack, Dry, Knorr*	1 Pack/61g	204	2.4	335	12	58.8	4	6.9
Minestrone, Sainsbury's*	½ Can/200g	66	0.8	33	1.1	6.3	0.4	0.9
Minestrone, Soupreme, Aldi*	½ Pot/300g	162	2.7	54	1.9	8.5	0.9	2.2
Minestrone, with Croutons in a Cup, Sainsbury's*	1 Sachet/225ml	72	0.9	32	0.9	6.3	0.4	0.5
Minestrone, with Croutons in a Mug, Tesco*	1 Sachet/23g	83	1.9	360	9	62.6	8.1	2.7
Minestrone, with Croutons, Dry, Soupreme, Aldi*	1 Serving/27g	94	1.7	349	7.6	65.3	6.4	4.4
Minestrone, with Pasta, Chunky, Co-Op*	1 Pack/400g	140	2.4	35	1	6	0.6	0.7
Miso, Barley, Mugi, Miso Tasty*	1 Sachet/20g	45	1.5	223	8.7	26	7.4	5.1
Miso, Japanese, Made Up, Yutaka*	1 Serving/250ml	24	0.7	10	0.6	1.1	0.3	0
Miso, Wakama*	1 Sachet/8g	27	0.6	336	18.7	48.6	7.6	0
Miso, with Tofu, Instant, Kikkoman*	1 Sachet/10g	35	1	350	30	30	10	0
More Bangalore, Skinnylicious, Skinny Soup, Glorious!*	½ Pot/300g	147	4.2	49	2	6.1	1.4	2.2
Moroccan, Inspired, Pot, Tesco*	½ Pack/266g	146	2.4	55	1.9	8.9	0.9	1.9
Moroccan, with Vegan Pieces, Quorn*	½ Pot/283g	136	1.7	48	4.2	4.4	0.6	3.7
Mulligatawny	*1 Serving/220g*	*213*	*15*	*97*	*1.4*	*8.2*	*6.8*	*0.9*
Mulligatawny, Canned, Tesco*	1 Can/400g	188	4	47	1.3	8.1	1	0.3
Mulligatawny, Classic, Heinz*	1 Can/400g	232	7.6	58	1.9	8	1.9	0.5
Mulligatawny, Slimming World*	1 Serving/200ml	82	0.6	41	2.3	6.5	0.3	1.6
Mushroom, & Chestnut, Fresh, Finest, Tesco*	1 Serving/250g	130	8.2	52	1.1	4.7	3.3	0.7
Mushroom, Roasted Garlic, Soup of the Day, Heinz*	½ Carton/200g	75	3	38	0.8	5.5	1.5	0.4
Mushroom, Canned, HL, Tesco*	1 Can/400g	132	5.6	33	0.5	4.4	1.4	0.2
Mushroom, Cream of, Canned, Tesco*	½ Can/200g	94	5.8	47	0.7	4.8	2.9	0.2
Mushroom, Cream of, Classics, Heinz*	1 Can/400g	208	11.2	52	1.5	5.2	2.8	0.1
Mushroom, Cream of, Condensed, Batchelors*	1 Can/295g	330	25.1	112	1.3	7.5	8.5	0.2
Mushroom, Cream of, Fresh, Finest, Tesco*	½ Pot/300g	238	19	79	1.9	3.5	6.3	0.5
Mushroom, Diet Chef Ltd*	1 Pack/300g	105	5.1	35	1.9	3.2	1.7	0.9
Mushroom, for One, Heinz*	1 Can/290g	148	7.8	51	1.4	5.1	2.7	0.1
Mushroom, Fresh, Average	*1 Serving/300g*	*146*	*9.3*	*49*	*1.3*	*4*	*3.1*	*0.8*
Mushroom, Fresh, M&S*	½ Pack/300g	165	11.7	55	1.8	3.5	3.9	0.9
Mushroom, Potage, Woodland Mushrooms, Baxters*	1 Can/415g	328	20.8	79	1.6	6.9	5	0.3
Mushroom, Three, Broth, Soupologie*	1 Serving/300g	48	0.6	16	0.7	2.4	0.2	0.7
Mushroom, Wild, New Covent Garden Food Co*	1 Carton/600g	162	8.4	27	1	1.9	1.4	1.5
Mushroom, with Croutons in a Cup, Waitrose*	1 Sachet/212g	102	4.2	48	0.6	6.8	2	0.5
Mushroom, with Croutons, Soup in a Mug, Tesco*	1 Serving/226ml	115	4.7	51	1	6.8	2.1	0.4
Noodle, Cantonese Hot & Sour, Baxters*	1 Serving/215g	133	2.8	62	1.4	11.1	1.3	0.5
Noodle, Cup, Shin, Nongshim*	1 Cup/75g	326	11.2	435	7	68	15	0
Onion, French	*1oz/28g*	*11*	*0.6*	*40*	*0.2*	*5.7*	*2.1*	*1*

S

SOUP

INFO/WEIGHT	Measure	per Measure KCAL	FAT	Nutrition Values per 100g / 100ml KCAL	PROT	CARB	FAT	FIBRE
Onion, French, & Cider, Waitrose*	1 Can/425g	94	0.4	22	0.5	4.8	0.1	0.4
Onion, French, & Gruyere Cheese, Fresh, Finest, Tesco*	½ Pot/300g	210	15.3	70	1.4	4.7	5.1	0.5
Onion, French, Chilled, M&S*	½ Pot/300g	150	4.5	50	2	7.2	1.5	1
Onion, French, Favourites, Baxters*	½ Can/200g	66	1.2	33	0.7	5.8	0.6	0.6
Oxtail, Average	*1 Can/400g*	*163*	*4.5*	*41*	*2*	*5.8*	*1.1*	*0.4*
Oxtail, Canned	*1 Serving/220g*	*97*	*3.7*	*44*	*2.4*	*5.1*	*1.7*	*0.1*
Oxtail, Classic, Heinz*	1 Can/400g	168	2	42	1.9	7.3	0.5	0.3
Oxtail, Favourites, Baxters*	1 Can/400g	192	4.4	48	1.8	6.8	1.1	0.5
Oxtail, For One, Heinz*	1 Can/300g	126	1.5	42	1.9	7.3	0.5	0.3
Oxtail, Soupreme, Aldi*	1 Can/400g	152	2	38	2.2	6	0.5	0.5
Parsnip, & Butternut Squash, The Best, Morrisons*	1 Can/400g	244	8.4	61	2.4	8.1	2.1	1.6
Parsnip, & Honey, Festive, New Covent Garden Food Co*	½ Carton/350g	217	7	62	0.9	9.2	2	1.9
Parsnip, & Honey, Fresh, Sainsbury's*	½ Carton/300g	192	12.6	64	1.1	5.4	4.2	1.5
Parsnip, & Orchard Apple, Duchy Originals*	1 Pack/350g	116	3.2	33	0.7	5.4	0.9	1
Parsnip, Spicy, Aldi*	1 Serving/250g	132	8.5	53	0.6	4.9	3.4	1.4
Parsnip, Spicy, Average	*1 Serving/400g*	*212*	*11.2*	*53*	*0.9*	*6*	*2.8*	*1.6*
Parsnip, Spicy, Vegetarian, Baxters*	1 Can/425g	212	10.6	50	0.7	5.3	2.5	1.7
Pea, & Ham	*1 Serving/220g*	*154*	*4.6*	*70*	*4*	*9.2*	*2.1*	*1.4*
Pea, & Ham, Canned, Favourites, Baxters*	1 Can/400g	218	4	55	3.3	7.1	1	2
Pea, & Ham, Canned, Tesco*	1 Can/400g	184	2	46	3.1	6.1	0.5	2.1
Pea, & Ham, CBY, Asda*	1 Pot/600g	282	6.6	47	2.9	5.6	1.1	1.4
Pea, & Ham, Classic, Heinz*	1 Can/400g	252	3.2	63	2.8	10.1	0.8	1.1
Pea, & Ham, Diet Chef Ltd*	1 Pack/300g	138	3.3	46	3.2	5.8	1.1	2.6
Pea, & Ham, Fresh, Sainsbury's*	½ Pack/300ml	120	1.5	40	1.9	7	0.5	0.3
Pea, & Ham, Fresh, Waitrose*	1 Serving/300g	196	10	65	2.9	6.2	3.3	1.6
Pea, & Ham, Petit Pois, Fresh, TTD, Sainsbury's*	½ Pot/300g	201	7.8	67	3.8	6.1	2.6	2.2
Pea, & Ham, Split, Asda*	1 Serving/300g	129	0.6	43	3.5	6.9	0.2	0.7
Pea, & Mint, Best of British, Crosse & Blackwell*	1 Can/400g	192	8.4	48	1.7	4.6	2.1	1.9
Pea, & Mint, Canned, M&S*	½ Can/200g	96	4.2	48	1.7	4.6	2.1	1.9
Pea, & Mint, Fresh, Co-Op*	½ Tub/300g	105	1.7	35	1.7	4.8	0.6	1.8
Pea, & Mint, Fresh, Finest, Tesco*	1 Serving/300g	165	7.2	55	1.3	6	2.4	1.5
Pea, & Mint, Fresh, M&S*	1 Serving/164g	49	0.2	30	1.8	6.3	0.1	1.5
Pea, & Mint, Fresh, Sainsbury's*	½ Pot/300g	102	2.7	34	1.4	5	0.9	1.9
Pea, & Mint, Fresh, Tesco*	½ Pot/300g	145	3.3	48	2.4	6	1.1	2.4
Pea, & Mint, Garden, Vegetarian, Baxters*	½ Can/200g	100	1.6	50	2.5	7.3	0.8	1.9
Pea, & Mint, Slimming World, Iceland*	1 Tub/500g	205	2	41	2.5	5.6	0.4	2.7
Pea, & Mint, with Leek, Fresh, Waitrose*	1 Serving/300g	123	4.5	41	1.7	4.4	1.5	1.5
Pea, Hearty, & Wiltshire Cured Ham Hock, Waitrose*	½ Carton/300g	165	4.2	55	3.1	6.6	1.4	1.8
Pea, Split, Yellow, Simply Organic*	1 Pot/600g	354	3	59	4.3	10.4	0.5	2.6
Pepper, & Chorizo, Canned, Sainsbury's*	1 Can/400ml	172	4	43	7	2	1	0
Pepper, Spicy, & Rice, Korean, Skinny Soup, Glorious!*	½ Tub/300g	108	2.7	36	1	5.4	0.9	1.1
Pepper, Sweetcorn Chilli, Mexican, TTD, Sainsbury's*	½ Pot/300g	190	6.6	63	2.4	7.2	2.2	3
Pepper, with Chilli, Italiamo, Lidl*	1 Can/390ml	222	9.4	57	0.6	7.6	2.4	1.3
Prawn, King, Glass Noodles, Pho, pot	*1 Pot/642g*	*212*	*2.6*	*33*	*1.8*	*5.4*	*0.4*	*0.5*
Prawn, Tom Yum, Cook*	1 Portion/335g	231	3	69	3.5	10.8	0.9	0
Pumpkin, & Chestnut, Cream of, Organic, Bio, La Potagere*	1 Pack/300ml	114	3.3	38	0.8	5.5	1.1	1.5
Pumpkin, Ginger, New Covent Garden Food Co*	1 Serving/300	128	4.8	43	0.7	5.7	1.6	1.5
Pumpkin, Coconut, Thai, New Covent Garden Food Co*	1 Carton/568ml	182	7.4	32	1.3	3.5	1.3	1.1
Pumpkin, Creamy, Very Special, Heinz*	1 Sm Can/290g	188	5.5	65	1.3	9.9	1.9	1.1
Pumpkin, Spiced, Spooky, New Covent Garden Food Co*	1 Serving/350g	168	5.2	48	1.8	6	1.5	1.6
Pumpkin, Spicy, Fresh, Sainsbury's*	½ Pot/300g	87	3	29	0.9	4.2	1	1.3
Pumpkin, Sweet Potato Red Pepper, SO, Sainsbury's*	½ Pot/300g	111	3.9	37	0.8	5.6	1.3	0.8
Red Pepper, & Wensleydale, Asda*	1 Carton /600g	306	12.6	51	2.5	5	2.1	0.8

S

SOUP

INFO/WEIGHT	Measure	per Measure KCAL	FAT	Nutrition Values per 100g / 100ml KCAL	PROT	CARB	FAT	FIBRE
Red Pepper, Roasted, & Tomato, Canned, Sainsbury's*	1 Can/400g	196	6	49	1	7.5	1.5	0.9
Red Pepper, Roasted, & Tomato, M&S*	1 Serving/150g	105	7.4	70	1.4	5	4.9	0.6
Red Pepper, Roasted, Fresh, Waitrose*	1 Pack/600g	172	9	29	0.8	3	1.5	1
Scotch Broth, Canned, Tesco*	½ Can/200g	85	2.6	42	1.3	5.9	1.3	0.8
Scotch Broth, Classic, Heinz*	1 Can/400g	156	2.4	39	1.4	6.7	0.6	0.6
Scotch Broth, Favourites, Baxters*	1 Can/400g	196	6	49	1.8	6.2	1.5	1.5
Seaweed, Spirulina & Quinoa, Supergreens, Tideford*	1 Pot/600g	198	3	33	2.5	3.9	0.5	1.3
Spinach, & Chickpea, Indian, Super, Glorious!*	½ Pot/300g	232	6.9	77	3.4	7.9	2.3	5.4
Spinach, & Green Lentil, Spiced, Asda*	½ Pot/250g	122	5	49	2.7	5	2	0
Spinach, & Watercress, New Covent Garden Food Co*	½ Carton/298g	60	1.2	20	1.3	2.8	0.4	0.8
Spinach, Creme Fraiche, Nutmeg, Organic, Waitrose*	½ Pot/300g	243	22.8	81	0.9	2.3	7.6	1.1
Steak, & Potato, Angus, Big Soup, Heinz*	½ Can/250g	120	2	48	3.1	6.8	0.8	0.6
Steak, Ale, Chunky, Asda*	1 Can/400g	188	4.4	47	3	5.9	1.1	0.6
Steak, Veg, Angus, Mighty, Big Soup, Heinz*	1 Can/500g	270	4.5	54	3.4	7.5	0.9	1
Stilton, Celery & Watercress, Morrisons*	1 Serving/250g	272	23	109	3.9	3.1	9.2	0.3
Super Grain, Brazilian, Glorious!*	½ Pot/300g	163	4.2	54	2.6	6.6	1.4	2.3
Sweet Potato, & Cauliflower, Super Soup, Bol*	½ Pot/250g	110	1.8	44	2.5	8.9	0.7	3.4
Sweet Potato, Lentil, Dahl, Yorkshire Provender*	1 Pot/600g	330	16.2	55	2.6	6.9	2.7	0
Sweet Potato, Coconut Chilli, TTD, Sainsbury's*	½ Pot/300g	176	5.7	59	0.9	8.5	1.9	1.8
Sweet Potato, Coconut, Chilli, Finest, Tesco*	½ Pot/300g	216	13.5	72	1.1	6.5	4.5	0.6
Sweetcorn, & Yellow Pepper, Blended, Heinz*	½ Can/200g	98	4.2	49	0.9	6.6	2.1	0.6
The Big Broth, Yorkshire Provender*	½ Pot/300g	159	6	53	2.9	5.6	2	0
Tomato, & Balsamic, Sicilian, Skinny Soup, Glorious!*	1 Carton/600g	216	11.4	36	1	3.3	1.9	0.7
Tomato, & Basil, CBY, Asda*	½ Pot/297g	89	2.4	30	1	4.3	0.8	0.7
Tomato, & Basil, Creamy, Cully & Sully*	1 Pack/400g	216	18.5	54	0.8	2.5	4.6	0.5
Tomato, & Basil, Cup a Soup, Made Up, GFY, Asda*	1 Serving/250ml	50	0.2	20	0.4	4.4	0.1	0.2
Tomato, & Basil, Cup, Co-Op*	1 Sachet/45g	158	1.8	350	2	76	4	4
Tomato, & Basil, Flavoured, CWP*	1 Sachet/54g	200	4.9	370	33.2	35.7	9.1	4.6
Tomato, & Basil, Fresh, Finest, Tesco*	½ Pot/300g	219	14.7	73	1	6.3	4.9	0.6
Tomato, & Basil, Fresh, Low Fat, Sainsbury's*	½ Carton/300ml	75	1.8	25	1.1	4.1	0.6	0.7
Tomato, & Basil, Fresh, M Kitchen, Morrisons*	½ Pot/300g	115	3.6	38	1	5.5	1.2	0.7
Tomato, & Basil, Fresh, M&S*	½ Pot/300g	120	5.1	40	1	5	1.7	1.3
Tomato, & Basil, Italian Plum, Finest, Tesco*	1 Pot/600g	360	13.8	60	1.3	7.2	2.3	0.6
Tomato, & Basil, Italian Plum, PB, Waitrose*	½ Pot/300g	69	1.5	23	0.9	3.8	0.5	0.9
Tomato, & Basil, Italian Style, Co-Op*	1 Pack/500g	200	10	40	1	4	2	0.6
Tomato, & Basil, Italian, 99% Fat Free, Baxters*	½ Can/208g	119	2.1	57	2.6	9.3	1	1.1
Tomato, & Basil, Italian, Vegetarian, Baxters*	1 Can/415g	170	3.7	41	1.4	5.7	0.9	0.6
Tomato, & Basil, M&S*	½ Pot/300g	105	4.2	35	0.7	4.5	1.4	1
Tomato, & Basil, Plum, New Covent Garden Food Co*	½ Carton/300g	132	6	44	1.3	5.2	2	1.3
Tomato, & Basil, Rich, Waitrose*	1 Serving/130g	53	1.3	41	1.3	6.3	1	0.7
Tomato, & Basil, Sun Dried, Heinz*	1 Serving/275ml	124	5.2	45	0.6	6.5	1.9	0.1
Tomato, & Basil, Weight Watchers*	1 Serving/295g	114	1.8	39	0.6	7.5	0.6	0.6
Tomato, & Brown Lentil, Healthy, Baxters*	1 Can/415g	199	0.8	48	2.6	9	0.2	2.7
Tomato, & Butter Bean, Classic, Heinz*	½ Can/200g	92	1.4	46	1.3	8.1	0.7	0.8
Tomato, & Lentil, Organic, Tideford*	1 Carton/300g	120	2.7	40	2.3	8.1	0.9	0.9
Tomato, & Lentil, Truly Irresistible, Co-Op*	½ Pot/300g	165	2.1	55	3.1	8	0.7	1.2
Tomato, & Red Pepper, Fire Roasted, Asda*	½ Tub/265g	114	6.9	43	0.7	4.1	2.6	1
Tomato, & Rice, with Sweetcorn, Spicy, Healthy, Baxters*	1 Can/414g	219	1.2	53	1.8	9.4	0.3	0.9
Tomato, & Roasted Red Pepper, COU, M&S*	1 Serving/415g	145	0.4	35	1	7.6	0.1	0.9
Tomato, & Three Bean, Canned, BGTY, Sainsbury's*	½ Can/200g	120	2.2	60	2.8	8.4	1.1	2.4
Tomato, & Three Bean, Co-Op*	½ Can/200g	130	1.8	65	3.7	10.2	0.9	2
Tomato, & Three Bean, Eat Smart, Morrisons*	1 Can/400g	228	4	57	2.8	8.2	1	2.2
Tomato, & Thyme, Organic, Duchy, Waitrose*	½ Pot/300g	140	8.9	47	1.2	3.3	3	1

S

SOUP

	Measure INFO/WEIGHT	per Measure KCAL	FAT	Nutrition Values per 100g / 100ml KCAL	PROT	CARB	FAT	FIBRE
Tomato, & Vegetable, Cup a Soup, Batchelors*	1 Serving/218g	107	2.6	49	1.1	8.5	1.2	0.6
Tomato, & Vegetable, Spicy, Healthy Living, Co-Op*	1 Can/400g	180	3.2	45	2	8	0.8	2
Tomato, & Vegetable, Mediterranean, Fresh, Tesco*	½ Pot/300g	105	2.1	35	1	6.2	0.7	0.7
Tomato, Balsamic, Finest, Tesco*	½ Pot/300g	116	4.2	38	1.2	4.9	1.4	0.7
Tomato, Basil, Quinoa, Musclefood*	1 Serving/400g	188	2.8	47	2.8	8	0.7	1.4
Tomato, Bean, Chipotle, New Covent Garden Food Co*	½ Carton/300g	138	1.5	46	2.7	6.5	0.5	2.2
Tomato, Big Red, Heinz*	½ Can/210g	63	0.8	30	0.5	6.4	0.4	0
Tomato, Borlotti Bean Kale, Fresh, M&S*	1 Pot/600g	318	10.2	53	2	6.3	1.7	2.1
Tomato, Canned, LC, Tesco*	½ Can/200g	90	3.8	45	0.9	5.9	1.9	0.4
Tomato, Cannellini Beans, Garlic, Heinz*	½ Can/200g	110	2.2	55	2.4	9.1	1.1	2.4
Tomato, Chunky, Organic, Canned, Amy's Kitchen*	1 Can/400g	212	5.6	53	1.2	8.6	1.4	1.2
Tomato, Cream of, Asda*	½ Can/200g	122	6.4	61	0.7	7.3	3.2	0.7
Tomato, Cream of, Canned, Average	**1 Can/400g**	**208**	**12**	**52**	**0.8**	**5.9**	**3**	**0.7**
Tomato, Cream of, Canned, Crosse & Blackwell*	1 Can/400g	228	10	57	0.9	7.4	2.5	0.8
Tomato, Cream of, Canned, Tesco*	½ Can/192g	115	4.8	60	0.9	7.4	2.5	0.8
Tomato, Cream of, Classic, Heinz*	½ Can/200g	118	6	59	0.9	6.7	3	0.4
Tomato, Cream of, Classics, Soupreme, Aldi*	1 Can/400g	192	8	48	0.8	6.4	2	0.8
Tomato, Cream of, Eat Well, M&S*	½ Pot/300g	189	9.9	63	0.8	7.1	3.3	0.6
Tomato, Cream of, Favourites, Baxters*	½ Can/200g	132	5.4	66	1.1	6.9	2.7	0.4
Tomato, Cream of, for One, Heinz*	1 Can/300g	189	10.8	63	0.8	6.9	3.6	0.4
Tomato, Cream of, Fresh, Sainsbury's*	1 Pot/600g	318	19.2	53	0.8	5.2	3.2	1.3
Tomato, Cream of, Sainsbury's*	1 Can/400g	244	12.8	61	0.7	7.3	3.2	0.7
Tomato, Cream Of, with a Hint of Basil, Heinz*	½ Can/200g	114	6	57	0.9	6.6	3	0.4
Tomato, Cream of, with Spanish Chorizo, Heinz*	1 Can/400g	244	12	61	1.4	6.9	3	0.4
Tomato, Fresh, Mediterranean, Organic, Sainsbury's*	1 Serving/250ml	78	3.5	31	1.3	3.3	1.4	1
Tomato, Gazpacho, Innocent*	1 Bowl/200g	80	4.6	40	0.6	2.8	2.3	2.4
Tomato, Herb Roasted, & Wheatberry, Waitrose*	1 Pot/400g	222	9.9	56	1.1	6.4	2.5	1.5
Tomato, Kale, Borlotti Bean, Italian, Asda*	½ Tub/300g	144	3.9	48	1.9	6.1	1.3	2.2
Tomato, Original, Cup a Soup, Batchelors*	1 Sachet/254g	104	2.3	41	0.6	7.3	0.9	0.5
Tomato, Red Lentil Pepper, CBY, Asda*	½ Pot/300g	177	3.3	59	3	8.8	1.1	0.9
Tomato, Roasted Garlic, & Black Pepper, Heinz*	½ Carton/200g	98	3.8	49	1.2	6.7	1.9	1.1
Tomato, Singapore Crushed, Skinny Soup, Glorious!*	½ Pot/300g	129	5.4	43	1	5.8	1.8	1.1
Tomato, Slow Roast, New Covent Garden Food Co*	½ Carton/350g	98	1.4	28	0.9	4.4	0.4	1.5
Tomato, Smart Price, Asda*	1 Can/400g	184	7.6	46	0.6	6.5	1.9	0.9
Tomato, Spicy, Lentil, Red Pepper, Fresh, Sainsbury's*	1 Pot/600g	390	7.8	65	3.7	8.8	1.3	1.8
Tomato, Spinach, Lentil, Heinz*	½ Can/200g	85	1.4	43	1.7	7.7	0.7	1.1
Tomato, Vine, Harissa & Mint, The Best, Morrisons*	1 Pot/600g	294	11.4	49	1.5	6.4	1.9	1.1
Tomato, Weight Watchers*	1 Can/295g	76	1.5	26	0.7	4.6	0.5	0.3
Tomato, Mediterranean, Slim a Soup, Cup, Batchelors*	1 Serving/208g	56	1.2	27	0.5	4.8	0.6	0.4
Tomato, Mediterranean, Vegetarian, Baxters*	1 Can/400g	126	0.4	32	0.9	5.6	0.1	0.8
Turkey, Broth, Canned, Baxters*	½ Can/208g	79	1.5	38	1.3	6.5	0.7	0.7
Vegetable, & Three Bean, Chunky, M&S*	1 Can/400g	228	3.6	57	3	7.7	0.9	3.1
Vegetable, Barley, Ready to Serve, Wattie's*	½ Can/262g	97	0.5	37	1.6	6.4	0.2	1.6
Vegetable, Balance, Reduced Salt, Canned, Heinz*	1 Can/400g	168	2.8	42	1.2	7.2	0.7	1.2
Vegetable, Broth, Best of British, Crosse & Blackwell*	1 Can/400g	135	1.6	34	1.1	5.9	0.4	1.1
Vegetable, Broth, Hearty, Weight Watchers*	1 Can/295g	135	0.6	46	2	8.2	0.2	1.4
Vegetable, Canned	**1oz/28g**	**13**	**0.2**	**48**	**1.4**	**9.9**	**0.6**	**1.5**
Vegetable, Canned, Essential, Waitrose*	½ Can/200g	103	1	52	1.9	9.2	0.5	1.4
Vegetable, Canned, Tesco*	½ Can/200g	70	1	35	1.1	5.9	0.5	1
Vegetable, Canned, Tesco*	½ Can/200g	100	2	50	1.4	8.1	1	1.3
Vegetable, Chunky, Canned, Sainsbury's*	1 Can/400g	184	2.8	46	1.5	8.3	0.7	1.2
Vegetable, Chunky, Canned, Soupreme, Aldi*	1 Can/400g	172	4	43	1.1	6.4	1	2.3
Vegetable, Chunky, Diet Chef Ltd*	1 Pack/300g	114	0.9	38	1.4	7.4	0.3	1.3

S

	Measure INFO/WEIGHT	per Measure KCAL	FAT	Nutrition Values per 100g / 100ml KCAL	PROT	CARB	FAT	FIBRE
SOUP								
Vegetable, Chunky, Fresh, CBY, Asda*	½ Pot/300g	117	2.1	39	1.6	5.9	0.7	1.1
Vegetable, Chunky, Fresh, Tesco*	½ Pot/300g	138	4.8	46	1.4	5.7	1.6	1.6
Vegetable, Chunky, Fresh, Waitrose*	½ Pot/300g	117	5.4	39	1.3	4.5	1.8	2.1
Vegetable, Classic, Heinz*	1 Can/400g	188	3.2	47	1.1	8.3	0.8	0.9
Vegetable, Country, Canned, Heinz, Weight Watchers*	1 Can/295g	97	0.6	33	1.2	5.9	0.2	1
Vegetable, Country, Chunky, Baxters*	1 Can/400g	188	2.4	47	1.6	7.2	0.6	2
Vegetable, Country, Fresh, Soupreme, Aldi*	1 Tub/600g	204	3.6	34	1.1	5.1	0.6	1.7
Vegetable, Country, Hearty, Canned, Baxters*	1 Can/400g	192	2.4	48	1.9	7.5	0.6	1.9
Vegetable, Country, Knorr*	1 Pack/500ml	160	3.5	32	0.9	5.5	0.7	1.2
Vegetable, Country, Weight Watchers*	1 Can/295g	97	0.3	33	1.2	6.3	0.1	1
Vegetable, Cully & Sully*	1 Pack/400g	204	14.4	51	0.6	4.2	3.6	0.9
Vegetable, Cup Soup, Dry, Heinz*	1 Sachet/16g	54	1.1	348	5.8	64.5	7.1	3.2
Vegetable, Cup Soup, Made Up, Heinz*	1 Cup/200g	62	0.6	31	0.5	6.3	0.3	0.3
Vegetable, Farmhouse, Thick, Co-Op*	1 Can/400g	140	1.6	35	1	7	0.4	0.3
Vegetable, Fresh, Average	*1 Serving/300g*	*118*	*4.1*	*40*	*1.4*	*5.4*	*1.4*	*1.3*
Vegetable, Fresh, Co-Op*	1 Pack/600g	150	6	25	0.6	4	1	1
Vegetable, Golden, Cup, GFY, Asda*	1 Sachet/217ml	52	1.1	24	0.5	4.4	0.5	0.2
Vegetable, Golden, Slim a Soup, Batchelors*	1 Sachet/207g	58	1.7	28	0.5	4.7	0.8	0.7
Vegetable, Golden, with Croutons Cup Soup, Co-Op*	1 Sachet/25g	120	6.5	480	4	56	26	2
Vegetable, Green, & Grains, Vegan, Waitrose*	1 Pot/400g	248	12	62	3.1	3.8	3	3.6
Vegetable, Gyoza, with Miso Broth, Everdine*	1 Serving/450g	369	5	82	2.9	13.3	1.1	3.6
Vegetable, in a Cup, HL, Tesco*	1 Sachet/18g	66	1.4	367	7.2	66.1	7.8	2.8
Vegetable, Instant, Cup, Average	*1 Pack/19g*	*69*	*2*	*362*	*8.7*	*57.1*	*10.5*	*5.5*
Vegetable, Lighter Life*	1 Serving/39g	150	4.9	381	31.7	32.2	12.5	6.3
Vegetable, Moroccan, Tagine, Yorkshire Provender*	½ Pot/300g	171	5.1	57	2.3	7.2	1.7	0.7
Vegetable, No Added Sugar, Canned, Heinz*	½ Can/200g	84	1.4	42	1.2	7.2	0.7	1.2
Vegetable, Root, & Turmeric, Baxters*	1 Can/400g	164	5.6	41	0.8	6.3	1.4	0.5
Vegetable, Soup In A Mug, Made Up, HL, Tesco*	1 Sachet/218ml	66	1.1	30	0.7	5.5	0.5	0.4
Vegetable, Spring, Classic, Heinz*	1 Can/400g	148	1.6	37	0.8	7	0.4	0.8
Vegetable, Spring, Florida, Dry, Knorr*	1 Pack/36g	104	2	290	7.8	52.2	5.6	5.2
Vegetable, Spring, Sainsbury's*	½ Can/200g	72	0.8	36	0.8	7.4	0.4	0.6
Vegetable, Ten, Broth, Morrisons*	1 Pot/600g	240	7.8	40	1.7	5.8	1.3	1.1
Vegetable, Winter, & Lentils, Mouline, Bio, La Potagere*	1 Pack/300ml	111	5.1	37	0.9	3.5	1.7	2.2
Vegetable, Winter, New Covent Garden Food Co*	½ Pack/300g	117	2.1	39	2	5.1	0.7	2.3
Vegetable, Roasted, Fresh, Sainsbury's*	½ Pot/300ml	78	1.5	26	0.5	4.8	0.5	1.2
Watercress, M&S*	½ Pot/300g	75	5.1	25	1.3	1.5	1.7	0.6
SOUP MIX								
Butternut Squash, Sainsbury's*	¼ Pack/147g	47	1	32	0.8	5.3	0.7	0.5
Leek Potato, As Sold, Good & Balanced, Asda*	¼ Pack/125g	69	0.4	55	1.7	10.5	0.3	1.7
Minestrone Bean, Cooks' Ingredients, Waitrose*	½ Pack/200g	118	1	59	2.7	9	0.5	3.6
Red Pepper, Carrot, Nature's Pick, Aldi*	1 Serving/100g	16	0.5	16	1.4	1.8	0.5	0.8
Soup Broth Mix, Dry, Wholefoods, Tesco*	¼ Pack/125g	456	2.4	365	14.7	71.4	1.9	7.3
Sweet Potato, Nature's Pick, Aldi*	1 Serving/100g	24	0.5	24	0.8	4.1	0.5	1.2
Vegetable, Kit, Morrisons*	1 Pack/500g	220	3.5	44	1.2	6.6	0.7	3
SOUTHERN COMFORT								
37.5% Volume	*1 Pub Shot/35ml*	*72*	*0*	*207*	*0*	*0*	*0*	*0*
SOYA								
Barbeque Chilli, Vegelicious, Tesco*	1 Portion/450g	450	15.8	100	3.1	12.9	3.5	2.7
Chunks, Dried, Cooked, Sainsbury's*	1oz/28g	27	0.1	98	14	9.8	0.3	1.1
Chunks, Protein, Natural, Nature's Harvest*	1 Serving/50g	172	0.5	345	50	35	1	4
Chunks, with Chilli, Coriander, Soy Marinade, M&S*	1 Pack/175g	180	1.6	103	18.6	1.7	0.9	6.8
Mince, Dry Weight, Sainsbury's*	1 Serving/50g	164	0.4	328	47.2	33.2	0.8	3.6
Mince, Granules	*1oz/28g*	*74*	*1.5*	*263*	*43.2*	*11*	*5.4*	*0*

INFO/WEIGHT	Measure	per Measure		Nutrition Values per 100g / 100ml				
		KCAL	FAT	KCAL	PROT	CARB	FAT	FIBRE

SOYA

Mince, Prepared, Sainsbury's*	1 Serving/200g	164	0.4	82	11.8	8.3	0.2	0.9

SPAGHETTI

50/50, Dry, Napolina*	1 Serving/75g	257	1.4	343	11.2	67	1.8	7.2
Bare Naked, Barenaked*	1 Serving/100g	17	0.1	17	0.3	0.9	0.1	3.4
Black Bean, Organic, Dry, Explore Asian*	1 Serving/56g	198	2	353	44	15	3.6	21
Brown Rice, GF, Organic, Dry, Dove's Farm*	1 Serving/70g	237	1	338	7.9	70.3	1.5	4.1
Cooked, Average	*1oz/28g*	*33*	*0.2*	*119*	*4.1*	*24.8*	*0.6*	*1.1*
Dry, Average	*1oz/28g*	*98*	*0.4*	*350*	*12.1*	*72.1*	*1.5*	*2.4*
Durum Wheat, Dry, Average	*1oz/28g*	*97*	*0.1*	*348*	*12.4*	*71.8*	*0.4*	*1.4*
Edamame, Organic, Dry, Explore Asian*	1 Serving/56g	204	2	365	45	18	3.6	20
Fresh, Cooked, Average	*1 Serving/125g*	*182*	*2.2*	*146*	*6.1*	*26.9*	*1.7*	*1.8*
Fresh, Dry, Average	*1 Serving/100g*	*278*	*3*	*278*	*10.8*	*53*	*3*	*2.2*
Hoops, Canned, Smart Price, Asda*	½ Can/205g	127	0.6	62	1.7	13	0.3	0.4
Hoops, in Tomato Sauce, Heinz*	½ Can/200g	106	0.4	53	1.7	11.1	0.2	0.5
Hoops, in Tomato Sauce, Snap Pot, Heinz*	1 Pot/190g	115	0.4	61	1.7	12.6	0.2	0.6
in Rich Tomato Sauce, Canned, Corale, Aldi*	½ Can/200g	114	1	57	2.1	10	0.5	2.6
in Tomato Sauce with Parsley, Weight Watchers*	1 Sm Can/200g	100	0.4	50	1.8	9.9	0.2	0.6
In Tomato Sauce, Basics, Sainsbury's*	1 Can/410g	197	1.2	48	1.4	10	0.3	0.7
in Tomato Sauce, Canned	*1oz/28g*	*18*	*0.1*	*64*	*1.9*	*14.1*	*0.4*	*0.7*
in Tomato Sauce, Heinz*	½ Can/200g	120	0.6	60	1.7	12.7	0.3	2.4
Lentil, Mushroom, Italian, Good Health, Waitrose*	1 Pack/373g	433	14.6	116	3.4	14	3.9	5.5
Marinara	*1 Serving/450g*	*675*	*18.9*	*150*	*8*	*19*	*4.2*	*0.9*
Pancetta, Smoked, & Mushroom, Creamy Sauce, Tesco*	1 Serving/350g	590	33.3	168	7	13	9.5	1.3
Whole Wheat, Cooked, Average	*1oz/28g*	*32*	*0.3*	*113*	*4.7*	*23.2*	*0.9*	*3.5*
Whole Wheat, Dry, Average	*1 Serving/100g*	*324*	*2.6*	*324*	*13.5*	*62.2*	*2.6*	*8*
with Sausages, in Tomato Sauce, Heinz*	1 Can/400g	352	14	88	3.4	10.8	3.5	0.5

SPAGHETTI & MEATBALLS

556, Wiltshire Farm Foods*	1 Serving/405g	456	22.5	112	4.4	10.8	5.6	1
American, Superbowl, Asda*	1 Pack/453g	594	17.7	131	11	13	3.9	1.1
Annabel Karmel*	1 Meal/200g	216	8	108	4.8	15.6	4	1.7
Beef Pork, Calorie Controlled, Love Life, Waitrose*	1 Pack/356g	342	9.3	96	5.5	11.9	2.6	1.3
Chicken, in Tomato Sauce, Heinz*	1 Can/400g	332	9.2	83	4.2	11.3	2.3	0.5
Frozen, Tesco*	1 Serving/368g	488	19	133	5.6	15	5.2	2
GFY, Asda*	1 Pack/400g	344	6	86	7	11	1.5	1.5
Italian Cuisine, Tesco*	1 Pack/413g	516	18.2	125	7.4	13	4.4	1.4
Little Dish*	1 Pack/200g	227	9.6	114	6.2	10.6	4.8	1.6
Low Fat, Co-Op*	1 Pack/390g	355	9	91	5.2	11	2.3	2
Meal for One, Microwaved, Iceland*	1 Meal/453g	421	4.5	93	4.4	15.7	1	1.8
Meatballs, Italian, As Prepared, Waitrose*	1 Pack/400g	520	23.8	131	6.1	12.8	6	0.8
Pork Beef, in Tomato Sauce, Prepared, Sainsbury's*	1 Pack/401g	566	27.3	141	7.3	11.9	6.8	1.6
Ready Mea, lHealthy Range, Average	*1 Serving/400g*	*375*	*8.3*	*94*	*5.7*	*12.9*	*2.1*	*1.7*

SPAGHETTI WITH

King Prawn, Italian, Cooked, Finest, Tesco*	1 Pack/390g	485	22.9	125	5	12.2	5.9	1.3
Pulled Beef, Ragu, Everdine*	1 Serving/450g	360	8.1	80	7.7	7.2	1.8	2.1
Tomato, & Basil, Parsley & Parmesan Cheese, M&S*	1 Pack/400g	584	29.2	146	3.8	15.1	7.3	2.2

SPAM*

Pork Ham, Chopped, Spam*	1 Serving/100g	289	24.3	289	15	3.2	24.3	0

SPICE MIX

Biryani, Schwartz*	1 Sachet/28g	89	2.9	318	15.4	29.8	10.4	21.6
Chicken Tikka, Blend, Parampara*	¼ Pack/20g	89	5	446	5.8	42.4	24.8	15
Chilli Con Carne, Tex Mex, Recipe Mix, Schwartz*	1 Sachet/35g	97	2.3	277	12.9	66.6	6.6	24.6
for Burritos, Old El Paso*	½ Pack/23g	68	0.9	304	13	54	4	0
for Fajitas, Old El Paso*	1 Pack/35g	107	2.1	306	9	54	6	0

S

	Measure INFO/WEIGHT	per Measure		Nutrition Values per 100g / 100ml				
		KCAL	FAT	KCAL	PROT	CARB	FAT	FIBRE
SPICE MIX								
for Mexican Fajitas, Discovery*	½ Pack/15g	34	1	230	8	35	6.5	17.5
Moroccan, Rub, Schwartz*	1 Serving/3g	9	0.3	309	15	36.4	11.4	19.5
Peri-Peri, Medium, Bag Bake, Nando's*	1 Serving/20g	57	0.2	286	4.6	60	1.2	0
Ras El Hanout, Al'fez*	1 Tsp/2g	4	0.2	217	9.8	25.7	8.3	17.5
Ras El Hanout, Blend, Finest, Tesco*	1 Tsp/5g	16	0.5	320	9.4	37.1	9.2	23.6
Thai, Blend, Sharwood's*	1 Pack 260g	424	30.9	163	1.8	12	11.9	1
Tikka, Blend, Sharwood's*	1 Pack/260g	263	14	101	2.7	10.2	5.4	1.7
Zaatar, Waitrose*	1 Serving/10g	42	3	416	14.7	8.2	30.2	26.1
SPICE PASTE								
Biryani, Patak's*	1 Serving/30g	77	5.9	257	4.5	8.2	19.6	10.5
SPINACH								
Baby, Average	*1 Serving/90g*	*22*	*0.7*	*25*	*2.8*	*1.6*	*0.8*	*2.1*
Boiled or Steamed, Average	*1 Serving/80g*	*17*	*0.6*	*21*	*2.6*	*0.9*	*0.8*	*2.1*
Canned, Average	*1 Serving/80g*	*16*	*0.4*	*20*	*2.8*	*1.3*	*0.5*	*2.7*
Mornay, Waitrose*	½ Pack/125g	112	8.6	90	3.3	3.6	6.9	1.6
Raw, Average	*1 Serving/80g*	*19*	*0.6*	*24*	*2.9*	*1.4*	*0.7*	*2.2*
SPIRALI								
Dry, Average	*1 Serving/50g*	*176*	*0.8*	*352*	*12.2*	*72.6*	*1.6*	*2.8*
SPIRITS								
37.5% Volume	*1 Pub Shot/35ml*	*72*	*0*	*207*	*0*	*0*	*0*	*0*
40% Volume	*1 Shot/35ml*	*78*	*0*	*222*	*0*	*0*	*0*	*0*
Non Alcoholic, Garden, Seedlip Ltd*	1 Serving/50ml	0	0	0	0	0	0	0
Non Alcoholic, Spice 94, Botanical, Seedlip Ltd*	1 Serving/50ml	0	0	0	0	0	0	0
SPLIT PEAS								
Dried, Average	*1oz/28g*	*89*	*0.5*	*319*	*22.1*	*57.4*	*1.7*	*3.2*
Green, Dried, Average	*1 Serving/80g*	*261*	*1.3*	*326*	*22.5*	*45*	*1.6*	*20*
Green, Dried, Boiled, Average	*1 Tbsp/35g*	*40*	*0.2*	*115*	*8.3*	*19.8*	*0.6*	*3.9*
Yellow, Dried, Uncooked, Sainsbury's*	1 Serving/40g	116	0.7	290	20	42.5	1.8	11.8
SPONGE FINGERS								
Almond Fingers, Tesco*	1 Finger/46g	174	6.1	379	5.3	58.8	13.2	1.7
Boudoir, Sainsbury's*	1 Finger/5g	20	0.2	396	8.1	82.8	3.6	0.4
Tesco*	1 Finger/5g	19	0.2	386	7.6	80.6	3.7	1
Trifle, Average	*1 Sponge/24g*	*77*	*0.5*	*319*	*5.2*	*69.9*	*2.2*	*0.8*
SPONGE PUDDING								
Average	*1 Portion/170g*	*578*	*27.7*	*340*	*5.8*	*45.3*	*16.3*	*1.1*
Blackberry & Apple, HE, Tesco*	1 Pot/103g	159	1.4	155	3.1	32.6	1.4	0.7
Blackcurrant, BGTY, Sainsbury's*	1 Serving/110g	155	1	141	2.5	30.7	0.9	3.2
Canned, Average	*1 Serving/75g*	*214*	*8.6*	*285*	*3.1*	*45.4*	*11.4*	*0.8*
Cherry & Almond Flavour, Sainsbury's*	¼ Pudding/110g	334	15.7	304	3.5	40.3	14.3	0.7
Cherry, Almond, Tesco*	1 Pudding/115g	427	17.4	372	3.5	55.1	15.2	0.5
Chocolate & Sauce, Co-Op*	1 Pack/225g	608	29.2	270	5	34	13	0.6
Chocolate, Cadbury*	1 Pack/370g	1276	73.3	345	4.9	36.7	19.8	0
Chocolate, Free From, Sainsbury's*	1 Pudding/110g	388	10.2	353	5.2	62	9.3	0.3
Chocolate, Less Than 3% Fat, BGTY, Sainsbury's*	1 Pudding/105g	180	2	171	4.5	34	1.9	0.9
Chocolate, M&S*	¼ Pudding/131g	524	32.2	400	6.1	38.6	24.6	1.8
Chocolate, M&S*	1 Pudding/105g	401	24.3	382	5.7	36	23.1	3.5
Chocolate, Sainsbury's*	¼ Pudding/110g	464	28.3	422	5.4	42.3	25.7	0.8
Chocolate, Tesco*	1 Serving/115g	430	19.2	374	3.7	50.8	16.7	2.7
Chocolate, Trufree*	1 Serving/115g	374	17.2	325	2.5	44	15	2
Chocolate, Waitrose*	1 Pudding/110g	400	22.5	363	3.6	41.4	20.4	1.7
Fruit, Co-Op*	1 Can/300g	1110	48	370	3	53	16	2

S

SPONGE PUDDING

INFO/WEIGHT	Measure	per Measure KCAL	per Measure FAT	per 100g KCAL	PROT	CARB	FAT	FIBRE
Fruited with Brandy Sauce, Sainsbury's*	1 Pudding/125g	261	8.4	209	3.6	33.6	6.7	0.8
Ginger with Plum Sauce, Waitrose*	1 Pudding/120g	424	17.9	353	3.1	51.7	14.9	0.7
Golden Syrup, Co-Op*	1 Can/300g	945	39	315	2	47	13	0.6
HoneyFig, M&S*	¼ Pudding/73g	225	12	310	3.6	34.8	16.6	3.4
Lemon Curd, Heinz*	¼ Can/78g	236	9.1	302	2.6	46.7	11.7	0.6
Lemon, COU, M&S*	1 Pudding/100g	157	2.3	157	2	32.1	2.3	1.9
Lemon, M&S*	1 Pudding/105g	326	16	310	4.3	39.4	15.2	2.3
Lemon, Waitrose*	1 Serving/105g	212	2.5	202	3.4	41.7	2.4	1.4
Milk Chocolate, Sticky Puds, Cadbury*	1 Pudding/95g	390	17.3	360	4.2	48.9	16	0.8
Mixed Berry, BGTY, Sainsbury's*	1 Pudding/110g	189	2.6	172	2.4	33.3	2.4	3.8
Pear & Ginger, COU, M&S*	1 Pudding/100g	175	0.7	175	1.9	39.8	0.7	1.1
Raspberry Jam, Asda*	½ Pudding/147g	481	16.2	327	3.1	54	11	4.1
Raspberry, Tesco*	1 Serving/100g	377	14.5	377	3.2	58.2	14.5	0.7
Salted Caramel, Specially Selected, Aldi*	1 Pudding/115g	459	20.7	399	3.6	54	18	1
Salted Caramel, Tesco*	1 Pudding/115g	464	21.6	404	3.2	55.2	18.8	0.6
Sticky Ginger, Really Good Puds, M Kitchen, Morrisons*	1 Pudding/110g	372	12	338	3.5	56.2	10.9	0.5
Sticky Toffee, Microwavable, Heinz*	1 Serving/75g	233	9	311	3.3	47.4	12	0.7
Strawberry Jam, Heinz*	¼ Can/82g	230	6.2	281	2.6	50.4	7.6	0.6
Sultana with Toffee Sauce, HL, Tesco*	1 Serving/80g	280	2.2	350	3.2	60.2	2.8	1
Summer Fruits, BGTY, Sainsbury's*	1 Serving/110g	243	4.7	221	2.7	42.9	4.3	1
Syrup & Custard, Morrisons*	1 Serving/125g	290	8.6	232	3.4	39.1	6.9	0.8
Syrup, BGTY, Sainsbury's*	1 Pudding/110g	338	4.5	307	2.8	64.6	4.1	0.4
Syrup, Finest, Tesco*	1 Pudding/115g	330	9	287	3.1	51.2	7.8	0.6
Syrup, GFY, Asda*	1 Sponge/105g	207	4.3	197	2	38	4.1	2.6
Syrup, Individual, Tesco*	1 Pudding/110g	390	14.5	355	3.1	55.6	13.2	0.5
Syrup, Pudding, with Golden Syrup Sauce, Tesco*	1 Serving/100g	394	15.6	394	2.9	59.8	15.6	1.4
Syrup, Sainsbury's*	¼ Pudding/110g	408	13	371	2.7	63.5	11.8	0.4
Syrup, Value, Tesco*	1 Serving/100g	307	10.2	307	2.1	51.7	10.2	0.6
Toffee Pecan	*½ Pudding/100g*	*395*	*18.4*	*395*	*4.3*	*52.3*	*18.4*	*1.4*
Toffee, Pecan, Finest, Tesco*	½ Sponge/100g	395	18.4	395	4.3	52.3	18.4	1.4
Treacle with Custard, Farmfoods*	1 Serving/145g	539	33.1	372	3.2	38.4	22.8	0.8
Treacle, Heinz*	1 Serving/160g	445	13	278	2.5	48.9	8.1	0.6
Treacle, Super Sticky, Heinz*	1 Pudding/110g	318	12.2	289	1.9	45.3	11.1	1.6
Treacle, Waitrose*	1 Pudding/105g	385	13.8	367	2.8	59.5	13.1	0.6
Vanilla, with Blackcurrant Sauce, Waitrose*	1 Pudding/105g	263	10.9	250	3.5	34.5	10.4	2.6
Very Fruity Cherry, M&S*	1 Pot/110g	286	11.3	260	3.5	38.6	10.3	1.8
with Custard	*1 Serving/200g*	*521*	*24.9*	*261*	*4.8*	*34.1*	*12.4*	*0.9*
with Dried Fruit	*1oz/28g*	*93*	*4*	*331*	*5.4*	*48.1*	*14.3*	*1.2*
with Jam or Treacle	*1oz/28g*	*93*	*4*	*333*	*5.1*	*48.7*	*14.4*	*1*
with Lyles Golden Syrup, Heinz*	½ Pudding/95g	368	14.4	386	3.1	53.3	15.1	0.5

SPOTTED DICK

INFO/WEIGHT	Measure	per Measure KCAL	per Measure FAT	per 100g KCAL	PROT	CARB	FAT	FIBRE
Average	*1 Serving/105g*	*343*	*17.5*	*327*	*4.2*	*42.7*	*16.7*	*1*
Individual, Tesco*	1 Pudding/121g	417	14.5	345	3.2	55.2	12	1.2
Pudding, Individual, Sainsbury's*	1 Serving/110g	346	12.9	315	3.8	48.7	11.7	2.2
with Custard	*1 Serving/210g*	*438*	*15.6*	*209*	*3.4*	*31.5*	*7.4*	*1.3*

SPRATS

INFO/WEIGHT	Measure	per Measure KCAL	per Measure FAT	per 100g KCAL	PROT	CARB	FAT	FIBRE
Fried	*1oz/28g*	*116*	*9.8*	*415*	*24.9*	*0*	*35*	*0*
Raw	*1oz/28g*	*33*	*2.1*	*117*	*12.4*	*0*	*7.5*	*0*

SPREAD

INFO/WEIGHT	Measure	per Measure KCAL	per Measure FAT	per 100g KCAL	PROT	CARB	FAT	FIBRE
Apple, Bramley, M&S*	1 Tsp/5g	8	0	169	0.3	40.2	0.8	0.1
Average	*1 Thin Spread/7g*	*51*	*5.7*	*726*	*0.1*	*0.5*	*81*	*0*
Butter Me Up, Light, Tesco*	1 Thin Spread/7g	24	2.7	350	0.3	0.5	38	0
Butter Me Up, Tesco*	1 Thin Spread/7g	35	3.8	503	0.7	1	55	0.5

SPREAD

	Measure INFO/WEIGHT	per Measure KCAL	per Measure FAT	Nutrition Values per 100g / 100ml KCAL	PROT	CARB	FAT	FIBRE
Butter Style, Average	*1 Thin Spread/7g*	*44*	*4.8*	*627*	*0.7*	*1.1*	*68.9*	*0*
Butterlicious, Vegetable, Sainsbury's*	1 Thin Spread/7g	44	4.8	628	0.6	1.1	69	0
Butterlicious, Vegetable, Sainsbury's*	1 Serving/10g	41	4.5	414	0.5	1.5	45	1
Buttersoft, Light, Reduced Fat, Sainsbury's*	1 Thin Spread/7g	38	4.2	544	0.4	0.5	60	0
Buttery Taste, Benecol*	1 Thin Spread/7g	40	4.4	575	0	0.8	63.3	0
Clover, Light, Dairy Crest Ltd*	1 Serving/7g	32	3.4	455	0.7	2.9	49	0
Cocoa, & Hazelnut, Butter, Nature's Energy, Meridian*	1 Tsp/5g	33	3	661	13.2	14.5	59.9	5.6
Dairy Free, Organic, Pure Spreads*	1 Thin Spread/7g	37	4.1	533	0.5	0	59	0
Enriched Olive, Tesco*	1 Thin Spread/7g	38	4.1	540	0.2	1.2	59	0
Fruit, Strawberry, Organic, Nature's Energy, Meridian*	1 Tsp/5g	6	0	129	0.6	29.6	0.3	1.4
Gold, Made with Buttermilk, Low Low, Kerry*	1 Spread/10g	48	5.3	483	0.6	0.8	53	0
Heart, Cholesterol Reducing, Dairygold	*1 Thin Spread/7g*	*24*	*2.5*	*338*	*0.7*	*2.8*	*36*	*0*
Lactofree Spreadable, Lactofree, Arla*	1 Serving/10g	68	7.5	679	0.5	0.5	75	0
Light, Benecol*	1 Thin Spread/7g	23	2.4	333	2.5	0	35	0
Lighter Than Light, Flora*	1 Serving/10g	19	1.8	188	5	1.6	18	0
Low Fat, Average	*1 Thin Spread/7g*	*27*	*2.8*	*390*	*5.8*	*0.5*	*40.5*	*0*
Olive Oil, 55% Reduced Fat, Benecol*	1 Thin Spread/7g	35	3.8	498	0.3	0.5	55	0
Olive Oil, Bertolli*	1 Serving/10g	53	5.9	532	0.5	0.5	59	0
Olive, Light, Tesco*	1 Spread/10g	28	3	278	0.1	0.6	30.5	0.5
Olive, Low Fat, Morrisons*	1 Thin Spread/7g	24	2.7	346	0.9	0	38	0
Olive, Reduced Fat, Asda*	1 Thin Spread/7g	38	4.1	536	0.2	1.1	59	0
Olive, Sainsbury's*	1 Thin Spread/7g	29	3.2	410	0.5	1	45	0.5
Olive, Tesco*	1 Thin Spread/7g	29	3.2	415	0.2	2	45	0.7
Olive, Waitrose*	1 Thin Spread/7g	37	4.1	534	0.2	0.5	59	0
Orange, Thick Cut, St Dalfour*	1 Spread/11g	23	0	211	0.6	52	0.1	1.6
Original, Made with Buttermilk, Low Low, Kerry*	1 Spread/10g	39	4.2	394	0.2	3	42	0
Pro Activ with Olive Oil, Flora*	1 Thin Spread/7g	23	2.4	331	0.1	4	35	0
Pro Activ, Light, Flora*	1 Thin Spread/7g	22	2.4	319	0.5	1.4	35	0
Pro Active, Becel*	1 Serving/7g	22	1.8	320	0	0	25	0
Prutella, Musclefood*	1 Tsp/15g	49	0.9	327	19.2	68.2	6.3	26.2
Reduced Fat, Average	*1 Thin Spread/7g*	*25*	*2.7*	*356*	*0.6*	*3*	*38*	*0*
Slightly Salted, M&S*	1 Thick Spread/12g	87	9.6	725	0.6	0.6	80	0.3
Soft, Reduced Fat, Smart Price, Asda*	1 Thin Spread/7g	32	3.5	455	0.2	1	50	0
Soft, Value, Tesco*	1 Thin Spread/7g	30	3.4	433	0	0	48.1	0
Sunflower, Average	*1 Thin Spread/7g*	*42*	*4.6*	*595*	*0.1*	*0.4*	*65.9*	*0.4*
Sunflower, Enriched, Tesco*	1 Thin Spread/7g	37	4.1	535	0.1	0.2	59	0
Sunflower, Light, BFY, Morrisons*	1 Thin Spread/7g	24	2.7	342	0	0	38	0
Sunflower, Light, Reduced Fat, Asda*	1 Thin Spread/7g	24	2.7	347	0.3	1	38	0.1
Sunflower, Low Fat, Aldi*	1 Thin Spread/7g	26	2.7	366	0.2	5.7	38	0
Sunflower, M&S*	1 Thin Spread/7g	44	4.9	630	0	0	70	3
Sunflower, Morrisons*	1 Thin Spread/7g	37	4.1	531	0	0.2	59	0
Sunflower, Sainsbury's*	1 Thin Spread/7g	37	4.1	532	0.1	0.2	59	0
Utterly Butterly*	1 Thin Spread/7g	32	3.4	452	0.3	2.5	49	0
Vegetable, Soft, Tesco*	1 Thin Spread/7g	46	5.1	661	0.1	1	73	0
Vitalite, Dairy Free, Dairy Crest Ltd*	1 Thin Spread/7g	35	3.9	503	0	0	56	0
with Soya, Dairy Free, Pure Spreads*	1 Thin Spread/7g	34	3.8	490	0.5	1	54	0
with Sunflower, Dairy Free, Organic, Pure Spreads*	1 Thin Spread/7g	38	4.1	537	0.5	1	59	0

SPRING ROLLS

	Measure INFO/WEIGHT	per Measure KCAL	per Measure FAT	Nutrition Values per 100g / 100ml KCAL	PROT	CARB	FAT	FIBRE
Chicken, Asda*	1 Roll/58g	115	5.2	199	4.6	25	9	3.4
Chicken, Oriental Snack Selection, Sainsbury's*	1 Roll/15g	38	1.5	256	11.5	30.3	9.9	1.7
Chinese Takeaway, Tesco*	1 Roll/50g	100	4.3	201	4.4	26.4	8.6	1.5
Duck, Hoisin , Sainsbury's*	1 Roll/20g	57	3	287	5.9	30.6	15.3	1.8
Duck, Mini, Asda*	1 Roll/18g	47	1.9	259	8.7	32.8	10.3	1.9

S

	Measure INFO/WEIGHT	per Measure KCAL	per Measure FAT	Nutrition Values per 100g / 100ml KCAL	PROT	CARB	FAT	FIBRE
SPRING ROLLS								
Duck, Party Bites, Sainsbury's*	1 Roll/20g	49	1.8	245	10.1	31.4	8.8	1
From Restaurant, Average	*1 Roll/140g*	*344*	*14.8*	*246*	*11.1*	*23.2*	*10.6*	*0*
M&S*	1 Roll/36g	66	2.3	183	4.6	25.6	6.4	2.2
Mini Vegetable, Co-Op*	1 Roll/18g	40	1.6	220	4.1	30.9	9.1	2.7
Mini, Asda*	1 Roll/20g	35	0.6	175	3.5	33.6	3	1.9
Mini, Sainsbury's*	1 Roll/12g	27	1.2	221	4.2	28.7	9.9	1.6
Oriental Vegetable, Tesco*	1 Roll/60g	148	7.4	248	3.6	29.7	12.4	1.4
Pork & Vegetable, Mini, Taste Thailand, Banquet Box, M&S*	½ Pack/51g	122	5.5	240	6.3	28.9	10.7	1.6
Prawn, Crispy, M&S*	1 Roll/34g	75	3.4	220	10	22.2	9.9	1.3
Thai, Sainsbury's*	1 Roll/30g	69	3.4	229	2.9	28.8	11.3	3.5
Vegetable, Asda*	1 Roll/62g	126	5.6	203	3.5	27	9	2.7
Vegetable, Cantonese, Large, Sainsbury's*	1 Roll/63g	130	6.3	205	3.6	25.3	9.9	1.5
Vegetable, Cantonese, Sainsbury's*	1 Roll/36g	84	4.2	233	3.6	28.1	11.7	1.4
Vegetable, Chilled, Tesco*	1 Roll/68g	149	7.6	221	4	25.9	11.3	1.6
Vegetable, Chinese Favourites Box, M&S*	½ Pack/70g	128	4.5	183	4.6	25.6	6.4	2.2
Vegetable, Chinese Selection, Frozen, Tesco*	1 Roll/17g	42	2	251	5.2	29	12.2	2.4
Vegetable, Chinese Takeaway, Sainsbury's*	1 Roll/59g	100	3.7	170	4	24.4	6.3	2.8
Vegetable, M&S*	1 Roll/37g	80	3.6	215	4.3	27.8	9.6	2
Vegetable, Meal for Two, Meal Box, Tesco*	2 Rolls/36g	94	4.1	264	5.5	33	11.4	3.5
Vegetable, Mini, Nirvana*	1 Roll/26g	54	2.7	208	3.5	25.1	10.4	1.7
Vegetable, Mini, Occasions, Sainsbury's*	1 Roll/24g	52	2.3	216	4.1	28.2	9.6	2.9
Vegetable, Mini, Party Food, M&S*	1 Roll/20g	40	1.6	200	3.7	26.2	8.1	2.7
Vegetable, Mini, Tesco*	1 Roll/16g	33	1.3	208	4	28.3	8.1	3
Vegetable, Oriental Selection, Party, Iceland*	1 Roll/15g	36	1.4	241	4.3	34.1	9.7	2.1
Vegetable, Oriental, Waitrose*	1 Roll/36g	90	4.3	249	5.7	27.1	12	4.8
Vegetable, Parcels, Snack Selection, Oriental, Waitrose*	1 Parcel/18g	48	2	267	4.5	34.6	11.3	4.6
Vegetable, Sainsbury's*	2 Rolls/84g	239	13.1	284	6	28.8	15.6	2.1
Vegetable, Tempura, M&S*	1 Pack/140g	280	12	200	2.8	27.9	8.6	1.8
SPRITE*								
Sprite*	1 Bottle/500ml	70	0	14	0	3.3	0	0
Zero, Lemon Lime, Sprite*	1 Bottle/500ml	6	0	1	0	0	0	0
Zero, Sprite*	1 Can/330ml	3	0	1	0	0	0	0
SPRITZER								
Red Grape, Non-Alcoholic, Extra Special, Asda*	1 Bottle/750ml	330	0	44	0	11	0	0
Rose Grape, Non Alcoholic, Extra Special, Asda*	1 Bottle/750ml	90	0	12	0	3	0	0
White Wine, Echo Falls*	1 Serving/125ml	78	0	39	0	0	0	0
with White Zinfandel, Echo Falls*	1 Serving/200ml	216	0	108	0	0	0	0
SQUASH								
Acorn, Raw, Average	*1 Serving/80g*	*32*	*0.1*	*40*	*0.8*	*10.4*	*0.1*	*1.5*
Apple & Blackcurrant, No Added Sugar, Tesco*	1 Serving/30ml	4	0	15	0.2	2	0	0
Apple & Blackcurrant, Special R, Diluted, Robinson's*	1 Serving/30ml	2	0	8	0.1	1.1	0.1	0
Apple & Blackcurrant, Special R, Robinson's*	1 Serving/30ml	2	0	8	0.1	1.1	0	0
Apple & Mango, High Juice, Diluted, Sainsbury's*	1 Serving/250ml	88	0	35	0	8.5	0	0.2
Apple & Strawberry High Juice, Sainsbury's*	1 Serving/250ml	82	0.2	33	0.1	8.2	0.1	0.1
Apple Blackcurrant, Fruit, Robinson's*	1 Glass/50ml	18	0	36	0.1	8	0	0
Apple, Blackcurrant, Low Sugar, Diluted, Sainsbury's*	1 Glass/250ml	5	0.2	2	0.1	0.2	0.1	0.1
Apple, Cherry & Raspberry, High Juice, Robinson's*	1 Serving/25ml	49	0	196	0.2	47.6	0.1	0
Blackcurrant, High Juice, M&S*	1 Glass/250ml	50	0	20	0.1	5.2	0	0.1
Blackcurrant, High Juice, Tesco*	1 Serving/75ml	215	0	287	0.3	70	0	0
Blackcurrant, No Added Sugar, Tesco*	1 Serving/25ml	4	0	14	0.4	1.7	0	0
Cherries & Berries, Tesco*	1 Serving/25ml	5	0	21	0.2	3.2	0	0
Cherries Berries, Sugar Free, Diluted, Tesco*	1 Glass/250ml	5	0	2	0	0.3	0	0
Cranberry, Light, Classic, Undiluted, Ocean Spray*	1 Serving/50ml	32	0	63	0.2	14.1	0	0

S

	Measure INFO/WEIGHT	per Measure KCAL	FAT	Nutrition Values per 100g / 100ml KCAL	PROT	CARB	FAT	FIBRE
SQUASH								
Delicata, Raw, Average	**1 Serving/80g**	**27**	**0**	**34**	**1**	**9**	**0**	**2**
Elderflower, 0%, No Added Sugar, Undiluted, Teisseire*	1 Serving/20ml	5	0	23	0.1	0.5	0.1	0
Fruit Barley Orange, Diluted, Robinson's*	1 Serving/50ml	6	0	12	0.2	1.7	0	0.1
Fruit Barley, No Added Sugar, Robinson's*	1 fl oz/30ml	4	0	14	0.3	2	0	0
Fruit Barley, Tropical, No Added Sugar, Robinson's*	1 Serving/60ml	7	0	12	0.2	1.6	0	0
Grape & Passion Fruit, High Juice, Diluted, Sainsbury's*	1 Serving/250ml	100	0.2	40	0.1	9.8	0.1	0.1
Grapefruit, High Juice, No Added Sugar, Sainsbury's*	1 Serving/25ml	2	0	6	0.1	1.1	0	0
Hubbard, Raw, Average	**1 Serving/80g**	**34**	**0.3**	**43**	**1.7**	**8.6**	**0.4**	**1.7**
Just A dash, Apple, Concentrate, MacB*	1 Serving/25ml	0	0	1	0.1	0	0	0
Just A dash, Peach, Concentrate, MacB*	1 Serving/25ml	0	0	1	0.1	0	0	0
Kobacha, Raw, Average	**1 Serving/80g**	**73**	**0.2**	**91**	**1.9**	**20.6**	**0.3**	**0**
Lemon Lime, Double Strength, No Added Sugar, Asda*	1 Glass/200ml	4	0	2	0	0	0	0
Lemon Barley Water, Made Up, Robinson's*	1 Serving/250ml	48	0	19	0.1	4.4	0	0
Lemon, Double Concentrate, Value, Tesco*	1 Serving/25ml	3	0	11	0.2	0.3	0	0
Lemon, High Juice, Diluted, Sainsbury's*	1 Glass /250ml	98	0.2	39	0.1	9.1	0.1	0.1
Lemon, No Added Sugar, Double Concentrate, Tesco*	1 Serving/25ml	4	0	16	0.3	0.7	0	0
Mixed Fruit, Diluted, Kia Ora*	1 Serving/250ml	5	0	2	0	0.3	0	0
Mixed Fruit, Low Sugar, Sainsbury's*	1 Glass/250ml	5	0.2	2	0.1	0.2	0.1	0.1
Mixed Fruit, Tesco*	1 Serving/75ml	13	0	17	0	3.5	0	0
Orange & Mandarin, Fruit Spring, Robinson's*	1 Serving/440ml	26	0	6	0.1	0.8	0	0
Orange & Mango, Low Sugar, Sainsbury's*	1 Serving/250ml	5	0.2	2	0.1	0.2	0.1	0.1
Orange & Mango, Special R, Diluted, Robinson's*	1 Serving/250ml	20	0	8	0.2	0.9	0	0
Orange & Pineapple, Original, Undiluted, Robinson's*	1 Serving/250ml	138	0	55	1	13	0	0
Orange Mango, No Added Sugar, Robinson's*	1 Serving/25ml	2	0	8	0.2	0.9	0	0
Orange Pineapple, No Sugar Added, Robinson's*	1 Serving/25ml	2	0	8	0.2	0.7	0	0.2
Orange, Hi Juice, Tesco*	1 Serving/75ml	140	0.1	187	0.3	45	0.1	0
Orange, High Juice, Undiluted, Robinson's*	1 Serving/200ml	364	0.2	182	0.3	44	0.1	0
Orange, No Added Sugar, Diluted, Kia Ora*	1 Serving/200ml	14	0	7	0	0.1	0	0
Orange, No Added Sugar, High Juice, Sainsbury's*	1 Serving/100ml	6	0.1	6	0.1	1.1	0.1	0.1
Orange, Special R, Diluted, Robinson's*	1fl oz/30ml	2	0	8	0.2	0.7	0.1	0
Peach & Apricot, Fruit & Barley, Diluted, CBY, Asda*	1 Serving/250ml	5	0	2	0	0.2	0	0.1
Pear Drop Flavour, Diluted, Tesco*	1 Serving/50ml	3	0	6	0.1	0.5	0	0
Pink Grapefruit, High Juice, Low Sugar, Tesco*	1 Serving/75ml	12	0.1	16	0.2	3.7	0.1	0
Pink Grapefruit, High Juice, Undiluted, Robinson's*	1 Glass/250ml	455	0.2	182	0.2	43.3	0.1	0
Puree, Cube, Ella's Kitchen*	2 Cubes/42g	13	0.2	31	0.7	6.1	0.5	1.6
Red Apple, No Added Sugar, Diluted, Ribena*	1 Serving/250ml	12	0	5	0	0.9	0	0
Spaghetti, Baked	**1oz/28g**	**6**	**0.1**	**23**	**0.7**	**4.3**	**0.3**	**2.1**
Spaghetti, Including Pips & Rind, Raw	**1oz/28g**	**5**	**0.1**	**20**	**0.4**	**3.4**	**0.4**	**1.7**
Strawberry, Kiwi, Creations, Diluted, Robinson's*	1 Serving/200ml	6	0	3	0	0.6	0	0
Summer Fruit, No Added Sugar, Sainsbury's*	1 Serving/250ml	5	0.2	2	0.1	0.2	0.1	0.1
Summer Fruits Barley, no Added Sugar, Tesco*	1 Serving/50ml	6	0	11	0.2	1.7	0	0
Summer Fruits, High Juice, Undiluted, Robinson's*	1fl oz/30ml	61	0	203	0.1	49	0.1	0
Summer Fruits, High Juice, Waitrose*	1 Serving/250ml	102	0	41	0	10	0	0
Summer Fruits, No Added Sugar, Double Strength, Asda*	1 Serving/50ml	1	0	2	0	0.2	0	0
Summer Fruits, No Added Sugar, Made Up, Morrisons*	1 Glass/200ml	3	0	2	0	0.2	0	0
Summer Fruits, No Added Sugar, Sun Quench, Aldi*	1 Serving/25ml	5	0.1	21	0.5	2.9	0.5	0.5
Summer Fruits, Robinson's*	1 Measure/25ml	14	0	56	0.1	13	0	0
Summer, All Varieties	**1 Sm/118g**	**19**	**0.2**	**16**	**1.2**	**3.4**	**0.2**	**1.1**
Summerfruits, High Juice, Tesco*	1 Serving/50ml	12	0	23	0.2	4.5	0	0
Tropical, Double Strength, No Added Sugar, CBY, Asda*	1 Serving/100ml	2	0	2	0	0.2	0	0
Tropical, No Added Sugar, Diluted, Tesco*	1 Glass/200ml	18	0	9	0.2	0.9	0	0
Winter, Acorn, Baked, Average	**1oz/28g**	**16**	**0**	**56**	**1.1**	**12.6**	**0.1**	**3.2**
Winter, Acorn, Raw, Average	**1oz/28g**	**9**	**0**	**30**	**0.6**	**6.8**	**0.1**	**1.7**

S

	Measure INFO/WEIGHT	per Measure KCAL	FAT	Nutrition Values per 100g / 100ml KCAL	PROT	CARB	FAT	FIBRE
SQUASH								
Winter, All Varieties, Flesh Only, Raw, Average	*1oz/28g*	*10*	*0*	*34*	*1*	*8.6*	*0.1*	*1.5*
SQUID								
in Batter, Fried in Blended Oil, Average	*1oz/28g*	*55*	*2.8*	*195*	*11.5*	*15.7*	*10*	*0.5*
Raw, Average	*1oz/28g*	*23*	*0.5*	*81*	*15.4*	*1.2*	*1.7*	*0*
Salt Pepper Chargrilled, Cooked, Tesco*	1 Pack/80g	78	2.3	98	17.9	0	2.9	0.1
STAR FRUIT								
Average, Tesco*	1oz/28g	9	0.1	31	0.5	7.1	0.3	1.3
STARBAR								
Cadbury*	1 Bar/53g	260	14.8	491	10.7	49	27.9	0
STARBURST								
Fruit Chews, Tropical, Mars*	1 Tube/45g	168	3.3	373	0	76.9	7.3	0
Mars*	1 Pack/45g	182	3.3	405	0	83.9	7.3	0
STEAK & KIDNEY PUDDING								
M&S*	1 Pudding/121g	260	13.4	215	9.2	19.4	11.1	3.2
Sainsbury's*	1 Pudding/435g	1135	62.6	261	10.5	22.3	14.4	0.8
Tesco*	1 Serving/190g	437	22.6	230	10	20.7	11.9	1.2
Waitrose*	1 Pudding/223g	497	26.1	223	8.9	20.4	11.7	1.2
STEW								
Beef & Dumplings, British Classics, Tesco*	1 Pack/450g	563	29.7	125	7.9	8.6	6.6	0.5
Beef Dumplings	*1 Serving/652g*	*766*	*32.7*	*117*	*7.4*	*10.7*	*5*	*0.8*
Beef with Dumplings, Classic British, Sainsbury's*	1 Pack/450g	657	29.2	146	8.4	12.9	6.5	1.2
Beef with Dumplings, COU, M&S*	1 Pack/454g	431	11.8	95	8.9	9.1	2.6	0.8
Beef with Dumplings, Sainsbury's*	1 Pack/450g	603	27.4	134	9.3	10.5	6.1	0.7
Beef, Chorizo, with Cheesy Polenta Mash, Tesco*	1 Pack/441g	549	27.9	124	7	8.9	6.3	1.9
Beef, Dumplings, Aldi*	1 Pack/450g	567	27.9	126	8	8.6	6.2	2
Beef, Dumplings, Frozen, Tesco*	1 Serving/400g	380	12.8	95	5.7	10.5	3.2	1.5
Beef, Dumplings, HFC, Tesco*	1 Pack/384g	347	7.7	90	7.1	9.6	2	2.6
Beef, Kidney, Mini, Oakhouse Foods Ltd*	1 Pack/250g	238	7.3	95	7.3	9	2.9	1.2
Beef, Asda*	½ Can/196g	178	4.9	91	10	7	2.5	1.5
Beef, Meal for One, M&S*	1 Pack/440g	350	8.4	80	7	8.7	1.9	2
Beef, Minced, Onion, Tesco*	1 Pack/300g	219	7.2	73	3.6	8.8	2.4	0.9
Beef, Value, Tesco*	1 Serving/200g	170	9.8	85	4	6.2	4.9	1
Chicken & Dumplings, Birds Eye*	1 Pack/320g	282	8.6	88	7	8.9	2.7	0.5
Chicken & Dumplings, Tesco*	1 Serving/450g	567	29.7	126	7.6	9.1	6.6	0.7
Chicken, Morrisons*	1 Pack/400g	492	7.6	123	17.6	8.9	1.9	0.5
Chickpea, Moroccan, Allplants*	½ Pack/380g	551	20.1	145	4.8	17	5.3	3.9
Chickpea, Roast Sweet Potato, Feta, Stewed!*	½ Pot/250g	188	7.2	75	3.3	8.8	2.9	2.7
Irish, Tesco*	1 Can/400g	308	11.2	77	7	5.9	2.8	0.8
Lentil & Vegetable, Organic, Simply Organic*	1 Pack/400g	284	6	71	3.5	11	1.5	1.3
Moroccan, Vegetable, Slimfree, Aldi*	1 Pack/500g	155	2.5	31	1.2	4.7	0.5	1.9
Roots, Hearty, Allplants*	½ Pack/380g	433	19.8	114	4.2	11	5.2	3
Tuscan Bean, Tasty Veg Pot, Innocent*	1 Pot/400g	320	7.6	80	3.1	12.5	1.9	3.6
Vegetable, Rainbow, & Dumplings, Sainsbury's*	1 Pack/385g	354	14.6	92	2.7	9.9	3.8	4
STIR FRY								
Bean Sprout Vegetable with Red Peppers, Asda*	1 Pack/350g	126	3.9	36	1.8	4.7	1.1	2.3
Beef, BGTY, Sainsbury's*	½ Pack/125g	156	5.1	125	22	0.1	4.1	0
Beef, Chilli, Spicy, Musclefood*	1 Serving/353g	314	8.8	89	13.4	2.5	2.5	1.6
Cabbage, Carrot, Broccoli Onion, Vegetable, Tesco*	1 Serving/100g	31	0.4	31	1.9	4.9	0.4	2.6
Chicken Chow Mein, Fresh, HL, Tesco*	1 Pack/400g	312	4.8	78	5.7	11.4	1.2	1.3
Chicken, Chinese, Meal Kit, Aldi*	½ Pack/210g	277	8.6	132	16	7.6	4.1	1.2
Chicken, Fajita, Musclefood*	1 Serving/358g	301	10.4	84	11.4	2	2.9	2.3
Chicken, Naked, Musclefood*	1 Serving/350g	217	4.2	62	9.9	2.5	1.2	1
Chicken, Thai, Musclefood*	1 Serving/336g	279	8.7	83	11.8	1.9	2.6	2.4

S

	INFO/WEIGHT	KCAL	FAT	KCAL	PROT	CARB	FAT	FIBRE
STIR FRY								
Chinese Chicken, As Consumed, Iceland*	½ Pack/371g	353	2.6	95	6.5	15.2	0.7	1
Chinese Prawn, Iceland*	1 Pack/340g	235	4.4	69	3.1	11.1	1.3	2.1
Chinese Style Rice with Vegetables, Tesco*	1 Serving/550g	495	13.8	90	2.2	14.8	2.5	0.3
Chinese Vegetables, Oriental Express*	½ Pack/200g	44	0.4	22	1.4	3.7	0.2	2.2
Edamame, Pea, M&S*	½ Pack/140g	64	1.4	46	3	3.8	1	5.1
Family Pack, Vegetables & Beansprouts, Fresh, Tesco*	1 Pack/600g	108	0.6	18	2	2.2	0.1	2.1
Green Vegetable, M&S*	1 Pack/220g	165	13	75	3.1	2.5	5.9	2.2
Hot Spicy, Mixed Vegetables, Cooked, Sainsbury's*	½ Pack/149g	85	4.6	57	1.2	4.9	3.1	2.2
Mixed Pepper, Sainsbury's*	1 Pack/300g	188	12.9	70	1.5	4.6	4.8	1.2
Mixed Pepper, Tesco*	1/3 Pack/100g	23	0.1	23	1.9	3.7	0.1	1.9
Mixed Vegetable Beansprout, Tesco*	1 Bag/320g	170	6.1	53	2.5	5.1	1.9	2.5
Noodles & Bean Sprouts, Tesco*	½ Pack/125g	131	2.6	105	4.2	16.1	2.1	0.7
Oriental Mix, Quick Easy, Frozen, Cooked, CBY, Asda*	1 Pack/500g	130	1	26	1.1	3.5	0.2	3
Oriental Style Pak Choi, M&S*	1 Pack/220g	165	12.5	75	2.2	3.5	5.7	2.4
Oriental Style, Vegetables, Sainsbury's*	1 Pack/300g	195	14.4	65	1.5	4.1	4.8	2.1
Pork, Chinese Style, Musclefood*	1 Serving/328g	282	8.9	86	11.6	2.7	2.7	1.9
Rice, Quinoa Vegetable, Waitrose*	½ Pack/134g	199	7.8	148	5.4	15.6	5.8	6
Singapore, Noodle, Iceland*	½ Pack/346g	294	10.7	85	5.4	8.2	3.1	1.5
Vegetable & Mushroom, Asda*	½ Pack/160g	59	2.4	37	2.4	3.4	1.5	3.4
Vegetable Mix, As Consumed, Tesco*	½ Pack/128g	72	3	56	1.9	5.5	2.3	3
Vegetable, Chop Suey, Chinese, Sharwood's*	1 Pack/310g	223	3.4	72	1.5	13.9	1.1	0.6
Vegetable, Oriental Mix, Tesco*	½ Pack/126g	88	4.4	70	2.6	5.7	3.5	2.7
Vegetable, Oriental, Just Stir Fry, Sainsbury's*	½ Pack/135g	94	7.2	70	2.2	3.4	5.3	1.3
Vegetable, Rainbow, Fresh Tastes, Asda*	½ Pack/225g	119	5	53	1.8	4.6	2.2	3.8
Vegetable, Ready Prepared, M&S*	½ Pack/150g	38	0.4	25	2.2	3.5	0.3	2.2
Vegetable, Sweet & Crunchy, Waitrose*	1 Pack/300g	69	0.3	23	1.8	3.6	0.1	1.4
Vegetable, Thai Style, Tesco*	½ Pack/135g	42	0.7	31	2.3	4.2	0.5	2.1
Vegetables, Frozen, Farm Foods*	1 Pack/650g	208	3.2	32	1.9	4.9	0.5	2.2
Vegetables, Mixed with Slices of Pepper, Cooked, Tesco*	½ Pack/125g	58	1.6	47	2.4	5.6	1.3	2.4
STOCK								
Beef, Cooks' Ingredients, Waitrose*	1 Jar/500g	110	2.5	22	3.2	0.9	0.5	0.5
Beef, Fresh, Sainsbury's*	¼ Pot/113g	27	0.6	24	5.1	0.5	0.5	0.5
Beef, Fresh, Tesco*	1 Serving/300ml	54	0.9	18	2.1	1.6	0.3	0.5
Beef, Frozen, Tesco*	¼ Pot/61g	27	0.1	44	2.3	8.1	0.2	0.6
Beef, Made Up, Stock Pot, Knorr*	1 Serving/100ml	10	0.4	10	0.2	1	0.4	0
Beef, Pots, Unprepared, Sainsbury's*	1 Pot/28g	31	1.7	112	4.1	8.5	6.2	2.9
Beef, Rich, Stock Pot, Knorr*	1 Pot/28g	42	1.1	150	3	27	4	0.8
Beef, Rich, with Onion & Rosemary, As Prepared, Oxo*	1 Serving/100ml	7	0.5	7	0.5	0.9	0.5	0.5
Beef, Simply Stock, Knorr*	1 Serving/100ml	6	0	6	1.4	0.1	0	0
Beef, Slow Cooked, Finest, Tesco*	¼ Pouch/113ml	18	0.2	16	2	1.6	0.2	0
Beef, Slowly Prepared, Sainsbury's*	1 Serving/100g	7	0.3	7	0.7	0.3	0.3	0.5
Chicken, As Sold, Stock Pot, Knorr*	1 Pot/28g	45	1.1	160	4	26	4	0.8
Chicken, Asda*	½ Pot/150g	26	1.4	17	1.8	0.7	0.9	0.2
Chicken, Concentrated, M&S*	1 Tsp/5g	16	0.9	315	25.6	12.2	18.1	0.8
Chicken, COOK!, M&S*	¼ Pack/125ml	10	0.2	8	1.4	0.1	0.2	0
Chicken, Cooks' Ingredients, Waitrose*	1 Pack/500ml	75	0.5	15	3.2	0.3	0.1	0.2
Chicken, Fresh, Sainsbury's*	½ Pot/142ml	23	0.1	16	3.7	0.1	0.1	0.3
Chicken, Fresh, Tesco*	1 Serving/300ml	27	0.3	9	1.6	0.5	0.1	0.5
Chicken, Frozen, Tesco*	¼ Pack/61g	31	0.5	50	1.7	8.6	0.8	0.6
Chicken, Granules, Knorr*	1 Tsp/4.5g	10	0.2	232	13.1	36.5	3.7	0.4
Chicken, Home Prepared, Average	**1fl oz/30ml**	**7**	**0.3**	**24**	**3.8**	**0.7**	**0.9**	**0.3**
Chicken, Made Up, Stock Pot, Knorr*	1 Serving/125ml	15	0.3	12	0.2	1.6	0.2	0
Chicken, Prepared, Tesco*	1 Serving/300ml	54	0.3	18	2.4	1.8	0.1	0.5

S

	Measure INFO/WEIGHT	per Measure		Nutrition Values per 100g / 100ml				
		KCAL	FAT	KCAL	PROT	CARB	FAT	FIBRE
STOCK								
Chicken, Roast, Diluted Concentrate, Finest, Tesco*	½ Pot/150g	39	0	26	4.9	1	0	1
Chicken, Slow Roasted, Fresh, Extra Special, Asda*	1 Serving/100g	21	0.5	21	4.2	0.5	0.5	0.5
Chicken, Slowly Prepared, Sainsbury's*	1 Pot/300g	27	0.3	9	0.6	1.3	0.1	0.5
Fish, Fresh, Finest, Tesco*	1 Serving/100g	10	0	10	0.6	1.8	0	0.5
Fish, Home Prepared, Average	*1 Serving/250ml*	*42*	*2*	*17*	*2.3*	*0*	*0.8*	*0*
Vegetable, 3 Peppercorn, Flavour Pot , Knorr*	1 Pot/9g	14	0.6	160	0.9	22	7	4.5
Vegetable, As Sold, Stock Pot, Knorr*	1 Serving/100ml	9	0.5	180	6	19	9	1.5
Vegetable, Campbell's*	1 Serving/250ml	38	1.8	15	0.3	2	0.7	0
Vegetable, Cooks Ingredients, Waitrose*	1 Pouch/500ml	15	0.5	3	0.2	0.4	0.1	0.5
Vegetable, Fresh, COOK!, M&S*	¼ Pouch/125ml	15	0.1	12	0.3	2.5	0.1	0.1
Vegetable, Frozen, Tesco*	¼ Pack/61g	36	0.2	58	0.9	12.6	0.3	0.6
Vegetable, Granules, Knorr*	2 Tsp/9g	18	0.1	199	8.5	39.9	0.6	0.9
Vegetable, Made Up, Stock Pot, Knorr*	1 Serving/100ml	10	0.5	10	0.4	1	0.5	0.1
STOCK CUBES								
Beef, Dry Weight, Bovril*	1 Cube/6g	12	0.2	197	10.8	29.3	4.1	0
Beef, Dry Weight, Oxo*	1 Cube/6g	15	0.3	265	17.4	38.4	4.9	4.2
Beef, Knorr*	1 Cube/10g	31	2.3	310	5	19	23	0
Beef, Knorr*	1 Cube/11ml	1	0.1	7	0.5	0.5	0.5	0.5
Beef, Made Up, Oxo*	1 Cube/189ml	17	0.4	9	0.6	1.3	0.2	0.1
Beef, Organic, Kallo*	1 Cube/12g	25	1	208	16.7	16.7	8.3	0
Beef, Smart Price, Asda*	1 Cube/11g	31	2.5	279	10	8	23	0
Beef, Tesco*	1 Cube/7g	17	0.2	260	9.7	48.9	2.8	1.3
Beef, Value, Tesco*	1 Cube/10g	14	0.4	135	11.1	12.9	3.9	6.6
Chicken	*1 Cube/6g*	*14*	*0.9*	*237*	*15.4*	*9.9*	*15.4*	*0*
Chicken, Dry, Average	*1 Cube/10g*	*29*	*1.8*	*293*	*7.3*	*25.5*	*18*	*0.4*
Chicken, Dry, Oxo*	1 Cube/7g	17	0.2	249	10.9	44	3.3	0.9
Chicken, Just Bouillon, Kallo*	1 Cube/12g	30	1.3	247	11.8	26.1	10.6	1
Chicken, Knorr*	1 Cube/10g	31	2	310	4	29	20	0
Chicken, Made Up, Average	*1 Pint/568ml*	*43*	*1*	*8*	*0.4*	*1.1*	*0.2*	*0.1*
Chicken, Made Up, Sainsbury's*	1 Cube/200ml	16	0.2	8	0.3	1.4	0.1	0.1
Chicken, Prepared, Oxo*	1 Cube/100ml	9	0.1	9	0.4	1.5	0.1	0.1
Chicken, Tesco*	1 Cube/11g	32	2.5	290	10.5	11.1	22.6	0.7
Chicken, Value, Tesco*	1 Cube/10g	15	0.6	150	9.4	14.3	5.9	0.8
Fish, Knorr*	1 Cube/10g	32	2.4	321	8	18	24	1
Fish, Sainsbury's*	1 Cube/11g	31	2.2	282	19.1	7.3	20	0.9
Ham, Knorr*	1 Cube/10g	31	1.9	313	11.8	24.4	18.7	0
Ham, Quixo*	1 Cube/450ml	18	2.2	4	0.5	0.5	0.5	0.5
Lamb, Made Up, Knorr*	1 Serving/100ml	5	0.6	5	0.3	0.3	0.6	0.1
Vegetable, Average	*1 Cube/7g*	*18*	*1.2*	*253*	*13.5*	*11.6*	*17.3*	*0*
Vegetable, Bouillon, Vegetarian, Amoy*	1 Cube/10g	30	2	300	0	20	20	0
Vegetable, Bouillon, Yeast Free, Made Up, Marigold*	1 Serving/250ml	19	1.6	8	0	0.5	0.6	0
Vegetable, Dry, Oxo*	1 Cube/6g	17	0.3	251	10.4	41.4	4.9	1.4
Vegetable, Knorr*	1 Cube/10g	33	2.4	330	10	25	24	1
Vegetable, Low Salt, Organic, Made Up, Kallo*	1 Serving/500ml	50	3.5	10	0.3	0.7	0.7	0.2
Vegetable, Made Up, Organic, Kallo*	2 Cubes/100ml	7	0.4	7	0.1	0.5	0.4	0.1
Vegetable, Made up, Oxo*	1 Cube/100ml	9	0.2	9	0.4	1.4	0.2	0.1
Vegetable, Organic, Yeast Free, Dry, Kallo*	1 Cube/11g	37	3.1	334	11.4	8.2	27.8	2.3
Vegetable, Smart Price, Asda*	1 Cube/11g	27	2.1	243	6	12	19	0
Vegetable, Value, Tesco*	1 Cube/10g	14	0.3	145	10.6	17.4	3.3	3.6
STOLLEN								
Bites, Betty's*	1 Bite/11g	46	2.5	420	7.3	41	23	0
Bites, Marzipan, Holly Lane, Aldi*	1 Bite/27g	111	4.8	412	5.9	55	18	1.9
Bites, with Jamaican Rum, Aldi*	1 Bite/23g	92	4.4	400	6.2	51	19	2.4

	Measure INFO/WEIGHT	per Measure KCAL	FAT	Nutrition Values per 100g / 100ml KCAL	PROT	CARB	FAT	FIBRE
STOVIES								
Chef Select, Lidl*	1 Pack/412g	346	3.7	84	4.6	13	0.9	2.9
STRAWBERRIES								
Dried, Urban Fresh Fruit*	1 Pack/35g	111	0.1	318	1.6	77	0.4	5.9
Fresh, Raw, Average	*1 Berry/12g*	*3*	*0*	*28*	*0.8*	*6*	*0.1*	*1.4*
Frozen, Average	*1 Serving/100g*	*30*	*0.2*	*30*	*0.8*	*6.3*	*0.2*	*1*
in Fruit Juice, Canned, Average	*1/3 Can/127g*	*58*	*0*	*46*	*0.4*	*11*	*0*	*1*
in Syrup, Canned, Average	*1 Serving/100g*	*63*	*0*	*63*	*0.4*	*15.2*	*0*	*0.6*
Lightly Yoghurt Coated, Bites, Yu!*	1 Bag/18g	70	1.8	389	3	61.3	9.9	10.2
STROGANOFF								
Beef, & Rice, TTD, Sainsbury's*	1 Pack/410g	595	20.9	145	9.6	15.2	5.1	1.7
Beef, 604, Wiltshire Farm Foods*	1 Serving/360g	466	22	129	6	11	6.1	0
Beef, Asda*	1 Serving/120g	276	20.4	230	16	3.3	17	0.6
Beef, Creamy, COOK!, M&S*	½ Pack/250g	292	17	117	10.3	3.5	6.8	0
Beef, Finest, Tesco*	½ Pack/200g	330	13.4	165	9.4	16.2	6.7	0.7
Beef, Steak, & Wild Rice, Slow Cooked, TTD, Sainsbury's*	1 Pack/450g	662	32.8	147	6.3	13.2	7.3	1.5
Beef, with White Wild Rice, Heated, Finest, Tesco*	1 Pack/426g	591	21.3	139	10.3	12	5	2.2
Chicken, with Rice, BGTY, Sainsbury's*	1 Pack/415g	448	5.4	108	7	17.1	1.3	1.1
Mushroom, Eat Smart, Morrisons*	1 Pack/400g	312	4.4	78	2.6	14.3	1.1	1
Mushroom, with Rice, BGTY, Sainsbury's*	1 Serving/450g	418	6.8	93	3.3	16.6	1.5	1
Pork, Classic Kitchen, Tesco*	½ Pack/222g	284	13.5	128	12.9	4.6	6.1	1.2
STRUDEL								
Apple & Mincemeat, Tesco*	1 Serving/100g	322	16.7	322	3.3	39.6	16.7	2
Apple with Sultanas, Tesco*	1/6 Strudel/100g	245	12	245	2.9	30.9	12	0.7
Apple, Co-Op*	1 Slice/100g	225	12	225	3	28	12	3
Apple, Ovenbaked, CBY, Asda*	1 Slice/100g	249	12	249	2.7	31.6	12	1.7
Apple, Plum Custard, Heavenly Desserts, Aldi*	1/6 Strudel/94g	265	13.2	282	4	35	14	2
Apple, Sainsbury's*	1 Serving/90g	233	11.7	259	2.8	31.6	13	1.9
Apple, Tesco*	1 Serving/94g	226	11.6	241	2.6	28.9	12.4	1.7
Berry, Frozen, Tesco*	1 Serving/94g	220	9.9	234	2.7	31.2	10.5	1.9
STUFFING								
Apple Apricot, Tray, As Sold, Mr Crumb *	1 Serving/45g	84	3	186	2.8	27.5	6.6	2.3
Leek, Pancetta Thyme, Parcels, Cooked, Finest, Tesco*	1 Parcel/39g	103	7.8	263	12.9	7.2	20	1.4
Olde English Chestnut, Sainsbury's*	1 Serving/110g	216	12.8	196	9.4	13.5	11.6	2.1
Parsley & Thyme, Co-Op*	1 Serving/28g	95	0.8	340	10	67	3	6
Pork, Chestnut Onion, Cooked, Finest, Tesco*	1/8 Pack/41g	108	6.9	263	12.9	13.6	16.8	2.4
Pork, Cranberry, Sage Onion, Tesco*	2 Balls/82g	140	4.2	170	11.3	18.5	5.1	2.3
Pork, with Chestnuts Leek, Waitrose*	1 Serving/100g	192	8.8	192	12.5	14.9	8.8	1.3
Sage Onion with Lemon, Paxo*	1 Serving/50g	61	0.6	122	3.4	24.2	1.2	1.9
Sage Onion, for Chicken, Paxo*	1 Serving/50g	60	0.6	120	3.4	22.8	1.3	1.7
Sausagemeat & Thyme, Made Up, Celebrations, Paxo*	1 Serving/50g	80	1.8	160	6.3	25.8	3.5	4
Sausagemeat, Pork, Gourmet, British, Cooked, Waitrose*	1 Serving/59g	134	6.4	229	20	12.7	10.9	0.5
Sausagemeat, Sainsbury's*	1 Serving/100g	175	4.2	175	7	27	4.2	2.3
STUFFING BALLS								
British Pork, Sage Onion, Cooked, Finest, Tesco*	2 Balls/49g	110	5	224	13.9	17.4	10.2	2.2
Pork, Sausagemeat, Aunt Bessie's*	1 Ball/26g	55	2.1	212	7.2	27.3	8.2	3
Sage & Onion, Aunt Bessie's*	1 Ball/26g	60	1.6	229	5.5	39	6.3	3.1
STUFFING MIX								
Apple & Herb, Special Recipe, Sainsbury's*	1 Serving/41g	68	0.9	165	3.8	32.4	2.2	2.2
Apple, Herb, Made Up, Tesco*	1 Serving/50g	87	0.8	173	3.6	34.7	1.5	3.3
Apricot Walnut, Made Up, Celebrations, Paxo*	1 Serving/50g	80	1.8	161	4.3	28	3.5	2.8
Chestnut & Cranberry, Celebration, Paxo*	1 Serving/25g	35	0.5	141	4	26.7	2	2.4
Chestnut, Morrisons*	1 Serving/20g	33	0.7	165	4.6	29.1	3.4	3.7
Dry, Average	*1 Serving/25g*	*84*	*1*	*338*	*9.6*	*70.1*	*3.8*	*5.3*

S

	Measure INFO/WEIGHT	per Measure KCAL	FAT	Nutrition Values per 100g / 100ml KCAL	PROT	CARB	FAT	FIBRE
STUFFING MIX								
Herb & Onion, GF, Allergycare*	1 Serving/12g	43	0.3	360	7.9	76.8	2.4	0
Parsley, Thyme & Lemon, Sainsbury's*	1 Pack/170g	240	2.2	141	4.2	28.2	1.3	1.3
Sage & Onion, Asda*	1 Serving/27g	29	0.2	107	3.4	22	0.6	1.3
Sage & Onion, Co-Op*	1 Serving/28g	94	0.6	335	10	68	2	6
Sage & Onion, Prepared, Tesco*	1 Serving/100g	50	0.4	50	1.5	10.1	0.4	0.9
Sage & Onion, Smart Price, Asda*	¼ Pack/75g	262	2.8	349	11	68	3.7	4.7
Sage Onion, Dry Weight, Tesco*	1 Std Pack/170g	578	4.1	340	10.3	69.3	2.4	6.3
Sage Onion, Free From, Tesco*	1 Pack/170g	197	18.5	116	0.8	3.6	10.9	0.3
Sage Onion, M&S*	1 Serving/30g	108	1	359	11.4	67.8	3.4	6
Sage Onion, Value, Tesco*	1 Ball/38g	133	1.1	350	10.2	70.7	2.9	5.1
Sage Onion, with Apple, Made Up, Paxo*	1 Serving/50g	69	0.8	138	3.8	26	1.6	2.2
Sausage Meat, Morrisons*	1 Serving/20g	35	0.5	174	6.8	30.8	2.6	2.9
SUET								
Beef, Tesco*	1 Serving/100g	854	91.9	854	0.6	6.2	91.9	0.1
Vegetable, Average	*1oz/28g*	*234*	*24.6*	*836*	*1.2*	*10.1*	*87.9*	*0*
SUGAR								
Brown, Soft, Average	*1 Tsp/4g*	*15*	*0*	*382*	*0*	*96.5*	*0*	*0*
Brown, Soft, Light, Average	*1 Tsp/5g*	*20*	*0*	*393*	*0.2*	*97.8*	*0.1*	*0*
Caster, Average	*1 Tsp/5g*	*20*	*0*	*399*	*0*	*99.8*	*0*	*0*
Cubes, Rogers*	2 Cubes/6g	22	0	375	0	100	0	0
Dark Brown, Muscovado, Average	*1 Tsp/7g*	*27*	*0*	*380*	*0.2*	*94.8*	*0*	*0*
Dark Brown, Soft, Average	*1 Tsp/5g*	*18*	*0*	*369*	*0.1*	*92*	*0*	*0*
Demerara, Average	*1 Tsp/5g*	*18*	*0*	*368*	*0.2*	*99.2*	*0*	*0*
Golden, Unrefined, Average	*1 Tsp/4g*	*16*	*0*	*399*	*0*	*99.8*	*0*	*0*
Granulated, Organic, Average	*1 Tsp/4g*	*16*	*0*	*398*	*0.2*	*99.7*	*0*	*0*
Icing, Average	*1 Tsp/4g*	*16*	*0*	*394*	*0*	*102.2*	*0*	*0*
Light Or Diet, Average	*1 Tsp/4g*	*16*	*0*	*394*	*0*	*98.5*	*0*	*0*
Maple, Average	*1 Tsp/5g*	*18*	*0*	*354*	*0.1*	*90.9*	*0.2*	*0*
Muscovado, Light, Average	*1 Tsp/5g*	*19*	*0*	*384*	*0*	*96*	*0*	*0*
White Plus Stevia Blend, Light at Heart, Tate & Lyle*	1 Serving/2g	8	0	398	0	99.6	0	0
White, Granulated, Average	*1 Tsp/5g*	*20*	*0*	*398*	*0*	*100*	*0*	*0*
SULTANAS								
Average	*1oz/28g*	*82*	*0.1*	*291*	*2.8*	*69.2*	*0.4*	*2*
SUNDAE								
Blackcurrant, M&S*	1 Sundae/53g	212	10.2	400	3	54.2	19.2	1.9
Caramel, From Restaurant, Average	*1 Sundae/155g*	*304*	*9.3*	*196*	*4.7*	*31.8*	*6*	*0*
Chocolate & Vanilla, HL, Tesco*	1 Sundae/120g	193	3.1	161	2.8	31.5	2.6	0.6
Chocolate & Vanilla, Tesco*	1 Sundae/70g	140	6	199	2.8	27.5	8.6	0.5
Chocolate Cookie, Weight Watchers*	1 Pot/82g	128	2.8	156	2.5	30.3	3.4	2.2
Chocolate Brownie, Finest, Tesco*	1 Serving/215g	778	56.5	362	2.7	28.7	26.3	2.3
Chocolate Mint, COU, M&S*	1 Pot/90g	108	2.3	120	5.4	17.8	2.6	0.5
Chocolate Nut	*1 Serving/70g*	*195*	*10.7*	*278*	*3*	*34.2*	*15.3*	*0.1*
Chocolate, Double, Belgian, COU, M&S*	1 Pot/130g	170	3.2	131	3.6	23.1	2.5	0.8
Chocolate, Sainsbury's*	1 Pot/140g	393	29.8	281	2.5	19.3	21.3	0.6
Hot Fudge, Two Scoop, Baskin Robbins*	1 Serving/203g	530	29	261	3.9	30.5	14.3	0
Ice Cream	*1 Serving/170g*	*482*	*15.4*	*284*	*5.9*	*45.3*	*9.1*	*0.3*
Raspberry, PB, Waitrose*	1 Pot/175ml	150	1	86	1.7	18.9	0.6	0
Strawberry & Vanilla, Tesco*	1 Serving/68g	120	3.9	177	2	29.5	5.7	0.1
Strawberry & Vanilla, Weight Watchers*	1 Pot/105g	148	2.2	141	1.2	29.1	2.1	0.3
Strawberry, M&S*	1 Sundae/45g	173	8	385	3.4	53.3	17.8	1
Strawberry, Tesco*	1 Sundae/48g	194	8.7	408	3.3	57.6	18.3	1.3
Toffee & Vanilla, Tesco*	1 Serving/70g	133	4.5	189	2.1	30.7	6.4	0.1
Toffee, Asda*	1 Serving/120g	322	19.2	268	2.1	29	16	0

	Measure INFO/WEIGHT	per Measure KCAL	FAT	Nutrition Values per 100g / 100ml KCAL	PROT	CARB	FAT	FIBRE
SUNDAE								
Toffee, Good Puds, M Kitchen, Morrisons*	1 Pot/138g	268	13.4	194	3.6	22.9	9.7	0.4
Toffee, Sainsbury's*	1 Sundae/140g	378	27.2	270	3.1	20.2	19.4	0.9
Vanilla Caramel, Aldi*	1 Sundae/72g	159	7.4	221	2.6	29.2	10.3	0.7
SUPPLEMENT								
BCAA Power Punch, Ultimate Sports Nutrition*	2 Tsp/13g	40	0	304	0	3	0	0
Blackcurrant, Flaxseed, & Cacao, Ceres Organic*	1 Serving/30g	146	11	485	17.5	9.4	36.8	26.1
Chocolate, Forever Lite, Ultra, Powder, Forever Living*	1 Scoop/25g	90	1	360	68	16	4	4
Fibre, Powder, Benefibre*	1 Tsp/3.2g	6	0	200	0.5	15	0	85
Green Apple, Vitamin Drink, Low Calorie, Vit Hit*	1 Serving/100ml	8	0.1	8	0.1	1.4	0.1	0.1
GU Energy Gel, Chocolate Outrage, TCL Sports*	1 Pack/32g	100	2	312	0	62.5	6.2	0
GU Energy Gel, Vanilla Bean, TCL Sports*	1 Pack/32g	100	0	312	0	78.1	0	0
High Protein Powder, Sanatogen*	2 Tsp/7g	25	0.1	360	81	5.8	1.2	0
Protein Shake, Coconut, Purition*	1 Serving/40g	192	12.8	480	41	7.8	32	17.2
Protein Shake, Macadamia Vanilla, Purition*	1 Serving/40g	198	14	495	39.1	8.6	35	15.6
Protein Shake, Pistachio, Purition*	1 Serving/40g	192	12.8	481	40.5	9.9	32	15.7
Protein Shake, Protein Haus*	1 Bottle/330ml	275	8	83	7.2	5.7	2.4	0
Protein Shake, Pumpkin Spice, Puriton*	1 Serving/40g	187	12.4	467	41.2	7.7	31	15.7
Protein Shake, Vegan Hemp, Chocolate, Purition*	1 Serving/40g	194	12.1	484	35.4	11.3	30.3	27.3
Protein, Total Gainer, Myprotein*	1 Serving/100g	411	9.8	411	34.7	46	9.8	3.3
Psyllium Husk, Average	*1 Tsp/5g*	*19*	*0*	*377*	*0.4*	*89*	*0.4*	*58*
Soya Protein Isolate Powder, Holland & Barrett*	1 Scoop/28g	109	1.3	391	86.6	1	4.5	0
Superfood, Fibre Blend, Organic, Cleanse, Neal's Yard*	1 Scoop/5g	12	0.2	236	7	41	4	50
Tablet, Berocca*	1 Tablet/4.5g	5	0	109	0	5.7	0.1	0
Total Superfood, Powder, Nutriseed*	1 Serving/10g	40	1.7	405	22.2	29.2	17.1	18.3
Vegan, Superfood Blend, Myprotein*	1 Serving/38g	135	2.7	354	41	22	7	19
Whey protein, Holland & Barrett*	1 Serving/24g	94	1.9	392	73.3	7.1	7.9	0
Whey, Chocolate, White, Diet, PhD Nutrition*	1 Serving/50g	195	2.5	390	70	12.5	5	3.7
Whey, High Protein, Cookies Cream, Whey Box*	1 Serving/20g	82	1.7	411	70	13	8.7	3.3
SUSHI								
California Rolls 8 Pack	*1 Pack/206g*	*354*	*9.3*	*172*	*5.1*	*27.5*	*4.5*	*1.4*
California Set, Waitrose*	1 Pack/120g	223	9.1	186	3.8	25.2	7.6	1.7
Californian Roll & Nigiri, Selection, M&S*	1 Pack/215g	355	5.8	165	7.1	28	2.7	1.1
Chicken Duck, Asian Inspired, Selection, Tesco*	1 Pack/205g	333	6.3	163	4.4	28.9	3.1	0.7
Fish Veg Selection, Tesco*	1 Pack/150g	248	3.4	165	6.7	29.2	2.3	0.4
Fish Roll, Nigiri & Maki Selection, M&S*	1 Pack/210g	315	4.8	150	6.5	25.8	2.3	1
Fish Selection, Large, Tesco*	1 Pack/218g	365	6.8	167	5.3	29	3.1	0.9
Fish, Selection, Asda*	1 Pack/153g	242	2.6	158	5.3	30	1.7	0.6
Fish, Snack Pack, On the Go, Sainsbury's*	1 Pack/96g	150	2.4	156	5.5	27.3	2.5	1.2
Fish, Snack, Tesco*	1 Pack/104g	159	2.6	153	4.5	28	2.5	1.5
Komachi Set with Salmon, Whiting Handroll, Waitrose*	1 Pack/257g	447	13.9	174	5.3	25.8	5.4	1.2
Medium Pack, Tesco*	1 Pack/139g	211	3.2	152	6.3	26.6	2.3	2.3
Naniwa, Box, Lidl*	1 Pack/190g	262	3.8	138	4.6	25	2	0.6
Nigiri Set, Taiko, Salmon Tuna, Waitrose*	1 Pack/113g	174	2.3	154	6.3	26	2	0.6
Roll Selection, Sainsbury's*	1 Pack/217g	363	8	167	5	28.4	3.7	0.5
Salmon & Roll Set, Sainsbury's*	1 Serving/101g	167	2.6	165	4.9	30.4	2.6	0.8
Salmon Prawn, Nigiri, M&S*	1 Pack/125g	186	1.4	149	7	27.2	1.1	1
Salmon Tuna, Tesco*	1 Pack/151g	248	5.6	164	6.9	25.6	3.7	0.5
Salmon Wrap, Taiko Foods*	1 Pack/200g	284	4.6	142	5.1	24.8	2.3	0
Salmon, Smoked, Snack Pack, Tesco*	1 Pack/69g	114	1.9	165	5	29.1	2.7	0.9
Snack Box, with Soy Sauce, Eat Well, M&S*	1 Box/78g	115	1.1	147	4.5	28.8	1.4	0.6
Taiko, California, Waitrose*	1 Pack/140g	246	10.1	176	4.1	22	7.2	4.1
Taiko, Fuji Set, Waitrose*	1 Pack /332g	515	10	155	5	28	3	1
Tuna, to Snack Selection, Food to Go, M&S*	1 Serving/150g	225	3.9	150	5.2	26.4	2.6	2.3

S

Measure INFO/WEIGHT	per Measure		Nutrition Values per 100g / 100ml				
	KCAL	FAT	KCAL	PROT	CARB	FAT	FIBRE

SUSHI

	Measure INFO/WEIGHT	KCAL	FAT	KCAL	PROT	CARB	FAT	FIBRE
Vegetable Selection Pack, M&S*	1 Pack/154g	215	2.8	140	2.8	28.1	1.8	1.3
Vegetable, Mixed, Pick Mix, Snack Pack, Tesco*	1 Pack/85g	132	2	155	3.7	28.6	2.4	1.4
Vegetable, Morrisons*	1 Pack/75g	126	2.9	168	3.4	29.2	3.9	1.4
Vegetable, Selection, Aldi*	1 Pack/149g	238	5.1	160	3.1	29	3.4	1.1
Vegetarian with Pickled Vegetables, Waitrose*	1 Pack/135g	244	4.9	181	5	27.8	3.6	1.7
Vegetarian, Snack Selection, Tesco*	1 Pack/85g	106	2.8	125	3.7	20.1	3.3	0.6
Yo!, Bento Box, Sainsbury's*	1 Pack/208g	530	6.2	255	8.4	48.7	3	0.9

SWEDE

	Measure INFO/WEIGHT	KCAL	FAT	KCAL	PROT	CARB	FAT	FIBRE
Boiled, Average	*1oz/28g*	*3*	*0*	*11*	*0.3*	*2.3*	*0.1*	*0.7*
Raw, Flesh Only, Peeled	*1 Serving/100g*	*24*	*0.3*	*24*	*0.7*	*5*	*0.3*	*1.6*
Raw, Unprepared, Average	*1oz/28g*	*5*	*0.1*	*18*	*0.7*	*3.8*	*0.3*	*1.6*

SWEET & SOUR

	Measure INFO/WEIGHT	KCAL	FAT	KCAL	PROT	CARB	FAT	FIBRE
Chicken, Noodles, Chinese Takeaway, Tesco*	1 Pack/350g	350	0.7	100	5.7	18.8	0.2	0.2
Chicken, Balls, Chinese Takeaway, Iceland*	1 Pack/255g	311	3.3	122	9.9	17.5	1.3	6
Chicken, Breaded, Fried, From Restaurant, Average	*6 Pieces/130g*	*346*	*18*	*266*	*13*	*22.3*	*13.8*	*0*
Chicken, Chinese Favourites Box, M&S*	½ Pack/125g	146	0.8	117	8.1	19.3	0.6	1.1
Chicken, Chinese Takeaway, Sainsbury's*	1 Pack/264g	515	16.9	195	13.1	21.3	6.4	1
Chicken, Crispy, with Sweet & Sour Sauce, Tesco*	½ Pack/165g	354	16.7	214	11.1	19.3	10.1	1
Chicken, in Batter, Cantonese, Chilled, Sainsbury's*	1 Pack/350g	560	21	160	8.9	22.4	6	0.9
Chicken, M&S*	1 Pack/300g	465	10.8	155	6.6	24.4	3.6	0.8
Chicken, Take It Away, M&S*	1 Pack/200g	200	1.6	100	9.4	13.2	0.8	1.2
Chicken, with Egg Fried Rice, Chilled, HL, Tesco*	1 Pack/400g	388	4	103	6.9	15.5	1.1	1.9
Chicken, with Noodles, Steamed, HE, Tesco*	1 Pack/370g	289	0.7	78	8.3	10.8	0.2	0.6
Chicken, with Rice, Chilled, BGTY, Sainsbury's*	1 Pack/400g	344	3.6	86	6	13.5	0.9	1
Chicken, with Rice, Weight Watchers, Heinz*	1 Pack/310g	360	3.1	116	5.2	21.2	1	0.4
Chicken, without Batter, Cantonese, Chilled, Sainsbury's*	1 Pack/350g	410	4.9	117	8.5	17.6	1.4	1
Pork	*1oz/28g*	*48*	*2.5*	*172*	*12.7*	*11.3*	*8.8*	*0.6*
Pork, Battered, Sainsbury's*	½ Pack/175g	306	8.8	175	7.3	25.1	5	0.6
Pork, with Rice, 229, Oakhouse Foods Ltd*	1 Meal/400g	484	12	121	5.1	18.4	3	0.7
with Long Grain Rice, Rice Time, Uncle Ben's*	1 Pot/300g	393	2.4	131	1.9	28.4	0.8	0.7

SWEET POTATO

	Measure INFO/WEIGHT	KCAL	FAT	KCAL	PROT	CARB	FAT	FIBRE
Baked, Flesh Only, Average	*1 Med/130g*	*150*	*0.5*	*115*	*1.6*	*27.9*	*0.4*	*2.8*
Boiled in Salted Water, Average	*1 Med/200g*	*168*	*0.6*	*84*	*1.1*	*20.5*	*0.3*	*2.3*
Lattices, As Sold, Aunt Bessie's*	¼ Pack/125g	231	13.8	185	2.4	18	11	3.9
Mash, Frozen, As Consumed, Aunt Bessie's*	1 Serving/80g	70	1.1	88	0.8	17	1.4	2.3
Mash, Tesco*	½ Pack/200g	181	3.6	90	1.4	16	1.8	2.2
Oven Baked, Strong Roots*	1 Serving/80g	130	4.6	162	2	24	5.7	3.4
Raw, Peeled, Average	*1 Sm/130g*	*112*	*0.1*	*86*	*1.6*	*20.1*	*0*	*2.1*
Raw, Unprepared, Average	*1 Potato/200g*	*174*	*0.6*	*87*	*1.2*	*21.3*	*0.3*	*3*
Roasted, So Organic, Sainsbury's*	1 Serving/176g	216	0.9	123	2.9	24.7	0.5	4.2
Steamed, Average	*1 Med/200g*	*168*	*0.6*	*84*	*1.1*	*20.4*	*0.3*	*2.3*
Wedges, Eat Well, M&S*	½ Pack/150g	123	2.2	82	1.4	14.5	1.5	2.6
Wedges, Sainsbury's*	1 Serving/125g	186	6.2	149	2.2	21.8	5	3.9
Wedges, Spicy Zesty Chilli Lime, Waitrose*	½ Pack/195g	205	7	105	1.3	15.2	3.6	3.5

SWEETBREAD

	Measure INFO/WEIGHT	KCAL	FAT	KCAL	PROT	CARB	FAT	FIBRE
Lamb, Fried	*1oz/28g*	*61*	*3.2*	*217*	*28.7*	*0*	*11.4*	*0*

SWEETCORN

	Measure INFO/WEIGHT	KCAL	FAT	KCAL	PROT	CARB	FAT	FIBRE
Baby, Frozen, Average	*1oz/28g*	*7*	*0.1*	*24*	*2.5*	*2.7*	*0.4*	*1.7*
Boiled, Average	*1oz/28g*	*31*	*0.6*	*111*	*4.2*	*19.6*	*2.3*	*2.2*
Canned with Sugar Salt, Average	*1 Lge Can/340g*	*369*	*4*	*108*	*3.2*	*21.5*	*1.2*	*1.9*
Frozen, Average	*1 Serving/80g*	*84*	*1.7*	*105*	*3.8*	*17.9*	*2.1*	*1.8*
No Sugar Salt, Canned, Average	*½ Can/125g*	*99*	*1.3*	*79*	*2.7*	*15*	*1.1*	*1.6*
with Peppers, Canned, Average	*1 Serving/50g*	*40*	*0.2*	*79*	*2.6*	*16.4*	*0.3*	*0.6*

INFO/WEIGHT	Measure	per Measure KCAL	FAT	Nutrition Values per 100g / 100ml KCAL	PROT	CARB	FAT	FIBRE

SWEETENER

Aspartamo, Artificial Sugar, Zen*	1 Tbsp/2g	8	0	383	1.8	94	0	0
Calorie Free, Truvia*	1 Sachet/1.5g	0	0	0	0	99	0	0
Canderel*	1 Tbsp/2g	8	0	379	24.7	7	0	5.3
Canderel, Spoonful, Canderel*	1 Tsp/0.5g	2	0	384	2.9	93	0	0
Granulated, Low Calorie, Splenda*	1 Tsp/0.5g	2	0	391	0	97.7	0	0
Granulated, Silver Spoon*	1 Tsp/0.5g	2	0	387	1	96.8	0	0
Granulated, Tesco*	1 Tsp/1g	4	0	383	1.8	94	0	0
Lucuma Powder, Navitas*	1 Tbsp/15g	60	0	400	6.7	86.7	0	0
Natural Syrup, Fruit, Dark, Sweet Freedom*	1 Tsp/5g	13	0	292	0	79	0	0
Silver Spoon*	1 Tablet/0.1g	0	0	325	10	71	0	0
Simply Sweet*	1 Tbsp/2g	8	0	375	1.4	92.3	0	0
Slendasweet, Sainsbury's*	1 Tsp/1g	4	0	395	1.8	97	0	0.1
Slendersweet, Sainsbury's*	1 Tsp/1g	4	0	395	1.8	97	0	0.1
Spoonfull, Low Calorie, SupaSweet*	1 Tsp/1g	4	0	392	3	95	0	0
Sweet' N Low*	1 Sachet/1g	3	0	368	0	92	0	0
Tablet, Average	*1 Tablet/0.1g*	*0*	*0*	*355*	*8.7*	*73*	*0*	*0.8*
Tablets, Low Calorie, Canderel*	1 Tablet/0.1g	0	0	342	13	72.4	0	0
Tablets, Splenda*	1 Tablet/0.1g	0	0	345	10	76.2	0	1.6
Tablets, Tesco*	1 Tablet/1g	0	0	20	2	2	0.5	0
The Pantry, Aldi*	1 Tsp1g	4	0	376	0.5	94	0.5	0.5
Xylosweet, Xylitol*	1 Serving/4g	10	0	240	0	100	0	0

SWEETS

Almonds, Sugared, Dragee*	1 Sweet/4g	17	0.6	472	10	68.3	17.9	2.5
Alphabet Candies, Asda*	1 Pack/80g	306	0	382	0.5	95	0	0
Banana Split Eclairs, Walker's Nonsuch Ltd*	1 Serving/40g	200	8.9	501	2.7	72.4	22.2	0
Banana, Baby Foam, M&S*	1/3 Pack/34g	131	0	385	4.1	92.7	0	0
Big Purple One, Quality Street, Nestle*	1 Sweet/39g	191	9.9	490	4.7	60.5	25.5	0.7
Black Jacks & Fruit Salad, Bassett's*	1 Serving/190g	760	11.8	400	0.7	84.9	6.2	0
Blackcurrant & Liquorice, M&S*	1 Sweet/8g	32	0.3	400	0.6	89	4.3	0
Blackcurrant Liquorice, Dark, Glacier, Fox's*	1 Sweet/5g	18	0	360	0	90.1	0	0
Blueberry, Bliss, Candy Kittens*	1 Sweet/6g	20	0	335	0.8	81	0.1	0
Body Parts, Rowntree's*	1 Pack/42g	146	0	348	4.3	82.9	0	0
Bon Bons, Strawberry, Classic Favourites, Asda*	1 Sweet/5g	20	0.3	402	0	88	5.6	0
Butter Candies, Original, Werther's*	1 Sweet/5g	21	0.4	424	0.1	85.7	8.9	0.1
Butterscotch Candies, Weight Watchers*	1 Box/42g	95	0	226	0	81.9	0	14.5
Candy Cane, Average	*1 Cane/13g*	*50*	*0*	*386*	*0*	*96*	*0*	*0.2*
Candy Cane, Peppermint, Sainsbury's*	1 Cane/12g	48	0	386	0	96.5	0	0
Candy Corn, Brachs*	19 Pieces/39g	140	0	359	0	92.3	0	0
Candy Floss, Asda*	1 Tub/75g	292	0	390	0	100	0	0
Candy Foam Shapes, Fun Fruits, Value, Tesco*	1 Serving/25g	94	0	374	3.1	90.3	0.1	0.5
Cherry Lips, Chewits*	1 Serving/100g	319	0.2	319	5.6	72.1	0.2	0
Chew	*1oz/28g*	*107*	*1.6*	*381*	*1*	*87*	*5.6*	*1*
Chewits, Blackcurrant, Leaf*	1 Chew/3g	12	0.1	385	0.2	87.5	3	0
Chewits, Cola, Leaf*	1 Chew/3g	12	0.1	385	0.2	87.5	3	0
Chewits, Fruit Salad, Leaf*	1 Chew/3g	12	0.1	385	0.2	87.5	3	0
Chewits, Strawberry, Leaf*	1 Chew/3g	12	0.1	385	0.2	87.5	3	0
Chewitts, Blackcurrant	*1 Pack/33g*	*125*	*0.9*	*378*	*0.3*	*86.9*	*2.7*	*0*
Chews, Calcium, Ellactiva*	1 Sweet/7g	24	1.1	350	1.4	51.4	15.7	0
Chews, Just Fruit, Fruit-tella*	1 Serving/43g	170	2.8	400	0.9	79.5	6.5	0
Chews, Spearmint, Victoria, Aldi*	1 Sweet/10g	40	0.8	405	0.3	83.8	7.6	0
Chews, Strawberry Mix, Starburst*	1 Sweet/4g	15	0.3	401	0	83.9	7.3	0
Choco Mint, Mentos*	1 Pack/38g	156	3.2	410	2.8	79	8.5	0
Choco Toffee, Sula*	1 Sweet/8g	21	1.2	267	3.3	31.7	15.8	0

SWEETS

INFO/WEIGHT	Measure	per Measure KCAL	FAT	Nutrition Values per 100g / 100ml KCAL	PROT	CARB	FAT	FIBRE
Chocolate Caramels, Milk, Tesco*	1 Sweet/3g	15	0.5	444	2.7	72.1	16.1	0.1
Chocolate Eclairs, Cadbury*	1 Sweet/8g	36	1.4	455	4.5	68.9	17.9	0
Chocolate Eclairs, Co-Op*	1 Sweet/8g	38	1.6	480	3	71	20	0.6
Chocolate Eclairs, Holland & Barrett*	1 Sweet/6g	18	0.7	306	1.8	81.9	11.3	1.4
Chocolate Limes, Pascall*	1 Sweet/8g	27	0.2	333	0.3	77.2	2.5	0
Cocoa Orange, Super Bites, Truffles, Good 4u*	1 Bag/40g	153	6.1	383	10.8	46.9	15.2	7.7
Cola Bottles, Asda*	1 Serving/100g	329	0.2	329	9	73	0.2	0
Cola Bottles, Barratt*	1 Sweet/10g	34	0	337	1.3	82	0.4	0.1
Cola Bottles, Fizzy Wizzy, Woolworths*	1 Bag/100g	336	0	336	3.5	77.2	0	0
Cola Bottles, Fizzy, M&S*	1 Pack/200g	650	0	325	6.4	75	0	0
Cough, Herbs, Swiss, Orginal, Ricola*	1 Pack/37g	148	0	400	0	98	0	0
Cream Caramel, Sula*	1 Sweet/3g	10	0	297	0.4	86.1	0	0
Creme Caramel, Sugar Free, Be Light, Aldi*	1 Sweet/3g	7	0.2	275	0.2	90.2	6.3	0.1
Crunchies, Fruit, Fruit-tella*	1 Box/23g	90	1.2	390	0.7	86	5	0
Dolly Mix, Bassett's*	1 Bag/45g	171	1.4	380	3	85.1	3.1	0.4
Dolly Mixtures, M&S*	1 Pack/115g	431	1.6	375	1.8	89.2	1.4	0
Dolly Mixtures, Sainsbury's*	1 Serving/10g	40	0.2	401	1.4	94.4	1.9	0.1
Dolly Mixtures, Smart Price, Asda*	1 Sweet/3g	11	0	380	0.5	91	1.6	0
Dolly Mixtures, Tesco*	1 Pack/100g	376	1.5	376	1.6	88.9	1.5	0
Double Lolly, Swizzels Matlow*	1 Lolly/10g	41	0.3	407	0	92.4	3.4	0
Drops, Lemon Orange, M&S*	1 Pack42g	97	0	230	0	61	0	0
Drumstick, Matlow's*	1 Pack/40g	164	2.2	409	0.4	88.3	5.5	0
Drumstick, Squashies, Swizzels*	1 Bag/160g	568	0.2	355	3.4	83.5	0.1	0
Edinburgh Rock, Gardiners of Scotland*	1 Piece/2g	8	0	380	0.1	94.4	0.3	0.8
Eton Mess, Candy Kittens*	1 Sweet/6g	20	0	340	1.4	82	0.2	0
Fizzy Mix, Tesco*	½ Bag/50g	166	0	332	5.2	75.2	0	0
Fizzy Pop, M&S*	1 Sweet/4g	14	0	352	0.1	88.7	0.5	0.5
Flumps, Bassett's*	1 Serving/5g	16	0	325	4	77	0	0
Flumps, Fluffy Mallow Twists, Fat Free, Bassett's*	1 Twist/13g	30	0	230	4.1	77.1	0	0
Flying Saucers, Tesco*	½ Pack/9g	34	0.1	380	1.3	90.8	1	1.2
Foamy Mushrooms, Chewy, Asda*	1 Sweet/2.6g	9	0	347	4.2	82	0.2	0
Fruit Gums & Jellies	**1 Tube/33g**	**107**	**0**	**324**	**6.5**	**79.5**	**0**	**0**
Fruit, Mentos*	1 Sweet/3g	10	0	333	0	100	0	0
Fruities, Lemon & Lime, Weight Watchers*	1 Sweet/2g	3	0	134	0	54	0	33
Fruity Chews, Starburst*	1 Sweet/8g	34	0.6	404	0	83.4	7.4	0
Fruity Frogs, Rowntree's*	1 Serving/40g	128	0.1	321	4.7	74.5	0.2	0
Fudge, Clotted Cream, Spar*	3 Sweets/30g	134	4.2	447	2	78.2	14	0.1
Gobstoppers, Everlasting, Wonka*	9 Pieces/15g	60	0	400	0	93.3	0	0
Gummy Bears	**10 Bears/25g**	**80**	**0**	**320**	**8**	**76**	**0**	**0**
Gummy Mix, Tesco*	1 Pack/100g	327	0.1	327	5.9	75.7	0.1	0
Gummy Worms	**10 Worms/74g**	**286**	**0**	**386**	**0**	**98.9**	**0**	**98.9**
Gummy Zingy Fruits, Bassett's*	1 Sm Bag/40g	135	0	337	5.1	79.2	0	0
Ice Cream Sundae, Asda*	1 Sweet/2g	9	0	387	4.9	70	0.5	0.5
Jellies, Fruit, Ringtons*	4 Jellies/44g	150	0.2	341	0.1	84	0.4	0.7
Jellies, Very Berry, Rowntrees*	1 Sweet/4g	12	0	326	5	74.8	0.2	0.1
Jelly Babies, Morrisons*	1 Serving/227g	781	0	344	5.3	80.7	0	0
Jelly Beans, Lucozade*	1 Pack/30g	111	0	370	0	92	0	0
Jelly Beans, Tesco*	¼ Bag/63g	243	0.2	385	0.1	94.5	0.3	0.3
Jelly Bears, Co-Op*	1 Sweet/3g	10	0	325	6	76	0.1	0
Jelly Bunnies, Bassetts, Maynards*	4 Sweets/26g	87	0	330	3.5	78	0.1	0
Jelly Tots, Rowntree's*	1 Pack/42g	145	0	346	0.1	86.5	0	0
Kisses, Hershey*	1 Sweet/5g	28	1.6	561	7	59	32	0
Laces, Apple Flavour, Tesco*	5 Laces/15g	52	0.5	347	3.6	74.8	3.2	2.1

SWEETS

INFO/WEIGHT	Measure	per Measure		Nutrition Values per 100g / 100ml				
		KCAL	FAT	KCAL	PROT	CARB	FAT	FIBRE
Laces, Strawberry, Sainsbury's*	1 Serving/25g	94	1.2	377	3.3	76.3	4.6	0.1
Laces, Strawberry, Tesco*	1 Serving/75g	260	2.4	347	3.6	74.8	3.2	2.1
Lances, Strawberry & Cream Flavour, Tesco*	1 Bag/75g	276	0.9	368	3.2	86.1	1.2	2.1
Lances, Strawberry Flavour, Fizzy, Tesco*	½ Pack/50g	177	1.3	354	2.8	79.8	2.6	1.8
Lemon Mint Flavour, Herb Drops, Sugar Free, Ricola*	1 Sweet/3g	7	0	235	0	96	0	0
Licorice, Sugar Free, Dominion, Aldi*	1 Serving/25g	56	0.1	224	0.5	77	0.5	1.6
Liquorice, Boiled, Sugar Free, Sula*	1 Sweet/3g	7	0	227	0.2	93	0	0.2
Liquorice, Gums, Lion*	1 Sweet/4g	14	0	351	8.5	77.7	0.6	0.7
Lovehearts, Giant, Swizzels*	1 Pack/42g	165	0	393	0	100	0	0
Lovehearts, Swizzels*	1oz/28g	100	0	359	0.7	88.2	0	0
Maoam Sour, Haribo*	1 Pack/22g	85	1.4	386	1.2	80	6.5	0.1
Maynards Sours, Bassett's*	1 Pack/52g	169	0	325	6.1	75	0	0
Midget Gems, Free From Fellows*	1 Sweet/2g	4	0	217	0	81	0.3	0
Midget Gems, Maynards*	1 Sweet/1g	3	0	340	8.7	76.2	0	0
Midget Gems, Value, Tesco*	1 Serving/40g	130	0.1	324	4.5	76.1	0.2	0
Milk Chocolate Eclairs, Sainsbury's*	1 Sweet/8g	33	1.1	442	2.1	75.7	14.5	0.5
Milk Chocolate Eclairs, Value, Tesco*	1 Bag/200g	918	32.6	459	2.6	75.2	16.3	1
Milk Duds, Hershey*	13 Pieces/33g	170	6	510	3	84	18	0
Mini Gums, Sugar Free, Dominion, Aldi*	1 Serving/25g	53	0.1	213	0.5	80	0.5	0.5
Mini Macs, CBY, Asda*	1 Pack/200g	437	13.1	218	1	38.8	6.6	0
Mini Marti, Mushrooms, Asda*	1 Sweet/3g	10	0	340	3.8	81.1	0.1	0
Original, Chocolate Soft Caramel, Speciality, Werther's*	1 Piece/6g	30	1.5	480	5.1	61.5	23.5	1
Paradise Fruits, Dominion, Aldi*	1 Sweet/6g	23	0	382	0	95.5	0	0
Parma Violets, Swizzlers*	1 Sm Tube/10g	41	0.3	414	0	94.9	3.3	0
Pear Drops, Free From Fellows*	1 Sweet/4g	11	0	273	0	97	0	0
Percy Pig Pals, Soft, M&S*	1 Sweet/8g	30	0	344	5.8	80	0.1	0
Pic 'n' Mix, Woolworths*	1 Serving/180g	750	6	417	0	96.7	3.3	0
Randoms, 30% Less Sugar, Rowntree's*	9 Sweets/35g	106	0	299	5	63	0.1	13
Randoms, Rowntree's*	1 Pack/50g	164	0.2	328	4.9	75.7	0.3	0.6
Refreshers, Candyland, Barratt*	1 Tube/34g	129	0.5	380	0	89.1	1.4	0
Rhubarb & Custard, Sainsbury's*	1 Sweet/8g	28	0	351	0.1	87.7	0	0
Rhubarb Custards, Tesco*	1 Sweet/8g	32	0	395	0.1	98.2	0.1	0.5
Rotella, Haribo*	1 Sweet/12.5g	43	0	343	1.5	84	0.2	0
Santa Babies, Berry Mix, Bassetts*	1 Bag/165g	544	0	330	3.5	78.5	0	0
Scary Mix, Tesco*	1 Bag/100g	327	0.5	327	9.5	71.1	0.5	0.3
Scary Sours, Rowntree's*	1 Serving/100g	321	0	321	3.5	74.7	0	0
Sherbert Dib Dab with Strawberry Lolly, Barratt*	1 Pack/23g	90	0	385	0.1	95.6	0.1	0
Sherbert Lemons, M&S*	1 Serving/20g	76	0	380	0	93.9	0	0
Sherbert Lemons, Weight Watchers*	1 Box/35g	84	0.2	239	0	94.7	0.5	0
Sherbet Lemons, Bassett's*	1 Sweet/7g	25	0	375	0	93.9	0	0
Shrimps & Bananas, Sainsbury's*	½ Pack/50g	188	0	376	2.5	91.3	0.1	0.5
Snakes, Bassett's*	1 Sweet/9g	30	0	320	3.5	76.8	0.1	0
Soft Fruits, Trebor*	1 Roll/45g	165	0	367	0	90.9	0	0
Sour Apple Sticks, Fizzy Wizzy, Woolworths*	1 Sweet/5g	18	0.1	358	2.8	79.8	2.7	0
Sour Supreme, Tweek*	1 Pack/80g	152	0.4	190	5.1	21	0.5	59
Strawberry Cream, Sugar Free, Sula*	1 Sweet/3g	9	0.2	267	0.2	90.5	5.4	0
Strawberry Laces, CBY, Asda*	1 Pack/50g	184	1.2	367	3.3	82	2.5	1.6
Strawberry, Wild, Candy Kittens*	1 Sweet/6g	20	0	334	0.8	81	0.1	0
Sugar Free, Sula*	1 Sweet/3g	7	0	231	0	96.1	0	0
Sweetshop Favourites, Bassett's*	1 Sweet/5g	17	0	340	0	84.3	0	0
Tangfastics, Mini, Haribo*	1 Pack/16g	55	0.1	346	6.6	80	0.5	0
Tic Tac, Cool Cherry, Ferrero*	1 Pack/18g	69	0.1	382	0.2	92.2	0.7	0
Tootsie Roll, Sm Midgees, Tootsie*	1 Sweet/7g	23	0.5	350	2.5	70	7.5	0

S

	Measure INFO/WEIGHT	per Measure KCAL	FAT	Nutrition Values per 100g / 100ml KCAL	PROT	CARB	FAT	FIBRE
SWEETS								
Tooty Frooties, Rowntree's*	1 Bag/28g	111	1	397	0.1	91.5	3.5	0
Wiggly Worms, Sainsbury's*	1 Serving/10g	32	0	317	5.6	72.7	0.4	0.2
Wine Gummies, Matlow, Swizzels*	1 Pack/16g	52	0	324	0	58.7	0	0
Yo Yo's, All Flavours, 100% Fruit, We Are Bear*	1 Roll/10g	28	0	275	1.9	63.4	0.2	12
Yo Yo's, Strawberry 100% Fruit, We Are Bear*	1 Roll/10g	28	0	275	1.9	63.4	0.2	12
York Fruits, Terry's*	1 Sweet/9g	29	0	320	0	78.5	0	0.5
SWORDFISH								
Grilled, Average	**1oz/28g**	**39**	**1.5**	**139**	**22.9**	**0**	**5.2**	**0**
Raw, Average	**1oz/28g**	**42**	**2**	**149**	**21.1**	**0**	**7.2**	**0**
SYRUP								
Amaretto, Sugar Free, Monin*	1 Serving/30ml	0	0	0	0	13.3	0	0
Artificial Maple Flavour, Sugar Free, Cary's*	1 Serving/60ml	30	0	50	0	20	0	0.5
Balsamic, Merchant Gourmet*	1 Tsp/5g	12	0	232	0.4	60	0.1	0
Black Forest, Premium, Monin*	1 Serving/30ml	100	0	334	0	82	0	0
Blueberry, Blackberry Patch*	1 Tbsp/15g	22	0.1	150	0.3	38.2	0.4	0
Blueberry, Sugar Free, Myprotein*	1 Serving/10g	0	0	5	0	0.2	0	0
Butterscotch, Monin*	1 Serving/30ml	100	0	333	0	80	0	0
Caramel, for Coffee, Lyle's*	2 Tsps/10ml	33	0	329	0	83	0	0
Caramel, Sugar Free, Monin*	1 Serving/30ml	0	0	0	0	13.3	0	0
Chocolate Mint, Monin*	1 Serving/30ml	100	0	333	0	80	0	0
Cinnamon, Monin*	1 Serving/30ml	100	0	333	0	80	0	0
Corn, Dark, Average	**1 Tbsp/20g**	**56**	**0**	**282**	**0**	**76.6**	**0**	**0**
Gingerbread, Monin*	1 Serving/30ml	90	0	300	0	76.7	0	0
Golden, Average	**1 Tbsp/20g**	**61**	**0**	**304**	**0.4**	**78.2**	**0**	**0**
Golden, M&S*	1 Tbsp/15ml	51	0	343	0.1	85.3	0.1	0.5
Hazelnut, Monin*	1 Serving/30ml	90	0	300	0	73.3	0	0
Maple, Average	**1 Tbsp/20g**	**52**	**0**	**262**	**0**	**67.2**	**0.2**	**0**
Maple, Flavour, Zero Calorie, Bulk Powders*	1 Tsp/5g	0	0	4	0	0	0	1.2
Maple, Pure, Vermont, 100%, Butternut Mountain Farm*	1 Tbsp/15ml	50	0	334	0	88	0	0
Organic Rice Malt, Clearspring*	2 Tbsp/42g	133	0.2	316	1.5	76.8	0.4	0
Passion Fruit, Premium, Monin*	1 Serving/30ml	103	0	343	0	84.9	0	0
Peppermint, Monin*	1 Serving/30ml	96	0	320	0	80	0	0
Praline, Monin*	1 Serving/30ml	94	0	313	0	76.7	0	0
Strawberry, Aardbeien Siroop, Plein Sud, Lidl*	1 Serving/20ml	56	0	280	0	71	0	0
Sugar	**1 Tbsp/20g**	**64**	**0**	**319**	**0**	**83.9**	**0**	**0**
Toffee Nut, Monin*	1 Serving/30ml	90	0	300	0	70	0	0
Vanilla, Fabbri*	1 Serving/20ml	70	0	349	0	86	0	0
Vanilla, Monin*	1 Shot/35ml	119	0	340	0	84.4	0	0
Vanilla, Sugar Free, Monin*	1 Serving/30ml	0	0	0	0	13.3	0	0

S

INFO/WEIGHT	Measure	per Measure		Nutrition Values per 100g / 100ml				
		KCAL	FAT	KCAL	PROT	CARB	FAT	FIBRE
TABOULEH								
Average	**1oz/28g**	**33**	**1.3**	**119**	**2.6**	**17.2**	**4.6**	**0**
TACO KIT								
Crispy Chicken, Soft, Stand 'N' Stuff, Old El Paso*	1 Taco/44g	100	1.5	227	7	41.1	3.4	2.5
Enchilada, Open, Stand 'N' Stuff, Old El Paso *	1 Enchilada/50g	102	2	204	5.5	34.7	4	3.4
Garlic Paprika, Crunchy, As Sold, Old El Paso *	1 Taco/26g	77	3.6	296	3.8	37.3	13.8	2.7
TACO SHELLS								
Corn, Crunchy, Old El Paso*	1 Taco/13g	66	3.5	509	5.4	59.2	27	3.6
Old El Paso*	1 Taco/12g	57	2.7	478	7.4	60.8	22.8	0
Traditional, Discovery*	1 Taco/11g	55	3.2	489	5.7	53.4	28.1	6
TAGINE								
Beef, Slow Cooked, Cook*	1 Portion/325g	462	15.6	142	13.5	11.2	4.8	1.3
Chicken, & Chickpeas, Men's Health *	1 Pack/422g	394	5.5	93	9	10.2	1.3	2.5
Chickpea, & Vegetable, Everdine*	1 Serving/450g	351	9	78	1.9	10.9	2	3.9
Chickpea, Creationz, Heinz*	½ Can/196g	176	5.1	90	4	11	2.6	3.4
Lamb, & Couscous, Finest, Tesco*	1 Pack/422g	570	16	135	7.2	17.1	3.8	1.8
Lamb, Frozen, Giraffe*	1 Pack/373g	421	8.6	113	7.1	15	2.3	1.6
Lamb, Moroccan Style with Couscous, COU, M&S*	1 Pack/400g	340	5.6	85	8.9	8.3	1.4	1.6
Lamb, Spiced, with Bulgur Wheat, Weight Watchers, Heinz*	1 Pack/399g	295	6.8	74	4	9.5	1.7	2.1
Moroccan, Allplants*	½ Pack/370g	370	16.3	100	3.3	9.3	4.4	5
Moroccan, Veggie Bowl, Birds Eye*	1 Serving/380g	433	11.4	114	4.9	15	3	3.3
Squash, Apricot, Chickpeas, Sunset, Allplants*	½ Pack/380g	353	11	93	3.8	11	2.9	3.5
TAGLIATELLE								
Dry, Average	**1 Serving/100g**	**356**	**1.8**	**356**	**12.6**	**72.4**	**1.8**	**1**
Egg, Dry, Average	**1 Serving/75g**	**272**	**2.5**	**362**	**14.2**	**68.8**	**3.3**	**2.3**
Egg, Fresh, Dry, Average	**1 Serving/125g**	**345**	**3.5**	**276**	**10.6**	**53**	**2.8**	**2.1**
Fresh, Dry, Average	**1 Serving/75g**	**211**	**2**	**281**	**11.4**	**53.3**	**2.6**	**2.6**
Ham Mushroom, BGTY, Sainsbury's*	1 Pack/400g	371	7.4	95	5.1	13.8	1.9	1.2
Ham Mushroom, Italian, Waitrose*	1 Pack/400g	585	24	151	7.1	16.3	6.2	1
Ham, Mushroom, Creamy, Meal for One, M&S*	1 Pack/400g	636	26.8	159	7.5	16.7	6.7	0.9
Ham, Mushroom, Sainsbury's*	1 Pack/396g	570	20.2	144	6.6	17.4	5.1	1.1
Ham, Mushroom, Taste of Italy, Tesco*	1 Pack/450g	460	15.5	110	6.5	11.5	3.7	2.1
Lamb Ragu, Slow Cooked, Finest, Tesco*	1 Pack/400g	560	19.2	140	8.5	14.9	4.8	1.1
Vegetables, Retail	**1oz/28g**	**21**	**0.8**	**74**	**1.6**	**11**	**3**	**0.7**
Verdi, Fresh, Average	**1 Serving/125g**	**171**	**1.8**	**137**	**5.5**	**25.5**	**1.5**	**1.8**
Wholewheat, Cooked, Co-Op*	1 Serving/100g	138	1.1	138	5.1	24	1.1	5.9
Wholewheat, Fresh, Uncooked, Essential, Waitrose*	1 Portion/125g	278	4.1	222	10.9	33.6	3.3	7.6
TAHINI PASTE								
Average	**1 Tsp/6g**	**36**	**3.5**	**607**	**18.5**	**0.9**	**58.9**	**8**
TANGERINES								
Fresh, Raw	**1oz/28g**	**10**	**0**	**35**	**0.9**	**8**	**0.1**	**1.3**
Fresh, Raw, Weighed with Peel, Average	**1 Med/70g**	**13**	**0.1**	**18**	**0.5**	**4.2**	**0.1**	**0.7**
TANGO*								
Cherry, Britvic*	1 Bottle/500ml	55	0	11	0	2.4	0	0
Orange, Britvic*	1 Can/330ml	63	0	19	0.1	4.4	0	0
Orange, Sugar Free, Britvic*	1 Can/330ml	13	0	4	0	0	0	0
TAPAS								
Basque Beef, (Estofado Vasco), Tapas at, Tesco*	½ Pack/80g	80	3.1	100	9.5	6.4	3.9	1.5
Champinones Al Ajillo, Tapas at, Tesco*	½ Pack/85g	123	11.6	145	2.3	2.5	13.6	1.5
Chorizo Cheese Croquettes, Tapas at, Tesco*	½ Pack/117g	263	11.1	225	5.4	28.6	9.5	2.6
TAPENADE								
Black Olive, M&S*	¼ Jar/33g	122	12.8	374	1.2	0.1	39.5	6.8
Black Olive, Specially Selected, Aldi*	1 Tbsp/20g	46	4.6	231	1.4	2.7	23	4.4

T

Food	Measure INFO/WEIGHT	per Measure KCAL	per Measure FAT	Nutrition Values per 100g / 100ml KCAL	PROT	CARB	FAT	FIBRE
TAPIOCA								
Creamed, Ambrosia*	½ Can/213g	159	3.4	75	2.6	12.6	1.6	0.2
Raw	*1oz/28g*	*101*	*0*	*359*	*0.4*	*95*	*0.1*	*0.4*
TARAMASALATA								
Average	*1 Tbsp/30g*	*143*	*14.4*	*478*	*4.2*	*7.9*	*47.9*	*1.1*
Reduced Fat, Waitrose*	1 Pack/170g	522	48.3	307	4	8.9	28.4	1.5
TARRAGON								
Dried, Ground	*1 Tsp/2g*	*5*	*0.1*	*295*	*22.8*	*42.8*	*7.2*	*0*
Fresh, Average	*1 Tbsp/3.8g*	*2*	*0*	*49*	*3.4*	*6.3*	*1.1*	*0*
TART								
Apple Custard, Asda*	1 Tart/84g	227	11	270	3.1	35	13.1	0.1
Apple, Salted Caramel, Tesco*	1 Slice/83g	222	7.9	267	3.1	41.5	9.5	1.9
Aubergine & Feta, Roast Marinated, Sainsbury's*	1 Serving/105g	227	15.2	216	4.8	16.6	14.5	1.7
Bacon, Maple, Extra Mature Cheddar, Finest, Tesco*	½ Pack/200g	642	42.8	321	10.5	21	21.4	1.4
Bakewell, Average	*1 Tart/50g*	*228*	*14.8*	*456*	*6.3*	*43.5*	*29.7*	*1.9*
Bakewell, Cherry, Free From, Tesco*	1 Tart/52g	225	8.8	434	1	68.7	17	1
Bakewell, Cherry, Morrisons*	1 Tart/46g	198	9.8	430	4.6	54.9	21.4	1.3
Bakewell, Individual, Bakery, Tesco*	1 Tart/78g	319	13.6	409	6.3	55.5	17.5	2
Bakewell, Large, Tesco*	1 Serving/57g	247	11.2	433	4.3	59.5	19.7	1.7
Bakewell, Lemon, Average	*1 Tart/46g*	*206*	*9.7*	*447*	*3.7*	*60.9*	*21.1*	*0.9*
Bakewell, Lyons*	1/6 Tart/52g	205	8.9	397	3.8	56.7	17.2	0.9
Bakewell, Raspberry, Tesco*	1 Slice/63g	269	14.6	428	5.2	48.3	23.3	2.2
Bakewell, Toffee, Morrisons*	1 Tart/47g	201	7.4	422	3	67.2	15.5	0.9
Beef, Pulled, Open, Gastropub, M&S*	½ Pack/152g	351	21.9	231	9.8	14.8	14.4	1.4
Blackcurrant Sundae, Asda*	1 Tart/55g	227	10.4	413	3.5	57	19	2.3
Blackcurrant, Sundae, Tesco*	1 Tart/55g	240	11	436	3	60	19.9	2.2
Brie, Pear Hazelnut Crowns, Luxury	*1 Serving/110g*	*242*	*14*	*220*	*8*	*18*	*12.7*	*1.2*
Caramel, Salted, & Chocolate, Waitrose*	1/12 Tart/79g	349	18.5	443	5.1	52.2	23.5	1.2
Chocolate, Co-Op*	1 Tart/22g	102	6.8	465	4	42	31	0.7
Chocolate, Dark, Cherry, Pecans, Graze*	1 Pack/40g	184	10	459	4.8	57	25	6.9
Custard, Individual, Average	*1 Tart/94g*	*260*	*13.6*	*277*	*6.3*	*32.4*	*14.5*	*1.2*
Custard, Portuguese, Tesco*	1 Tart/55g	157	6	286	3.6	42.8	10.8	1.3
Date, Pecan & Almond, Sticky, Sainsbury's*	1/8 Tart/75g	298	10.3	397	5	63.5	13.7	1.7
Ecclefechan, Mince, Mini, TTD, Sainsbury's*	1 Tart/27g	113	4.3	417	3.4	63.9	15.9	2.2
Egg Custard, Asda*	1 Tart/80g	215	10.4	269	9	29	13	1.2
Egg Custard, Free Range, Sainsbury's*	1 Tart/85g	232	10	273	6.3	35	11.8	0.9
Egg Custard, Twin Pack, Tesco*	1 Tart/85g	229	10.5	270	6.1	33.1	12.4	0.8
Feta Cheese & Spinach, Puff Pastry, Tesco*	1 Tart/108g	306	19.2	283	7.1	23.5	17.8	0.9
Frangipane, Apple, The Best, Morrisons*	1/6 Tart/75g	264	12.7	352	5.1	43.9	16.9	1.7
Fruit, & Almond, Seriously Fruity, Waitrose*	1 Slice/64g	195	10	303	4.9	34.3	15.6	2.7
Gruyere Pancetta Balsamic Onion, Finest, Tesco*	¼ Tart/106g	320	21.9	301	7.7	21.3	20.6	3.3
Jam, Assorted, Free From, Sainsbury's*	1 Tart/43g	180	6	417	2.4	69.5	13.9	1.9
Jam, Assorted, Tesco*	1 Tart/30g	121	4.4	405	3.8	63.6	14.6	1.9
Jam, Average	*1 Slice/90g*	*342*	*13.4*	*380*	*3.3*	*62*	*14.9*	*1.6*
Jam, Free From, Tesco*	1 Tart/35g	142	5.5	408	1.3	63.9	15.9	1.9
Jam, Real Fruit, Mr Kipling*	1 Tart/35g	139	4.7	396	3.5	64.5	13.4	1.5
Jam, Real Fruit, Sainsbury's*	1 Tart/37g	142	5.2	383	3.4	60.9	14	1.4
Lemon Curd, Asda*	1 Tart/30g	121	4.5	402	2.8	64	15	2.2
Lemon Curd, Tesco*	1 Tart/30g	128	4.7	428	3.4	67	15.8	2
Lemon, & Raspberry, Finest, Tesco*	1 Tart/120g	360	16.8	300	5.2	38.4	14	2.9
Lemon, M&S*	1/6 Tart/50g	208	14.6	415	5	32.7	29.3	0.9
Lemon, Sainsbury's*	1/8 Tart/56g	258	15.8	459	4.4	47	28.1	0.6
Lemon, Zesty, Iced, Tesco*	1 Tart/50g	211	8.2	423	3.2	64.7	16.5	1.5
Lemon, Zesty, Tesco*	1/6 Tart/64g	260	15.5	405	5.3	41	24.2	0.7

	Measure INFO/WEIGHT	per Measure KCAL	FAT	Nutrition Values per 100g / 100ml KCAL	PROT	CARB	FAT	FIBRE
TART								
Mandarin, Peach, Tesco*	1 Tart/135g	354	17.3	262	3.5	32.8	12.8	1.1
Millionaires, Toffee, Chocolate, Thorntons*	1 Serving/77g	353	20.1	459	4.2	50.5	26.2	2.2
Mince, Gluten Wheat Free, Florentines, Lovemore*	1 Tart/45g	183	8.3	407	4.5	55.7	18.4	2.5
Mixed Fruit, Fresh, Waitrose*	1 Tart/129g	351	17.4	272	4.2	32.8	13.5	1.5
Pea, Crushed, with Carrot, Cumin, GF, Clive's*	1 Tart/190g	382	23.8	201	3.6	16.8	12.5	0
Pineapple, Individual, Waitrose*	1 Tart/54g	216	6.1	400	2.2	77.2	11.3	0.5
Plum, Seriously Fruity, Waitrose*	1/6 Tart/95g	183	5.9	192	2.9	30.2	6.2	1.9
Raspberry, & Blueberry, Tesco*	1 Serving/85g	168	7.5	198	2.7	27	8.8	2.8
Spinach, & Ricotta, Individual, TTD, Sainsbury's*	1 Quiche/170g	466	33.7	274	7.5	16.5	19.8	1.4
Strawberry, & Fresh Cream, Finest, Tesco*	1 Tart/129g	350	19.1	271	3.3	31.1	14.8	1.2
Strawberry, Custard, Asda*	1 Tart/100g	335	15	335	3.1	47	15	0
Strawberry, Fresh, M&S*	1 Tart/120g	305	18.4	255	3.1	26.4	15.4	2.4
Toffee, & Pecan, Waitrose*	¼ Tart/133g	564	19.1	423	4.3	69.3	14.3	1.6
Tomato, & Mascarpone, Cherry, Asda*	1 Tart/160g	290	18	181	4.4	15.6	11.2	1.1
Tomato, Olive, Provencale, GF, Clive's*	1 Tart/190g	361	25.1	190	2.8	13.8	13.2	0
Treacle, Average	***1 Portion/125g***	***460***	***17.6***	***368***	***3.7***	***60.4***	***14.1***	***1.1***
Treacle, Tesco*	1 Slice/63g	249	10.3	396	4.3	57	16.4	1.4
Treacle, Waitrose*	¼ Tart/106g	302	11	285	2.8	45	10.4	0.6
Treacle, with Custard	***1 Serving/251g***	***586***	***23.5***	***233***	***3.1***	***36.1***	***9.4***	***0.8***
Vegetable Feta, Deli, M&S*	½ Tart/115g	315	18.4	274	5	20	16	6
Vegetable, Roasted, Finest, Tesco*	¼ Tart/113g	213	10.4	188	2.9	22.5	9.2	2.1
Vegetables, Bombay, with Daal, GF, Clive's*	1 Tart/191g	416	22.5	218	6	19.9	11.8	0
TARTE								
Au Chocolat, Seriously Chocolatey, Waitrose*	1/6 Tarte/70g	348	22.8	497	6	43.8	32.6	2.6
Au Citron, Frozen, TTD, Sainsbury's*	1/6 Tarte/80g	232	13.4	290	4.7	40.7	16.8	7.7
Au Citron, Waitrose*	1 Tarte/100g	325	18.1	325	4.9	35.7	18.1	1
Bacon, Leek Roquefort, Bistro, Waitrose*	¼ Tarte/100g	277	18.2	277	8.4	19.8	18.2	0.6
Tatin, 1, Waitrose*	1 Segment/50g	106	4.6	212	1.9	29.9	9.1	1.6
TARTLETS								
Brie Cranberry, Filo, Waitrose*	1 Tartlet/16g	44	2.2	275	8.9	26.9	13.9	3.5
Brie, Cranberry, Party Food, M&S*	1 Tartlet/19g	56	3.2	295	7.8	26.9	17.1	1.3
Butternut Squash Goats Cheese, Linda McCartney*	1 Tartlet/150g	405	25	270	6.3	24.2	16.7	1.2
Goats Cheese Caramelised Onion, Aldi*	1 Tartlet/150g	402	26	268	7.3	20.7	17.3	1.2
Lemon, Petit, Bonne Maman*	1 Tartlet/14g	61	2.4	439	5	66	17	0
Raspberry, Mini, M&S*	1 Tartlet/27g	90	5.4	330	4.3	34.4	19.6	0.5
Red Onion Goats Cheese, Sainsbury's*	1 Tartlet/113g	335	21.8	297	7	23.7	19.3	1.5
Tomato & Goats Cheese, Waitrose*	1 Tartlet/130g	295	19	227	6.6	17.4	14.6	2
TEA								
A Moment of Calm, herbal Infusion, Brewed, Twinings*	1 Mug/200ml	4	0	2	0	0.3	0	0
Apple Cinnamon, Made Up, Heath And Heather*	1 Serving/250ml	8	0	3	0.1	0.7	0	0
Assam, Blended, TTD, Sainsbury's*	1 Serving/2g	0	0	0	0	0	0	0
Blackberry Nettle, Twinings*	1 Cup/250ml	5	0	2	0	0.3	0	0
Blackcurrant, Fruit Creations, Typhoo*	1 Sm Cup/100ml	5	0	5	0.2	0.8	0	0.2
Camomile, Pure, Classic Herbal, Twinings*	1 Serving/200ml	4	0	2	0	0.3	0	0
Chai Latte, Skinny Blend, Drink Me Chai*	1 Serving/15g	62	1.2	415	7.5	77.7	8	1.3
Chai, Twinings*	1 Cup/200ml	2	0	1	0.1	0	0	0
Chamomile Spiced Apple, Warming, Twinings*	1 Cup/100ml	2	0	2	0	0.3	0	0
Cranberry Elderflower, Boost, Tetley*	1 Serving/225ml	5	0	2	0.1	0.6	0	0
Damask, Rose, Chinese, Choi Time*	1 Mug/500ml	0	0.3	0	0	0	0.1	0
Darjeeling Infusion, with Raspberry Juice, M&S*	1 Bottle/500ml	170	0	34	0	8.5	0	0
Decaf, Tetley*	1 Cup/100ml	1	0	1	0	0.3	0	0
Earl Grey, Green, Twinings*	1 Cup/200ml	2	0	1	0	0.2	0	0
Earl Grey, Infusion with Water, Average	***1 Mug/250ml***	***2***	***0***	***1***	***0***	***0.2***	***0***	***0***

T

INFO/WEIGHT	Measure	per Measure		Nutrition Values per 100g / 100ml				
		KCAL	FAT	KCAL	PROT	CARB	FAT	FIBRE

TEA

Fruit Or Herbal, Made with Water, Twinings*	1 Mug/200ml	8	0	4	0	1	0	0
Fruit, Green, Infusion, Eat Well, M&S*	½ Pack/150g	80	1.2	53	1.4	9.8	0.8	0.6
Fruit, Twinings*	1 Mug/227ml	4	0	2	0	0.4	0	0
Fruits of the Forest, Westminster Tea*	1 Bag/250ml	5	0	2	0	0.6	0	0
Ginger, Herbal, Brit Tang*	1 Tea Bag/2g	5	0	278	0	55.6	0	0
Green Tea, Apple Cucumber, Super, Beauty, Tetley*	1 Teabag/200ml	2	0	1	0	0.3	0	0
Green with Citrus, Twinings*	1 Serving/200ml	2	0	1	1	0.2	0	0
Green with Jasmine, Twinings*	1 Serving/100ml	1	0	1	0	0.2	0	0
Green with Jasmine, Wellbeing Selection, Flavia*	1 Cup/200ml	0	0	0	0	0	0	0
Green with Lemon, Jackson's*	1 Serving/200ml	2	0	1	0	0.2	0	0
Green with Mango, Brewed with Water, Twinings*	1 Cup/200ml	2	0	1	0	0.2	0	0
Green with Mint, Whittards of Chelsea*	1 Cup/100ml	1	0	1	0.2	0.1	0	0
Green with Pomegranate, Twinings*	1 Serving/200ml	2	0	1	0	0.2	0	0
Green, Caramelised Apple, Twinings*	1 Mug/250ml	2	0	1	0	0.2	0	0
Green, Powder, Matcha*	1 Serving/10g	30	0	300	0	50	0	30
Green, Pure, Tetley*	1 Serving/250ml	2	0	1	0	0.3	0	0
Green, Rooibos, Naturally Caffeine Free, Tick Tock*	1 Serving/250ml	0	0	0	0	0	0	0
Green, with Yerba Mate Honey, Herbal Mist*	1 Serving/240ml	80	0	33	0	8.3	0	0
Herbal, Wellbeing Blends, Infusions, Twinings*	1 Serving/200ml	4	0	2	0	0.3	0	0
Ice with Lemon, Lipton*	1 Bottle/325ml	91	0	28	0	6.9	0	0
Ice with Mango, Lipton*	1 Bottle/500ml	165	0	33	0	8.1	0	0
Ice with Peach, Lipton*	1 Bottle/500ml	140	0	28	0	6.8	0	0
Iced, Green, Orange, Lipton*	1 Bottle/500ml	100	0	20	0	5	0	0
Iced, No Sugar Peach Flavour, Nestle*	1 Glass/100ml	1	0	1	0	0.1	0	0
Iced, Peach, Low Calories, Lipton*	1 Bottle/505ml	96	2.5	19	0.5	4.7	0.5	0
Iced, Peach, Twinings*	1 Serving/200ml	60	0.2	30	0.1	7.3	0.1	0
Iced, Raspberry, Bottle, Lipton*	1 Serving/250ml	48	1.3	19	0.5	4.6	0.5	0
Lemon Earl Grey Flavour, Sainsbury's*	1 Serving/250ml	7	1.2	3	0.5	0.7	0.5	0.5
Lemon Ginger, Lipton*	1 Cup/200ml	8	0	4	0.5	0.5	0	0
Lemon, Ginger, Manuka Honey, Pukka Herbs*	1 Serving/200ml	6	0	3	0	0	0	0
Lemon, Iced, Diet, Nestea*	1 Glass/250ml	3	0	1	0	0	0	0
Lemon, Instant, Original, Lift*	1 Serving/15g	53	0	352	0	87	0	0
Lemon, Instant, Tesco*	1 Serving/7g	23	0	326	1	80.5	0	0
Lemon, with Yerba Mate, Herbal Mist*	1 Serving/240ml	80	0	33	0	8.8	0	0
Light Delicate, Green with Lemon, Twinings*	1 Cup/100ml	1	0.1	1	0.1	0.2	0.1	0.1
Made with Water	*1 Mug/227ml*	*0*	*0*	*0*	*0.1*	*0*	*0*	*0*
Made with Water with Semi-Skimmed Milk, Average	*1 Cup/200ml*	*14*	*0.4*	*7*	*0.5*	*0.7*	*0.2*	*0*
Made with Water with Skimmed Milk, Average	*1 Mug/270ml*	*16*	*0.5*	*6*	*0.5*	*0.7*	*0.2*	*0*
Made with Water with Whole Milk, Average	*1 Cup/200ml*	*16*	*0.8*	*8*	*0.4*	*0.5*	*0.4*	*0*
Mango, with Yerba Mate, Herbal Mist*	1 Serving/240ml	70	0	29	0	7.5	0	0
Morning Detox, Twinings*	1 Serving/200ml	5	0	2	0	0.3	0	0
Nettle Peppermint, Twinings*	1 Cup/200ml	2	0	1	0	0.2	0	0
Nettle Sweet Fennel, Twinings*	1 Cup/200ml	4	0	2	0	0.3	0	0
Oolong, Average	*1 Serving/200ml*	*5*	*0.2*	*2*	*0.1*	*0.2*	*0.1*	*0.2*
Orange Mango, Herbal, Organic, Honest, Coca-Cola*	1 Bottle/500ml	96	0	19	0	4.7	0	0
Peach, with Yerba Mate, Herbal Mist*	1 Serving/240ml	80	0	33	0	9.2	0	0
Peppermint, Made with Water, Average	*1 Serving/200ml*	*3*	*0*	*2*	*0*	*0.2*	*0*	*0*
Raspberry & Cranberry, T of Life, Tetley*	1 Serving/100ml	36	0	36	0	9	0	0
Raspberry, with Yerba Mate, Herbal Mist*	1 Serving/240ml	80	0	33	0	9.2	0	0
Red Berries, Brewed, PG Tips*	1 Cup/200ml	5	0	2	0	0.6	0	0
Red Bush, Made with Water, Tetley*	1 Mug/250ml	2	0	1	0	0.1	0	0
Sleep, Herbal Infusion, Brewed, Twinings*	1 Mug/200ml	4	0	2	0	0.3	0	0
Turmeric, Spiced, Infusions, Sainsbury's*	1 Teabag/2g	1	0.1	65	5	0	5	0

	Measure INFO/WEIGHT	per Measure KCAL	FAT	Nutrition Values per 100g / 100ml KCAL	PROT	CARB	FAT	FIBRE
TEACAKES								
Average	*1 Teacake/60g*	*178*	*4.5*	*296*	*8*	*52.5*	*7.5*	*0*
Caramel, Highlights, Mallows, Cadbury*	1 Teacake/15g	61	1.9	408	6.2	69.1	12.4	3.6
Cinnamon, Raisin, Irish, Rankin Selection*	1 Teacake/60g	172	3.5	287	5.8	68.5	5.8	2.5
Fruit, Sunblest*	1 Teacake/75g	212	2.6	282	6.2	55.4	3.4	2.3
Fruited, Co-Op*	1 Teacake/62g	160	2	258	9.7	46.8	3.2	3.2
Fruity, Warburton's*	1 Teacake/63g	164	1.9	262	8.7	48	3	3.2
Large, Sainsbury's*	1 Teacake/73g	212	3.6	291	7.6	52.4	4.9	3.4
Marshmallow, Milk Chocolate, Tunnock's*	1 Teacake/24g	106	4.6	440	4.9	61.9	19.2	2.4
Mini Bites, M&S*	1 Bite/6g	29	1.2	484	3.2	72.6	20.3	2.1
Morrisons*	1 Teacake/61g	168	2.1	275	7.8	51.6	3.5	3.1
Richly Fruited, Waitrose*	1 Teacake/72g	205	2.7	285	7.8	55	3.7	2.2
Tesco*	1 Teacake/73g	201	2.6	276	7.7	51.4	3.6	3.4
Toasted, Average	*1 Teacake/60g*	*197*	*5*	*329*	*8.9*	*58.3*	*8.3*	*0*
with Orange Filling, M&S*	1 Teacake/20g	80	2.8	410	4.5	66.6	14.2	0.9
TEMPEH								
Average	*1oz/28g*	*46*	*1.8*	*166*	*20.7*	*6.4*	*6.4*	*4.3*
Barbecue, Slices, Oasis*	1 Serving/30g	58	4.2	193	12.4	2.9	14	0
TEQUILA								
Average	*1 Pub Shot/35ml*	*78*	*0*	*224*	*0*	*0*	*0*	*0*
TERRINE								
Ham Hock, M&S*	1 Slice/70g	98	4.1	140	22.5	0.1	5.8	0.5
Lobster & Prawn, Slices, M&S*	1 Serving/55g	107	7.4	195	18.2	0.7	13.4	0.7
Salmon & King Prawn, Waitrose*	1 Serving/75g	98	4	130	19.3	1.3	5.3	0
Salmon Crayfish, Slice, Finest, Tesco*	1 Serving/110g	148	5.7	135	21.9	0.1	5.2	0.1
Salmon Lemon, Luxury, Tesco*	1 Serving/50g	98	7.8	196	10.6	3.2	15.7	0.8
Salmon, Poached, Tesco*	1 Pack/113g	349	30.6	309	15.5	0.8	27.1	0
Salmon, Three, M&S*	1 Serving/80g	168	12.2	210	17.6	0.8	15.3	0.9
THYME								
Dried, Average	*1 Tsp/1g*	*3*	*0.1*	*276*	*9.1*	*45.3*	*7.4*	*0*
Fresh, Average	*1 Tsp/1g*	*1*	*0*	*95*	*3*	*15.1*	*2.5*	*0*
TIA MARIA								
Original	*1 Pub Shot/35ml*	*105*	*0*	*300*	*0*	*0*	*0*	*0*
TIC TAC								
Extra Strong Mint, Ferrero*	2 Tic tacs/1g	4	0	381	0	95.2	0	0
Fresh Mint, Ferrero*	2 Tic Tacs/1g	4	0	390	0	97.5	0	0
Lime & Orange, Ferrero*	2 Tic Tacs/1g	4	0	386	0	95.5	0	0
Orange, Ferrero*	2 Tic Tacs/1g	4	0	385	0	95.5	0	0
Spearmint, Ferrero*	1 Box/16g	62	0	390	0	97.5	0	0
TIKKA MASALA								
Chicken, & Pilau Basmati Rice, Frozen, Patak's*	1 Pack/400g	580	20	145	9.9	15.1	5	0.2
Chicken, & Pilau Rice, BGTY, Sainsbury's*	1 Pack/400g	380	4.8	95	8.1	13	1.2	1.1
Chicken, & Pilau Rice, Waitrose*	1 Pack/400g	644	32.4	161	6.8	13.4	8.1	3.8
Chicken, & Rice, Ready Meal, Healthy Range, Average	*1 Serving/400g*	*390*	*6.4*	*98*	*6.6*	*14.3*	*1.6*	*1.1*
Chicken, Pilau Rice, Meal for One, M&S*	1 Pack/400g	592	20.4	148	8.9	15.3	5.1	2.7
Chicken, Rice, Be Light, Aldi*	1 Pack/400g	516	10	129	9.8	16	2.5	1.5
Chicken, Rice, Finest, Tesco*	1 Pack/450g	637	18.6	154	8.6	19.1	4.5	1.2
Chicken, Rice, Pot, Musclefood*	1 Serving/309g	334	5.6	108	12.5	9.4	1.8	1.7
Chicken, Breast, GFY, Asda*	1 Pack/380g	486	14.4	128	19	4.5	3.8	0.2
Chicken, Chef Select, Lidl*	1 Pack/450g	707	31	157	8.7	13.1	6.9	4
Chicken, Curry Kit, Musclefood*	1 Serving/385g	285	6.9	74	11.3	3.2	1.8	0.1
Chicken, Frozen, Annabel Karmel*	1 Pack/200g	238	7.6	119	5.9	14.6	3.8	1.5
Chicken, Frozen, Microwaved, Slimzone, Asda*	1 Pack/443g	350	5.8	79	13	3.3	1.3	1.2
Chicken, Hot, Sainsbury's*	1 Pack/400g	604	37.2	151	13.2	3.6	9.3	1.5

T

	Measure INFO/WEIGHT	per Measure KCAL	FAT	Nutrition Values per 100g / 100ml KCAL	PROT	CARB	FAT	FIBRE
TIKKA MASALA								
Chicken, Hot, Takeaway, Tesco*	½ Pack/194g	244	13.9	126	9	5.3	7.2	2
Chicken, Indian Takeaway, Iceland*	1 Pack/400g	484	28.4	121	8.9	6	7.1	1.9
Chicken, Indian, Medium, Sainsbury's*	1 Pack/400g	848	61.2	212	13.2	5.3	15.3	0.1
Chicken, M&S*	½ Pack/200g	288	15.6	144	13.5	4.7	7.8	0.7
Chicken, with Long Grain Rice, Kirstys*	1 Meal/309g	315	13.6	102	4.6	10.3	4.4	1.5
Chicken, with Pilau Rice, Frozen, Waitrose*	1 Pack/400g	676	32.4	169	9.3	14.6	8.1	2.1
Chicken, with Pilau Rice, Serves 1, Sainsbury's*	1 Pack/450g	724	24.8	161	7.5	18.7	5.5	3.3
Chicken, with White Rice, Good Choice, Iceland*	1 Serving/400g	356	4	89	5.4	14.7	1	0.6
Spicy, with Long Grain Rice, Rice Time, Uncle Ben's*	1 Tub/300g	328	4.8	109	2	21.1	1.6	0.8
Vegetable, Waitrose*	1 Serving/196g	149	4.3	76	3.6	10.5	2.2	3.8
Vegetarian, Chef's Selection, Quorn*	½ Pack/170g	274	17	161	6	10	10	3.5
TILAPIA								
Raw, Average	*100g*	*95*	*1*	*95*	*20*	*0*	*1*	*0*
TIME OUT								
Break Pack, Cadbury*	1 Serving/20g	108	6.3	530	6.2	58.3	30.7	0
Chocolate Fingers, Cadbury*	2 Fingers/35g	186	10.6	530	7.1	57.3	30.3	1.1
TIRAMISU								
Asda*	1 Pot/100g	252	11	252	4.3	34	11	0.5
Classic, Sainsbury's*	1 Serving/84g	209	8.5	250	4.2	31.7	10.2	1.1
Dine in Dessert, M&S*	½ Dessert/145g	515	36.7	355	2.6	28.8	25.3	0.7
Family Size, Tesco*	1 Serving/125g	356	18.1	285	4.3	34.5	14.5	4.3
Morrisons*	1 Pot/90g	248	9.9	276	4	38	11	0
Single Size, Tesco*	1 Pot/100g	290	12.9	290	3.8	35.1	12.9	4.5
Twin, Frozen, Bella Italia*	1 Serving/93g	285	21.2	306	3.1	8.3	22.8	0.5
Waitrose*	1 Pot/90g	221	11.2	246	6.4	27.2	12.4	0
TOAD IN THE HOLE								
Average	*1 Serving/231g*	*640*	*40.2*	*277*	*11.9*	*19.5*	*17.4*	*1.1*
Classic Kitchen, Tesco*	1 Pack/340g	859	49.3	268	12.2	19	15.4	2.4
Frozen, Cooked, CBY, Asda*	1 Slice/72g	168	7.5	232	9.2	24.2	10.4	2.6
HFC, Tesco*	1 Pack/223g	463	18.3	208	9.5	23.3	8.2	1.4
Large, Great Value, Asda*	¼ Pack/81g	238	13.8	293	10	25	17	2.3
Mini, Aunt Bessie's*	1 Serving/62g	118	6.8	191	11	12	11	3.6
Mini, Christmas, Ovenbaked, Asda*	1 Toad/20g	57	2.8	283	13	25	14	2.5
with Three Sausages, Asda*	1 Pack/150g	435	27	290	10	22	18	1
TOASTIE								
All Day Breakfast, M&S*	1 Serving/174g	375	13.8	215	11.2	25	7.9	1.7
Cheese & Pickle, M&S*	1 Toastie/136g	320	9.1	235	10.4	33.5	6.7	2.6
Cheese Ham, Tayto*	1 Serving/50g	260	14.8	519	6.8	58	29.7	0
Cheese Onion, Ginsters*	1 Toastie/122g	330	12.3	269	10.9	33.1	10	1.5
Cheese, Tomato, Spinach, Frozen, Tesco*	1 Pack/134g	291	6.6	218	9.4	32.4	4.9	3.1
Chicken, Bacon, Three Cheese, Greggs*	1 Toastie/223g	617	29	277	19	20	13	0
Ham & Cheddar, British, M&S*	1 Pack/128g	269	8.6	210	15.5	22.3	6.7	1.3
Ham & Cheese, Tesco*	1 Pack/124g	349	10.4	282	13.2	37.2	8.4	2.4
Ham Cheese, White Bread	*1 Toastie/150g*	*409*	*14.9*	*273*	*14.5*	*31.3*	*9.9*	*0.9*
Ham, Three Cheese, Greggs*	1 Toastie/175g	451	19.2	258	16	25	11	0
TOFFEE APPLE								
Average	*1 Apple/141g*	*188*	*3*	*133*	*1.2*	*29.2*	*2.1*	*2.3*
TOFFEE CRISP								
Biscuit, Nestle*	1 Biscuit/19g	99	5.3	519	3.9	62.3	27.8	1.4
Bitesize, Nestle*	1 Serving/20g	101	5.4	518	3.8	63	27.6	1.3
TOFFEES								
Assorted, Bassett's*	1 Toffee/8g	35	1.1	434	3.8	73.1	14	0
Assorted, Sainsbury's*	1 Sweet/8g	37	1.3	457	2.2	76.5	15.8	0.2

T

	Measure INFO/WEIGHT	per Measure KCAL	per Measure FAT	Nutrition Values per 100g / 100ml KCAL	PROT	CARB	FAT	FIBRE
TOFFEES								
Brazil Nut, Diabetic, Thorntons*	1 Serving/20g	93	7	467	3.2	49	35.1	0.5
Butter, Smart Price, Asda*	1 Toffee/8g	37	1.3	440	1.3	75	15	0
Chewy, Werther's*	1 Toffee/5g	22	0.8	436	3.5	71.3	15.2	0.1
Dairy, Smart Price, Asda*	1 Sweet/9g	37	1.3	407	1.3	68.4	14.2	0
Dairy, Waitrose*	1 Toffee/8g	37	1.1	458	2	80.2	14.3	0.5
Devon Butter, Thorntons*	1 Sweet/9g	40	1.5	444	1.7	72.2	16.7	0
English Butter, Co-Op*	1 Toffee/8g	38	1.6	470	2	71	20	0
Everyday Value, Tesco*	3 Toffees/23g	101	3.3	450	2.1	77.3	14.8	0.3
Liquorice, Thorntons*	1 Bag/100g	506	29.4	506	1.9	58.8	29.4	0
Milk Chocolate Covered, Thorntons*	1 Bag/215g	1120	66	521	4.1	57.2	30.7	0.9
Milk Chocolate Smothered, Thorntons*	1 Pack/125g	655	38.5	524	4.3	57.5	30.8	1.1
Mixed, Average	*1oz/28g*	*119*	*5.2*	*426*	*2.2*	*66.7*	*18.6*	*0*
Original, Thorntons*	1 Bag/100g	514	30.1	514	1.8	59.3	30.1	0
Squares, No Added Sugar, Russell Stover*	1 Piece/15g	57	3.9	380	6	49.3	26	1.3
TOFU								
Average	*1 Pack/250g*	*297*	*16.5*	*119*	*13.4*	*1.4*	*6.6*	*0.1*
Beech Smoked, Organic, Cauldron Foods*	½ Pack/110g	124	7.8	113	10.9	1	7.1	0.5
Fried, Average	*1oz/28g*	*75*	*4*	*268*	*28.6*	*9.3*	*14.1*	*0*
Original, Cauldron Foods*	1 Pack/396g	467	28.1	118	12.6	1	7.1	1.9
Pieces, Marinated, Organic, Cauldron Foods*	1 Pack/160g	363	27.2	227	17.5	1	17	2.7
Smoked, Organic, Evernat*	1oz/28g	36	1.8	127	16.3	0.8	6.6	0
TOMATILLOS								
Raw	*1 Med/34g*	*11*	*0.3*	*32*	*1*	*5.8*	*1*	*1.9*
TOMATO PASTE								
Average	*1 Tbsp/20g*	*19*	*0*	*96*	*5*	*19.2*	*0.2*	*1.5*
Sun Dried, Average	*1 Hpd Tsp/10g*	*38*	*3.5*	*385*	*3.2*	*13.8*	*35.2*	*0*
TOMATO PUREE								
Average	*1 Tsp/5g*	*4*	*0*	*76*	*4.5*	*14.1*	*0.2*	*2.3*
Double Concentrate, Average	*1 Tbsp/15g*	*13*	*0*	*85*	*4.9*	*14.9*	*0.2*	*3.6*
Garlic, Double Concentrate, Morrisons*	1 Tbsp/15g	13	0	86	3.9	14.9	0.3	3.8
Sun Dried, & Olive Oil & Herbs, GIA*	1 Tsp/5g	10	1.1	204	2.6	0.5	21.6	0
TOMATOES								
Cherry, Average	*1 Tomato/15g*	*3*	*0*	*18*	*0.7*	*3*	*0.3*	*0.5*
Cherry, Canned, TTD, Sainsbury's*	½ Can/204g	47	0.4	23	1.4	4	0.2	0.9
Cherry, on the Vine, Average	*1 Serving/80g*	*15*	*0.3*	*18*	*0.7*	*3.1*	*0.3*	*1.2*
Chopped, Canned, Branded Average	*1 Serving/130g*	*27*	*0.2*	*21*	*1.1*	*3.8*	*0.1*	*0.8*
Chopped, Italian, Average	*½ Can/200g*	*47*	*0.2*	*23*	*1.3*	*4.4*	*0.1*	*0.9*
Chopped, with Garlic, Average	*½ Can/200g*	*43*	*0.3*	*21*	*1.2*	*3.8*	*0.1*	*0.8*
Chopped, with Herbs, Average	*½ Can/200g*	*42*	*0.3*	*21*	*1.1*	*3.8*	*0.1*	*0.8*
Chopped, with Olive Oil & Roasted Garlic, Sainsbury's*	1 Pack/390g	187	8.2	48	1.3	5.9	2.1	1
Fresh, Raw, Average	*1 Med/123g*	*22*	*0.2*	*18*	*0.9*	*3.9*	*0.2*	*1.2*
Fried in Blended Oil	*1 Med/85g*	*77*	*6.5*	*91*	*0.7*	*5*	*7.7*	*1.3*
Grilled, Average	*1 Med/85g*	*17*	*0.3*	*20*	*0.8*	*3.5*	*0.3*	*1.5*
Marinated, with Garlic Oregano, The Deli, Aldi*	½ Pack/75g	68	3.5	90	2.8	7.8	4.7	2.7
Plum, Baby, Average	*1 Serving/50g*	*9*	*0.2*	*18*	*1.5*	*2.3*	*0.3*	*1*
Plum, in Tomato Juice, Average	*1 Can/400g*	*71*	*0.4*	*18*	*1*	*3.3*	*0.1*	*0.7*
Plum, in Tomato Juice, Premium, Average	*1 Can/400g*	*93*	*1.2*	*23*	*1.3*	*3.8*	*0.3*	*0.7*
Pome Dei Moro, Waitrose*	1 Serving/80g	16	0.2	20	0.7	3.1	0.3	1.2
Pomodorino, TTD, Sainsbury's*	1 Tomato/8g	1	0	17	0.7	3.1	0.4	1.3
Ripened on the Vine, Average	*1 Med/123g*	*22*	*0.4*	*18*	*0.7*	*3.1*	*0.3*	*0.7*
Santini, M&S*	1 Serving/80g	16	0.2	20	0.7	3.1	0.3	1
Stuffed with Rice Based Filling, Average	*1oz/28g*	*59*	*3.8*	*212*	*2.1*	*22.2*	*13.4*	*1.1*
Sugardrop, Finest, Tesco*	1 Tomato/14g	3	0	20	0.7	3.1	0.3	1

T

	Measure INFO/WEIGHT	per Measure KCAL	FAT	Nutrition Values per 100g / 100ml KCAL	PROT	CARB	FAT	FIBRE
TOMATOES								
Sun Dried in Oil	*100g*	*301*	*24.8*	*301*	*5.8*	*13.5*	*24.8*	*7*
Sun Dried, Average	*3 Pieces/20g*	*43*	*3.2*	*214*	*4.7*	*13*	*15.9*	*3.3*
Sweet, Baby, Mixed, Finest, Tesco*	½ Pack/125g	25	0.4	20	0.7	3.1	0.3	1
Tri-Colour, On the Vine, Finest, Tesco*	8 Tomatoes/80g	21	0.4	26	1.1	3.6	0.5	1.2
Vine Ripened, Sweet, Raw, Tesco*	2 Tomatoes/90g	18	0.3	20	0.7	3.1	0.3	1
TONGUE								
Lunch, Average	*1oz/28g*	*51*	*3*	*181*	*20.1*	*1.8*	*10.6*	*0*
Ox, Deli Counter, Sainsbury's*	1 Serving/100g	195	13.3	195	18.3	0.5	13.3	0.1
Slices, Average	*1oz/28g*	*56*	*3.9*	*201*	*18.7*	*0*	*14*	*0*
TONIC WATER								
Average	*1 Glass/250ml*	*82*	*0*	*33*	*0*	*8.8*	*0*	*0*
Diet, Asda*	1 Glass/200ml	2	0	1	0	0	0	0
Indian with Lime, Low Calorie, Tesco*	1 Glass/250ml	5	0	2	0	0	0	0
Indian, Britvic*	1 Mini Can/150ml	39	0.2	26	0.1	6.2	0.1	0.1
Indian, Diet, Schweppes*	1 Glass/100ml	1	0	1	0	0	0	0
Indian, Fever-Tree*	1 Bottle/200ml	72	0	36	0	8.9	0	0
Indian, Schweppes*	1 Serving/500ml	110	0	22	0	5.1	0	0
Indian, Slimline, Schweppes*	1 Serving/188ml	3	0	2	0.4	0	0	0
Low Calorie, Tesco*	1 Serving/200ml	4	0	2	0	0.5	0	0
Quinine, Schweppes*	1 Glass/125ml	46	0	37	0	9	0	0
TONIC WINE								
Original, Sanatogen*	1 Bottle/700ml	889	0	127	0	124.4	0	0
TOPIC								
Mars*	1 Bar/47g	234	12.3	498	6.2	59.6	26.2	1.7
TORTE								
Chocolate Pecan Brownie, Gu*	1/6 Torte/67g	292	17.7	436	5.3	45.1	26.4	3.1
Chocolate Brownie, Belgian, TTD, Sainsbury's*	1 Slice/90g	360	24.6	400	5.6	32.5	27.3	0.8
Chocolate Fondant, Gu*	1/8 Torte/62g	264	18.9	423	5.7	32	30.2	1.8
Chocolate Orange Almond, Gu*	1 Serving/65g	273	19.8	420	5	28.2	30.5	2.7
Chocolate Truffle, Waitrose*	1 Serving/116g	359	20.1	309	4.6	30.1	17.3	1.4
Chocolate, Tesco*	1 Serving/50g	126	6	251	3.6	32.3	11.9	1
Lemon & Mango, Waitrose*	1 Serving/80g	142	2.4	177	3.9	33.6	3	0.6
Salted Caramel Chocolate, Weight Watchers, Heinz*	1 Dessert/65g	164	3.8	252	4.1	45	5.8	1.8
TORTELLINI								
Beef, & Red Wine, Italian, Asda*	½ Pack/150g	242	4.2	161	9	25	2.8	0
Beef, & Red Wine, Italiano, Tesco*	1 Serving/150g	324	4.8	216	11.7	35.3	3.2	3.3
Cheese, & Ham, Italiano, Tesco*	½ Pack/150g	396	12.3	264	12.8	34.8	8.2	3
Cheese, Tomato Basil, Cooked, Tesco*	1 Serving/270g	551	15.1	204	6.7	30.5	5.6	2.5
Ham, & Cheese, Fresh, Asda*	½ Pack/150g	255	9	170	6	23	6	1.7
Meat, Italian, Tesco*	1 Serving/125g	332	9.5	266	10.6	38.9	7.6	2.3
Mushroom, Asda*	1 Serving/125g	218	5.2	174	6	28	4.2	2.3
Pepperoni, Spicy, Asda*	½ Pack/150g	252	6	168	7	26	4	0
Pesto, & Goats Cheese, Fresh, Sainsbury's*	½ Pack/150g	310	12.2	207	8.9	24.6	8.1	2.6
Ricotta, & Spinach, Giovanni Rana*	½ Pack/125g	319	10	255	9	35.5	8	10
Sausage, & Ham, Italiano, Tesco*	1 Pack/300g	816	27.9	272	13.1	34	9.3	3.7
Spinach, & Ricotta, Italian, Asda*	½ Pack/150g	189	3.6	126	5	21	2.4	0.6
Tomato, & Mozzarella, Fresh, Sainsbury's*	½ Pack/150g	291	12	194	7.5	23	8	3.4
TORTELLONI								
Arrabiata, Sainsbury's*	½ Pack/210g	407	11.8	194	7.1	28.8	5.6	2.6
Cheese, & Smoked Ham, As Consumed, Tesco*	½ Pack/270g	535	17.3	198	8.4	25.8	6.4	1.8
Cheese, Tomato, Italian, Cooked, Asda*	½ Pack/209g	454	13.4	217	7.9	31	6.4	2.1
Chicken Bacon, As Consumed, Italiano, Tesco*	½ Pack/280g	567	14	202	6.8	30.7	5	3.7
Chicken, Mushroom, Italian, Cooked, Asda*	½ Pack/209g	427	8.6	204	7.5	33	4.1	2.3

	Measure INFO/WEIGHT	per Measure		Nutrition Values per 100g / 100ml				
		KCAL	FAT	KCAL	PROT	CARB	FAT	FIBRE
TORTELLONI								
Chicken, Prosciutto, Buitoni*	1 Serving/109g	330	9	302	14.7	42.2	8.2	1.8
Cream Cheese, Garlic & Herb, Fresh, Morrisons*	1 Serving/150g	400	9	267	10.3	46.1	6	3.2
Mushroom, Fresh, Sainsbury's*	1 Pack/400g	656	10.8	164	5.9	27.9	2.7	2.3
Sausage, & Ham, As Consumed, Italiano, Tesco*	1/3 Pack/180g	355	12.6	197	8.6	23.8	7	2
Spinach, & Ricotta Cheese, Co-Op*	½ Pack/126g	315	6.3	250	10	41	5	4
Spinach, & Ricotta, Fresh, Waitrose*	½ Pack/150g	239	5.3	159	6.3	24.4	3.5	2.5
Spinach, & Ricotta, Sainsbury's*	½ Pack/150g	326	10.8	217	7.8	30.2	7.2	2.4
Tomato, & Mozzarella, Sainsbury's*	1 Serving/175g	340	14	194	7.5	23	8	3.4
Wild Mushroom, Italian, Sainsbury's*	½ Pack/150g	309	12.3	206	7.7	25.4	8.2	2.3
TORTIGLIONI								
Dry, Average	*1 Serving/75g*	*266*	*1.4*	*355*	*12.5*	*72.2*	*1.9*	*2.1*
TORTILLA								
Chorizo, Roasted Vegetables, Morrisons*	1 Tortilla/130g	238	15.2	183	9.1	10	11.7	1
Onion, Caramelised, & Potato, Eat Well, M&S*	½ Pack/110g	148	6	135	5.9	13.5	5.5	3.7
Potato Caramelised Onion, Good Life, Co-Op*	1 Slice/112g	175	9.9	156	5.8	12	8.8	2.2
Red Pepper Chorizo, Slices, Waitrose*	1 Slice/113g	180	10.3	160	10	8.6	9.2	1.6
Vegetable, Roasted, Mediterranean, M&S*	½ Pack/110g	138	5.9	125	6.9	11.1	5.4	2.3
TORTILLA CHIPS								
Aldi*	¼ Pack/50g	234	9.5	469	6.3	66	19	4.2
Cheddar, Food Should Taste Good*	9 Chips/28g	130	6	464	7.1	60.7	21.4	7.1
Chilli, with Chopped Jalapeno, Tyrrells*	1 Serving/30g	154	8.3	512	5.9	57.3	27.5	0
Cool Flavour, BGTY, Sainsbury's*	1 Pack/22g	94	2.7	425	7.1	71.4	12.3	4.5
Cool Flavour, Sainsbury's*	1 Serving/50g	232	9.4	463	5.7	68.1	18.7	3.7
Cool, Tesco*	1 Serving/40g	190	9.9	474	6.3	56.7	24.7	7.8
Easy Cheesy!, Sainsbury's*	1 Serving/50g	249	13	498	7.1	58.7	26.1	4.5
Guacamole, Food Should Taste Good*	10 Chips/28g	130	5	464	7.1	64.3	17.9	7.1
Jalapeno, Food Should Taste Good*	12 Chips/28g	130	6	464	7.1	64.3	21.4	7.1
Kimchi, Food Should Taste Good*	12 Chips/28g	140	7	500	7.1	60.7	25	3.6
Lightly Salted, M&S*	1 Serving/20g	98	4.8	490	7.2	61.5	24.1	4.5
Lightly Salted, Smart Price, Asda*	¼ Bag/50g	251	13	502	7	60	26	5
Lightly Salted, Tesco*	1 Serving/50g	248	13.8	495	4.8	56.8	27.6	7.5
Lightly Salted, Waitrose*	1 Serving/40g	187	8.6	468	7.1	61.2	21.6	6.5
Lighty Salted, Basics, Sainsbury's*	½ Pack/50g	242	11.9	483	6.5	60.7	23.8	5.3
Multigrain, Black Bean, Food Should Taste Good*	10 Chips/28g	130	6	464	14.3	57.1	21.4	14.3
Nacho Cheese Flavour, Morrisons*	1 Serving/25g	126	6.6	504	7.2	59.4	26.4	3.6
Olive, Food Should Taste Good*	10 Chips/28g	140	7	500	7.1	64.3	25	7.1
Plain	*1 Serving/100g*	*486*	*21.1*	*486*	*6.8*	*62*	*21.1*	*4.2*
Salsa, M&S*	½ Bag/75g	364	18.8	485	5.7	59.1	25.1	6.1
Sweet Potato, Food Should Taste Good*	12 Chips/28g	140	7	500	7.1	64.3	25	3.6
Tortilla Rolls, Texan Barbecue, The Best, Morrisons*	1 Serving/25g	127	6.2	508	5.2	63.6	24.9	4.5
Tortillas, Nacho Cheese Flavour, Weight Watchers*	1 Pack/18g	78	2.9	433	6.1	66.7	16.1	3.9
Tortillas, Sour Cream, Lime, TTD, Sainsbury's*	1 Serving/30g	148	6.9	495	5.7	63.9	23.1	4.4
Veggie, Lightly Salted, Co-Op*	1 Serving/33g	165	8.3	499	5.9	60	25	4.8
with Guacamole	*1 Serving/100g*	*515*	*30.8*	*515*	*6*	*53*	*30.8*	*6.3*
TREACLE								
Black, Average	*1 Tbsp/20g*	*51*	*0*	*257*	*1.2*	*67.2*	*0*	*0*
TRIFLE								
Average	*1 Portion/170g*	*272*	*10.7*	*160*	*3.6*	*22.3*	*6.3*	*0.5*
Black Forest, Asda*	1 Serving/100g	237	9	237	3.1	36	9	0
Chocolate , Tesco*	1 Pot/120g	238	13	198	3.2	21.7	10.8	0.7
Fruit Cocktail, Individual, M&S*	1 Pot/135g	205	9.2	150	2.7	19.3	6.7	0.7
Fruit Cocktail, Individual, Tesco*	1 Pot/113g	175	8.8	155	1.7	19.6	7.8	0.6
Peach & Zabaglione, COU, M&S*	1 Glass/130g	150	3	115	2.8	20.6	2.3	0.8

T

	Measure INFO/WEIGHT	per Measure KCAL	FAT	Nutrition per 100g KCAL	PROT	CARB	FAT	FIBRE
TRIFLE								
Raspberry Sherry, Waitrose*	1 Pot/120g	223	14.3	186	2.5	16.9	11.9	0.7
Raspberry, Co-Op*	1 Trifle/125g	206	10	165	2	22	8	0.3
Raspberry, Pot, Sainsbury's*	1 Pot/125g	181	7.6	145	2.1	19.9	6.1	1.3
Raspberry, Tesco*	1 Pot/145g	188	8.8	130	1.7	16.8	6.1	0.6
Strawberry, Aldi*	1/3 Trifle/153g	193	8	126	1.9	18	5.2	0.7
Strawberry, Co-Op*	1 Serving/120g	175	9.1	146	1.7	16.7	7.6	1.4
Strawberry, Everyday Value, Tesco*	1/4 Trifle/118g	157	6.4	133	1.4	18.5	5.4	2.4
Strawberry, Individual, Waitrose*	1 Pot/150g	206	8.6	137	1.8	19.7	5.7	1
Strawberry, Low Fat, COU, M&S*	1 Pot/140g	148	3.5	106	2.9	17.6	2.5	0.8
Strawberry, Tesco*	1 Trifle/605g	998	55.7	165	1.5	19.1	9.2	0.8
TRIPE								
Onions, Stewed	*1oz/28g*	*26*	*0.8*	*93*	*8.3*	*9.5*	*2.7*	*0.7*
Ox, Real Lancashire*	1 Serving/100g	36	0.7	36	7.2	0.1	0.7	0
TROMPRETTI								
Fresh, Waitrose*	1 Serving/125g	339	3	271	11.7	50.6	2.4	2
TROUT								
Brown, Steamed, Average	*1 Serving/120g*	*162*	*5.4*	*135*	*23.5*	*0*	*4.5*	*0*
Fillets, with Juniper Berries, Ocean Sea, Lidl*	1 Serving /63g	87	3.5	138	22	0	5.5	0
Grilled, Weighed with Bones Skin	*1 Serving/100g*	*98*	*3.9*	*98*	*15.7*	*0*	*3.9*	*0*
Rainbow, Grilled, Average	*1 Serving/120g*	*162*	*6.5*	*135*	*21.5*	*0*	*5.4*	*0*
Rainbow, Raw, Average	*1oz/28g*	*33*	*1.3*	*118*	*19.1*	*0*	*4.7*	*0*
Rainbow, Smoked, Average	*1 Pack/135g*	*190*	*7.6*	*140*	*21.7*	*0.8*	*5.6*	*0*
Raw, Average	*1 Serving/120g*	*159*	*6.5*	*132*	*20.6*	*0*	*5.4*	*0*
Smoked, Average	*2 Fillets/135g*	*187*	*7.1*	*138*	*22.7*	*0.3*	*5.2*	*0.1*
TUMS								
Extra 750, Sugar Free, Tums*	2 Tablets/2g	5	0	250	0	50	0	0
Extra 750, Tums*	2 Tablets/2g	10	0	500	0	100	0	0
Reg, Tums*	1 Tablet/2g	2	0	125	0	25	0	0
Smoothies, Extra Strength 750, Tums*	2 Tablets/2g	10	0	500	0	100	0	0
TUNA								
Bluefin, Cooked, Dry Heat, Average	*1 Serving/100g*	*184*	*6.3*	*184*	*29.9*	*0*	*6.3*	*0*
Chipotle, No Drain, Infusions, John West*	1 Pot/80g	165	8.4	206	24.4	3.3	10.5	0
Chunks, in Brine, Average, Drained	*1 Can/130g*	*141*	*0.7*	*108*	*25.9*	*0*	*0.5*	*0*
Chunks, in Brine, Drained, Average	*1 Can/130g*	*141*	*0.7*	*108*	*25.9*	*0*	*0.5*	*0*
Chunks, in Spring Water, Average, Drained	*1 Sm Can/56g*	*60*	*0.4*	*108*	*25.4*	*0*	*0.6*	*0.1*
Chunks, in Sunflower Oil, Average, Drained	*1 Can/138g*	*260*	*12.6*	*188*	*26.5*	*0*	*9.2*	*0*
Chunks, Skipjack, in Brine, Average	*1 Can/138g*	*141*	*0.8*	*102*	*24.3*	*0*	*0.6*	*0*
Coronation Style, Canned, Average	*1 Can/80g*	*122*	*7.6*	*152*	*10.2*	*6.5*	*9.5*	*0.6*
Flakes, in Brine, Average	*1oz/28g*	*29*	*0.2*	*104*	*24.8*	*0*	*0.6*	*0*
in a Light Mayonnaise, Slimming World, Princes*	1 Can/80g	96	3.3	120	17.3	3.6	4.1	0
in a Tomato Herb Dressing, Weight Watchers*	1 Can/80g	79	2.9	99	11.6	5.1	3.6	0.5
in Coronation Style Dressing, Weight Watchers*	1 Can/80g	75	2	94	9.3	8.7	2.5	0.4
in Water, Average	*1 Serving/120g*	*126*	*1*	*105*	*24*	*0.1*	*0.8*	*0*
Jalapeno, & Spicy Couscous, Infusions, John West*	1 Serving/285g	390	7.7	137	9.9	17.7	2.7	1.7
Jalapeno, Infusions, John West*	1 Can/80g	142	6.1	177	24.1	3	7.6	0
Lime & Black Pepper, John West*	1 Serving/85g	134	7	158	18	2	8.2	2.1
Mexican Style, Spreadables, John West*	1 Can/80g	149	9.8	186	13.1	5.6	12.3	1.3
Mexican, Filler, Princes*	1 Pot/85g	134	8.2	158	13.9	3.7	9.7	0.2
Steaks, in Brine, Average	*1 Sm Can/99g*	*106*	*0.5*	*107*	*25.6*	*0*	*0.6*	*0*
Steaks, in Olive Oil, Average	*1 Serving/111g*	*211*	*10.7*	*190*	*25.8*	*0*	*9.6*	*0*
Steaks, in Sunflower Oil, Average	*1 Can/150g*	*269*	*12.6*	*179*	*26*	*0*	*8.4*	*0*
Steaks, in Water, Average	*1 Serving/200g*	*215*	*0.8*	*107*	*25.6*	*0*	*0.4*	*0*
Steaks, Raw, Average	*1 Serving/140g*	*179*	*2.7*	*128*	*27.6*	*0.1*	*1.9*	*0.2*

	Measure INFO/WEIGHT	per Measure KCAL	FAT	Nutrition Values per 100g / 100ml KCAL	PROT	CARB	FAT	FIBRE
TUNA								
Steaks, Skipjack, in Brine, Average	½ Can/75g	73	0.4	98	23.2	0	0.6	0
with Basil, & Sun-Dried Couscous, John West*	1 Pot/285g	430	13.4	151	9.7	16.9	4.7	0
with Lemon Black Pepper, Tesco*	1 Can/85g	144	6.5	170	21.2	4	7.6	0.5
with Soy, Ginger, & Mushroom, Couscous, John West*	1 Pot/285g	413	10	145	10	17.9	3.5	0
Yellowfin, Cooked, Dry Heat, Average	1 Serving/100g	139	1.2	139	30	0	1.2	0
TUNA MAYONNAISE								
with Sweetcorn, Spreadable, John West*	1 Serving/20g	45	3.5	227	12.7	4.6	17.4	0.5
TUNA WITH								
Wild Rice Lentils, Indian Style, Creations, John West*	1 Sachet/180g	250	8.5	139	9.5	14	4.7	1.2
TURBOT								
Grilled	1oz/28g	34	1	122	22.7	0	3.5	0
Raw	1oz/28g	27	0.8	95	17.7	0	2.7	0
TURKEY								
Breast, Butter Basted, Average	1 Serving/75g	110	3.6	146	23.7	1.9	4.9	0.4
Breast, Butter Basted, Joint, with Stuffing, Roasted, Tesco*	¼ Joint/150g	294	15	196	24.3	2.1	10	0.2
Breast, Diced, Healthy Range, Average	1oz/28g	30	0.4	108	23.8	0	1.3	0
Breast, Honey Roast, Sliced, Average	1 Serving/50g	57	0.7	114	24	1.6	1.4	0.2
Breast, Joint, Raw, Average	1 Serving/125g	134	2.6	108	21.3	0.7	2.1	0.6
Breast, Raw, Average	1oz/28g	33	0.6	117	24.1	0.5	2	0.1
Breast, Roasted, Average	1oz/28g	37	0.9	131	24.6	0.7	3.3	0.1
Breast, Roll, Cooked, Average	1 Slice/10g	9	0.1	92	17.6	3.5	0.8	0
Breast, Slices, Cooked, Average	1 Slice/20g	23	0.3	114	24	1.2	1.4	0.3
Breast, Smoked, Sliced, Average	1 Slice/20g	23	0.4	113	23.4	0.7	2	0
Breast, Steaks, in Crumbs, Average	1 Steak/76g	217	14.1	286	13.7	16.4	18.5	0.2
Breast, Steaks, Raw, Average	1oz/28g	30	0.3	107	24.3	0	1.1	0
Breast, Strips, for Stir Fry, Average	1 Serving/175g	205	2.7	117	25.6	0.1	1.6	0
Dark Meat, Raw, Average	1oz/28g	29	0.7	104	20.4	0	2.5	0
Escalope, Average	1 Escalope/138g	341	19.3	247	13.5	16.7	14	0.6
Escalope, Lemon & Pepper, Average	1 Escalope/143g	371	22.6	260	12.6	16.7	15.8	0.4
Leg, Dark Meat, Raw, Average, Weighed with Bone	1 Serving/100g	73	1.8	73	14.3	0	1.8	0
Light Meat, Raw, Average	1oz/28g	29	0.2	105	24.4	0	0.8	0
Light Meat, Roasted	1 Cup/140g	163	3.3	116	22.1	0	2.4	0
Mince, Average	1oz/28g	45	2	161	23.9	0	7.2	0
Mince, Lean, Healthy Range, Average	1oz/28g	33	1.1	118	20.3	0	4.1	0
Pudding, Christmas	1 Serving/175g	312	10.9	178	26.4	3.7	6.2	1
Rashers, Average	1 Rasher/26g	26	0.4	101	19.1	2.3	1.6	0
Rashers, Smoked, Average	1 Serving/75g	76	1.4	101	19.8	1.5	1.8	0
Roast, Meat & Skin, Average	1oz/28g	48	1.8	171	28	0	6.5	0
Roast, Meat Only, Average	1 Serving/100g	157	3.2	157	29.9	0	3.2	0
Smoked, Applewood, 1, Waitrose*	½ Pack/40g	48	0.4	121	27.3	0.5	1.1	0.1
Strips, Stir-Fried, Average	1oz/28g	46	1.3	164	31	0	4.5	0
Thigh, Diced, Average	1oz/28g	33	1.2	117	19.6	0	4.3	0
Vegetarian, Slices, Deli, with Stuffing, Quorn*	½ Pack/50g	60	1.2	120	16	8.9	2.3	4
Vegetarian, Slices, with Sage, Meat Free, Quorn*	¼ Pack/25g	32	0.6	128	16	8.9	2.3	4
Wafer Thin, Cooked, Average	1 Slice/10g	12	0.4	122	19	3.2	3.7	0
Wafer Thin, Honey Roast, Average	1 Slice/10g	11	0.2	109	19.2	4.2	1.7	0.2
Wafer Thin, Smoked, Average	1 Slice/10g	12	0.4	119	18.1	3.6	3.7	0
TURKEY DINNER								
Roast Dinner, 105, Oakhouse Foods Ltd*	1 Dinner/430g	624	16.3	145	7	9.4	3.8	1.4
Roast, Asda*	1 Pack/400g	344	6.4	86	7	11	1.6	2
Roast, Meal for One, M&S*	1 Pack/370g	462	16.3	125	9.1	12.4	4.4	2.7
Roast, Sainsbury's*	1 Pack/450g	354	9	79	6.8	8.4	2	1.9
Traditional, Birds Eye*	1 Pack/340g	292	7.8	86	6.1	10.3	2.3	1.7

T

	Measure INFO/WEIGHT	per Measure KCAL	FAT	Nutrition Values per 100g / 100ml KCAL	PROT	CARB	FAT	FIBRE
TURKEY HAM								
Average	*1 Serving/75g*	*81*	*2.9*	*108*	*15.6*	*2.8*	*3.9*	*0*
TURKISH DELIGHT								
Fry's*	1 Bar/51g	185	3.4	363	1.2	74	6.7	1.2
Milk Chocolate, M&S*	1 Pack/55g	220	4.7	400	1.6	79	8.5	0
with Rose, Hazer Baba*	1 Square/18g	70	0.3	389	1.6	88.6	1.7	0
TURMERIC								
Powder	*1 Tsp/3g*	*11*	*0.3*	*354*	*7.8*	*58.2*	*9.9*	*0*
TURNIP								
Boiled, Average	*1oz/28g*	*3*	*0.1*	*12*	*0.6*	*2*	*0.2*	*1.9*
Greens, Leaves, Cooked	*1 Serving/80g*	*16*	*0.2*	*20*	*1.1*	*4.4*	*0.2*	*3.5*
Mashed, Mash Direct*	½ Pack/200g	84	0.8	42	0.8	7.4	0.4	3.1
Raw, Unprepared, Average	*1oz/28g*	*5*	*0.1*	*17*	*0.7*	*3.5*	*0.2*	*1.8*
TURNOVER								
Apple, Bramley Cream, Sainsbury's*	1 Turnover/78g	243	13.6	312	3.9	34.3	17.4	1.3
Apple, Co-Op*	1 Turnover/77g	308	20.8	400	4	35	27	1
Apple, Puff Pastry, Bakery, Tesco*	1 Turnover/83g	263	13	317	4.3	38.6	15.7	1.8
Raspberry, Fresh Cream, Asda*	1 Turnover/100g	411	23	411	6	45	23	2.1
Raspberry, Fresh Cream, Tesco*	1 Turnover/74g	244	15.6	330	4.4	29.9	21.1	1.6
TWIGLETS								
Original, Jacob's*	1 Sm Bag/25g	104	3	414	13.3	57.3	12	11.5
TWIRL								
Cadbury*	1 Finger/22g	118	6.8	535	7.6	56	30.9	0.8
Treat Size, Cadbury*	1 Bar/21g	115	6.6	535	7.6	56	30.9	0.8
TWIX								
'Xtra, Mars*	1 Pack/85g	416	20.1	490	4.7	65.5	23.7	1.5
Fun Size, Mars*	1 Bar/20g	99	4.8	495	4.5	64.6	24	1.5
Standard, Mars*	1 Pack/58g	284	13.7	490	4.7	65.5	23.7	1.5
Top, Mars*	1 Bar/28g	143	7.8	511	5.2	60.2	27.7	0
TZATZIKI								
Average	*1 Tbsp/15g*	*11*	*0.8*	*76*	*3.4*	*3.4*	*5.5*	*0.2*

T

	Measure INFO/WEIGHT	per Measure KCAL	FAT	Nutrition Values per 100g / 100ml KCAL	PROT	CARB	FAT	FIBRE
VANILLA								
Bean, Average	*1 Pod/2g*	*6*	*0*	*288*	*0*	*13*	*0*	*0*
VANILLA EXTRACT								
Average	*1 Tbsp/13g*	*37*	*0*	*288*	*0.1*	*12.6*	*0.1*	*0*
VEAL								
Chop, Loin, Raw, Weighed with Bone, Average	*1 Chop/195g*	*317*	*17.8*	*163*	*18.9*	*0*	*9.1*	*0*
Diced, Lean, British, Waitrose*	1 Pack/275g	300	7.4	109	21.1	0	2.7	0
Escalope, Breaded, M&S*	1 Escalope/130g	292	13.9	225	13.6	18.7	10.7	0.4
Escalope, Fried, Average	*1oz/28g*	*55*	*1.9*	*196*	*33.7*	*0*	*6.8*	*0*
Mince, Raw, Average	*1oz/28g*	*40*	*2*	*144*	*20.3*	*0*	*7*	*0*
Shoulder, Lean & Fat, Roasted, Average	*1oz/28g*	*41*	*1.8*	*145*	*20.1*	*0*	*6.5*	*0*
Shoulder, Lean Only, Roasted, Average	*1oz/28g*	*35*	*1.3*	*125*	*19.9*	*0*	*4.4*	*0*
Sirloin, Lean & Fat, Roasted, Average	*1oz/28g*	*43*	*2.2*	*152*	*18.9*	*0*	*7.8*	*0*
Sirloin, Lean Only, Roasted, Average	*1oz/28g*	*33*	*1.2*	*118*	*18.4*	*0*	*4.4*	*0*
VEGAN								
Fillets, Quorn*	1 Fillet/63g	58	0.4	92	14.2	3.5	0.6	7.8
NoChicken, Chunks, The Vegetarian Butcher*	½ Pack/80g	131	3.8	164	21.4	4.7	4.8	8
Pieces, Vegan, Quorn*	¼ Pack/76g	79	1.1	104	16	4.3	1.4	5.3
Strips, No Chick, Iceland*	½ Pack/160g	200	5	125	19	0.8	3.1	7.4
VEGEMITE								
Australian, Kraft*	1 Tsp/5g	9	0	173	23.5	19.7	0	0
VEGETABLE CHIPS								
As Sold, Aunt Bessie's*	1 Serving/125g	189	11	151	2.1	13	8.8	5.3
Cassava, Average	*1oz/28g*	*99*	*0.1*	*353*	*1.8*	*91.4*	*0.4*	*4*
Oven Cooked, Aunt Bessie's*	1 Serving/125g	205	11.9	164	2.2	14	9.5	5.8
VEGETABLE FINGERS								
Crispy Crunchy, Dalepak*	1 Finger/28g	62	3.1	223	4.2	26.7	11	15
Crispy, Birds Eye*	2 Fingers/60g	107	4.8	179	3.2	23.5	8	2.3
Indian Platter, Tesco*	1 Finger/12g	24	1.4	204	3	18.4	12.2	4.7
Sainsbury's*	3 Fingers/79g	191	8.4	243	4.6	30	10.7	4.1
Sweetcorn, Tesco*	1 Finger/28g	66	3.5	236	7.7	23	12.6	3
Tesco*	1 Finger/25g	52	2.2	206	4.1	26.4	8.6	3.3
VEGETABLE MEDLEY								
Carrots, Sweetcorn, Peas, Broccoli, Four, Tesco*	¼Pack/84g	51	0.9	61	3.6	7.2	1.1	3.9
Frozen, M&S*	1 Pack/500g	175	4	35	3.4	3.9	0.8	3.1
Green, Peas, Broccoli, Beans & Leek, Mint Butter, Co-Op*	½ Pack/130g	99	5.8	76	2.9	4.2	4.5	3.7
Green, Sainsbury's*	1 Pack/220g	178	14.3	81	3	2.5	6.5	2.9
Green, with Jersey Butter, The Best, Morrisons*	½ Pack/119g	64	2.3	54	3.5	4.4	1.9	2.7
Roasted, Waitrose*	½ Pack/200g	282	15.6	141	1.2	16.4	7.8	3.7
VEGETABLE MIX								
Carrot, Broccoli, Sweetcorn, Iceland*	1 Pack/300g	150	3	50	2.5	6.1	1	3.6
Fajita, Ready to Cook, Tesco*	½ Pack/139g	82	2.4	59	1.1	8.5	1.7	2.4
Mixed Greens, Corn, Steam Bags, Tesco*	1 Bag/160g	90	1.9	56	3.9	5.4	1.2	4
Soup, Quinfresh*	1 Serving/80g	26	0.4	33	1.1	4.4	0.5	2.8
VEGETABLES								
Avocado Houmous, Boots*	1 Pot/90g	76	5.2	84	1.4	5.4	5.8	2.3
Bean, Stew Mix, Cooks' Ingredients, Waitrose*	½ Pack /200g	166	3.8	83	4.2	10.2	1.9	4.3
Haricot Bean, Cobbler, Tesco*	1 Pack/200g	255	9.9	128	3	16.5	4.9	2.5
Balls, Mushroom, Lentil, Vegetarian, Tesco*	½ Pack/131g	173	4.5	132	7.2	15	3.4	6.4
Broccoli, Leek Cabbage, Prepared Fresh, Waitrose*	1 Serving/80g	29	0.6	36	3.2	2.7	0.8	2.8
Carrots Peas, Chilled, Fresh Tastes, Asda*	1 Serving/200g	76	0.8	38	2.4	4.8	0.4	2.9
Casserole, Cooks' Ingredients, Waitrose*	¼ Pack/138g	48	0.4	35	0.9	6	0.3	2.5
Chilli Mix, Tesco*	1 Serving/50g	50	1	99	3.3	13.8	2.1	5.7
Chunky Mediterranean, Cooked, Sainsbury's*	¼ Pack/119g	56	2	47	1.1	5.9	1.7	2

VEGETABLES

Measure INFO/WEIGHT		per Measure		Nutrition Values per 100g / 100ml				
		KCAL	FAT	KCAL	PROT	CARB	FAT	FIBRE
Collard Greens, Raw, Average*	1 Serving/80g	26	0.5	32	3	5	0.6	4
Colourful, Ribbon, Stir Fry, Waitrose*	½ Pack/116g	57	2.4	49	1.3	5	2.1	2.3
Farmhouse, Mixed, Frozen, Boiled in Salted Water, Tesco*	1 Portion/80g	41	0.7	51	3.2	5.7	0.9	3.5
Grilled Mix, Frozen, Essential, Waitrose*	1 Serving/80g	34	0.2	42	1.8	8.1	0.3	2.4
Grilled, Frozen, Sainsbury's*	1 Serving/80g	42	2.9	52	1.2	3.8	3.6	1.5
Indian Spiced, HL, Tesco*	1 Pack/347g	267	5.5	77	3	11.5	1.6	2.7
Layered, Super Green, with Minted Butter, M&S*	1 Serving/80g	51	2.2	64	3.6	4.4	2.7	3.6
Layered, with Butter, Waitrose*	1 Pack/280g	207	16.2	74	1.7	3.6	5.8	2.4
Mediterranean Style, Roast, Nature's Pick, Aldi*	½ Pack/200g	114	6.4	57	1.2	5.2	3.2	1.5
Mediterranean, Ready to Roast, Waitrose*	1 Serving/200g	128	8	64	1.3	5.6	4	1.6
Medley, Tender, Green, Sainsbury's*	1 Pack/160g	62	0.8	39	2.9	4.3	0.5	3.6
Mixed, Farmhouse, Frozen, Four Seasons, Aldi*	1oz/28g	10	0.2	34	2.8	4.3	0.7	0
Peas Leeks, with a Lemon Herb Butter, Cook*	1 Portion/145g	202	17.1	139	3.1	5.3	11.8	3.2
Peas, Spinach, Spring Greens, Samphire, M&S*	½ Pack/105g	85	4.4	81	3.8	4.7	4.2	4.6
Roasted Root, Extra Special, Asda*	½ Pack/205g	160	3.1	78	1.1	15	1.5	6
Roasted Root, Ready to Roast, Mash Direct*	1 Pack/350g	200	7.4	57	0.8	5.8	2.1	5.9
Roasted, Italian, M&S*	1 Serving/95g	218	20	230	1.8	7.1	21	1.7
Roasting, with Rosemary, Thyme, Tesco*	1 Serving/100g	119	3.1	119	1.3	18	3.1	7
Root, for Mashing, Eat Fresh, Tesco*	1 Pack/720g	238	2.9	33	0.7	5.4	0.4	2.7
Root, Mashed, Microwaved, Growers Selection, Asda*	½ Pack/200g	116	4.4	58	0.7	7.2	2.2	2.7
Root, Rainbow, Collection, M&S*	½ Pack/176g	67	2.5	38	0.7	3.9	1.4	3.6
Selection, Lightly Buttered Seasoned, M&S*	½ Pack/150g	122	7.5	81	1.5	6.2	5	2.6
Selection, Roasted, COU, M&S*	1 Pack/250g	88	2	35	1.2	6.1	0.8	0.6
Stir Fry, Frozen, Sainsbury's*	1 Serving/80g	19	0.2	24	1.3	3.9	0.3	2
Stir Fry, Hot, Spicy, Natures Pick, Aldi*	1 Serving/100g	37	0.5	37	1.6	5.3	0.5	2.3
Stir Fry, Tesco*	1 Serving/150g	38	0.2	25	0.9	5	0.1	1.4
Tenderstem, Mixed Vegetables, Tesco*	1 Serving/80g	54	0.6	34	2.1	4.2	0.4	2.6
Thai Style, Aldi*	1 Serving/80g	46	1.8	57	1.9	6.1	2.2	2.4
Thai Style, Frozen, Four Seasons, Aldi*	1 Serving/100g	57	2.2	57	1.9	6.1	2.2	2.4
Vibrant, Super Bright, Stir Fry, Love Life, Waitrose*	¼ Pack/75g	37	1.2	49	2.5	5.5	1.6	12
Winter Soup Mix, Sainsbury's*	1 Portion/149g	61	0.3	41	1.1	7.9	0.2	1.7

VEGETABLES MIXED

Carrot, Cauliflower, Broccoli, Meadow Fresh, Lidl*	1 Serving/80g	213	2.7	266	13.3	38	3.3	14
Carrots, Peas, Cauliflower, & Broccoli, Frozen, Tesco*	1 Serving/80g	36	0.6	45	2.4	5.4	0.8	3.1
Mediterranean, Ovenbaked, Growers Selection, Asda*	1 Pack/400g	260	9.6	65	1.9	7.1	2.4	3.6
Mix, Steamer, Love Life, Waitrose*	1 Bag/160g	83	1.8	52	2.8	7.7	1.1	2.8
Mixed, Baby, Steam, Fresh, Tesco*	1 Pack/160g	72	1.3	45	2.7	6.7	0.8	3.8
Mixed, Bag, M&S*	1 Serving/200g	70	0.4	35	2.9	5.6	0.2	0
Mixed, Broccoli Cauliflower Florets, Baby Carrots, Asda*	1 Serving/113g	28	0.7	25	2.2	2.6	0.6	2.4
Mixed, Broccoli, Peas Green Beans, Co-Op*	1 Serving/80g	36	0.3	45	4.8	3.8	0.4	3.6
Mixed, Broccoli, Sweetcorn & Peas, Rice, Birds Eye*	1 Bag/160g	181	5.3	113	3.5	17.3	3.3	2.1
Mixed, Carrot, Cauliflower Broccoli, Prepared, Co-Op*	1 Pack/250g	100	1.5	40	2.4	5	0.6	2.7
Mixed, Carrot, Cauliflower, Broccoli, Fresh, Tesco*	1 Serving/80g	26	0.2	32	2.6	3.9	0.2	2.8
Mixed, Carrots, Broccoli & Sweetcorn, Sainsbury's*	1 Pack/120g	67	1.4	56	2.6	8.7	1.2	2
Mixed, Carrots, Broccoli Sweetcorn, Steam Veg, Tesco*	1 Sachet/160g	80	1.8	50	2.5	7.5	1.1	3
Mixed, Carrots, Cauliflower Broccoli, Waitrose*	1 Serving/80g	32	0.5	40	2.4	4.9	0.6	2.9
Mixed, Carrots, Peas, Green Beans & Sweetcorn, Tesco*	1 Serving/80g	45	0.6	56	3.1	7.3	0.7	3.9
Mixed, Casserole with Baby Potatoes, Fresh, M&S*	½ Pack/350g	140	1	40	1.2	7.8	0.3	2.1
Mixed, Casserole, Tesco*	1 Serving/80g	35	0.2	44	1	7.9	0.3	2.7
Mixed, Fresh, Asda*	1oz/28g	7	0.2	26	1.9	3	0.7	1
Mixed, Freshly Frozen, Asda*	1 Serving/80g	42	0.6	52	3.2	8	0.8	3
Mixed, Freshly Frozen, Iceland*	1 Serving/100g	54	0.8	54	3.3	8.3	0.8	3.7
Mixed, Frozen, Cooked, Sainsbury's*	1 Serving/80g	45	0.6	56	2.9	7.5	0.7	4

V

	Measure INFO/WEIGHT	per Measure KCAL	FAT	Nutrition Values per 100g / 100ml KCAL	PROT	CARB	FAT	FIBRE
VEGETABLES MIXED								
Mixed, Layered, Classics, M&S*	½ Pack/160g	112	6.2	70	1.2	7.3	3.9	1.2
Mixed, Peas Carrots, Buttery Tender, Tesco*	½ Pack/150g	138	6.1	92	3.7	7.9	4.1	4.5
Mixed, Roast, Four Seasons*	1 Serving/187g	79	0.4	42	1.2	8.8	0.2	0
Mixed, Special, Sainsbury's*	1 Serving/120g	68	1.2	57	3.2	8.9	1	2.9
Peas, Sweetcorn, Broccoli, Spinach, Steam Bags, Ocado*	1 Bag/153g	121	1.1	79	3.5	13	0.7	3.2
Red Pepper, Butternut, Courgette, Red Onion, M&S*	½ Pack/143g	48	0.3	34	1.2	5.9	0.2	1.9
Roasting, Selection, Sweet Colourful, Waitrose*	½ Pack/300g	147	3	49	1	7.5	1	2.8
VEGETARIAN								
Mixed Vegie Bites, Australian Eatwell*	½ Pack/112g	171	1.5	153	6	22	1.3	6.5
Nut Date Roast with Gravy, Asda*	1 Serving/196g	300	12.7	153	4.7	16.1	6.5	5.5
Schnitzel, Breaded, Tivall*	1 Schnitzel/100g	202	9.5	202	16	11	9.5	4
Slices, Sage Onion, Vegi Deli, The Redwood Co*	1 Slice/10g	23	1.4	233	21.4	5	14.1	0.5
Slices, Vegetable, Tesco*	1 Slice/165g	452	30.5	274	5.6	21.4	18.5	3.3
Smokey BBQ Pulled Veggie, Vivera*	½ Pack/88g	98	0.4	111	14.6	10	0.4	4.4
Steak, Beef Style, Quorn*	1 Steak/86g	126	4.5	146	16	5.3	5.2	6.9
Steak, Vivera*	1 Steak/100g	222	13	222	17	7.8	13	3.6
VEGETARIAN MINCE								
Chicken Style Pieces, Realeat*	¼ Pack/88g	119	1.4	136	29	1.5	1.6	4.4
Easy Cook, Linda McCartney*	1oz/28g	35	0.1	126	21.4	9.3	0.4	1.7
Frozen, Meatfree, Improved Recipe, Sainsbury's*	1 Serving/77g	131	3.9	170	18.6	11.7	5	2
Meat Free, Boiled, CBY, Asda*	1 Serving/75g	83	2.5	111	13.7	6.7	3.3	4.4
Simply, Garden Gourmet*	1 Serving/80g	119	2.4	149	19.3	6.9	3	8.8
Vegan, Meat Free, Ocado*	¼ Pack/128g	115	0.6	90	15	3.7	0.5	5.8
Vegemince, Realeat*	1 Serving/125g	218	12.5	174	18	3	10	3
Vegetarian, Mince, Frozen Chilled, Quorn*	1 Serving/87g	91	1.7	105	14.5	4.5	2	5.5
Vivera*	1 Pack/220g	240	0.2	109	21	3.3	0.1	5.9
VENISON								
Grill Steak, Average	*1 Steak/150g*	*178*	*3.8*	*119*	*19*	*5*	*2.5*	*1*
in Red Wine Port, Average	*1oz/28g*	*21*	*0.7*	*76*	*9.8*	*3.5*	*2.6*	*0.4*
Minced, Cooked, Average	*1 Serving/100g*	*187*	*8.2*	*187*	*26.4*	*0*	*8.2*	*0*
Minced, Raw, Average	*1 Serving/100g*	*157*	*7.1*	*157*	*21.8*	*0*	*7.1*	*0*
Raw, Haunch, Meat Only, Average	*1 Serving/100g*	*103*	*1.6*	*103*	*22.2*	*0*	*1.6*	*0*
Roasted, Average	*1oz/28g*	*46*	*0.7*	*165*	*35.6*	*0*	*2.5*	*0*
Steak, Raw, Average	*1oz/28g*	*30*	*0.5*	*108*	*22.8*	*0*	*1.9*	*0*
VERMICELLI								
Dry	*1oz/28g*	*99*	*0.1*	*355*	*8.7*	*78.3*	*0.4*	*0*
Egg, Cooked, Average	*1 Serving/185g*	*239*	*2.6*	*129*	*5*	*24*	*1.4*	*1*
VERMOUTH								
Dry	*1 Shot/50ml*	*54*	*0*	*109*	*0.1*	*3*	*0*	*0*
Sweet	*1 Shot/50ml*	*76*	*0*	*151*	*0*	*15.9*	*0*	*0*
VIMTO*								
Cordial, No Added Sugar, Diluted, Vimto*	1 Glass/250ml	6	0.2	2	0.1	0.4	0.1	0
Cordial, No Added Sugar, Undiluted, Vimto*	1 Serving/50ml	2	0	4	0	0.7	0	0
Cordial, Original, Diluted, Vimto*	1 Serving/200ml	60	0	30	0	7.4	0	0
Cordial, Original, Undiluted, Vimto*	1 Serving/50ml	49	0	98	0	23.6	0	0
Grape, Blackcurrant Raspberry Drink, Fizzy, Vimto*	1 Can/330ml	147	0	44	0	11	0	0
Mango, Strawberry Pineapple, Remix, Diluted, Vimto*	1 Serving/200ml	4	0	2	0	0.2	0	0
Raspberry, Orange & Passionfruit, Remix, Vimto*	1 Serving/200ml	4	0	2	0	0.2	0	0
Still, Vimto*	1 Bottle/500ml	95	0	19	0	4.8	0	0
VINAIGRETTE								
Balsamic Vinegar & Pistachio, Finest, Tesco*	1 Tbsp/15ml	56	5.9	370	0.2	2.8	39.2	0
Balsamic, Hellmann's*	1 Tbsp/15ml	12	0.4	82	0.1	9.6	2.7	0.6
Cider Vinegar, Maille*	1 Tsp/5ml	20	2	400	0.5	7	40	0

V

	Measure INFO/WEIGHT	per Measure KCAL	per Measure FAT	Nutrition Values per 100g / 100ml KCAL	PROT	CARB	FAT	FIBRE
VINAIGRETTE								
Fat Free, Hellmann's*	1 Serving/15ml	8	0	50	0.1	11	0	0.3
French Style, Finest, Tesco*	1 Tbsp/15ml	93	9.8	620	0.6	6.3	65.3	0.2
French, Real, Briannas*	2 Tbsp/30ml	150	17	500	0	0	56.7	0
Luxury French, Hellmann's*	1 Tsp/5ml	15	1.3	305	0.8	16	26.1	0.4
Olive Oil & Lemon, Amoy*	½ Sachet/15ml	38	3.6	250	0.3	3	24	0
PB, Waitrose*	1 Tsp/5ml	4	0	89	0.4	20.9	0.4	0.5
Raspberry, Fat Free, Love Life, Waitrose*	1 Serving/15ml	9	0.1	62	0.8	13.2	0.5	0.5
VINDALOO								
Chicken, Pilau Rice, Taste of India, Tesco*	1 Pack/427g	516	14.9	121	5.9	15.3	3.5	2.3
Chicken, Average	**1 Serving/410g**	**787**	**51.2**	**192**	**18.5**	**2.6**	**12.5**	**0.3**
Chicken, Sainsbury's*	1 Pack/400g	460	16.8	115	14.6	4.8	4.2	0.6
Chicken, Scorching Hot, Microwaved, CBY, Asda*	1 Pack/450g	414	14.4	92	7.4	7.5	3.2	1.8
Chicken, Waitrose*	1 Pack/340g	398	18.4	117	10.6	6.4	5.4	1.6
VINE LEAVES								
Stuffed with Rice	**1oz/28g**	**73**	**5**	**262**	**2.8**	**23.8**	**18**	**0**
VINEGAR								
Apple Cider, Ginger Spice, Bragg*	½ Bottle/240ml	0	0	0	0	0	0	0
Balsamic, Average	**1 Tsp/5ml**	**6**	**0**	**115**	**0.9**	**26**	**0**	**0**
Cider	**1 Tbsp/15ml**	**2**	**0**	**14**	**0**	**5.9**	**0**	**0**
Malt, Average	**1 Tbsp/15g**	**1**	**0**	**4**	**0.4**	**0.6**	**0**	**0**
Red Wine, Average	**1 Tbsp/15ml**	**3**	**0**	**19**	**0**	**0.3**	**0**	**0**
Rice Wine, Shaoxing, Waitrose*	1 Tbsp/15ml	18	0	121	1.6	4.1	0	0
VODKA								
Diet Coke, Average	**1 Serving/150ml**	**68**	**0**	**45**	**0**	**0**	**0**	**0**
Tonic, Ready Mixed, M&S*	1 Can/250ml	202	0	81	0	6.3	0	0
37.5% Volume	**1 Pub Shot/35ml**	**72**	**0**	**207**	**0**	**0**	**0**	**0**
40% Volume	**1 Pub Shot/35ml**	**78**	**0**	**222**	**0**	**0**	**0**	**0**
Bullett Cola, Premixed, Canned, Diageo*	1 Can/250ml	218	0	87	0	10.6	0	0
Cookies Cream, Sidekick, Halewood International Ltd*	1 Serving/30ml	48	0.5	160	0.3	7.7	1.6	0
Rhubarb, Average	**1 Single/25ml**	**57**	**0**	**229**	**0**	**0**	**0**	**0**
Smirnoff Cola, Premixed, canned, Diageo*	1 Can/250ml	178	0	71	0	8.9	0	0
Smirnoff Cranberry, Premixed, Canned, Diageo*	1 Can/250ml	175	0	70	0	8.5	0	0
Smirnoff Diet Cola, Premixed, Canned, Diageo*	1 Can/250ml	100	0	40	0	0	0	0
Smirnoff Schweppes Tonic, Premixed, Canned, Diageo*	1 Can/250ml	158	0	63	0	6.4	0	0
VOL AU VENTS								
Chicken & Mushroom, M&S*	1oz/28g	98	6.8	350	7.7	25.2	24.3	2.1
Deluxe, Lidl*	1 Pastry/7g	40	2.8	567	7.8	41.5	40.7	1.5
Garlic Mushroom, Mini, Asda*	1 Serving/17g	59	4.6	347	5	21	27	0
Mushroom & Roast Garlic, M&S*	1 Serving/19g	65	4.6	345	6.2	25.2	24.3	1.9
Mushroom, Sainsbury's*	1 Serving/14g	49	3.1	350	6.9	30.8	22.1	1.4
Seafood, Party, Youngs*	1 Serving/17g	60	4.2	354	8.3	26	24.8	1

Measure INFO/WEIGHT	per Measure KCAL	FAT	Nutrition Values per 100g / 100ml KCAL	PROT	CARB	FAT	FIBRE

WAFERS

	Measure	KCAL	FAT	KCAL	PROT	CARB	FAT	FIBRE
Cafe Curls, Rolled, Askeys*	1 Wafer/5g	21	0.4	422	5.8	80.3	8.6	0
Caramel Log, Tunnock's*	1 Wafer/32g	150	6.7	468	4.2	65.7	21	3.4
Caramel, Dark Chocolate, Tunnock's*	1 Wafer/26g	128	6.6	492	5.2	60.7	25.4	0
Caramel, Milk Chocolate, Basics, Sainsbury's*	1 Wafer/18g	88	3.9	489	6.2	66.5	21.6	2
Caramel, Tunnock's*	1 Wafer/26g	116	4.5	448	3.6	69.2	17.4	2.5
Chewy Caramel, Tesco*	1 Bar/28g	132	5.6	472	5	66.7	20	2.6
Filled, Average	*1oz/28g*	*150*	*8.4*	*535*	*4.7*	*66*	*29.9*	*0*
for Ice Cream, Askeys*	1 Wafer/2g	6	0	388	11.4	79	2.9	0
Hazelnut, Elledi*	1 Wafer/8g	38	1.9	493	6.3	62.4	24.3	0
Timeout, Cadbury*	1 Bar/21g	111	6	524	6.7	60	28.3	2.1

WAFFLES

Belgian Sugar, Aldi*	1 Waffle/55g	249	12.6	452	5.7	54	23	2
Belgian, TTD, Sainsbury's*	1 Waffle/25g	122	7.3	490	6	50.6	29.3	1.2
Caramel, Asda*	1 Waffle/8g	37	1.8	459	3.3	62	22	1.1
Classic, Frozen, Hello Morning, Birds Eye*	1 Waffle/30g	97	4.3	319	7	40	14	2.6
GF, Schar*	1 Waffle/25g	120	7	478	4.8	52	28	1.1
Stroopwafel, Caramel, Daelmans*	1 Wafel/29g	131	6.1	452	3	62	21	1.5
Sweet, American Style, Sainsbury's*	1 Waffle/35g	160	8.9	457	7.2	50.6	25.3	1.1
Toasting, McVitie's*	1 Waffle/25g	115	6.3	461	5.7	52.6	25.5	0.8
Toffee, Tregroes, Aldi*	1 Waffle/35g	160	6.2	463	3.5	71.7	18	2.2

WAGON WHEEL

Chocolate, Original, Epic Inside, Burton's*	1 Biscuit/39g	172	5.7	441	5.1	68.7	14.5	2.1
Jammie, Burton's*	1 Biscuit/40g	168	5.6	420	5.1	67.7	14.1	1.9

WAHOO

Fresh, Raw	*1 Serving/113g*	*110*	*1*	*97*	*23*	*0*	*0.9*	*0*

WALNUT WHIP

Classic, M&S*	1 Whip/28g	144	8.1	515	6.8	55.8	28.9	2
Nestle*	1 Whip/35g	173	8.8	494	5.3	61.3	25.2	0.7

WALNUTS

Average	*1 Nut/7g*	*48*	*4.8*	*688*	*14.7*	*3.3*	*68.5*	*3.5*
Halves, Average	*1 Half/3g*	*23*	*2.3*	*669*	*17.4*	*6.3*	*65*	*4.7*
Pickled, in Malt Vinegar, Drained, Opies*	1 Walnut/25g	23	0	92	0.8	23	0	3.4

WASABI

Paste, Ready Mixed, Japanese, Yutaka*	1 Tsp/5g	14	0.4	286	2.7	53	7	0

WATER

Apple Raspberry Flavour, Sparkling, Spar*	1 Glass/250ml	2	0	1	0	0	0	0
Apple Strawberry Flavoured, Morrisons*	1 Serving/200ml	3	0	2	0.2	0.1	0	0
Blackberry Strawberry, Sparkling, Strathmore*	1 Glass/250ml	45	0	18	0	4.3	0	0
Cactus, Truenopal*	1 Serving/330ml	30	0	9	0	2.2	0	0
Coconut, Not From Concentrate, Coco Loco, Aldi*	1 Serving/250ml	48	1.2	19	0.5	4.5	0.5	0.5
Cranberry Raspberry Flavoured, Morrisons*	1 Serving/200ml	3	0	2	0.2	0.1	0	0
Elderflower Pear, Detox, V Water*	1 Bottle/500ml	40	0	8	0	1.9	0	0
Elderflower Presse, Bottle Green*	1 Serving/250ml	88	0	35	0	8.9	0	0
Elderflower, Presse, Sparkling, M&S*	1 Bottle/330ml	99	0.3	30	0.1	7.4	0.1	0.5
Grapefruit, Slightly Sparkling, Tesco*	1 Serving/200ml	4	0	2	0	0.2	0	0
Juicy Spring, Blackcurrant Apple, Drench*	1 Serving/250ml	98	0	39	0	9.2	0	0
Lemon & Lime, Sugar Free, Touch of Fruit, Volvic*	1 Bottle/150ml	2	0	1	0	0	0	0
Lemon Lime Flavour Sparkling Spring, Co-Op*	1 Serving/200ml	2	0	1	0	0	0	0
Lemon Lime Flavoured, Strathmore*	1 Bottle/500ml	85	0	17	0	4	0	0
Lemon Lime, Sparkling, M&S*	1 Bottle/500ml	15	0	3	0	0.4	0	0
Lemon Lime, Still, M&S*	1 Bottle/500ml	5	0	1	0	0.2	0	0
Lemon, Vittel*	1 Bottle/500ml	6	0	1	0	0	0	0
Lemons Limes, Spring Water, This Juicy Water*	1 Bottle/420ml	164	0	39	0	9.7	0	0

W

	Measure INFO/WEIGHT	per Measure KCAL	per Measure FAT	Nutrition Values per 100g / 100ml KCAL	PROT	CARB	FAT	FIBRE
WATER								
Mango Lime, Carbonated, Henniez, Nestle*	1 Bottle/50ml	7	0	14	0	3.2	0	0
Mineral Or Tap	*1 Glass/200ml*	*0*	*0*	*0*	*0*	*0*	*0*	*0*
Mineral, Apple & Elderflower, Hedgerow*	1 Serving/250ml	85	0	34	0	8.2	0	0
Orange Passion Fruit, Vital V, V Water*	1 Bottle/500ml	45	0	9	0	2.1	0	0
Orange, Passionfruit, Still, Refresh'd, Robinson's*	1 Bottle/500ml	35	0	7	0	1.3	0	0
Peach & Raspberry, Still, M&S*	1 Bottle/500ml	10	0	2	0	0	0	0
Peach Orange Flavoured, Morrisons*	1 Serving/200ml	3	0	2	0.2	0.1	0	0
Peach, Slightly Sparkling, Tesco*	1 Serving/200ml	4	0	2	0	0.2	0	0
Raspberries, Blackcurrants, SPring Water, Juicy Water*	1 Bottle/420ml	155	0	37	0	9.3	0	0
Raspberry & Apple, Still, Shapers, Boots*	1 Serving/250ml	10	0	4	0	0.8	0	0
Sparkling, Fruit, Aqua Libra*	1 Glass/200ml	54	0	27	0	5.1	0	0
Sparkling, San Pellegrino*	1 Glass/200ml	0	0	0	0	0	0	0
Sparkling, Smart Price, Asda*	1 Glass/300ml	0	0	0	0	0	0	0
Sparkling, Strawberry Kiwi, Sugar Free, Perfectly Clear*	1 Glass/250ml	2	0	1	0	0	0	0
Sparkling, Strawberry Flavoured, Spring, Tesco*	1 Serving/250ml	4	0	2	0	0.2	0	0
Spring, Apple Cherry Flavoured, Sparkling, Sainsbury's*	1 Glass/250ml	5	0.2	2	0.1	0.2	0.1	0.1
Spring, Apple Mango, Sparkling, Asda*	1 Glass/200ml	2	0	1	0	0.2	0	0
Spring, Apple Raspberry, Sparkling, Tesco*	1 Glass/330ml	7	0	2	0	0.5	0	0
Spring, Cranberry Raspberry, Drench*	1 Bottle/440ml	146	0.4	33	0.1	7.7	0.1	0
Spring, Lemon Lime Flavoured, Sparkling, Sainsbury's*	1 Glass/250ml	4	0.2	2	0.1	0.1	0.1	0.1
Spring, Lemon Lime, Slightly Sparkling, Tesco*	1 Serving/200ml	4	0.2	2	0.1	0.2	0.1	0.1
Spring, Orange Passionfruit, Drench*	1 Serving/250ml	95	0.5	38	0.1	9	0.2	0
Spring, Strawberry & Aloe Vera, Botanical, M&S*	1 Bottle/500ml	5	0	1	0	0.2	0	0
Spring, Strawberry & Kiwi, Still, Shapers, Boots*	1 Glass/250ml	2	0	1	0	0.1	0	0.9
Spring, Strawberry, Sparkling, Tesco*	1 Bottle/1000g	20	0	2	0	0.2	0	0
Spring, White Grape & Blackberry, Tesco*	1 Glass/200ml	4	0	2	0	0.5	0	0
Spring, with a Hint of Orange, Slightly Sparkling, Tesco*	1 Serving/250ml	5	0	2	0	0.2	0	0
Still Raspberry Apple Spring, WaterVit, Shapers, Boots*	1 Bottle/500ml	5	0	1	0	0	0	0
Still, Cranberry Apple, Sugar Free, Blue Keld*	1 Serving/200ml	2	0	1	0	0.1	0	0
Still, Highland Spring*	1 Bottle/750ml	0	0	0	0	0	0	0
Still, Pure, Artesian, Spring, Water Within*	1 Bottle/500ml	5	0	1	0	0	0	0
Still, Raspberry Mango, Shapers, Boots*	1 Bottle/500g	5	0	1	0	0	0	0
Strawberry & Guava, Still, M&S*	1 Glass/250ml	5	0	2	0	0.1	0	0
Strawberry Kiwi, Flavoured, Loved by Us, Co-Op*	1 Serving/250ml	2	0	1	0	0	0	0
Strawberry, Original, Touch of Fruit, Volvic*	1 Bottle/500ml	99	0	20	0	4.8	0	0
Strawberry, Sugar Free, Touch of Fruit, Volvic*	1 Bottle/500ml	7	0	1	0	0.1	0	0
Tonic, Indian, Low Calorie, Vive, Aldi*	1 Serving/250ml	3	0	1	0	0	0	0
Vitamin, XXX, Triple Berry, Glaceau, Coca-Cola*	1 Bottle/500ml	65	0	13	0	3	0	0
WaterVit, Refresh Revive, Shapers, Boots*	1 Bottle/500ml	10	0	2	0	0.2	0	0
WATER CHESTNUTS								
Raw, Average	*1oz/28g*	*8*	*0*	*29*	*0.8*	*6.6*	*0*	*0.1*
with Bamboo Shoots, Sainsbury's*	1 Serving/50g	29	0.1	58	2	12	0.2	1.1
WATERCRESS								
Raw, Trimmed, Average	*1 Sprig/2.5g*	*1*	*0*	*22*	*3*	*0.4*	*1*	*1.5*
WATERMELON								
Flesh Only, Average	*1 Serving/250g*	*75*	*0.8*	*30*	*0.4*	*7*	*0.3*	*0.4*
Raw	*1 Wedge/286g*	*48*	*0.6*	*17*	*0.3*	*3.7*	*0.2*	*0.3*
Raw, Weighed with Skin, Average	*1 Wedge/286g*	*49*	*0.5*	*17*	*0.2*	*4*	*0.2*	*0.2*
WELLINGTON								
Portabello Mushroom, Vegetarian, Tesco*	¼ Pack/117g	268	12.2	229	5.1	27.6	10.4	2
Salmon, Scottish, Frozen, Finest, Tesco*	¼ Pack/157g	400	25.9	254	10	15.6	16.5	1.8
WHEAT								
Whole Grain, Split, Average	*1 Serving/60g*	*205*	*1*	*342*	*11.3*	*75.9*	*1.7*	*12.2*

W

	Measure INFO/WEIGHT	per Measure KCAL	FAT	Nutrition Values per 100g / 100ml KCAL	PROT	CARB	FAT	FIBRE
WHEAT BRAN								
Average	*1 Tbsp/7g*	*14*	*0.4*	*206*	*14.1*	*26.8*	*5.5*	*36.4*
WHEAT GERM								
Average	*1oz/28g*	*100*	*2.6*	*357*	*26.7*	*44.7*	*9.2*	*15.6*
WHELKS								
Boiled, Weighed without Shell	*1oz/28g*	*25*	*0.3*	*89*	*19.5*	*0*	*1.2*	*0*
WHISKEY								
Irish, Jameson*	1 Shot/25ml	58	0	233	0	0	0	0
Jack Daniel's*	1 Pub Shot/35ml	78	0	222	0	0	0	0
WHISKY								
37.5% Volume	*1 Pub Shot/35ml*	*72*	*0*	*207*	*0*	*0*	*0*	*0*
40% Volume	*1 Pub Shot/35ml*	*78*	*0*	*222*	*0*	*0*	*0*	*0*
Scots, 37.5% Volume	*1 Pub Shot/35ml*	*72*	*0*	*207*	*0*	*0*	*0*	*0*
Scots, 40% Volume	*1 Pub Shot/35ml*	*78*	*0*	*224*	*0*	*0*	*0*	*0*
Teacher's*	1 Pub Shot/35ml	78	0	222	0	0	0	0
WHITE PUDDING								
Average	*1oz/28g*	*126*	*8.9*	*450*	*7*	*36.3*	*31.8*	*0*
WHITEBAIT								
in Flour, Fried	*1oz/28g*	*147*	*13.3*	*525*	*19.5*	*5.3*	*47.5*	*0.2*
Raw, Average	*1 Serving/100g*	*172*	*11*	*172*	*18.3*	*0*	*11*	*0*
WHITING								
in Crumbs, Fried in Blended Oil	*1 Serving/180g*	*344*	*18.5*	*191*	*18.1*	*7*	*10.3*	*0.2*
Raw	*1oz/28g*	*23*	*0.2*	*81*	*18.7*	*0*	*0.7*	*0*
Steamed	*1 Serving/85g*	*78*	*0.8*	*92*	*20.9*	*0*	*0.9*	*0*
WIENER SCHNITZEL								
Average	*1oz/28g*	*62*	*2.8*	*223*	*20.9*	*13.1*	*10*	*0.4*
WINE								
Diet, Lambrini*	1 Glass/125ml	29	0	23	0	0	0	0
Fruit, Average	*1 Glass/125ml*	*115*	*0*	*92*	*0*	*5.5*	*0*	*0*
Light, made with Italian Pinot Grigio, First Cape*	1 Serving/125ml	51	0	41	0	0	0	0
Madeira, Henriques Henriques*	1 Glass/100ml	130	0	130	0	0	0	0
Mulled, Homemade, Average	*1 Glass/125ml*	*245*	*0*	*196*	*0.1*	*25.2*	*0*	*0*
Mulled, Sainsbury's*	1 Glass/125ml	112	0	90	0	8.6	0	0
Mulled, Vinglogg, Average*	1 Glass/125ml	162	0	130	0	14	0	0
Original, Lambrini*	1 Glass/125ml	88	0	70	0	0	0	0
Red, Alcohol Free, Winemakers' Selection, Sainsbury's*	1 Glass/125ml	32	0	26	0.5	6	0	0.5
Red, Amarone, Average	*1 Glass/125ml*	*120*	*0*	*96*	*0.1*	*3*	*0*	*0*
Red, Average	*1 Glass/125ml*	*104*	*0*	*83*	*0*	*2*	*0*	*0*
Red, Burgundy, 12.9% Abv, Average	*1 Glass/125ml*	*110*	*0*	*88*	*0.1*	*3.7*	*0*	*0*
Red, Cabernet Sauvignon, 13.1% Abv, Average	*1 Glass/125ml*	*105*	*0*	*84*	*0.1*	*2.6*	*0*	*0*
Red, Cabernet Sauvignon, Non Alcoholic, Eisberg*	1 Glass/125ml	26	0	21	0	4.5	0	0
Red, California, Blossom Hill*	1 Glass/175ml	132	0	75	0	0.9	0	0
Red, Claret, 12.8% Abv, Average	*1 Glass/125ml*	*105*	*0*	*84*	*0.1*	*3*	*0*	*0*
Red, Gamay, 12.3% Abv, Average	*1 Glass/125ml*	*99*	*0*	*79*	*0.1*	*2.4*	*0*	*0*
Red, Merlot, 13.3% Abv, Average	*1 Glass/125ml*	*105*	*0*	*84*	*0.1*	*2.5*	*0*	*0*
Red, Non Alcoholic, Ame*	1 Glass/125ml	42	0	34	0	5.7	0	0
Red, Petit Sirah, 13.5% Abv, Average	*1 Glass/125ml*	*108*	*0*	*86*	*0.1*	*2.7*	*0*	*0*
Red, Pinot Noir, 13% Abv, Average	*1 Glass/125ml*	*104*	*0*	*83*	*0.1*	*2.3*	*0*	*0*
Red, Sangiovese, 13.6% Abv, Average	*1 Glass/125ml*	*109*	*0*	*87*	*0.1*	*2.6*	*0*	*0*
Red, Syrah, 13.1% Abv, Average	*1 Glass/125ml*	*105*	*0*	*84*	*0.1*	*2.6*	*0*	*0*
Red, Willow Stone*	1 Serving/200ml	127	0	63	0	1.7	0	0
Red, Zinfandel, 13.9% Abv, Average	*1 Glass/125ml*	*111*	*0*	*89*	*0.1*	*2.9*	*0*	*0*
Rose, Alcohol Free, Eisberg*	1 Glass/200ml	52	0	26	0	5.9	0	0
Rose, Garnacha, Low Alcohol	*1 Glass/125ml*	*58*	*0*	*46*	*0*	*10.9*	*0*	*0*

W

	Measure INFO/WEIGHT	per Measure KCAL	FAT	Nutrition Values per 100g / 100ml KCAL	PROT	CARB	FAT	FIBRE
WINE								
Rose, Medium, Average	*1 Glass/125ml*	*98*	*0*	*79*	*0*	*2.1*	*0*	*0*
Rose, Muscat, Non Alcoholic, Co-Op*	1 Serving/200ml	88	0	44	0	11	0	0
Rose, Sparkling, Average	*1 Glass/125ml*	*102*	*0*	*82*	*0*	*2.5*	*0*	*0*
Rose, The Pink Chill, Co-Op*	1 Glass/125ml	85	0	68	0	0	0	0
Rose, White Grenache, Blossom Hill*	1 Glass/125ml	105	0	84	0	3.2	0	0
Rose, White Zinfandel, Ernest Julio Gallo*	1 Glass/125ml	101	0	81	0.2	2.7	0	0
Sangria, Average	*1 Glass/125ml*	*95*	*0*	*76*	*0.1*	*9.9*	*0*	*0.1*
Sauvignon Blanc, Low Alcohol, Featherweight*	1 Serving/200ml	88	0	44	0	0	0	0
Strong Ale Barley	*1 Can/440ml*	*290*	*0*	*66*	*0.7*	*6.1*	*0*	*0*
Vie, Rose, Low Alcohol, Blossom Hill*	1 Glass/175ml	93	0	53	0	3.9	0	0
White, Average	*1 Glass/125ml*	*95*	*0*	*76*	*0*	*2.4*	*0*	*0*
White, Chardonnay, Southern Australia, Kissing Tree*	1 Bottle/185ml	85	0	46	0	0	0	0
White, Chenin Blanc, 12% Abv, Average	*1 Glass/125ml*	*101*	*0*	*81*	*0.1*	*3.3*	*0*	*0*
White, Dry, Average	*1 Glass/125ml*	*88*	*0*	*70*	*0.1*	*0.6*	*0*	*0*
White, Fume Blanc, 13.1% Abv, Average	*1 Glass/125ml*	*104*	*0*	*83*	*0.1*	*2.3*	*0*	*0*
White, Gewurztraminer, 12.6% Abv, Average	*1 Glass/125ml*	*102*	*0*	*82*	*0.1*	*2.6*	*0*	*0*
White, Late Harvest, 10.6% Abv, Average	*1 Glass/125ml*	*141*	*0*	*113*	*0.1*	*13.4*	*0*	*0*
White, Medium, Average	*1 Glass/125ml*	*92*	*0*	*74*	*0.1*	*3*	*0*	*0*
White, Muller-Thurgau, 11.3% Abv, Average	*1 Glass/125ml*	*96*	*0*	*77*	*0.1*	*3.5*	*0*	*0*
White, Muscat, 11% Abv, Average	*1 Glass/125ml*	*104*	*0*	*83*	*0.1*	*5.2*	*0*	*0*
White, Pinot Blanc, 13.3% Abv, Average	*1 Glass/125ml*	*102*	*0*	*82*	*0.1*	*0*	*0*	*0*
White, Pinot Grigio, 13.4% Abv, Average	*1 Glass/125ml*	*105*	*0*	*84*	*0.1*	*2.1*	*0*	*0*
White, Pinot Grigio, Wave Break, 12% Abv, M&S*	1 Glass/125ml	89	0	71	0	0	0	0
White, Riesling, 11.9% Abv, Average	*1 Glass/125ml*	*101*	*0*	*81*	*0.1*	*3.7*	*0*	*0*
White, Sauvignon Blanc, 13.1% Abv, Average	*1 Glass/125ml*	*102*	*0*	*82*	*0.1*	*2*	*0*	*0*
White, Semillon, 12.5% Abv, Average	*1 Glass/125ml*	*104*	*0*	*83*	*0.1*	*3.1*	*0*	*0*
White, Sparkling, Average	*1 Glass/125ml*	*92*	*0*	*74*	*0.3*	*5.1*	*0*	*0*
White, Sweet, Average	*1 Glass/120ml*	*113*	*0*	*94*	*0.2*	*5.9*	*0*	*0*
WINE GUMS								
Average	*1 Sweet/6g*	*19*	*0*	*315*	*5*	*73.4*	*0.2*	*0.1*
Haribo*	1 Pack/175g	609	0.4	348	0.1	86.4	0.2	0.4
Mini, Rowntree's*	1 Sm Bag/36g	125	0	348	6.7	80.5	0	0
Sour, Bassett's*	¼ Bag/50g	160	0	319	3.7	78	0	0
WISPA								
Cadbury*	1 Bar/40g	220	13.6	550	7.3	52.5	34	1
Gold, Cadbury*	1 Bar/52g	265	15.1	510	5.3	56	29	0.7
WONTON								
Prawn, Crispy from Selection, Modern Asian, M&S*	1 Wonton/25g	65	3.3	250	9.5	23.4	12.7	2
Prawn, Dim Sum Selection, Sainsbury's*	1 Wonton/10g	26	1.2	259	11.3	26.8	11.8	1.3
Prawn, Oriental Selection, Waitrose*	1 Wonton/18g	45	2	252	9.1	29.2	11	1.1
Prawn, Oriental Snack Selection, Sainsbury's*	1 Wonton/20g	53	2.7	265	10.6	25.6	13.4	2
Vegetable, Sweet Sour, Tesco*	1 Wonton/14g	39	1.9	281	4.5	33.6	13.5	3.6
WOTSITS								
Baked, Really Cheesy, Walkers*	1 Bag/23g	123	7.4	546	5.5	56	33	1.1
Really Cheesy, Big Eat, Walkers*	1 Bag/36g	197	11.9	547	5.5	56	33	1.1
WRAP								
Bean, Spicy, with Cheese, Tesco*	1 Pack/198g	423	15.8	213	7.6	25.8	8	3.9
Carrot, & Pastrami, Inspired, Wicked Kitchen, Tesco*	1 Pack/265g	389	15.1	147	4	18.5	5.7	2.9
Cheese, Bean, Tesco*	1 Pack/105g	235	9.4	224	7	28.6	9	1
Chicken, & Bacon, Caesar, Just Tasty, Aldi*	1 Pack/196g	459	18	234	12.8	24	9.2	1.5
Chicken, Bacon, Caesar Salad, Asda*	1 Pack/160g	565	35.2	353	18	20.8	22	0.9
Chicken, Bacon, Caesar, COU, M&S*	1 Pack/205g	607	31	296	13.3	26	15.1	1.3
Chicken, Bacon, Simple Solutions, Tesco*	1 Pack/300g	474	23.4	158	20.7	1.2	7.8	0.5

W

WRAP

INFO/WEIGHT	Measure	per Measure		Nutrition Values per 100g / 100ml				
		KCAL	FAT	KCAL	PROT	CARB	FAT	FIBRE
Chicken, Bacon, Tesco*	1 Pack/175g	448	19.8	256	13.8	23.9	11.3	1.8
Chicken, BBQ, No Mayo, Tesco*	1 Pack/154g	353	8.6	229	12.2	31.7	5.6	1.7
Chicken, BBQ, Shapers, Boots*	1 Wrap/156g	278	4.5	178	11	26	2.9	1.8
Chicken, Caesar, Ginsters*	1 Pack/180g	440	21.1	244	11.1	23.5	11.7	1.8
Chicken, Cajun, Sandwich King*	1 Pack/138g	386	19.9	279	12.3	25	14.4	0
Chicken, Cajun, Tesco*	1 Pack/175g	310	10	177	6.3	24.6	5.7	1.1
Chicken, Coronation , Waitrose*	1 Pack/164g	283	8.3	173	10.1	21.3	5.1	2.2
Chicken, Curry, Thai Green, Tesco*	1 Pack/175g	390	14.9	223	9.3	26.5	8.5	1.9
Chicken, Fajita, M&S*	1 Pack/213g	394	15.1	185	8.8	20.1	7.1	2.5
Chicken, Fajita, Morrisons*	1 Pack/214g	430	16.5	201	9.5	22.5	7.7	1.9
Chicken, Fajita, Omelette, Tesco*	1 Pack/161g	289	16.6	179	16.7	4	10.3	1.5
Chicken, Fajita, PB, Waitrose*	1 Serving/218g	368	5.7	169	10.5	26	2.6	1.9
Chicken, Fillets, with Cheese, Bacon, Asda*	1 Pack/164g	366	21.3	223	25	1.4	13	0
Chicken, Korma, Rainbow, Co-Op*	1 Wrap/198g	348	8.5	176	8.6	24	4.3	2.4
Chicken, Lemon, Garlic, Tesco*	1 Pack/185g	411	14.6	222	10.1	27.2	7.9	1.1
Chicken, Lemon, Herb, Delicious, Boots*	1 Pack/173g	351	13.1	203	7.9	24	7.6	3
Chicken, M&S*	1 Pack/247g	530	24.9	215	8.2	23.4	10.1	1.6
Chicken, Mexican Style, Co-Op*	1 Pack/163g	367	14.7	225	11	26	9	3
Chicken, Moroccan, BGTY, Sainsbury's*	1 Pack/207g	315	3.1	152	9.4	25.3	1.5	0
Chicken, Piri Piri, No Mayonnaise, Tesco*	1 Pack/185g	352	9.3	190	8.6	26.6	5	2.1
Chicken, Salad, Free From Gluten, CBY, Asda*	1 Pack/187g	352	11	188	9.6	23	5.9	2.3
Chicken, Salad, Roast, Sainsbury's*	1 Pack/214g	443	19.9	207	10	20.9	9.3	2.5
Chicken, Southern Fried, CBY, Asda*	1 Pack/210g	452	17	215	7.1	27	8.1	2.7
Chicken, Sweet Chilli , Sainsbury's*	1 Pack/209g	434	11.5	208	8.5	30.1	5.5	1.8
Chicken, Sweet Chilli, Shapers, Boots*	1 Pack/195g	302	3.7	155	10	24	1.9	3
Chicken, Tikka, Average	*1 Wrap/200g*	*403*	*15.1*	*202*	*9.5*	*23.6*	*7.6*	*4.4*
Duck, Hoisin, Delicious, Boots*	1 Pack/160g	295	4.3	184	11	28	2.7	2
Duck, Hoisin, GF, M&S*	1 Pack/183g	285	6	156	10.2	17.5	3.3	7.6
Duck, Hoisin, M&S*	1 Pack/225g	405	8.3	180	8.4	27.7	3.7	1.5
Duck, Hoisin, No Mayo, Tesco*	1 Pack/178g	361	10	203	9.8	27.7	5.6	1.2
Feta, Beetroot, Spiced Butternut Squash, Co-Op*	1 Pack/232g	421	17	181	5.6	22.4	7.3	1.9
Feta, Salad, Greek , Shapers, Boots*	1 Pack/158g	241	5.7	153	6.4	24	3.6	1.2
Frijoles, Spicy, Wicked Kitchen, Tesco*	1 Pack/238g	431	14	181	4.3	26.2	5.9	2.8
Ham, Mozzarella, Smoked, Soft Olive Oil Wrap, M&S*	1 Pack/203g	465	14	229	10.3	30.4	6.9	1.9
Ham, Cheese, Pickle Tortilla, Weight Watchers*	1 Pack/170g	296	4.8	174	10.9	26.4	2.8	1.2
Lamb, Minted, Darwins Deli*	1 Pack/250g	287	6.3	115	3.2	19.9	2.5	0
Pork, Mexican, Tesco*	1 Pack/237g	448	17.3	189	7.9	22	7.3	1.6
Pork, Pulled, Mexican Spiced, Good to Go, Waitrose*	1 Pack/189g	339	14.2	179	7.2	19.8	7.5	1.8
Prawn, Sweet Chilli, King, M&S*	1 Pack/155g	225	3.1	145	8	24.2	2	2.1
Salmon, Smoked, Prawn, Finest, Tesco*	1 Serving/59g	84	5.3	143	14.3	1	9.1	0
Sausage, Bacon, Cooked, Sainsbury's*	1 Wrap/12g	38	2.6	315	17.7	12.1	21.7	0
Soft Cheese, Spinach, to Go*	1 Serving/250g	278	6.7	111	4.5	17.4	2.7	0
Sushi Rice, & Vegetables, Japanese, Vegan, Morrisons*	1 Pack/189g	401	9.8	212	5.1	32.5	5.2	2.2
Tuna, Sweetcorn, Red Pepper, BGTY, Sainsbury's*	1 Pack/178g	306	8.2	172	11.5	21.2	4.6	2.1
Turkey, Bacon, Cranberry, COU, M&S*	1 Pack/144g	230	2.2	160	9.6	27.1	1.5	2.3
Turkey, Feast, Sainsbury's*	1 Pack/212g	502	18.2	237	11.3	27.6	8.6	1.8
Turkey, Ranch, & Bacon, Roast, Arby's*	1 Wrap/279g	620	31	222	13.3	14	11.1	1.4

W

	Measure INFO/WEIGHT	per Measure KCAL	FAT	Nutrition Values per 100g / 100ml KCAL	PROT	CARB	FAT	FIBRE
YAM								
Baked	**1oz/28g**	**43**	**0.1**	**153**	**2.1**	**37.5**	**0.4**	**1.7**
Boiled, Average	**1oz/28g**	**37**	**0.1**	**133**	**1.7**	**33**	**0.3**	**1.4**
Raw	**1oz/28g**	**26**	**0.1**	**92**	**1.2**	**22.8**	**0.2**	**1.1**
YEAST								
Extract	**1 Tsp/9g**	**16**	**0**	**180**	**40.7**	**3.5**	**0.4**	**0**
Extract, Reduced Salt, Sainsbury's*	1 Tsp/4g	10	0	246	41.2	17.6	0.5	4.3
Flakes, Nutritional, Whole Food Earth*	1 Tbsp/5g	17	0.2	341	53	34.8	5	21
Quick, Doves Farm*	1 Serving/8g	24	0.5	301	43.5	19	5.7	27
YOGHURT								
0.1% Fat, Lidl*	1 Pot/150g	118	0.2	79	4	15.6	0.1	0
Activia, Danone*	1 Pot/132g	125	4.2	94	3.5	12.8	3.2	2
After Dinner Mint, Limited Edition, Mullerlight, Muller*	1 Pot/165g	91	0.8	55	4.3	7.6	0.5	0
Apple, & Berry Pie, Dessert Recipe, Weight Watchers*	1 Pot/120g	58	0.1	49	4.1	6.8	0.1	0.3
Apple, & Peach, Bircher Muesli, Moma Foods*	1 Pot/170g	224	4.1	132	4.3	24.3	2.4	1.7
Apple, & Pear, Low Fat, Sainsbury's*	1 Pot/125g	115	1.9	92	4.3	15.2	1.5	0.2
Apple, & Prune, Fat Free, Yeo Valley*	1 Pot/125g	98	0.1	78	5.1	14.1	0.1	0.2
Apple, Quince, Spiced, Yeo Valley*	¼ Pot/113g	115	4.3	102	4.6	12.3	3.8	0
Apple, Spiced, 6% Fat, TTD, Sainsbury's*	1 Pot/15g	16	0.6	107	2.7	15.6	3.8	0.5
Apricot, & Mango, Thick & Creamy, Sainsbury's*	1 Pot/150g	178	5.4	119	4.3	17.3	3.6	0.2
Apricot, & Passion Fruit, Fat Free, Yeo Valley*	1 Pot/125g	94	0.1	75	5.3	13.2	0.1	0.1
Apricot, Bio Activia, Danone*	1 Pot/125g	121	4	97	3.7	13.3	3.2	1.7
Apricot, Fat Free, Weight Watchers*	1 Pot/110g	45	0.1	41	4	5	0.1	0.2
Apricot, Low Fat, Brooklea, Aldi*	1 Pot/125g	99	1	79	2.8	15.1	0.8	0
Apricot, Low Fat, Sainsbury's*	1 Pot/124g	108	1.6	87	4.2	14.3	1.3	0.5
Apricot, Low Fat, Tesco*	1 Pot/125g	112	2.2	90	4.3	14.1	1.8	0
Banana, & Custard, Smooth, Mullerlight, Muller*	1 Pot/175g	94	0.2	54	4.1	8.6	0.1	0.6
Banana, & Custard, Yeo Valley*	1 Serving/100g	109	4.3	109	4.6	13	4.3	0
Banana, Choco Flakes, Crunch Corner, Muller*	1 Pot/135g	193	6.9	143	4.3	19.3	5.1	0.3
Banana, Low Fat, Average	**1 Serving/100g**	**98**	**1.4**	**98**	**4.6**	**16.7**	**1.4**	**0.1**
Banoffee, Snackpot, Activia, Danone*	1 Pot/155g	116	0.2	75	5	13.3	0.1	0.3
Berry, & Apple, Low Fat, Breakfast Pot, Tesco*	1 Pot/215g	233	2.6	108	0	14.5	1.2	2.4
Bio, Low Fat, Spelga*	1 Pot/125g	125	2.1	100	3.9	17	1.7	0
Blackberry, & Raspberry, Fruit Corner, Muller*	1 Pot/150g	158	5.8	105	3.8	13.1	3.9	0.9
Blackberry, Soya, Alpro*	1 Pot/125g	94	2.4	75	3.6	9.7	1.9	1.1
Blackberry, Wild, Seriously Fruity, Waitrose*	1 Pot/125g	120	1.3	96	4.4	17.2	1	0.4
Blackcurrant, Elderflower, Soya, Alpro*	1 Pot/125g	92	2.4	74	3.6	9.5	1.9	1.1
Blackcurrant, Garden Fruits, Low Fat, Tesco*	1 Pot/125g	120	2.4	95	3.8	15.1	1.9	0.3
Blackcurrant, Probiotic, Organic, Yeo Valley*	1 Pot/150g	152	5.8	101	4.1	12.4	3.9	0.2
Blackcurrant, Soya, Go On, Alpro*	1 Pot/150g	122	4.2	81	5.1	7.5	2.8	2
Blueberry, & Cream, Made Up, Easiyo*	1 Serving/100g	105	4.1	105	3.9	13.7	4.1	0
Blueberry, Blast, Skyr, Icelandic, Light & Free, Danone*	1 Pot/150g	81	0.8	54	9.1	3.8	0.5	0.5
Blueberry, Bursting, Intensely Creamy, Activia, Danone*	1 Pot/110g	112	3.3	102	5	13.4	3	0.5
Blueberry, Fruit Corner, Muller*	1 Pot/150g	156	5.7	104	3.8	12.9	3.8	0.4
Blueberry, Icelandic Style, Skyr, Brooklea, Aldi*	1 Pot/150g	122	0.8	81	7.7	12	0.5	0.5
Blueberry, Longley Farm*	1 Pot/150g	168	8	112	4.1	12.8	5.3	0
Blueberry, Protein, Arla*	1 Pot/200g	140	0.4	70	10	6.5	0.2	0
Blueberry, Soya, Alpro*	1 Pot/125g	91	2.5	73	3.6	9.4	2	1.2
Blueberry, Soya, Free From, Tesco*	1 Pot/100g	76	2.1	76	3.7	10.5	2.1	0.3
Blueberry, with Crunchy Granola, Organic, Yeo Valley*	1 Yoghurt/135g	217	7.7	161	5.6	21.1	5.7	0
Bramble, & Apple, Virtually Fat Free, Longley Farm*	1 Pot/150g	118	0.2	79	5.5	13.9	0.1	0
Caramel, Indulgent Layered, Specially Selected, Aldi*	1 Pot/150g	276	16.5	184	2.3	19	11	1.4
Caramel, Salted, Cheesecake, Greek Style Whipped, Muller	1 Pot/100g	180	7.9	180	4.2	21.8	7.9	0
Caramel, Salted, Greek Style, Luxury, Oykos, Danone*	1 Pot/110g	172	9.2	157	2.7	17.6	8.4	0

Y

YOGHURT

INFO/WEIGHT	Measure	per Measure KCAL	per Measure FAT	Nutrition Values per 100g / 100ml KCAL	PROT	CARB	FAT	FIBRE
Cereals, Fibre, Bio Activia, Danone*	1 Pot/120g	119	4.1	99	3.7	13.5	3.4	3
Cherry, Black, & Cream, The Best, Morrisons*	1 Pot/150g	218	9.4	146	3.2	19	6.3	0
Cherry, Black, 0%, Greek Style, Yeo Valley*	1 Serving/150g	108	0	72	6.6	10.7	0	0
Cherry, Black, Average	*1 Serving/100g*	*96*	*2.2*	*96*	*3.4*	*16.5*	*2.2*	*0.1*
Cherry, Black, Extremely Fruity, Bio, M&S*	1 Pot/150g	165	2.2	110	4.9	18.4	1.5	0.2
Cherry, Black, Garden Fruits, Fat Free, Benecol*	1 Pot/125g	79	0.6	63	3	11	0.5	2.1
Cherry, Black, Greek Style, Corner, Muller*	1 Pot/150g	172	4.5	115	5	16.2	3	0.1
Cherry, Black, Low Fat, Average	*1 Serving/100g*	*69*	*0.6*	*69*	*3.8*	*12.2*	*0.6*	*0.3*
Cherry, Black, Swiss, Finest, Tesco*	1 Pot/150g	195	8.8	130	3.5	15.7	5.9	0.5
Cherry, Black, Thick & Creamy, Waitrose*	1 Pot/125g	139	3.1	111	3.7	18.3	2.5	0.4
Cherry, Charmer, Greek Style, Light Free, Danone*	1 Pot/115g	59	0.1	51	4.7	7.7	0.1	0.1
Cherry, Fat Free, Activia, Danone*	1 Pot/125g	64	0.1	51	4.7	7.7	0.1	0.1
Cherry, Fruit, Biopot, Onken*	1 Serving/100g	107	2.7	107	3.7	16.7	2.7	0.2
Cherry, Fruity, Mullerlight, Muller*	1 Pot/175g	86	0.2	49	4.3	7	0.1	0.2
Cherry, Greek Style, Fruitopolis, Mullerlight, Muller*	1 Pot/130g	65	0.1	50	4.7	7.2	0.1	0
Cherry, Light, Fat Free, Muller*	1 Pot/175g	88	0.2	50	3.9	7.9	0.1	0.2
Cherry, Low Fat, CBY, Asda*	1 Pot/125g	90	1.6	72	3.6	11.4	1.3	0.3
Cherry, Luscious, Intensely Creamy, Activia, Danone*	1 Pot/110g	109	3.3	99	5	12.8	3	0.2
Cherry, Morello, Specially Selected, Aldi*	1 Pot/150g	171	7.5	114	2.5	15	5	0.5
Cherry, Red, Fruit Corner, Muller*	1 Pot/150g	158	5.8	105	3.8	13	3.9	0.5
Cherry, Red, Summer Fruits, Benecol*	1 Pot/120g	103	2	86	3.7	14	1.7	0.1
Cherry, Soya, Alpro*	1 Pot/125g	91	2.5	73	3.6	9.4	2	1.2
Coconut, & Lemon, Dairy Free, Koko*	1 Pot/125g	141	6.9	113	0.7	15.1	5.5	0.3
Coconut, & Vanilla, Greek Style, Fat Free, Brooklea, Aldi*	1 Pot/125g	74	0.6	59	5.9	7.6	0.5	0.5
Coconut, Greek Style, Brooklea, Aldi*	1 Serving/150g	212	12.9	141	3.7	12	8.6	0.5
Coconut, Greek Style, Milbona, Lidl*	1 Pot/150g	236	14.7	157	3.9	13	9.8	0.5
Coconut, Low Fat, Tesco*	1 Portion/150g	150	4	100	5	13.8	2.7	0.1
Coconut, Protein, Arla*	1 Pot/200g	144	1	72	10	6.2	0.5	0
Cranberry, Bio Activia, Danone*	1 Pot/125g	115	4	92	3.6	12.3	3.2	1.7
Fig, Bio, Activia, Danone*	1 Pot/125g	124	4.2	99	3.6	13.4	3.4	0.2
Forest Fruits, Soya, Dairy Free, Alpro*	1 Serving/100g	79	2.2	79	3.8	10.1	2.2	1.2
French, Set, Low Fat, Iceland*	1 Pot/125g	100	1.5	80	3.6	13.6	1.2	0
Fruit, Fat free, Average	*1 Sm Pot/125g*	*67*	*0.1*	*54*	*4.8*	*8.2*	*0.1*	*0.8*
Fruit, Low Fat, Average	*1 Pot/125g*	*112*	*0.9*	*90*	*4.1*	*17.9*	*0.7*	*0*
Fruity, Favourites, Organic, Yeo Valley*	1 Pot/125g	126	4.9	101	4.1	12.4	3.9	0.2
Fudge, Devonshire Style, Finest, Tesco*	1 Pot/150g	206	9.2	137	4	16.4	6.1	0.4
Fudge, Devonshire Style,, Specially Selected, Aldi*	1 Pot/150g	234	12	156	3.2	18	8	0.5
Fudge, Gourmet, Moo!, Aldi*	¼ Pot/113g	143	6.4	127	4.2	15	5.7	0.5
Ginger, Greek Style, Bio, Live, Rachel's Organic*	1 Serving/100g	137	7.4	137	3.2	14.4	7.4	0
Goat's Milk, Natural, Fat Free, St Helen's Farm*	1 Serving/150g	63	0.2	42	6	4.3	0.1	0
Goat's Milk, Natural, St Helen's Farm*	1 Serving/150g	158	11	105	5.5	4.3	7.3	0
Goats Whole Milk	*1 Carton/150g*	*94*	*5.7*	*63*	*3.5*	*3.9*	*3.8*	*0*
Gooseberry, & Elderflower, Fragrant, Creamy, Waitrose*	1 Pot/150g	188	9.9	125	2.6	13.8	6.6	0.5
Gooseberry, Garden Fruits, Low Fat, Tesco*	1 Pot/125g	115	2.4	90	3.3	14.9	1.9	0.3
Gooseberry, Low Fat, Average	*1 Serving/100g*	*90*	*1.4*	*90*	*4.5*	*14.5*	*1.4*	*0.2*
Gooseberry, Virtually Fat Free, Longley Farm*	1 Pot/150g	122	0.2	81	4.2	15.7	0.1	0
Greek Style, Fat Free, Counted, Eat Smart, Morrisons*	¼ Pot/125g	95	0.6	76	7	10.9	0.5	0
Greek Style, Low Fat, M&S*	1 Serving/100g	71	2.6	71	5.2	6.6	2.6	0.5
Greek Style, Natural, Llaeth Y Llan, Village Dairy*	½ Pot/225g	209	8.3	93	6.3	8.7	3.7	0.1
Greek Style, Natural, Milbona, Lidl*	1 Serving/150g	183	15	122	4.6	3.2	10	0
Greek Style, Natural, Organic, M&S*	1 Pot/150g	186	13.8	124	4.6	5.6	9.2	0.5
Greek Style, Raspberry, Light, Fat Free, Brooklea, Aldi*	1 Pot/125g	72	0.6	58	5.8	8.2	0.5	0.5
Greek Style, Strained, 0%, Glenisk Organic Dairy Co*	1 Pot/150g	84	0	56	10	4	0	0

YOGHURT

INFO/WEIGHT	Measure	per Measure KCAL	FAT	Nutrition Values per 100g / 100ml KCAL	PROT	CARB	FAT	FIBRE
Greek Style, Vanilla, 0% Fat, COU, M&S*	1 Pot/140g	81	0.3	58	6.8	7.2	0.2	0.5
Greek Style, Whipped, Strawberry, Bliss, Corner, Muller*	1 Pot/110g	142	6.5	129	4.1	14.3	5.9	0
Greek Style, with Blueberry Layer, Luxury, Oykos, Danone*	1 Pot/110g	152	9.4	138	2.7	12.5	8.5	0.4
Greek Style, with Honey, Tesco*	1 Pot/100g	144	8	144	4.2	13.7	8	0
Greek, 0% Fat, Strained, Authentic, Total, Fage*	1 Sm Pot/170g	92	0	54	10.3	3	0	0
Greek, 0%, Mevgal*	1 Serving/100g	52	0	52	8	5	0	0
Greek, 2% Fat, Strained, Authentic, Total, Fage*	1 Pot/170g	119	3.4	70	9.9	3	2	0
Greek, Authentic, Natural, Strained, Waitrose*	1 Serving/125g	164	12.8	131	5.9	3.7	10.2	0.3
Greek, with Blueberries, Total 0%, Total, Fage*	1 Serving/150g	123	0	82	8.3	12.3	0	0
Greek, with Espresso, Finest, Tesco*	1 Pot/150g	133	0.2	88	8.6	13.1	0.2	0
Hazelnut, Longley Farm*	1 Pot/150g	201	8.5	134	5.5	16	5.7	0
Hazelnut, Low Fat, Deliciously Nutty, Waitrose*	1 Pot/150g	153	4.2	102	6.1	12.9	2.8	0.5
Hazelnut, Sainsbury's*	1 Serving/150g	183	3.4	122	5	20.3	2.3	0.2
Homey, Icelandic Style, Strained, Fat Free, Skyr, Arla*	1 Serving/150g	110	0.2	73	9.4	7.8	0.1	0
Honey, & Ginger, West Country, Luxury, M&S*	1 Pot/150g	219	11.6	146	3.6	15.6	7.7	0
Honey, Breakfast Pot, Activia, Danone*	1 Pot/160g	192	4.2	120	4.9	18.8	2.6	0.7
Honey, Golden, Greek Style, Activia, Danone*	1 Pack/126g	122	3.5	97	5	13	2.8	0.1
Honey, Greek Style, 0% Fat, Tesco*	1/3 Pot/150g	122	0.3	81	6.8	13.1	0.2	0
Honey, Greek Style, Milbona, Lidl*	1 Yoghurt/100g	145	8.3	145	3.8	13.5	8.3	0.5
Honey, Greek Style, Morrisons*	1/3 Pot/150g	236	14.3	157	4.1	13.5	9.5	0.7
Honey, Greek Style, Strained, 0% Fat, Liberte, Yoplait*	1 Pot/100g	92	0.1	92	7.7	14.1	0.1	0.1
Kefir, Coconut, Honey, The Great Dairy Collective*	1 Serving/250g	143	6.5	57	3	8.2	2.6	0
Kefir, Natural, Organic, Yeo Valley*	1 Pot/350g	224	7.4	64	4.7	6.4	2.1	0
Kiwi, Bio, Activia, Danone*	1 Pot/125g	122	4.2	98	3.6	12.9	3.4	0.3
Latte, Skinny, Fat Free, Mullerlight, Muller*	1 Pot/165g	84	0.2	51	4.1	7.7	0.1	0
Lemon Curd, West Country, Extra Special, Asda*	1 Pot/150g	252	13	168	3.2	19	8.7	0
Lemon Curd, West Country, TTD, Sainsbury's*	1 Pot/150g	243	10	162	3.7	21.6	6.7	0.5
Lemon Curd, Whole Milk, Yeo Valley*	1 Pot/120g	149	5.3	124	4.7	16.3	4.4	0
Lemon, Cheesecake, Average	*1 Serving/100g*	*55*	*0.2*	*55*	*4.3*	*8.8*	*0.2*	*0.2*
Lemon, Greek Style, Whipped, Bliss Corner, Muller*	1 Pot/110g	177	6.5	161	4	22.2	5.9	0
Lemon, Lavish, Greek Style, Light Free, Danone*	1 Pot/115g	56	0.1	49	4.9	7.1	0.1	0.1
Lemon, Longley Farm*	1 Pot/150g	159	5.6	106	5	13.4	3.7	0
Lemon, Luscious, Greek Style, Mullerlight, Muller*	1 Pot/125g	75	0.2	60	6.3	7.5	0.2	0
Lemon, Sicilain, The Best, Morrisons*	1 Pot/150g	235	12.1	157	3.4	17.5	8.1	0
Lemon, Sicilian, Italian Dream, Corner, Muller*	1 Pot/150g	170	5.7	113	3.9	15.1	3.8	0
Low Calorie	*1 Pot/120g*	*49*	*0.2*	*41*	*4.3*	*6*	*0.2*	*0*
Mandarin, Fat Free, Mullerlight, Muller*	1 Pot/175g	95	0.2	54	4.2	8.5	0.1	0
Mandarin, Llaeth Y Llan, Village Dairy*	1 Pot/125g	130	3.5	104	5.6	14.3	2.8	0.1
Mandarin, Longley Farm*	1 Pot/150g	141	5.7	94	4.9	13.3	3.8	0
Mango, & Passion Fruit, Low Fat, Sainsbury's*	1 Pot/125g	105	1.6	84	4.2	13.5	1.3	0.5
Mango, Bio, Activia, Danone*	1 Pot/125g	124	4.2	99	3.5	13.5	3.4	0.2
Mango, Soya, Go On, Alpro*	1 Pot/150g	129	4.2	86	5	9.1	2.8	1.3
Muesli, Bircher, Summer Berry, M&S*	1 Pot/195g	277	13.1	142	3.7	15	6.7	3.4
Muesli, Nut, Low Fat	*1 Pot/120g*	*134*	*2.6*	*112*	*5*	*19.2*	*2.2*	*0*
Natural, Almond Milk, Dairy Free, Nush Foods*	1 Pot/125g	165	10	132	4	3	8	0
Natural, Bio Activia, Individual Pots, Danone*	1 Pot/125g	86	4.2	69	4.2	5.5	3.4	0
Natural, Bio Live, Low Fat, Organic, Waitrose*	¼ Pot/125g	81	1.2	65	5.8	8.3	1	0
Natural, Bio Set, Low Fat, Sainsbury's*	1 Pot/150g	78	2.2	52	3.9	5.7	1.5	0
Natural, Bio, Lancashire Farm*	3 Dstsps/40g	32	1.4	80	5.2	7	3.5	0.5
Natural, Danone*	1 Pot/125g	71	3.6	57	3.2	3.8	2.9	0
Natural, Fat Free, Eat Smart, Morrisons*	1 Pot/150g	88	0.3	59	7	7.2	0.2	0
Natural, Fat Free, Lancashire Farm Dairies*	1 Serving/100g	48	0.1	48	5	7.3	0.1	0.9
Natural, Fat Free, Llaeth Y Llan, Village Dairy*	1 Serving/100g	57	0.2	57	5.7	7.9	0.2	0.1

Y

YOGHURT

Measure INFO/WEIGHT	per Measure KCAL	per Measure FAT	Nutrition Values per 100g / 100ml KCAL	PROT	CARB	FAT	FIBRE
Natural, Fat Free, Onken*	1 Serving/150g	63	0	42	5.6	3.1	0	0
Natural, Greek Style, Average	**1 Serving/100g**	**138**	**10.6**	**138**	**4.7**	**6.1**	**10.6**	**0**
Natural, Greek Style, Bio Live, Rachel's Organic*	1 Pot/450g	518	40.5	115	3.6	4.9	9	0
Natural, Greek Style, Bio Live, Tims Dairy*	1 Serving/50g	65	5	130	5.7	4.9	10	0
Natural, Greek Style, Fat Free, CBY, Asda*	1 Serving/30g	16	0.2	55	7.4	5.3	0.5	0
Natural, Greek Style, Fat Free, Essential, Waitrose*	1 Serving/125g	68	0.5	54	7.8	4.8	0.4	0
Natural, Greek Style, Fat Free, Tesco*	1 Pot/100g	55	0.2	55	7.5	4.8	0.2	0.4
Natural, Greek Style, Low Fat, Average	**1 Serving/100g**	**77**	**2.7**	**77**	**6.1**	**7.3**	**2.7**	**0.2**
Natural, Greek Style, Low Fat, Tesco*	1 Serving/100g	77	3	77	5.5	7	3	0
Natural, Greek Style, Milbona, Lidl*	1 Pot/125g	135	10.6	108	3.2	4.3	8.5	0.5
Natural, Greek Style, Strained, 0% Fat, Liberte, Yoplait*	¼ Pot/125g	70	0.1	56	9.6	3.2	0.1	0.1
Natural, Icelandic Style, Strained, Fat Free, Skyr, Arla*	1 Serving/150g	98	0.3	65	11	4	0.2	0
Natural, Icelandic Style, Strained, Fat Free, Skyr, Arla*	1 Serving/150g	98	0.3	65	11	4	0.2	0
Natural, Longley Farm*	1 Pot/150g	118	5.2	79	4.8	7	3.5	0
Natural, Low Fat, Average	**1 Med Pot/125g**	**75**	**1.6**	**60**	**5.4**	**7**	**1.3**	**0**
Natural, Low Fat, Everyday Value, Tesco*	1 Pot/125g	78	1.9	62	5	7.2	1.5	0
Natural, Low Fat, Live, Waitrose*	1 Pot/175g	114	1.8	65	5.8	8.2	1	0
Natural, Low Fat, Organic, Average	**1 Serving/100g**	**87**	**1.2**	**87**	**5.7**	**7.7**	**1.2**	**0**
Natural, Probiotic, Fat Free, Organic, Yeo Valley*	1 Pot/150g	87	0.2	58	5.9	8.4	0.1	0
Natural, Probiotic, Organic, Yeo Valley*	1 Pot/120g	98	5.4	82	5.1	5.6	4.5	0
Natural, Whole Milk, Set, Biopot, Onken*	1 Serving/125g	85	4.4	68	4.5	4.1	3.5	0
Natural, Wholemilk, Live Bio, Organic, Waitrose*	1 Serving/100g	88	4.4	88	5.1	7.1	4.4	0
Natural, with Honey, Greek Style, Sainsbury's*	1 Sm Pot/125g	174	9.8	139	3.7	13.4	7.8	0.5
Natural, with Oat Clusters, Chocolate, Nomadic*	1 Pot/169g	326	12.5	193	4.9	25.5	7.4	2.2
Nectarine, Fat Free, Weight Watchers*	1 Pot/110g	45	0.1	41	4.1	4.8	0.1	0.3
Orange, Sprinkled with Dark Chocolate, Brooklea, Aldi*	1 Pot/165g	73	0.8	44	3.5	6.9	0.5	0.5
Orange, Sprinkled with Dark Chocolate, Light, Muller*	1 Pot/165g	91	0.8	55	4.3	7.4	0.5	0.1
Orange, with Chocolate Flakes, Fat Free, Brooklea, Aldi*	1 Pot/165g	84	0.8	51	3.5	8.3	0.5	0.5
Original, Dairy Free, Koko*	1 Serving/100g	79	4.9	79	0.6	8	4.9	0.2
Passion Fruit, Gourmet, Live, The Great Dairy Collective*	1 Pot/150g	190	8.2	127	5.1	14.2	5.5	0
Passion Fruit, Greek Style, Luxury, Oykos, Danone*	1 Pot/110g	163	9.1	148	2.9	15.4	8.3	0.1
Passion Fruit, Light & Fruity, 0% Fat, Onken*	1 Serving/150g	76	0	51	4.9	6.3	0	0
Passion Fruit, Soya, Go On, Alpro*	1 Pot/150g	126	4.4	84	5.2	8.5	2.9	1.4
Peach, & Apricot, Fruit Corner, Muller*	1 Pot/150g	160	5.7	107	3.9	13.5	3.8	0.5
Peach, & Apricot, HL, Tesco*	1 Bottle/100g	70	1.2	70	2.3	12.4	1.2	0.2
Peach, & Cream, Intensely Creamy, Activia, Danone*	1 Pot/120g	118	3.6	98	4.8	13	3	0.3
Peach, & Mango, Thick & Creamy, Waitrose*	1 Pot/125g	136	3.1	109	3.7	17.8	2.5	0.3
Peach, & Pineapple, Fat Free, Mullerlight, Muller*	1 Pot/175g	89	0.2	51	4.3	7.7	0.1	0.2
Peach, Pear, Soya, No Bits, Alpro*	1 Pot/125g	99	2.5	79	3.7	10.7	2	1
Peach, Bio, Activia, Fat Free, Danone*	1 Sm Pot/125g	71	0.1	57	4.7	9.3	0.1	1
Peach, Greek Style, Luxury, Oykos, Danone*	1 Pot/110g	154	8.9	140	3.1	13.4	8.1	0.3
Peach, Low Fat, Average	**1 Serving/100g**	**86**	**1.1**	**86**	**4.5**	**14.6**	**1.1**	**0.2**
Peach, Melba, Low Fat, Average	**1 Serving/100g**	**75**	**0.7**	**75**	**2.6**	**14.5**	**0.7**	**0**
Peach, Summer Fruits, Weight Watchers*	1 Pot/120g	58	0.1	48	4.1	6.8	0.1	0.2
Pineapple, & Peach, Fruity, Mullerlight, Muller*	1 Pot/175g	89	0.2	51	4.2	7.7	0.1	0.2
Pineapple, Average	**1 Serving/100g**	**73**	**1.1**	**73**	**4.4**	**11.3**	**1.1**	**0.5**
Pineapple, Low Fat, Average	**1 Serving/100g**	**89**	**1.2**	**89**	**4.6**	**14.7**	**1.2**	**0**
Plain, Go On, Alpro*	1 Portion/100g	71	3.6	71	6.2	2.5	3.6	1.5
Plain, Low Fat, Average	**1 Serving/100g**	**63**	**1.6**	**63**	**5.2**	**7**	**1.6**	**0**
Plain, Soya, Average	**1oz/28g**	**20**	**1.2**	**72**	**5**	**3.9**	**4.2**	**0**
Plain, Soya, Simply, Alpro*	1 Tbsp/20g	10	0.5	50	4	2.1	2.3	1
Plain, Whole Milk, Average	**1oz/28g**	**22**	**0.8**	**79**	**5.7**	**7.8**	**3**	**0**
Plain, with Almond, Soya, Alpro*	1 Tbsp/20g	11	0.6	54	3.9	2.3	2.8	1.1

YOGHURT

	Measure INFO/WEIGHT	per Measure KCAL	FAT	Nutrition Values per 100g / 100ml KCAL	PROT	CARB	FAT	FIBRE
Plain, with Coconut, Soya, Alpro*	1 Tbsp/20g	11	0.6	55	3.9	2.3	3	0.8
Plum, Custard, Greek Style, 0% Fat, COU, M&S*	1 Pot/141g	83	0.3	59	6.4	8	0.2	0.5
Pomegranate, Soya, Alpro*	1 Pot/125g	92	2.4	74	3.6	9.5	1.9	1.1
Protein Greens, Mango, Kale, Lime, 20g, Arla*	1 Pot /200g	155	1.2	77	10.1	8	0.6	0
Prune, Bio, Activia, Danone*	1 Pot/125g	122	4.1	98	3.6	13.1	3.3	0.8
Prune, Live, M&S*	1 Pack/159g	254	6.5	160	5.4	24.4	4.1	1.7
Raspberry, & Cranberry, Fat Free, Milbona, Lidl*	1 Yoghurt/174g	87	0.2	50	4.2	7.8	0.1	0.5
Raspberry, & Cranberry, Fat Free, Mullerlight, Muller*	1 Pot/175g	91	0.2	52	4.3	7.8	0.1	0.5
Raspberry, & Cream, The Best, Morrisons*	1 Pot/150g	205	9.7	137	3.2	16.2	6.5	0.3
Raspberry, Cranberry, Skyr, Arla*	1/3 Pot/150g	118	0.8	79	9.2	8.1	0.5	0.3
Raspberry, Cranberry, Soya, Alpro*	1 Pot/125g	94	2.4	75	3.6	9.7	1.9	1.1
Raspberry, Bio Live, Low Fat, Rachel's Organic*	1 Pot/125g	114	2	91	4.1	15.1	1.6	0.1
Raspberry, Bio, Activia, Fat Free, Danone*	1 Pot/125g	68	0.1	54	4.7	7.2	0.1	2.6
Raspberry, Biopot, Onken*	1 Serving/150g	150	3.9	100	3.8	14	2.6	0
Raspberry, Fat Free, Average	*1 Serving/100g*	*64*	*0.1*	*64*	*4.9*	*11*	*0.1*	*1.7*
Raspberry, Fat Free, Probiotic, Organic, Yeo Valley*	1 Pot/125g	98	0.1	78	5.2	14	0.1	0.4
Raspberry, Intensely Creamy, Juicy, Activia, Danone*	1 Pot/110g	109	3.3	99	4.8	12.7	3	0.6
Raspberry, Lactose Free, Lactofree, Arla*	1 Pot/125g	130	3.4	104	3.3	16.5	2.7	0.7
Raspberry, Low Fat, Average	*1 Serving/100g*	*83*	*1.1*	*83*	*4.1*	*14.1*	*1.1*	*0.8*
Raspberry, Low Fat, Deliciously Fruity, Waitrose*	1 Pot/125g	99	1.4	79	4.5	12.6	1.1	0.5
Raspberry, Low Fat, Stapleton*	1 Serving/150g	105	0.8	70	3.3	13.6	0.5	2
Raspberry, or Strawberry, Smooth (No Bits), Ski, Nestle*	1 Pot/120g	118	3.2	98	3.9	13.6	2.7	0
Raspberry, Organic, Yeo Valley*	1 Pot/150g	152	5.8	101	4.2	12.3	3.9	0.4
Raspberry, Protein, Arla*	1 Pot/200g	140	0.4	70	10	6.5	0.2	0
Raspberry, Razzle, Greek Style, Light Free, Danone*	1 Pot/115g	61	0.1	53	4.7	7.8	0.1	1.1
Raspberry, Scottish, The Best, Morrisons*	1 Pot/150g	208	10.4	139	3.6	15.6	6.9	1.3
Raspberry, Squidgy Pouches, Brooklea, Aldi*	1 Puch/80g	67	2.3	84	3.4	11	2.9	0.5
Raspberry, Summer Fruits, Benecol*	1 Pot/120g	109	2	91	3.7	15	1.7	0.4
Raspberry, Summer, Biopot, Onken*	1/5 Pot/90g	91	2.4	101	3.8	15	2.7	0.6
Red Berry, Vitality, Low Fat, with Omega 3, Muller*	1 Pot/150g	138	2.8	92	4.3	13.8	1.9	0.7
Rhubarb, & Beetroot, Icelandic Style, Skyr, Arla*	1 Tub/149g	103	0.3	69	9.4	7.1	0.2	0.6
Rhubarb, & Champagne, Finest, Tesco*	1 Pot/150g	212	11.6	141	3.4	14.1	7.7	0.7
Rhubarb, & Fiery Ginger, Greek Style , Brooklea, Aldi*	1/3 Pot/150g	207	11	138	3	15	7.3	0.5
Rhubarb, & Vanilla, Gourmet, The Collective Dairy*	1 Bowl/100g	124	5	124	4.9	14.7	5	0
Rhubarb, Bio Live, Low Fat, Luscious, Rachel's Organic*	1 Pot/125g	104	2	83	4	13.1	1.6	0.1
Rhubarb, British, Yeo Valley*	1 Serving/100g	95	3.8	95	4.1	11.1	3.8	0
Rhubarb, Crumble, Inspired, Mullerlight, Muller*	1 Pot/172g	86	0.2	50	4.1	7.5	0.1	0
Rhubarb, Fruity, Mullerlight, Muller*	1 Pot/175g	91	0.2	52	4.2	7.9	0.1	0
Rhubarb, Layer, Bonne Maman*	1 Pot/125g	134	5.1	107	2.3	15	4.1	0.6
Rhubarb, Longley Farm*	1 Pot/150g	165	5.6	110	4.9	14.3	3.7	0
Rhubarb, Low Fat, Average	*1 Serving/100g*	*83*	*1.2*	*83*	*4.6*	*13.3*	*1.2*	*0.2*
Rhubarb, Low Fat, Garden Fruits, Tesco*	1 Pot/125g	119	2.4	95	3	15.5	1.9	0.3
Rhubarb, Spiced, Thick & Creamy, COU, M&S*	1 Pot/170g	68	0.2	40	4.3	5.8	0.1	0.5
Rhubarb, Timperley, TTD, Sainsbury's*	1 Pot/150g	170	9.9	113	3.2	10.1	6.6	0.5
Soya, Plain, Unsweetened, Free From, Asda*	¼ Pot/124g	57	3.6	46	4.8	0	2.9	0.5
Strawberry, & Cream, 0.06% Fat, TTD, Sainsbury's*	1 Pot/150g	183	8.2	122	3.5	14.7	5.5	0.4
Strawberry, & Cream, Finest, Tesco*	1 Pot/150g	206	10.4	137	3.4	15.4	6.9	0.5
Strawberry, & Raspberry, High In Protein , Go On, Alpro*	1 Pot/150g	128	4.2	85	5.1	8.8	2.8	1.2
Strawberry, Banana, Bircher Muesli, Moma Foods*	1 Pot/220g	306	4.8	139	4.5	24	2.2	0
Strawberry, Banana, Soya, No Bits, Alpro*	1 Pot/125g	99	2.5	79	3.7	10.7	2	1
Strawberry, Active, Fat Free, Optifit, Aldi*	1 Tub/125g	54	0.5	43	3	7.1	0.4	0.4
Strawberry, Bio, Activia, Danone*	1 Pot/125g	124	4.1	99	3.6	13.6	3.3	0.2
Strawberry, Breakfast Crunch, Corner, Muller*	1 Pot/135g	163	3.5	121	5.5	0	2.6	0

YOGHURT

Measure INFO/WEIGHT	per Measure KCAL	FAT	Nutrition Values per 100g / 100ml KCAL	PROT	CARB	FAT	FIBRE
Strawberry, Crumble, Crunch Corner, Muller*	1 Pot/150g	234	8.4	156	3.6	22.9	5.6	0.5
Strawberry, Everyday Low Fat, Co-Op*	1 Pot/125g	88	0.9	70	3	13	0.7	0
Strawberry, Fat Free, Average	*1 Serving/100g*	*66*	*0.1*	*66*	*4.9*	*11.1*	*0.1*	*0.6*
Strawberry, Greek Style, 0% Fat, Liberte, Yoplait*	1 Pot/100g	79	0.2	79	8	11	0.2	0.4
Strawberry, Greek Style, Fat Free, Brooklea, Aldi*	1 Pot/125g	72	0.3	57	4.9	8.8	0.2	0.2
Strawberry, Greek Style, Fruitopolis, Mullerlight, Muller*	1 Pot/130g	84	0.1	65	4.8	10.8	0.1	0
Strawberry, Greek Style, Luxury, Oykos, Danone*	1 Pot/110g	159	8.9	145	3.2	14.6	8.1	0.3
Strawberry, Greek Style, Milbona, Lidl*	1 Pot/125g	160	7.8	128	2.4	15.5	6.2	0.5
Strawberry, Icelandic Style, Strained, Fat Free, Skyr, Arla*	1 Pot/150g	112	0.3	75	9.4	8	0.2	0.2
Strawberry, Lactose Free, Lactofree, Arla*	1 Pot/125g	126	3.2	101	3.5	15.9	2.6	0.4
Strawberry, Layer, Bonne Maman*	1 Pot/125g	139	5.1	111	2.3	16	4.1	0.4
Strawberry, Light Free, Skyr, Danone*	1 Pot/150g	81	0.8	54	9.1	3.8	0.5	0.5
Strawberry, Light, Brooklea, Aldi*	1 Pot/200g	154	0.2	77	6.1	12.9	0.1	0.4
Strawberry, Low Fat, Average	*1 Serving/100g*	*81*	*1*	*81*	*4.5*	*13.6*	*1*	*0.2*
Strawberry, Milbona, Lidl*	1 Pot/175g	175	5.2	100	3	15	3	0
Strawberry, Organic, Yeo Valley*	1 Pot/120g	114	40.6	95	4.5	10.5	33.8	0
Strawberry, Probiotic, Organic, Yeo Valley*	1 Pot/125g	125	5	100	4.4	11.7	4	0.1
Strawberry, Protein 20g, Arla*	1 Pot/200g	140	0.4	70	10	6.5	0.2	0
Strawberry, Rice, Low Fat, Muller*	1 Pot/180g	193	4.1	107	3.2	18.4	2.3	0.4
Strawberry, Shortcake, Crunch Corner, Muller*	1 Pot/135g	212	8	157	4.1	21.2	5.9	0.1
Strawberry, Smooth Set French, Low Fat, Sainsbury's*	1 Pot/125g	112	4	90	3.7	11.8	3.2	0
Strawberry, Soya, Alpro*	¼ Pot/125g	92	2.4	74	3.6	9.4	1.9	1
Strawberry, Squidgy Pouches, Brooklea, Aldi*	1 Pouch/80g	67	2.4	84	3.5	11	3	0.5
Strawberry, Suckies, The Great Dairy Collective*	1 Pack/100g	77	3.1	77	3.2	9.2	3.1	0
Strawberry, Summer Fruits, Benecol*	1 Pot/120g	102	2	85	3.7	13	1.7	0.2
Strawberry, Thick & Creamy, Co-Op*	1 Pot/150g	182	6.9	121	3.6	16.4	4.6	0.1
Strawberry, Totally, Low Fat, CBY, Asda*	1 Pot/125g	104	1.2	83	4.1	14.2	1	0.4
Strawberry, Virtually Fat Free, Average	*1 Serving/100g*	*65*	*0.2*	*65*	*4.7*	*11.3*	*0.2*	*0.2*
Strawberry, Yoplait*	1 Pot/125g	61	0.2	49	4.2	7.6	0.2	0.9
Toffee, & Vanilla, Fat Free, Multipack, Weight Watchers*	1 Vanilla/110g	50	0.1	45	4.1	6	0.1	0.1
Toffee, Low Fat, Average	*1 Pot/125g*	*136*	*3.1*	*109*	*4.3*	*19.5*	*2.4*	*0.1*
Toffee, Low Fat, Deliciously Silky, Waitrose*	1 Pot/151g	143	3	95	4.6	14.5	2	0.5
Toffee, Smooth, Fat Free, Mullerlight, Muller*	1 Pot/175g	89	0.2	51	4.1	7.9	0.1	0
Toffee, Tempting, Greek Style, Muller Light *	1 Pot/120g	84	0.1	70	6.3	10.1	0.1	0
Toffee, with Chocolate Hoops, Crunch Corner, Muller*	1 Pot/135g	209	7.8	155	4.2	20.8	5.8	0.2
Tropical Fruit, Bio, Granola, Corner, Muller*	1 Pot/135g	161	3.2	119	5.4	18.2	2.4	0.6
Tropical, Granola, Duo, Brooklea, Aldi*	1 Pot/135g	177	6.2	131	3.6	18.5	4.6	0.8
Turkish Cream, Yayla*	1 Serving/100g	83	6	83	3.6	3.7	6	0
Turkish Delight, Mullerlight, Muller*	1 Pot/165g	91	0.8	55	4.5	7.4	0.5	0
Vanilla, Chocolate Sprinkles, Fat Free, Milbona, Lidl*	1 Pot/175g	93	0.9	53	3.9	7.6	0.5	0.1
Vanilla, Average	*1 Serving/120g*	*100*	*5.4*	*83*	*4.5*	*12.4*	*4.5*	*0.8*
Vanilla, Breakfast Topper, Activia, Danone*	1 Pot/160g	165	4	103	4.9	15.1	2.5	0
Vanilla, Cashew Milk, Dairy Free, Nush Foods*	1 Pot/125g	88	5.2	70	2	3	4.2	0
Vanilla, Choco Balls, Crunch Corner, Snack Size, Muller*	1 Pot/85g	118	4.1	139	3.8	20.2	4.8	0
Vanilla, Creamy, with Mini Smarties, Nestle*	1 Pot/120g	182	6.5	152	3.6	21.5	5.4	0
Vanilla, Fat Free, Onken*	½ Pot/225g	166	0.2	74	4.4	12.6	0.1	0.3
Vanilla, Intensely Creamy, Velvety, Activia, Danone*	1 Pot/120g	116	3.6	97	4.8	12.7	3	0.1
Vanilla, Low Fat, Probiotic, Organic, M&S*	1 Serving/100g	85	1.8	85	6.2	10.9	1.8	0
Vanilla, Madagascan, Deluxe, Lidl*	1 Pot/150g	212	10.2	141	2.7	17	6.8	0.5
Vanilla, Madagascan, West Country, TTD, Sainsbury's*	1 Pot/150g	197	11.8	132	3.1	11.9	7.9	0.5
Vanilla, Non Dairy, The Coconut Collaborative*	1 Pot/350g	508	42	145	1.4	7.9	12	0
Vanilla, Onken*	1 Serving/100g	100	2.7	100	3.1	15.9	2.7	0
Vanilla, Organic, Probiotic, Fat Free, Yeo Valley*	1 Pot/500g	400	0.5	80	5.4	14.2	0.1	0

	Measure INFO/WEIGHT	per Measure KCAL	FAT	Nutrition Values per 100g / 100ml KCAL	PROT	CARB	FAT	FIBRE
YOGHURT								
Vanilla, Smooth, Light, Fat Free, Mullerlight, Muller*	1 Pot/175g	88	0.2	50	4.3	7.2	0.1	0
Vanilla, Soya, Alpro*	1oz/28g	21	0.6	75	3.7	9.5	2.2	1
Vanilla, Soya, Pots, Eat Well, M&S*	1 Pot/86g	74	1.9	86	4	12.6	2.2	0.1
Vanilla, Sprinkled with Dark Chocolate, Brooklea, Aldi*	1 Pot/165g	82	0.8	50	3.5	8.2	0.5	0.5
Vanilla, Thick & Creamy, Channel Island, M&S*	1 Pot/150g	188	6.6	125	4.5	17.5	4.4	1
Vanilla, Virtually Fat Free, Yeo Valley*	1 Pot/150g	122	0.2	81	5.1	15	0.1	0
Vanilla, with Oreo Pieces, Muller*	1 Pot/120g	186	7.1	155	3.5	21.3	5.9	0
YOGHURT DRINK								
Actimel, Blueberry, Danone*	1 Bottle/100g	74	1.5	74	2.6	11.8	1.5	0.5
Average	*1fl oz/30ml*	*19*	*0*	*62*	*3.1*	*13.1*	*0*	*0*
Blueberry Blackcurrant, Skyr, Arla*	1 Bottle/350ml	214	0.7	61	5.8	8.1	0.2	0
Blueberry, Cholesterol Reducing, Tesco*	1 Bottle/100g	49	1.5	49	2.5	6.2	1.5	0.1
Cholesterol Lowering, Asda*	1 Bottle/100g	76	1.4	76	2.9	13	1.4	1
Cholesterol Reducing, Strawberry, Brooklea, Aldi*	1 Bottle/100g	38	1.3	38	0	0	1.3	0
Fruit, Mixed, Actimel, Danone*	1 Bottle/100ml	88	1.5	88	2.7	16	1.5	0
Light, Benecol*	1 Bottle/68g	40	1.4	60	2.8	7.3	2.1	0.1
Light, Yakult*	1 Bottle/65ml	27	0	42	1.4	10.2	0	1.8
Multi Fruit, Actimel, Danone*	1 Bottle/100g	85	1.5	85	2.7	14.4	1.5	0.1
Orange, Pro Activ, Cholesterol, Flora*	1 Bottle/100g	45	1.5	45	3.2	5.6	1.5	1.1
Original, 0.1% Fat, Actimel, Danone*	1 Bottle/100g	27	0.1	27	2.7	3	0.1	0.2
Original, No Added Sugar, Benecol*	1 Bottle/68g	32	1.4	47	2.8	4.3	2	0
Peach & Apricot, Benecol*	1 Bottle/68g	33	1.4	49	2.9	4.8	2	0
Strawberry, Actimel, Danone*	1 Bottle/100g	74	1.5	74	2.9	11.5	1.5	0
Strawberry, Benecol*	1 Bottle/68g	38	1.4	56	3.2	6.2	2	0
Strawberry, Cholesterol Reducing, Tesco*	1 Bottle/100g	46	1.7	46	2.7	4.7	1.7	0.8
Yakult*	1 Pot/65ml	43	0.1	66	1.3	14.7	0.1	0
YORKIE								
King Size, Nestle*	1 Bar/83g	445	26.1	537	6.1	57.3	31.5	0
Original, Nestle*	1 Bar/55g	302	17.4	546	6.2	57.9	31.5	1.9
Raisin Biscuit, Nestle*	1 Bar/67g	338	16.9	508	5.3	61.9	25.4	1.7
YORKSHIRE PUDDING								
3", Baked, Aunt Bessie's*	1 Pudding/36g	91	2.8	252	9	36.4	7.9	1.7
Average	*1 Pudding/30g*	*62*	*3*	*208*	*6.6*	*24.7*	*9.9*	*0.9*
Baked, Frozen, 4 Pack, Morrisons*	1 Pudding/34g	82	2.3	241	8.4	36.7	6.7	1.6
Batters, in Foils, Ready to Bake, Frozen, Aunt Bessie's*	1 Pudding/17g	47	1.8	276	9.1	32.6	10.8	1.4
Beef Dripping, Cooked, Specially Selected, Aldi*	1 Pudding/44g	129	5.7	293	9.4	32	13	3
Beef, Mini, Waitrose*	1 Pudding/14g	33	1.3	234	13.5	23.2	9.4	1.3
Frozen, Ovenbaked, Iceland*	1 Pudding/20g	53	1.8	262	7.4	36.8	8.8	3.1
Fully Prepared, M&S*	1 Pudding/22g	63	2.9	285	9.4	31.6	13.2	1.2
Giant, As Consumed, Morrisons*	1 Pudding/104g	264	7.9	254	9.1	36.3	7.6	2.1
Giant, Aunt Bessie's*	1 Pudding/97g	260	7.5	269	8.6	42	7.8	2.6
Home Bake, Aunt Bessie's*	1 Pudding/47g	78	2.1	165	6.1	25	4.4	1
Home Bake, Rise in 20 Minutes, Baked, Aunt Bessie's*	1 Pudding/25g	43	1.7	174	6	20	7	3.1
Mini, Co-Op*	1 Serving/16g	50	2	312	6.2	43.8	12.5	2.5
Mini, Farmfoods*	1 Pudding/3g	8	0.2	281	9.6	43.2	7.7	1.9
Ready to Bake, Baked, Aunt Bessie's*	1 Pudding/17g	42	1.4	246	8.5	35.1	8	1.7
Ready to Bake, Sainsbury's*	1 Pudding/18g	48	1.6	263	9.9	35.9	8.9	1.3
YULE LOG								
Belgian Chocolate, Finest, Tesco*	1 Slice/93g	294	14.6	316	4.7	38.2	15.7	1.8
Chocolate, Frozen, Tesco*	1 Serving/80g	251	14.6	315	7.5	28.8	18.3	2.3
Chocolate, Iceland*	1 Serving/75g	243	14.4	324	7.1	29.7	19.2	2.3
Chocolate, Sainsbury's*	1 Slice/35g	153	7.7	432	5	51.6	21.8	4.6
Chocolate, Tesco*	1 Slice/30g	133	6.7	439	5.3	52.6	22.2	3.6

Y

YULE LOG

	Measure INFO/WEIGHT	per Measure KCAL	FAT	Nutrition Values per 100g / 100ml KCAL	PROT	CARB	FAT	FIBRE
Christmas Range, Tesco*	1 Serving/30g	131	6.4	442	4.9	56.8	21.7	2.8
Mini, M&S*	1 Cake/36g	165	8.4	460	5.7	56.9	23.3	1.1
Penguin, Mini, McVitie's*	1 Roll/24g	107	5.3	453	5.2	58.6	22.3	1.6

ALL BAR ONE

BEEF
	KCAL
Steak, & Frites	1089

BREAD
Rustic, with Olive Oil	711

BREAKFAST
Sausage, Egg, Beans, & Toast, Sm Appetites	469
Vegetarian	838

BREAKFAST - FULL ENGLISH
& Toasted Sourdough	1005
with Spinach & Potato Hash, & Toasted Sourdough	1419

BREAKFAST - PROTEIN POWER UP
Salmon, Egg, Avocado, & Grapefruit, with Salad	372

BREAKFAST CEREAL
Bircher, Blueberry	528

BROWNIES
Chocolate, with Bourbon Vanilla Ice Cream	727
Chocolate, with Vanilla Ice Cream, Sm Appetites	459

BRUSCHETTA
Avocado, & Tomato, Crushed	545

BURGERS
Beef, Classic	967
Beef, Sliders, Sm Appetites	303
Beef, The Californian	1267
Beef, The French	1166
Beef, The Hipster	1243
Beef, The Skinny	549
Beef, The Smoky	1399
Beef, The Spanish	1205
Beef, The Wagyu	1403
Chicken, Grilled, Classic	850
Chicken, Grilled, Sm Appetites	187
Chicken, Grilled, The Californian	1150
Chicken, Grilled, The French	1049
Chicken, Grilled, The Hipster	1126
Chicken, Grilled, The Skinny	432
Chicken, Grilled, The Smoky	1282
Chicken, Grilled, The Spanish	1089

BURGERS VEGETARIAN
Tomato, Beetroot, & Mozzarella	905
Tomato, Beetroot, & Mozzarella, The Californian	1205
Tomato, Beetroot, & Mozzarella, The French	1104
Tomato, Beetroot, & Mozzarella, The Hipster	1181
Tomato, Beetroot, & Mozzarella, The Skinny	487
Tomato, Beetroot, & Mozzarella, The Smoky	1337
Tomato, Beetroot, & Mozzarella, The Spanish	1144

BURRITO
Chicken	776
Chicken, with Fries	1179
Chicken, with House Salad	967

CAKE
Chocolate, Mascarpone, & Orange, Mousse	250
Raspberry, & Pistachio, Traybake	150

ALL BAR ONE

CHEESECAKE
	KCAL
Lemon, Sicilian, with Blueberry Compote, Baked	558

CHICKEN
Skewers, Teriyaki, Ginger	335
Wings, Buttermilk	657

CHICKEN KATSU
Main	702

CHICKEN PIRI PIRI
Half	450
Half, with Fries	853
Half, with House Salad	641

CROISSANT
with Butter, & Jam	662

DOUGHNUTS
Churros	867

DUMPLINGS
Duck, Crispy	400

EGGS
Benedict	733
Benedict, with Avocado	1009
Florentine	728
Florentine, with Avocado	1004
Poached, with Mushrooms, on Toasted Sourdough	461
Royale	807
Royale, with Avocado	1083

EGGS - SCRAMBLED ON TOAST
with Smoked Salmon, on Toasted Sourdough	722

FISH & CHIPS
Main	918

FISH - BATTERED COD
with Mushy Peas, & Tartare Sauce, Sm Appetites	301

FISH CAKES
Haddock, Smoked, & Mustard	291
Haddock, Smoked, & Mustard, with Fries	694
Haddock, Smoked, & Mustard, with House Salad	482

FLATBREAD
Garlic, Stonebaked	1053
Houmous, & Kale	615

FRIES
Potato	403
Potato, Sm Appetites	177
Sweet Potato	505
Trio	1180

FRUIT
Strawberries, & Bananas, Fresh, Sm Appetites	128

HASH
Potato, Spinach, & Onion, Pan Fried	414

HOUMOUS
Duo	715

ICE CREAM
Trio	318
Vanilla, 2 Scoops, Sm Appetites	243

	KCAL

ALL BAR ONE

KEBAB
Chorizo, & Halloumi, Skewers	515

LAMB
Kibbeh	553

MEZZE
Little, Sm Appetites	738

MUFFIN
Blueberry Cheesecake	463
Carrot Cake	459
Chocolate, Triple	505
Lemon, & White Chocolate	462

NACHOS
Original	912
with BBQ Pulled Pork	1425

NOODLES
Pad Thai	523
Pad Thai, Little, Sm Appetites	391
Pad Thai, with Chicken Breast	808
Pad Thai, with Pan Fried King Prawns	707
Pad Thai, with Sliced Beef Fillet	775

ONION RINGS
Tempura	861

PAIN AU CHOCOLAT
Pastry	425

PANCAKES - BUTTERMILK
with Maple Syrup, Banana, & Berries	491
with Maple Syrup, & Smoked Bacon	568

PASTRY
Spinach & Feta, Bourek	303

PIE
Pecan, Bourbon, with Cinnamon Ice Cream	540

PLATTER
Brunch Board, for Two, Breakfast, ½ Board	1137
Deli Board, Sharing, Whole Board	1826
Grazing Board, Sharing, Whole Board	2074
Mezze Board, Sharing, Whole Board	1645

POTATOES
Patatas Bravas	283

PRAWNS
King, Pan Fried, Add On	104
King, Pan Fried	410

QUESADILLA
Chicken	423

RIBS
BBQ, Smoked	1494

RICE
Miso, Bowl	474
Miso, Bowl, with Chicken Breast	670
Miso, Bowl, with Pan Fried King Prawns	585
Miso, Bowl, with Sliced Beef Fillet	726
Steamed, Sm Appetites	179

ROLL
Bacon, Sour Cream, Chilli Tomato Jam, & Coriander	716

	KCAL

ALL BAR ONE

SALAD
Chicken, & Avocado, Chargrilled	618
Duck, Crispy	568
Feta, Carrot, & Quinoa	626
House	191
Side	191
Small Appetites	96
Superfood	440
Superfood, with Chicken Breast	634
Superfood, with Garlic & Lemon Marinated Halloumi	634
Superfood, with Pan Fried King Prawns	654

SANDWICH
Chicken, Grilled, Focaccia	610
Steak, Fillet	606

SORBET
Raspberry, 2 Scoops, Sm Appetites	158
Raspberry	236

SOUP
Tomato, Vegetable, & Quinoa	122

SQUID
Calamari, Salt & Pepper	404

TOAST
Sourdough, with Avocado, & Feta	446

TORTE
Chocolate, Salted Caramel, with Hazelnut Ice Cream	535

TORTILLA
Huevos Rancheros	585

WRAP
Fish Finger	553

ASK ITALIAN

ARANCINI
	KCAL
Pumpkin, Risotto, with Tomato Dip	285

AUBERGINE
Melanzane Al Forno, Main	578
Melanzane Al Forno, Starter	301

BOLOGNESE
Spaghetti, Vegan	849

BREADS / NIBBLES
Fonduta, with Dough Sticks	771
Garlic Bread	588
Garlic Bread Speciale - with Balsamic Onions	838
Garlic Bread Speciale - with Purple Pesto	801
Garlic Bread with Mozzarella	784
Italian Olives	204
Rosemary, & Sea Salt	499

BREADSTICKS
& Tomato, Dip, Tiny Tums, Kids Menu	159

CAKE
Pistachio, & Olive Oil, Vanilla Gelato	452

CALZONE
Con Carne Piccante	970
Pollo	899

CANNELLONI
Sausage, Ragu, Baked, with Creme Fraiche	658

CARBONARA
Linguine	1060
Tagliatelle	882

CHEESECAKE
Honeycomb. with Vanilla Gelato	719

CHICKEN
Pollo, Milanese	480
Pollo, Milanese, with Chips	1051

DESSERTS
Fruity Ice Lolly - Apple, & Raspberry, Kids Menu	43
Panna Cotta	190
Tiramisu	419
Chocolate, Eton Mess, Melting	472
Chocolate Etna	767
Frutti, Kids Menu	14
Fruity Ice Lolly - Orange & Apple, Kids Menu	45
Chocolate Pizza, Kids Menu	244

DESSERTS - GELATO
Chocolate, 2 Scoops	225
Hazelnut	283
Pistachio, 2 Scoops	273
Salted Caramel	252
Strawberry	266
Vanilla	242
Gelato Gondola, Chocolate, & Nut	628
Gelato Gondola, Salted Caramel	536

DESSERTS - MAKE YOUR OWN SUNDAE
Ice Cream, Chocolate, Kids Menu	109
Sauce, Chocolate, Kids Menu	302

ASK ITALIAN

DESSERTS - MAKE YOUR OWN SUNDAE
	KCAL
Ice Cream, Strawberry, Kids Menu	102
Ice Cream, Vanilla, Kids Menu	117
Sauce, Choconut, Kids Menu	57
Sauce, Strawberry, Kids Menu	22

DESSERTS - SORBET
Mango	179
Rasperry	166

FETTUCCINE
Bolognese	692

GIRASOLE
Spinach, & Ricotta	743

GNOCCHI
Chocolate, Baked	473

LASAGNE
Beef, & Pork, Ragu	717

LINGUINE
Seafood, Con Frutti Di Mare	703

NUTS
Chilli, Nuts	291

PASTA
with Tomato Sauce, & Cheese, Dip, & Dunk	459
in Tomato Sauce, Tiny Tums, Kids Menu	201
with Butter, Tiny Tums, Kids Menu	245

PASTA CARTWHEELS
in Bolognese Sauce, Kids Menu	424
in Cheese Sauce, Kids Menu	504
in Perfect Pesto Sauce, Kids Menu	509
in Tomato Sauce, Kids Menu	396

PENNE
Arrabiata	759
Arrabiata, with Chicken	869
Chicken, Al Pollo Della Casa	842
in Bolognese Sauce, Kids Menu	452
in Cheese Sauce, Kids Menu	352
in Perfect Pesto Sauce, Kids Menu	537
in Tomato Sauce, Kids Menu	424

PIZZA
Beef, & Gorgonzola, Prima	948
Black Olives, & Chicken, Kids Menu	480
Black Olives, & Extra Cheese, Kids Menu	594
Black Olives, & Ham, Kids Menu	470
Black Olives, & Mushrooms, Kids Menu	450
Black Olives, & Pepperoni, Kids Menu	529
Black Olives, & Roasted Red Peppers, Kids Menu	444
Black Olives, Kids Menu	136
Caprina, Prima	973
Chicken, & Extra Cheese, Kids Menu	625
Chicken, & Ham, Kids Menu	501
Chicken, & Mushrooms, Kids Menu	481
Chicken, & Pepperoni, Kids Menu	560
Chicken, & Roasted Red Pepper, Kids Menu	475
Chicken, Kids Menu	467

ASK ITALIAN

PIZZA

Ham, & Extra Cheese, Kids Menu	615
Ham, & Roasted Red Peppers, Kids Menu	465
Ham, & Smoked Scarmorza Cheese, Prima	1082
Ham, Kids Menu	457
Margherita, Classic	802
Margherita, Extra Cheese, Red Peppers, Kids Menu	589
Margherita, Extra Cheese, Kids Menu	581
Margherita, No Topping, Kids Menu	423
Margherita, Speciale, Alto Base	1137
Margherita, Vegan, Prima	535
Mushrooms, & Extra Cheese, Kids Menu	595
Mushrooms, & Ham, Kids Menu	471
Mushrooms, & Roasted Red Pepper, Kids Menu	445
Mushrooms, Kids Menu	437
Pepperoni, & Extra Cheese, Kids Menu	674
Pepperoni, & Ham, Kids Menu	550
Pepperoni, & Mushrooms, Kids Menu	530
Pepperoni, & Roasted Red Pepper, Kids Menu	524
Pepperoni, Alto Base	1338
Pepperoni, Kids Menu	516
Pollo Picante Con Pancetta, Prima	878
Roasted Red Peppers, Kids Menu	431
Salami, Misti, Prima	1011
Salsiccia, Sausage, Spicy, Prima	1116
Stromboli, Classic	881
Verdure, Classic	793

PORK

Belly, Porchetta	1143

RIGATONI

Meatballs, Ragu, Mozzarella, Al Manzo Piccante	718

RISOTTO

Con Pollo E Funghi	818

SALAD

Caesar, Chicken	815
Cheese, Burrata, Tomatoes, Rocket, Caprese	303
Insalata Di Pollo E Pancetta	743
Mozzarella, & Mixed Grain	501
Salmon, Roast, & Mixed Grain	624

SEA BASS

Al Forno	584

SEAFOOD

Calamari, Breaded	476

SIDES

Baked Broccoli with Chilli Cheese Crumb	147
Chips Garlic & Cheese	892
Mixed Salad	18
Plum Tomatoes, Kids Menu	4
Broccoli, Kids Menu	13
Side Salad, Kids Menu	44
Courgette Sticks, Battered	281

SORBET

Lemon	144

ASK ITALIAN

SPAGHETTI

Al Pomodoro, with Mozzarella	672
in Bolognese Sauce, Kids Menu	483
in Cheese Sauce, Kids Menu	563
in Perfect Pesto Sauce, Kids Menu	568
in Tomato Sauce, Kids Menu	455

STARTERS & SHARES

Mushrooms Al Forno	540
Chicken Lecca-Lecca	675
Bruschetta, Marinated Tomatoes, Basil, & Ricotta	321
Baked Dough Ball - Fontal Cheese and Chilli	711
Antipasti - Fritto	1105
Butterfly King Prawns	416
Plain	550
Meatballs Picante	718
Antipasti - Classico, The Mixed One	1310
Tuscan Bean Soup	433

TAGLIATELLE

Beef, Brisket, Rago	630
Lobster, & Prawn, Aragosta E Gamberoni	652
Pesto, Genovese, Purple	926

TART

Chocolate, & Blood Orange	451
Pear, with Raspberries, & Cream	415

TORTELLINI

Cheese, & Vegetable, with Tomato Sauce, & Cheese	281

VEGETABLES

Vegetable Sticks with Bread Soldiers, Kids Menu	175

BEEFEATER RESTAURANT

BEANS

Baked, in Tomato Sauce, Side, Kids Menu	51
BBQ, Spiced, Side	157

BEEF

Duo	1437
Slow Cooked, Kids, Sunday Lunch Menu	644
Slow Cooked, Sunday Lunch Menu	897

BEEF - STEAK

Fillet, 8oz, with Chips	813
Fillet, 8oz, with Chips & Salad	831
Fillet, 8oz, with Side Salad	461
Fillet, 8oz, with Veg Medley	505
Flat Iron, 6oz, with Chips	747
Flat Iron, 6oz, with Chips & Salad	765
Flat Iron, 6oz, with Side Salad	395
Flat Iron, 6oz, with Veg Medley	439
Porterhouse, 18oz, with Chips	1503
Porterhouse, 18oz, with Chips & Salad	1521
Porterhouse, 18oz, with Side Salad	1151
Porterhouse, 18oz, with Veg Medley	1197
Rib-eye, 10oz, with Chips	975
Rib-eye, 10oz, with Chips & Salad	993
Rib-eye, 10oz, with Side Salad	624
Rib-eye, 10oz, with Veg Medley	668
Ribs, & Prawn, Combo	1720
Rump, 10oz, Daytime Saver Menu	898
Rump, 10oz, Daytime Saver Menu	898
Rump, 10oz, with Chips	947
Rump, 10oz, with Chips & Salad	966
Rump, 10oz, with Veg Medley	651
Rump. 10oz, with Side Salad	595
Sirloin, 8oz, Daytime Saver Menu	758
Sirloin, 8oz, with Chips	789
Sirloin, 8oz, with Chips & Salad	808
Sirloin, 8oz, with Salad	437
Sirloin, 8oz, with Veg Medley	482
with Chips, Kids Menu	461

BREAD

Brown, Buttered, Extra	257
Flatbread, Garlic, & Dips	912
Flatbread, Garlic, Strips	1013
Garlic	218
Garlic, Kids Menu	112
White, Buttered, Extra	254

BROWNIES

Chocolate	557
Chocolate, Daytime Saver Menu	570

BURGERS

Beef, Bacon & Cheese, Double	1373
Beef, Bacon & Cheese, Triple	1697
Beef, Kids Menu	587
Steak, Daytime Saver Menu	939
Steak, Double, Daytime Saver Menu	1152

BEEFEATER RESTAURANT

BURGERS

Steak, with Cheese & Bacon, Daytime Saver Menu	1080
Steak, with Cheese & Bacon	1081
Chicken, Tabasco, Crispy	1059
Steak, Smoky BBQ, Summer BBQ Specials	1463

BURGERS VEGETARIAN

Main	910

CAKE

Trio of Sponges, with Custard	695

CAULIFLOWER CHEESE

Sunday Lunch Menu	281

CHEESECAKE

Vanilla, Baked	675

CHICKEN

BBQ, with Half Rack Of Ribs	1025
BBQ, with Whole Rack Of Ribs	1432
Breast, Kids, Sunday Lunch Menu	471
Breast, Plain	693
Breast, Smoky Paprika, Grilled	724
Breast, Smoky Paprika, Grilled, Daytime Saver Menu	632
Escalope, Breast, Breaded	1309
Goujons, Buttermilk, Summer BBQ Specials	742
Half, Roasted, Sunday Lunch Menu	1121
Melt, BBQ Sauce, Grilled	858
Poppin, with Chips, & Beans, Kids Menu	400
Wings, with BBQ, Spicy, 3, Side	160
Wings, with BBQ, Crispy, 5	260
Wings, with BBQ, Crispy, 8	401
Wings, with Piri Piri, Crispy, 5	252
Wings, with Piri Piri, Crispy, 8	394
Wings, with Piri Piri, Spicy, 3, Side	153

CHIPS

Side, Kids Menu	187
Triple Cooked, Side	418
Triple Cooked, Spicy, Side	420

COD

Bites, Breaded, Kids Menu	517

CORN

Cob, Mini, Side	61
Cob, Mini, Side, Kids Menu	29

CRUMBLE

Apple, Toffee, Salted	596

DESSERT

Caramel Apple Betty, with Custard	454
Caramel Apple Betty, with Ice Cream	446
Caramel Apple Betty, with Pouring Cream	488
Caramel Apple Betty, with Whipped Cream	413
Chocolate Challenge, Mini, Kids Menu	342
Mississippi Mud Pie	991

DOUGHNUTS

Mini, Kids Menu	249

FISH & CHIPS

Beer Battered, Daytime Saver Menu	1197

BEEFEATER RESTAURANT

FRIES

Skinny, Side	328
Skinny, Spicy, Side	329

FROZEN YOGHURT

Strawberry	235
Strawberry, Kids Menu	197

FRUIT SALAD

Mixed, Kids Menu	49

GAMMON

Blackened, with Egg, Daytime Saver Menu	751
Blackened, with Pineapple, Daytime Saver Menu	729
Steak, Blackened, in Spicy Rub	1034
Steak, Chargrilled, with Egg & Pineapple	1026
Steak, with Egg, Daytime Saver Menu	746
Steak, with Pineapple, Daytime Saver Menu	723

HADDOCK

Beer Battered, with Chips & Mushy Peas	1031
Beer Battered, with Chips & Peas	993

ICE CREAM

Vanilla, with Caramel Sauce, Kids Menu	254
Vanilla, with Chocolate Sauce, Kids Menu	253
Vanilla, with Raspberry Sauce, Kids Menu	253
with Chocolate Sauce	279
with Chocolate Sauce, Sunday Lunch Menu	275

KEBAB

Pork & Beef, Kofta, Grilled	444

LAMB

Rump, Minted, Grilled	720
Rump, Sunday Lunch Menu	901

LASAGNE

Beef, & Pork, with Chips, Daytime Saver Menu	860
Beef, & Pork, with Salad, Daytime Saver Menu	530

LINGUINE

Roast Vegetable, in Tomato Sauce	563
Roast Vegetable, In Tomato Sauce, with Chicken	718
Roast Vegetable, in Tomato Sauce, with Salmon	1010

MEATBALLS

Arrabiata, Linguine	821

MIXED GRILL

Rump Steak, Chicken Breast, Gammon, Sausage	1741
Flat Iron Steak, Chicken Breast, Gammon, Sausage	1498
Sirloin Steak, Chicken Breast, Gammon, Sausage	1583

MUSHROOMS

Crispy, Flat Cap, in Breadcrumbs	489

NACHOS

with Cheesy Yoghurt Dip, Kids Menu	235

ONION RINGS

Beer Battered, Crispy, Side	221

PASTA

Penne, in Tomato Sauce, Kids Menu	347

PATE

Duck, with Ciabatta	430

BEEFEATER RESTAURANT

PEAS

Side, Kids Menu	47

PIE

Banoffee	701
Beef, & Cheddar, with Mash & Gravy	1397

PLATTER

The Beefeater, Sharing, ½ Platter	700
The Beefeater, with Ribs, Sharing, ½ Platter	904

POTATO MASH

Side, Kids Menu	131

POTATOES

Crushed, Garlic, Side	344
Dauphinoise, Sunday Lunch Menu	320
Dippers, With Cheese, & Bacon, Loaded	587
Dippers, with Cheese, Loaded	482
Dippers, with Cheese, Sharing	1262
Dippers, with Cheese & Spring Onion, Loaded	517
Jacket, Side	438

PRAWN COCKTAIL

Classic, with Ciabatta	423

PRAWNS

Garlic, with Ciabatta	371
King, Garlic, 3, Side	151

PROFITEROLES

Main Menu	490
Daytime Saver Menu	504

RIBS

BBQ, Sticky, Summer BBQ Specials	451
Pork, Sticky Bourbon BBQ, Grill	1320

RISOTTO

Chicken, & Mushroom, Creamy	833
Chicken, & Mushroom, Daytime Saver Menu	831
Mushroom, Creamy	678
Mushroom, Daytime Saver Menu	676

SALAD

BLT, with Egg, Daytime Saver Menu	328
Caesar, Chicken, Goujons, Summer BBQ Specials	986
Caesar, Salmon, Blackened, Summer BBQ Specials	1076
Caesar, Summer BBQ Specials	421
Chicken, Jerk, Mango, Summer BBQ Specials	323
Chunky Slaw, Side	149
Greek, Crunchy, Side	173
Halloumi, Jerk, Mango, Summer BBQ Specials	421
Mixed, Large, Side	68
Mixed Bean	604
Salmon, Jerk, Mango, Summer BBQ Specials	621
Side, Kids Menu	6
Steak, with Pear	778

SALMON

Grilled	1014

SANDWICH

Steak, Open, with Fries, Daytime Saver Menu	1066

BEEFEATER RESTAURANT

SAUCE
Bearnaise, Steak Sauces	135
Beef, Rich, Steak Sauces	42
Cheddar, Pulled Ham, & Mushroom, Steak Sauces	98
Peppercorn, Triple, Steak Sauces	41
Prawn & Lobster, Steak Sauces	67

SAUSAGE & MASH
Bangers, Kids Menu	391
Main	835
Vegetarian, Bangers, Kids Menu	361

SEA BASS
Oven Baked, with Crunchy Greek Salad	451

SORBET
Lemon Curd	242

SOUP
Tomato	368

SPAGHETTI BOLOGNESE
Kids Menu	345

SPINACH
Creamy, Side	123

SUNDAE
Cookie Dough	694
Funny Face, Kids Menu	265
Rocky Road	791

TRIFLE
Strawberry, Pimms, Summer BBQ Specials	699

VEGETABLE MEDLEY
Side	112

VEGETABLES
Sticks, Side, Kids Menu	28
Sticks, with Yoghurt Dip	51

WAFFLES
Apple, Salted, Toffee, Summer BBQ Specials	881

WELLINGTON
Vegetable, Sunday Lunch Menu	1179

WRAP
Chicken Breast, Cheese, Vegetables, Kids Menu	540
Quorn Sausage, Cheese, Vegetables, Kids Menu	540
Salmon, Cheese, Vegetables, Kids Menu	605

YOGHURT
Strawberry, Kids Menu	127

BILL'S

BEEF
Steak, Flat Iron	694
Steak, Minute, with Chips, & Egg, & Garlic Butter	950
Steak, Minute, with Chips, & Garlic Butter	785
Steak, no Chips, Kids	359
Steak, Ribeye, 14oz	830
Steak, Sirloin, 10oz	617
Steak, with Chips, Kids	534

BREAD
Basket, with Butters, ½ Basket	730
Basket, without Butters, Whole Basket	956
Flatbread, Smoky, Italian, ½ Bread	333
Garlic, & Herb, Flatbread, ½ Bread	237
Tortilla, Corn, Spiced, with Guacamole	516
Tortilla, Corn, Spiced, without Guacamole	441

BREAKFAST
with Toast	807
Garden, No Hollandaise	746
Kids	598

BREAKFAST - BAKED EGGS
with Spicy Beans, & Chorizo	444
with Spicy Beans, & Chorizo, & Flatbread	564

BREAKFAST - FULL ENGLISH
with Toast	1110

BROCCOLI
Long Stem	121

BROWNIES
Chocolate, Warm, no Ice Cream	617
Chocolate, Warm, no Ice Cream, Kids	218
Chocolate, Warm, with Ice Cream	724
Chocolate, Warm, with Ice Cream, Kids	325

BUNS
Bacon, Breakfast	584
Sausage, Cumberland, Breakfast	565

BURGERS
Chicken, Buttermilk, no Chipotle Mayo	772
Chicken, Buttermilk, with Chipotle Mayo	986
Chicken, Fillet, Kids	365
Halloumi	888
Hamburger	696
Hamburger, no Mayo, Kids	372
Hamburger, with Mayo, Kids	522
Lamb, no Tzatziki	804
Lamb, with Tzatziki	833
Naked, with Salad, & Tzatziki, no Bun	525

CAKE
Victoria Sponge	598

CAULIFLOWER CHEESE
for Two, ½ Portion	119

CHEESE
Halloumi, Sticks, Crispy, with Lemon Garlic Mayo	962
Halloumi, Sticks, Crispy, no Lemon Garlic Mayo	675

BILL'S

CHEESECAKE
Banana, & Honeycomb	827

CHICKEN
Milanese, with Salad	738
Paillard	596
Mojo Marinated, with Dressed Salad	619

CHICKEN - SKEWERS
Dakkochi	462
Mojo Marinated, with Dressed Salad, & Flatbread	771
Mojo Marinated, with Salad, & Flatbread	674
Mojo Marinated, with Salad	522

CHOCOLATES
Truffles, Salted Caramel, 3 Truffles	168

CRAB CAKES
Baked, with Tartare Sauce	567
Baked, without Tartare Sauce	417
with Egg, & Asparagus	655

CREME BRULEE
Coconut, & Orange Rice	344

CRUMBLE
Plum, & Apple, no Ice Cream	606
Plum, & Apple, with Ice Cream	713

CURRY
Chicken, Thai Green, with Rice	790
Chicken, Thai Green, without Rice	563

DESSERT
Chocolate Bombe, Meltin	862

DHAL - AUBERGINE
Lentil, & Chickpea, Roasted	543
Lentil, & Chickpea, Roasted, with Flatbread	695

DOUGHNUTS - CINNAMON
Mini, Warm, no Sauce	483
Mini, Warm, Salted Caramel & Chocolate Sauce	649

DUMPLINGS
Pork, Sesame, Golden Fried, with Dipping Sauce	451

EGGS
Benedict, with Hollandaise	863
Benedict, without Hollandaise	549
on Toast, Kids	333
Royale, with Hollandaise	909
Royale, without Hollandaise	595
Scrambled, on Toast	555
Scrambled, on Toast, with Bacon	745
Scrambled, on Toast, with Salmon	698

FISH FINGERS
Cod, Kids	271

FRIES
Potato	349
Potato, Kids	175
Sweet Potato	510

FRUIT
Strawberries, & Banana, no Sauce, Kids	93
Strawberries, & Banana, Chocolate Sauce, Kids	198

BILL'S

GNOCCHI
Diablo	928

KALE
Sauteed	104

MACARONI
Kids	502

MACARONI CHEESE
with Mushroom, & Leek	1167

MAYONNAISE
Chipotle	216

MERINGUE
Eton Mess, Lemon	690

MEZZE
Sharing, for 4, ¼ Mezze	302
Veggie, Sharing, for 4, ¼ Mezze	275

MUSHROOMS
Garlic, Sauteed, Chestnut	180

OLIVES
Green, Giant, Gordal	161

OMELETTE
Summer	488

PANCAKES - BUTTERMILK
Kids	326
with Bacon, & Syrup, 3 Stack	844
with Bacon, & Syrup, 5 Stack	932
with Banana, Berries, with Syrup, 3 Stack	548
with Banana, Berries, with Syrup, 5 Stack	820

PATE
Chicken Liver, Oak Smoked, Parfait, with Toast	809
Chicken Liver, Oak Smoked, Parfait, without Toast	528

PIE
Fish	942

RIBS
BBQ, Kids	305
Main	791

SALAD
Caesar, Chicken, without Dressing	627
Halloumi, Grilled, & Pesto Toast, with Dressing	706
Halloumi, Grilled, with Dressing	548
Halloumi, Grilled, no Dressing	356
Halloumi, Grilled, & Pesto Toast, no Dressing	514
Mixed, no Dressing	24
Mixed, with Dressing	121
Salmon, Seared	728
Summer	695
Summer, with Flatbread	815

SANDWICH
Bacon, Kids	512
Fish Finger	725
Sausage, Kids	482

SAUCE
Bearnaise, for Steak	267
Chimichuri, for Steak	173

BILL'S

SAUCE
	KCAL
Garlic Butter, for Steak	193
Hollandaise	224
Peppercorn, for Steak	46

SAUSAGE
Cumberland, Mini, Glazed	696
Cumberland, Kids	619

SCONE
with Jam, & Clotted Cream, Warm	709
with Jam, Warm	562

SEA BASS
Pan Fried, with Rosti	147
Pan Fried, without Rosti	465

SOUP
Tomato, Roasted, with Cream	209
Tomato, Roasted, with Cream & Pesto Toast	367
Tomato, Roasted, with Pesto Toast	250
Tomato, Roasted, without Cream & Pesto Toast	92

SQUID
Calamari, Crispy, with lemon Garlic Mayonnaise	756
Calamari, Crispy, without lemon Garlic Mayonnaise	469

SUNDAE
Granola, Breakfast	412
Ice Cream, Vanilla, Kids	292

TART
Ricotta, Red Pepper, & Cheddar, no Dressing	664
Ricotta, Red Pepper, & Cheddar, with Dressing	761

TEACAKES
Toasted, no Butter	267
Toasted, with Butter	527

TOAST
& Butter, Bloomer	356
with Avocado, & Bacon	687
with Avocado, & Poached Eggs	676
with Avocado, & Salmon	640
with Avocado	497
with Beans, Kids	220

TOASTIE
Ham, & Cheese, Kids	478

TORTILLA CHIPS
Corn, Crispy, Kids	247

YOGHURT
Strawberries, Banana, & Honey, Kids	108

BREWERS FAYRE

BEANS
	KCAL
Baked, in Tomato Sauce, Side, Kids Menu	51

BEEF
Steak, Rib-eye, BBQ	1372
Steak, Rib-eye, with Hollandaise Sauce	1443
Steak, Rib-eye, with Peppercorn Sauce	1361
Steak, Rib-eye, with Tennessee Whisky Sauce	1425
Steak, Rump, Grilled	920
Steak, Sirloin, Grilled	933
Steak & Eggs	1041

BHAJI
Sweet Potato	58

BREAD
Garlic, Kids Menu	110
Garlic, Side, Kids Menu	106
Garlic, with Cheese, Side	316

BROWNIES
Chocolate, with Ice Cream	562

BUBBLE & SQUEAK
Side	348

BURGERS
Beef, Bash Street, Kids Menu	697
Beef, Black & Blue, with Chips	1379
Beef, Black & Blue, with Sweet Potato Fries	1312
Beef, Cheese, & Mushroom	1157
Beef, Extra	303
Brie, & Bacon	1443
Chicken, Breaded, The South Western	980
Chicken, Extra	211
Cluck 'N' Ale, with Chips	1563
Cluck 'N' Ale, with Sweet Potato Fries	1497
Halloumi, Heaven, with Chips	1136
Halloumi Heaven, with Sweet Potato Fries	1069
Smash 'N' Stack, with Chips	1010
Smash 'N' Stack, with Sweet Potato Fries	943
The New Yorker	1161

BURGERS VEGETARIAN
Hot 'N' Spicy, Nacho Burger	1233

BURRITO
Bowl, with Salad	550
Chicken, Bowl	705

CAULIFLOWER CHEESE
Side	281

CHEESE
Brie, Breaded, Bites	326
Halloumi, & Red Pepper, Grilled	235
Mozzarella, Sticks, Side	330

CHEESECAKE
Raspberry, & Prosecco	502

BREWERS FAYRE

CHICKEN

	KCAL
BBQ, with Full Rack of Ribs, Combo	1743
BBQ, with Half Rack of Ribs, Combo	1375
Bites, Breaded, Kids Menu	525
Breast, Garlic, Breaded	1326
Breast, Smoky Paprika, Grilled	430
Breast, Smothered, BBQ Sauce,	953
Goujons, Southern Fried	477
Half, Roasted, with Chips, BBQ	954
Half, Roasted, with Chips	974
Skewers, Jerk	292

CHICKEN & RIBS COMBO

Full Rack Ribs, with Chips, Coleslaw, & Salad	1637
Half Rack Ribs, with Chips, Coleslaw, & Salad	1322

CHICKEN KATSU

Curry	1037

CHICKEN TIKKA

with Rice	863

CHILLI

Beef, Mexican, with Rice	716

CHIPS

Side	416
Smothered, Creamy Cheese Sauce, Side	551
Smothered, Curry Sauce, Side	467
Smothered, Gravy, Side	436

COD

Bites, Breaded, Kids Menu	642

COLESLAW

Side	139
Side, Kids Menu	40

CORN

Cob, Mini, Side, Kids Menu	29

CRUMBLE

Apple, Toffee, Salted	670

DESSERT

Caramel Apple Betty	454
Chocolate, Mini, Mash Up, Kids Menu	344
Dirty Mud Pie	995
Fondue, Chocolate Fudge, ½ Portion, Sharing	854

DIP

Dessicated Coconut	158

DOUGHNUTS

Cinnamon	547

EMPANADAS

Cheese	401

FISH & CHIPS

with Mushy Peas	1286
with Peas	1248

FISH CAKES

Single	126

FRIES

Sweet Potato, Side	350

BREWERS FAYRE

FROZEN YOGHURT

Strawberry	274

FRUIT SALAD

Kids Menu	49

GAMMON

Steak, With Egg, Grilled	917
Steak, with Egg & Pineapple, Grilled	895
Steak, with Pineapple, Grilled	873

GRILLS

Ultimate, Summer	1781
Ultimate, Summer, with Prawns	1983

HADDOCK

Battered, with Chips & Mushy Peas, Atlantic, Giant	1113
Battered, with Chips & Peas, Atlantic, Giant	1075

HOT DOG

The Big Bad Dog, Kids Menu	612

ICE CREAM

Vanilla, with Caramel Sauce, Kids Menu	259
Vanilla, with Chocolate Sauce, Kids Menu	256
Vanilla, with Raspberry Sauce, Kids Menu	256

LAMB

Shank, Slow Cooked, in Gravy	623

LASAGNE

Beef, & Pork, with Side Salad	634
Sweet Potato & Feta, with Side Salad	742

MIXED GRILL - FLAT ITRON STEAK

Gammon, Chicken Breast, & Sausage	1413

MIXED GRILL - RUMP STEAK

Gammon, Chicken Breast, & Sausage, Ultimate	1657

MUSHROOMS

Garlic, & Herb, Breaded	389

NACHOS

with Cheesy Yoghurt Dip, Kids Menu	230

ONION RINGS

Battered, Side	442

PASTA

in Tomato Sauce, Kids Menu	344
Penne, Tomato, & Roasted Vegetable, with Chicken	731

PATE

Chicken Liver, with Toast	388

PEAS

Side, Kids Menu	47

PIE

Chicken, & Chorizo, Creamy Sauce	536
Fish	823
Lemon Meringue, with Cream	606

PIZZA

Chocolate, Kids Menu	375

POPPADOMS

Single	32

BREWERS FAYRE

	KCAL
POTATOES	
Dippers, Crispy	488
Dippers, Loaded, Sharing, ½ Portion	526
Dippers, Spicy Cheese, Loaded, Sharing, ½ Portion	494
PRAWN COCKTAIL	
Starter	343
PRAWNS	
King, Tempura, with Sweet Chilli	475
PROFITEROLES	
with Salted Caramel Sauce	422
PUDDING	
Beef, & Doom Bar Ale	1300
Bread & Butter, Summer Berry	587
Jaffa, Sharing	1034
Sticky Toffee	671
RIBS	
Full Rack, BBQ	1261
Pork, Full Rack, in Whisky Glaze	1160
SALAD	
Chicken, & Bacon, Grilled	434
Chicken, Coronation	549
Halloumi, Grilled	396
Mixed, Side	51
Prawn, Sweet Chilli, Battered	718
Salmon	384
SALMON	
Baked, with Hollandaise Sauce	754
SAMOSAS	
Vegetable	191
SANDWICH	
Chicken, Strip, Spicy, Brown Bread	688
Chicken, Strip, Spicy, White Bread	682
Fish, Goujons, Brown Bread	682
Fish, Goujons, White Bread	676
Ham, & Cheese, Brown Bread	630
Ham, & Cheese, White Bread	624
Prawn, Brown Bread	589
Prawn, White Bread	583
SAUCE	
Hollandaise	128
Peppercorn	46
Tennessee Whisky Glaze, Jack Daniels	84
SAUSAGE	
Egg, & Chips	996
Pork, Battered	159
SAUSAGES & MASH	
Bangers, Kids Menu	391
Vegetarian, Bangers, Kids Menu	364
SCAMPI	
Wholetail, Breaded, with Mushy Peas	966
Wholetail, Breaded, with Peas	928
SOUP	
Tomato	234

BREWERS FAYRE

	KCAL
SPAGHETTI BOLOGNESE	
Beano-ese, Kids Menu	320
SUNDAE	
Choc-a-block, Cadbury	709
Funny Face, Kids Menu	268
Salted Caramel, Brownie, & Popcorn	714
TRIFLE	
Strawberry Pimms	634
VEGETABLES	
Green, Medley, Side	112
Sticks, & Cucumber Yoghurt Dip, Kids Menu	49
Sticks, Side, Kids Menu	28
WAFFLES	
Belgian, with Chocolate Honeycomb Ice Cream	604
Belgian, with Salted Caramel Ice Cream	604
WRAP	
Chicken, Build Your Own, Kids Menu	491
Salmon, Build Your Own, Kids Menu	495
Sausage, Quorn, Build Your Own, Kids Menu	491
YORKSHIRE PUDDING	
with Sausage & Mash, Giant	1335

	KCAL

BURGER KING

BITES
Cheese, Chilli, 4 Bites	238

BREAKFAST - CROISSAN'WICH
Bacon, Egg, & Cheese	404
Sausage, Bacon, Egg, Cheese, Double	540
Sausage, Egg, & Cheese	600

BROWNIES
Chocolate, Hottie, with Real Ice Cream	449

BURGERS
Angus, Angry	760
Angus, Classic	579
Bacon, Double Cheese, XL	890
Big King, Long	620
Big King, XL	1010
Cheeseburger	303
Cheeseburger, Double	431
Cheeseburger, Kids	301
Cheeseburger. Bacon, Double	380
Chicken	392
Chicken, Royale, Bacon, & Cheese	680
Chicken, Tendercrisp, Angry	660
Chicken, Tendercrisp	639
Chicken Royale	567
Chilli Cheese, Long	480
Hamburger	263
Hamburger, Kids	260
King Fish	440
Steakhouse	760
Steakhouse	760
Texas BBQ, Long	540
Veggie, Kids	330
Whopper, Angry	710
Whopper	500
Whopper, Double	840
Whopper, JR	330

BURGERS VEGETARIAN
Veggie Bean	547

CHEESE
Mozzarella, Sticks, 5	340
Mozzarella, Sticks,3	210

CHICKEN
Nuggets, 4	190
Nuggets, 6	290
Nuggets, 9	440
Strips, Crispy	410

COFFEE
Cappuccino, Frappe, Iced	360
Cappuccino, Large	360
Cappuccino, Reg	280
Latte	140

DOUGHNUTS
Chocolate	330
Glazed	210

	KCAL

BURGER KING

FRIES
Apple	28
Large	395
Reg	277
Small	222
Super	469

HASH BROWNS
Single	276

ICE CREAM
Cone	120
Oreo, Fusions	264

MILK SHAKE
Chocolate	430
Oreo	570
Strawberry	430

MUFFIN
Bacon, King	320
Blueberry Filled	430
Chocolate Filled	482
Sausage, King	428

ONION RINGS
Large, 12	535
Reg, 5	232
Super, 16	713

PANCAKE
& Maple Syrup, Mini	268
& Maple Syrup, Mini, 9	360

SALAD
Garden, Side	15

SANDWICH
Bacon, Butty	210

SMOOTHIE
Strawberry, Banana, Iced Fruit, Large	279
Strawberry, Banana, Iced Fruit, Reg	208
Tropical Mango, Iced Fruit, Large	295
Tropical Mango, Iced Fruit, Reg	221

SUNDAE
Caramel	90
Chocolate	237
Strawberry	223

WAFFLES - WARM BELGIAN
with Real Dairy Ice Cream, & Chocolate Sauce	400
with Whipped Cream, & Chocolate Sauce	364

WRAP
Chicken, BLT	384

CAFFE NERO

BARS

Granola, Organic	278
Oat, with Fruit Seeds & Honey	259
Rocky Road	268

BISCUITS

Amaretti	40
Biscotti, Almond, Organic	147
Biscotti, Chocolate, Organic	136
Double Chocolate	126
Rocco Reindeer, Christmas Special	338
Stem Ginger	264

BOLOGNESE

Pasta, Beef, Oven Bake	521

BREAD

Ciabatta, Roll	180

BREAKFAST CEREAL

Porridge, with Semi Skimmed Milk, no Topping	234
Porridge, with Skimmed Milk, no Topping	210
Porridge, with Soya Milk, no Topping	232

BROWNIES

Chocolate, Belgian	324
Chocolate, Double, GF	319

CAKE

Banana & Walnut Loaf, Wheat Free	236
Blackcurrant & Earl Grey	502
Bruno Bear, Milk & White Chocolate	250
Cappuccino	486
Carrot, & Raisin, Organic, Wrapped	290
Carrot	531
Carrot & Raisin, Wheat Free	292
Chocolate Crunch	308
Chocolate Fudge	500
Chocolate Fudge, Festive	547
Lemon Drizzle, Organic	247
Lemon Drizzle, Slice, Organic, Wrapped	248
Panettone, Classic, Mini	374
Panettone, Mini Chocolate	404
Raspberry & Vanilla Sponge	385
Red Velvet	414
Red Velvet	408

CHEESECAKE

Lemon, Sicilian	341
White & Dark Chocolate	420

CHOCOLATE

Bar, Dark, 50% Cocoa	213
Bar, Milk	223
Bar, Milk, with Hazelnuts	229
Coins	109
Dark, Venezuelan Gold, Willies Cacao, Bar	139
Milk, of the Gods, Willies Cacao, Bar	146
White, El Blanco, Willies Cacao, Bar	159

CAFFE NERO

COFFEE - CAPPUCCINO

Semi Skimmed, Grande	92
Skimmed Milk, Grande	68
Soya Milk, Grande	90
Semi Skimmed, Reg	37
Skimmed Milk, Reg	27
Soya Milk, Reg	36

COFFEE - LATTE

Amaretto, No Cream, Skimmed Milk, Reg	143
Amaretto, Whipped Cream, Skimmed Milk, Reg	315
Caramel, Semi Skimmed Milk	274
Semi Skimmed Milk, Grande	138
Skimmed Milk, Grande	102
Soya Milk, Grande	135
Iced, Semi Skimmed	155
Iced, with Sugar Free Vanilla Syrup	84
Iced, with Vanilla Syrup	205
Praline, No Cream, Skimmed Milk, Reg	154
Praline, with Whipped Cream, Skimmed Milk, Reg	325
Semi Skimmed, Shot of Syrup, Reg	191
Semi Skimmed Milk, Reg	69
Semi Skimmed Milk, Shot Sugar Free Syrup, Reg	74
Skimmed Milk, Reg	51
Soya Milk, Reg	68
Spiced Orange, Reg	155
Spiced Orange, with Cream, Reg	326
Winter Berry, Grande	557
Winter Berry, Reg	488

COFFEE - MOCHA

Semi Skim Milk, no Cream, Reg	150
Skimmed Milk, no Cream, Reg	132
Soya Milk, no Cream, Reg	148
Semi Skimmed Milk, with Whipped Cream, Reg	302
White Chocolate, Semi Skimmed Milk	414

COFFEE BEANS

Chocolate Coated	133

COOKIES

Chocolate, Triple	336
Chocolate Chip, Wrapped	266
Chocolate Chunk, Milk	344
Oat & Raisin	332
Oat & Raisin, Wrapped	241

CRISPS

Cheddar & Spring Onion, Mature	202
Sea Salt	205
Sea Salt & Balsamic Vinegar	199

CROISSANT

Almond	350
Apricot	260
Butter	204
Cheddar & Tomato	305
Cheese Twist	316
Chocolate Twist	320

CAFFE NERO

	KCAL
CROISSANT	
Ham & Cheddar Cheese	336
Pain au Raisin	320
CUPCAKES	
Chocolate	311
Lemon	340
Raspberry	295
DANISH PASTRY	
Maple Pecan	312
DESSERT	
Triple Chocolate Cup, Luxury	315
DRIED FRUIT & NUTS	
Pack	236
FLATBREAD	
Mozzarella, & Chargrilled Vegetable	274
Mozzarella, Tomato, & Pesto	306
FRUIT SALAD	
Fresh	78
GINGERBREAD	
Man, Ginger Giovanni, Iced	189
Man, Gino, Christmas Special	289
HOT CHOCOLATE	
Amaretto, No Cream, Reg	284
No Cream, Semi Skimmed Milk, Reg	288
Amaretto, with Whipped Cream, Reg	456
with Whipped Cream, Semi Skimmed Milk, Reg	460
Luxury, No Cream, Reg	199
Luxury, with Cream, Reg	352
Milano, with Whipped Cream	424
Mint, Reg, Whipped Cream, Semi Skimmed Milk	437
No Cream, Semi Skimmed Milk, Reg	235
No Cream, Skimmed Milk, Reg	217
No Cream, Soya Milk, Reg	229
Whipped Cream, Semi Skimmed Milk, Reg	352
with Whipped Cream, Reg	388
No Cream, Semi Skimmed Milk, Reg	290
with Whipped Cream, Semi Skimmed Milk, Reg	462
Spiced Orange, Reg	285
with Cream, Reg	457
JUICE	
Apple, Organic, Carton	94
Mango & Passionfruit, Booster	220
Orange, 100% Squeezed, Fresh	95
Orange, Lemon & Lime, Booster	207
Raspberry & Orange, Booster	236
Strawberry & Raspberry, Booster	206
LEMONADE	
Crushed Raspberry, Iced	96
Iced, Italian	328
MARSHMALLOWS	
for Hot Chocolate	20

CAFFE NERO

	KCAL
MILK SHAKE	
Banana	315
Banana, Skimmed Milk	284
Banana, with Cream & Sprinkles	402
Chocolate	386
Coffee & Caramel, Creme	367
Double Chocolate, Cream, & Sprinkles	411
Double Chocolate, Skimmed Milk	290
Latte, Caramel	274
Latte, Caramel, Cream, & Sprinkles	369
Latte, Cream, & Sprinkles	334
Latte, Semi Skimmed Milk	225
Mocha Latte, Skimmed Milk	290
Raspberry & White Chocolate, Creme	452
Strawberry	285
Strawberry, with Cream, & Chocolate Sprinkles	403
MILK SHAKE - FRAPPE	
Latte, Skimmed Milk	198
Latte, Soya Milk	101
Mint	399
Mint, Semi Skimmed Milk	310
Mint, Skimmed Milk	281
Mocha Latte, Cream, & Sprinkles	386
Mocha Latte, Semi Skimmed Milk	317
Vanilla	266
Vanilla, Skimmed Milk	285
Vanilla, with Cream, & Chocolate Sprinkles	402
Creme, Banana & Caramel	460
Creme, Coconut & Chocolate	516
Creme, Strawberry & Vanilla	469
MINTS	
Peppermints, Sugar Free	35
MUFFIN	
Apple, & Pecan, Spiced	522
Bacon, & Tomato Sauce, English	277
Blueberry	415
Blueberry, Reduced Fat	351
Chocolate, Triple	503
Chocolate Orange, Filled	486
Cranberry & Orange, Reduced Fat	322
Egg Mayo, with Cheese & Mustard, English	314
Gingerbread Filled	516
Ham, & Egg Mayo, with Cheese, English	314
Lemon Poppyseed	461
Raisin, Multiseed	475
Raspberry & White Chocolate	422
PAIN AU CHOCOLAT	
Pastry	270
PANINI	
All Day Breakfast	480
Bacon, & Tomato Sauce, Breakfast	263
Brie, & Smoked Bacon	505
Brie, Bacon, & Caramelised Onion	624

CAFFE NERO

PANINI

Brie & Cranberry, Christmas Special	489
Chicken, Bacon, & Arrabiata Sauce	422
Chicken, Pesto Genovese	400
Chicken, Piri Piri, Seasonal Special	353
Chicken Milanese	428
Chorizo, & Mozzarella, Spicy	461
Four Cheese, & Cranberry Chutney	544
Goats Cheese & Grilled Red Pepper	426
Ham, & Egg Mayo, Breakfast	326
Ham, & Mature Cheddar, Tostati	213
Ham, & Mozzarella	394
Ham, Mozzarella, & Emmental, Tostati	225
Il Genovese	424
Meatball, & Mozzarella, Napoletana	511
Mozzarella, & Tomato, with Pesto	438
Mozzarella, Cheddar, & Tomato, Tostati	418
Mozzarella, Red Pepper, & Roast Tomato	432
Mushroom, & Mascarpone, Tostati	395
Mushroom, Mozzarella & Cheddar	348
Mushroom, with Gorgonzola Cheese	377
Pepperoni, Mozzarella, & Tomato	472
Salami, & Grilled Peppers	451
Three Cheese, & Roasted Tomato, Tostati	170
Tuna, & Mozzarella, Melt	431
Turkey, Stuffing & Cranberry	409

PASTA

Chicken Pesto, Oven Bake	524
Vegetable Arrabiata	434

PIE

Lemon Meringue	299
Mince	361

POPCORN

Sea Salt, Propercorn	88
Sea Salt & Sweet Brown Sugar, Propercorn	129

RISOTTO

Mushroom & Spinach, Creamy	384

ROLL

Ham, & Egg, GF	283

SALAD

Chicken with Caesar Dressing	156
Falafel & Tabbouleh	390
Mozzarella & Cherry Tomato, Red Pesto Dressing	276

SANDWICH

Bacon, on Bloomer Bread	365
BLT	442
Cheddar & Pickle, Mature, Malted Wheatgrain Bread	434
Chicken, Salad, & pesto, Roll, GF	359
Chicken, Salad, Malted Wheatgrain Bread	309
Chicken, with Rosemary Mayonnaise	309
Egg, Bacon & Sausage, on Bloomer Bread	410
Egg Mayonnaise, Free Range	323
Brie & Cranberry, & Turkey & Cranberry, Festive	412

CAFFE NERO

SANDWICH

Ham, & Cheddar, Malted Wheatgrain Bread	454
Salmon, Smoked, & Soft Cheese	294
Tuna Mayo, & Cucumber, Less Than 300 Calories	258
Tuna Salad	268

SAUCE

Berry Compote, Topping, for Porridge	47
Maple, Topping, for Porridge	94

SCONE

Fruit, Sultana	287

SHORTBREAD

Bars, Crunchy, All Butter	264

SLICES

Caramel Shortcake	330
Coconut & Raspberry, Gluten & Dairy Free	286
Tiramisu	378

SOUP

Carrot & Coriander	150
Chicken, Cream Of	75
Potato & Leek, Low Fat	129
Spanish Chorizo & Lentil	233
Tomato, & Mascarpone	163
Tomato, Sundried, & Basil	192

SYRUP

Vanilla	122
Vanilla, Sugar Free	5

TART

Apple & Blackcurrant	279
Custard, Portuguese	184
Lemon	331

TEA

Chai Latte, Semi Skimmed Milk	281
Chai Latte, Skimmed Milk	239

TEACAKES

Rich Fruit, Toasted, with Butter	302

WAFFLES

Caramel	356

WRAP

Chicken, Fajita	418
Chicken Caesar	434
Houmous, & Falafel	455
Spicy Bean Fajita	382

YOGHURT

Berry & Granola	223
Blackcurrant, Greek Style, Bio	224
Blueberry, Greek Style, Brunch Pot	198
Blueberry Bircher Muesli, Greek Style, Half Fat	236
Honey, Greek Style, Bio	264
Raspberry, Greek Style	236

COSTA	KCAL
APPLES	
Fresh	43
BANANA	
Fresh	51
BARS	
Granola, Square, Traybake	335
BISCUITS	
Biscotti, Almond	77
Fruit, & Oat	224
Ginger, Stem	248
Gingerbread	162
Jammy, Ultimate	310
BREAD	
Focaccia, Halloumi, & Roasted Pepper	411
BREAKFAST	
Bacon, Roll	389
Bloomer	493
Croissant, Ham, & Emmenthal	358
Muffin, Scrambled Egg, & Mushroom	298
Oats, Instant, Porridge Pot	294
Porridge	219
BROWNIES	
Chocolate	373
Chocolate, GF	418
Mocha, Mini	160
BUTTER	
Salted, Extra	48
CAKE	
Brioche, Maple, & Pecan, Swirl	267
Caramel, Crisp, Traybake	410
Carrot, Layered	593
Chocolate, & Hazelnut, Shimmer	524
Chocolate, Tiffin	457
Fruity, Caramel, Crispie, Bites	536
Lemon, Drizzle, Loaf	322
Orange, & Polenta	363
Peach, Melba, Loaf	332
Raspberry, & Almond, Traybake	465
Raspberry, Brioche, Fingers	141
Sponge, Victoria	537
Sticky Toffee, Brownie, Cakesplosion	501
CHAI	
Powder	50
CHICKEN	
Chorizo, & Roasted Pepper, Rice, Box	327
CHOCOLATE	
Belgian, Lattice	32
Dark, Blossoms	52
Dusting	8
Flake	44
Gianduja, Milk	47
Magic Dust, Powder	8

COSTA	KCAL
CHOCOLATES	
Dark, Belgian, Stirrer	55
COFFEE - AMERICANO	
No Milk, Massimo	10
No Milk, Medio	8
No Milk, Primo	6
Skimmed Milk, Massimo	27
Skimmed Milk, Medio	16
Skimmed Milk, Primo	12
Soya Milk, Massimo	27
Soya Milk, Medio	21
Soya Milk, Primo	15
Whole Milk, Massimo	38
Whole Milk, Medio	29
Whole Milk, Primo	18
COFFEE - BABYCCINO	
Chocolate, with Flake, Skimmed Milk	143
Chocolate, with Flake, Soya Milk	121
Chocolate, with Flake, Whole Milk	143
Chocolate, with Marshmallow, Skimmed Milk	93
Chocolate, with Marshmallow, Soya Milk	102
Chocolate, with Marshmallow, Whole Milk	124
with Marshmallow, Skimmed Milk	64
with Marshmallow, Soya Milk	73
with Marshmallow, Whole Milk	95
COFFEE - CAPPUCCINO	
Whole Milk, Massimo, Iced	150
Whole Milk, Medio, Iced	119
Whole Milk, Primo, Iced	85
Popcorn, Full Fat Milk, Medio, Iced	127
Popcorn, Full Fat Milk, Primo, Iced, Costa	92
Popcorn, Skimmed Milk, Massimo, Iced	119
Popcorn, Skimmed Milk, Medio, Iced	95
Popcorn, Skimmed Milk, Primo, Iced	69
Popcorn, Soya Milk, Massimo, Iced	133
Popcorn, Soya Milk, Medio, Iced	106
Popcorn, Soya Milk, Primo, Iced	77
Salted Caramel, Skimmed Milk, Massimo	114
Salted Caramel, Skimmed Milk, Medio	91
Salted Caramel, Skimmed Milk, Primo	61
Salted Caramel, Soya Milk, Massimo	143
Salted Caramel, Soya Milk, Medio	114
Salted Caramel, Soya Milk, Primo	75
Salted Caramel, Whole Milk, Massimo	212
Salted Caramel, Whole Milk, Medio	169
Salted Caramel, Whole Milk, Primo	110
Skimmed Milk, Massimo	111
Skimmed Milk, Massimo, Takeaway	120
Skimmed Milk, Medio	90
Skimmed Milk, Medio, Takeaway	90
Skimmed Milk, Primo	60
Skimmed Milk, Primo, Takeaway	70
Soya Milk, Massimo, Takeaway	150

COSTA
COFFEE - CAPPUCCINO
Soya Milk, Massimo	139
Soya Milk, Massimo, Iced	128
Soya Milk, Medio	112
Soya Milk, Medio, Iced	100
Soya Milk, Medio, Takeaway	112
Soya Milk, Primo	74
Soya Milk, Primo, Iced	71
Soya Milk, Primo, Takeaway	87
Whole Milk, Massimo	209
Whole Milk, Massimo, Takeaway	223
Whole Milk, Medio	168
Whole Milk, Medio, Takeaway	168
Whole Milk, Primo	109
Whole Milk, Primo, Takeaway	129

COFFEE - CORTADO
Whole Milk, Solo, Iced	75
Skimmed Milk, Solo	42
Skimmed Milk, Solo, Iced	46
Skimmed Milk, Solo, Takeaway	53
Soya Milk, Solo	55
Soya Milk, Solo, Iced	56
Soya Milk, Solo, Takeaway	69
Whole Milk, Solo	85
Whole Milk, Solo, Takeaway	108

COFFEE - CORTADO, CARAMEL
Skimmed Milk	73
Skimmed Milk, Takeaway	84
Soya Milk	84
Soya Milk, Takeaway	98
Whole Milk	111
Whole Milk, Takeaway	132

COFFEE - ESPRESSO
Decaff, Doppio	6
Decaff, Solo	3
Doppio, Iced	40
Ristretto, Doppio, Iced	38
Ristretto, Solo, Iced	19
Shot	4
Solo, Iced	20
Old Paradise Street, Doppio	6
Old Paradise Street, Solo	3

COFFEE - ESPRESSO, MACCHIATO
Whole Milk, Doppio, Iced	41
Whole Milk, Solo, Iced	21
Skimmed Milk, Doppio, Iced	40
Skimmed Milk, Solo, Iced	20
Soya Milk, Doppio, Iced	41
Soya Milk, Solo, Iced	21

COFFEE - FLAT WHITE
Skimmed Milk, Primo	75
Skimmed Milk, Primo, Takeaway	89
Soya Milk, Primo	98

COSTA
COFFEE - FLAT WHITE
Soya Milk, Primo, Takeaway	116
Whole Milk, Primo	152
Whole Milk, Primo, Takeaway	178

COFFEE - LATTE
Skimmed Milk, Massimo	132
Skimmed Milk, Massimo, Takeaway	139
Skimmed Milk, Medio	102
Skimmed Milk, Medio, Takeaway	102
Skimmed Milk, Primo	66
Skimmed Milk, Primo, Takeaway	75
Soya Milk, Massimo	175
Soya Milk, Massimo, Takeaway	184
Soya Milk, Medio	135
Soya Milk, Medio, Takeaway	135
Soya Milk, Primo	86
Soya Milk, Primo, Takeaway	97
Whole Milk, Massimo	269
Whole Milk, Massimo, Takeaway	283
Whole Milk, Medio	207
Whole Milk, Medio, Takeaway	207
Whole Milk, Primo	133
Whole Milk, Primo, Takeaway	149
Coconut Milk, Massimo	137
Caffe Latte, Coconut Milk, Massimo, Takeaway	144
Caffe Latte, Coconut Milk, Medio	106
Caffe Latte, Coconut Milk, Medio, Takeaway	106
Caffe Latte, Coconut Milk, Primo	68
Caffe Latte, Coconut Milk, Primo, Takeaway	77
Soya Milk, Medio, Takeaway	258
Whole Milk, Massimo, Iced	263
Whole Milk, Medio, Iced	205
Whole Milk, Primo, Iced	152
Skimmed Milk, Massimo, Iced	179
Skimmed Milk, Medio, Iced	129
Skimmed Milk, Primo, Iced	94
Soya Milk, Massimo, Iced	200
Soya Milk, Medio, Iced	156
Soya Milk, Primo, Iced	115

COFFEE - LATTE, BILLIONAIRE
Skimmed Milk, Medio	341
Skimmed Milk, Medio, Takeaway	351
Soya Milk, Medio	363
Soya Milk, Medio, Takeaway	376
Whole Milk, Medio	416
Whole Milk, Medio, Takeaway	436

COFFEE - LATTE, CARAMEL
Skimmed Milk, Massimo, Speciality	190
Skimmed Milk, Massimo, Speciality, Takeaway	355
Skimmed Milk, Medio, Speciality	147
Skimmed Milk, Medio, Speciality, Takeaway	147
Skimmed Milk, Primo, Speciality	96
Skimmed Milk, Primo, Speciality, Takeaway	106

COSTA

COFFEE - LATTE, CARAMEL

Skimmed Milk, Primo, Speciality, Takeaway	125
Soya Milk, Massimo, Speciality	228
Soya Milk, Massimo, Speciality, Takeaway	240
Soya Milk, Medio, Speciality	176
Soya Milk, Medio, Speciality, Takeaway	176
Soya Milk, Primo, Speciality	114
Soya Milk, Medio, Takeaway	136
Whole Milk, Massimo, Speciality	319
Whole Milk, Massimo, Speciality	267
Whole Milk, Massimo, Speciality, Takeaway	335
Whole Milk, Medio, Speciality	246
Whole Milk, Medio, Speciality, Takeaway	246
Whole Milk, Primo, Speciality	160
Whole Milk, Primo, Speciality, Takeaway	175

COFFEE - LATTE, CARAMEL, ICED

Skimmed Milk, Massimo, Speciality	161
Skimmed Milk, Primo, Speciality	84
Soya Milk, Massimo, Speciality	195
Soya Milk, Medio, Speciality	151
Soya Milk, Primo, Speciality	112
Whole Milk, Massimo, Speciality	257
Whole Milk, Medio, Speciality	203
Whole Milk, Primo, Speciality	150

COFFEE - LATTE, CARAMEL, ICED, SUGAR FREE

Whole Milk, Massimo, Speciality	199
Whole Milk, Medio, Speciality	157
Whole Milk, Primo, Speciality	120
Skimmed Milk, Massimo, Speciality	103
Skimmed Milk, Medio, Speciality	81
Skimmed Milk, Primo, Speciality	62
Soya Milk, Massimo, Speciality	137
Soya Milk, Medio, Speciality	108
Soya Milk, Primo, Speciality	83

COFFEE - LATTE, CARAMEL, SUGAR FREE

Skimmed Milk, Massimo	138
Skimmed Milk, Massimo, Takeaway	168
Skimmed Milk, Medio	106
Skimmed Milk, Medio, Takeaway	106
Skimmed Milk, Primo	68
Skimmed Milk, Primo, Takeaway	78
Soya Milk, Massimo	176
Soya Milk, Massimo, Takeaway	185
Soya Milk, Medio	136
Soya Milk, Primo	87
Soya Milk, Primo, Takeaway	97
Whole Milk, Massimo	267
Whole Milk, Massimo, Takeaway	280
Whole Milk, Medio	206
Whole Milk, Medio, Takeaway	206
Whole Milk, Primo	132
Whole Milk, Primo, Takeaway	147

COSTA

COFFEE - LATTE, CINNAMON, ICED

Whole Milk, Massimo, Speciality	261
Whole Milk, Medio, Speciality	204
Whole Milk, Primo, Speciality	151
Skimmed Milk, Massimo, Speciality	164
Skimmed Milk, Medio, Speciality	127
Skimmed Milk, Primo, Speciality	93
Soya Milk, Massimo, Speciality	199
Soya Milk, Medio, Speciality	154
Soya Milk, Primo, Speciality	114

COFFEE - LATTE, GINGERBREAD

Skimmed Milk, Massimo	268
Skimmed Milk, Massimo, Speciality	195
Skimmed Milk, Massimo, Speciality, Takeaway	205
Skimmed Milk, Massimo, Takeaway	244
Skimmed Milk, Medio	217
Skimmed Milk, Medio, Speciality	150
Skimmed Milk, Medio, Speciality, Takeaway	150
Skimmed Milk, Medio, Takeaway	227
Skimmed Milk, Primo	165
Skimmed Milk, Primo, Speciality	96
Skimmed Milk, Primo, Speciality, Takeaway	106
Skimmed Milk, Primo, Takeaway	180
Soya Milk, Massimo	301
Soya Milk, Massimo, Speciality	233
Soya Milk, Massimo, Speciality, Takeaway	245
Soya Milk, Massimo, Takeaway	279
Soya Milk, Medio	245
Soya Milk, Medio, Speciality	180
Soya Milk, Medio, Speciality, Takeaway	180
Soya Milk, Primo	183
Soya Milk, Primo, Speciality	116
Soya Milk, Primo, Speciality, Takeaway	128
Soya Milk, Primo, Takeaway	201
Whole Milk, Massimo	380
Whole Milk, Massimo, Speciality	324
Whole Milk, Massimo, Speciality, Takeaway	340
Whole Milk, Massimo, Takeaway	364
Whole Milk, Medio	312
Whole Milk, Medio, Speciality	250
Whole Milk, Medio, Speciality, Takeaway	250
Whole Milk, Medio, Takeaway	332
Whole Milk, Primo	227
Whole Milk, Primo, Speciality	160
Whole Milk, Primo, Speciality, Takeaway	178
Whole Milk, Primo, Takeaway	253

COFFEE - LATTE, GINGERBREAD, ICED

Whole Milk, Massimo, Speciality	264
Whole Milk, Medio, Speciality	206
Whole Milk, Primo, Speciality	152
Skimmed Milk, Massimo, Speciality	167
Skimmed Milk, Medio, Speciality	129
Skimmed Milk, Primo, Speciality	95

COSTA

COFFEE - LATTE, GINGERBREAD, ICED

Soya Milk, Massimo, Speciality	201
Soya Milk, Medio, Speciality	156
Soya Milk, Primo, Speciality	115

COFFEE - LATTE, GINGERBREAD, ICED, SUGAR FREE

Sugar Free, Full Fat Milk, Massimo, Speciality	198
Sugar Free, Full Fat Milk, Medio, Speciality	156
Sugar Free, Full Fat Milk, Primo, Speciality	120
Sugar Free, Skimmed Milk, Massimo, Speciality	102
Sugar Free, Skimmed Milk, Medio, Speciality	80
Sugar Free, Skimmed Milk, Primo, Speciality	62
Sugar Free, Soya Milk, Massimo, Speciality	136
Sugar Free, Soya Milk, Medio, Speciality	107
Sugar Free, Soya Milk, Primo, Speciality	82

COFFEE - LATTE, HONEYCOMB

Skimmed Milk, Massimo	392
Skimmed Milk, Massimo, Takeaway	387
Skimmed Milk, Medio	309
Skimmed Milk, Medio, Takeaway	338
Skimmed Milk, Primo	248
Skimmed Milk, Primo, Takeaway	269
Soya Milk, Massimo	419
Soya Milk, Massimo, Takeaway	422
Soya Milk, Medio	331
Soya Milk, Medio, Takeaway	369
Soya Milk, Primo	264
Soya Milk, Primo, Takeaway	290
Whole Milk, Massimo	483
Whole Milk, Massimo, Takeaway	508
Whole Milk, Medio	384
Whole Milk, Medio, Takeaway	443
Whole Milk, Primo	303
Whole Milk, Primo, Takeaway	342

COFFEE - LATTE, ROASTED HAZELNUT

Skimmed Milk, Massimo, Speciality	190
Skimmed Milk, Massimo, Speciality, Takeaway	200
Skimmed Milk, Medio, Speciality	147
Skimmed Milk, Medio, Speciality, Takeaway	147
Skimmed Milk, Primo, Speciality	78
Soya Milk, Massimo, Speciality	228
Soya Milk, Massimo, Speciality, Takeaway	240
Soya Milk, Medio, Speciality	176
Soya Milk, Medio, Speciality, Takeaway	176
Soya Milk, Primo, Speciality	114
Soya Milk, Primo, Speciality, Takeaway	125
Whole Milk, Massimo, Speciality	319
Whole Milk, Massimo, Speciality, Takeaway	335
Whole Milk, Medio, Speciality	246
Whole Milk, Medio, Speciality, Takeaway	246
Whole Milk, Primo, Speciality	160
Whole Milk, Primo, Speciality, Takeaway	175

COSTA

COFFEE - LATTE, ROASTED HAZELNUT, ICED

Full Fat Milk, Massimo, Speciality	259
Full Fat Milk, Medio, Speciality	202
Full Fat Milk, Primo, Speciality	150
Skimmed Milk, Massimo, Speciality	162
Skimmed Milk, Medio, Speciality	125
Skimmed Milk, Primo, Speciality	92
Soya Milk, Massimo, Speciality	202
Soya Milk, Medio, Speciality	152
Soya Milk, Primo, Speciality	112

COFFEE - LATTE, VANILLA

Skimmed Milk, Massimo, Speciality	195
Skimmed Milk, Massimo, Speciality, Takeaway	205
Skimmed Milk, Medio, Speciality	150
Skimmed Milk, Medio, Speciality, Takeaway	150
Skimmed Milk, Primo, Speciality	98
Skimmed Milk, Primo, Speciality, Takeaway	106
Soya Milk, Massimo, Speciality	233
Soya Milk, Massimo, Speciality, Takeaway	245
Soya Milk, Medio, Speciality	180
Soya Milk, Medio, Speciality, Takeaway	180
Soya Milk, Primo, Speciality	116
Soya Milk, Primo, Speciality, Takeaway	128
Whole Milk, Massimo, Speciality	324
Whole Milk, Massimo, Speciality, Takeaway	340
Whole Milk, Medio, Speciality	250
Whole Milk, Medio, Speciality, Takeaway	250
Whole Milk, Primo, Speciality	162
Whole Milk, Primo, Speciality, Takeaway	178

COFFEE - LATTE, VANILLA, ICED

Whole Milk, Massimo, Speciality	260
Whole Milk, Medio, Speciality	203
Whole Milk, Primo, Speciality	151
Skimmed, Massimo, Speciality	164
Skimmed, Medio, Speciality	127
Skimmed, Primo, Speciality	93
Soya, Massimo, Speciality	198
Soya, Medio, Speciality	154
Soya, Primo, Speciality	113

COFFEE - MACCHIATO

Skimmed Milk, Solo	9
Soya Milk, Solo	10
Whole Milk, Solo	13

COFFEE - MOCHA

Italia, Espresso, Doppio	6
Italia, Espresso, Solo	3
Skimmed Milk, Massimo	362
Skimmed Milk, Massimo, Takeaway	367
Skimmed Milk, Medio	237
Skimmed Milk, Medio, Takeaway	237
Skimmed Milk, Primo	159
Skimmed Milk, Primo, Takeaway	168
Soya Milk, Massimo	390

COSTA

COFFEE - MOCHA

	KCAL
Soya Milk, Massimo, Takeaway	396
Soya Milk, Medio	261
Soya Milk, Medio, Takeaway	261
Soya Milk, Primo	175
Soya Milk, Primo, Takeaway	186
Whole Milk, Massimo	456
Whole Milk, Massimo, Takeaway	469
Whole Milk, Medio	317
Whole Milk, Medio, Takeaway	317
Whole Milk, Primo	209
Whole Milk, Primo, Takeaway	228

COFFEE - MOCHA CORTADO

Skimmed Milk	53
Skimmed Milk, Takeaway	71
Skimmed Milk, Takeaway	84
Soya Milk	85
Soya Milk, New Recipe	61
Soya Milk, Takeaway	85
Soya Milk, Takeaway	100
Whole Milk	114
Whole Milk	82
Whole MilkTakeaway	118
Whole Milk, Takeaway	138

COFFEE - MOCHA CORTADO, ICED

Whole Milk, Solo	102
Skimmed Milk, Solo	77
Soya Milk, Solo	86

COFFEE - MOCHA LATTE

Skimmed Milk, Massimo	390
Skimmed Milk, Massimo, Takeaway	396
Skimmed Milk, Medio	261
Skimmed Milk, Medio, Takeaway	261
Skimmed Milk, Primo	177
Skimmed Milk, Primo	162
Skimmed Milk, Primo, Takeaway	189
Soya Milk, Massimo	342
Soya Milk, Massimo, Takeaway	441
Soya Milk, Medio	289
Soya Milk, Medio, Takeaway	289
Soya Milk, Primo	197
Soya Milk, Primo, Takeaway	215
Whole Milk, Massimo	523
Whole Milk, Massimo, Takeaway	536
Whole Milk, Medio	362
Whole Milk, Medio, Takeaway	362
Whole Milk, Primo	243
Whole Milk, Primo, Takeaway	271

COFFEE - MOCHA LATTE, ICED

Whole Milk, Massimo	399
Whole Milk, Medio	307
Whole Milk, Primo	220
Skimmed Milk, Massimo	302

COSTA

COFFEE - MOCHA LATTE, ICED

	KCAL
Skimmed Milk, Medio	231
Soya Milk, Massimo	336
Soya Milk, Medio	258
Soya Milk, Primo	183

COFFEE - MOCHA, ICED

Whole Milk, Massimo	347
Whole Milk, Medio	269
Whole Milk, Primo	190
Skimmed Milk, Massimo	279
Skimmed Milk, Medio	213
Skimmed Milk, Primo	148
Soya Milk, Massimo	303
Soya Milk, Medio	233
Soya Milk, Primo	163

COFFEE BEANS

Chocolate Coated	221

COOKIES

Chocolate, Belgian, All Butter	428
Chocolate Chip	377
Chocolate Chip, Triple	368

CREAM

Clotted, Extra	234
Whipping	80

CROISSANT

Almond	351
Plain	314

CRUMBLE

Fruity, Gluten, & Dairy Free	282

CRUMPETS

No Butter, Breakfast	210

CUPCAKES

Banoffee	431

DOUGHNUTS

Choc O Crunch, Milk	275
Choc O Crunch, White	262

DRIED FRUIT

Mango	120

FLAPJACK

Fruity	380
Nutty	425

FROSTINO

Billionaire, Skimmed Milk, No Coffee, Medio	459
Billionaire, Skimmed Milk, with Coffee, Medio	465
Billionaire, Soya Milk, No Coffee, Medio	476
Billionaire, Soya Milk, with Coffee, Medio	482
Billionaire, Whole Milk, No Coffee, Medio	517
Billionaire, Whole Milk, with Coffee, Medio	523
Black Forest, Soya Milk, Medio	466
Black Forest, Whole Milk, Medio	507
Latte, Caramel, Skimmed, Milk, Primo	155
Latte, Caramel, Skimmed Milk, Medio	210

COSTA

FRUIT & NUT
Mix	204

FRUIT COMPOTE
Mixed Berry, Topping	38

FRUIT SALAD
Breakfast	80

HONEY
Extra	64

HOT CHOCOLATE
Billionaire, Skimmed Milk, Medio	439
Billionaire, Skimmed Milk, Medio, Takeaway	449
Billionaire, Skimmed Milk, Primo	294
Billionaire, Skimmed Milk, Primo, Takeaway	306
Billionaire, Soya Milk, Medio	465
Billionaire, Soya Milk, Medio, Takeaway	478
Billionaire, Soya Milk, Primo	312
Billionaire, Soya Milk, Primo, Takeaway	327
Billionaire, Whole Milk, Medio	528
Billionaire, Whole Milk, Medio, Takeaway	547
Billionaire, Whole Milk, Primo	356
Billionaire, Whole Milk, Primo, Takeaway	379
Black Forest, Skimmed Milk, Primo	287
Black Forest, Soya Milk, Medio	402
Black Forest, Soya Milk, Primo	309
Black Forest, Whole Milk, Medio	477
Black Forest, Whole Milk, Primo	363
Lindt	329
Lindt, Takeaway	348
Mint, Skimmed Milk, Medio	394
Mint, Skimmed Milk, Primo	297
Mint, Soya Milk, Medio	425
Mint, Soya Milk, Primo	319
Mint, Whole Milk, Medio	499
Mint, Whole Milk, Primo	373
Powder, Costa*	49
Skimmed Milk, Massimo	353
Skimmed Milk, Massimo, Takeaway	355
Skimmed Milk, Medio	232
Skimmed Milk, Medio, Takeaway	232
Skimmed Milk, Primo	150
Skimmed Milk, Primo, Takeaway	162
Skimmed Milk, Primo, Takeaway	162
Soya Milk, Massimo	387
Soya Milk, Massimo, Takeaway	395
Soya Milk, Medio	258
Soya Milk, Medio, Takeaway	258
Soya Milk, Primo	168
Soya Milk, Primo, Takeaway	183
Whole Milk, Massimo	476
Whole Milk, Massimo	476
Whole Milk, Massimo, Takeaway	488
Whole Milk, Medio	328
Whole Milk, Medio, Takeaway	328

COSTA

HOT CHOCOLATE
Whole Milk, Primo	210
Whole Milk, Primo, Takeaway	233

HOT CHOCOLATE - WITH CREAM & MARSHMALLOWS
Skimmed Milk, Primo, Takeaway	283
Medio, Takeaway	477
Skimmed Milk, Massimo	576
Skimmed Milk, Massimo, Takeaway	542
Skimmed Milk, Medio	380
Skimmed Milk, Medio, Takeaway	392
Skimmed Milk, Primo	276
Soya Milk, Massimo	609
Soya Milk, Massimo, Takeaway	574
Soya Milk, Medio	408
Soya Milk, Medio, Takeaway	416
Soya Milk, Primo	294
Soya Milk, Primo, Takeaway	303
Whole Milk, Massimo	690
Whole Milk, Massimo, Takeaway	656
Whole Milk, Medio	472
Whole Milk, Primo	334
Whole Milk, Primo, Takeaway	480

JAM
Strawberry, Extra	75

JUICE
Apple, Spiced, Winter Warmer, Medio	122
Apple, Spiced, Winter Warmer, Medio, Takeaway	136
Apple, Spiced, Winter Warmer, Primo	79
Apple, Spiced, Winter Warmer, Primo, Takeaway	93

JUICE DRINK
Blackberry, & Raspberry, Fruit Cooler, Massimo	310
Blackberry, & Raspberry, Fruit Cooler, Medio	250
Blackberry, & Raspberry, Fruit Cooler, Primo	189
Cherry, & Orange, Cooler, Massimo	292
Cherry, & Orange, Cooler, Medio	230
Cherry, & Orange, Cooler, Primo	172
Mango & Passionfruit, Fruit Cooler, Massimo	295
Mango & Passionfruit, Fruit Cooler, Medio	234
Mango & Passionfruit, Fruit Cooler, Primo	177
Tropical, Cooler, Massimo	257
Tropical, Cooler, Medio	205
Tropical, Cooler, Primo	156

KETCHUP
Sachet, Extra	7

LEMON
Slices	32

LEMONADE
Original, Massimo	145
Original, Medio	115
Original, Primo	87
Raspberry, Massimo	145
Raspberry, Medio	115
Raspberry, Primo	87

COSTA

MACARONI CHEESE
Box	598

MARMALADE
Extra	75

MARMITE*
Extra	20

MILK
Full Fat, Whole	25
Skimmed	13
Soya	18

MILK DRINK
Chocolate, Full Fat Milk, Massimo, Iced	351
Chocolate, Full Fat Milk, Medio, Iced	271
Chocolate, Full Fat Milk, Primo, Iced	194
Chocolate, Skimmed Milk, Massimo, Iced	275
Chocolate, Skimmed Milk, Medio, Iced	210
Chocolate, Skimmed Milk, Primo, Iced	147
Chocolate, Soya Milk, Massimo, Iced	302
Chocolate, Soya Milk, Medio, Iced	232
Chocolate, Soya Milk, Primo, Iced	163

MIXED NUTS
Chilli, & Lime, Mix	204

MUFFIN
Banana & Pecan Breakfast Loaf	442
Blueberry	448
Caramel, Salted	483
Chocolate, Triple	422
Gingerbread	496
Lemon	454
Mini, Chocolate, & Raspberry & White Chocolate	75

NUTELLA
Extra	81

PANETTONE
Classic	374

PANINI
Bacon, British, & Brie	499
Goats Cheese, & Sweet Chilli, Chutney	420
Ham, British, & Cheese	427
Mozzarella, Tomato, & Basil	519
Salami, & Tomato	449
Tuna, Melt	483

PASTA
Meatball	466

PASTRY
Chocolate, Twist	396
Pain Aux Chocolat	266
Pain Aux Raisins	292

PEANUT BUTTER
Extra	92

SALAD
Chicken, Roast	196
Cous Cous, Moroccan Styles	392
Pasta, Feta, Tomato	472

COSTA

SALAD
Tuna, Nicoise	219

SANDWICH
BLT	384
Chicken, Salad, Roast	352
Chicken, Salad, Roast, GF	355
Chicken, Salad, Roast, GF	355
Egg, Free Range	342
Salmon, Smoked, & Soft Cheese	388
Selection	436

SAUCE
Belgian Chocolate	54
Brown, Sachet, Extra	12
Cherry	82
White Chocolate	214

SAUSAGE
Bap, Breakfast	488

SCONE
Fruit	258

SHORTBREAD
Bites, Mini	52
Caramel, Traybake	404

SMOOTHIE
Coffee, Oats, & Banana, Superday	258
Passion Fruit, Mango, & Peach, Superday	206
Spinach, Mango, Pineapple, & Banana, Superday	154
Strawberry, & Banana, Superday	136

SOUP
Chicken, & Vegetable	110

SPREAD
Sunflower, Extra	43

SUGAR
Brown	10
White, Granulated	10

SWEETENER
Sweet 'n' Low	4

SYRUP
Amaretto, No Added Sugar	1
Caramel	16
Caramel, Sugar Free	2
Cinnamon	32
Gingerbread	33
Gingerbread, No Added Sugar	1
Gomme	17
Honeycomb	15
Maple, Sachet	62
Marshmallow	1
Popcorn	32
Roasted Hazelnut	16
Vanilla	17

TART
Apple, & Blackberry, Crumble	266
Bakewell, Cherry	392

COSTA

TART

Bakewell, Mini	137
Lemon	351

TEA

Chai Latte, Skimmed Milk, Massimo	352
Chai Latte, Skimmed Milk, Medio	221
Chai Latte, Skimmed Milk, Primo	141
Chai Latte, Soya Milk, Massimo	402
Chai Latte, Soya Milk, Medio	254
Chai Latte, Whole Milk, Massimo	522
Chai Latte, Whole Milk, Medio	334
Chai Latte, Whole Milk, Primo	209
Citrus, & Ginger, Twist	6
English Breakfast, Decaff	3
Everyday	3
Green, Simply Sencha	3
Iced, Lemon, Massimo	181
Iced, lemon, Medio	136
Iced, Lemon, Primo	91
Iced, Peach, Massimo	175
Iced, Peach, Medoi	131
Iced, Peach, Primo	88
Chai Latte, Whole Milk, Massimo, Iced	426
Chai Latte, Whole Milk, Medio, Iced	327
Chai Latte, Whole Milk, Primo, Iced	231
Chai Latte, Skimmed, Massimo, Iced	350
Chai Latte, Skimmed, Medio, Iced	266
Chai Latte, Skimmed, Primo, Iced	184
Chai Latte, Soya Milk, Massimo, Iced	376
Chai Latte, Soya Milk, Medio, Iced	288
Chai Latte, Soya Milk, Primo, Iced	201
The Earl	3
Thoroughly Minted	3

TEACAKES

Fruit, No Butter, Breakfast	311

TOAST

Brown, Seeded	350
Fruit	288
White, No Butter	251

TOASTIE

Cheddar, & Tomato, Slow Roasted	443
Chicken, & Bacon	418
Emmenthal, & Mushroom	443
Ham, British, & Cheese	307
Ham, Wiltshire, & Mature Cheddar	409
Sausage, Cumberland, with Red Onion	493

VANILLA

Powder	26

WRAP

Chicken, Fajita, Roast	428
Meatball	582

YOGHURT

with Raspberry, & Strawberry, Compote, Breakfast	109

DOMINO'S PIZZA

BREAD

Garlic, Italiano, ¼ Bread	228
Garlic, Pizza, 1 Slice	156

BROWNIES

Chocolate	147

CAKE

Chocolate Melt	374

CHICKEN

Chick n Mix Box, ½ Box	324
Kickers, Combo Box, ¼ Box	177
Kickers, 1 Kicker	53
Strippers, Combo Box, ¼ Box	160
Strippers, 1 Stripper	43
Wings, Combo Box, ¼ Box	220
Wings, 1 Wing	78
Wings, Red Hot, Franks, 1 Wing	65
Wings, Spicy BBQ, 1 Wing	72

COLESLAW

Half Pot	155

COOKIES

Warm, 1 Cookie	182

DIP

BBQ, Big	188
BBQ	47
Garlic & Herb	169
Honey & Mystard	109
Red Hot, Franks, Big	24
Red Hot, Franks	6
Salsa, Tangy	41

DIP & DIPPERS

Cinni, ½ Box	400

DOUGH BALLS

Twisted, Pepperoni, ½ Box	305
Twisted, with Cheese and Herb Sauce, ½ Box	326

MEATBALLS

Meltin', ½ Box	191

NACHOS

no Jalapenos, ½ Box	243
with Jalapenos, ½ Boxs	244

OIL

Chilli Infused	127

PIZZA

Chocolate, Lotta, ½ Pizza	204

PIZZA - AMERICAN HOT

BBQ Stuffed Crust, Delight Mozzarella, Large	236
BBQ Stuffed Crust, Delight Mozzarella, Medium	222
BBQ Stuffed Crust, Large	251
BBQ Stuffed Crust, Medium	245
Classic Crust, Delight Mozzarella, Large	189
Classic Crust, Delight Mozzarella, Medium	175
Classic Crust, Delight Mozzarella, Personal	130
Classic Crust, Delight Mozzarella, Small	157
Classic Crust, Large	196

DOMINO'S PIZZA

PIZZA - AMERICAN HOT

Classic Crust, Medium	181
Classic Crust, Personal	134
Classic Crust, Small	160
Double Decadence, Delight Mozzarella, Large	261
Double Decadence, Delight Mozzarella, Medium	239
Double Decadence, Large	265
Double Decadence, Medium	243
GF Crust, Delight Mozzarella, Small	138
GF Crust, Small	134
Italian Style Crust, Delight Mozzarella, Large	173
Italian Style Crust, Delight Mozzarella, Medium	155
Italian Style Crust, Delight Mozzarella, Small	137
Italian Style Crust, Large	153
Italian Style Crust, Medium	58
Italian Style Crust, Small	122
Stuffed Crust, Delight Mozzarella, Large	230
Stuffed Crust, Delight Mozzarella, Medium	216
Stuffed Crust, Large	255
Stuffed Crust, Medium	240
Thin & Crispy, Delight Mozzarella, Large	160
Thin & Crispy, Delight Mozzarella, Medium	149
Thin & Crispy, Large	168
Thin & Crispy, Medium	157

PIZZA - AMERICANO

BBQ Stuffed Crust, Delight Mozzarella, Large	269
BBQ Stuffed Crust, Delight Mozzarella, Medium	246
BBQ Stuffed Crust, Large	269
BBQ Stuffed Crust, Medium	253
Classic Crust, Delight Mozzarella, Large	213
Classic Crust, Delight Mozzarella, Medium	197
Classic Crust, Delight Mozzarella, Personal	147
Classic Crust, Delight Mozzarella, Small	182
Classic Crust, Large	221
Classic Crust, Medium	204
Classic Crust, Small	183
Double Decadence, Delight Mozzarella, Large	287
Double Decadence, Delight Mozzarella, Medium	263
Double Decadence, Large	288
Double Decadence, Medium	264
GF Crust, Delight Mozzarella, Small	159
GF Crust, Small	166
Italian Style Crust, Delight Mozzarella, Large	192
Italian Style Crust, Delight Mozzarella, Medium	172
Italian Style Crust, Delight Mozzarella, Small	153
Italian Style Crust, Large	197
Italian Style Crust, Medium	176
Italian Style Crust, Small	156
Stuffed Crust, Delight Mozzarella, Large	256
Stuffed Crust, Delight Mozzarella, Medium	240
Stuffed Crust, Large	263
Stuffed Crust, Medium	247
Thin & Crispy, Delight Mozzarella, Large	183

DOMINO'S PIZZA

PIZZA - AMERICANO

Thin & Crispy, Delight Mozzarella, Medium	171
Thin & Crispy, Large	191
Thin & Crispy, Medium	179
Classic Crust, Personal	152

PIZZA - BACON DOUBLE CHEESE

BBQ Stuffed Crust, Delight Mozzarella, Large	249
BBQ Stuffed Crust, Delight Mozzarella, Medium	230
BBQ Stuffed Crust, Large	267
BBQ Stuffed Crust, Medium	256
Classic Crust, Delight Mozzarella, Large	202
Classic Crust, Delight Mozzarella, Medium	183
Classic Crust, Delight Mozzarella, Personal	140
Classic Crust, Delight Mozzarella, Small	160
Classic Crust, Large	212
Classic Crust, Medium	192
Classic Crust, Personal	146
Classic Crust, Small	165
Double Decadence, Delight Mozzarella, Large	274
Double Decadence, Delight Mozzarella, Medium	247
Double Decadence, Large	281
Double Decadence, Medium	254
GF Crust, Delight Mozzarella, Small	141
GF Crust, Small	140
Italian Style Crust, Delight Mozzarella, Large	185
Italian Style Crust, Delight Mozzarella, Medium	163
Italian Style Crust, Delight Mozzarella, Small	140
Italian Style Crust, Large	169
Italian Style Crust, Medium	149
Italian Style Crust, Small	128
Stuffed Crust, Delight Mozzarella, Large	242
Stuffed Crust, Delight Mozzarella, Medium	224
Stuffed Crust, Large	271
Stuffed Crust, Medium	251
Thin & Crispy, Delight Mozzarella, Large	173
Thin & Crispy, Delight Mozzarella, Medium	158
Thin & Crispy, Large	184
Thin & Crispy, Medium	168

PIZZA - CHEESE & TOMATO

BBQ Stuffed Crust, Delight Mozzarella, Large	197
BBQ Stuffed Crust, Delight Mozzarella, Medium	183
BBQ Stuffed Crust, Large	214
BBQ Stuffed Crust, Medium	208
Classic Crust, Delight Mozzarella, Large	150
Classic Crust, Delight Mozzarella, Medium	136
Classic Crust, Delight Mozzarella, Personal	112
Classic Crust, Delight Mozzarella, Small	133
Classic Crust, Large	159
Classic Crust, Medium	145
Classic Crust, Personal	118
Classic Crust, Personal	118
Classic Crust, Small	139
Double Decadence, Delight Mozzarella, Large	220

DOMINO'S PIZZA

PIZZA - CHEESE & TOMATO

	KCAL
Double Decadence, Delight Mozzarella, Medium	199
Double Decadence, Large	227
Double Decadence, Medium	205
GF Crust, Delight Mozzarella, Small	115
GF Crust, Small	113
Italian Style Crust, Delight Mozzarella, Large	132
Italian Style Crust, Delight Mozzarella, Medium	115
Italian Style Crust, Delight Mozzarella, Small	105
Italian Style Crust, Large	119
Italian Style Crust, Medium	103
Italian Style Crust, Small	88
Stuffed Crust, Delight Mozzarella, Large	191
Stuffed Crust, Delight Mozzarella, Medium	178
Stuffed Crust, Large	217
Stuffed Crust, Medium	202
Thin & Crispy, Delight Mozzarella, Large	116
Thin & Crispy, Delight Mozzarella, Medium	106
Thin & Crispy, Large	126
Thin & Crispy, Medium	115

PIZZA - CHICKEN & RASHER BACON

	KCAL
BBQ Stuffed Crust, Delight Mozzarella, Large	228
BBQ Stuffed Crust, Delight Mozzarella, Medium	211
BBQ Stuffed Crust, Large	243
BBQ Stuffed Crust, Medium	235
Classic Crust, Delight Mozzarella, Large	181
Classic Crust, Delight Mozzarella, Medium	165
Classic Crust, Delight Mozzarella, Personal	127
Classic Crust, Delight Mozzarella, Small	145
Classic Crust, Large	188
Classic Crust, Medium	171
Classic Crust, Personal	174
Classic Crust, Small	147
Double Decadence, Delight Mozzarella, Large	253
Double Decadence, Delight Mozzarella, Medium	144
Double Decadence, Large	257
Double Decadence, Medium	233
GF Crust, Delight Mozzarella, Small	126
GF Crust, Small	121
Italian Style Crust, Delight Mozzarella, Large	164
Italian Style Crust, Delight Mozzarella, Medium	144
Italian Style Crust, Delight Mozzarella, Small	124
Italian Style Crust, Large	145
Italian Style Crust, Medium	128
Italian Style Crust, Small	110
Stuffed Crust, Delight Mozzarella, Large	222
Stuffed Crust, Delight Mozzarella, Medium	206
Stuffed Crust, Large	247
Stuffed Crust, Medium	230
Thin & Crispy, Delight Mozzarella, Large	152
Thin & Crispy, Delight Mozzarella, Medium	139
Thin & Crispy, Large	160
Thin & Crispy, Medium	147

DOMINO'S PIZZA

PIZZA - CHICKEN FEAST

	KCAL
BBQ Stuffed Crust, Delight Mozzarella, Large	223
BBQ Stuffed Crust, Delight Mozzarella, Medium	208
BBQ Stuffed Crust, Large	238
BBQ Stuffed Crust, Medium	232
Classic Crust, Delight Mozzarella, Large	177
Classic Crust, Delight Mozzarella, Medium	161
Classic Crust, Delight Mozzarella, Personal	121
Classic Crust, Delight Mozzarella, Small	141
Classic Crust, Large	184
Classic Crust, Medium	167
Classic Crust, Personal	125
Classic Crust, Small	143
Double Decadence, Delight Mozzarella, Large	249
Double Decadence, Delight Mozzarella, Medium	225
Double Decadence, Large	253
Double Decadence, Medium	229
GF Crust, Delight Mozzarella, Small	122
GF Crust, Small	117
Italian Style Crust, Delight Mozzarella, Lge	160
Italian Style Crust, Delight Mozzarella, Medium	141
Italian Style Crust, Delight Mozzarella, Small	120
Italian Style Crust, Lge	141
Italian Style Crust, Medium	124
Italian Style Crust, Small	106
Stuffed Crust, Delight Mozzarella, Large	217
Stuffed Crust, Delight Mozzarella, Medium	202
Stuffed Crust, Large	243
Stuffed Crust, Medium	226
Thin & Crispy, Delight Mozzarella, Large	147
Thin & Crispy, Delight Mozzarella, Medium	136
Thin & Crispy, Large	156
Thin & Crispy, Medium	143

PIZZA - CHIPOTLE PULLED PORK

	KCAL
BBQ Stuffed Crust, Delight Mozzarella, Large	218
BBQ Stuffed Crust, Delight Mozzarella, Medium	204
BBQ Stuffed Crust, Large	233
BBQ Stuffed Crust, Medium	227
Classic Crust, Delight Mozzarella, Large	172
Classic Crust, Delight Mozzarella, Medium	157
Classic Crust, Delight Mozzarella, Personal	117
Classic Crust, Delight Mozzarella, Small	139
Classic Crust, Large	178
Classic Crust, Medium	163
Classic Crust, Personal	121
Classic Crust, Small	141
Delight Mozzarella, Large	244
Double Decadence, Delight Mozzarella, Medium	221
Double Decadence, Large	248
Double Decadence, Medium	225
GF Crust, Delight Mozzarella, Small	120
GF Crust, Small	116
Italian Style Crust, Delight Mozzarella, Large	155

DOMINO'S PIZZA

PIZZA - CHIPOTLE PULLED PORK

	KCAL
Italian Style Crust, Delight Mozzarella, Medium	137
Italian Style Crust, Delight Mozzarella, Small	118
Italian Style Crust, Large	136
Italian Style Crust, Medium	120
Italian Style Crust, Small	104
Stuffed Crust, Delight Mozzarella, Large	212
Stuffed Crust, Delight Mozzarella, Medium	198
Stuffed Crust, Large	238
Stuffed Crust, Medium	222
Thin & Crispy, Delight Mozzarella, Large	142
Thin & Crispy, Delight Mozzarella, Medium	131
Thin & Crispy, Large	151
Thin & Crispy, Medium	139

PIZZA - DELUXE

	KCAL
BBQ Stuffed Crust, Delight Mozzarella, Large	234
BBQ Stuffed Crust, Delight Mozzarella, Medium	220
BBQ Stuffed Crust, Large	249
BBQ Stuffed Crust, Medium	244
Classic Crust, Delight Mozzarella, Large	188
Classic Crust, Delight Mozzarella, Medium	174
Classic Crust, Delight Mozzarella, Personal	129
Classic Crust, Delight Mozzarella, Small	156
Classic Crust, Large	195
Classic Crust, Medium	180
Classic Crust, Personal	132
Classic Crust, Small	158
Double Decadence, Delight Mozzarella, Large	260
Double Decadence, Delight Mozzarella, Medium	238
Double Decadence, Large	264
Double Decadence, Medium	241
GF Crust, Delight Mozzarella, Small	137
GF Crust, Small	133
Italian Style Crust, Delight Mozzarella, Large	171
Italian Style Crust, Delight Mozzarella, Medium	153
Italian Style Crust, Delight Mozzarella, Small	135
Italian Style Crust, Large	152
Italian Style Crust, Medium	137
Italian Style Crust, Small	121
Stuffed Crust, Delight Mozzarella, Large	228
Stuffed Crust, Delight Mozzarella, Medium	215
Stuffed Crust, Large	254
Stuffed Crust, Medium	239
Thin & Crispy, Delight Mozzarella, Large	158
Thin & Crispy, Delight Mozzarella, Medium	148
Thin & Crispy, Large	167
Thin & Crispy, Medium	156

PIZZA - EXTRAVAGANZA

	KCAL
BBQ Stuffed Crust, Delight Mozzarella, Large	253
BBQ Stuffed Crust, Delight Mozzarella, Medium	237
BBQ Stuffed Crust, Large	271
BBQ Stuffed Crust, Medium	263
Classic Crust, Delight Mozzarella, Large	207

DOMINO'S PIZZA

PIZZA - EXTRAVAGANZA

	KCAL
Classic Crust, Delight Mozzarella, Medium	190
Classic Crust, Delight Mozzarella, Personal	148
Classic Crust, Delight Mozzarella, Small	168
Classic Crust, Large	217
Classic Crust, Medium	199
Classic Crust, Personal	153
Classic Crust, Small	174
Double Decadence, Delight Mozzarella, Large	279
Double Decadence, Delight Mozzarella, Medium	254
Double Decadence, Large	286
Double Decadence, Medium	261
GF Crust, Delight Mozzarella, Small	150
GF Crust, Small	148
Italian Style Crust, Delight Mozzarella, Large	190
Italian Style Crust, Delight Mozzarella, Medium	170
Italian Style Crust, Delight Mozzarella, Small	148
Italian Style Crust, Large	174
Italian Style Crust, Medium	156
Italian Style Crust, Small	136
Stuffed Crust, Delight Mozzarella, Large	247
Stuffed Crust, Delight Mozzarella, Medium	231
Stuffed Crust, Large	276
Stuffed Crust, Medium	258
Thin & Crispy, Delight Mozzarella, Large	177
Thin & Crispy, Delight Mozzarella, Medium	164
Thin & Crispy, Large	189
Thin & Crispy, Medium	175

PIZZA - FARMHOUSE

	KCAL
BBQ Stuffed Crust, Delight Mozzarella, Large	216
BBQ Stuffed Crust, Delight Mozzarella, Medium	197
BBQ Stuffed Crust, Large	226
BBQ Stuffed Crust, Medium	220
Classic Crust, Delight Mozzarella, Large	164
Classic Crust, Delight Mozzarella, Medium	150
Classic Crust, Delight Mozzarella, Personal	113
Classic Crust, Delight Mozzarella, Small	132
Classic Crust, Large	171
Classic Crust, Medium	156
Classic Crust, Personal	117
Classic Crust, Small	135
Double Decadence, Delight Mozzarella, Large	236
Double Decadence, Delight Mozzarella, Medium	214
Double Decadence, Large	240
Double Decadence, Medium	218
GF Crust, Delight Mozzarella, Small	113
GF Crust, Small	109
Italian Style Crust, Delight Mozzarella, Large	148
Italian Style Crust, Delight Mozzarella, Medium	130
Italian Style Crust, Delight Mozzarella, Small	112
Italian Style Crust, Large	128
Italian Style Crust, Medium	113
Italian Style Crust, Small	97

DOMINO'S PIZZA
PIZZA - FARMHOUSE

	KCAL
Stuffed Crust, Delight Mozzarella, Large	205
Stuffed Crust, Delight Mozzarella, Medium	191
Stuffed Crust, Large	230
Stuffed Crust, Medium	215
Thin & Crispy, Delight Mozzarella, Large	135
Thin & Crispy, Delight Mozzarella, Medium	124
Thin & Crispy, Large	143
Thin & Crispy, Medium	132

PIZZA - FOUR VEGI

	KCAL
BBQ Stuffed Crust, Delight Mozzarella, Large	205
BBQ Stuffed Crust, Delight Mozzarella, Medium	192
BBQ Stuffed Crust, Large	220
BBQ Stuffed Crust, Medium	216
Classic Crust, Delight Mozzarella, Large	159
Classic Crust, Delight Mozzarella, Medium	145
Classic Crust, Delight Mozzarella, Personal	110
Classic Crust, Delight Mozzarella, Small	126
Classic Crust, Large	166
Classic Crust, Medium	152
Classic Crust, Personal	115
Classic Crust, Small	129
Double Decadence, Delight Mozzarella, Large	231
Double Decadence, Delight Mozzarella, Medium	210
Double Decadence, Large	235
Double Decadence, Medium	213
GF Crust, Delight Mozzarella, Small	107
GF Crust, Small	103
Italian Style Crust, Delight Mozzarella, Large	142
Italian Style Crust, Delight Mozzarella, Medium	125
Italian Style Crust, Delight Mozzarella, Small	106
Italian Style Crust, Large	123
Italian Style Crust, Medium	108
Italian Style Crust, Small	91
Stuffed Crust, Delight Mozzarella, Large	199
Stuffed Crust, Delight Mozzarella, Medium	186
Stuffed Crust, Large	225
Stuffed Crust, Medium	210
Thin & Crispy, Delight Mozzarella, Large	129
Thin & Crispy, Delight Mozzarella, Medium	120
Thin & Crispy, Large	138
Thin & Crispy, Medium	127

PIZZA - FULL HOUSE

	KCAL
BBQ Stuffed Crust, Delight Mozzarella, Large	235
BBQ Stuffed Crust, Delight Mozzarella, Medium	220
BBQ Stuffed Crust, Large	250
BBQ Stuffed Crust, Medium	244
Classic Crust, Delight Mozzarella, Large	188
Classic Crust, Delight Mozzarella, Medium	174
Classic Crust, Delight Mozzarella, Personal	137
Classic Crust, Delight Mozzarella, Small	155
Classic Crust, Large	195
Classic Crust, Medium	180

DOMINO'S PIZZA
PIZZA - FULL HOUSE

	KCAL
Classic Crust, Personal	142
Classic Crust, Small	158
Double Decadence, Delight Mozzarella, Large	260
Double Decadence, Delight Mozzarella, Medium	238
Double Decadence, Large	264
Double Decadence, Medium	241
GF Crust, Delight Mozzarella, Small	136
GF Crust, Small	132
Italian Style Crust, Delight Mozzarella, Large	172
Italian Style Crust, Delight Mozzarella, Medium	153
Italian Style Crust, Delight Mozzarella, Small	135
Italian Style Crust, Large	153
Italian Style Crust, Medium	136
Italian Style Crust, Small	120
Stuffed Crust, Delight Mozzarella, Large	229
Stuffed Crust, Delight Mozzarella, Medium	215
Stuffed Crust, Large	255
Stuffed Crust, Medium	238
Thin & Crispy, Delight Mozzarella, Large	159
Thin & Crispy, Delight Mozzarella, Medium	148
Thin & Crispy, Large	167
Thin & Crispy, Medium	156

PIZZA - HAM & PINEAPPLE

	KCAL
BBQ Stuffed Crust, Delight Mozzarella, Large	212
BBQ Stuffed Crust, Delight Mozzarella, Medium	198
BBQ Stuffed Crust, Large	227
BBQ Stuffed Crust, Medium	221
Classic Crust, Delight Mozzarella, Large	165
Classic Crust, Delight Mozzarella, Medium	151
Classic Crust, Delight Mozzarella, Personal	114
Classic Crust, Delight Mozzarella, Small	133
Classic Crust, Large	172
Classic Crust, Medium	157
Classic Crust, Personal	118
Classic Crust, Small	136
Double Decadence, Delight Mozzarella, Large	237
Double Decadence, Delight Mozzarella, Medium	215
Double Decadence, Large	241
Double Decadence, Medium	219
GF Crust, Delight Mozzarella, Small	114
GF Crust, Small	110
Italian Style Crust, Delight Mozzarella, Large	149
Italian Style Crust, Delight Mozzarella, Medium	131
Italian Style Crust, Delight Mozzarella, Small	136
Italian Style Crust, Large	129
Italian Style Crust, Medium	114
Italian Style Crust, Small	98
Stuffed Crust, Delight Mozzarella, Large	206
Stuffed Crust, Delight Mozzarella, Medium	192
Stuffed Crust, Large	231
Stuffed Crust, Large	231
Stuffed Crust, Medium	216

DOMINO'S PIZZA

PIZZA - HAM & PINEAPPLE

Thin & Crispy, Delight Mozzarella, Large	136
Thin & Crispy, Delight Mozzarella, Medium	125
Thin & Crispy, Large	144
Thin & Crispy, Medium	133

PIZZA - HAMROCK

BBQ Stuffed Crust, Delight Mozzarella, Large	228
BBQ Stuffed Crust, Delight Mozzarella, Medium	212
BBQ Stuffed Crust, Large	243
BBQ Stuffed Crust, Medium	236
Classic Crust, Delight Mozzarella, Large	181
Classic Crust, Delight Mozzarella, Medium	162
Classic Crust, Delight Mozzarella, Personal	122
Classic Crust, Delight Mozzarella, Small	144
Classic Crust, Large	188
Classic Crust, Medium	172
Classic Crust, Personal	126
Classic Crust, Small	144
Classic Crust, Small	146
Double Decadence, Delight Mozzarella, Large	253
Double Decadence, Delight Mozzarella, Medium	229
Double Decadence, Large	257
Double Decadence, Medium	233
GF Crust, Delight Mozzarella, Small	125
GF Crust, Small	121
Italian Style Crust, Delight Mozzarella, Large	165
Italian Style Crust, Delight Mozzarella, Medium	165
Italian Style Crust, Delight Mozzarella, Medium	145
Italian Style Crust, Delight Mozzarella, Small	123
Italian Style Crust, Large	146
Italian Style Crust, Medium	128
Italian Style Crust, Small	109
Stuffed Crust, Delight Mozzarella, Large	222
Stuffed Crust, Delight Mozzarella, Medium	206
Stuffed Crust, Large	248
Stuffed Crust, Medium	230
Thin & Crispy, Delight Mozzarella, Large	152
Thin & Crispy, Delight Mozzarella, Medium	140
Thin & Crispy, Large	160
Thin & Crispy, Medium	143

PIZZA - HAWAIIAN

BBQ Stuffed Crust, Delight Mozzarella, Large	212
BBQ Stuffed Crust, Delight Mozzarella, Medium	198
BBQ Stuffed Crust, Large	227
BBQ Stuffed Crust, Medium	222
Classic Crust, Delight Mozzarella, Large	166
Classic Crust, Delight Mozzarella, Medium	152
Classic Crust, Delight Mozzarella, Personal	114
Classic Crust, Delight Mozzarella, Small	133
Classic Crust, Large	173
Classic Crust, Medium	158
Classic Crust, Personal	119
Classic Crust, Small	136

DOMINO'S PIZZA

PIZZA - HAWAIIAN

Double Decadence, Delight Mozzarella, Large	238
Double Decadence, Delight Mozzarella, Medium	216
Double Decadence, Large	242
Double Decadence, Medium	219
GF Crust, Delight Mozzarella, Small	115
GF Crust, Small	110
Italian Style Crust, Delight Mozzarella, Large	149
Italian Style Crust, Delight Mozzarella, Medium	131
Italian Style Crust, Delight Mozzarella, Small	113
Italian Style Crust, Large	130
Italian Style Crust, Medium	115
Italian Style Crust, Small	99
Stuffed Crust, Delight Mozzarella, Large	206
Stuffed Crust, Delight Mozzarella, Medium	193
Stuffed Crust, Large	232
Stuffed Crust, Medium	217
Thin & Crispy, Delight Mozzarella, Large	136
Thin & Crispy, Delight Mozzarella, Medium	126
Thin & Crispy, Large	145
Thin & Crispy, Medium	134

PIZZA - HOT & SPICY

BBQ Stuffed Crust, Delight Mozzarella, Large	207
BBQ Stuffed Crust, Delight Mozzarella, Medium	193
BBQ Stuffed Crust, Large	222
BBQ Stuffed Crust, Medium	217
Classic Crust, Delight Mozzarella, Large	161
Classic Crust, Delight Mozzarella, Medium	146
Classic Crust, Delight Mozzarella, Personal	111
Classic Crust, Delight Mozzarella, Small	128
Classic Crust, Large	504
Classic Crust, Medium	152
Classic Crust, Personal	115
Classic Crust, Small	130
Double Decadence, Delight Mozzarella, Large	233
Double Decadence, Delight Mozzarella, Medium	210
Double Decadence, Large	237
Double Decadence, Medium	214
GF Crust, Delight Mozzarella, Small	109
GF Crust, Small	105
Italian Style Crust, Delight Mozzarella, Large	144
Italian Style Crust, Delight Mozzarella, Medium	126
Italian Style Crust, Delight Mozzarella, Small	107
Italian Style Crust, Large	125
Italian Style Crust, Medium	109
Italian Style Crust, Small	93
Stuffed Crust, Delight Mozzarella, Large	201
Stuffed Crust, Delight Mozzarella, Medium	187
Stuffed Crust, Large	227
Stuffed Crust, Medium	211
Thin & Crispy, Delight Mozzarella, Large	131
Thin & Crispy, Delight Mozzarella, Medium	120
Thin & Crispy, Large	140

DOMINO'S PIZZA

PIZZA - HOT & SPICY

Thin & Crispy, Medium	128

PIZZA - HOUSE SPECIAL ROAST CHICKEN

BBQ Stuffed Crust, Delight Mozzarella, Large	268
BBQ Stuffed Crust, Delight Mozzarella, Medium	250
BBQ Stuffed Crust, Large	286
BBQ Stuffed Crust, Medium	277
Classic Crust, Delight Mozzarella, Large	221
Classic Crust, Delight Mozzarella, Medium	203
Classic Crust, Delight Mozzarella, Personal	160
Classic Crust, Delight Mozzarella, Small	180
Classic Crust, Large	231
Classic Crust, Medium	213
Classic Crust, Personal	166
Classic Crust, Small	186
Double Decadence, Delight Mozzarella, Large	293
Double Decadence, Delight Mozzarella, Medium	268
Double Decadence, Large	300
Double Decadence, Medium	274
GF Crust, Delight Mozzarella, Small	162
GF Crust, Small	160
Italian Style Crust, Delight Mozzarella, Large	205
Italian Style Crust, Delight Mozzarella, Medium	183
Italian Style Crust, Delight Mozzarella, Small	160
Italian Style Crust, Large	189
Italian Style Crust, Medium	169
Italian Style Crust, Small	148
Stuffed Crust, Delight Mozzarella, Large	262
Stuffed Crust, Delight Mozzarella, Medium	244
Stuffed Crust, Large	291
Stuffed Crust, Medium	271
Thin & Crispy, Delight Mozzarella, Large	192
Thin & Crispy, Delight Mozzarella, Medium	178
Thin & Crispy, Large	203
Thin & Crispy, Medium	188

PIZZA - HOUSE SPECIAL TANDOORI

BBQ Stuffed Crust, Delight Mozzarella, Medium	251
BBQ Stuffed Crust, Large	287
BBQ Stuffed Crust, Medium	278
Classic Crust, Delight Mozzarella, Large	222
Classic Crust, Delight Mozzarella, Medium	204
Classic Crust, Delight Mozzarella, Personal	158
Classic Crust, Delight Mozzarella, Small	174
Classic Crust, Large	233
Classic Crust, Medium	214
Classic Crust, Personal	163
Classic Crust, Small	177
Double Decadence, Delight Mozzarella, Large	294
Double Decadence, Delight Mozzarella, Medium	269
Double Decadence, Large	302
Double Decadence, Medium	275
GF Crust, Delight Mozzarella, Small	155
GF Crust, Small	152

DOMINO'S PIZZA

PIZZA - HOUSE SPECIAL TANDOORI

Italian Style Crust, Delight Mozzarella, Large	206
Italian Style Crust, Delight Mozzarella, Medium	184
Italian Style Crust, Delight Mozzarella, Small	153
Italian Style Crust, Large	222
Italian Style Crust, Medium	170
Italian Style Crust, Small	140
Stuffed Crust, Delight Mozzarella, Large	263
Stuffed Crust, Delight Mozzarella, Medium	246
Stuffed Crust, Large	292
Stuffed Crust, Medium	272
Thin & Crispy, Delight Mozzarella, Large	193
Thin & Crispy, Delight Mozzarella, Medium	179
Thin & Crispy, Large	205
Thin & Crispy, Medium	189

PIZZA - MEAT LOVERS

BBQ Stuffed Crust, Delight Mozzarella, Large	249
BBQ Stuffed Crust, Delight Mozzarella, Medium	233
BBQ Stuffed Crust, Large	264
BBQ Stuffed Crust, Medium	256
Classic Crust, Delight Mozzarella, Large	202
Classic Crust, Delight Mozzarella, Medium	186
Classic Crust, Delight Mozzarella, Personal	136
Classic Crust, Delight Mozzarella, Small	167
Classic Crust, Large	209
Classic Crust, Medium	192
Classic Crust, Personal	141
Classic Crust, Small	170
Double Decadence, Delight Mozzarella, Large	274
Double Decadence, Delight Mozzarella, Medium	250
Double Decadence, Large	278
Double Decadence, Medium	254
GF Crust, Delight Mozzarella, Small	148
GF Crust, Small	144
Italian Style Crust, Delight Mozzarella, Large	185
Italian Style Crust, Delight Mozzarella, Medium	166
Italian Style Crust, Delight Mozzarella, Small	147
Italian Style Crust, Large	166
Italian Style Crust, Medium	149
Italian Style Crust, Small	132
Stuffed Crust, Delight Mozzarella, Large	243
Stuffed Crust, Delight Mozzarella, Medium	227
Stuffed Crust, Large	268
Stuffed Crust, Medium	251
Thin & Crispy, Delight Mozzarella, Large	173
Thin & Crispy, Delight Mozzarella, Medium	160
Thin & Crispy, Large	181
Thin & Crispy, Medium	168

PIZZA - MEATEOR

BBQ Stuffed Crust, Delight Mozzarella, Large	280
BBQ Stuffed Crust, Delight Mozzarella, Medium	255
BBQ Stuffed Crust, Large	280
BBQ Stuffed Crust, Medium	262

DOMINO'S PIZZA

PIZZA - MEATEOR

Classic Crust, Delight Mozzarella, Large	224
Classic Crust, Delight Mozzarella, Medium	207
Classic Crust, Delight Mozzarella, Personal	170
Classic Crust, Delight Mozzarella, Small	191
Classic Crust, Large	232
Classic Crust, Medium	214
Classic Crust, Personal	175
Classic Crust, Small	192
Double Decadence, Delight Mozzarella, Large	298
Double Decadence, Delight Mozzarella, Medium	273
Double Decadence, Large	298
Double Decadence, Medium	273
GF Crust, Delight Mozzarella, Small	169
GF Crust, Small	175
Italian Style Crust, Delight Mozzarella, Large	203
Italian Style Crust, Delight Mozzarella, Medium	182
Italian Style Crust, Delight Mozzarella, Small	162
Italian Style Crust, Large	207
Italian Style Crust, Medium	186
Italian Style Crust, Small	166
Stuffed Crust, Delight Mozzarella, Large	266
Stuffed Crust, Delight Mozzarella, Medium	250
Stuffed Crust, Large	274
Stuffed Crust, Medium	257
Thin & Crispy, Delight Mozzarella, Large	194
Thin & Crispy, Delight Mozzarella, Medium	181
Thin & Crispy, Large	202
Thin & Crispy, Medium	188

PIZZA - MEATILICIOUS

BBQ Stuffed Crust, Delight Mozzarella, Large	242
BBQ Stuffed Crust, Delight Mozzarella, Medium	226
BBQ Stuffed Crust, Large	257
BBQ Stuffed Crust, Medium	250
Classic Crust, Delight Mozzarella, Large	195
Classic Crust, Delight Mozzarella, Medium	180
Classic Crust, Delight Mozzarella, Personal	144
Classic Crust, Large	202
Classic Crust, Medium	186
Classic Crust, Personal	198
Classic Crust, Small	164
Double Decadence, Delight Mozzarella, Large	267
Double Decadence, Delight Mozzarella, Medium	244
Double Decadence, Large	271
Double Decadence, Medium	247
GF Crust, Delight Mozzarella, Small	142
GF Crust, Small	138
Italian Style Crust, Delight Mozzarella, Large	179
Italian Style Crust, Delight Mozzarella, Medium	159
Italian Style Crust, Delight Mozzarella, Medium	141
Italian Style Crust, Large	160
Italian Style Crust, Medium	143
Italian Style Crust, Small	126

DOMINO'S PIZZA

PIZZA - MEATILICIOUS

Stuffed Crust, Delight Mozzarella, Large	236
Stuffed Crust, Delight Mozzarella, Medium	221
Stuffed Crust, Large	262
Stuffed Crust, Medium	245
Thin & Crispy, Delight Mozzarella, Large	166
Thin & Crispy, Delight Mozzarella, Medium	154
Thin & Crispy, Large	174
Thin & Crispy, Medium	162

PIZZA - MEATZZA

BBQ Stuffed Crust, Delight Mozzarella, Large	245
BBQ Stuffed Crust, Delight Mozzarella, Medium	231
BBQ Stuffed Crust, Large	260
BBQ Stuffed Crust, Medium	254
Classic Crust, Delight Mozzarella, Large	198
Classic Crust, Delight Mozzarella, Medium	184
Classic Crust, Delight Mozzarella, Personal	134
Classic Crust, Delight Mozzarella, Small	166
Classic Crust, Large	205
Classic Crust, Medium	190
Classic Crust, Personal	138
Classic Crust, Small	168
Double Decadence, Delight Mozzarella, Large	270
Double Decadence, Delight Mozzarella, Medium	248
Double Decadence, Large	274
Double Decadence, Medium	252
GF Crust, Delight Mozzarella, Small	147
GF Crust, Delight Mozzarella, Small	147
GF Crust, Small	143
Italian Style Crust, Delight Mozzarella, Large	182
Italian Style Crust, Delight Mozzarella, Medium	163
Italian Style Crust, Delight Mozzarella, Small	145
Italian Style Crust, Large	162
Italian Style Crust, Medium	249
Italian Style Crust, Small	131
Stuffed Crust, Delight Mozzarella, Large	239
Stuffed Crust, Delight Mozzarella, Medium	225
Stuffed Crust, Large	265
Stuffed Crust, Medium	249
Thin & Crispy, Delight Mozzarella, Large	169
Thin & Crispy, Delight Mozzarella, Medium	158
Thin & Crispy, Large	177

PIZZA - MEXICAN HOT

BBQ Stuffed Crust, Delight Mozzarella, Large	242
BBQ Stuffed Crust, Delight Mozzarella, Medium	227
BBQ Stuffed Crust, Large	260
BBQ Stuffed Crust, Medium	253
Classic Crust, Delight Mozzarella, Large	196
Classic Crust, Delight Mozzarella, Medium	180
Classic Crust, Delight Mozzarella, Personal	128
Classic Crust, Delight Mozzarella, Small	159
Classic Crust, Large	206
Classic Crust, Medium	189

DOMINO'S PIZZA

PIZZA - MEXICAN HOT

Classic Crust, Personal	134
Classic Crust, Personal	134
Classic Crust, Small	164
Double Decadence, Delight Mozzarella, Large	268
Double Decadence, Delight Mozzarella, Medium	244
Double Decadence, Large	275
Double Decadence, Medium	251
GF Crust, Delight Mozzarella, Small	140
GF Crust, Small	138
Italian Style Crust, Delight Mozzarella, Large	179
Italian Style Crust, Delight Mozzarella, Medium	160
Italian Style Crust, Delight Mozzarella, Small	139
Italian Style Crust, Large	163
Italian Style Crust, Medium	146
Italian Style Crust, Small	127
Stuffed Crust, Delight Mozzarella, Large	236
Stuffed Crust, Delight Mozzarella, Medium	221
Stuffed Crust, Large	265
Stuffed Crust, Medium	248
Thin & Crispy, Delight Mozzarella, Large	166
Thin & Crispy, Delight Mozzarella, Medium	154
Thin & Crispy, Large	178
Thin & Crispy, Medium	165

PIZZA - MIGHTY MEATY

BBQ Stuffed Crust, Delight Mozzarella, Large	247
BBQ Stuffed Crust, Delight Mozzarella, Medium	232
BBQ Stuffed Crust, Large	262
BBQ Stuffed Crust, Medium	256
Classic Crust, Delight Mozzarella, Large	200
Classic Crust, Delight Mozzarella, Medium	186
Classic Crust, Delight Mozzarella, Personal	135
Classic Crust, Delight Mozzarella, Small	167
Classic Crust, Large	207
Classic Crust, Medium	192
Classic Crust, Personal	139
Classic Crust, Small	170
Double Decadence, Delight Mozzarella, Large	272
Double Decadence, Delight Mozzarella, Medium	250
Double Decadence, Large	276
Double Decadence, Medium	253
GF Crust, Delight Mozzarella, Small	148
GF Crust, Small	144
Italian Style Crust, Delight Mozzarella, Large	184
Italian Style Crust, Delight Mozzarella, Medium	165
Italian Style Crust, Delight Mozzarella, Small	147
Italian Style Crust, Large	164
Italian Style Crust, Medium	148
Italian Style Crust, Small	133
Stuffed Crust, Delight Mozzarella, Large	241
Stuffed Crust, Delight Mozzarella, Medium	227
Stuffed Crust, Large	266
Stuffed Crust, Medium	250

DOMINO'S PIZZA

PIZZA - MIGHTY MEATY

Thin & Crispy, Delight Mozzarella, Large	171
Thin & Crispy, Delight Mozzarella, Medium	160
Thin & Crispy, Large	179
Thin & Crispy, Medium	168

PIZZA - MIXED GRILL

BBQ Stuffed Crust, Delight Mozzarella, Large	244
BBQ Stuffed Crust, Delight Mozzarella, Medium	229
BBQ Stuffed Crust, Large	259
BBQ Stuffed Crust, Medium	252
Classic Crust, Delight Mozzarella, Large	197
Classic Crust, Delight Mozzarella, Medium	182
Classic Crust, Delight Mozzarella, Personal	138
Classic Crust, Delight Mozzarella, Small	163
Classic Crust, Large	204
Classic Crust, Medium	188
Classic Crust, Personal	143
Classic Crust, Small	166
Double Decadence, Delight Mozzarella, Large	269
Double Decadence, Delight Mozzarella, Medium	246
Double Decadence, Large	273
Double Decadence, Medium	250
GF Crust, Delight Mozzarella, Small	144
GF Crust, Small	140
Italian Style Crust, Delight Mozzarella, Large	181
Italian Style Crust, Delight Mozzarella, Medium	162
Italian Style Crust, Delight Mozzarella, Small	143
Italian Style Crust, Large	161
Italian Style Crust, Medium	145
Italian Style Crust, Small	129
Stuffed Crust, Delight Mozzarella, Large	238
Stuffed Crust, Delight Mozzarella, Medium	223
Stuffed Crust, Large	264
Stuffed Crust, Medium	247
Thin & Crispy, Delight Mozzarella, Large	168
Thin & Crispy, Delight Mozzarella, Medium	156
Thin & Crispy, Large	176
Thin & Crispy, Medium	164

PIZZA - NEW YORKER

BBQ Stuffed Crust, Delight Mozzarella, Large	242
BBQ Stuffed Crust, Delight Mozzarella, Medium	227
BBQ Stuffed Crust, Large	257
BBQ Stuffed Crust, Medium	251
Classic Crust, Delight Mozzarella, Large	196
Classic Crust, Delight Mozzarella, Medium	180
Classic Crust, Delight Mozzarella, Personal	132
Classic Crust, Delight Mozzarella, Small	162
Classic Crust, Large	203
Classic Crust, Medium	187
Classic Crust, Medium	164
Classic Crust, Personal	136
Double Decadence, Delight Mozzarella, Large	268
Double Decadence, Delight Mozzarella, Medium	245

DOMINO'S PIZZA

PIZZA - NEW YORKER

	KCAL
Double Decadence, Large	272
Double Decadence, Medium	248
GF Crust, Delight Mozzarella, Small	143
GF Crust, Small	139
Italian Style Crust, Delight Mozzarella, Large	179
Italian Style Crust, Delight Mozzarella, Medium	160
Italian Style Crust, Delight Mozzarella, Small	141
Italian Style Crust, Large	160
Italian Style Crust, Medium	143
Italian Style Crust, Small	127
Stuffed Crust, Delight Mozzarella, Large	236
Stuffed Crust, Delight Mozzarella, Medium	221
Stuffed Crust, Large	262
Stuffed Crust, Medium	245
Thin & Crispy, Delight Mozzarella, Large	166
Thin & Crispy, Delight Mozzarella, Medium	155
Thin & Crispy, Large	175
Thin & Crispy, Medium	163

PIZZA - PEPPERONI PASSION

	KCAL
BBQ Stuffed Crust, Delight Mozzarella, Large	263
BBQ Stuffed Crust, Delight Mozzarella, Medium	248
BBQ Stuffed Crust, Large	281
BBQ Stuffed Crust, Medium	274
Classic Crust, Delight Mozzarella, Large	216
Classic Crust, Delight Mozzarella, Medium	201
Classic Crust, Delight Mozzarella, Personal	150
Classic Crust, Delight Mozzarella, Small	180
Classic Crust, Large	226
Classic Crust, Medium	210
Classic Crust, Personal	156
Classic Crust, Small	185
Double Decadence, Delight Mozzarella, Large	288
Double Decadence, Delight Mozzarella, Medium	265
Double Decadence, Large	295
Double Decadence, Large	295
Double Decadence, Medium	272
GF Crust, Delight Mozzarella, Small	161
GF Crust, Small	160
Italian Style Crust, Delight Mozzarella, Large	200
Italian Style Crust, Delight Mozzarella, Medium	181
Italian Style Crust, Delight Mozzarella, Small	160
Italian Style Crust, Large	184
Italian Style Crust, Medium	167
Italian Style Crust, Medium	178
Stuffed Crust, Delight Mozzarella, Large	257
Stuffed Crust, Delight Mozzarella, Medium	242
Stuffed Crust, Large	286
Stuffed Crust, Medium	269
Thin & Crispy, Delight Mozzarella, Large	187
Thin & Crispy, Delight Mozzarella, Medium	175
Thin & Crispy, Large	198
Thin & Crispy, Medium	186

DOMINO'S PIZZA

PIZZA - RANCH BBQ

	KCAL
BBQ Stuffed Crust, Delight Mozzarella, Large	273
BBQ Stuffed Crust, Delight Mozzarella, Medium	248
BBQ Stuffed Crust, Large	273
BBQ Stuffed Crust, Medium	255
Classic Crust, Delight Mozzarella, Large	217
Classic Crust, Delight Mozzarella, Medium	199
Classic Crust, Delight Mozzarella, Personal	148
Classic Crust, Delight Mozzarella, Small	183
Classic Crust, Large	225
Classic Crust, Medium	207
Classic Crust, Personal	153
Classic Crust, Small	184
Double Decadence, Delight Mozzarella, Large	291
Double Decadence, Delight Mozzarella, Medium	265
Double Decadence, Large	292
Double Decadence, Medium	266
GF Crust, Delight Mozzarella, Small	160
GF Crust, Small	167
Italian Style Crust, Delight Mozzarella, Large	196
Italian Style Crust, Delight Mozzarella, Medium	174
Italian Style Crust, Delight Mozzarella, Small	154
Italian Style Crust, Large	201
Italian Style Crust, Medium	178
Italian Style Crust, Small	157
Stuffed Crust, Delight Mozzarella, Large	260
Stuffed Crust, Delight Mozzarella, Medium	242
Stuffed Crust, Large	267
Stuffed Crust, Medium	249
Thin & Crispy, Delight Mozzarella, Large	187
Thin & Crispy, Delight Mozzarella, Medium	173
Thin & Crispy, Large	196
Thin & Crispy, Medium	181

PIZZA - SCRUMMY

	KCAL
BBQ Stuffed Crust, Delight Mozzarella, Large	273
BBQ Stuffed Crust, Delight Mozzarella, Medium	256
BBQ Stuffed Crust, Large	288
BBQ Stuffed Crust, Medium	280
Classic Crust, Delight Mozzarella, Large	227
Classic Crust, Delight Mozzarella, Medium	209
Classic Crust, Delight Mozzarella, Personal	166
Classic Crust, Delight Mozzarella, Small	189
Classic Crust, Large	234
Classic Crust, Medium	216
Classic Crust, Personal	169
Classic Crust, Small	192
Double Decadence, Delight Mozzarella, Large	299
Double Decadence, Delight Mozzarella, Medium	274
Double Decadence, Large	303
Double Decadence, Medium	277
GF Crust, Delight Mozzarella, Small	170
GF Crust, Small	166
Italian Style Crust, Delight Mozzarella, Large	210

DOMINO'S PIZZA
PIZZA - SCRUMMY

Italian Style Crust, Delight Mozzarella, Medium	189
Italian Style Crust, Delight Mozzarella, Small	169
Italian Style Crust, Large	191
Italian Style Crust, Medium	172
Italian Style Crust, Small	154
Stuffed Crust, Delight Mozzarella, Large	267
Stuffed Crust, Delight Mozzarella, Medium	250
Stuffed Crust, Large	293
Stuffed Crust, Medium	274
Thin & Crispy, Delight Mozzarella, Large	197
Thin & Crispy, Delight Mozzarella, Medium	184
Thin & Crispy, Large	206
Thin & Crispy, Medium	191

PIZZA - SIZZLER

BBQ Stuffed Crust, Delight Mozzarella, Large	246
BBQ Stuffed Crust, Delight Mozzarella, Medium	231
BBQ Stuffed Crust, Large	263
BBQ Stuffed Crust, Medium	247
Classic Crust, Delight Mozzarella, Large	206
Classic Crust, Delight Mozzarella, Medium	190
Classic Crust, Delight Mozzarella, Personal	141
Classic Crust, Delight Mozzarella, Small	169
Classic Crust, Large	212
Classic Crust, Medium	195
Classic Crust, Personal	145
Classic Crust, Small	174
Double Decadence, Delight Mozzarella, Large	280
Double Decadence, Delight Mozzarella, Medium	256
Double Decadence, Large	275
Double Decadence, Medium	252
GF Crust, Delight Mozzarella, Small	150
GF Crust, Small	158
Italian Style Crust, Delight Mozzarella, Large	184
Italian Style Crust, Delight Mozzarella, Medium	165
Italian Style Crust, Delight Mozzarella, Small	145
Italian Style Crust, Large	187
Italian Style Crust, Medium	167
Italian Style Crust, Small	146
Stuffed Crust, Delight Mozzarella, Large	240
Stuffed Crust, Delight Mozzarella, Medium	226
Stuffed Crust, Large	258
Stuffed Crust, Medium	242
Thin & Crispy, Delight Mozzarella, Large	174
Thin & Crispy, Delight Mozzarella, Medium	162
Thin & Crispy, Large	182
Thin & Crispy, Medium	170

PIZZA - SPANISH SIZZLER

BBQ Stuffed Crust, Delight Mozzarella, Large	238
BBQ Stuffed Crust, Delight Mozzarella, Medium	220
BBQ Stuffed Crust, Large	253
BBQ Stuffed Crust, Medium	244
Classic Crust, Delight Mozzarella, Large	191

DOMINO'S PIZZA
PIZZA - SPANISH SIZZLER

Classic Crust, Delight Mozzarella, Medium	174
Classic Crust, Delight Mozzarella, Personal	129
Classic Crust, Delight Mozzarella, Small	153
Classic Crust, Large	198
Classic Crust, Medium	180
Classic Crust, Personal	133
Classic Crust, Small	156
Double Decadence, Delight Mozzarella, Large	263
Double Decadence, Delight Mozzarella, Medium	238
Double Decadence, Large	267
Double Decadence, Medium	241
GF Crust, Delight Mozzarella, Small	134
GF Crust, Small	130
Italian Style Crust, Delight Mozzarella, Large	175
Italian Style Crust, Delight Mozzarella, Medium	153
Italian Style Crust, Delight Mozzarella, Small	133
Italian Style Crust, Large	155
Italian Style Crust, Medium	137
Italian Style Crust, Small	119
Stuffed Crust, Delight Mozzarella, Large	232
Stuffed Crust, Delight Mozzarella, Medium	215
Stuffed Crust, Large	257
Stuffed Crust, Medium	239
Thin & Crispy, Delight Mozzarella, Large	162
Thin & Crispy, Delight Mozzarella, Medium	148
Thin & Crispy, Large	170
Thin & Crispy, Medium	156

PIZZA - TANDOORI HOT

BBQ Stuffed Crust, Delight Mozzarella, Large	215
BBQ Stuffed Crust, Delight Mozzarella, Medium	200
BBQ Stuffed Crust, Large	230
BBQ Stuffed Crust, Medium	224
Classic Crust, Delight Mozzarella, Large	168
Classic Crust, Delight Mozzarella, Medium	153
Classic Crust, Delight Mozzarella, Personal	115
Classic Crust, Delight Mozzarella, Small	134
Classic Crust, Large	175
Classic Crust, Medium	160
Classic Crust, Personal	119
Classic Crust, Small	137
Double Decadence, Delight Mozzarella, Large	240
Double Decadence, Delight Mozzarella, Medium	218
Double Decadence, Large	244
Double Decadence, Medium	221
GF Crust, Delight Mozzarella, Small	115
GF Crust, Small	111
Italian Style Crust, Delight Mozzarella, Large	152
Italian Style Crust, Delight Mozzarella, Medium	133
Italian Style Crust, Delight Mozzarella, Small	114
Italian Style Crust, Large	133
Italian Style Crust, Medium	116
Italian Style Crust, Small	99

DOMINO'S PIZZA

PIZZA - TANDOORI HOT

	KCAL
Stuffed Crust, Delight Mozzarella, Large	209
Stuffed Crust, Delight Mozzarella, Medium	194
Stuffed Crust, Large	235
Stuffed Crust, Medium	218
Thin & Crispy, Delight Mozzarella, Large	139
Thin & Crispy, Delight Mozzarella, Medium	128
Thin & Crispy, Large	147
Thin & Crispy, Medium	136

PIZZA - TEXAS BBQ

	KCAL
BBQ Stuffed Crust, Large	247
BBQ Stuffed Crust, Medium	230
Classic Crust, Large	199
Classic Crust, Medium	181
Classic Crust, Personal	139
Classic Crust, Small	158
Double Decadence, Large	266
Double Decadence, Medium	240
GF Crust, Small	141
Italian Style Crust, Large	175
Italian Style Crust, Medium	153
Italian Style Crust, Small	132
Stuffed Crust, Large	241
Stuffed Crust, Medium	224
Thin & Crispy, Large	169
Thin & Crispy, Medium	155

PIZZA - TUNA DELIGHT

	KCAL
BBQ Stuffed Crust, Delight Mozzarella, Large	217
BBQ Stuffed Crust, Delight Mozzarella, Medium	201
BBQ Stuffed Crust, Large	232
BBQ Stuffed Crust, Medium	225
Classic Crust, Delight Mozzarella, Large	170
Classic Crust, Delight Mozzarella, Medium	154
Classic Crust, Delight Mozzarella, Personal	116
Classic Crust, Delight Mozzarella, Small	135
Classic Crust, Large	177
Classic Crust, Medium	161
Classic Crust, Personal	120
Classic Crust, Small	137
Double Decadence, Delight Mozzarella, Large	242
Double Decadence, Delight Mozzarella, Medium	218
Double Decadence, Large	246
Double Decadence, Medium	222
GF Crust, Delight Mozzarella, Small	116
GF Crust, Small	112
Italian Style Crust, Delight Mozzarella, Large	154
Italian Style Crust, Delight Mozzarella, Large	134
Italian Style Crust, Delight Mozzarella, Medium	134
Italian Style Crust, Delight Mozzarella, Small	114
Italian Style Crust, Large	134
Italian Style Crust, Medium	117
Italian Style Crust, Small	100
Stuffed Crust, Delight Mozzarella, Large	211

DOMINO'S PIZZA

PIZZA - TUNA DELIGHT

	KCAL
Stuffed Crust, Delight Mozzarella, Medium	195
Stuffed Crust, Large	236
Stuffed Crust, Medium	219
Thin & Crispy, Delight Mozzarella, Large	141
Thin & Crispy, Delight Mozzarella, Medium	129
Thin & Crispy, Large	149
Thin & Crispy, Medium	136

PIZZA - VEG-A-ROMA

	KCAL
BBQ Stuffed Crust, Delight Mozzarella, Large	212
BBQ Stuffed Crust, Delight Mozzarella, Medium	197
BBQ Stuffed Crust, Large	229
BBQ Stuffed Crust, Medium	213
Classic Crust, Delight Mozzarella, Large	171
Classic Crust, Delight Mozzarella, Medium	156
Classic Crust, Delight Mozzarella, Personal	125
Classic Crust, Delight Mozzarella, Small	137
Classic Crust, Large	177
Classic Crust, Medium	161
Classic Crust, Personal	126
Classic Crust, Small	142
Double Decadence, Delight Mozzarella, Large	245
Double Decadence, Delight Mozzarella, Medium	222
Double Decadence, Large	241
Double Decadence, Medium	218
GF Crust, Delight Mozzarella, Small	117
GF Crust, Small	125
Italian Style Crust, Delight Mozzarella, Large	150
Italian Style Crust, Delight Mozzarella, Medium	131
Italian Style Crust, Large	152
Italian Style Crust, Medium	133
Italian Style Crust, Small	113
Stuffed Crust, Delight Mozzarella, Large	206
Stuffed Crust, Delight Mozzarella, Medium	191
Stuffed Crust, Large	223
Stuffed Crust, Medium	208
Thin & Crispy, Delight Mozzarella, Large	139
Thin & Crispy, Large	147
Thin & Crispy Crust, Medium	136

PIZZA - VEGI SUPREME

	KCAL
BBQ Stuffed Crust, Delight Mozzarella, Large	205
BBQ Stuffed Crust, Delight Mozzarella, Medium	191
BBQ Stuffed Crust, Large	220
BBQ Stuffed Crust, Large	215
Classic Crust, Delight Mozzarella, Large	159
Classic Crust, Delight Mozzarella, Medium	144
Classic Crust, Delight Mozzarella, Personal	109
Classic Crust, Delight Mozzarella, Small	126
Classic Crust, Large	166
Classic Crust, Medium	151
Classic Crust, Personal	113
Classic Crust, Small	128
Double Decadence, Delight Mozzarella, Large	231

DOMINO'S PIZZA
PIZZA - VEGI SUPREME

Double Decadence, Delight Mozzarella, Medium	208
Double Decadence, Large	235
Double Decadence, Medium	212
Double Decadence, Medium	212
GF Crust, Delight Mozzarella, Small	107
GF Crust, Small	103
Italian Style Crust, Delight Mozzarella, Large	142
Italian Style Crust, Delight Mozzarella, Medium	124
Italian Style Crust, Delight Mozzarella, Small	105
Italian Style Crust, Large	123
Italian Style Crust, Medium	107
Italian Style Crust, Small	91
Stuffed Crust, Delight Mozzarella, Large	199
Stuffed Crust, Delight Mozzarella, Medium	185
Stuffed Crust, Large	225
Stuffed Crust, Medium	209
Thin & Crispy, Delight Mozzarella, Large	129
Thin & Crispy, Delight Mozzarella, Medium	119
Thin & Crispy, Large	138
Thin & Crispy, Medium	126

PIZZA - VEGI VOLCANO

BBQ Stuffed Crust, Delight Mozzarella, Large	220
BBQ Stuffed Crust, Large	238
BBQ Stuffed Crust, Large	231
Classic Crust, Delight Mozzarella, Large	173
Classic Crust, Delight Mozzarella, Medium	157
Classic Crust, Delight Mozzarella, Personal	117
Classic Crust, Delight Mozzarella, Small	136
Classic Crust, Large	183
Classic Crust, Medium	167
Classic Crust, Personal	123
Classic Crust, Small	142
Double Decadence, Delight Mozzarella, Large	245
Double Decadence, Delight Mozzarella, Medium	222
Double Decadence, Large	252
Double Decadence, Medium	228
GF Crust, Delight Mozzarella, Small	118
GF Crust, Small	116
Italian Style Crust, Delight Mozzarella, Large	157
Italian Style Crust, Delight Mozzarella, Medium	137
Italian Style Crust, Delight Mozzarella, Small	116
Italian Style Crust, Large	140
Italian Style Crust, Medium	123
Italian Style Crust, Small	93
Stuffed Crust, Delight Mozzarella, Large	214
Stuffed Crust, Delight Mozzarella, Medium	198
Stuffed Crust, Large	243
Stuffed Crust, Medium	225
Thin & Crispy, Delight Mozzarella, Large	144
Thin & Crispy, Delight Mozzarella, Medium	132
Thin & Crispy, Large	155
Thin & Crispy, Medium	142

DOMINO'S PIZZA
POTATO WEDGES

Half Box	168

RIBS

BBQ, 1 Rib	140

SALAD

Caesar, ½ Box	95

WRAP

Chicken, & Bacon, Wrapzz	192
Meatball Feast, Wrapzz	302
Meatball Mayhem, 6, Wrapzz	208
Meatball Mayhem, 8, Wrapzz	246
Pepperoni Passion, 12, Wrapzz	242
Pepperoni Passion, 8, Wrapzz	195
Tandoori Hot, Wrapzz	121
Texas BBQ, Wrapzz	180
Veggie Supreme, Wrapzz	91

EAT

BAGEL
	KCAL
Smoked Salmon & Cream Cheese	444

BAGUETTE
Brie, Tomato, & Basil	455
Chicken, Bacon & Avocado	552
Chicken, Herb, & Avocado	552
Chicken, Pulled, BBQ, The Brooklyn	421
Ham, & Emmental	566
Ham, & Emmental, Half	282
Ham, & Emmental, Rustic	622
Ham, Brie, & Chilli Jam	588
Ham, Brie, & Cranberry	634
Ham Hock, & Egg, The Bronx, Breakfast	439
Prosciutto, Italian	435
Red Pepper Tapenade, Avocado, & Feta, Rustic	526
Reuben, Veggie, The Staten	418
Salmon, & Egg, The Manhattan, Breakfast	484
Tuna, & Cucumber	583
Turkey, Stuffing, & Crispy Onion	635

BARS
Dried Fruit, Nuts, & Seeds, GF	237

BEANS
Fava, Chickpea, & Pumpkin Seeds	156

BISCUITS
Milk Chocolate, Tiffin, Tin	346

BREAD
Banana	349

BREAKFAST
Mango, & Coconut, Chia, Pot	309
Poached Egg, & Avocado, with Feta, Pot	313
Poached Egg, & Avocado, with Ham Hock, Pot	307
Poached Egg, BBQ Beans, & Smoked Ham, Hot Pot	334

BREAKFAST CEREAL
Muesli, Apple, & Berry, Bircher	312
Porridge, Plain, Sm	137
Porridge, Quinoa, & Coconut	441
Porridge, with Banana, & Honey, Big	284
Porridge, with Banana, & Honey, Small	210
Porridge, with Banana, Big	234
Porridge, with Banana, Small	162

BROWNIES
Chocolate, GF	310

BUTTER
Almond, Porridge Topping	95

CAKE
Jaffa	253

CROISSANT
All Butter	347
Almond	365
Chocolate	380
Egg, & Bacon	444
Ham, & Emmental Cheese	513

EAT

CURRY
	KCAL
Chicken, Red Thai, with Noodles	292

DESSERT
Avocado, & Chocolate, Pot	213
Bakewell, Slice	408
Carrot, Cake	265
Carrot, Caramel, & Pecan, Cake	443
Cheesecake, Sicilian Lemon	284
Coffee, & Walnut, Cake	371
Cookie, Oat, & Fruit	329
Cookie, Triple Chocolate	394
Lemon Drizzle Cake	555
Mincemeat, Merry, Crumble, Slice	350
Red Velvet, Cake	263
Tiffin, Milk Chocolate & Brazil Nut	374

EGGS
Free Range, & Chilli Greens	116

FLAPJACK
with Sultanas, Apricots, & Orange, GF	263

FLATBREAD
Butternut, Chickpea, & Harissa	506
Chilli, Beef, & Cheese	509
Chipotle, Cheddar, & Black Bean	499

FRUIT
Grape, Bag	80
Mango, & Lime, Pot	86

FRUIT COMPOTE
Apple, & Cinnamo, Porridge Topping	55

FRUIT SALAD
Clementine, Blackberry, & Redcurrant	70
Rainbow	95

FUDGE
Scottish, Handmade	194

HOT POT
Mac 'N' Cheese, Kids	232
Mac 'N' Cheese, Large	790
Mac 'N' Cheese, Reg	544
Pigs in Blankets, Mash, & Gravy	498
Pigs in Blankets	237
Turkey, Festive, Full Works	504

HOUMOUS
Turmeric, & Dip Sticks	237

MISO
Wakame, Mushroom, & Noodles	147

NOODLES
Chicken, Ramen	262

NUT & SEED MIX
Chocolate Almonds, Raisins, Sunflower Seeds	380

NUTS
Natural, Mix	222

PAIN AU RAISIN
Pastry	383

EAT

PEANUTS

Honey Coated, with Chilli	204

PIE

Cauliflower, & Kale, Cheese, Pie Only	678
Cauliflower, & Kale, Cheese, with Mash, & Gravy	926
Chicken, & Mushroom, Pie Only	685
Chicken, & Mushroom, with Mash, & Gravy	931
Mince, Famous	310
Steak, & Ale, Pie Only	553
Steak, & Ale, with Mash, & Gravy	799

PIZZA

Chicken, Grill	533

POPCORN

Salted, Rock Salt	105
Sweet, & Salty	136

ROLL

Bacon, British Back, Rustic	321
Bacon, Poached Egg, British Back, Rustic	336

SALAD

Beetroot, Squash, & Feta	359
Chicken, Caeser Mayonnaise, Four Leaf Salad	347
Chicken, Noodle, Spicy, Less Than 5% Fat	429
Crayfish, Spicy, Noodles, Less Than 5% Fat	380
Houmous, & Falafel, Mezze, with Dressing	473
Houmous, & Falafel, Mezze, without Dressing	371
Jerk Chicken, with Dressing	313
Jerk Chicken, without Dressing	266
Miso, & Beef, Tahini, with Dressing	463
Miso, & Beef, Tahini, without Dressing	335
Quinoa, Black Rice, & Nuts, Super Nutty, Fit Box	342
Salmon, Smoked, & Egg, Fit Box	260
Tuna, Nicoise, with Dressing	345
Tuna, Nicoise, & without Dressing	188

SANDWICH

Butternut Squash, Stuffing, & Slaw	445
Cheese, Marmite, Morning Melt	458
Cheese, Tomato, Soft Grain	391
Chicken, & Bacon	457
Chicken, Roast, Salad	616
Chicken, Smoked, & Basil, on Stonebaked Ciabatta	458
Chicken & Chorizo	371
Egg Mayo, & Watercress, Chunky, Malted Bread	403
Emmenthal, Simple, Kids	435
Full Works, Festive, White Bloomer	599
Ham, & Egg, Free Range	567
Ham, & Mature Cheddar	474
Ham, Simple, Kids, on Malted Granary Bread	326
Pastrami, New York	525
Salmon, Smoked, Soft Cheese, Malted Granary	367
Tuna, Mayonnaise, & Cucumber	365
Turkey, & Cranberry, Less Than 5% Fat	359

SHORTBREAD

Millionaires	441

EAT

SOUP

Bacon, & Potato, Fully Loaded, Sm	250
Beef, Rendang, Malaysian, without Garnish, Sm	261
Beef Ragu, Reg	283
Beef Ragu, Small	217
Beef Ragu, Very Big	425
Broth, Shot	33
Butternut Squash, Thai, Sm	168
Cauliflower Cheese, Sm	219
Chicken, & Garden Vegetable, Sm	123
Chicken, & Kale Dahl, Big	251
Chicken, & Kale Dahl, Small	192
Chicken & Kale Dahl, Very Big	405
Chicken, Chipotle, & Black Bean	247
Chicken, Jerk, without Garnish, Sm	282
Chicken, Laksa, without Salad Garnish, Sm	256
Chicken, Mushroom, & Barley, with Garnish, Sm	216
Chicken, Pot Pie, no Pastry, Sm	216
Chicken, Pot Pie, with Pastry, Big	413
Chicken, Pot Pie, with Pastry, Small	343
Chicken, Pot Pie, with Pastry, Very Big	576
Chicken, Thai Green Curry, no Garnish, Sm	243
Chicken Noodle, Coconut, Sm	313
Duck, Hoi Sin, Gyoza, Pho, Pot	392
French Onion with Garnish	267
Leek, & Potato, Sm	210
Lentil, Spiced, Spinach, & Sweet Potato	279
Meatball, Italian, without Garnish, Sm	228
Mushroom, Wild, & Chestnut, Sm	240
Red Pepper, & Goats Cheese, Fire Roasted, Sm	141
Sweet Potato, & Chilli, Sm	261
Sweetcorn, Creamy, Sm	315
Tomato, & Basil, Spicy, Sm	78
Tomato, Slow Roasted, Creamy, Sm	240
Vegetable Gyoza, Wok Pot, Broth	300

SPONGE

Chocolate, Cookie Buttercream, & Chocolate Button	451

SWEETS

Midget Gems	174

TOAST

Avocado, Sourdough	338
Avocado, with Feta, Sourdough	392
Avocado, with Ham Hock, Sourdough	376
Ham, Cheese, Dijon Mustard, Stonebaked Ciabatta	551
Mozzarella, Pesto, & Tomato, Stonebaked Ciabatta	539
Sourdough, with Butter	218

TOASTIE

British Beef & English Mustard Grill	506
Tuna, & Cheddar Melt, on Ciabatta Bread	650

TORTILLA CHIPS

Guacamole, Creamy, & Chipotle Bean Salsa	233

EAT

WRAP

	KCAL
Beetroot, & Feta	401
Chicken, Mexican	427
Chicken, Salad	491
Duck, Hoisin	421
Houmous, & Falafel	492
Houmous, & Falafel, Half	246
Simple Houmous, & Salad	377

YOGHURT

	KCAL
Honey, Grapenuts, & Banana	349
with Berry Compote	136
with Granola, & Berry Compote	303

YULE LOG

	KCAL
Festive	173

FARMHOUSE INNS

	KCAL
BACON	
Cheese, & BBQ Sauce, New York, Steak Topper	415
BEANS	
Extra	109
BEEF	
Steak, Rib-eye, 10oz, with Sides	1465
Steak, Rump, 14oz, with Sides	1537
Steak, Rump, 5oz, Mix & Match	181
Steak, Rump, 8oz, with Sides	1319
Steak, Sirloin, 8oz, with Sides	1317
BEEF DINNER	
Rib, Roast	1104
BHAJI	
Onion, Sides	798
BITES	
Jalapeno, Crispy, Sides	176
BLACK PUDDING	
Tower, with Bacon, Smoked	1200
BREAD	
& Butter, Sides	89
Ciabatta, Garlic, Cheesy	705
Ciabatta, Garlic, Sides	438
BREAKFAST	
All Day	1374
BUNS	
Sides	196
BURGERS	
Cheese, & Gammon, Ploughmans, Chips, Coleslaw	2033
Classic, with Chips, & Coleslaw	1733
Giant, The Farm, with Chips, & Coleslaw	2504
Cheese, & Jalapeno Melt, with Chips, & Coleslaw	2220
Cheese, Smoked Bacon, with Chips, & Coleslaw	1849
Cheese, with Chips, & Coleslaw	1759
Chicken, Southern Fried, Mix & Match	322
Chicken, Tex Mex, with Chips, & Coleslaw	2238
Mixed Grill, Giant, with Chips, & Coleslaw	2390
Vegetarian, Spicy, with Chips, & Coleslaw	1624
CHEESE	
Extra	164
Parmigiana, Topper	158
Stilton, Extra	107
CHICKEN	
Breast, Roasted, Mix & Match	204
Goujons, Southern Fried, with BBQ Dip	114
Medley, Crispy	1648
Smothered	1256
Wings, Mix & Match	420
Wings, with Sour Cream	813
CHICKEN DINNER	
Roast	1214
CHILLI	
Bean, Smoky, Vegetarian	632
Bean, Smoky, Vegetarian, with Rice, & Chips	1135

FARMHOUSE INNS

CHILLI

Bean, Smoky, Vegetarian, with Rice	1017
Bean, Smoky, Vegetarian, with Chips	1253
Beef, Farmhouse	710
Beef, Farmhouse, with Basmati Rice, & Chips	1213
Beef, Farmhouse, with Basmati Rice	1095
Beef, Farmhouse, with Chips	1331

CHIPS

BLANK	621
Peas, Onion Rings, Mushrooms, Tomato, Mix Match	995
Seasoned, Sides	621

COD

Beer Battered, with Chips, & Garden Peas	1812
Beer Battered, with Chips, & Garden Peas, Large	1670
Beer Battered, with Chips, & Mushy Peas	1857
Beer Battered, with Chips, & Mushy Peas, Large	1715
Beer Battered, with Chips	1750
Beer Battered, with Chips, Large	1608

COLESLAW

Extra	154
Homemade, Sides	205

CORN

Cob, Mini, Sides	348

CURRY

Sweet Potato, & Chickpea	1084
Sweet Potato, & Chickpea, with Chips	1705
Sweet Potato, & Chickpea, with Pilau Rice, & Chips	1616
Sweet Potato, & Chickpea, with Pilau Rice	1527

EGGS

Fried, Free Range	120

FRIES

Sides	874

GAMMON

Steak, 5oz, Mix & Match	221
Steak, with Chips, & Peas	913

GRAVY

Extra	9

GUACAMOLE

Side Serving	129

HAM

Hand Carved, & Eggs, with Chips, & Peas	1099

KORMA

Chicken	1159
Chicken, with Chips	1780
Chicken, with Pilau Rice, & Chips	1691
Chicken, with Pilau Rice	1602

LAMB

Shank, Minted, with Mash, & Veg	651

LAMB DINNER

Shank, Roast	655

LASAGNE

Beef, with Chips, & Garlic Bread	1404

FARMHOUSE INNS

LINGUINE

Seafood	1144

MACARONI CHEESE

Luxury	807
Luxury, with Streaky Bacon	942

MAYONNAISE

Citrus	643
Muddy	512

MIXED GRILL

Farmhouse	1988

MUSHROOMS

Button, Breaded, Garlic, with Garlic Mayonnaise	494
Button, Sides	290

NACHOS

Cheesy	982
Cheesy, with Beef Chilli	1180
Cheesy, with Smoky Bean Chilli	1141

ONION RINGS

Sides	532

PATE

Chicken, Liver, with Bread, Onion Chutney, & Salad	649

PIE

Beef, & Ale, Slow Cooked	1740
Cheese, Onion, & Potato	1999
Fish	1165
Ham Hock	968
Lamb, Shank	782
Shepherds	1240
Steak, & Kidney, Suet, Pudding	1703
Steak, & Kidney, Suet, Pudding, with Garden Peas	1765
Steak, & Kidney, Suet, Pudding, with Mushy Peas	1810

PINEAPPLE

Slices, in Syrup, for Gammon, 2 Slices	31

PLATTER

Chicken, Sharer, ½ Platter	1430
Farmhouse, Sharing, ½ Platter	1244
Ploughmans, Ultimate, ½ Platter	782

POTATO WEDGES

Sides	638

POTATOES

Jacket, with Baked Beans	368
Jacket, with Beef Chilli	411
Jacket, with Cheddar Cheese	375
Jacket, with Coleslaw	539
Jacket, with Prawn Cocktail	399
Jacket, with Smoky Bean Chilli	373
Jacket, with Tuna Mayonnaise	449
Thyme, Saute, Sides	158

PRAWN COCKTAIL

Starter	454

RIBS

Rack, Half, BBQ, Mix & Match	271
Rack, Half, BBQ, Sides	271

FARMHOUSE INNS

	KCAL
SALAD	
Bowl, Starter	1057
Caesar, No Extra Topping	407
Caesar, with Chicken, & Bacon	701
Caesar, with Salmon, Grilled	703
Caesar, with Steak, Rump, 5oz	588
Chicken, & Bacon, Hot	1062
Side	64
SALMON	
Smoked	768
Tail, Fillet, Poached	427
Tail, Fillet, Poached, with Hollandaise Sauce	600
SALSA	
Side or Extra	41
SANDWICH	
Beef, & Stilton, Ciabatta	1138
Beef, Hand Carved	259
Carvery, Bap	715
Chicken, & Bacon, Club	844
Chicken, Hunters, Melt, Ciabatta	1184
Ham, Hand Carved	163
Ham, Tomato, & Melted Cheese, Ciabatta	1105
Prawn Cocktail	232
Tuna, Melt, Ciabatta	1126
SAUCE	
BBQ	162
Diane	32
Peppercorn	37
Piri Piri	43
Piri Piri, for Chicken Wings	22
Sour Cream	185
Sweet Chilli	0
SAUSAGE & MASH	
Main	1412
SCAMPI	
Wholetail, Breaded	1297
Wholetail, Breaded, Mix & Match	589
SOUP	
Of The Day, Homemade	434
TART	
Beetroot, & Camembert	1878
TIKKA MASALA	
Chicken	1172
Chicken, with Chips	1793
Chicken, with Pilau Rice, & Chips	1704
Chicken, with Pilau Rice	1615
WRAP	
Chicken, Goujons, Southern Fried	502
Tuna, Mayonnaise, & Lettuce	534
YORKSHIRE PUDDING	
& Pigs in Blanket, Extra	409
Extra	100
Giant, Sides	490

FIVE GUYS

	KCAL
BURGERS	
Bacon, Bunless	628
Bacon	888
Bacon, Little, Bunless	383
Bacon, Little	643
Cheeseburger, Bacon, Bunless	708
Cheeseburger, Bacon	968
Cheeseburger, Bacon, Little, Bunless	423
Cheeseburger, Bacon, Little	683
Cheeseburger, Bunless	570
Cheeseburger	830
Cheeseburger, Little, Bunless	285
Cheeseburger, Little	545
Hamburger, Bunless	490
Hamburger, Bunless, Little	245
Hamburger	750
Hamburger, Little	505
FRIES	
Large	1314
Little	526
Reg	953
HOT DOG	
Bacon, & Cheese, Bunless	388
Bacon, & Cheese	648
Bacon, Bunless	348
Bacon	608
Cheese, Bunless	250
Cheese	510
Original, Bunless	210
Original	470
SANDWICH	
BLT	642
Cheese, Grilled	470
Veggie, Cheese	372
Veggie	292
TOPPING	
BBQ Sauce	45
Green Peppers	4
Jalapenos	2
Lettuce	4
Mayonnaise	93
Mushrooms	6
Onions	9
Relish	18
Tomatoes	9

GOURMET BURGER KITCHEN

	KCAL
BACON	
Crispy, Extras	54
BURGERS	
Beef, Avocado, & Bacon	875
Beef, Blue Cheese, with Blue Cheese Mayo	935
Beef, Blue Cheese, with Blue Cheese Mayo, Small	645
Beef, Blue Cheese, with Cheese Slice	817
Beef, Blue Cheese, with Cheese Slice, Small	582
Beef, Bourbon Street	885
Beef, Cheese, & Bacon, with American Cheese	942
Beef, Cheese, & Bacon, with Cheddar	982
Beef, Cheese, & Bacon, with Red Leicester	980
Beef, Cheese, & Bacon, with Smoked Applewood	982
Beef, Classic	692
Beef, Classic, Small	533
Beef, Classic, with American Cheese	815
Beef, Classic, with American Cheese, Small	595
Beef, Classic, with Cheddar	855
Beef, Classic, with Cheddar, Small	614
Beef, Classic, with Red Leicester	853
Beef, Classic, with Red Leicester, Small	613
Beef, Classic, with Smoked Applewood	855
Beef, Classic, with Smoked Applewood, Small	696
Beef, Gourmet, Simply Seasoned	292
Beef, Habanero	839
Beef, Junior	538
Beef, Kiwiburger	996
Beef, Major Tom	922
Beef, Taxidriver	875
Beef, the Don	867
Beef, The Mighty	1328
Beef, The Stack	1010
Buffalo	811
Chicken, & Bacon, Pesterella	860
Chicken, & Bacon, Pesterella, Panko	1041
Chicken, Cajun Blue	583
Chicken, Cajun Blue, Panko	757
Chicken, Cam & Cranberry	622
Chicken, Cam & Cranberry, Panko	803
Chicken, Classic	445
Chicken, Classic, Panko	627
Chicken, Classic, Panko, Small	579
Chicken, Classic, Small	360
Chicken, Grilled, Junior	348
Chicken, Panko, Junior	499
Chicken, Satay	552
Chicken, Satay, Panko	795
Lamb, Herman the Lamb	845
Lamb, Psychobilly	676
BURGERS VEGETARIAN	
Californian	802
Classic, Small	406
Classic	513

GOURMET BURGER KITCHEN

	KCAL
BURGERS VEGETARIAN	
Classic, with American Cheese	635
Classic, with American Cheese, Small	468
Classic, with Cheddar	676
Classic, with Cheddar, Small	488
Classic, with Red Leicester	674
Classic, with Red Leicester, Small	487
Classic, with Smoked Applewood Cheese	676
Classic, with Smoked Applewood Cheese, Small	489
Dippy Hippy	598
Falafel	550
Johnny Be Goat	485
Junior	467
CHEESE	
American, Extras	123
Cheddar, Extras	163
Halloumi, Bites	418
Red Leicester, Extras	161
Smoked Applewood, Extras	163
CHICKEN	
Bites, Chilli Fried	289
Skewers, with Smoked Chilli Mayo	466
COLESLAW	
Blue Cheese Slaw	412
Homeslaw	49
FRIES	
Chunky	635
Skinny	454
Sweet Potato	405
Sweet Potato, with Baconnaise	632
Truffle Cheese	756
MILK SHAKE	
Banana	627
Banana, Junior	313
Chocolate	752
Chocolate, Junior	376
Honeycomb	722
Honeycomb, Junior	361
Lime	640
Lime, Junior	320
Oreo	850
Oreo, Junior	425
Peanut Butter	912
Peanut Butter, Junior	456
Salted Caramel	681
Salted Caramel, Junior	340
Strawberry	631
Strawberry, Junior	315
The Nutter	1034
The Nutter, Junior	517
Vanilla	624
Vanilla, Junior	312

GOURMET BURGER KITCHEN	KCAL
MUSHROOMS	
Bourbon Glazed, Extras	30
ONION RINGS	
Extras	171
House	514
PEPPERS	
Jalapeno, Extras	22
PICKLE	
Dill, Extras	13
PINEAPPLE	
Extras	48
SALAD	
Chicken, Chilli Chick	507
Simple	81
Siperfood	669
SAUCE	
Chilli Salsa	37
Mayo, Baconnaise	227
Mayo, Basil	245
Mayo, Blue Cheese	225
Mayo, Garlic	241
Mayo, Smoked Chilli	202
Mayo, Sriracha	219
SWEETCORN	
with Butter, 1 Piece	73

GREGGS	KCAL
BAGUETTE	
Bacon, & Egg, Omelette, Free Range, Hot	544
Bacon, & Sausage, Hot	617
Bacon, Hot	540
Cheese, & Ham	541
Cheese, & Ham, Hot	542
Cheese, & Salad	492
Chicken, Club	491
Chicken, Southern Fried, Hot	585
Chicken, Tandoori	494
Chicken Mayonnaise	488
Egg, Omelette, Free Range, Hot	454
Meatball, Spicy, Aberdeen Angus, Hot	558
Prawn Mayonnaise	473
Sausage, & Egg, Omelette, Free Range, Hot	593
Sausage, Hot	604
Tuna, Crunch	462
BAKE	
Chicken	426
Sausage, Bean, & Cheese, Melt	453
Steak	405
BARS	
Granola	296
BISCUITS	
Bunny	269
Gingerbread, Man	180
Jammy Heart	285
Shortbread, Caramel	297
BREAD	
Brown, Bloomer	98
Oatmeal, Loaf	190
Rolls, Corn Topped	190
Rolls, Oval Bite	230
Rolls, Sub, Seeded	270
Rolls, Sub, White	230
Stottie	347
White, Bloomer, Loaf	138
BREAKFAST CEREAL	
Porridge, Creamy Oats, Simply	253
Porridge, Golden Syrup	248
Porridge, Red Berry	250
BROWNIES	
Chocolate, Mini	90
BUNS	
Belgian	403
Cinnamon	425
Easter Ring	246
Hot Cross	176
Iced, Christmas Ring	210
Iced, Finger	111
Ring, Novelty	243

	KCAL
GREGGS	
CAKE	
Christmas Slice	360
Crispy Cornfake	280
Easter, Crispy nest	326
Raspberry, & Almond, Bake	63
Rocky Road, Belgian Chocolate	362
Vanilla Slice	359
Victoria Sponge, Mini	497
COFFEE	
Americano, Large	11
Americano, Reg	9
Black, Decaf, Large	7
Black, Decaf, Reg	6
Cappuccino, No Chocolate Topping, Large	111
Cappuccino, No Chocolate Topping, Reg	90
Espresso, Double	11
Espresso, Shot	8
Latte, Large	133
Latte, Reg	111
Mocha, Large	300
Mocha, Reg	233
White, Decaf, Large	24
White, Decaf, Reg	19
White, Large	45
White, Reg	34
COLA	
Coca-Cola	139
Coke Zero, Coca-Cola	3
Diet, Coca-Cola	3
COOKIES	
Chocolate, Chunk, Triple	374
Chocolate, Milk	380
Chocolate, White	382
Fruit & Oat	341
CROISSANT	
All Butter	298
Almond	343
CUPCAKES	
Chocolate	280
Easter	393
Foundation	320
Ice Cream	270
Sweet Lemon	380
DOUGHNUTS	
Caramel	303
Chocolate, & Vanilla, Triple	341
Chocolate, Milk, Ring	223
Cream, Finger	334
Cream, Toffee, Finger	379
Glazed, Ring	191
Iced, Ring	226
Jam	242
Mini	64

	KCAL
GREGGS	
DOUGHNUTS	
Pink, Jammie	334
Sugar Strand	246
Yum Yum	291
Yum Yum, Mini	120
DRIED FRUIT	
Sweet Mango	88
DRIED FRUIT MIX	
Berries & Cherries	81
ECLAIR	
with Cream Filling	347
FANTA	
Fanta	150
FLAPJACK	
Fruity, Mini	110
FRUIT	
Medley	72
Summer Berry Pot	91
Tropical, Fingers	70
GRAPES	
Mixed	92
HOT CHOCOLATE	
Large	281
Reg	219
IRN BRU	
Diet	2
Original	215
JUICE	
Apple, Fairtrade	220
Orange, Fairtrade	220
JUICE DRINK	
Citrus Punch, Oasis	90
Summer Fruits, Oasis	90
LEMONADE	
Raspberry, Sparkling	10
LUCOZADE	
Energy Orange	350
Sport	140
MIXED NUTS	
Naked	156
MUFFIN	
Chocolate, Triple	507
Jam & Toast, Breakfast	381
Lemon, Sicilian	500
Sticky Toffee	530
PAIN AU CHOCOLAT	
Pastry	297
with Belgian Chocolate	393
PASTA	
Cheese & Tomato, with Mixed Herbs, Pot	381
Fajita Chicken, in Tomato Sauce, Spicy, Pot	345

GREGGS

KCAL	
PASTA SALAD	
Cheese, & Tomato	399
Cheese, Tomato, & Basil	328
Chicken, Mexican	375
Tuna, Crunch	283
PASTRY	
Greggsnut, Caramel & Pecan	457
PASTY	
Beef, & Vegetable	509
Cheese, & Onion	434
Steak, & Cheese, Roll	340
PIE	
Mince, Sweet	290
Mince, Sweet, Iced	230
PIZZA	
Margherita, Thin & Crispy, Slice	365
Pepperoni, Thin & Crispy, Slice	444
PUDDING	
Bread	118
RIBENA*	
Original	215
ROLL - CORN TOPPED	
Bacon, & Egg, Omelette, Free Range, Hot	363
Bacon, & Sausage, Hot	437
Bacon, Hot	359
Sausage, & Egg, Omelette, Free Range	394
Sausage, Hot	407
ROLL - OVAL BITES	
Chicken, & Salad, Honey Mustard Mayo, Seeded	389
Chicken, Mexican, & Salad, Fajita Mayo, Seeded	393
Egg, Omelette, Free Range, Hot	380
SALAD	
Chicken, & Bacon, Layered	327
Chicken, Chargrill	200
Chicken, Coconut, Lime & Chilli	220
Chicken, Chargrill, Roasted Vegetables, & Grains	285
Chicken, Oriental, with Sticky Rice	340
Chicken, Teriyaki, & Noodle	256
Falafel, & Houmous	316
Ham, & Egg, Honey Roast	238
SANDWICH	
Cheese, & Onion	366
Egg Mayonnaise, Free Range	348
Ham, & Egg, with Salad, Honey Roast	347
Ham, Honey Roast, & Egg, Sub, Roll	332
Tuna Mayonnaise, & Cucumber	350
SAUSAGE ROLL	
Freshly Baked	349
Mini	81
SCONE	
Cheese	349
Derby	268

GREGGS

KCAL	
SEED MIX	
Super	135
SLICES	
Toffee Apple, Lattice	277
SMOOTHIE	
Mango & Orange	145
Raspberry & Banana	135
SOUP	
Tomato, Cream of	213
Tomato	240
SPRITE*	
Original	220
SUBS	
Chicken Mayonnaise	342
Ham, & Salad	737
Tuna Mayonnaise	336
TART	
Egg Custard	257
Strawberry	180
Strawberry, with Fresh Cream	300
TEA	
White, Large	12
White, Reg	9
TEACAKES	
Bakery	206
TURNOVER	
Apple, Fresh Cream	540
WATER	
Cranberry or Raspberry	5
WRAP	
Bacon, & Cheese	320
Chicken, & Bacon, Caesar	450
Chicken, Chargrilled	410
Chicken, Chilli, Coconut, & Lime	340
Chicken, Katsu	394
Moroccan Tagine Chicken	354
YOGHURT	
Mango, & Passionfruit	162
Strawberry, & Granola, Natural	226
Strawberry, & Granola, with Almonds & Seeds	194

KCAL

HARVESTER RESTAURANT

BEANS
Baked, Extra	64

BEEF
Short Rib, Big Shorty, with Apple & Fennel Slaw	1119

BEEF - STEAK
Bulls Head, Mushroom, Tomato, Onion Rings, ½	828
Fillet, 8oz, with Mushroom, Tomato, & Onion Rings	440
Ribeye, 16oz, with Mushroom, Tomato, & Onion	821
Sirloin, 10oz, with Mushroom, Tomato, & Onion Rings	675

BITES
Mac & Cheese, Smoked Applewood, Starter	428

BREAD
Garlic, Cheesy, Side	354
Garlic, Side	165
Garlic, Starter	331
Garlic, with Cheese, Starter	695

BREAKFAST
Boho	524
Boho, Kids	347
Hipster	974
Hispter, Kids	278
Signature	1077
Signature, Kids	300

BROCCOLI
Tenderstem, Chargrilled, Side	31

BROWNIES
Chocolate, with Chocolate Drizzle, Belgian, Mini	286
Chocolate, with Ice Cream	731

BUNS
Fish Finger	815
Steak	610

BURGERS
Bean, Patty, Extra	333
Beef, Patty, Extra	329
The Angry Bird	937
The BBQ King	1026
The Big One	1512
The Boho	970
The Classic	823
The Cowboy	916
The Frenchie	889

CAKE
Chocolate, Fudge, Chocolate Sauce, & Ice Cream	997

CHEESE
Camembert, & Garlic Bread, Sharer, Starter, ½	602
Extra	65

CHEESECAKE
Caramel, Biscuit, with Toffee Fudge Sauce, Mini	334

CHICKEN
Breast, Burger Extra	196
Breast, Southern Fried, Burger Extra	392
Grilled, with Buttered Peas, Simply	399
Peri Peri, Starter	324

KCAL

HARVESTER RESTAURANT

CHICKEN
Rotisserie, Half, with Gravy, & Buttered Corn	477
Stack, BBQ, with Apple & Fennel Slaw, & Corn Cob	918
Strips, Buttermilk Fried, Starter	511
Wings, BBQ, Sticky, Starter	306

CHICKEN CARIBBEAN
Salsa, with Golden Rice	556

CHICKEN CHASSEUR
Breast, with Vegetable Medley	294
Rotisserie, Half, with Vegetable Medley	361

CHICKEN PIRI PIRI
Spit	541

CHILLI
Beef, Chipotle, Pulled	328

CHIPS
Chunky, Triple Cooked, Side	436

COD & CHIPS
Battered, with Tartare Sauce	635

COLESLAW
Apple & Fennel	277

CORN
Buttered, Side	214

DESSERT
Mini Combo	750

EGGS
Benedict	668
Mediterranean	758

FRIES
Halloumi, with Spiked Maple Sauce, Starter	444
Sage & Onion Seasoned, Side	400
Side	399
Sweet Potato, Side	503

FRITTERS
Sweetcorn, Spicy, with Avocado, & Eggs	613

GAMMON - 7OZ
Egg, Mushroom, Tomato, & Onion Rings	454
Egg, Pineapple, Mushroom, Tomato, Onion Rings	482
Pineapple, Mushroom, Tomato, & Onion Rings	396

GAMMON - DOUBLE UP
Egg, Mushroom, Tomato, & Onion Rings	719
Egg, Pineapple, Mushroom, Tomato, Onion Rings	747
Pineapple, Mushroom, Tomato, & Onion Rings	661

HASH
Steak	884

KATSU
Vegetable, Jamaican, Vegan	796

KEBAB
Tofu, Lemon & Herb, Peri Peri, Skewers	519

MACARONI CHEESE
Side	276

HARVESTER RESTAURANT

MILK SHAKE

	KCAL
Cookie Monster, Freak Shake	1067
Salted Caramel Waffle, Freak Shake	753
Strawberry, Fun Fair, Freak Shake	762

MIXED GRILL

Ultimate, with Mushroom, Tomato, & Onion Rings	1785
with Mushroom, Tomato, & Onion Rings	900

MUSHROOMS

Breaded, with Garlic Mayo Dip, Starter	392
Garlic, Oven Baked, with Garlic Bread, Starter	392

NACHOS

Sharer, Starter, ½	992
Starter	579
Vegan, Sharer, Starter, ½	878
Vegan, Starter	522
with BBQ Pulled Pork, Sharer, Starter, ½	1232
with BBQ Pulled Pork, Starter	999

ONION RINGS

Side	312

PANCAKE

Buttermilk, & Bacon, with Syrup	752
Buttermilk, with Fruit, & Syrup	623

PASTA

Spinach, & Artichoke, with Garlic Bread	831

PEAS

Garden, Side	132
Mushy, Side	73
Smash, Kickin', Side	120

PIE

Cherry, Sugar Dusted	567
Fish, Cheddar Mash Topped	437

PORK

Belly, Bourbon Glazed	1762

POTATO SKINS

with Cheese, & Bacon, Loaded, Starter	322
with Cheese, Loaded, Starter	254

POTATOES

Jacket, Side	273
Jacket, with Sour Cream, Side	355
Mashed, Side	187

PRAWNS

Crackerjack, with Spiked Maple Sauce, Starter	416
in Garlic & Chilli Butter, with Garlic Bread, Starter	358

QUESADILLA

Pork, BBQ, Pulled, with Apple & Fennel Slaw	568

RIBS - BBQ RACK

Jerk, with Apple & Fennel Slaw, & Corn Cob	725
Large, with Apple & Fennel Slaw, & Corn Cob	1046
with Apple & Fennel Slaw, & Corn Cob	814

RICE

Golden, & Beans, Side	229

HARVESTER RESTAURANT

RICE PUDDING

	KCAL
Coconut, & Black Cherry	388

ROULADE

Butternut Squash, Spinach, & Cheese	405

SALAD - FEEL GOOD BOWL

No Extras	308
with Cajun Chicken, Half Portion	409
with Cajun Chicken	510
with Chicken, Half Portion	396
with Chicken	485
with Halloumi, 2 Pieces	573
with Halloumi, 3 Pieces	706
with Lemon & Herb Tofu Skewers, Three	663
with Lemon & Herb Tofu Skewers, Two	545
with Rump Steak, 4oz	497
with Rump Steak, 8oz	637
with Salmon	686

SALMON

Sweet & Sticky Salsa, Golden Rice, Corn, & Slaw	690

SCAMPI

Wholetail, Whitby, Dozen	707
Wholetail, with Tartare Sauce	647
Wholetail, with Tartare Sauce	647

SEA BASS

Fillets, Grilled, with Lobster & Prosecco Sauce	464

SPONGE PUDDING

Treacle	474

SQUID

Calamari, Strips, with Garlic Mayo, Starter	322

TAGINE

Aubergine, & Red Lentil, with Couscous, & Flatbread	1077

TART

Camembert, & Cherry Tomato, with Slaw	643

VEGETABLES MIXED

Carrots, Peas, & Beans, Buttered, Side	94

WAFFLES

Chicken, Buttermilk Fried, Bacon, Syrup, Breakfast	1252

WRAP

Chicken, Breast, Plain, Grilled	455
Chicken, Buttermilk Fried	618
Chicken, Cajun, Grilled	480
Halloumi	543

HUNGRY HORSE

BACON
	KCAL
Streaky, Side, Extra	66

BEANS
Baked, Jacket Potato Topping	63
Baked, Side, Extra	63

BEEF
Steak, Rump, 12oz, Big Plate Specials	1698
Steak, Rump, 12oz, Side, Extra	434
Steak, Rump, 5oz, Pub Favourites	1131
Steak, Rump, 8oz, Mix it Up, Big Plate Specials	289
Steak, Rump, 8oz, Pub Favourites	1239
Steak, Sirloin, 9oz, Big Plate Specials	1658
Steak, Smothered, 8oz, Sizzler, Big Plate Specials	1661

BEEF DINNER
Roast, Sunday	982
Sunday Roast, Big Plate Specials	1609
Sunday Roasts, Kids	530

BHAJI
Onion, Extra Portion	541

BREAD
Brown, & Butter, Side	272
Garlic, Ciabatta, Cheesy	521
Garlic, Ciabatta	358
Naan	172
White, & Butter, Side	299
Tortilla, Super Soft, Mix it Up, Big Plate Specials	82

BREAKFAST
All Day, Big Plate Specials	1513
Full English, Pub Favourites	835

BURGERS
Beef, & Chicken, Quadzilla	2795
Beef, B.E.S.T	2075
Beef, Classic, Double	1460
Beef, Classic	1103
Beef, Double Daddy	2497
Beef, Extra Patty	357
Beef, Sizzler, Combo, Big Plate Specials	2507
Beef, Smokin' Jack	3318
Beef, with Cheese, & Bacon, Double	1565
Beef, with Cheese, & Bacon	1208
Beef, with Cheese, Double	1499
Beef, with Cheese, Double	1499
Beef, with Cheese	1142
Chicken, Extra Fillet	266
Chicken, Southern Fried, Double	1467
Chicken, Southern Fried	1106
Falafel, Double	1094
Falafel, Extra Patty	253
Falafel	841

BUTTER
Portion	29

HUNGRY HORSE

CAKE
	KCAL
Chocolate, Fudge, Warm	918
Freakshake	1063

CHEESE
Grated, Side, Extra	164
Halloumi, Fingers	771
Halloumi, Mexican, Big Plate Specials	2011
Mozzarella, White Cheddar, Jacket Potato Topping	164

CHEESECAKE
Millionaires	633

CHICKEN
Breast, Extra Portion	204
Crispy, Jumbo, Curry Sauce Topper	2074
Crispy, Jumbo, Parmigiana Topper	2131
Fingers, Coated, Mix it Up, Big Plate Specials	935
Fingers, Plain, Starter	607
Fingers, with Franks Red Hot Pepper Sauce, Starter	619
Fingers, with Piri Piri Sauce. Starter	631
Fingers, with Sweet Chilli Sauce, Starter	689
Fingers, with Texan BBQ Sauce, Starter	697
Mexican, Big Plate Specials	1398
New Yorker, & Salad, Light Bites	502
New Yorker, Big Plate Specials	1805
New Yorker, Pub Favourites	1210
Roast, Half, Flattened, Mix it Up, Big Plate Specials	304
Wings, Plain, Starter	925
Wings, with Franks Red Hot Pepper Sauce, Starter	937
Wings, with Piri Piri Sauce, Starter	949
Wings, with Sweet Chilli Sauce, Starter	1007
Wings, with Texan BBQ Sauce, Starter	1015

CHICKEN DINNER
Breast, Sunday Roasts, Kids	528
Fillets, Sunday Roast, Big Plate Specials	1514
Fillets, Sunday Roast	905

CHILLI
Con Carne, Jacket Potato Topping	198

CHIPS
Cheesy, Side	798
Mix it Up, Big Plate Specials	870
Side	634
Side, Lunch Menu	634

COD & CHIPS
Jumbo, Chunky, with Baked Beans	1965
Jumbo, Chunky, with Garden Peas	1962
Jumbo, Chunky, with Mushy Peas	2022
Jumbo, Chunky, with Salad	1909

COLESLAW
Jacket Potato Topping	75
Mix it Up, Big Plate Specials	100
Side	75

CORN
Cobs, Mini, Mix it Up, Big Plate Specials	112
on the Cob, Side	141

HUNGRY HORSE

	KCAL
CRUMBLE	
Apple	653
CURRY	
Chickpea, & Sweet Potato, Big Plate Specials	2354
Chickpea, & Sweet Potato, Pub Favourites	696
CUSTARD	
Extra	89
DESSERT	
Candymania, Big, The Ultimate	2203
EGGS	
Fried, Side, Extra	118
FISH & CHIPS	
Fillets, Vegan, with Baked Beans	990
Fillets, Vegan, with Garden Peas	987
Fillets, Vegan, with Mushy Peas	1047
Fillets, Vegan, with Salad	934
Hand Battered, Chunky, with Baked Beans	1612
Hand Battered, Chunky, with Garden Peas	1609
Hand Battered, Chunky, with Mushy Peas	1669
Hand Battered, Chunky, with Salad	1556
FRIES	
Dirty, Mac & Bacon Topper, Side	910
Dirty, Mac Cheese Topper	778
Dirty, Nacho Cheesy Bacon, Side	752
Dirty, Pizza Topper, Side	691
Mix it Up, Big Plate Specials	546
Side	546
Sweet Potato, Mix it Up, Big Plate Specials	410
Sweet Potato, Side	410
GAMMON	
15oz, Grilled, Big Plate Specials	1799
Grilled, 5oz, Pub Favourites	998
GRAVY	
Extra Portion	26
ICE CREAM	
Bubblegum	133
Chocolate	112
Vanilla	110
KEBAB	
Chicken, Skewer, Breast, Plain, Mix it Up	611
Chicken, Skewer, Plain, Side, Extra	189
Chicken, Skewer, Southern Fried, Mix it Up	844
Chicken, Skewer, Southern Fried, Side, Extra	294
Chicken, Skewer, Tandoori	461
LASAGNE	
& Salad, Light Bites	554
Beef, Pub Favourites	687
MACARONI CHEESE	
Pub Specials	755
Side	281

HUNGRY HORSE

	KCAL
MIXED GRILL	
Full Monty, Big Plate Specials	2293
Mini, with Egg, Pub Favourites	1668
Mini, with Pineapple, Pub Favourites	1616
MUSHROOMS	
Breaded, Garlic	686
Side, Extra	57
NACHOS	
Muchos Nachos Grande, Chilli, ½	622
Muchos Nachos Grande, ½	523
ONION RINGS	
5, Side	392
Horseshoe Stacker, 20, ½	892
Mix it Up, Big Plate Specials	311
PEAS	
Mushy, Side, Extra	120
Side, Extra	60
PEPPERS	
Jalapeno, Battered, Crispy, Side	92
PIE	
Beef, with Steak, Steak on a Pie	2193
Chicken, Roasted Woodland, with Chips	1626
Chicken, Roasted Woodland, with Mash	1241
PLATTER	
Chip Shop, with Garden Peas	2657
Chip Shop, with Mushy Peas	2717
Ultimate, Big Combo, Starter, ½	1260
POPPADOMS	
& Chutney, Extra Portion	190
POTATOES	
Jacket, Mix it Up, Big Plate Specials	272
Jacket, Plain, Add Toppings Seperately	337
Jacket, Plain, Side	272
Mashed, Side, Extra	249
Roast, Extra	335
PRAWN COCKTAIL	
Popcorn	560
RIBS	
St Louis, Full Rack, Big Plate Special	3505
St Louis, Mix it Up, Big Plate Specials	1148
RICE	
Dirty, Mix it Up, Big Plate Specials	192
ROULADE	
Red Cabbage, & Apple, Vegetarian, Big Plate Specials	1782
Red Cabbage, & Apple, Vegetarian	961
Red Cabbage, & Apple, Vegetarian, Kids	692

	KCAL		KCAL

HUNGRY HORSE

SALAD
	KCAL
Chicken Fillets, Bowl	238
Chicken Tikka, Bites, Bowl	268
Dressed, Side	17
Falafel Burger, Bowl, Vegan	287
Halloumi, Bowl	434
Steak, Rump, 5oz, Bowl	215

SAUCE
	KCAL
BBQ, Texan, Mix it Up, Big Plate Specials	180
BBQ, with Jack Daniels	146
Curry	141
Garlic, & Lemon, Mix it Up, Big Plate Specials	160
Hot, Pepper, Franks, Mix it Up, Big Plate Specials	23
Lemon & Garlic	193
Parmigiana, Side	35
Peppercorn	52
Piri Piri, Hot, Mix it Up, Big Plate Specials	48
Piri Piri	24
Sour Cream	103
Sweet Chilli	82
Sweet Chilli, Mix it Up, Big Plate Specials	164

SAUSAGE
	KCAL
Quorn*, Extra	76
Side, Extra	348

SAUSAGE & MASH
	KCAL
Pork, Pub Favourites	953
Vegetarian, Quorn*, Pub Favourites	648

SCAMPI
	KCAL
Breaded, Wholetail, & Salad, Light Bites	491
Breaded, Wholetail, & Baked Beans, Pub Favourites	1219
Breaded, Wholetail, & Garden Peas, Pub Favourites	1216
Breaded, Wholetail, & Mushy Peas, Pub Favourites	1276
Breaded, Wholetail, & Salad, Pub Favourites	1163
Jumbo, & Baked Beans, Big Plate Specials	1902
Jumbo, & Garden Peas, Big Plate Specials	1899
Jumbo, & Mushy Peas, Big Plate Specials	1959
Jumbo, & Salad, Big Plate Specials	1846

SOUP
	KCAL
Tomato, Roasted	280
Tomato, Roasted, Vegan	171

SPONGE PUDDING
	KCAL
Syrup	665

SUNDAE
	KCAL
Candymania	1044
Trifle-tastic	424

TART
	KCAL
Bakewell, with Custard	546
Bakewell, with Ice Cream, Vegan	530

TIKKA MASALA
	KCAL
Chicken, Big Plate Specials	2587
Chicken, Pub Favourites	815

YORKSHIRE PUDDING
	KCAL
Extra	100

ITSU

BEANS
	KCAL
Edamame	124
Edamame, Yoghurt Coated, ½ Pack	110

BREAD
	KCAL
Wrap, Khobez, for Salad & Sandwich Box	178

CHICKEN &
	KCAL
Coconut, Noodle Pot	299

CHICKEN TERIYAKI
	KCAL
On a Bed, Low Carb	423
Potsu, Hot	446

DRESSING
	KCAL
Caesar	57
for Salad Boxes	41
Green Herb	37
Peanut, Bang Bang	53
Sesame	60
Teriyaki	39

DRIED FRUIT & NUTS
	KCAL
Superseeds, Frogo	359

DUCK
	KCAL
Peek'ing, & Watermelon	240

DUMPLINGS
	KCAL
Vegetable, with Rice	382

EGGS
	KCAL
Benedict, with Brown & Red Rice	363
Florentine, with Brown & Red Rice	289

FRUIT
	KCAL
Fresh, Pot	102

FRUIT COCKTAIL
	KCAL
Melon, Pineapple, Mango, Apple & Red Grapes	80

FRUIT SALAD
	KCAL
Hawaii 5 0	113

MIXED FRUIT
	KCAL
Yoghurt Fruit & Goji Berries	211

NOODLES
	KCAL
Pot, Chicken	409
Vegetable Festival, Crystal Noodle Cup	160

POPCORN
	KCAL
Sea Salt Flavour	115
Wasabi	121

POTSU
	KCAL
Ricebowl, Superbowl, Large	525
Superbowl, 7 Vegetables with Rice	525

PUDDING
	KCAL
Lemon Zinger	234
White Chocolate Dream, Pot	293

RICE CAKES
	KCAL
Chocolate, Dark	85
Chocolate, Milk	249
Yoghurt	240

RICE CRACKERS
	KCAL
Peanut, Snack	239

	KCAL
ITSU	
SALAD	
Chicken, Avocado, & Hard Boiled Egg, Low Carb	345
Chicken, Avocado, & Poached Egg	355
Chicken, Avocado, Low Carb, No Dressing	359
Chicken, Bento, Perfect, No Dressing	462
Chicken, Smoked, Box	425
Chicken, Smoked, Low Carb, Box	269
Duck Hoisin & Quinoa	488
Egg, Avo & Quinoa, with Spicy Sauce, Go Go Pot	192
Egg & Muki 'Go .Go'	149
Greens & Beans, with Zero Noodles	176
Ham Hock	404
Hip & Healthy, Box	230
Lobster, Freshwater & Poached Egg, Go Go Pot	79
Low Carb Salmon & Tuna Tartar, Box	173
Miso Salmon, with Zero Noodles, & Green Beans	198
Poke, On a Bed	558
Roast Beef Vietnam, Double Bed	618
Salmon & Tuna Tartare, Low Carb	160
Salmon Supreme, Omega 3	367
Satay Chicken, Zero Noodles	191
Special Salmon	402
Special Salmon & Poached Egg	314
Tokyo Caesar, on a Bed	352
Tuna, Low Carb	169
Tuna, No Lettuce	169
Tuna Rice Oise	333
SALMON	
& Avocado, Spicy, Maki Box	458
& Egg, Special, Go Go Pot	219
Poached, Cooked Rare	370
Sashimi, Muki Beans, Wakame & Wasabi	198
SANDWICH	
Crab, California, Maki Boxes & Sushi Sandwiches	327
Duck & Pomegranate, without Khobez Bread	163
Salmon Supreme, Sushi	202
Tangy Tuna, Salad, No Mayo	256
Tuna Sushi, Sushi	179
Veggie Club, Sushi	175
SAUCE	
Hot Su Potsu	6
SEAWEED	
Crispy Thins, Snack	24
Crispy Thins, Wasabi Flavour	22
Thins, Sweet Soy & Sea Salt Flavour	22
SMOOTHIE	
Fruit, Superssed, Dairy Free	363
Raw Veg Cleanse	162
SOUP	
Chicken Noodle, Classic	219
Miso	96
Miso, Noodle, Detox	157
Miso, Original, from Supermarket	44

	KCAL
ITSU	
SOUP	
Teriyaki Chicken with Rice, Potsu	627
Thai Duck Hot, Potsu	397
SUSHI	
Best of Its	413
Collection, Veggie	561
Crab, California Rolls	194
Health & Happiness, Box	584
It Box	284
Maki, Spicy Tuna	151
Maki Roll, Duck Hoisin	197
Omega 3 Salmon Supreme	459
Salad, Box	488
Salmon, Sashimi	177
Salmon, Super, Light	403
Salmon & Avo, Maki Rolls	242
Salmon & Salmon	518
Salmon & Tuna, Junior Pack	165
Salmon Sushi	203
Slim Salmon	288
Super Salmon 3 Ways	586
Tuna, Lots of Ginger	141
Tuna & Salmon, Sashimi Box	240
Tuna & Salmon Junior	174
Tuna & Salmon Sushi	245
TOFU	
Smoked, Organic, Greens	234
WATER	
Vitsu Water, Lemon Ninja	60
WRAP	
Chicken, Satay, Tokyo	455
Falafel, Quinoa, & Greens, Tokyo	486
Pork, Spicy, Tokyo	405
Salmon, Teriyaki, Tokyo	443
YOGHURT	
Strawberry & Blueberry, Coulis, Greek Style, Pot	141
Chocolate with GF Brownie, Greek Style, Geisha	255
Frozen, Fruitifix, Fro-Go	113
Frozen, Naked, Fro-Go	99
with, Superseeds & Blueberries, Pot	375
with, Superseeds & Strawberries, Pot	374

J D WETHERSPOON

AVOCADO
Add on, Chicken Club	86
Burger Topping	86

BACON
Maple Cured, Extra	86

BAGEL
Avocado, Smashed, Breakfast	457
Avocado, Smashed, Deli Deals	547
Avocado, Smashed, with Bacon, & Egg, Deli Deals	606
Avocado, Smashed, with Bacon, Deli Deals	543
Avocado, Smashed, with Egg, Deli Deals	520
Cheese, Cream, Breakfast	396
Salmon, Smoked, & Cream Cheese, Breakfast	460
Salmon, Smoked, & Cream Cheese, Deli Deals	460

BEANS
on Toast	503
on Toast, Wholemeal	498

BEEF - STEAK, RUMP
& Eggs, Brunch	703
14oz, Steak Club	1449
with Peas, Tomato, & Mushrooms, & Chips	1395
with Peas, Tomato, & Mushrooms, & Jacket Potato	1063

BEEF - STEAK, RUMP, SURF & TURF
with Peas, Tomato, & Mushrooms, & Chips	1625
with Peas, Tomato, & Mushrooms, & Jacket Potato	1293

BEEF - STEAK, SIRLOIN
& Eggs, Brunch	1158
8oz, Skinny, with Quinoa Salad	698
8oz, Steak Club	1198
with Peas, Tomato, & Mushrooms, with Chips	1160
with Peas, Tomato, & Mushrooms, with Jacket Potato	828

BEEF - STEAK, SIRLOIN, SURF & TURF
with Peas, Tomato, & Mushrooms, with Chips	1390

BHAJI
Onion, 1, Curry Club	165
Onion, 2, Curry Club	331

BLACK PUDDING
BLANK	246

BOLOGNESE
Spaghetti, Kids	318

BREAD
& Butter, Side, Pub Classics	450
Garlic, Ciabatta, Plait, Side	405
Garlic, Ciabatta, with Cheese, Side	571
Garlic, Pizza, Large	658
Garlic, Pizza, Large, Sm Plates	658
Garlic, Pizza, Small	347
Garlic, Pizza, with Mozzarella, Large	846
Garlic, Pizza, with Mozzarella, Small	538
Naan, Garlic, Curry Club	272

BREAKFAST
All Day, Brunch, Pub Classics	1256
All Day, Brunch, vegetarian, Pub Classics	1055

J D WETHERSPOON

BREAKFAST
All Day, Brunch, with Black Pudding, Pub Classics	1502
American	1486
GF	373
Large	1499
Small	469
Traditional	860
Vegan	638
Vegetarian	919
Vegetarian, Large	1324
Vegetarian, Small	377

BREAKFAST CEREAL
Porridge, with Banana, & Honey MOMA!*	462
Porridge, with Blueberries, & Brown Sugar, MOMA!*	313

BROWNIES
Chocolate, with Ice Cream, Warm	770
Chocolate, with Ice Cream, Warm, Mini	438

BUNS
Chicken, Pulled, Chicken Club	526

BURGERS
Beef, 6oz Classic	588
Beef, BBQ	1769
Beef, Drive Thru	1882
Beef, Empire State	2032
Beef, Hardy;s Shiraz, & Mushroom, Gourmet	1375
Beef, Pulled, Gourmet	1664
Beef, Tennessee	1678
Beef, Ultimate, Gourmet	2058
Chicken, BBQ	1625
Chicken, Breast, Grilled	438
Chicken, Breast, Grilled, Skinny	452
Chicken, Buttermilk, BBQ	1785
Chicken, Buttermilk, Breaded, Fried	598
Chicken, Buttermilk, Drive Thru	1893
Chicken, Buttermilk, Gourmet	843
Chicken, Buttermilk, Tennessee	1688
Chicken, Buttermilk, with Brie, & Smoky Chilli	1740
Chicken, Grilled, Drive Thru	1733
Chicken, Grilled, Gourmet	683
Chicken, Grilled, with Brie, & Smoky Chilli	1560
Chicken, Tennessee	1529
Vegetable, Gourmet	1689
Vegetable	1099

CAKE
Carrot	382
Chocolate, Fudge, with Ice Cream, Warm	924

CHEESE
American, Burger Topping	82
Cheddar, Burger Topping	83
Halloumi, Grilled, Add on, Chicken Club	477
Halloumi, Grilled, Extra	416
Halloumi, Grilled, Sm Plates	477

J D WETHERSPOON

	KCAL
CHICKEN	
Breast, Buttermilk, Fried, Chicken Club	447
Breast, Grilled, Chicken Club	287
CHICKEN & RIBS COMBO	
Breast, with Coleslaw, Onion Rings, & Chips	1885
Triple, with Coleslaw, Chips, & Corn on the Cob	1731
Wings, with Coleslaw, Chips, & Onion Rings	2204
CHICKEN - BBQ MELT	
with Cheese, Bacon, & BBQ Sauce, Steak Club	1121
with Peas, Tomato, & Mushrooms, & Chips	1718
with Peas, Tomato, & Mushrooms, & Jacket Potato	1386
CHICKEN - BBQ MELT, SURF & TURF	
with Peas, Tomato, & Mushrooms, & Chips	1948
with Peas, Tomato, & Mushrooms, & Jacket Potato	1616
CHICKEN - BITES	
Breast, Battered, 10, Chicken Club	405
Breast, Battered, with Sticky Soy Sauce	411
Breast, with Sticky Soy Sauce, Add on	155
CHICKEN - STRIPS	
Southern Fried, with Smoky Chipotle Mayo	655
Southern Fried, 5, Chicken Club	559
Southern Fried, JD Honey Glaze, Add on	348
Southern Fried, JD Honey Glaze, Coleslaw, & Chips	1225
CHICKEN - TRIPLE FEAST	
Coleslaw, Chips, Corn Cob, BBQ Sauce	1731
CHICKEN - WINGS	
Spicy, 10, Chicken Club	1166
with Sriracha Sauce, & Blue Cheese Dip, Sm Plates	1296
with Sriracha Sauce, Add on, Chicken Club	594
CHICKEN STUFFED	
Bacon Wrapped, with Mash, Peas, & Gravy	872
CHILLI	
Beef, Burger Topping	178
Beef, with Rice, Tortilla Chips, & Sour Cream	777
Five Bean, Burger Topping	107
Five Bean, with Rice, & Tortilla Chips	512
CHIPS	
Bowl, Side	955
Bowl, with Curry Sauce, Side	1057
Dish Add On	597
CHIPS - TOPPED	
BBQ Pulled Chicken, & Cheese, Sm Plates	1324
Beef Chilli, & Sour Cream, British, Sm Plates	1233
Curry Sauce, Chip Shop Style, Sm Plates	1057
Five Bean Chilli, British, Sm Plates	1062
Loaded, Cheese, Bacon, & Sour Cream, Sm Plates	1316
COLESLAW	
Burger Extra	95
Side	95
CORN	
Cobs, Mini, Side or Add on	86

J D WETHERSPOON

	KCAL
CRUMBLE	
Apple, Bramley, with Custard	498
Apple, Bramley, with Ice CReam	659
CURRY	
Cauliflower, & Spinach, Roasted, Mangolorean	895
Chicken, Flaming Dragon, Curry Club	827
Sweet Potato, Chickpea, & Spinach, Curry Club	850
Sweet Potato, Spinach, & Chickpea, Pub Classics	850
DESSERT	
Cookie Dough Sandwich, & Ice Cream, Warm	718
Cookie Dough Sandwich, & Ice Cream, Warm, Mini	428
DOUGHNUTS	
Dipping, with Chocolate Sauce, & Caramel Sauce	530
EGGS	
Benedict	551
Benedict, Small	355
Benedict, with Mushroom	502
Benedict, with Mushroom, Small	337
Fried, Burger Topping	72
Fried	72
Royale	536
Royale, Small	354
Scrambled, on Toast	551
Scrambled, on Toast, Wholemeal	546
FISH & CHIPS	
Cod, Battered, Fresh, with Mushy Peas	1289
Cod, Battered, Fresh, with Mushy Peas, Small	890
Cod, Battered, Fresh, with Peas	1236
Cod, Battered, Fresh, with Peas, Small	841
Cod, Oven Baked, with Mushy Peas	936
Cod, Oven Baked, with Peas	887
Haddock, Battered, Fresh, with Mushy Peas	1309
Haddock, Battered, Fresh, with Mushy Peas, Small	869
Haddock, Battered, Fresh, with Peas	1257
Haddock, Battered, Fresh, with Peas, Small	819
FRIES	
Skinny, Deli Deals	263
Skinny, Grill Option	263
FRUIT	
Fresh, & Ice CReam	433
Fresh, Breakfast	174
GAMMON & EGGS, 10OZ	
with Peas, Tomato, & Mushrooms, & Chips	1360
with Peas, Tomato, & Mushrooms, & Jacket Potato	1028
GAMMON & EGGS, 10OZ, SURF & TURF	
with Peas, Tomato, & Mushrooms, & Chips	1590
with Peas, Tomato, & Mushrooms, & Jacket Potato	1258
GAMMON & EGGS, 5OZ	
with Chips	993
GAMMON WITH	
Eggs, Steak Club	1395

J D WETHERSPOON

HAM

Egg, & Chips, Wiltshire Cured, Pub Classics	866
Egg, & Chips, Wiltshire Cured, Small, Pub Classics	453

HOUMOUS

& Falafel, Sm Plates	451
& Tortilla Chips, Sm Plates	605

JALFREZI

Chicken, Curry Club	896

KORMA

Chicken, Curry Club	1040

LAMB

Shank, Mash, Vegetables, & Gravy, Pub Classics	1217

LASAGNE

Beef, British, with Dressed Side Salad	768
Beef, Irish, with Dressed Side Salad	796
Vegetable, Mediterranean, with Dressed Side Salad	615

MADRAS

Beef, Curry Club	1136

MAKHANI

Chicken, & Paneer, Curry Club	1301

MIXED GRILL

Large, Steak Club	2086
Steak Club	1499
with Peas, Tomato, Mushrooms, & Chips	1194
with Peas, Tomato, Mushrooms, & Chips, Lge	2112
with Peas, Tomato, Mushrooms, Jacket Potato	1194
with Peas, Tomato, Mushrooms, Jacket Potato, Lge	1780

MIXED GRILL - SURF & TURF

with Peas, Tomato, Mushrooms, & Chips	1756
with Peas, Tomato, Mushrooms, & Chips, Lge	2342
with Peas, Tomato, Mushrooms, Jacket Potato	1424
with Peas, Tomato, Mushrooms, Jacket Potato, Lge	2010

MUFFIN

Avocado, Smashed	348
Avocado, Smashed, with Bacon, & Egg	497
Avocado, Smashed, with Bacon, & Halloumi	850
Avocado, Smashed, with Bacon, Egg, & Halloumi	913
Avocado, Smashed, with Bacon	434
Avocado, Smashed, with Egg, & Halloumi	827
Avocado, Smashed, with Egg	411
Avocado, Smashed, with Halloumi	764

NACHOS

Cheese, Guacamole, Salsa, Sour Cream, & Chilli's	657

NOODLES

Teriyaki, Pub Classics	389
Teriyaki, with Pulled Chicken	581

ONION RINGS

Battered, Beer, 12, Side or Add on	675
Battered, Beer, 6, Side or Add on	338
Battered, Beer	338

J D WETHERSPOON

PANCAKES - AMERICAN STYLE

with Bacon, & Maple Flavour Syrup, Breakfast	632
with Maple Flavour Syrup, & Ice Cream	507
with Maple Flavour Syrup, Breakfast	546

PANINI

Brie, Bacon, & Smoky Chilli Jam, Deli Deals	606
Cheese, & Tomato, Deli Deals	564
Chicken, Bacon, & Cheese, BBQ, Deli Deals	575
Ham, & Cheese, Wiltshire Cured, Deli Deals	530
Tuna, Cheese, & Mayo, Melt, Deli Deals	708

PEAS

Mushy, Side	248
Side	149

PIE - BEEF & DOOM BAR ALE

with Chips, Mushy Peas, & Gravy, Pub Classics	1457
with Chips, Peas, & Gravy, Pub Classics	1407
with Mash, Mushy Peas, & Gravy, Pub Classics	1128
with Mash, Peas, & Gravy, Pub Classics	1078

PIE - COTTAGE

with Peas, & Gravy, British, Pub Classics	528

PIZZA

Chicken, BBQ	1085
Chicken, Pulled, with Avocado, & Bacon	1343
Goat's Cheese, & Spiced Red Onion Chutney	955
Haggis	940
Ham, & Mushroom	943
Ham, & Pineapple	971
Margherita, Classic	869
Meat Feast, Spicy	1147
Pepperoni	1107
Vegetable, Gourmet	490

PIZZA TOPPING

BBQ Sauce	83
Chicken, Breast	96
Chillies, Sliced	4
Ham, Wiltshire Cured	56
Mushrooms	8
Onion, Red	10
Pepperoni	120
Pineapple	24

POTATOES - JACKET

Grill Option	299
with Beans, & Salad, Deli Deals	433
with Beef Chilli, & Sour Cream, with Salad, Deli Deals	538
with Cheese, & Salad, Deli Deals	572
with Coleslaw, & Salad, Deli Deals	595

POTATOES - JACKET

with Five Bean Chilli, & Salad, Deli Deals	417
with Roasted Vegetables, Deli Deals	395
with Tuna Mayo, & Salad, Deli Deals	543

PRAWNS

Coated, Spicy, with Sweet Chilli Dip, Add on	474
King, Spicy Coated, with Sweet Chilli Sauce	474

	KCAL

J D WETHERSPOON

PUDDING
Steak & Kidney, with Chips, Peas, & Gravy	1347

RIBS
Pork, BBQ, Half Rack, Side or Add on	581
Pork, BBQ, Half Rack, with Onion Rings, Sm Plates	918
Pork, BBQ, with Coleslaw, Onions Rings, & Chips	2191

RICE
Mexican Style, Chicken Club	202
Naan, & Poppadoms, Side or Add on, Curry Club	455

RISOTTO
Mushroom, Creamy	470
Mushroom, Creamy, with Pulled Chicken	662

ROGAN JOSH
Lamb, Curry Club	1076

ROLL
Bacon, Breakfast	293
Sausage, Breakfast	546
Sausage, Quorn*, Breakfast	442

SALAD
Caesar, Chicken	474
Caesar, Chicken, with Maple Cured Bacon	560
Chicken, Avocado, & Bacon, Balsamic Vinaigrette	450
Halloumi, Falafel, & Houmous, with Tortilla	926
Houmous, & Roasted Vegetable, Bowl, Deli Deals	328
Mozzarella, Tomato, Rocket, & Balsamic Glaze	402
Quinoa, Side or Add on	242
Quinoa, with Falafel, & Kale Dressing	583
Quinoa, with Halloumi, & Kale Dressing	935
Quinoa, with Kale Dressing	519
Quinoa, with Pulled Chicken, & Kale Dressing	711
Quinoa, with Roasted Vegetables, & Kale Dressing	608
with Dressing, Side or Add on	84

SAMOSAS
Vegetable, 1, Curry Club	105
Vegetable, 2, Curry Club	209
Vegetable, Sm Plates	534

SANDWICH
Bacon, Butty	510
Sausage, Butty	665
Sausage, Butty, Quorn*	494

SAUCE
Baconnaise, Burger Topping	191
Baconnaise, Chicken Club	191
BBQ, Burger Topping	83
BBQ, Chicken Club	83
Blue Cheese, Burger Topping	167
Cheese, & Leek, Caerphilly, Burger Topping	144
Garlic & Parsley Butter	97
Honey Glaze, Jack Daniels Honey, Chicken Club	70
Honey Glaze, with Jack Daniels Honey	70
Peppercorn, Creamy	74
Red Wine, Shiraz, Hardy's	48
Soy, Sticky, Chicken Club	101

	KCAL

J D WETHERSPOON

SAUCE
Sriracha, Chicken Club	58

SAUSAGE & MASH
Lincolnshire, with Peas, & Gravy	893
Vegetarian, with Peas, & Gravy, Quorn*	754

SCAMPI
Breaded, Whitby, with Chips, & Peas	905
Breaded, Whitby, with Chips, & Peas, Small	667

SOUP
Potato & Leek, with Bread & Butter, Sm Plates	556
Vegetable, Broth, with Bread & Butter, Sm Plates	306

TIKKA MASALA
Chicken, Curry Club	964
Chicken, Pub Classics	964

TOAST
& Preserves	466
& Preserves, Wholewheat Bloomer	461

VEGETABLES
Roasted, Burger Topping	89
Roasted, Side	89

VINDALOO
Chicken, Curry Club	953

WRAP
Breakfast	750
Breakfast, Vegetarian	876
Breakfast, with Black Pudding	996
Chicken, & Avocado, with Mayonnaise	381
Chicken, Breast, Pulled, & Sweet Chilli Sauce	481
Chicken, Southern Fried, with Smokey Chipotle Mayo	614
Falafel, & Houmous, with Mango Chutney	560
Halloumi, Grilled, with Avocado, & Sweet Chilli Sauce	804
Halloumi, Grilled, with Sweet Chilli Sauce	718
Houmous, & Roasted Vegetable	488

KCAL

KFC

BEANS

Baked, BBQ, Large	165
Baked, BBQ, Reg	70

BURGERS

Chicken, Big Daddy, Box Meal	1450
Chicken, Big Daddy	686
Chicken, Fillet, Bacon & Cheese	585
Chicken, Fillet, Bacon & Cheese, Meal	890
Chicken, Fillet, Box Meal	1100
Chicken, Fillet	475
Chicken, Fillet, Meal	780
Chicken, Fillet, Mini, Streetwise	290
Chicken, Fillet, Tower	620
Chicken, Fillet, Tower, Meal	925
Chicken, Kids	265
Chicken, Louisiana Dirty, Box Meal	1270
Chicken, Louisiana Dirty	750
Chicken, Louisiana Dirty, Meal	1050
Chicken, Meal, Kids	455
Chicken, Zinger, Box Meal	920
Chicken, Zinger	450
Chicken, Zinger, Meal	755
Chicken, Zinger, Tower	595
Chicken, Zinger, Tower, Meal	900
Chicken. Fillet, with Bacon & Cheese, Box Meal	1215

BURRITO

Chicken, Fillet	670
Chicken, Fillet, Meal	970
Chicken, Zinger	645
Chicken, Zinger, Meal	950

CHICKEN

Boneless, 3 Piece, Dips Meal	820
Boneless, 4 Piece, Dips Meal	950
Boneless, Banquet, Box Meal	975
Boneless, Feast, Dipping, 12 Piece	965
Boneless, Feast, Dipping, 8 Piece	835
Bucket, Bargain, 10 Piece	905
Bucket, Bargain, 14 Piece	1145
Bucket, Bargain, 6 Piece	665
Bucket, Mighty, For One	970
Bucket, Party, 14 Piece	1280
Drumstick, Original Recipe	170
Family Feast, 10 Piece	990
Family Feast, 14 Piece	1235
Family Feast, 6 Piece	750
Fillet, Mini	130
Fillet, Mini, Snackbox	735
Keel, Original recipe	265
Lunchbox	930
Megabox, with Gravy	1105
Original Recipe, 2 Piece, Meal	785
Original Recipe, 3 Piece, Meal	1025
Original Recipe, Meal, Kids	430

KCAL

KFC

CHICKEN

Original Recipe, Snackbox	845
Popcorn, Large	465
Popcorn, Meal	590
Popcorn, Meal, Kids	325
Popcorn, Meal, Large	770
Popcorn, Reg	285
Popcorn, Small	135
Popcorn, Snackbox	740
Rib, Original Recipe	325
Thigh, Original Recipe	285
Variety, 2 Piece, Meal	1085
Variety, 3 Piece, Meal	1320
Variety, Pack, Mini	710
Wicked Variety, 10 Piece	1200
Wicked Variety, 6 Piece	960
Wing, Hot, 1 Wing	85
Wing, Original Recipe	175
Wings, Hot, 6, Meal	800

COFFEE

Americano, Black, Large	10
Americano, Black, Reg	5
Americano, White, Large	70
Americano, White, Reg	50
Cappuccino, Large	110
Cappuccino, Reg	95
Espresso, Single	5
Latte, Caramel, Large	220
Latte, Caramel, Reg	175
Latte, Large	110
Latte, Reg	85
Latte, Vanilla, Large	170
Latte, Vanilla, Reg	125
Mocha, Large	390
Mocha, Reg	295

COLA

Pepsi*, Diet or Max, Kids	2
Pepsi*, Diet or Max, Large	3
Pepsi*, Diet or Max, Reg	2
Pepsi*, Kids	100
Pepsi*, Large	180
Pepsi*, Reg	130

COLESLAW

Large	320
Reg	160

COOKIES

Chocolate, Milk	375
Chocolate, White	380

CORN

Cobette	85
Cobette, Lge Portion	165

KFC
DESSERT
Kream Ball, Caramel Fudge	325
Kream Ball, Indulgent Chocolate	345
Krushems, Malteser	280
Krushems, Milky Bar	400
Krushems, Oreo	350
Krushems, Skittles	295

FRIES
Large	440
Reg	305

GRAVY
Large	110
Reg	45

HOT CHOCOLATE
with Cream, Large	435
with Cream, Reg	355

JUICE
Apple, Copella*	115
Orange, Tropicana*	120

JUICE DRINK
Apple, & Blackcurrant, Robinsons*, Kids	5
Apple, & Blackcurrant, Robinsons*, Large	10
Apple, & Blackcurrant, Robinsons*, Reg	5
Blackvurrant, & Apple, Fruit Shoot	10
Orange, Fruit Shoot	10

LEMONADE
7up*, Free, Kids	5
7up*, Free, Large	10
7up*, Free, Reg	5

MUFFIN
Chocolate	555
Lemon	540

ONION RINGS
BLANK	400

POTATOES
Mashed	97

RICE
Chicken, Fillet, Ricebox, Meal	800
Chicken, Zinger, Ricebox	490
Chicken, Zinger, Ricebox, Meal	790
Veggie, Ricebox	375
Veggie, Ricebox, Meal	675

SALAD
Chicken, Fillet	405
Chicken, Fillet, Meal	710
Chicken, Zinger	380
Chicken, Zinger, Meal	685
Veggie	270
Veggie, Meal	570

SAUCE
BBQ, Kentucky Smoky, Dip Pot	50
Curry, Large	175
Curry, Reg	75

KFC
SAUCE
Garlic Buttermilk Mayo, Dip Pot	110
Hot, Original, Dip Pot	40
HP, BBQ, Heinz, Sachet	15
HP, Brown, Heinz, Sachet	15
Ketchup, Heinz, Sachet	10
Mayonnaise, Light, Heinz, Sachet	30
Sweet Chilli, Sticky, Dip Pot	75
Tomato Sauce, Real, Dip Pot	40

SUNDAE
Strawberry	170
Toffee	175

TANGO*
Apple, Kids	90
Apple, Large	165
Apple, Reg	120
Orange, Kids	60
Orange, Large	105
Orange, Reg	75

TEA
Black	0
Iced, Lipton*, Kids	20
Iced, Lipton*, Large	60
Iced, Lipton*, Reg	45

WRAP
Chicken, BBQ, All Stars, Streetwise, Meal	735
Chicken, BBQ, Streetwise	300
Chicken, Fillet, Twister	510
Chicken, Fillet, Twister, Meal	810
Chicken, Flamin', All Stars, Streetwise, Meal	770
Chicken, Flamin', Streetwise	335
Chicken, Zinger, Twister	440
Chicken, Zinger, Twister, Meal	745

YOGHURT
Much Bunch	100

	KCAL
KRISPY KREME	
DOUGHNUTS	
Apple Pie	296
Blueberry, Powdered, Filled	307
Butterscotch Fudge	372
Chocolate, Glazed, Ring	237
Chocolate	340
Chocolate Dreamcake	351
Chocolate Iced, Creme Filled	372
Chocolate Iced, Custard Filled	289
Chocolate Iced, Ring, Glazed	278
Chocolate Iced, with Creme Filling	350
Chocolate Iced, with Sprinkles	262
Chocolate Praline Fudge Cake	346
Cinnamon Apple, Filled	269
Cookie Crunch	261
Cookies & Kreme	379
Cruller, Glazed	353
Glazed, Original	200
Glazed, with a Creme Filling	309
Lemon Filled, Glazed	218
Maple Iced, Crunch	250
Millionaires Shortbread	349
Orange Sundae Gloss	338
Raspberry, Glazed	324
Salted Caramel, Cheesecake	367
Strawberries & Kreme	326
Strawberry Filled, Powdered	248
Strawberry Gloss	244
Vanilla	315
White Chocolate & Almond	421

	KCAL
LOCH FYNE	
ANCHOVIES	
Smoked, Hot	129
AVOCADO	
& Smoked Salmon	620
with Pink Grapefruit, & Chilli	550
BACON	
Crispy, Breakfast Extra	144
Crispy, Side	144
BEEF - STEAK, FLAT IRON	
Flat Iron	550
BEEF - STEAK, RIBEYE	
28 Day Aged, 10oz, British	1618
28 Day Aged, 10oz, British, with ƒ š½ Lobster	1873
BEEF - STEAK, SIRLOIN	
28 Day Aged, 8oz, Scottish	1311
28 Day Aged, 8oz, Scottish, with ƒ š½ Lobster	1516
BEETROOT	
Baked, with Creme Fraiche, & Chives	168
Roast, Fish Bar	168
BLACK PUDDING	
Breakfast Extra	230
BREAD	
Basket, ½ Basket	334
BREAKFAST	
Full, with Fried Eggs, & Country Malt Bloomer	1463
Full, with Fried Eggs, & No Gluten Rolls	1614
Full, with Fried Eggs, & White Bloomer	1464
Full, with Poached Eggs, & Malt Bloomer	1305
Full, with Poached Eggs, & No Gluten Roll	1456
Full, with Poached Eggs, & White Bloomer	1306
Full, with Scrambled Egg, & Malt Bloomer	1545
Full, with Scrambled Egg, & No Gluten Roll	1696
Full, with Scrambled Egg, & White Bloomer	1546
BREAKFAST CEREAL	
Porridge, with Bananas	453
Porridge, with Blossom Honey	482
Porridge, with Maple Syrup	471
Porridge. Plain	405
BRILL	
Whole, Grilled, Fish Bar	424
Whole, Pan Fried, Fish Bar	461
Whole, Pan Fried, Fish Bar	461
Whole, Steamed, Fish Bar	424
BURGERS	
Chargrilled, 8oz, British	1741
Chargrilled, 8oz, British, Set Menu	1125
Chargrilled, 8oz, British, with ½ Lobster	1942
Chargrilled, 8oz, Scottish, with ½ Lobster	2009
BUTTER	
Lobster, Fish Bar	133
Lobster	133

LOCH FYNE

CHEESE

Goats, Baked, Crottin	333
Goats, Baked, with Heritage Potatoes, & Beetroot	321
Selection, British	534

CHEESECAKE

Passion Fruit	534

CHILLI

Sin Carne	769

CHIPS

Twice Cooked, Fish Bar	526
Twice Cooked	526
Twice Cooked, Set Menu Side	478

COD

Grilled, Line Caught, Fish Bar	318
Pan Fried, Line Caught, Fish Bar	361
Steamed, Line Caught, Fish Bar	323

COURGETTE

Chargrilled, with Lemon, Garlic, & Parsley	209

CREME BRULEE

BLANK	403
Set Menu	453

CROISSANT

BLANK	824

CURRY

Malabar, King Prawn	750

DESSERT

Delice, Spiced Rum & Chocolate	2857
Eton Mess	614

EGGS

Benedict	933
Dippy, with Toast, Malt Bloomer	412
Dippy, with Toast, No Gluten Roll	563
Dippy, with Toast, White Bloomer	413
Florentine	656
Fried, Breakfast Extra	268
Poached, Breakfast Extra	110
Royale	719
Scrambled, Breakfast Extra	350

FISH & CHIPS

Cod, Takeaway	1745
Haddock, Takeaway	1448
BLANK	1680

FISH CAKES

Salmon, Wilted Spinach, Provencale Sauce	683

FISH FINGERS

BLANK	789

FRIES

French, Fish Bar	616
French	460
Halloumi, with Tomato Ketchup	469

HADDOCK

Smoked, Poached	580
Smoked, Poached, with Soft Poached Egg	754

LOCH FYNE

HADDOCK WITH

Chips, Mushy Peas, & Tartar Sauce, Loin, Battered	1348

HAGGIS

Breakfast Extra	230

HAKE

Grilled, Line Caught, Fish Bar	327
Pan Fried, Line Caught, Fish Bar	461
Pan Fried	933
Steamed, Line Caught, Fish Bar	322

HALIBUT

Grilled, Fish Bar	312
Pan Fried, Fish Bar	392
Steamed, Fish Bar	318

HAM

& Piccalilli, Flaked	643

ICE CREAM

Amaretti Amaretto, Luxury	136
Chocolate, Luxury	123
Mint Chocolate, Luxury	122
Rum & Raisin, Luxury	98
Strawberry, Luxury	82
Vanilla, Luxury	110
Walnut, Luxury	130

KALE

Curly, Blanched, with Garlic Butter, Fish Bar	183
Curly, with Garlic Butter	183

KIPPER

Grilled, Pair, Malt Bloomer	897
Grilled, Pair, No Gluten Roll	1048
Grilled, Pair, White Bloomer	898

LEMON SOLE

Whole, Grilled, Fish Bar	353
Whole, Pan Fried, Fish Bar	427
Whole, Steamed, Fish Bar	353

LOBSTER

Benedict	736
Half, Side	264
Whole, Baked	1490

MACKEREL

Peppered, Potted, Scottish	355
Whole, Roasted, with Lemon & Thyme	854

MONKFISH

Grilled, Supreme, Fish Bar	287
Pan Fried, Supreme, Fish Bar	361
Steamed, Supreme, Fish Bar	387

MUSHROOMS

Breakfast Extra	101

MUSSELS

Scottish, Rope Grown	363
Scottish, Rope Grown, Main	1174
with Chilli, & Coriander	423
with Chilli, & Coriander, with French Fries	1243
with Provencale	323

LOCH FYNE

MUSSELS
with Provencale, Main	1051

OIL
Chilli, Roasted, Fish Bar	93
Chilli, Roasted	93

OLIVES
Mixed, Marinated	160

OYSTERS
Garlic, in Breadcrumbs, 1	97
Garlic, in Breadcrumbs, 12	1145
Garlic, in Breadcrumbs, 3	286
Garlic, in Breadcrumbs, 6	573
My First Oyster	61
Tequila & Lime, 1	60
Tequila & Lime, 12	716
Tequila & Lime, 3	179
Tequila & Lime, 6	358
with Vinegar, Tabasco, & Lemon, 1	61
with Vinegar, Tabasco, & Lemon, 12	690
with Vinegar, Tabasco, & Lemon, 3	175
with Vinegar, Tabasco, & Lemon, 6	345

PANCAKE
Bacon, & Maple Syrup	1381
Banana, & Cream	873

PEAS
Mushy	82

PLAICE
Fillet, Breaded, with Tartar Sauce	960
Whole, Grilled, Fish Bar	565
Whole, Pan Fried, Fish Bar	602
Whole, Steamed, Fish Bar	565

PLATTER
Meat Charcuterie, for One	378
Shellfish, Hot, ½ Platter	1254
Shellfish, with Lobster, ½ Platter	917
Shellfish, with Whole Crab, ½ Platter	902

POTATOES
Heritage, Sauteed, Fish Bar	355
Heritage, Sauteed	355
Heritage, with Minted Butter, Fish Bar	236
Heritage, with Minted Butter	236
Mashed	123
Mashed, Premium, Fish Bar	123

PRAWN COCKTAIL
Starter	537

PRAWNS
King, Chilli & Garlic, Pan Fried	835

PUDDING
Toffee, with Butterscotch Sauce, & Ice Cream	857

RISOTTO
Butternut Squash, with Sweet Potato Crisps	966
Summer Spelt	569

LOCH FYNE

ROE
Cod, Smoked, with Oat Cakes, & Sesame Seeds	533

SALAD
Chicken Caesar, Bowl	716
Fennel, Braised, with Quinoa	888
Greek, Fish Bar	375
Greek, Side	375
Green, Fish Bar	120
Green, Side	120
Herring, Beetroot, Egg, & Horseradish, with Madeira	655

SALMON
Grilled, Scottish, Fish Bar	535
Pan Fried, Scottish, Fish Bar	609
Steamed, Scottish, Fish Bar	535

SALMON - SMOKED
Gin & Beetroot Cured, Bradan Orach, for Two, ½	268
Gin & Beetroot Cured, Bradan Orach	288
with Scrambled Eggs, Malt Bloomer	548
with Scrambled Eggs, No Gluten Roll	699
with Scrambled Eggs, White Bloomer	549

SALSA
Verde, Fish Bar	139
Verde	139

SAMPHIRE
Fish Bar	37
with Garlic Butter	101

SARDINES
Chargrilled, with Chilli Oil, & Yoghurt	497
Grilled, with Parsley & Lemon	600

SAUCE
Gribiche, Fish Bar	165
Gribiche	165
Hollandaise, Fish Bar	233
Hollandaise	388
Pesto, Lovage, Fish Bar	159
Pesto, Lovage	159

SAUSAGE
Breakfast Extra	271

SCALLOPS
Grilled, with Chorizo, & Garlic Butter, 3	382
King, Grilled, Scottish	302

SEA BASS
Whole, Roasted	791

SEA BREAM
Grilled, Gilt Head, Fish Bar	273
Pan Fried, Gilt Head, Fish Bar	310
Steamed, Gilt Head, Fish Bar	273

SEAFOOD
Grill	1031

SORBET
Lemon	62
Pear	63
Raspberry	85

LOCH FYNE	KCAL
SOUP	
Courgette, Lemon, & Rosemary	493
Fish	469
Fish	469
Onion, Roast, with Cumin, & Yoghurt	309
SPAGHETTI WITH	
Prawns, King	981
SPINACH	
Buttered	50
Fish Bar	50
SPRATS	
Crispy	804
SQUID	
Salt & Pepper	511
STEW	
Fishermans	871
Fishermans, to Share, ½	1055
TAGINE	
Bean, Mixed	458
TAGLIATELLE	
Seafood	875
TART	
Chocolate	586
Treacle	552
Treacle, with Clotted Cream, & Orange	552
TOAST	
Granary, Breakfast Extra	362
White Bloomer, Breakfast Extra	363
TOAST & AVOCADO	
& Bacon. Malt Bloomer	1162
& Bacon. No Gluten Roll	1313
& Bacon. White Bloomer	1163
& Poached Eggs, Loch Muffin	1451
& Poached Eggs, Malt Bloomer	917
& Poached Eggs, on No Gluten Roll	1068
& Poached Eggs, White Bloomer	918
Bacon, & Poached Eggs, Malt Bloomer	1123
Bacon, & Poached Eggs, No Gluten Roll	1274
Bacon, & Poached Eggs, White Bloomer	1124
Malt Bloomer	615
No Gluten Roll	766
White Bloomer	616
TOMATOES	
Breakfast Extra	52
TUNA	
Chargrilled, Fish Bar	374
Grilled, Fish Bar	369
Pan Fried, Fish Bar	412
TURBOT	
Grilled, Supreme, Fish Bar	391
Pan Fried, Supreme, Fish Bar	471
Steamed, Supreme, Fish Bar	396

MCDONALD'S	KCAL
BAGEL	
with Bacon, Egg & Cheese	480
with Sausage, Egg & Cheese	562
BITES	
Cheese, Monterey Jack, Melts	212
BREAD	
Bagel, Plain, Toasted	216
BREAKFAST CEREAL	
Porridge, Oat So Simple, Apple & Cherry	228
Porridge, Oat So Simple, Plain	194
BURGERS	
Beef, & Cheese, Feast	833
Beef, Signature Collection, The BBQ	782
Beef, Signature Collection, The Classic	698
Beef, Signature Collection, The Spicy	635
Big Mac	508
Cheeseburger, Double	445
Cheeseburger	301
Chicken, BLC	399
Chicken, Christmas Warmer	560
Chicken, The Ranch, California	652
Chicken Legend, with Bacon, & BBQ Sauce	535
Chicken Legend, with Bacon, & Hot & Spicy Mayo	569
Chicken Legend, with Bacon, Cool Mayo	580
Chicken Legend, with BBQ Sauce	484
Chicken Legend, with Cool Mayo	529
Chicken Legend, with Hot & Spicy Mayo	519
Filet-O-Fish	329
Hamburger	250
Mayo Chicken	319
McChicken Sandwich	388
McKrocket	349
Quarter Pounder, with Cheese	518
BURGERS VEGETARIAN	
Vegetable, Deluxe	400
Vegetable Deluxe, Spicy	412
CARROTS	
Sticks	34
CHEESE	
Melt, Dippers	257
CHICKEN	
McNuggets, 6 Pieces	259
McNuggets, 9 Pieces	388
Nuggets, Sharebox, 20	863
Selects, 3 Pieces	359
Selects, 5 Pieces	599
COFFEE	
Black, Large	8
Black, Medium	6
Cappuccino, Large	124
Cappuccino, Medium	94
Espresso, Double Shot	1
Espresso, Single Shot	1

MCDONALD'S

COFFEE

Flat White, Semi Skimmed Milk	86
Latte, Large	192
Latte, Medium	142
Latte, Spiced Cookie, Large	219
Latte, Spiced Cookie, Medium	174
Latte, Toffee, Large	227
Latte, Toffee	183
Mocha, McCafe	340
White, Large	40
White, Medium	30

COLA

Coca-Cola, Diet	2
Coca-Cola	170
Coke, Zero	1

COOKIES

Triple Chocolate	368

DOUGHNUTS

Chocolate Donut	254
Sugared Donut	189

DRESSING

Balsamic, for Shaker Side Salad	26

FANTA

Orange	48

FLATBREAD

Cheesy, Bacon	298

FRIES

French, Large	444
French, Medium	337
French, Small	237

FRUIT

Bag, Apple & Grape	46
Bag, Happy Meal	46

FRUIT SHOOT

Robinsons	10

HAPPY MEAL

Cheeseburger with Carrot Sticks	335
Cheeseburger with Fruit Bag	347
Cheeseburger with Sm Fries	538
Chicken McNuggets with Carrot Sticks	207
Chicken McNuggets with Fruit Bag	219
Chicken McNuggets with Sm Fries	410
Crispy Chicken Wrap, with Carrot Sticks	277
Crispy Chicken Wrap, with Fruit Bag	289
Crispy Chicken Wrap, with Sm Fries	480
Fish Fingers with Carrot Sticks	228
Fish Fingers with Fruit Bag	240
Fish Fingers with Sm Fries	431
Hamburger with Carrot Sticks	284
Hamburger with Fruit bag	296
Hamburger with Sm Fries	487

HASH BROWNS

Single	136

MCDONALD'S

HOT CHOCOLATE

Large	231
BLANK	173

ICE CREAM CONE

BLANK	145
with Flake	190

IRN BRU

BLANK	170

JUICE

Tropicana	108

JUICE DRINK

Oasis	42

LEMONADE

Sprite, Zero	5

MCFLURRY

Chocolate Orange	408
Crunchie	323
Dairy Milk	332

MCMUFFIN

Bacon & Egg, Double	401
Bacon & Egg	348
Egg, & Cheese	295
Sausage & Egg, Double	565
Sausage & Egg	430

MILK SHAKE

Banana, Large	495
Banana, Medium	386
Banana, Small	203
Chocolate, Large	488
Chocolate, Medium	380
Chocolate, Small	200
Strawberry, Large	488
Strawberry, Medium	379
Strawberry, Small	200
Vanilla, Large	483
Vanilla, Medium	377
Vanilla, Small	198

MUFFIN

Blueberry	401
Chocolate	515

PANCAKE

& Sausage, with Syrup	670
& Syrup	535

PIE

Apple, Hot	250

ROLL

Bacon, with Brown Sauce	323
Bacon, with Tomato Ketchup	319

SALAD

Chicken, No Bacon, Grilled	133
Chicken, with Bacon, Grilled	184
Crispy Chicken, No Bacon	265
Crispy Chicken, with Bacon	316

MCDONALD'S

SALAD

	KCAL
Side, Shaker	18

SMOOTHIE

Berry Burst, Large	208
Berry Burst, Medium	159
Mango & Pineapple, Iced, Large	236
Mango & Pineapple, Iced, Medium	187

SUNDAE

Strawberry	292
Toffee	344

TEA

with Milk, Large	12
with Milk	6

WRAP

Breakfast, Bacon, & Egg Snack, Brown Sauce	281
Breakfast, Bacon, & Egg Snack, Ketchup	279
Breakfast, Egg, & Cheese, Snack, Brown Sauce	256
Breakfast, Egg, & Cheese, Snack, Ketchup	253
Breakfast, Sausage, & Egg Snack, Brown Sauce	323
Breakfast, Sausage, & Egg Snack, Ketchup	321
Breakfast, with Brown Sauce	609
Breakfast, with Tomato Ketchup	605
Chicken, Spicy, Snack	322
Chicken & Bacon One, Crispy, BBQ	500
Chicken & Bacon One, Grilled, BBQ	366
Chicken One, Crispy, Garlic Mayo	479
Chicken One, Crispy, Hot Peri Peri	488
Chicken One, Crispy, Sweet Chilli	474
Chicken One, Grilled, Garlic Mayo	345
Chicken One, Grilled, Hot Peri Peri, Big Flavour	353
Chicken One, Grilled, Sweet Chilli	340

NANDO'S

AVOCADO

	KCAL
Burger Add-On	80
Salad Extra	161

BREAD

Garlic, Roll, Kids Menu	218
Garlic, Large, Side	672
Garlic, Side	336

BROWNIES

Salted Caramel	389

BURGERS

Beanie, Peri Peri, Extra Hot	614
Beanie, Peri Peri, Hot	573
Beanie, Peri Peri, Lemon & Herb	542
Beanie, Peri Peri, Mango & Lime	555
Beanie, Peri Peri, Medium	552
Beanie, Plain	532
Chicken, Breast, Peri-Peri, Extra Hot	449
Chicken, Breast, Peri-Peri, Hot	408
Chicken, Breast, Peri-Peri, Lemon & Herb	377
Chicken, Breast, Peri-Peri, Mango & Lime	390
Chicken, Breast, Peri-Peri, Medium	387
Chicken, Breast, Plain, Kids Menu	289
Chicken, Breast, Plain	367
Chicken, Butterfly Burger, Peri Peri, Extra Hot	629
Chicken, Butterfly Burger, Peri Peri, Hot	588
Chicken, Butterfly Burger, Peri Peri, Lemon & Herb	557
Chicken, Butterfly Burger, Peri Peri, Mango & Lime	570
Chicken, Butterfly Burger, Peri Peri, Medium	567
Chicken, Butterfly Burger, Plain	547
Chicken, Double, Peri Peri, Extra Hot	579
Chicken, Double, Peri Peri, Hot	538
Chicken, Double, Peri Peri, Lemon & Herb	507
Chicken, Double, Peri Peri, Mango & Lime	520
Chicken, Double, Peri Peri, Medium	517
Chicken, Double, Plain	497
Chicken, Sunset Burger, Peri Peri, Extra Hot	683
Chicken, Sunset Burger, Peri Peri, Hot	642
Chicken, Sunset Burger, Peri Peri, Lemon & Herb	611
Chicken, Sunset Burger, Peri Peri, Mango & Lime	624
Chicken, Sunset Burger, Peri Peri, Medium	621
Chicken, Sunset Burger, Plain	601
Mushroom, & Halloumi, Peri Peri, Extra Hot	729
Mushroom, & Halloumi, Peri Peri, Hot	688
Mushroom, & Halloumi, Peri Peri, Lemon & Herb	657
Mushroom, & Halloumi, Peri Peri, Mango & Lime	670
Mushroom, & Halloumi, Peri Peri, Medium	667
Mushroom, & Halloumi, Plain	647
Supergreen, Peri Peri, Extra Hot	484
Supergreen, Peri Peri, Hot	443
Supergreen, Peri Peri, Lemon & Herb	412
Supergreen, Peri Peri, Mango & Lime	425
Supergreen, Peri Peri, Medium	422
Supergreen, Plain	402

NANDO'S

BURGERS

Sweet Potato, & Butternut, Kids Menu	333
Sweet Potato, & Butternut, Pattie Only, Kids Menu	219
Sweet Potato, & Butternut, Peri Peri, Extra Hot	511
Sweet Potato, & Butternut, Peri Peri, Hot	470
Sweet Potato, & Butternut, Peri Peri, Lemon & Herb	439
Sweet Potato, & Butternut, Peri Peri, Mango & Lime	452
Sweet Potato, & Butternut, Peri Peri, Medium	449
Sweet Potato, & Butternut, Plain	429

CAKE

Carrot, Four High	711
Choc-A-Lot	535

CHEESE

Cheddar, Burger Add-on	78
Halloumi, Grilled, Burger Add-On	177

CHEESECAKE

Gooey Caramel	434
Raspberrry	508

CHICKEN

Butterfly, Crispy, Peri Peri, Extra Hot	392
Butterfly, Crispy, Peri Peri, Hot	351
Butterfly, Crispy, Peri Peri, Lemon & Herb	320
Butterfly, Crispy, Peri Peri, Mango & Lime	333
Butterfly, Crispy, Peri Peri, Medium	330
Butterfly, Crispy, Plain	310
Half, Peri-Peri, Extra Hot	639
Half, Peri-Peri, Hot	598
Half, Peri-Peri, Lemon & Herb	567
Half, Peri-Peri, Mango & Lime	580
Half, Peri-Peri, Med	577
Half, Plain	557
Quarter, Breast, & Wing, Peri-Peri, Extra Hot	360
Quarter, Breast, & Wing, Peri-Peri, Hot	319
Quarter, Breast, & Wing, Peri-Peri, Lemon & Herb	288
Quarter, Breast, & Wing, Peri-Peri, Mango & Lime	301
Quarter, Breast, & Wing, Peri-Peri, Medium	298
Quarter, Breast, & Wing, Plain	278
Quarter, Leg, & Thigh, Peri-Peri, Extra Hot	361
Quarter, Leg, & Thigh, Peri-Peri, Hot	320
Quarter, Leg, & Thigh, Peri-Peri, Lemon & Herb	289
Quarter, Leg, & Thigh, Peri-Peri, Mango & Lime	302
Quarter, Leg, & Thigh, Peri-Peri, Medium	299
Quarter, Leg, & Thigh, Plain	279
Strips, Plain, Kids Menu	130
Thighs, Deboned, Peri-Peri, Extra Hot	653
Thighs, Deboned, Peri-Peri, Hot	612
Thighs, Deboned, Peri-Peri, Lemon & Herb	581
Thighs, Deboned, Peri-Peri, Mango & Lime	594
Thighs, Deboned, Peri-Peri, Medium	591
Thighs, Deboned, Plain	571
Thighs 2, Salad Extra, Peri Peri, Extra Hot	368
Thighs 2, Salad Extra, Peri Peri, Hot	327
Thighs 2, Salad Extra, Peri Peri, Lemon & Herb	296

NANDO'S

CHICKEN

Thighs 2, Salad Extra, Peri Peri, Mango & Lime	309
Thighs 2, Salad Extra, Peri Peri, Medium	306
Thighs 2, Salad Extra, Plain	286
Whole, Peri-Peri, Extra Hot	1196
Whole, Peri-Peri, Hot	1155
Whole, Peri-Peri, Lemon & Herb	1124
Whole, Peri-Peri, Mango & Lime	1137
Whole, Peri-Peri, Medium	1134
Whole, Plain	1114
Wings, Peri-Peri, Extra Hot, 10	1017
Wings, Peri-Peri, Extra Hot, 3	362
Wings, Peri-Peri, Extra Hot, 5	549
Wings, Peri-Peri, Hot, 10	976
Wings, Peri-Peri, Hot, 3	321
Wings, Peri-Peri, Hot, 5	508
Wings, Peri-Peri, Lemon & Herb, 10	945
Wings, Peri-Peri, Lemon & Herb, 3	290
Wings, Peri-Peri, Lemon & Herb, 5	477
Wings, Peri-Peri, Mango & Lime, 10	958
Wings, Peri-Peri, Mango & Lime, 3	303
Wings, Peri-Peri, Mango & Lime, 5	490
Wings, Peri-Peri, Medium, 10	955
Wings, Peri-Peri, Medium, 3	300
Wings, Peri-Peri, Medium, 5	487
Wings, Plain, 10	935
Wings, Plain, 3	280
Wings, Plain, 5	467

CHIPS

Kids Menu	336
Large, Side	1256
Peri Salted, Large, Side	1260
Peri Salted, Reg, Side	467
Reg, Side	465

COFFEE

Americano	0
Cappuccino	73
Espresso	0
Latte	63

COLESLAW

Large, Side	535
Side	268

CORDIAL

Green, Kids Menu	29

CORN

Cob, Kids Menu	72
Cob, Flame-Grilled, 2, Side	288
Cob, Flame-Grilled, Side	144

DIP

Red Pepper, & Chilli, with Pitta	462

DRINK

Mango Quencher	129
Rubro	92

NANDO'S

FROZEN YOGHURT

Chocolate	91
Mango	71
Strawberry	70
Vanilla	71

HOT CHOCOLATE

Original	291

HOUMOUS

Peri Drizzle, & Pitta	800

ICE CREAM

Chocolate	145
Coconut	161
Mango	95
Vanilla, Kids Menu	158
Vanilla	161

ICE LOLLY

Chilly Billy	29

JUICE

Orange	118

LEMONADE

Cloudy	137

MASH

Creamy, Side	294
Large, Side	588
Sweet Potato, Kids Menu	124
Sweet Potato, Side	248

MILK

Organic, Kids Menu	113

MUSHROOMS

Portabello, Roasted, Burger Add-On	105

NUTS

Peri-Peri	793

OLIVES

Mixed, Spicy	138

PEAS

Macho, Large, Side	283
Macho, Side	141

PINEAPPLE

Slice, Grilled, Burger Add-On	37

POTATO WEDGES

Sweet Potato, Kids Menu	87
Sweet Potato, Side	330
Sweet Potato, with Peri Peri Salt, Side	333

RELISH

Chilli, Jam, Burger Add-On	59

RICE

Portuguese, Large, Side	453
Portuguese, Side	227

ROLL - CHICKEN, LIVER

Portuguese, Peri Peri, Extra Hot	551
Portuguese, Peri Peri, Hot	510
Portuguese, Peri Peri, Lemon & Herb	479
Portuguese, Peri Peri, Mango & Lime	492

NANDO'S

ROLL - CHICKEN, LIVER

Portuguese, Peri Peri, Medium	489
Portuguese, Plain	469

ROLL - STEAK, FILLET

Prego, Peri Peri, Extra Hot	446
Prego, Peri Peri, Hot	405
Prego, Peri Peri, Lemon & Herb	374
Prego, Peri Peri, Mango & Lime	387
Prego, Peri Peri, Medium	384
Prego, Plain	364

SALAD

Mixed Leaf, Side, Large	25

SALAD - CAESAR

no Chicken	334

SALAD - CAESAR, CHICKEN

& Extra Grilled Chicken, Peri-Peri, Extra Hot	546
& Extra Grilled Chicken, Peri-Peri, Hot	505
& Extra Grilled Chicken, Peri-Peri, Lemon & Herb	474
& Extra Grilled Chicken, Peri-Peri, Mango & Lime	487
& Extra Grilled Chicken, Peri-Peri, Med	484
Chicken	464

SALAD - MEDITERRANEAN

Plain	288
with Grilled Chicken, Peri-Peri, Extra Hot	499
with Grilled Chicken, Peri-Peri, Hot	458
with Grilled Chicken, Peri-Peri, Lemon & Herb	427
with Grilled Chicken, Peri-Peri, Mango & Lime	440
with Grilled Chicken, Peri-Peri, Medium	437
with Grilled Chicken	417

SALAD - MIXED LEAF

with Chicken Breast, Peri Peri, Extra Hot	236
with Chicken Breast, Peri Peri, Hot	195
with Chicken Breast, Peri Peri, Lemon & Herb	164
with Chicken Breast, Peri Peri, Mango & Lime	177
with Chicken Breast, Peri Peri, Medium	174
with Chicken Breast, Plain	154

SALAD - QUINOA & AVOCADO

Plain	460
with Grilled Chicken, Peri-Peri, Extra Hot	672
with Grilled Chicken, Peri-Peri, Hot	631
with Grilled Chicken, Peri-Peri, Lemon & Herb	600
with Grilled Chicken, Peri-Peri, Mango & Lime	613
with Grilled Chicken, Peri-Peri, Med	610
with Grilled Chicken	590

SALAD - SUPERGRAIN

Kids Menu	114
Plain	377
Side, Large	359
Side, Reg	188
with Chicken Breast, Peri Peri, Extra Hot	589
with Chicken Breast, Peri Peri, Hot	548
with Chicken Breast, Peri Peri, Lemon & Herb	517
with Chicken Breast, Peri Peri, Mango & Lime	530

NANDO'S

SALAD - SUPERGRAIN

with Chicken Breast, Peri Peri, Medium	527
with Chicken Breast, Plain	507

SANDWICH - BEANIE

Peri Peri, Extra Hot, Pitta	628
Peri Peri, Hot, Pitta	587
Peri Peri, Lemon & Herb, Pitta	556
Peri Peri, Mango & Lime, Pitta	569
Peri Peri, Medium, Pitta	566
Plain, Pitta	546

SANDWICH - CHICKEN

Breast, Peri-Peri, Extra Hot, Pitta	463
Breast, Peri-Peri, Hot, Pitta	422
Breast, Peri-Peri, Lemon & Herb, Pitta	391
Breast, Peri-Peri, Mango & Lime, Pitta	404
Breast, Peri-Peri, Medium, Pitta	401
Breast, Plain, Pitta	381
Double, Pitta, Peri Peri, Extra Hot	592
Double, Pitta, Peri Peri, Hot	551
Double, Pitta, Peri Peri, Lemon & Herb	520
Double, Pitta, Peri Peri, Mango & Lime	533
Double, Pitta, Peri Peri, Medium	530
Thigh, Fino Pitta, Peri Peri, Extra Hot	875
Thigh, Fino Pitta, Peri Peri, Hot	834
Thigh, Fino Pitta, Peri Peri, Lemon & Herb	803
Thigh, Fino Pitta, Peri Peri, Mango & Lime	816
Thigh, Fino Pitta, Peri Peri, Medium	813
Thigh, Fino Pitta, Plain	793

SANDWICH - HALLOUMI & MUSHROOM

Peri Peri, Pitta, Extra Hot	719
Peri Peri, Pitta, Hot	678
Peri Peri, Pitta, Lemon & Herb	647
Peri Peri, Pitta, Mango & Lime	660
Peri Peri, Pitta, Medium	657
Pitta, Plain	637

SANDWICH - STEAK

Fillet, & Veg, Peri Peri, Extra Hot	496
Fillet, & Veg, Peri Peri, Hot	455
Fillet, & Veg, Peri Peri, Lemon & Herb	424
Fillet, & Veg, Peri Peri, Mango & Lime	437
Fillet, & Veg, Peri Peri, Medium	434
Fillet, & Veg, Plain	414

SANDWICH - SUPERGREEN

Peri Peri, Pitta, Extra Hot	526
Peri Peri, Pitta, Hot	485
Peri Peri, Pitta, Lemon & Herb	454
Peri Peri, Pitta, Mango & Lime	467
Peri Peri, Pitta, Medium	464
Pitta, Plain	444

SANDWICH - SWEET POTATO & BUTTERNUT

Peri Peri, Extra Hot, Pitta	552
Peri Peri, Hot, Pitta	511
Peri Peri, Lemon & Herb, Pitta	480

NANDO'S

SANDWICH - SWEET POTATO & BUTTERNUT

Peri Peri, Mango & Lime, Pitta	493
Peri Peri, Medium, Pitta	490
Plain, Pitta	470

SAUCE

Peri Peri Drizzle, Side	97
Perinaise, Condiments	159

TART

Custard, Naughty Natas	180

TEA

Infusions, All Flavours	0
Organic, Everyday	23

TOMATOES

Kids Menu	13

VEGETABLES

Roasted, Side	98

WRAP

Double, Peri Peri, Mango & Lime	721

WRAP - BEANIE

Peri Peri, Extra Hot	815
Peri Peri, Hot	774
Peri Peri, Lemon & Herb	743
Peri Peri, Mango & Lime	756
Peri Peri, Medium	753
Plain	733

WRAP - CHICKEN

Breast, Peri-Peri, Extra Hot	650
Breast, Peri-Peri, Hot	609
Breast, Peri-Peri, Lemon & Herb	578
Breast, Peri-Peri, Mango & Lime	591
Breast, Peri-Peri, Medium	588
Breast, Plain	568
Double, Peri Peri, Extra Hot	780
Double, Peri Peri, Hot	739
Double, Peri Peri, Lemon & Herb	708
Double, Peri Peri, Medium	718
Double, Plain	698

WRAP - HALLOUMI & MUSHROOM

Peri-Peri, Extra Hot	847
Peri-Peri, Hot	806
Peri-Peri, Lemon & Herb	775
Peri-Peri, Mango & Lime	788
Peri-Peri, Medium	785
Plain	765

WRAP - STEAK

Fillet, & Veg, Peri Peri, Extra Hot	600
Fillet, & Veg, Peri Peri, Hot	559
Fillet, & Veg, Peri Peri, Lemon & Herb	528
Fillet, & Veg, Peri Peri, Mango & Lime	541
Fillet, & Veg, Peri Peri, Medium	538
Fillet, & Veg, Plain	518

NANDO'S

WRAP - SUPERGREEN

	KCAL
Peri Peri, Extra Hot	713
Peri Peri, Hot	672
Peri Peri, Lemon & Herb	641
Peri Peri, Mango & Lime	654
Peri Peri, Medium	651
Plain	631

WRAP - SWEET POTATO & BUTTERNUT

	KCAL
Peri Peri, Extra Hot	740
Peri Peri, Hot	699
Peri Peri, Lemon & Herb	668
Peri Peri, Mango & Lime	681
Peri Peri, Medium	678
Plain	658

PIZZA EXPRESS

ANTIPASTO

	KCAL
Italian, Classic	795

BOLOGNESE

Penne, Al Forno	674
Penne, Piccolo	353

BREAD

Garlic, with Mozzarella	356

BROWNIES

Chocolate, Dolcetti	206
Chocolate, Piccolo	206
Chocolate, with Ice Cream	519

BRUSCHETTA

Originale	362

CAKE

Carrot, Vegan, Dolcetti	336
Chocolate, Fudge	312
Sticky Toffee, Bundt	494

CANNELLONI

Spinach, & Ricotta, Al Forno	798

CHEESE

Mascarpone, Side	118

CHEESECAKE

Lotus Biscoff, Dolcetti	319
Raspberry, Honeycomb, Cream, Slice	466
Vanilla, Reduced Fat & Sugar	377

CHICKEN

Wings, Lemon & Herb	556

CHIPS

Polenta	454

COLESLAW

Side	330

COULIS

Fruit, Side	25

CREAM

Side	139

DESSERT

Posset, Lemon, Crunch, Dolcetti	195

DOUGH BALLS

Doppio	828
GF, with Garlic Butter	370
Plain	396
Sticks, Side	263
with Balsamic Vinegar, & Olive Oil, Piccolo	160
with Butter, Piccolo	189

DRESSING

Caesar	157
Honey & Mustard	196
House, Classic	191
House, Light	135

FIGS

Caffe Reale, Dolcetti	208

PIZZA EXPRESS

ICE CREAM
Affogato, no Coffee	337
Caramel, Salted, & Chocolate Straw, Coppa Gelato	287
Strawberry, & Chocolate Straw, Coppa Gelato	211
Vanilla, & Chocolate Straw, Coppa Gelato	247
Vanilla, Gelato, Side	114

ICE LOLLY
Fruit, Organic, Pip	18
Rainbow, Organic, Pip	20

JUICE DRINK
Apple, & Pear, Cawston	54
Apple, & Summer Berries, Cawston	50

LASAGNE
Classica, Al Forno	712

MILK
Piccolo	82

OLIVES
Marinate	137

PENNE
Bianca, Piccolo	355
Napoletana, Piccolo	284
Pepperonata, Al Forno	542

PESTO
Pollo, Al Forno, GF	1082

PIZZA
American, Classic	1019
American, Hot, Leggera, Wholemeal	548
American, Hot, Romana	1010
American, Piccolo	510
Calabrese	1275
Carbonara, Romana	1420
Diavlo, Romana	167
Fiorentina, Classic	942
Giardiniera, Classic, Vegan	843
Giardiniera, Leggera, Wholemeal, Vegan	556
Giardiniera, Romana, Vegan	970
La Reine, Classic	898
La Reine, Piccolo	509
Margherita, Bufala, Romana	1051
Margherita, Classic	834
Margherita, Piccolo	448
Padana, Leggera, Wholemeal	587
Padana, Romana	1108
Pollo, ad Astra, Leggera, Wholemeal	599
Pollo, ad Astra, Romana	1145
Pollo, Forza, Romana	1253
Pollo, Piccolo	456
Puttanesca, Romana, Vegan	844
Ragu, Romana	1181
Sloppy Giuseppe, Classic	897
Veneziana, Classic	938

PROFITEROLES
Salted Caramel, Dolcetti	257

PIZZA EXPRESS

SALAD
Caesar, Chicken, Grand, no Dressing	477
Caesar, Chicken, Grand, Dressing, & Dough Sticks	894
Caesar, Chicken, Grand, with Dressing	636
Caesar, with Dressing, Restaurant	341
Caesar, without Dressing	238
Mixed, Side, no Dressiing	74
Mixed, Side, with House Dressing	202
Mozzarella, & Tomato, Buffalo	336
Nicoise, no Dressing	366
Nicoise, with Dressing, & Dough Sticks	820
Nicoise, with Dressing	558
Pollo, Milanese, Caesar	768
Pollo, Milanese, Rucola	787
Pollo, no Dressing	502
Pollo, with Dough Balls, Piccolo	283
Pollo, with Dressing, & Dough Sticks	954
Pollo, with Dressing	693
Pollo, with Polenta Chips, Piccolo	265
Side, Piccolo	16
Superfood, Leggera	446
Superfood, Pizza Addition	171
Superfood, with Anchovies, Leggera	497
Superfood, with Chicken, Leggera	593

SORBET
Coconut, Coppa Gelato	201
Raspberry, Coppa Gelato	122

SQUID
Calamari	504

SUNDAE
Ic Cream, with Chocolate Sauce, Piccolo	149
Ice Cream, with Fruit Sauce, Piccolo	131

TART
Lemon	351

TIRAMISU
Classic	412

TOMATOES
Roasted	67

PIZZA HUT	KCAL
APPLES	
Salad Station	10
BACON	
Bits, Salad Station	104
BEETROOT	
Diced, Salad Station	5
BITES	
Cheese, & Onion, Fried	361
Cheese, & Onion, Oven Baked	334
BREAD	
Garlic	511
Garlic, with Cheese	689
BREADSTICKS	
Salad Station	87
CARROTS	
Shredded, Salad Station	10
CHEESECAKE	
Chocolate, Chunk	438
CHICKEN	
Bites, BBQ	441
Bites, Plain	381
Bites, Sweet Chilli	468
Wings	612
COLESLAW	
Salad Station	38
COOKIES	
Dough, Chocolate Chip, Hot	596
Dough, S'mores, Hot	676
Dough, Salted Caramel, Hot	579
COUS COUS	
Tomato, & Basil, Salad Station	28
CRISPS	
with Cheese Sauce, & Onions, Fried	1730
with Cheese Sauce, & Onions, Microwaved	1687
CROUTONS	
Salad Station	85
CUCUMBER	
Salad Station	2
DIP	
Blue Cheese, Salad Station	68
DRESSING	
Caesar, Salad Station	48
French, Low Fat, Salad Station	18
Olive Oil, & Balsamic Vinegar, Salad Station	134
Thousand Island, Salad Station	45
DRINK	
Mango, Slush	206
FLATBREAD	
BBQ Steak	540
Chicken Delight	443
Shrimply Delicious	433
Tuna Nicoise	513
Virtuous Veg	375

PIZZA HUT	KCAL
FRIES	
Cheesy, Fried, Side	1069
Cheesy, Oven Baked, Side	680
Fried, Side	888
Oven Baked, Side	498
Sweet Potato, Side	772
ICE CREAM	
Chocolate	163
Strawberry	174
Vanilla, Extra	81
ICE CREAM FLOAT	
Cream Soda, Black Cherry	320
Cream Soda	320
Cream Soda	320
KETCHUP	
Pot	99
LASAGNE	
Beef	790
Beef	790
LETTUCE	
Mix, Salad Station	2
MACARONI CHEESE	
Main	824
MAYONNAISE	
Garlic, Salad Station	97
Light, Salad Station	74
MILK SHAKE	
Chocolate, & Orange	680
Chocolate	515
Oreo	804
Salted Caramel	530
Strawberry	482
MUSTARD	
Creamy	261
OIL	
Garlic, & Chilli, Salad Station	166
ONION RINGS	
Fried, Side	520
Oven Baked, Side	338
ONIONS	
Crispy, Salad Station	125
Red, Salad Station	7
PASTA	
BBQ, Salad Station	27
Cheesy, Sweetcorn, Salad Station	37
PEPPERS	
Jalapeno, Poppers, Fried	438
Jalapeno, Poppers, Oven Baked	312
Jalapeno, Salad Station	2
Mixed, Salad Station	3
PIZZA	
BBQ Americano, Cheesy Bites Crust	324
BBQ Americano, Deep Pan, Large	315

PIZZA HUT
PIZZA

BBQ Americano, Deep Pan, Reg	202
BBQ Americano, GF	184
BBQ Americano, Stuffed Crust, Large	324
BBQ Americano, Stuffed Crust, Reg	233
BBQ Americano, Thin Crust, Large	231
BBQ Americano, Thin Crust, Reg	178
BBQ Mac n' Cheese, Stuffed Crust, Large	398
BBQ Mac n' Cheese, Stuffed Crust, Reg	277
Californian King Of the Coast, Cheesy Bites Crust	292
Californian King Of the Coast, Deep Pan, Large	283
Californian King Of the Coast, Deep Pan, Reg	184
Californian King Of the Coast, GF	166
Californian King Of the Coast, Stuffed Crust, Large	292
Californian King Of the Coast, Stuffed Crust, Reg	215
Californian King Of the Coast, Thin Crust, Large	199
Californian King Of the Coast, Thin Crust, Reg	170
Chicken Supreme, Cheesy Bites Crust	295
Chicken Supreme, Deep Pan, Big Sharer	265
Chicken Supreme, Deep Pan, Large	286
Chicken Supreme, Deep Pan, Reg	183
Chicken Supreme, GF	165
Chicken Supreme, Stuffed Crust, Large	295
Chicken Supreme, Stuffed Crust, Reg	214
Chicken Supreme, Thin Crust, Big Sharer	147
Chicken Supreme, Thin Crust, Large	202
Chicken Supreme, Thin Crust, Reg	159
Hawaiian, Cheesy Bites Crust	281
Hawaiian, Deep Pan, Big Sharer	263
Hawaiian, Deep Pan, Large	272
Hawaiian, Deep Pan, Reg	176
Hawaiian, GF	158
Hawaiian, Stuffed Crust, Large	281
Hawaiian, Stuffed Crust, Reg	207
Hawaiian, Thin Crust, Big Sharer	145
Hawaiian, Thin Crust, Large	188
Hawaiian, Thin Crust, Reg	135
Heavenly Veg, Cheesy Bites Crust	313
Heavenly Veg, Deep Pan, Large	304
Heavenly Veg, Deep Pan, Reg	196
Heavenly Veg, GF	177
Heavenly Veg, Stuffed Crust, Large	313
Heavenly Veg, Stuffed Crust, Reg	226
Heavenly Veg, Thin Crust, Large	220
Heavenly Veg, Thin Crust, Reg	171
Mac n' Cheese, Stuffed Crust, Large	399
Mac n' Cheese, Stuffed Crust, Reg	278
Margherita, Cheesy Bites Crust	289
Margherita, Deep Pan, Big Sharer	272
Margherita, Deep Pan, Large	280
Margherita, Deep Pan, Reg	182
Margherita, GF	164
Margherita, Stuffed Crust, Large	289

PIZZA HUT
PIZZA

Margherita, Stuffed Crust, Reg	213
Margherita, Thin Crust, Big Sharer	155
Margherita, Thin Crust, Large	196
Margherita, Thin Crust, Reg	158
Meat Feast, Cheesy Bites Crust	336
Meat Feast, Deep Pan, Big Sharer	303
Meat Feast, Deep Pan, Large	327
Meat Feast, Deep Pan, Reg	203
Meat Feast, GF	196
Meat Feast, Stuffed Crust, Large	336
Meat Feast, Stuffed Crust, Reg	233
Meat Feast, Thin Crust, Big Sharer	185
Meat Feast, Thin Crust, Large	242
Meat Feast, Thin Crust, Reg	178
New Orleans Chicken Sizzler, Cheesy Bites Crust	292
New Orleans Chicken Sizzler, Deep pan, Big Sharer	357
New Orleans Chicken Sizzler, Deep pan, Large	287
New Orleans Chicken Sizzler, Deep Pan, Reg	178
New Orleans Chicken Sizzler, GF	165
New Orleans Chicken Sizzler, Stuffed Crust, Large	292
New Orleans Chicken Sizzler, Stuffed Crust, Reg	206
New Orleans Chicken Sizzler, Thin Crust, Big Sharer	239
New Orleans Chicken Sizzler, Thin Crust, Large	199
New Orleans Chicken Sizzler, Thin Crust, Reg	159
Pepperoni, Cheesy Bites Crust	307
Pepperoni, Deep Pan, Large	298
Pepperoni, Deep Pan, Reg	194
Pepperoni, GF	175
Pepperoni, Stuffed Crust, Large	307
Pepperoni, Stuffed Crust, Reg	224
Pepperoni, Thin Crust, Large	216
Pepperoni, Thin Crust, Reg	169
Philly Cheese Steak, Cheesy Bites Crust	370
Philly Cheese Steak, Deep Pan, Large	365
Philly Cheese Steak, Deep Pan, Reg	241
Philly Cheese Steak, GF	223
Philly Cheese Steak, Stuffed Crust, Large	373
Philly Cheese Steak, Stuffed Crust, Reg	271
Philly Cheese Steak, Thin Crust, Large	280
Philly Cheese Steak, Thin Crust, Reg	217
Supreme, Cheesy Bites Crust	331
Supreme, Deep Pan, Large	322
Supreme, Deep Pan, Reg	205
Supreme, GF	188
Supreme, Stuffed Crust, Large	331
Supreme, Stuffed Crust, Reg	236
Supreme, Thin Crust, Large	238
Supreme, Thin Crust, Reg	181
Texas Meat Meltdown, Cheesy Bites Crust	358
Texas Meat Meltdown, Deep Pan, Large	349
Texas Meat Meltdown, Deep Pan, Reg	229
Texas Meat Meltdown, GF	173

PIZZA HUT

PIZZA

	KCAL
Texas Meat Meltdown, Stuffed Crust, Large	358
Texas Meat Meltdown, Stuffed Crust, Reg	256
Texas Meat Meltdown, Thin Crust, Large	264
Texas Meat Meltdown, Thin Crust, Reg	201
Triple Pepperoni, Deep Pan, Big Sharer	339
Triple Pepperoni, Thin Crust, Big Sharer	224
Veggie, Cheesy Bites Crust	276
Veggie, Deep Pan, Big Sharer	273
Veggie, Deep Pan, Large	267
Veggie, Deep Pan, Reg	171
Veggie, GF	152
Veggie, Stuffed Crust, Large	276
Veggie, Stuffed Crust, Reg	201
Veggie, Thin Crust, Big Sharer	155
Veggie, Thin Crust, Large	183
Veggie, Thin Crust, Reg	146

POTATO SALAD

Salad Station	27

RIBS

BBQ	562
Rack, Meal, Fried	1473
Rack, Meal, Oven Baked	1182

SALSA

Salad Station	14

SAUCE

BBQ	119
Chocolate, Extra	71
Hot & Spicy	65
Hut House Seasoning	322
Mayonnaise, Garlic	243
Mayonnaise, Light	186
Salted Caramel, Extra	70
Sweet Chilli	175

SHRIMP

Popcorn	305

SORBET

Mango	179

SULTANAS

Salad Station	55

SWEETCORN

Salad Station	15

TOMATOES

Cherry, Salad Station	3

TORTILLA CHIPS

Salad Station	96

WAFFLES

Chocolate	685

PRET A MANGER

APPLES

	KCAL
Chopped	86
Juice, Sparkling, Pure Pret	139
Spiced, Infusion	45

BAGUETTE

Artichoke, Olives, & Tapenade, Vegan	454
Avocado, Olives, & Tomato, with Rocket	531
Bacon, Posh, Airports Only	518
Bahn Mi, Crunchy, Veggie	418
Beetroot, Smashed, Pistachios, & Feta	531
Brie, Tomato, & Basil, White	432
Brie & Cranberry	579
Butternut Squash, Wensleydale, & Cranberry	542
Cheese, Prosciutto, Tomatoes, Mayo, & Basil, White	531
Cheese, Cheddar, & Pickle, Cheddar, Posh, White	620
Chicken, & Bacon, Caesar, White	598
Egg Mayo, & Bacon, Breakfast	337
Egg Mayo, & Roasted Tomatoes, Breakfast	309
Egg Mayo, Asparagus, Watercress, & Parmesan	528
Ham, & Greve Cheese, Mustard Mayo, White	588
Ham, & Egg, Mustard Mayo, Classic, White	560
Ham, & Pickles, Jambon Beurre, White	355
Ham Hock, Stuffing, & Apple	597
Italian Veggie	539
Mozzarella, Chipotle, Hot	468
Salmon, & Soft Cheese, Smoked, White	454
Salmon, Smoked, & Free Range Egg, Breakfast	325
Tuna, Nicoise	531
Tuna Mayo, & Cucumber, Pole & Line Caught, White	540

BANANA

Fresh	62

BARS

Chocolate Brownie	305
Dairy Free Chocolatey Coconut Bite	205
Love Bar	329
Orange, Cardamom, Milk Chocolate	134
Pret Bar	266
Raw, Fruit, Seed	202

BEANS

Baked, with Avocado, Power Pot	251

BEEF

Short Rib, Korean, in Brioche Roll	527

BERRIES

Wild, Infusion	25

BITES

Almond Butter	142

BREAD

Baguette, Losange, for Soup	177
Baguette, Stone Baked, Mini	204

BREAKFAST

Acai, & Almond Butter, Bowl	380
Bacon Brioche	420
Bacon & Egg Brioche	490

PRET A MANGER

BREAKFAST

Egg Mayo, & Avocado	344
Ham & Egg Brioche	412
Poached Egg, Sausage & Beans, Power Pot	327
Sausage & Egg Brioche	546
Veggie Brioche	346

BREAKFAST CEREAL

Bircher, Dairy Free, Bowl	252
Bircher Muesli Bowl	308
Honey & Granola Pret Pot	281
Porridge, Coconut	198
Porridge, No Topping	242

BROWNIES

Chocolate, Salted Caramel Vegan	223

CAKE

Banana, Slice	224
Carrot, Slice	321
Choc Bar	355
Chocolate, Triple, Pioneer	598
Fruit Teacake, Pioneer	279
Lemon Drizzle, Slice, Pioneer	698
Mince Pie	315
Pecan Slice	436
Pistachio, & Mandarin	507
Sticky Toffee, & Pecan	558
Tiffin, Christmas	410
Victoria Sponge, Pioneer	641
Victoria Sponge, Pret a Manger*	503

CHEESECAKE

Lemon, Pot	406

CHOCOLATE

Dark with Sea Salt	136

CLEMENTINES

Fresh	63

COCONUT

Chips, Roasted	105
Water, Pret Pure	66

COFFEE

Americano, Black	1
Americano, White, Iced	36
Americano White, Semi Skimmed Milk	14
Cappuccino	92
Cappuccino, Soya	92
Cappucino, Oat Milk	96
Espresso	0
Filter Coffee	0
Filter Coffee, Semi Skimmed Milk	14
Flat White, Almond Milk	56
Flat White, Coconut	102
Flat White, Festive	135
Flat White, Oat Milk	81
Flat White	80
Flat White, Pumpkin Spiced	104

PRET A MANGER

COFFEE

Flat White, Soya	77
Frappe, Chocolate	439
Frappe, Classic	251
Latte, Coconut	150
Latte, Love Bar	145
Latte, Oat Milk	132
Latte, Skimmed Milk	118
Latte, Soya, Iced	114
Latte, Soya	113
Macchiato	5
Mocha, Coconut	216
Mocha, Mint	220
Mocha, Oat Milk	186
Mocha, Semi Skimmed Milk	185
Mocha, Soya	181

COOKIES

Chocolate Chunk	327
Chocolate Praline, Melt in the Middle	319
Double Chocolate Orange	389
Fruit, Oat & Spelt	339

CORN CAKES

Chocolate Covered	80

CRANBERRIES

in Coats, Yoghurt Coating	241

CRISPS

Croxton Manor Cheese & Red Onion	210
Kale	67
Maldon Sea Salt	203
Sea Salt & Organic Cider Vinegar Crisps	196
Smokey Chipotle	203

CROISSANT

Almond	366
Chocolate & Hazelnut	379
French, Butter	304
Ham, Cheese, Tomato & Bacon	298
Mozzarella & Tomato	329

DANISH PASTRY

Cinnamon	398

DHAL

Cauliflower, & Sweet Potato, Hot Pot	429

DRESSING

Dijon, Small	144
Green, Zingy	85
Teriyaki	36
Yoghurt, Lemon, & Mayo, Large	138

DRIED FRUIT & NUTS

Mango & Seeds	122

DRINK

Cucumber Seltzer	56

FLATBREAD

Artichokes, Olive Tapenade, Rocket, & Basil	422
Chicken, Lebanese	496

PRET A MANGER

FLATBREAD
Chicken, Pesto, & Rocket	486
Falafel	529
Greek, Green	402
Mediterranean Tuna	533
Mexican Avocado	508
Plain	211
Squash, with Feta & Mint	337
Super-Veg Rainbow	353
Sweet Potato Falafel, Coconut, & Cashew	455

FRUIT
British Berries	5
Five Berry Bowl	364
Five Berry Pot	158
Fruit Salad, Pret's	112
Mango & Lime	91
Seedless Grapes	109
Superfruit Salad, Pot, Pret a Manger*	107

FRUIT & NUT
Mix	175
Mix, with Chocolate Covered Raisins	177

FRUIT COMPOTE
Topping, Breakfast	26

GINGER BEER
Pure Pret	139

GINGERBREAD
Godfrey, Pret's Gingerbread Man	201
Melvin the Melting Snowman	257

HONEY
Breakfast Topping	107

HOT CHOCOLATE
Coconut	288
Oat Milk	256
Original	256
Soya	251

HOT POT
Chicken, & Butternut Squash	427

JUICE
Apple	125
Blood Orange	132
Carrot	50
Clementine	110
Daily Greens	92
Ginger & Apple, Shot	55
Green Goodness	176
Hot Shot	47
Orange, Lge	168
Pomegranate, & Hibiscus, Still, Pure Pret	108

JUICE DRINK
Beet Beautiful	188
Cranberry & Raspberry, Still	159
Ginseng & Echinacea, Sparking, Yoga Bunny	135
Grape & Elderflower, Sparkling, Pure Pret	129

PRET A MANGER

JUICE DRINK
Mandarin & Lychee, Pure, Still	106
Mango & Passion Fruit, Still	209
Melon, & Basil	171
Orange, & Passion Fruit, Still	133
Super Greens	269

KOMBUCHA
Lemon, & Ginger, Organic	37

LEMON
& Ginger, Infusion	15

LEMONADE
& Ginger, Still	160
Sparkling	109
Stll, Lemon & Ginger, Pure	153

MACARONI CHEESE
& Greens, Vegan	558
Beef, Short Rib, & Cauliflower	709
Ham Hock & Sprout	631
Kale & Cauli	553
Lasagne	572
Prosciutto	590

MANGO
Fresh	116

MILK
Babyccino, with Chocolate Sprinkles	14
British Organic, Kids	94
Coconut	150
Oat	118

MOUSSE
Chocolate	453

MUFFIN
Breakfast	431
Double Berry	442
Prets Christmas	466

NUTS
Naked	259

OMELETTE
Egg White	167
Ham, & Spinach	382
Mushroom, Tomato, & Cheddar	435

PAIN AU RAISIN
Pain au Raisin	361

POPCORN
Bar	176
Rock Salt, Light	143
Sweet & Salt, Light	163

PRETZELS
Plain	304

SADA SEV
Smashed Beetroot, & Feta, Pot	176

SALAD
Asian Greens, Veggie Pot	170
Avocado, Super-Greens, Pot	171

PRET A MANGER

SALAD

Cauliflower, & Turmeric, Super-Veg	306
Chicken, Italian, Chef's	345
Chicken, Pesto, & Mozzarella, Buffalo	365
Crayfish, & Avocado, No Bread	379
Egg, & Avocado, Protein Pot	224
Egg, & Spinach, Protein Pot	104
Egg, Poached, & Avocado, Protein Pot	197
Falafel, Mezze	359
Greens, Grains & Chicken	258
Rainbow Veggie, Pot	186
Roast Beets, Squash, & Feta, Box	421
Super Beans, Brocolli, & Turmeric Cauli, no Dressing	209
Sweet Potato Falafel & Smashed Beets, Box	334
Teriyaki Salmon Sushi, without Dressing	316
Tuna, Nicoise	471
Tuna, Nicoise, without Dressing	176

SALMON

Sesame, & Black Rice	369

SANDWICH

Aubergine, & Halloumi, Brioche	492
Cheese, Kids	422
Chicken, & Cucumber, Granary Bread	390
Chicken Avocado	485
Chickpeas, Curried, & Mango Chutney	476
Chipotle Pulled Chicken, Brioche	398
Christmas Lunch	482
Christmas Lunch, Veggie	531
Classic Super Club	528
Crayfish, & Avocado	383
Egg Mayo, Coronation	520
Free Range Egg Mayo	367
Cracking Egg Salad	375
Falafel, Halloumi, & Pickles, Brioche	520
Falafel & Red Tapenade	540
Ham, & Cheese	547
Ham, Kids	300
Mature Cheddar & Pret Pickle	520
New Yorker, on Rye, Veggie	582
Scottish Smoked Salmon	421
Super Greens & Reds	449
Tuna, & Cucumber	448
Very Merry Christmas Lunch	525

SEEDS

Tamari Pumpkin	186

SHORTBREAD

Plain	396

SMOOTHIE

Acai Super Berry	255
Almond, Protein Power	450
Berry Blast	239
Blueberry, Protein Power	425
Coconut Crush	168

PRET A MANGER

SMOOTHIE

Green, Breakfast Bowl	311
Mango Smoothie	145
Rhubarb	185
Strawberry Smoothie	211
Vitamin Volcano Smoothie	163

SOUP

Bean, Tuscan	148
Bean, Tuscan, Side	86
Broth, Dried Chilli, Extra	1
Butternut Squash, Spiced	240
Carrot, & Coriander, Lightly Spiced	181
Chicken, & Chorizo, Smoky	234
Chicken, & Vegetable, Red Thai	235
Chicken, Broccoli & Brown Rice	137
Chicken, Cream of, No Cream	141
Chicken, Curry, Coconut	222
Chicken, Edamame, & Ginger	226
Chilli, Vegan, Soup Of The Day	216
Kale, Lentil, & Roasted Spices	217
Miso, Veggie	44
Pea, & Mint	189
Pork, & Lentil, Ragu	218
Tomato, Souper	198
Vegetable, Tagine	187

SYRUP

Shot, Caramel	49
Shot, Hazelnut	47
Shot, Love Bar	46
Shot, Mince Pie	50
Shot, Mint	63
Shot, Pumpkin Spice	49
Shot, Vanilla	49

TART

Pret's Bakewell Tart	410

TEA

Black, Iced	0
Black, Iced, with Strawberry, Cucumber, & Mint	55
Ceylon, Breakfast	14
Chamomile	0
Earl Grey, Black	14
Fennel, & Mint	0
Green, & Peach	88
Green, Iced	0
Green, Iced, with Blood Orange, & Pomegranate	50
Green, White Matcha, Oolong	0
Latte, Chai, Iced	180
Latte, Chai	182
Latte, Golden Turmeric	111
Latte, Matcha	108
Peppermint	0
Rooibos Cacao	0
Tropical Green Tea	0

	KCAL
PRET A MANGER	
TEA	
Turmeric Tonic	0
TOASTIE	
Brie, Avocado & Tomato	562
Chicken, Basil, & Red Pepper	564
Egg, Cheddar, & Tomato	595
Egg Florentine	575
Halloumi & Red Pepper	556
Ham, Cheese & Mustard	570
Tuna Melt Toastie	552
TORTILLA	
Avocado, Beans, Toasted	435
Avocado, Cheddar, & Chipotle, Toasted	578
Banana, Blueberry, & Almond Butter	387
Chicken, Chipotle, Toasted	497
Egg, Bacon, & Avocado, Toasted	555
Eggs Florentine, Toasted	527
Mushroom, Florentine, Toasted	432
VEG POT	
Courgetti, Veggie	132
WATER	
Spring, Sparkling	0
WRAP	
Avocado, & Chipotle Chickpeas, Salad	444
Avocado, & Herb Salad	514
Butternut, & Pistachio, Spicy	313
Chakalaka, Beans, & Vegetables	340
Chana Chaat, Mint, & Mango Chutney	453
Chicken, Spicy, Hot	496
Falafel, & Halloumi, Hot	659
Hoisin Duck Wrap	457
Houmous, & Crunchy Vegetables, Vegan	386
Miso, Aubergine, & Edamame	365
Nicoise Salad, Veggie	500
Ragu, & Red Pepper, Vegan, Hot	421
Summer Salad	339
Swedish Meatball, Hot	666
YOGHURT	
Coconut, Mango Chia Pot	190
Dark Chocolate, & Toasted Coconut, Pot	362
Mango, Chia, Pot	137
YOGHURT - DAIRY FREE	
Chocolate, Coconut, Chia, Blueberries, Pomegranate	162

	KCAL
STARBUCKS	
BAGEL	
Beef, Salt, New York	490
BARS	
Fruit & Nut, Cranberry, Pumpkin seed & Blueberry	235
BREAKFAST CEREAL	
Berry Good Bircher	253
BROWNIES	
Burnt Caramel	370
CAKE	
Carrot, Loaf	323
White Chocolate, & Raspberry, Bundt	292
COFFEE - AMERICANO	
Grande	17
Short	6
Tall	11
Venti	23
COFFEE - AMERICANO, ICED	
Grande	17
Tall	11
Venti	23
COFFEE - CAPPUCCINO	
Almond Milk, Grande	74
Almond Milk, Short	35
Almond Milk, Tall	67
Almond Milk, Venti	104
Coconut Milk, Grande	120
Coconut Milk, Short	57
Coconut Milk, Tall	108
Coconut Milk, Venti	168
Oat Milk, Grande	213
Oat Milk, Short	100
Oat Milk, Tall	191
Oat Milk, Venti	297
Semi Skimmed Milk, Grande	143
Semi Skimmed Milk, Short	68
Semi Skimmed Milk, Tall	129
Semi Skimmed Milk, Venti	201
Skimmed Milk, Grande	103
Skimmed Milk, Short	49
Skimmed Milk, Tall	93
Skimmed Milk, Venti	144
Soy, Grande	119
Soy, Short	56
Soy, Tall	107
Soy, Venti	167
Whole Milk, Grande	181
Whole Milk, Short	85
Whole Milk, Tall	163
Whole Milk, Venti	253
COFFEE - CAPPUCCINO, ICED	
Almond Milk, Grande	70
Almond Milk, Tall	58
Almond Milk, Venti	83

STARBUCKS

COFFEE - CAPPUCCINO, ICED

Coconut Milk, Grande	113
Coconut Milk, Tall	92
Coconut Milk, Venti	131
Oat Milk, Grande	201
Oat Milk, Tall	162
Oat Milk, Venti	230
Semi Skimmed Milk, Grande	136
Semi Skimmed Milk, Tall	110
Semi Skimmed Milk, Venti	156
Skimmed Milk, Grande	97
Skimmed Milk, Tall	80
Skimmed Milk, Venti	113
Soy, Grande	113
Soy, Tall	92
Soy, Venti	131
Whole Milk, Grande	171
Whole Milk, Tall	138
Whole Milk, Venti	196

COFFEE - COLD BREW

Skimmed Milk, Solo	6
Festive Grande	33
Festive Tall	25
Festive Venti	41

COFFEE - CORTADO

Almond Milk	27
Coconut Milk	41
Oat Milk	84
Semi Skimmed Milk	47
Skimmed Milk	36
Soy	40
Whole Milk	60

COFFEE - ESPRESSO

Con Panna, Doppio	36
Con Panna, Solo	31
Doppio	48
Solo	6
Oat Milk, Doppio	23
Oat Milk, Solo	9

COFFEE - ESPRESSO, MACCHIATO

Almond Milk, Doppio	10
Almond Milk, Solo	6
Coconut Milk, Doppio	11
Coconut Milk, Solo	6
Semi Skimmed Milk, Doppio	11
Semi Skimmed Milk, Solo	7
Skimmed Milk, Doppio	11
Soy, Doppio	11
Soy, Solo	6
Whole Milk, Doppio	12
Whole Milk, Solo	7

STARBUCKS

COFFEE - FILTER

Grande	5
Short	3
Tall	4
Venti	6

COFFEE - FLAT WHITE

Skimmed Milk, Short	60
Whole Milk, Short	119

COFFEE - LATTE

Almond Milk, Grande	100
Almond Milk, Short	50
Almond Milk, Tall	74
Almond Milk, Venti	126
Coconut Milk, Venti	204
Coconut Milk, Grande	163
Coconut Milk, Short	81
Coconut Milk, Tall	121
Oat Milk, Grande	269
Oat Milk, Short	127
Oat Milk, Tall	212
Oat Milk, Venti	350
Semi Skimmed Milk, Grande	188
Semi Skimmed Milk, Short	95
Semi Skimmed Milk, Tall	143
Semi Skimmed Milk, Venti	248
Skimmed Milk, Grande	131
Skimmed Milk, Short	67
Skimmed Milk, Tall	102
Skimmed Milk, Venti	174
Soy, Grande	148
Soy, Short	75
Soy, Tall	110
Soy, Venti	185
Whole Milk, Grande	223
Whole Milk, Short	113
Whole Milk, Tall	172
Whole Milk, Venti	299
Eggnog, Grande	344
Eggnog, Short	169
Eggnog, Tall	271
Gingerbread, Almond Milk, Grande	254
Gingerbread, Almond Milk, Short	144
Gingerbread, Almond Milk, Tall	198
Gingerbread, Coconut Milk, Grande	313
Gingerbread, Coconut Milk, Short	171
Gingerbread, Coconut Milk, Tall	238
Gingerbread, Semi Skimmed Milk, Grande	343
Gingerbread, Semi Skimmed Milk, Short	185
Gingerbread, Semi Skimmed Milk, Tall	258
Gingerbread, Skimmed Milk, Grande	291
Gingerbread, Skimmed Milk, Short	161
Gingerbread, Skimmed Milk, Tall	223
Gingerbread, Soy, Grande	312

STARBUCKS

COFFEE - LATTE

Gingerbread, Soy, Short	171
Gingerbread, Soy, Tall	237
Gingerbread, Whole Milk, Grande	392
Gingerbread, Whole Milk, Short	208
Gingerbread, Whole Milk, Tall	291
Toffee Nut, Almond Milk, Grande	260
Toffee Nut, Almond Milk, Short	150
Toffee Nut, Almond Milk, Tall	203
Toffee Nut, Coconut Milk, Grande	318
Toffee Nut, Coconut Milk, Short	177
Toffee Nut, Coconut Milk, Tall	243
Toffee Nut, Semi Skimmed Milk, Grande	348
Toffee Nut, Semi Skimmed Milk, Short	191
Toffee Nut, Semi Skimmed Milk, Tall	264
Toffee Nut, Skimmed Milk, Grande	296
Toffee Nut, Skimmed Milk, Short	166
Toffee Nut, Skimmed Milk, Tall	228
Toffee Nut, Soy, Grande	317
Toffee Nut, Soy, Short	176
Toffee Nut, Soy, Tall	242
Toffee Nut, Whole Milk, Grande	397
Toffee Nut, Whole Milk, Short	213
Toffee Nut, Whole Milk, Tall	297

COFFEE - LATTE, ICED

Almond Milk, Grande	73
Almond Milk, Tall	57
Almond Milk, Venti	90
Coconut Milk, Grande	78
Coconut Milk, Tall	65
Coconut Milk, Venti	102
Oat Milk, Grande	185
Oat Milk, Tall	149
Oat Milk, Venti	214
Semi Skimmed Milk, Grande	87
Semi Skimmed Milk, Tall	77
Semi Skimmed Milk, Venti	126
Skimmed Milk, Grande	63
Skimmed Milk, Tall	56
Skimmed Milk, Venti	90
Soy, Tall	64
Soy, Venti	104
ISoy, Grande	71
Whole Milk, Grande	104
Whole Milk, Tall	100
Whole Milk, Venti	149

COFFEE - LATTE, TURMERIC

Oat Milk, Grande	347
Oat Milk, Short	164
Oat Milk, Tall	244
Oat Milk, Venti	441

STARBUCKS

COFFEE - MACCHIATO

Caramel, Almond Milk, Grande	172
Caramel, Almond Milk, Short	86
Caramel, Almond Milk, Tall	123
Caramel, Soy, Grande	207
Caramel, Soy, Short	104
Caramel, Whole Milk, Short	137

COFFEE - MACCHIATO, CARAMEL

Oat Milk, Grande	308
Oat Milk, Short	145
Oat Milk, Tall	243
Oat Milk, Venti	377

COFFEE - MACCHIATO, CARAMEL, ICED

Almond Milk, Grande	162
Almond Milk, Tall	121
Almond Milk, Venti	188
Skimmed Milk, Tall	142

COFFEE - MACCHIATO, ICED

Caramel, Oat Milk, Grande	259
Caramel, Oat Milk, Tall	205
Caramel, Oat Milk, Venti	307

COFFEE - MACHIATO, CARAMEL

Almond Milk, Venti	211
Coconut Milk, Grande	250
Coconut Milk, Short	124
Coconut Milk, Tall	183
Coconut Milk, Venti	308
Semi Skimmed Milk, Grande	240
Semi Skimmed Milk, Short	122
Semi Skimmed Milk, Tall	209
Semi Skimmed Milk, Venti	329
Skimmed Milk, Grande	193
Skimmed Milk, Short	97
Skimmed Milk, Tall	165
Skimmed Milk, Venti	261
Soy, Tall	167
Soy, Venti	280
Whole Milk, Grande	269
Whole Milk, Tall	240
Whole Milk, Venti	376

COFFEE - MACHIATO, CARAMEL, ICED

Coconut Milk, Grande	207
Coconut Milk, Tall	154
Coconut Milk, Venti	236
Semi Skimmed Milk, Grande	230
Semi Skimmed Milk, Tall	171
Semi Skimmed Milk, Venti	261
Skimmed Milk, Venti	219
Soy, Grande	205
Soy, Tall	153
Soy, Venti	235
Whole Milk, Grande	271
Whole Milk, Tall	202

STARBUCKS

COFFEE - MACHIATO, CARAMEL, ICED

Whole Milk, Venti	306
Skimmed Milk, Grande	191

COFFEE - MISTO

Almond Milk, Grande	59
Almond Milk, Short	30
Almond Milk, Tall	45
Almond Milk, Venti	75
Coconut Milk, Grande	95
Coconut Milk, Short	48
Coconut Milk, Tall	73
Coconut Milk, Venti	120
Oat Milk, Grande	149
Oat Milk, Short	76
Oat Milk, Tall	102
Oat Milk, Venti	200
Semi Skimmed Milk, Grande	106
Semi Skimmed Milk, Short	54
Semi Skimmed Milk, Tall	81
Semi Skimmed Milk, Venti	134
Skimmed Milk, Grande	73
Skimmed Milk, Short	37
Skimmed Milk, Tall	56
Skimmed Milk, Venti	92
Soy, Grande	82
Soy, Short	42
Soy, Tall	63
Soy, Venti	104
Whole Milk, Grande	126
Whole Milk, Short	65
Whole Milk, Tall	97
Whole Milk, Venti	160

COFFEE - MOCHA

& Whip Cream, Coconut Milk, Tall	298
& Whipped Cream, Almond Milk, Grande	317
& Whipped Cream, Almond Milk, Short	180
& Whipped Cream, Almond Milk, Tall	253
& Whipped Cream, Coconut Milk, Grande	374
& Whipped Cream, Coconut Milk, Short	208
& Whipped Cream, Oat Milk, Grande	346
& Whipped Cream, Oat Milk, Short	176
& Whipped Cream, Oat Milk, Tall	265
& Whipped Cream, Oat Milk, Venti	395
& Whipped Cream, Semi Skimmed Milk, Grande	403
& Whipped Cream, Semi Skimmed Milk, Short	222
& Whipped Cream, Semi Skimmed Milk, Tall	321
& Whipped Cream, Skimmed Milk, Grande	353
& Whipped Cream, Skimmed Milk, Short	198
& Whipped Cream, Skimmed Milk, Tall	282
& Whipped Cream, Soy, Grande	371
& Whipped Cream, Soy, Short	207
& Whipped Cream, Soy, Tall	297
& Whipped Cream, Whole Milk, Grande	456

STARBUCKS

COFFEE - MOCHA

& Whipped Cream, Whole Milk, Short	249
& Whipped Cream, Whole Milk, Tall	363

COFFEE - MOCHA, ICED

& Whipped Cream, Almond Milk, Grande	313
& Whipped Cream, Almond Milk, Tall	230
& Whipped Cream, Almond Milk, Venti	351
& Whipped Cream, Coconut Milk, Grande	341
& Whipped Cream, Coconut Milk, Tall	253
& Whipped Cream, Coconut Milk, Venti	382
& Whipped Cream, Oat Milk, Grande	398
& Whipped Cream, Oat Milk, Tall	306
& Whipped Cream, Oat Milk, Venti	447
& Whipped Cream, Semi Skimmed Milk, Grande	355
& Whipped Cream, Semi Skimmed Milk, Tall	265
& Whipped Cream, Semi Skimmed Milk, Venti	398
& Whipped Cream, Skimmed Milk, Grande	331
& Whipped Cream, Skimmed Milk, Tall	245
& Whipped Cream, Skimmed Milk, Venti	371
& Whipped Cream, Soy, Grande	340
& Whipped Cream, Soy, Tall	252
& Whipped Cream, Soy, Venti	381
& Whipped Cream, Whole Milk, Grande	381
& Whipped Cream, Whole Milk, Tall	286
& Whipped Cream, Whole Milk, Venti	426

COFFEE - MOCHA, WHITE CHOC

Whipped Cream, Almond Milk, Grande	371
Whipped Cream, Almond Milk, Short	203
Whipped Cream, Almond Milk, Tall	288
Whipped Cream, Coconut Milk, Grande	425
Whipped Cream, Coconut Milk, Short	230
Whipped Cream, Coconut Milk, Tall	326
Whipped Cream, Oat Milk, Grande	466
Whipped Cream, Oat Milk, Short	235
Whipped Cream, Oat Milk, Tall	369
Whipped Cream, Semi Skim Milk, Grande	453
Whipped Cream, Semi Skimmed Milk, Short	244
Whipped Cream, Semi Skimmed Milk, Tall	346
Whipped Cream, Skimmed Milk, Grande	406
Whipped Cream, Skimmed Milk, Short	221
Whipped Cream, Skimmed Milk, Tall	313
Whipped Cream, Soy, Grande	423
Whipped Cream, Soy, Short	229
Whipped Cream, Soy, Tall	325
Whipped Cream, Whole Milk, Grande	503
Whipped Cream, Whole Milk, Short	269
Whipped Cream, Whole Milk, Tall	383

FRAPPUCCINO - CARAMEL

with Whipped Cream, Almond Milk, Grande	380
with Whipped Cream, Almond Milk, Mini	218
with Whipped Cream, Almond Milk, Tall	274
with Whipped Cream, Coconut Milk, Grande	373
with Whipped Cream, Coconut Milk, Mini	251

STARBUCKS
FRAPPUCCINO - CARAMEL

	KCAL
with Whipped Cream, Coconut Milk, Tall	278
with Whipped Cream, Oat Milk, Grande	410
with Whipped Cream, Oat Milk, Mini	217
with Whipped Cream, Oat Milk, Tall	303
with Whipped Cream, Semi Skimmed Milk, Grande	374
with Whipped Cream, Semi Skimmed Milk, Mini	256
with Whipped Cream, Semi Skimmed Milk, Tall	275
with Whipped Cream, Skimmed Milk, Grande	358
with Whipped Cream, Skimmed Milk, Mini	247
with Whipped Cream, Skimmed Milk, Tall	262
with Whipped Cream, Soy, Grande	364
with Whipped Cream, Soy, Tall	267
with Whipped Cream, Soy Milk, Mini	250
with Whipped Cream, Whole Milk, Grande	379
with Whipped Cream, Whole Milk, Mini	266
with Whipped Cream, Whole Milk, Tall	280

FRAPPUCCINO - CARAMEL CREAM

	KCAL
with Whipped Cream, Almond Milk, Grande	300
with Whipped Cream, Almond Milk, Mini	164
with Whipped Cream, Almond Milk, Tall	224
with Whipped Cream, Coconut Milk, Grande	321
with Whipped Cream, Coconut Milk, Mini	175
with Whipped Cream, Coconut Milk, Tall	242
with Whipped Cream, Oat Milk, Grande	374
with Whipped Cream, Oat Milk, Mini	203
with Whipped Cream, Oat Milk, Tall	283
with Whipped Cream, Semi Skimmed Milk, Grande	332
with Whipped Cream, Semi Skimmed Milk, Mini	181
with Whipped Cream, Semi Skimmed Milk, Tall	251
with Whipped Cream, Skimmed Milk, Grande	314
with Whipped Cream, Skimmed Milk, Mini	171
with Whipped Cream, Skimmed Milk, Tall	236
with Whipped Cream, Soy, Grande	320
with Whipped Cream, Soy, Tall	241
with Whipped Cream, Soy Milk, Mini	175
with Whipped Cream, Whole Milk, Grande	353
with Whipped Cream, Whole Milk, Mini	192
with Whipped Cream, Whole Milk, Tall	267

FRAPPUCCINO - CARAMEL LIGHT

	KCAL
No Whip, Skimmed Milk, Grande	134
No Whip, Skimmed Milk, Mini	59
No Whip, Skimmed Milk, Tall	96

FRAPPUCCINO - CHAI TEA

	KCAL
with Whipped Cream, Almond Milk, Grande	293
with Whipped Cream, Almond Milk, Mini	156
with Whipped Cream, Almond Milk, Tall	211
with Whipped Cream, Coconut Milk, Grande	313
with Whipped Cream, Coconut Milk, Mini	167
with Whipped Cream, Coconut Milk, Tall	228
with Whipped Cream, Oat Milk, Grande	365
with Whipped Cream, Oat Milk, Mini	195
with Whipped Cream, Oat Milk, Tall	268

STARBUCKS
FRAPPUCCINO - CHAI TEA

	KCAL
with Whipped Cream, Semi Skimmed Milk, Grande	324
with Whipped Cream, Semi Skimmed Milk, Mini	173
with Whipped Cream, Semi Skimmed Milk, Tall	236
with Whipped Cream, Skimmed Milk, Grande	306
with Whipped Cream, Skimmed Milk, Mini	163
with Whipped Cream, Skimmed Milk, Tall	222
with Whipped Cream, Soy, Grande	313
with Whipped Cream, Soy, Mini	167
with Whipped Cream, Soy, Tall	227
with Whipped Cream, Whole Milk, Grande	343
with Whipped Cream, Whole Milk, Mini	184
with Whipped Cream, Whole Milk, Tall	252

FRAPPUCCINO - CHOCOLATE CREAM

	KCAL
with Whipped Cream, Almond Milk, Grande	317
with Whipped Cream, Almond Milk, Mini	165
with Whipped Cream, Almond Milk, Tall	226
with Whipped Cream, Coconut Milk, Grande	325
with Whipped Cream, Coconut Milk, Mini	177
with Whipped Cream, Coconut Milk, Tall	235
with Whipped Cream, Oat Milk, Grande	399
with Whipped Cream, Oat Milk, Mini	265
with Whipped Cream, Oat Milk, Tall	283
with Whipped Cream, Semi Skimmed Milk, Grande	336
with Whipped Cream, Semi Skimmed Milk, Mini	183
with Whipped Cream, Semi Skimmed Milk, Tall	243
with Whipped Cream, Skimmed Milk, Grande	317
with Whipped Cream, Skimmed Milk, Mini	173
with Whipped Cream, Skimmed Milk, Tall	229
with Whipped Cream, Soy, Grande	324
with Whipped Cream, Soy, Mini	176
with Whipped Cream, Soy, Tall	234
with Whipped Cream, Whole Milk, Grande	339
with Whipped Cream, Whole Milk, Mini	193
with Whipped Cream, Whole Milk, Tall	247

FRAPPUCCINO - COFFEE

	KCAL
No Whip, Almond Milk, Grande	191
No Whip, Almond Milk, Mini	111
No Whip, Almond Milk, Tall	137
No Whipped Cream, Coconut Milk, Grande	207
No Whip, Coconut Milk, Mini	122
No Whipped Cream, Coconut Milk, Tall	151
No Whip, Oat Milk, Grande	256
No Whip, Oat Milk, Mini	123
No Whip, Oat Milk, Tall	190
No Whipped Cream, Semi Skimmed Milk, Grande	215
No Whip, Semi Skimmed Milk, Mini	127
No Whipped Cream, Semi Skimmed Milk, Tall	157
No Whipped Cream, Skimmed Milk, Grande	201
No Whip, Skimmed Milk, Mini	118
No Whipped, Skimmed Milk, Tall	146
No Whipped Cream, Soy, Grande	206
No Whip, Soy, Mini	121

STARBUCKS

FRAPPUCCINO - COFFEE

No Whipped Cream, Soy, Tall	150
No Whipped Cream, Whole Milk, Grande	230
No Whip, Whole Milk, Mini	137
No Whipped Cream, Whole Milk, Tall	170
Light, No Whipped Cream, Skimmed Milk, Grande	118
Light, No Whip, Skimmed Milk, Mini	59
Light, No Whipped Cream, Skimmed Milk, Tall	83

FRAPPUCCINO - DOUBLE CHOC CHIP CREAM

with Whipped Cream, Almond Milk, Grande	380
with Whipped Cream, Almond Milk, Mini	225
with Whipped Cream, Almond Milk, Tall	273
with Whipped Cream, Coconut Milk, Grande	391
with Whipped Cream, Coconut Milk, Mini	231
with Whipped Cream, Coconut Milk, Tall	288
with Whipped Cream, Oat Milk, Grande	434
with Whipped Cream, Oat Milk, Mini	222
with Whipped Cream, Oat Milk, Tall	318
with Whipped Cream, Semi Skimmed Milk, Grande	402
with Whipped Cream, Semi Skimmed Milk, Mini	238
with Whipped Cream, Semi Skimmed Milk, Tall	297
with Whipped Cream, Skimmed Milk, Grande	383
with Whipped Cream, Skimmed Milk, Mini	220
with Whipped Cream, Skimmed Milk, Tall	280
with Whipped Cream, Soy, Grande	390
with Whipped Cream, Soy, Mini	230
with Whipped Cream, Soy, Tall	287
with Whipped Cream, Whole Milk, Grande	421
with Whipped Cream, Whole Milk, Mini	250
with Whipped Cream, Whole Milk, Tall	313

FRAPPUCCINO - ESPRESSO

No Whip, Almond Milk, Grande	175
No Whip, Almond Milk, Mini	91
No Whip, Almond Milk, Tall	116
No Whipped Cream, Coconut Milk, Grande	186
No Whip, Coconut Milk, Mini	100
No Whipped Cream, Coconut Milk, Tall	124
No Whip, Oat Milk, Grande	246
No Whip, Oat Milk, Mini	126
No Whip, Oat Milk, Tall	174
No Whipped Cream, Semi Skimmed Milk, Grande	191
No Whip, Semi Skimmed Milk, Mini	104
No Whipped Cream, Semi Skimmed Milk, Tall	128
No Whipped Cream, Skimmed Milk, Grande	182
No Whip, Skimmed Milk, Mini	97
No Whipped Cream, Skimmed Milk, Tall	121
No Whipped Cream, Soy, Grande	185
No Whip, Soy, Mini	99
No Whipped Cream, Soy, Tall	124
No Whipped Cream, Whole Milk, Grande	201
No Whip, Whole Milk, Mini	112
No Whipped Cream, Whole Milk, Tall	135

STARBUCKS

FRAPPUCCINO - ESPRESSO LIGHT

No Whip, Skimmed Milk, Grande	111
No Whip, Skimmed Milk, Mini	62
No Whip, Skimmed Milk, Tall	78

FRAPPUCCINO - GREEN TEA

with Whipped Cream, Almond Milk, Grande	286
with Whipped Cream, Almond Milk, Mini	183
with Whipped Cream, Almond Milk, Tall	200
with Whipped Cream, Coconut Milk, Grande	301
with Whipped Cream, Coconut Milk, Mini	192
with Whipped Cream, Coconut Milk, Tall	210
with Whipped Cream, Oat Milk, Grande	443
with Whipped Cream, Oat Milk, Mini	217
with Whipped Cream, Oat Milk, Tall	317
with Whipped Cream, Semi Skimmed Milk, Grande	310
with Whipped Cream, Semi Skimmed Milk, Mini	196
with Whipped Cream, Semi Skimmed Milk, Tall	216
with Whipped Cream, Skimmed Milk, Grande	296
with Whipped Cream, Skimmed Milk, Mini	189
with Whipped Cream, Skimmed Milk, Tall	207
with Whipped Cream, Soy, Grande	301
with Whipped Cream, Soy, Mini	192
with Whipped Cream, Soy, Tall	210
with Whipped Cream, Whole Milk, Grande	325
with Whipped Cream, Whole Milk, Mini	204
with Whipped Cream, Whole Milk, Tall	225

FRAPPUCCINO - JAVA CHIP

with Whipped Cream, Almond Milk, Grande	354
with Whipped Cream, Almond Milk, Mini	221
with Whipped Cream, Almond Milk, Tall	256
with Whipped Cream, Coconut Milk, Grande	435
with Whipped Cream, Coconut Milk, Mini	229
with Whipped Cream, Coconut Milk, Tall	314
with Whipped Cream, Oat Milk, Grande	474
with Whipped Cream, Oat Milk, Tall	343
with Whipped Cream, Semi Skimmed Milk, Grande	442
with Whipped Cream, Semi Skimmed Milk, Mini	234
with Whipped Cream, Semi Skimmed Milk, Tall	320
with Whipped Cream, Skimmed Milk, Grande	429
with Whipped Cream, Skimmed Milk, Mini	226
with Whipped Cream, Skimmed Milk, Tall	310
with Whipped Cream, Soy, Grande	434
with Whipped Cream, Soy, Mini	229
with Whipped Cream, Soy, Tall	314
with Whipped Cream, Whole Milk, Grande	457
with Whipped Cream, Whole Milk, Mini	242
with Whipped Cream, Whole Milk, Tall	332

FRAPPUCCINO - JAVA CHIP LIGHT

No Whip, Skimmed Milk, Grande	211
No Whip, Skimmed Milk, Mini	113
No Whip, Skimmed Milk, Tall	148

STARBUCKS

FRAPPUCCINO - MANGO PASSION

	KCAL
Tea, Grande	191
Tea, Mini	84
Tea, Tall	157

FRAPPUCCINO - MOCHA

	KCAL
with Whipped Cream, Almond Milk, Grande	361
with Whipped Cream, Almond Milk, Mini	208
with Whipped Cream, Almond Milk, Tall	258
with Whipped Cream, Coconut Milk, Grande	377
with Whipped Cream, Coconut Milk, Mini	219
with Whipped Cream, Coconut Milk, Tall	271
with Whipped Cream, Oat Milk, Grande	390
with Whipped Cream, Oat Milk, Mini	208
with Whipped Cream, Oat Milk, Tall	290
with Whipped Cream, Semi Skimmed Milk, Grande	385
with Whipped Cream, Semi Skimmed Milk, Mini	224
with Whipped Cream, Semi Skimmed Milk, Tall	278
with Whipped Cream, Skimmed Milk, Grande	371
with Whipped Cream, Skimmed Milk, Mini	215
with Whipped Cream, Skimmed Milk, Tall	267
with Whipped Cream, Soy, Grande	376
with Whipped Cream, Soy, Mini	218
with Whipped Cream, Soy, Tall	271
with Whipped Cream, Whole Milk, Grande	400
with Whipped Cream, Whole Milk, Mini	234
with Whipped Cream, Whole Milk, Tall	290
No Whip, Skimmed Milk, Grande	143
No Whip, Skimmed Milk, Mini	81
No Whip, Skimmed Milk, Tall	96

FRAPPUCCINO - MOCHA, WHITE CHOCOLATE

	KCAL
with Whipped Cream, Almond Milk, Grande	379
with Whipped Cream, Almond Milk, Mini	197
with Whipped Cream, Almond Milk, Tall	275
with Whipped Cream, Coconut Milk, Grande	394
with Whipped Cream, Coconut Milk, Mini	206
with Whipped Cream, Coconut Milk, Tall	288
with Whipped Cream, Oat Milk, Grande	445
with Whipped Cream, Oat Milk, Mini	233
with Whipped Cream, Oat Milk, Tall	329
with Whipped Cream, Semi Skimmed Milk, Grande	402
with Whipped Cream, Semi Skimmed Milk, Mini	211
with Whipped Cream, Semi Skimmed Milk, Tall	294
with Whipped Cream, Skimmed Milk, Grande	389
with Whipped Cream, Skimmed Milk, Mini	203
with Whipped Cream, Skimmed Milk, Tall	283
with Whipped Cream, Soy, Grande	393
with Whipped Cream, Soy, Mini	206
with Whipped Cream, Soy, Tall	287
with Whipped Cream, Whole Milk, Grande	416
with Whipped Cream, Whole Milk, Mini	219
with Whipped Cream, Whole Milk, Tall	306

FRAPPUCCINO - MOCHA, WHITE CHOCOLATE, LIGHT

	KCAL
No Whip, Skimmed Milk, Grande	155

STARBUCKS

FRAPPUCCINO - MOCHA, WHITE CHOCOLATE, LIGHT

	KCAL
No Whip, Skimmed Milk, Mini	78
No Whip, Skimmed Milk, Tall	98

FRAPPUCCINO - STRAWBERRIES & CREAM

	KCAL
with Whipped Cream, Almond Milk, Grande	321
with Whipped Cream, Almond Milk, Mini	217
with Whipped Cream, Almond Milk, Tall	235
with Whipped Cream, Coconut Milk, Grande	341
with Whipped Cream, Coconut Milk, Mini	234
with Whipped Cream, Coconut Milk, Tall	251
with Whipped Cream, Oat Milk, Grande	389
with Whipped Cream, Oat Milk, Mini	210
with Whipped Cream, Oat Milk, Tall	288
with Whipped Cream, Semi Skimmed Milk, Grande	351
with Whipped Cream, Semi Skimmed Milk, Mini	242
with Whipped Cream, Semi Skimmed Milk, Tall	259
with Whipped Cream, Skimmed Milk, Grande	334
with Whipped Cream, Skimmed Milk, Mini	228
with Whipped Cream, Skimmed Milk, Tall	245
with Whipped Cream, Soy, Grande	340
with Whipped Cream, Soy, Mini	233
with Whipped Cream, Soy, Tall	250
with Whipped Cream, Whole Milk, Grande	370
Strawith Whipped Cream, Whole Milk, Mini	257
with Whipped Cream, Whole Milk, Tall	275

FRAPPUCCINO - VANILLA CREAM

	KCAL
with Whipped Cream, Almond Milk, Grande	292
with Whipped Cream, Almond Milk, Mini	148
with Whipped Cream, Almond Milk, Tall	207
with Whipped Cream, Coconut Milk, Grande	296
with Whipped Cream, Coconut Milk, Mini	160
with Whipped Cream, Coconut Milk, Tall	221
with Whipped Cream, Oat Milk, Grande	366
with Whipped Cream, Oat Milk, Mini	186
with Whipped Cream, Oat Milk, Tall	262
with Whipped Cream, Semi Skimmed Milk, Grande	316
with Whipped Cream, Semi Skimmed Milk, Mini	165
with Whipped Cream, Semi Skimmed Milk, Tall	225
with Whipped Cream, Skimmed Milk , Tall	208
with Whipped Cream, Skimmed Milk, Grande	294
with Whipped Cream, Skimmed Milk, Mini	156
with Whipped Cream, Soy, Grande	302
with Whipped Cream, Soy, Mini	159
with Whipped Cream, Whole Milk, Grande	329
with Whipped Cream, Whole Milk, Mini	176
with Whipped Cream, Whole Milk, Tall	236

FRAPPUCCINO - WHITE CHOC CREAM

	KCAL
with Whipped Cream, Almond Milk, Grande	336
with Whipped Cream, Almond Milk, Mini	173
with Whipped Cream, Almond Milk, Tall	245
with Whipped Cream, Coconut Milk, Grande	358
with Whipped Cream, Coconut Milk, Mini	184
with Whipped Cream, Coconut Milk, Tall	262

KCAL KCAL

STARBUCKS

FRAPPUCCINO - WHITE CHOC CREAM

with Whipped Cream, Oat Milk, Grande	408
with Whipped Cream, Oat Milk, Mini	211
with Whipped Cream, Oat Milk, Tall	303
with Whipped Cream, Semi Skimmed Milk, Grande	369
with Whipped Cream, Semi Skimmed Milk, Mini	190
with Whipped Cream, Semi Skimmed Milk, Tall	271
with Whipped Cream, Skimmed Milk, Grande	350
with Whipped Cream, Skimmed Milk, Mini	180
with Whipped Cream, Skimmed Milk, Tall	256
with Whipped Cream, Soy, Grande	357
with Whipped Cream, Soy, Mini	184
with Whipped Cream, Soy, Tall	262
with Whipped Cream, Whole Milk, Grande	389
with Whipped Cream, Whole Milk, Mini	201
with Whipped Cream, Whole Milk, Tall	287

FRAPPUCCINO - ZEN TEA

Raspberry, Blackcurrant, Grande	192
Raspberry, Blackcurrant, Mini	87
Raspberry, Blackcurrant, Tall	158

HOT CHOCOLATE

Classic with Whipped Cream, Oat Milk, Grande	343
Classic with Whipped Cream, Oat Milk, Short	174
Classic with Whipped Cream, Oat Milk, Tall	282
Classic with Whipped Cream, Oat Milk, Venti	433
Classic with Whipped Cream, Soy, Venti	433
Kids with Whipped Cream, Oat Milk	174
Signature with Whipped Cream, Oat Milk, Short	273
Signature with Whipped Cream, Oat Milk, Tall	223

HOT CHOCOLATE - CLASSIC

with Whipped Cream, Almond Milk, Grande	286
with Whipped Cream, Almond Milk, Short	173
with Whipped Cream, Almond Milk, Tall	241
with Whipped Cream, Almond Milk, Venti	363
with Whipped Cream, Coconut Milk, Grande	343
with Whipped Cream, Coconut Milk, Short	201
with Whipped Cream, Coconut Milk, Tall	285
with Whipped Cream, Coconut Milk, Venti	435
with Whipped Cream, Semi Skimmed Milk, Grande	372
with Whipped Cream, Semi Skimmed Milk, Short	215
with Whipped Cream, Semi Skimmed Milk, Tall	307
with Whipped Cream, Semi Skimmed Milk, Venti	473
with Whipped Cream, Skimmed Milk, Grande	323
with Whipped Cream, Skimmed Milk, Short	191
with Whipped Cream, Skimmed Milk, Venti	410
with Whipped Cream, Soy, Grande	341
with Whipped Cream, Soy, Short	200
with Whipped Cream, Soy, Tall	283
with Whipped Cream, Whole Milk, Grande	426
with Whipped Cream, Whole Milk, Short	242
with Whipped Cream, Whole Milk, Tall	348
with Whipped Cream, Whole Milk, Venti	540
with Whippped Cream, Skimmed Milk, Tall	269

STARBUCKS

HOT CHOCOLATE - FUDGE

Grande	315
Short	198
Tall	257

HOT CHOCOLATE - KIDS

with Whipped Cream, Almond Milk	173
with Whipped Cream, Coconut Milk	201
with Whipped Cream, Semi Skimmed Milk	215
with Whipped Cream, Skimmed Milk	191
with Whipped Cream, Soy	200
with Whipped Cream, Whole Milk	242

HOT CHOCOLATE - SIGNATURE

with Whipped Cream, Almond Milk, Short	271
with Whipped Cream, Almond Milk, Tall	396
with Whipped Cream, Coconut Milk, Short	275
with Whipped Cream, Coconut Milk, Tall	399
with Whipped Cream, Semi Skimmed Milk, Short	283
with Whipped Cream, Semi Skimmed Milk, Tall	418
with Whipped Cream, Skimmed Milk, Short	267
with Whipped Cream, Skimmed Milk, Tall	393
with Whipped Cream, Soy, Short	272
with Whipped Cream, Soy, Tall	401
with Whipped Cream, Whole Milk, Short	293
with Whipped Cream, Whole Milk, Tall	433

MILK

Steamed, Almond Milk, Grande	89
Steamed, Almond Milk, Short	44
Steamed, Almond Milk, Tall	68
Steamed, Almond Milk, Venti	113
Steamed, Coconut, Venti	191
Steamed, Coconut Milk, Grande	151
Steamed, Coconut Milk, Short	74
Steamed, Coconut Milk, Tall	115
Steamed, Semi Skimmed Milk, Grande	182
Steamed, Semi Skimmed Milk, Short	89
Steamed, Semi Skimmed Milk, Tall	139
Steamed, Semi Skimmed Milk, Venti	531
Steamed, Skimmed Milk, Grande	129
Steamed, Skimmed Milk, Short	63
Steamed, Skimmed Milk, Tall	98
Steamed, Skimmed Milk, Venti	163
Steamed, Soy, Grande	148
Steamed, Soy, Short	73
Steamed, Soy, Tall	113
Steamed, Soy, Venti	188
Steamed, Whole Milk, Grande	240
Steamed, Whole Milk, Short	118
Steamed, Whole Milk, Tall	184
Steamed, Whole Milk, Venti	305

SALAD

Chicken, House	330

SANDWICH

Cheddar, & Marmite	367

STARBUCKS

SANDWICH

	KCAL
Chicken, California	393
Sure As Eggs Is Eggs	388

SYRUP

Bar Mocha, 1 Pump - ½ fl oz - 17 g	26
Bar Mocha, 2 Pumps - 1 fl oz - 34 g	53
Bar Mocha, 3 Pumps - 1½ fl oz - 51 g	79
Bar Mocha, 4 Pumps - 2 fl oz - 68 g	106
Bar Mocha, 5 Pumps - 2 ½ fl oz - 85 g	132
Flavoured, 1 Pump - ¼ fl oz 10g	20
Flavoured, 2 Pumps - ½ fl oz - 20 g	40
Flavoured, 3 Pumps - 3/4 fl oz - 30 g	60
Flavoured, 4 Pumps - 1 fl oz - 40 g	81
Sugar Free	0

TEA

Chai, Grande	0
Chai, Latte, Almond Milk, Grande	183
Chai, Latte, Almond Milk, Short	92
Chai, Latte, Almond Milk, Tall	139
Chai, Latte, Almond Milk, Venti	230
Chai, Latte, Coconut Milk, Grande	192
Chai, Latte, Coconut Milk, Short	96
Chai, Latte, Coconut Milk, Tall	143
Chai, Latte, Coconut Milk, Venti	239
Chai, Latte, Oat Milk, Grande	292
Chai, Latte, Oat Milk, Short	143
Chai, Latte, Oat Milk, Tall	227
Chai, Latte, Oat Milk, Venti	389
Chai, Latte, Semi Skimmed Milk, Grande	236
Chai, Latte, Semi Skimmed Milk, Short	119
Chai, Latte, Semi Skimmed Milk, Tall	179
Chai, Latte, Semi Skimmed Milk, Venti	297
Chai, Latte, Skimmed Milk, Grande	204
Chai, Latte, Skimmed Milk, Short	103
Chai, Latte, Skimmed Milk, Tall	154
Chai, Latte, Skimmed Milk, Venti	256
Chai, Latte, Soy, Grande	213
Chai, Latte, Soy, Short	108
Chai, Latte, Soy, Tall	162
Chai, Latte, Soy, Venti	268
Chai, Latte, Whole Milk, Grande	255
Chai, Latte, Whole Milk, Short	129
Chai, Latte, Whole Milk, Tall	194
Chai, Latte, Whole Milk, Venti	322
Chai, Tall	0
Chai, Venti	0
Chamomile, Grande	0
Chamomile, Tall	0
Chamomile, Venti	0
Earl Grey, Grande	0
Earl Grey, Tall	0
Earl Grey, Venti	0
Emperor's Clouds & Mist, Grande	0

STARBUCKS

TEA

	KCAL
Emperor's Clouds & Mist, Tall	0
Emperor's Clouds & Mist, Venti	0
English Breakfast, Grande	0
English Breakfast, Tall	0
English Breakfast, Venti	0
Green, Latte, Almond Milk, Grande	154
Green, Latte, Almond Milk, Short	65
Green, Latte, Almond Milk, Tall	113
Green, Latte, Almond Milk, Venti	204
Green, Latte, Coconut Milk, Grande	210
Green, Latte, Coconut Milk, Short	93
Green, Latte, Coconut Milk, Tall	158
Green, Latte, Coconut Milk, Venti	277
Green, Latte, Oat Milk, Grande	292
Green, Latte, Oat Milk, Short	119
Green, Latte, Oat Milk, Tall	199
Green, Latte, Oat Milk, Venti	369
Green, Latte, Semi Skimmed Milk, Grande	239
Green, Latte, Semi Skimmed Milk, Short	107
Green, Latte, Semi Skimmed Milk, Tall	181
Green, Latte, Semi Skimmed Milk, Venti	315
Green, Latte, Skimmed Milk, Grande	190
Green, Latte, Skimmed Milk, Short	83
Green, Latte, Skimmed Milk, Tall	142
Green, Latte, Skimmed Milk, Venti	251
Green, Latte, Soya Milk, Short	92
Green, Latte, Soya Milk, Grande	208
Green, Latte, Soya Milk, Tall	156
Green, Latte, Soya Milk, Venti	275
Green, Latte, Whole Milk, Grande	291
Green, Latte, Whole Milk, Short	133
Green, Latte, Whole Milk, Tall	223
Green, Latte, Whole Milk, Venti	384
Hibiscus, Grande	0
Hibiscus, Tall	0
Hibiscus, Venti	0
Iced, Black Tea, Shaken, Grande	0
Iced, Black Tea, Shaken, Tall	0
Iced, Black Tea, Shaken, Venti	0
Iced, Chai, Latte, Almond Milk, Grande	181
Iced, Chai, Latte, Almond Milk, Tall	136
Iced, Chai, Latte, Almond Milk, Venti	227
Iced, Chai, Latte, Coconut, Tall	164
Iced, Chai, Latte, Coconut, Venti	274
Iced, Chai, Latte, Coconut Milk, Grande	217
Iced, Chai, Latte, Oat Milk, Grande	197
Iced, Chai, Latte, Oat Milk, Tall	155
Iced, Chai, Latte, Oat Milk, Venti	260
Iced, Chai, Latte, Semi Skimmed Milk, Grande	236
Iced, Chai, Latte, Semi Skimmed Milk, Tall	179
Iced, Chai, Latte, Semi Skimmed Milk, Venti	298
Iced, Chai, Latte, Skimmed Milk, Grande	204

STARBUCKS
TEA

	KCAL
Iced, Chai, Latte, Skimmed Milk, Tall	154
Iced, Chai, Latte, Skimmed Milk, Venti	257
Iced, Chai, Latte, Soy, Grande	216
Iced, Chai, Latte, Soy, Tall	163
Iced, Chai, Latte, Soy, Venti	272
Iced, Chai, Latte, Whole Milk, Grande	270
Iced, Chai, Latte, Whole Milk, Tall	205
Iced, Chai, Latte, Whole Milk, Venti	341
Iced, Green Tea, Shaken, Grande	0
Iced, Green Tea, Shaken, Tall	0
Iced, Green Tea, Shaken, Venti	0
Iced, Hibiscus, Shaken, Grande	0
Iced, Hibiscus, Shaken, Tall	0
Iced, Hibiscus, Shaken, Venti	0
Jasmine Pearls, Grande	0
Jasmine Pearls, Tall	0
Jasmine Pearls, Venti	0
Mango, Black, Tea Lemonade, Grande	127
Mango, Black, Tea Lemonade, Tall	96
Mango, Black, Tea Lemonade, Venti	158
Mint Blend, Grande	0
Mint Blend, Tall	0
Mint Blend, Venti	0
Mint Citrus, Green Tea, Grande	0
Mint Citrus, Green Tea, Tall	0
Mint Citrus, Green Tea, Venti	0
Peach, Green, Tea Lemonade, Grande	127
Peach, Green, Tea Lemonade, Tall	96
Peach, Green, Tea Lemonade, Venti	158
Youthberry, Grande	0
Youthberry, Tall	0
Youthberry, Venti	0

TOASTIE

	KCAL
Cheese, & Ham, Mini, Grilled	331
Cheese, & Tomato, Mini, Grilled	305

TOPPING

	KCAL
Whipped Cream, Cold, Grande, Beverage	114
Whipped Cream, Cold, Venti, Beverage	104
Caramel - 4 g	15
Chocolate - 4 g	6
Sprinkles - 1 g	4
Whipped Cream, Cold, Tall, Beverage	81
Whipped Cream, Hot, Grande/Venti Beverage	72
Whipped Cream, Hot, Short, Beverage	52
Whipped Cream, Hot, Tall, Beverage	62

WRAP

	KCAL
Chicken, California	292
Falafel, & Slaw, Vegan	261

YOGHURT

	KCAL
Greek Style, with Berry Crunch	207

SUBWAY
BACON

	KCAL
2 Strips	40

BEEF

	KCAL
Patty, Big	142
Steak, Portion	94

BREAD

	KCAL
Flatbread	220
Rolls, Submarine, 9 Grain Honey Oat, 6"	218
Rolls, Submarine, 9 Grain Wheat, 6"	205
Rolls, Submarine, Hearty Italian, 6"	209
Rolls, Submarine, Italian Herb & Cheese, 6"	242
Rolls, Submarine, Italian White, 6"	198

CHEESE

	KCAL
Cheddar, Processed	40
Monterey Cheddar	57
Peppered	39

CHICKEN

	KCAL
Breast, Portion	35
Strips, Teriyaki Glazed, Portion	101
Tikka, Portion	89

COOKIES

	KCAL
Chocolate Chip Candy	211
Chocolate Chunk	216
Double Choc Chip	215
Oatmeal Raisin	195
Raspberry Cheesecake	207

DANISH PASTRY

	KCAL
Apricot Crown	419
Cinnamon Swirl	207
Vanilla Crown	329

DOUGHNUTS

	KCAL
Chocolate	351
Sugared	352

EGGS

	KCAL
Patty, Portion	55

FLATBREAD

	KCAL
Bacon, Egg, & Cheese, with Salad, Breakfast	352
Bacon, with Salad, Breakfast	345
Beef, Big Beef Melt, with Salad	418
Chicken, & Bacon, Ranch Melt, with Salad	518
Chicken, Breast, with Salad, Low Fat	321
Chicken, Teriyaki, with Salad, Low Fat	337
Chicken, Tikka, with Salad, Low Fat	325
Egg, & Cheese, wiith Salad, Breakfast	316
Ham, with Salad, Low Fat	305
Italian BMT, with Salad	427
Meatball Marinara, with Salad	454
Mega Melt, with Salad, Breakfast	529
Sausage, Egg, & Cheese, with Salad, Breakfast	492
Sausage, with Salad, Breakfast	396
Spicy Italian, with Salad	498
Steak, & Cheese, with Salad	370
Subway Melt, with Salad	388

SUBWAY

FLATBREAD

Tuna, with Salad	371
Turkey, & Ham, with Salad, Low Fat	308
Turkey, Breast, with Salad, Low Fat	292
Veggie Delite, with Salad, Low Fat	236
Veggie Patty, with Salad	396

HAM

Portion	69

MEATBALLS

Bowl	314
Marinara, Sub Portion	218

MUFFIN

Blueberry	394
Chocolate Chunk	243
Double Chocolate Chip	351
Raspberry, & White Chocolate	389

NACHOS

Cheese, Melted	403

PEPPERONI

Salami, & Cheese, Spicy Italian, Portion	262
Salami, & Ham, Italian BMT, Portion	192

SALAD

Beef, Big Beef Melt, without Dressing	234
Chicken, & Bacon, Ranch Melt, without Dressing	334
Chicken, Breast, without Dressing	137
Chicken, Pizziola, without Dressing	274
Chicken, Teriyaki, without Dressing	141
Ham, without Dressing	153
Italian BMT, without Dressing	244
Meatball, Marinara, without Dressing	270
Spicy Italian, without Dressing	314
Steak, & Cheese, without Dressing	186
Subway Melt, with Cheese, without Dressing	205
Tuna, without Dressing	187
Turkey, & Ham, without Dressing	124
Turkey, Breast, without Dressing	108
Veggie Delite, without Dressing	52
Veggie Patty, without Dressing	212

SAUCE

Barbecue	39
Caesar	84
Chilli, Hot	48
Chilli, Sweet	46
Chipotle Southwest	90
Deli Mustard	48
Honey Mustard	32
Mayonnaise, Lite	50
Ranch	43
Sweet Onion	34

SAUSAGE

Portion	176

SUBS

All Day Mega Melt, Sub of the Day, Standard 6"	550

SUBWAY

SUBS

Cheese & Onion, Sub of the Day, Standard 6"	406
Christmas Cracker, Hearty Italian Bread, 6"	432
Fiery Tuna, Sub of the Day, Standard 6"	263
Mango Chicken Tikka, Sub of the Day, Standard 6"	360
Meat Feast, Sub of the Day, Standard 6"	416
Nacho Chicken Salsa, Sub of the Day, Standard 6"	500
Pepperoni Pizza, Sub of the Day, Standard 6"	444

SUBS - BACON

9 Grain Honey Oat Bread, Breakfast, 6"	291
9 Grain Wheat Bread, Breakfast, 6"	278
Hearty Italian Bread, Breakfast, 6"	282
Italian Herb & Cheese Bread, Breakfast, 6"	315
Italian White Bread, Breakfast, 6"	271

SUBS - BACON, EGG, & CHEESE

9 Grain Honey Oat Bread, Breakfast, 6"	350
9 Grain Wheat Bread, 6"	337
Hearty Italian Bread, Breakfast, 6"	361
Italian Herb & Cheese Bread, Breakfast, 6"	374
Italian White Bread, Breakfast, 6"	330

SUBS - BIG BEEF MELT

with Salad, 9 Grain Honey Oat Bread, 6"	416
with Salad, 9 Grain Wheat Bread, 6"	403
with Salad, Hearty Italian Bread, 6"	407
with Salad, Italian Herb & Cheese Bread, 6"	440
with Salad, Italian White Bread, 6"	396

SUBS - CHICKEN & BACON RANCH MELT

with Salad, 9 Grain Honey Oat Bread, 6"	516
with Salad, 9 Grain Wheat Bread, 6"	503
with Salad, Hearty Italian Bread, 6"	507
with Salad, Italian Herb & Cheese Bread, 6"	540
with Salad, Italian White Bread, 6"	496

SUBS - CHICKEN BREAST

with Salad, 9 Grain Honey Oat Bread, Low Fat, 6"	319
with Salad, 9 Grain Wheat Bread, Low Fat, 6"	306
with Salad, Hearty Italian Bread, Low Fat, 6"	310
with Salad, Italian Herb & Cheese Bread, Low Fat, 6"	343
with Salad, Italian White Bread, Low Fat, 6"	299

SUBS - CHICKEN PIZZIOLA

with Salad, 9 Grain Honey Oat Bread, 6"	456
with Salad, 9 Grain Wheat Bread, 6"	443
with Salad, Hearty Italian Bread, 6"	447
with Salad, Italian Herb & Cheese Bread, 6"	480
with Salad, Italian White Bread, 6"	436

SUBS - CHICKEN TERIYAKI

with Salad, 9 Grain Honey Oat Bread, Low Fat, 6"	335
with Salad, 9 Grain Wheat Bread, Low Fat, 6"	321
with Salad, Hearty Italian Bread, Low Fat, 6"	326
with Salad, Italian Herb & Cheese Bread, Low Fat, 6"	359
with Salad, Italian White Bread, Low Fat, 6"	315

SUBS - CHICKEN TIKKA

with Salad, 9 Grain Honey Oat Bread, Low Fat, 6"	323
with Salad, 9 Grain Wheat Bread, Low Fat, 6"	310

SUBWAY

SUBS - CHICKEN TIKKA
	KCAL
with Salad, Hearty Italian Bread, Low Fat, 6"	314
with Salad, Italian Herb & Cheese Bread, Low Fat, 6"	347
with Salad, Italian White Bread, Low Fat, 6"	303

SUBS - EGG & CHEESE
9 Grain Honey Oat Bread, Breakfast, 6"	314
9 Grain Wheat Bread, Breakfast, 6"	301
Hearty Italian Bread, Breakfast, 6"	305
Italian Herb & Cheese Bread, Breakfast, 6"	338
Italian White Bread, Breakfast, 6"	294

SUBS - HAM
with Salad, 9 Grain Honey Oat Bread, Low Fat, 6"	303
with Salad, 9 Grain Wheat Bread, Kids Pak, 4"	182
with Salad, Hearty Italian Bread, Low Fat, 6"	294
with Salad, Italian Herb & Cheese Bread, Low Fat, 6"	327
with Salad, Italian White Bread, Kids Pak, 4"	177

SUBS - ITALIAN BMT
with Salad, 9 Grain Honey Oat Bread, 6"	425
with Salad, 9 Grain Wheat Bread, 6"	412
with Salad, Hearty Italian Bread, 6"	416
with Salad, Italian Herb & Cheese Bread, 6"	449
with Salad, Italian White Bread, 6"	405

SUBS - MEATBALL MARINARA
with Salad, 9 Grain Honey Oat Bread, 6"	452
with Salad, 9 Grain Wheat Bread, 6"	439
with Salad, Hearty Italian Bread, 6"	443
with Salad, Italian Herb & Cheese Bread, 6"	476
with Salad, Italian White Bread, 6"	432

SUBS - MEGA MELT
9 Grain Honey Oat Bread, Breakfast, 6"	527
9 Grain Wheat Bread, Breakfast, 6"	514
Hearty Italian Bread, Breakfast, 6"	518
Italian Herb & Cheese Bread, Breakfast, 6"	551
Italian White Bread, Breakfast, 6"	507

SUBS - SAUSAGE
9 Grain Honey Oat Bread, Breakfast, 6"	394
9 Grain Wheat Bread, Breakfast, 6"	381
Hearty Italian Bread, Breakfast, 6"	385
Italian Herb & Cheese Bread, Breakfast, 6"	418
Italian White Bread, Breakfast, 6"	374

SUBS - SAUSAGE, EGG & CHEESE
9 Grain Honey Oat Bread, 6"	490
9 Grain Wheat Bread, 6"	477
Hearty Italian Bread, Breakfast, 6"	481
Italian Herb & Cheese Bread, Breakfast, 6"	514
Italian White Bread, Breakfast, 6"	470

SUBS - SPICY ITALIAN
with Salad, 9 Grain Honey Oat Bread, 6"	495
with Salad, 9 Grain Wheat Bread, 6"	482
with Salad, Hearty Italian Bread, 6"	486
with Salad, Italian Herb & Cheese Bread, 6"	519
with Salad, Italian White Bread, 6"	475

SUBWAY

SUBS - STEAK & CHEESE
	KCAL
with Salad, 9 Grain Honey Oat Bread, 6"	368
with Salad, 9 Grain Wheat Bread, 6"	363
with Salad, Hearty Italian Bread, 6"	359
with Salad, Italian Herb & Cheese Bread, 6"	392
with Salad, Italian White Bread, 6"	348

SUBS - SUBWAY MELT
with Salad, 9 Grain Honey Oat Bread, 6"	386
with Salad, 9 Grain Wheat Bread, 6"	376
with Salad, Hearty Italian Bread, 6"	377
with Salad, Italian Herb & Cheese Bread, 6"	410
with Salad, Italian White Bread, 6"	366

SUBS - TUNA
with Salad, 9 Grain Honey Oat Bread, 6"	369
with Salad, 9 Grain Wheat Bread, 6"	356
with Salad, Hearty Italian Bread, 6"	360
with Salad, Italian Herb & Cheese Bread, 6"	393
with Salad, Italian White Bread, 6"	349

SUBS - TURKEY & HAM
with Salad, 9 Grain Honey Oat Bread, Low Fat, 6"	306
with Salad, 9 Grain Wheat Bread, Low Fat, 6"	293
with Salad, Hearty Italian Bread, Low Fat, 6"	297
with Salad, Italian Herb & Cheese Bread, Low Fat, 6"	330
with Salad, Italian White Bread, Low Fat, 6"	286

SUBS - TURKEY BREAST
with Salad, 9 Grain Honey Oat Bread, Low Fat, 6"	290
with Salad, 9 Grain Wheat Bread, 6"	275
with Salad, 9 Grain Wheat Bread, Kids Pak, 4"	184
with Salad, Hearty Italian Bread, Low Fat, 6"	281
with Salad, Italian Herb & Cheese Bread, Low Fat, 6"	314
with Salad, Italian White Bread, Kids Pak, 4"	180

SUBS - VEGGIE DELITE
with Salad, 9 Grain Honey Oat Bread, Low Fat, 6"	234
with Salad, 9 Grain Wheat Bread, 6"	219
with Salad, 9 Grain Wheat Bread, Kids Pak, 4"	147
with Salad, Hearty Italian Bread, Low Fat, 6"	258
with Salad, Italian Herb & Cheese Bread, Low Fat, 6"	258
with Salad, Italian White Bread, Kids Pak, 4"	142

SUBS - VEGGIE PATTY
with Salad, 9 Grain Honey Oat Bread, 6"	394
with Salad, 9 Grain Wheat Bread, 6"	381
with Salad, Hearty Italian Bread, 6"	385
with Salad, Italian Herb & Cheese Bread, 6"	418
with Salad, Italian White Bread, 6"	373

TOASTIE
Cheese	214
Pepperoni Pizza	254

TUNA
Portion	135

TURKEY
Breast, & Ham, Portion	72
Breast, Portion	56

SUBWAY
VEGETARIAN

	KCAL
Veggie Patty, Portion	160

WRAP

	KCAL
Chicken, & Bacon, Caesar, Signature, Halal	617
Chicken, & Bacon, Caesar, Signature, Standard	656
Chicken, Caesar, Rotisserie-Style, Signature, Halal	596
Chicken, Caesar, Rotisserie-Style, Signature, Standard	596
Steak, Chipotle, & Cheese, Signature, Halal	661
Steak, Chipotle, & Cheese, Signature, Standard	661
Turkey, Bacon, & Guacamole, Signature, Halal	523
Turkey, Bacon, & Guacamole, Signature, Standard	554

TABLE TABLE

	KCAL
BACON	
Back, Cooked, Breakfast	165
BAGEL	
Cinnamon, & Raisin, Breakfast	293
BEANS	
Baked, Breakfast	91
BEEF	
Steak, 6oz, Ranch, Great Grills	411
Steak, Rib Eye, 10oz, Great Grills	1018
Steak, Rump, 8oz, Great Grills	820
BEEF DINNER	
Topside, Roast	1060
BITES	
Cheesy Jalapeno, Side	378
Chicken, & Bacon, Hunter's, Side	408
BLACK PUDDING	
Slice, Breakfast	122
BREAD	
Garlic, Flatbread	265
Garlic, Flatbread, with Cheese	415
BROCCOLI	
Tenderstem, Side	139
BROWNIES	
Chocolate, Dark, & Black Cherry	672
Chocolate, Warm	533
BUBBLE & SQUEAK	
Breakfast	169
BURGERS	
Beef, Wagyu	1286
Chicken, Buttermilk, & Stilton	1217
Fish & Chip Shop	1010
Lamb, & Feta	1164
Prawn, Double Stack	1482
Sloppy Jo	1393
Steak, with Cheese, & Bacon, Double Stack	1276
Steak, with Cheese, Double	1213
Steak, with Cheese, Double Stack	1213
Steak, with Cheese	902
Tandoori	1160
Vegan, BBQ	925
BUTTER	
Salted, Portion, Breakfast	48
CAKE	
Chocolate, Fudge, Sensation	810
CAULIFLOWER CHEESE	
BLANK	282
CHEESECAKE	
Strawberry, Mini	223
CHICKEN	
Breast, Topped, Bacon & Cheese, with Chips	742
Breast, Topped, Bacon & Cheese, with Jacket Potato	755
Escalope	1303
Forestiere	726

TABLE TABLE

CHICKEN

Goujons, Buttermilk, & Rosemary	406
Paprika	522
Wings, Buttermilk	561

CHICKEN DINNER

Half, Roast	1171

CHIPS

Side	363

CROISSANT

Breakfast	161

CRUMBLE

Apple, Slice	299
Summer Fruit	596

CRUMPETS

Sourdough, Breakfast	91

CURRY

Thai, Green	787
Thai, Green, with Chicken Breast	942

EGGS

Boiled, Single, Breakfast	82
Fried, Single, Breakfast	61
Poached, Single, Breakfast	79
Scrambled, Breakfast	172

FISH & CHIPS

Haddock, Hand Battered, with Mushy Peas	1095
Haddock, Hand Battered, with Peas	1057

FRIES

Halloumi, Side	623
Skinny Cut, Side	329
Sweet Potato, Side	350

FROZEN YOGHURT

Strawberry	164

FRUIT MIX

Berry, Breakfast	23

FRUIT SALAD

Breakfast	49

GAMMON

Steak, with Chips, & Eggs	817
Steak, with Chips, & Pineapple	772
Steak, with Chips, Egg, & Pineapple	794
Steak, with Jacket Potato, & Eggs	830
Steak, with Jacket Potato, & Pineapple	785
Steak, with Jacket Potato, Egg, & Pineapple	808

HAM

Egg, & Chips	701

HASH BROWNS

Single, Breakfast	94

ICE CREAM

Dairy, with Caramel Sauce	146
Dairy, with Chocolate Sauce	145
Dairy, with Raspberry Sauce	143

TABLE TABLE

LAMB

Pulled, Spiced, with Houmous, Slow Cooked	595
Rump	716

LASAGNE

Beef	645
Sweet Potato, & Feta	676

LINGUINE

Vegetable, Roasted	459
Vegetable, Roasted, with Chicken	614

MAKHANI

Chicken, Curry	934

MIXED GRILL

BLANK	1292
with Rump Steak	1328

MUFFIN

Blueberry, Breakfast	114

MUSHROOMS

Breaded, Garlic & Herb	276
with Butter, Breakfast	169

NACHOS

Loaded	729

OMELETTE

Breakfast	311

ONION RINGS

Battered, Beer, Side	221

PAIN AU CHOCOLAT

Mini, Breakfast	146

PAIN AU RAISIN

Mini, Breakfast	118

PANCAKE

Reduced Sugar, Breakfast	96

PATE

Pork, with Red Onion Chutney	483

PIE

Apple, Caramel, with Cream	522
Apple, Caramel, with Custard	454
Apple, Caramel, with Ice Cream	421
Beef, & Stout	1268
Chicken, & Chorizo	568
Chicken, & Ham	1142

PLATTER

Sharing, ½ Platter	830
Sharing, with Buttermilk Chicken Wings, ½ Platter	1039

PORK

Trio	1505

PORK DINNER

Loin, Roast	1147

POTATOES

Dippers, Lunch Club	421
Jacket, with Cheese, & Beans	807
Jacket, with Prawns, & Marie Rose Sauce	554

TABLE TABLE
PRAWN COCKTAIL
Classic	457

PUDDING
Sticky Toffee	842

RIBS
Half Rack, & Smoky Paprika Chicken	968
Whole Rack, & Smoky Paprika Chicken	1332

SALAD
Chicken, Grilled	230
Halloumi, Grilled	357
Mixed, Side	37
Salmon, Fillet, Grilled	361

SALMON
Teriyaki	592

SANDWICH
Chicken, & Bacon, Club	842

SAUCE
Bearnaise	122
Diane	73
Peppercorn, Creamy	29

SAUSAGE
Breakfast	137
Quorn*, Breakfast	78

SCAMPI
Breaded, & Chips, with Mushy Peas	857
Breaded, & Chips, with Peas	829

SEA BASS
Fillet	579

SORBET
Gin Fizz	140

SOUP
Tomato	307

SPREAD
Sunflower, Portion, Breakfast	43

STEW
Beef, & Dumplings	793

SUNDAE
with Cadbury Dairy Milk	590
with Terry's Chocolate Orange	603

TART
Cheddar, & Sticky Onion	289
Cheese, Cheshire, & Bramley Apple	799

TOAST
GF, Breakfast	84
Malted, Breakfast	92
White, Breakfast	90

TOMATOES
Half, Breakfast	10

TORTE
Chocolate, Greek Yoghurt, Mini	295

VEGETABLES
Green, Mixed, Side	112

TABLE TABLE
WAFFLES
Chicken, & Bacon, Buttermilk	1006
Toffee Apple, Salted	566

WELLINGTON
Vegetable, Root, Roast	1416

THE REAL GREEK FOOD COMPANY LTD

ASPARAGUS
Grilled, Hot Meze	140

CHEESE
Halloumi, Grilled, Hot Meze	151
Halloumi, Skewers, Hot Meze	118
Halloumi, Skewers, Kids Menu	118

CHICK PEAS
Revithia, Cold Meze	286

CHICKEN
Skewers, Hot Meze	177
Skewers, Kids Menu	88

CHIPS
Side	528

COD
Salt, Hot Meze	346

CRUDITES
Cold Meze	37

DESSERT
Watermelon, Sweet & Salty	124
Yoghurt, Greek with Raspberries	223

DIP
Aioli, Parsley	176
Dip, Selection	589
Mayonnaise, Lemon, Preserved	279
Melitzanasalata, Cold Meze	236
Relish, Chilli, Smoked	42
Relish, Sun-Dried Tomato & Roast Red Pepper	92

DOLMADES
Cold Meze	254

FLATBREAD
Greek, Cold Meze	615
Greek, with Olive & Dukkah, Nibbles	538

HOUMOUS
Cold Meze	298

LAMB
Cutlets, Hot Meze	881
Kefte, Hot Meze	344
Skewers, Hot Meze	255

NUTS
Mixed, Athenian, Nibbles	479

OCTOPUS
Grilled, Hot Meze	447

OLIVES
Nibbles	317

PARCELS
Tiropitakia, Filo Pastry, Hot Meze	416

PORK
Skewers, Hot Meze	281

POTATOES
New, in Olive Oil & Lemon Juice, Hot Meze	293

RICE
Saffron, Hot Meze	406

THE REAL GREEK FOOD COMPANY LTD

SALAD
Cos	42
Tabouleh, Cold Meze	117
Watermelon, Mint & Feta, Cold Meze	102

SARDINES
Grilled, Hot Meze	619

SOUVLAKI
Lamb, Kefte	730
Lamb	607
Pork	633
Souvlaki, Halloumi & Vegetable	451

SQUID
Kalamari, Grilled, Hot Meze	286

TARAMASALATA
Cold Meze	913

TZATZIKI
Cold Meze	163

TOBY CARVERY

ANGEL DELIGHT

Strawberry, Mini, Kids Menu	79
Strawberry, with Popping Candy, Kids Menu	73

BEANS

Green	17
Romano	17

BEEF DINNER

Roast, Kids Menu	229
Roast, King Size	609
Roast	458

BOLOGNESE

Spaghetti, with Veggie Sticks, Kids Menu	263

BROCCOLI

Side	20

BROWNIES - CHOCOLATE

Whipped Cream, White Chocolate, & Rasperries	889
Mini, Whipped Cream, Kids Menu	370

CABBAGE

Red, with Cranberry, & Orange	12
with Onions	8

CAKE

Chocolate, Fudge	669
Chocolate, Fudge, with Custard	759
Chocolate, Fudge, with Ice Cream	804
Chocolate, Fudge, with Whipped Cream	1039

CARROTS

Side	24

CAULIFLOWER CHEESE

Side	17

CHEESE

Dorset, Bites, Chilli Seasoning	265
Fondue, Blue, with Bread, & Crudites	526

CHEESECAKE

Blueberry, & Vanilla, Strawberry Compote, Baked	742

CHICKEN

Breast, Roast, & Giant Yorkshire Pudding, Kids Menu	196
Wings, Honey, & Mustard	274

CRUMBLE - APPLE

Bramley, & Cinnamon, Mini	170
Mango, & Passion Fruit, Custard, Mini, Kids Menu	343
Plum, & Damson, Mini, Kids Menu	301
Plum, & Damson, with Custard	454
with Custard, Mini, Kids Menu	314

DESSERT

Bananas, & Custard, Kids Menu	223
Eton Mess, Strawberry, & Passion Fruit	914

EGGS

Scrambled, Breakfast, All You Can Eat	119

GAMMON

Cheddar, Salad, Chutney & Baguette	795
Pomegranate Glaze, King Size	422
Pomegranate Glaze	317
Roast, Kids Menu	158

TOBY CARVERY

GRATIN

Potato, Carrot, Garlic, Creamy	121

GRAVY

Beef, & Onion	21
Onion, Vegetarian	23
Poultry	21

ICE CREAM

Kids Menu	190

ICE LOLLY

Frozen Yoghurt, Strawberry, Greek Style, Kids Menu	55

JELLY

Orange, with Mandarins, Kids Menu	100

LEEKS

Side	8

MEATBALLS

Pork, & Beef, with Gravy	356

MUSHROOMS

Creamy, Cheddar Sauce, with Bread	346

MUSTARD

Original	29
Wholegrain	32

ONIONS

in Gravy	30

PARCELS

Broccoli, & Brie	492

PARSNIP

Side	134

PEAS

Side	46

PIE

Allotment, House Salad, & Steamed Potatoes	455
Shepherds, with Carrot & Swede Mash, Kids Menu	228

PORK

Riblets, Pomegranate glaze	210
Roast, Kids Menu	212
Roast, with Crackling, King Size	564
Roast, with Crackling	424

PORK CRACKLING

& Apple Sauce	1033
Homemade	670

POTATO MASH

Side	46

POTATOES

Roast, Roasties	375
Roast, Roasties, with Cheese	494
Roast, 3 Potatoes	258

PRAWN COCKTAIL

King, with Bread	528
King, with Wholemeal Bread, Mini, Kids Menu	291

PROFITEROLES

with Belgian Chocolate Sauce, & Whipped Cream	645

RICE PUDDING

Vanilla, with Raspberries	350

TOBY CARVERY

SALAD

Superfood, with French Dressing	158
Superfood, with Roast Chicken, & French Dressing	543
Superfood, with Salmon, & French Dressing	526

SALMON

En Pappillote	368

SANDWICH

Beef, & Horseradish, Crispy Baguette, Roast	989
Beef, & Horseradish, Homebaked Bap, Roast	931
Cheddar, Apple, & Chutney, Crispy Baguette	1097
Cheddar, Apple, & Chutney, Homebaked Bap	1039
Full Feast, Crispy Baguette	936
Full Feast, Homebaked Bap	878
Gammon, Lettuce, & Tomato, Crispy Baguette	936
Gammon, Lettuce, & Tomato, Homebaked Bap	878
Pork, Stuffing, & Apple Sauce, Crispy Baguette	986
Pork, Stuffing, & Apple Sauce, Homebaked Bap	928
Prawns, King, Seafood Sauce, Crispy Baguette	1175
Prawns, King, Seafood Sauce, Homebaked Bap	1117
Turkey, Stuffing, & Cranberry Sauce, Baguette	895
Turkey, Stuffing, & Cranberry Sauce, Bap	837

SAUCE

Apple	20
Bread	36
Cranberry	34
Horseradish	26
Mint	21

SAUSAGE

& Yorkshire Pudding, Kids Menu	274
Pigs, In Blankets	520

SAUSAGE & MASH

Bangers, with Gravy	1182

SOUP

Of The Day, with Bread	263
Tomato, with Wholemeal Bread, Kids Menu	232

SPONGE

Treacle	482
Treacle, with Custard	572
Treacle, with Ice Cream	617
Treacle, with Whipped Cream	852

SPROUTS

Side	26

STUFFING

Sage, & Onion	73

SUNDAE - CHOCOLATE BROWNIE

Kids Menu	353

SUNDAE - ICE CREAM

Munchies, Chocolate, & Caramel Sauce, Sharing	1020
Munchies, Chocolate, & Caramel Sauce	582

SUNDAE - ICE CREAM, CHOCOLATE BROWNIE

Sensation	675

SUNDAE - ICE CREAM, HONEYCOMB

Toffee, Fudge, & Chocolate Sauce	509

TOBY CARVERY

SUNDAE - ICE CREAM, PEACH MELBA

Raspberries, with Demarara Crumb, Sharing	742
Raspberries, with Demerara Crumb	535

SWEDE

Side	20

SWEETCORN

Side	61

TART

Lemon, Creamy, with Strawberries, Whipped Cream	596
Pepper, & Pomegranate	520
Portabello, Bulls-eye	522

TERRINE

Pork, Apple, & Cider	369

TOAD IN THE HOLE

Main	463

TURKEY

Roast, Kids Menu	126
Roast, King Size	337
Roast	253

VEGETABLES

Sticks, & Cheesy, BBQ, Dip, Kids Menu	103

WELLINGTON

Carrot, & Chickpea, Spiced	749

YORKSHIRE PUDDING

with Ice Cream, Kids Menu	425

VINTAGE INNS

ASPARAGUS

& Pulled Ham, with Egg, & Hollandaise, Starter	366

AUBERGINE

Miso Sesame Glazed, Side	156
Roll, Chipotle Dip, & Kale & Cauliflower Cous Cous	644

BACON

Streaky, Sweetcure, Burger Add On	101

BEANS

Baked, Side, Kids	80

BEEF - STEAK, FILLET

Triple Cooked Chips, Onion Rings, & Tomato	998
Rossini, with Asparagus, & Dauphinoise Potato	764

BEEF - STEAK, RIBEYE

Triple Cooked Chips, Onion Rings, & Tomato	1278

BEEF - STEAK, RUMP

Triple Cooked Chips, Onion Rings, & Tomato	1241

BEEF - STEAK, SIRLOIN

Triple Cooked Chips, Onions Rings, & Tomato	1280

BEEF DINNER

Roast, Kids Meal	842
Roast, Yorkshire Pudding, Potatoes, Veg, & Gravy	1536

BREAD

Garlic, Side, Kids	373

BREADSTICKS

with Dips, Sharers/Grazing	1048

BROCCOLI - TENDERSTEM

with Blacksticks Blue Cheese Sauce	123
with Chipotle Dressing, & Toasted Pumpkin Seeds	107

BROWNIES - CHOCOLATE

Chocolate Sauce, & Irish Liqueur Ice Cream	654
Chocolate Sauce, & Irish Liqueur Ice Cream, Mini	619
with Vanilla Ice Cream, Kids	428

BURGERS - BEEF

Cheddar, Bacon Chutney, Onion Rings, & Chips	1391
no Sides, Kids	343
Wagyu, Tomato Salsa, Salad, Onion Rings, & Chips	1033

BURGERS - CHICKPEA, AUBERGINE & SPINACH

with Triple Cooked Chips, Vegetarian	757
with Kale & Cauliflower Cous Cous, Vegan	515

CHEESE

Brie, Crispy Panko Crumb, Starter	482
Camembert, with Celery, & Bread, Sharers/Grazing	1021
Cheddar, Smoked, Burger Add On	83
Cheeseboard, with Biscuits, Grapes, & Chutney	1047
Duo, Camembert, & Brie, & Bread, Sharers/Grazing	1525

CHEESECAKE

Raspberry, Milkshake, & Cornish Clotted Cream	731

CHICKEN

Hunter's, with 4oz Gammon Steak, & Chips	1123
Half, in White Wine & Cider Sauce, with Potatoes	534
Topped, with Bacon, & BBQ Sauce, no Sides, Kids	365

VINTAGE INNS

CHIPS

Side, Kids	310
Triple Cooked	484

CHUTNEY

Bacon, Burger Add On	142

COD

Battered, Fillet, no Sides, Kids	392

CRAB CAKES

Lemon & Chive Mayo, & Mini Prawn Cocktail, Starter	314

CREME BRULEE

Vanilla, Classic, with Butter Biscuits	384

CRUMBLE

Apple, & Blackberry, with Custard	719
Apple, & Rhubarb, with Custard	715

CURRY

Vegetable, Coconut, with Sticky Jasmine Rice	658

CUSTARD

BLANK	90

DESSERT

Eton Mess	372
Melba Mallow Mess, Mini	300
Trio, Toffee & Nut	660

FALAFEL

with Spiced Red Pepper Dip, & Toasted Ciabatta	397

FISH & CHIPS - BEER BATTERED COD

with Chips, Mushy Peas, & Tartare Sauce, Main	1097
with Chips, Mushy Peas, & Tartare Sauce, Sm Main	910

FISH CAKES - SALMON & SPRING ONION

with Broccoli, Veg, & Basil Dressing, Lge Main	846
with Broccoli, Veg, & Basil Dressing, Sm Main	573

FLATBREAD

Garlic Butter, Sharers/Grazing	731
Garlic Butter, with Cheese, Sharers/Grazing	864

FRIES

Stealth	310
Sweet Potato, Side, Kids	391
Sweet Potato	503

HAM

& Egg, with Triple Cooked Chips, Lge Main	1178
& Egg, with Triple Cooked Chips, Sm Main	903
Hock, Glazed, & Carrots, Mash, White Wine Sauce	1085

ICE CREAM

Chocolate, Kids	218
Vanilla, Kids	176

ICE LOLLY

Tropical Fruit, Kids	20

JELLY

Orange, Kids	100

KEBAB

Lamb Kofta, with Tzatziki, & Dressed Slaw, Starter	339
Vegetable, Skewer, no Sides, Kids	83

VINTAGE INNS

LAMB

	KCAL
Duo, with Seasonal Veg, & Red Wine Jus, Main	896
Shank, Yorkshire Pudding, Potatoes, Veg, & Gravy	1319

MUSHROOMS

Garlic, & Cheese, Oven Baked, Side	140
Garlic, & Cheese, Oven Baked, Steak Add On	246
Garlic, & Cheese, Oven Baked, with Bread, Starter	356

OLIVES

Mixed, Marinated, Sharers/Grazing	163

ONION RINGS

Homemade	471
BLANK	664

PANNA COTTA

Coconut, with Passionfruit, & red Berries, Vegan	312
Creme Caramel, Mini	262

PASTA

Tomato, Kids	362

PATE

Duo, with Rustic Bread, Starter	357

PEAS

Side, Kids	45

PIE - APPLE

Bramley, Mini, with Custard	241
Bramley, with Custard, & Vanilla Pod Ice Cream	735
Bramley, with Raspberry Coulis, Vegan	510

PIE - BEEF & MERLOT

with Thyme Roasted Carrots, & Seasonal Greens	753

PIE - CHICKEN & GAMMON

with Thyme Roasted Carrots, & Seasonal Greens	971

PIE - CHICKEN & LEEK

with Thyme Roasted Carrots, & Seasonal Greens	748

PIE - CHICKEN & THYME

with Spring Onion Mash, & Seasonal Veg, Main	952
with Thyme Roasted Carrots, & Seasonal Greens	818

PIE - GAME

with Thyme Roasted Carrots, & Seasonal Greens	782

PIE - STEAK & MUSHROOM

with Mash, Seasonal Veg, & a Jug of Gravy, Main	957
with Thyme Roasted Carrots, & Seasonal Greens	870

PIE - TURKEY & SAGE

with Thyme Roasted Carrots, & Seasonal Greens	964

PIZZA

Four Cheese, Stonebaked	1203
Margherita, Kids	414
Margherita, Stonebaked	990
Meat Feast, Stonebaked	1274
Spicy Cajun, Stonebaked	1291
Vegetable, Roasted, with Pesto, Stonebaked	1212

PLATTER

Pudding, Tasting	1358
Sticky, Sharers/Grazing	989

VINTAGE INNS

PORK DINNER

	KCAL
Yorkshire Pudding, Roast Potatoes, Veg, & Gravy	1690
Roast, Kids Meal	793

POTATOES

Baby, Side, Kids	77
Mashed, Side, Children's	142
Roast	454

PRAWN COCKTAIL

with Lobster, with Rustic Bread, Starter	383

PRAWNS

Garlic, Steak Add On	186

PUDDING - GAME

Suet, with Thyme Roasted Carrots, & Greens	925

PUDDING - STICKY TOFFEE

& Apple, with Toffee Sauce, & Custard	1190
with Toffee Sauce, & Pouring Cream	523

RICE

Sticky, Side, Kids	179

RISOTTO

Seafood, &Thyme Roasted Potatoes, Basil Dressing	1207

SALAD - CAESAR

Chargrilled Chicken, & Garlic Flatbread, Lge Main	964
with Garlic Flatbread, Lge Main	763
Halloumi, & Garlic Flatbread, Lge Main	1326
Salmon Fillet, & Garlic Flatbread, Lge Main	1194

SALAD - KALE, & CAULIFLOWER COUS COUS

Vegan, Main	234
Chicken, & Pineapple Ginger Dressing, Lge Main	423
Chicken, & Pineapple Ginger Dressing, Sm Main	328
Halloumi, & Pineapple Ginger Dressing, Lge Main	633
Halloumi, & Pineapple Ginger Dressing, Sm Main	538
Lamb Kofta, & Pineapple Ginger Dressing, Lge Main	475
Lamb Kofta, & Pineapple Ginger Dressing, Sm Main	380
Pineapple Ginger Dressing, Lge Main	236
Pineapple Ginger Dressing, Sm Main	141
Pineapple Ginger Dressing, Starter	140
Salmon, & Pineapple Ginger Dressing, Lge Main	664
Salmon, & Pineapple Ginger Dressing, Sm Main	569

SALAD - SIDE

Kids	48
Dressed	34

SALMON

with Butternut Squash, Peppers, Beans, & Potatoes	853

SANDWICH - BEEF

Roast, on a Rustic Roll, without Chips	1392

SANDWICH - CHICKEN BLT

on a Rustic Roll, without Chips	1007

SANDWICH - FISH FINGER

Cod, on a Rustic Roll, without Chips	1131

SANDWICH - HAM & CHEDDAR

Melt, on a Rustic Roll, without Chips	1338

SANDWICH - STEAK, 4OZ

Horseradish Mayo, & Fried Onions, without Chips	1068

VINTAGE INNS

SANDWICH - STEAK, 8OZ
Horseradish Mayo, & Fried Onions, without Chips	1270

SAUCE
Bearnaise, for Steak	178
Beef Dripping, for Steak	162
Cheese, Blacksticks, & Blue, for Steak	273
Peppercorn, for Steak	60

SAUSAGE
in Duvet, Extra	160
Pork, with Gravy, no Sides, Kids	290

SAUSAGE & MASH
with Cabbage, & Red Wine Onion Gravy, Main	1106

SCALLOPS - BLACK PEARL
& Prawns, in Garlic Butter, with Bread, Starter	474
with Black Pudding, Pea Puree, & Bacon, Starter	497

SCAMPI
Breaded, with Chips, Salad, & Tartare Sauce, Main	895

SEA BASS
Potatoes, Asparagus, Lobster & Samphire Sauce	572

SEAFOOD
Fritto Misto, Chips, Chipotle Mayo, & Tartare Sauce	1533

SORBET
Coconut Milk	466
Coconut Milk, with Raspberries &Strawberries	665

SOUP
Broccoli, & Stilton	204
Parsnip, Spiced	273
Pea, Mint, & Ham	292
Pea & Mint	195
Tomato, & Basil	129

SQUID - SALT & PEPPER CALAMARI
& Tempura Prawns, with Chiptole Mayo, Starter	273

SQUID - SALT & PEPPER CALAMARI
with Chorizo Seasoning, & Chipotle Mayo, Starter	801

SWEET POTATO & BUTTERNUT SQUASH
Roasted with Thyme, Orange, & Spices	178

TART - CHOCOLATE
Rich, with Chocolate Sauce, & Strawberries, Vegan	323
Rich, with Cornish Clotted Cream, & Strawberries	581

TART - TREACLE & PECAN
Mini	243
with Coconut Milk Sorbet, & Rosehip Syrup	719

TART - VEGETABLE, ROAST
Kids Meal	894
with Yorkshire Pudding, Roast Potatoes, Veg, Gravy	1597
with Kale & Thyme Pastry, & Leek Sauce, Vegan	741
Kale & Thyme Pastry, Main	545

TURKEY DINNER
& Sausage, Kids Meal	724
Yorkshire Pudding, Roast Potatoes, Veg, Gravy	1263

VEGETABLES
Seasonal	84
Sticks, Side, Kids	37

VINTAGE INNS

VENISON
Mushroom, Asparagus, Dauphinoise, Red Wine Jus	765

WRAP
Vegetable, Spicy, with Asian Slaw, without Chips	800

YORKSHIRE PUDDING
Extra	99

WAGAMAMA

BANANA
Katsu, & Caramel Ice Cream	312

BEANS
Edamame, with Chilli	280
Edamame, with Salt	280

BEEF
Tataki, Chilled	165
Teriyaki, & Rice, Donburi	973

BROCCOLI
& Bok Choi, Wok-Fried	181

BUNS
Beef, Korean BBQ, & Red Onion, Steamed, Hirata	354
Chicken, Crispy, & Tomato, Steamed, Hirata	464
Mushroom, & Panko Aubergine, Steamed, Hirata	385
Pork, Belly, & Panko Apple, Steamed, Hirata	550

CAKE
Chocolate, Layer, & Ice Cream	485

CAULIFLOWER
Bang Bang	480

CHEESECAKE
Coconut, & Fig	394
White Chocolate, & Ginger	455

CHICKEN
Katsu, Breaded, & Sticky Rice, Amai Sauce, Kids	496
Katsu, Breaded, & Sticky Rice, Curry Sauce, Kids	496
Katsu, Grilled, & Sticky Rice, Amai Sauce, Kids	445
Katsu, Grilled, & Sticky Rice, Curry Sauce, Kids	445
Crispy, with Sesame, & Soy Sauce, Tori Kara Age	440
Grilled, & Soba Noodles, Kids Menu	419
Rice, Egg, Stir Fry, Cha Han, Kids Menu	433
Teriyaki, & Rice, Donburi	784

CHILLI
Side	2

COD
Cubes, Breaded, & Sticky Rice, Amai Sauce, Kids	610
Cubes, Breaded, & Sticky Rice, Curry Sauce, Kids	610

CURRY
Chicken, & White Rice, Raisukaree	1371
Chicken, & White Rice, Samla	1135
Chicken, Katsu, & Sticky Rice	1145
Chicken, Firecracker, & Steamed Rice	1229
Prawn, & White Rice, Raisukaree	1282
Prawns, Firecracker, & Steamed Rice	1110
Tofu, & Mushrooms, Yasai Samla	1108
Vegetable, Katsu, & Sticky Rice	1174

DESSERT
Mango, Spiced, & Coconut, Parfait	299

DUCK
Grilled, Teriyaki, with Rice, Donburi	1133
Lettuce, Wraps	339
Wrap, with Cucumber, & Hoisin Sauce	451

WAGAMAMA

DUMPLINGS
Chicken, Steamed, Gyoza	223
Duck, Fried, Gyoza	377
Pork, Pulled, Steamed, Gyoza	236
Prawn, Fried, Gyoza	232
Yasai, Steamed, Gyoza	210

EGGS
Tea Stained, Side	94

FISH
White, Grilled, with Soba Noodles, Kids Menu	353

ICE CREAM
Caramel, Salted	496
Chocolate, & Shichimi	393
Coconut, Passion Fruit Sauce, & Coconut Flakes	449
Coffee, Vietnamese	471
Vanilla, Pod, Kids Menu	137
Yuzu	251

ICE LOLLY
Fruit, & Berry, Kids Menu	83

JUICE
Blueberry, Spice	193
Carrot	72
Fruit	146
Green, Clean	174
Green, Super	128
Orange	110
Positive	159
Power	160
Raw	97
Repair	188
Tropical	167

KIMCHI
Side	18

NOODLES
Plain, Side	323

NOODLES - BEEF
Short Rib, Bone In, Ramen	1097
Steak, Sirloin, Chilli, Ramen	665
Steak, Sirloin, Teriyaki, Soba, Teppanyaki	813
Steak, Bulgogi, Soba, Omakase	778

NOODLES - CHICKEN
& Prawn, Pad-Thai, Teppanyaki	741
& Prawn, Yaki Soba, Teppanyaki	715
& Prawn, Yaki Udon, Teppanyaki	744
Coconut & Lemongrass Soup, Itame	820
Ginger, Udon, Teppanyaki	767
GF, Ramen	513
Grilled, Chilli, Ramen	590
Grilled, Ramen, Kids Menu	368
Grilled, Ramen	476
Pork, Prawns, & Mussels, Wagamama, Ramen	686
Soba, Teppanyaki, Kids Menu	374

WAGAMAMA

	KCAL
NOODLES - DUCK	
Grilled, Ramen	990
NOODLES - LAMB	
Teriyaki, Soba, Omakase	890
NOODLES - PORK	
Belly, Shirodashi, Ramen	959
NOODLES - PRAWN	
Coconut & Lemongrass Soup, Itame	718
NOODLES - SALMON	
Grilled, Teriyaki, Soba, Teppanyaki	803
NOODLES - SEAFOOD	
GF, Ramen	821
Ramen	821
NOODLES - TOFU	
& Vegetable, Pad-Thai, Teppanyaki	831
& Vegetables, Soba, Teppanyaki, Kids Menu	396
Vegetable Broth, Kare Burosu	629
Vegetable, Coconut Lemongrass Soup, Yasai Itame	842
Yasai Pad-Thai	765
NOODLES - VEGETABLE	
Yasai, Ramen, Kids Menu	324
Yasai Yaki Soba, Teppanyaki	696
Yasai Yaki Soba	564
OMELETTE	
Shiitake Mushroom, & Broccoli, with Rice, Donburi	725
PICKLE	
Japanese, Side	30
PORK BELLY	
in Breadcrumbs, & Sticky Rice, Tonkatsu, Omakase	1033
Sticky, with Miso Aubergine, Omakase	1394
PRAWNS	
in Breadcrumbs, Crispy, Chilli Sauce, Ebi Katsu	298
Skewers, Lollipop, Kushiyaki	142
RIBS	
Pork, Korean BBQ	698
RICE	
Brown, Side	543
Steamed, Side	543
Sticky, Side	543
SALAD	
Beef, Sirloin, & Shiitake Mushrooms	434
Chicken, & Prawn, Pad-Thai	342
Chicken, Chilli, Warm	487
Raw	108
Tofu, Chili, Warm	502
SORBET	
Lemongrass, & Lime	152
Lemongrass, & Lime	152
Pink Guava, & Passionfruit	162
SOUP	
Miso, & Japanese Pickles, Side	66
SQUID	
Chilli	534

WAGAMAMA

	KCAL
TART	
Yuzu, & Lemon	306
TOFU	
Rice, Egg, Stir Fry, Cha Han, Kids Menu	454
TUNA	
Steak, Seared, with Quinoa, Omakase	522
VEGETABLES	
Katsu, Breaded, & Sticky Rice, Amai Sauce, Kids	468
Katsu, Breaded, & Sticky Rice, Curry Sauce, Kids	468

WIMPY

BURGERS

	KCAL
Kingsize	821
Mega	873
Open, Chicken, Gourmet	542
Open, Jalapeno	627
Open, Smoky BBQ	725
Quarterpounder, BBQ Bacon	710
Quarterpounder, Club	735
Quarterpounder, Hawaiian	679
Quarterpounder, Jalapeno	616
Quarterpounder, Original	613
Quarterpounder, Patty	264
Quarterpounder, with Cheese, & Bacon, Original	621
Quarterpounder, with Cheese, Original	613

BURGERS VEGETARIAN

	KCAL
Bean, Spicy	542
Mushroom, Open	664
Quorn, Lemon & Pepper	554

CAKE

	KCAL
Chocolate Fudge	522

CHEESE

	KCAL
Grated, Burger Extra	51
Mozzarella, Melts, 4 Melts	260
Slice, Burger Extra	41

CHICKEN

	KCAL
Chunks, with Chips, Kids	422
Chunks, with Salad, Kids	243
Platter, Gourmet	531

CHICKEN WITH

	KCAL
Chips, Chunks	745

CHIPS

	KCAL
Reg	267

COFFEE

	KCAL
Americano, Large	12
Americano, Reg	6
Cappuccino, Large	134
Cappuccino, Reg	109
Esspresso	6
Latte, Large	194
Latte, Reg	160
Mocha, Large	303
Mocha, Reg	213

COLESLAW

	KCAL
Side	130

CREAM

	KCAL
Side	72

CUSTARD

	KCAL
Side	125

DOUGHNUTS - BROWN DERBY

	KCAL
with Ice Cream, Chocolate Sauce, & Chopped Nuts	426

DRESSING

	KCAL
Caesar	219
French	60

WIMPY

DRESSING

	KCAL
Wimpy Mayo	199

EGGS

	KCAL
Fried, Burger Extra	90
Fried, on Toast, Brekkie Bites	350
Scrambled, on Toast, Brekkie Bites	304
Scrambled, on Toast, Kids	226

FISH & CHIPS

	KCAL
Cod	783
Scampi	616

FISH FINGERS

	KCAL
with Chips, Kids	359
with Salad, Kids	180

GRILLS

	KCAL
All Day Breakfast	896
Bender Sausage	679
Breakfast Sausage	567
International	1077
Wimpy	856

HASH BROWNS

	KCAL
Extra	98

HOT CHOCOLATE

	KCAL
with Cream, Large	283
with Cream, Reg	202

ICE CREAM

	KCAL
Soft, Portion	159
with Chocolate Sauce, Kids	176
with Strawberry Sauce, Kids	175

ICE CREAM FLOAT

	KCAL
7 Up	182
Pepsi, Diet	96
Pepsi	181
Pepsi Max	96
Tango Orange	135

JELLY

	KCAL
Orange, Pot, Kids	3
Strawberry, Pot, Kids	5

MILK SHAKE

	KCAL
Banana, Ice Cream	236
Banana, Thick	296
Chocolate, Ice Cream	267
Chocolate, Thick	297
Strawberry, Ice Cream	257
Strawberry, Thick	295
Vanilla, Ice Cream	215
Vanilla, Thick	262

MUFFIN

	KCAL
British, Breakfast	404
Hashbrown	404
Sausage, & Hashbrown	502

MUSHROOMS

	KCAL
Burger Extra	133

	KCAL			KCAL

WIMPY

ONION RINGS
Side, 6 Rings	238

PEAS
Kids	86

PEPPERS
Jalapeno, Burger Extras	2

PINEAPPLE
Extra	40

POTATO FILLING
Bacon	65
Beans, Baked, Heinz	93
Cheese, Grated	171
Coleslaw	148
Mushrooms, Grilldled	133

POTATOES
Jacket, with Butter, & Salad	523

SALAD
Chicken, Breaded	345
Chicken, Gourmet	303
Fish	463
Scampi	376
Side, Kids	8
Side	56

SAUCE
BBQ	40
Chocolate	81
Firecracker	29
Ketchup	30
Mango	29
Maple Flavoured	86
Special	114
Strawberry	80
Wimpy Mayo	100

SAUSAGES
with Chips, Kids	398
with Salad, Kids	219

SMOOTHIE
Mango	233

SPONGE PUDDING
Sticky Toffee, with Cream	589
Sticky Toffee, with Custard	642
Sticky Toffee, with Ice Cream	612
Syrup, with Cream	529
Syrup, with Custard	581
Syrup, with Ice Cream	551

SUNDAE
Brownie	717
Eton Mess	301
Fruit Nut	207
Knickerbocker Glory	374
Rocky Road	396

WIMPY

SYRUP
Caramel, for Coffee	26
Hazlenut, for Coffee	25
Vanilla, for Coffee	27

TEA
Herbal	2
with Milk	23

TEACAKES
Toasted, with Butter	295

TOAST
with Butter, & Jam, 2 Slices	318
with Butter, & Marmalade, 2 Slices	318

TOASTIE
Cheese, & Ham, White	388
Cheese, & Red Onion, White	343
Cheese, & Tomato, White	338
Cheese, with Chips, Kids	474
Cheese, with Salad, Kids	298
Chicken, BBQ, White	475
Hawaiian, White	403

TOPPING
Flake, Crushed, for Drinks	44
Fruit	18
Marshmallows, Mini, for Drinks	32
Marshmallows, Mini	32
Nuts, Chopped	30
Oreo Minis	118
Strawberries	9

TORTE
Apple, with Cream	385
Apple, with Custard	438
Apple, with Ice Cream	408

VEGETABLES
Carrot & cucumber Pot, Kids	24

WAFFLES
Chocolate, with Cream, Kids	402
Chocolate, with Ice Cream, Kids	386
Eskimo, with Chocolate Sauce	746
Eskimo, with Maple Flavoured Syrup	757
Eskimo, with Strawberry Sauce	746

YO! SUSHI

AUBERGINE
Fried, in Garlic, Ginger, Sesame, & Soy, Harusame	108

BEANS
Edamame, Side	134

BEEF
Tataki	96

BEEF TERIYAKI
Large	897
Standard	312

BROCCOLI
Tenderstem, & Sesame	135

BROWNIES
Chocolate	363

BURGERS
Chicken, Katsu	476
Chicken, Teriyaki	268
Mushroom, Teriyaki	210

CAULIFLOWER
Pepper, Spicy	146

CHEESECAKE
Japanese	195

CHICKEN
Fried, Japanese	382
Fried, Korean	386

CHICKEN TERIYAKI
Large	785
Standard	246

DESSERT
Mochi, Chocolate	236
Mochi, Strawberry Cheesecake	188
Platter	610

DOUGH BALLS
Takoyaki	195

DUMPLINGS
Gyoza, Chicken	140
Gyoza, Prawn	148
Gyoza, Vegetable	132

FRIES
Japanese Style	412

FRUIT
Fresh, Plate	61

KATSU
Chicken, Curry, with Rice, Large	936
Chicken, Curry, with Rice	530
Chicken	225
Prawn, Curry, with Rice, Large	757
Prawn, Curry, with Rice	440
Prawn	173
Pumpkin, Curry, with Rice, Large	789
Pumpkin, Curry, with Rice	410
Pumpkin	152
Tofu, Curry, with Rice, Large	862
Tofu, Curry, with Rice	530

YO! SUSHI

KATSU
Tofu	190

MOUSSE
Chocolate, Pot	246

NOODLES
Chicken, Curry, Ramen	415
Chicken, Yakisoba	232
Seafood, Spicy, Ramen, Large	423
Seafood, Spicy, Ramen	256
Shitake, Ramen, Large	414
Shitake, Ramen	222
Side	187
Vegetable, Yakisoba	202

PAK CHOI
& Garlic, Stir Fried	86

PANCAKE
Dorayaki	138

RICE
Brown, Side	198
Chicken, Fried	355
Salmon, Fried	356
Vegetable, Fried	351
White, Side	303

SALAD
Chicken, & Tangerine	149
Leaf, Side	35

SEAWEED
Kaiso	175

SHRIMP
Popcorn	355

SOUP
Miso	53

SQUID
Pepper, Spicy	207

SUSHI
Aubergine, Glazed, Nigiri	70
Avocado, Maki	204
Avocado, Nigiri	110
Beef, Seared, Nigiri	108
Chicken, & Avocado, Roll, Platter	605
Chicken, & Avocado, Roll	198
Chicken, Katsu, Spicy, Roll, Platter	454
Chicken, Katsu, Spicy, Roll	155
Cucumber, Maki	150
Duck, Aromatic, Roll	218
Mixed, Maki, Plate	196
Mixed, Nigiri, Platter	303
Prawn, & Tuna, Blossom, Roll	201
Prawn, Panko Nigiri	121
Prawn, Star, Roll	240
Salmon, & Avocado, Dynamite, Roll	200
Salmon, & Avocado, Temaki, Hand Roll	164
Salmon, Aburi, Nigiri	112

YO! SUSHI

SUSHI

	KCAL
Salmon, Beetroot Cured, Sashimi	111
Salmon, Cream Cheese, & Cucumber, Ginza, Roll	204
Salmon, Dragon, Roll	202
Salmon, Kickin', Roll, Platter	615
Salmon, Kickin', Roll	212
Salmon, Maki	189
Salmon, Nigiri	99
Salmon, Ponzu Salsa, Sashimi	104
Salmon, Sashimi	112
Salmon, Selection, Platter	568
Salmon, Yo! Roll	157
Surimi, & Avocado, Californian, Crunchy, Roll, Platter	680
Surimi, & Avocado, Californian, Crunchy, Roll	277
Surimi, & Avocado, Temaki, Californian Roll	233
Tofu, Inari, & Avocado, Roll, Platter	497
Tofu, Inari, & Avocado, Roll	165
Tofu, Inari, & Avocado, Temaki, Hand Roll	145
Tuna, Coriander Seared, Sashimi	94
Tuna, maki	190
Tuna, Mayo, Roll	127
Tuna, Nigiri	90
Tuna, Sashimi	86

TACO

	KCAL
Tofu, Inari	170

Useful Resources

Weight Loss
Weight Loss Resources is home to the UK's largest calorie and nutrition database along with diaries, tools and expert advice for weight loss and health.
Tel: 01733 345592 Email: helpteam@weightlossresources.co.uk
Website: www.weightlossresources.co.uk

Products to Help You Keep Track
From food diaries to weight graphs and calorie counted recipe books visit the wlr shop.
Tel: 01733 345592 Email: helpteam@weightlossresources.co.uk
Website: www.weightlossresources.co.uk/shop

Dietary Advice
The British Dietetic Association has helpful food fact leaflets and information on how to contact a registered dietitian.
Tel: 0121 200 8080 Email: info@bda.uk.com
Website: www.bda.uk.com

Healthy Eating
The British Nutrition Foundation has lots of in depth scientifically based nutritional information, knowledge and advice on healthy eating for all ages.
Tel: 0207 7557 7930 Email: postbox@nutrition.org.uk
Website: www.nutrition.org.uk

Healthy Heart
The British Heart Foundation provides advice and information for all on all heart aspects from being healthy, to living with heart conditions, research and fundraising.
Tel: 0207 554 000 Email: via their website
Website: www.bhf.org.uk

Cancer Research
Cancer Research UK is the leading UK charity dedicated to research, education and fundraising for all forms of cancer.
Tel: 0300 123 1022 Email: via their website
Website: www.cancerresearchuk.org

Diabetes Advice
Diabetes UK is the leading charity working for people with diabetes. Their mission is to improve the lives of people with diabetes and to work towards a future without diabetes
Tel : 0345 123 2399 Email: info@diabetes.org.uk
Website: www.diabetes.org.uk

Beating Bowel Cancer
Beating Bowel Cancer is a leading UK charity for bowel cancer patients, working to raise awareness of symptoms, promote early diagnosis and encourage open access to treatment choice for those affected by bowel cancer.Tel: 08450 719301   Email: nurse@beatingbowelcancer.org
Website: www.beatingbowelcancer.org

Safety and Standards
The Food Standards Agency is an independent watchdog, set up to protect the public's health and consumer interests in relation to food.
Tel: 0207 276 8829 Email: helpline@foodstandards.gsi.gov.uk
Website: www.food.gov.uk

Feedback

If you have any comments or suggestions about The Calorie, Carb & Fat Bible, or would like further information on Weight Loss Resources, please call, email, or write to us:

Tel:	01733 345592
Email:	helpteam@weightlossresources.co.uk
Address:	Rebecca Walton,
	Weight Loss Resources Ltd,
	2C Flag Business Exchange,
	Vicarage Farm Road,
	Peterborough,
	PE1 5TX.

Reviews for The Calorie Carb & Fat Bible

'What a brilliant book. I know I'll be sinking my teeth into it.'
GMTV Nutritionist Amanda Ursell, BSc RD

'To help you make low-cal choices everyday, invest in a copy.'
ZEST magazine

'There is no doubt that the food listings are extremely helpful
for anyone wishing to control their calorie intake in order to lose
pounds or maintain a healthy weight.'
Women's Fitness magazine

'Useful if you don't want to exclude any overall food groups.'
Easy Living magazine

'Quite simply an astonishing achievement by the authors.'
Evening Post, Nottingham

'The book gives you all the basic information so you can work out
your daily calorie needs.'
Woman magazine

'This is a welcome resource in view of the 'national epidemic of obesity.'

Bryony Philip, Bowel Cancer UK

'The authors seem to understand the problems of slimming.'

Dr John Campion

'Jam-packed with info on dieting, and full to bursting point with the calorie, carbohydrate and fat values of thousands of different foods, it's the perfect weight loss tool.'

Evening Express, Aberdeen

'Excellent resource tool - used by myself in my role as a Practice Nurse.'

Pam Boal, Sunderland

'I recently bought your book called the Calorie, Carb & Fat Bible and would love to tell you what a brilliant book it is. I have recently started a weight management programme and I honestly don't know where I'd be without your book. It has helped me a lot and given me some really good advice.'

Rachel Mitchell

About Weight Loss Resources

If you want to lose weight in a healthy, sustainable way, you'll find all the tools and support you need at wlr. Available on your phone, tablet, or PC.

HERE'S THE HIGHLIGHTS:

- Track calories: how many you need, how many you've consumed and burned, and how many you have left

- New Visual Food Diary, a more relaxed way to track. Enables you to reflect on choices and gain insights about your relationship with food

- The best kept online UK food database

- 1000s of recipes and meal ideas that you can add to your online diary and adapt to suit yourself

- Create and calorie count your own recipes and diet plans

- Set a weight loss goal, see how many calories you need to get there, and the date you can expect to reach it

- Fantastic support from our knowledgeable Helpteam, available 7 days a week

You can take a free trial at www.weightlossresources.co.uk or give us a call on 01733 345592